Clinical Echocardiography

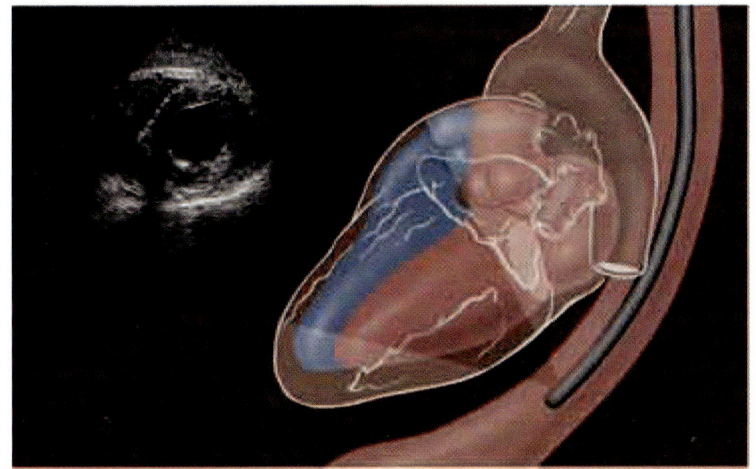

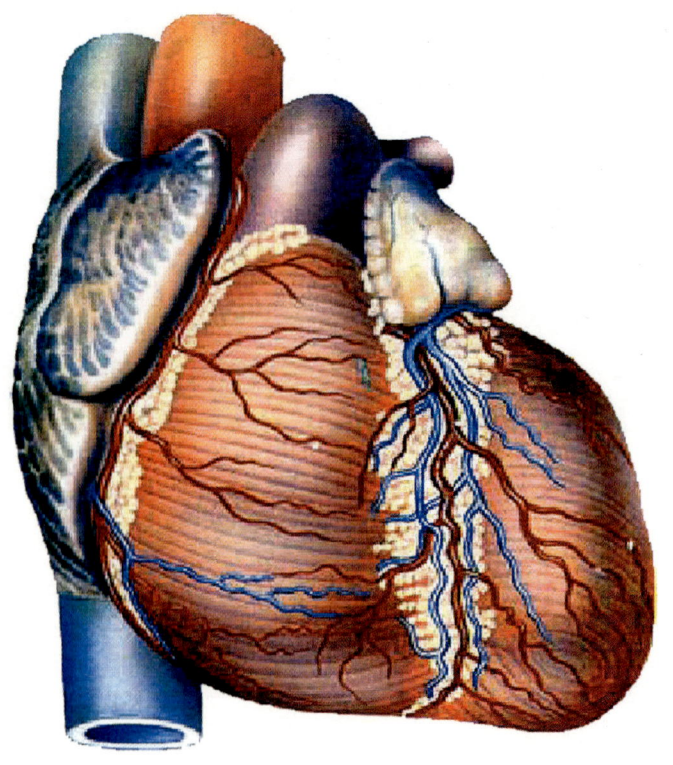

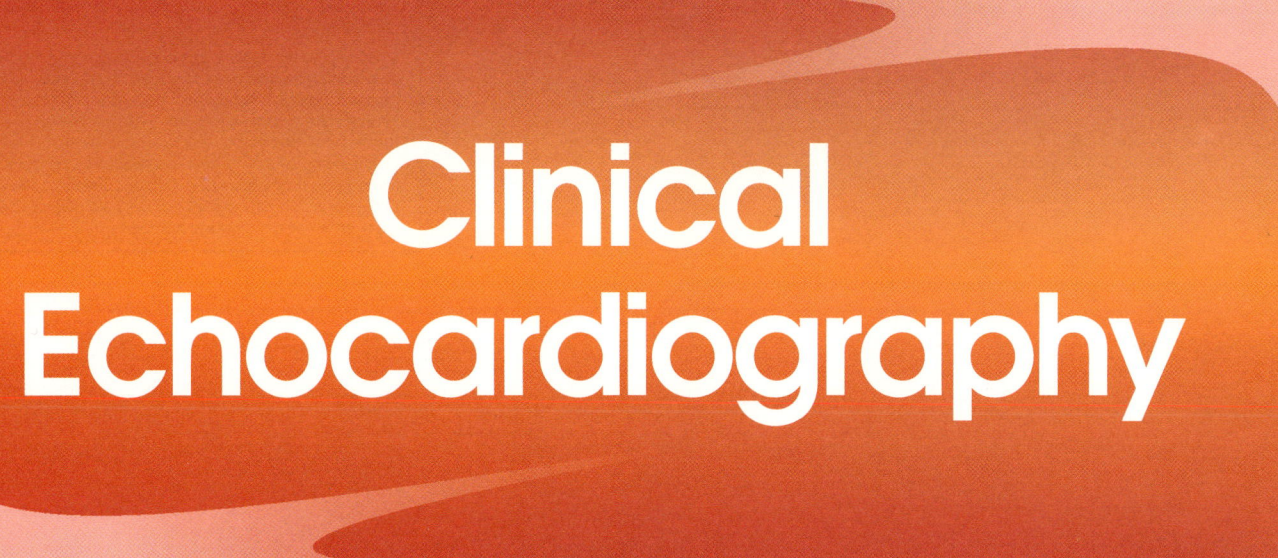

Clinical Echocardiography

K.C. VERMA

MBBS, DCH, MD, DM (Cardiology)
FICP (USA), FRSM&H (UK), FCSI (Medalist)

Former Professor in Cardiovascular and Thoracic Unit
Chest Diseases Hospital and Medical College
Jammu (J&K), India

SOURABH VERMA

MBBS, MD (General Medicine)

Former Senior Resident in Internal Medicine
Departments of Medicine
Government Medical College and
Batra Hospital, Jammu (J&K), India

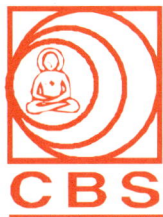

CBS

CBS Publishers & Distributors Pvt Ltd

New Delhi • Bangalore • Pune • Chennai • Cochin

Clinical Echocardiography

ISBN: 978-81-239-1789-4

Copyright © Authors and Publishers

First Edition: 2010

Published by Satish Kumar Jain and produced by Vinod K. Jain for
CBS Publishers & Distributors Pvt Ltd
4819/XI Prahlad Street, 24 Ansari Road, Daryaganj,
New Delhi 110 002, India.   Website: www.cbspd.com
Ph: 23289259, 23266861, 23266867   Fax: 011-23243014   e-mail: delhi@cbspd.com

Branches

• Bangalore: Seema House 2975, 17th Cross, K.R. Road,
  Banasankari 2nd Stage, Bangalore 560 070, Karnataka
  Ph: 26771678/79   Fax: 080-26771680   e-mail: cbsbng@gmail.com

• Pune: Shaan Brahmha Complex, 631/632 Basement, Appa Balwant Chowk,
  Budhwar Peth, next to Ratan Talkies, Pune 411 002, Maharashtra
  Ph: 020-24464057/58   Fax: 020-24464059   e-mail: pune@cbspd.com

• Cochin: 36/14 Kalluvilakam, Lissie Hospital Road,
  Cochin 682018, Kerala
  Ph: 0484-4059061-65   Fax: 0484-4059065   e-mail: cochin@cbspd.com

• Chennai: 20, West Park Road, Shenoy Nagar, Chennai 600030, TN
  Ph: 044-26260666, 26202620   Fax: 044-45530020   email: chennai@cbspd.com

Printed at Paras Offset Pvt. Ltd., C-176, Naraina Industrial Area Phase-1, New Delhi

Preface

This book begins with the fundamentals of echocardiography describing historical background of ultrasound, instrumentation, various modes in practice, examination of normal cardiac structures with M-mode, 2-D, Doppler and colour flows. This chapter is considered as the sheet anchor of basic clinical echocardiography, most useful to cardiac fellows and technical officers of cardiovascular medicine.

As it proceeds further, it highlights the importance of M-mode, 2-D and colour Doppler echocardiography in the assessment of rheumatic and congenital cardiac defects which is the main bulk load of any diagnostic echocardiographic laboratory in South East Asia including India.

Newer concepts of differential blood supply of IVS has been highlighted to prove that there exist two parts of IVS with different coronary arterial supply with central demarcating line. Echocardiographic evaluation of intracardiac mass lesions, pericardial diseases, A–V prolapse, infective endocarditis and right heart dysfunctions secondary to cardiorespiratory disorders have been lucidly depicted.

Readers are provided with the state of the art and in-depth reviews of selective transesophageal (TEE) echocardiography 3-D technology in the better understanding of both normal and diseased cardiac structures. Intracardiac echocardiography is of special interest to both the echocardiographer and interventional cardiologist to have clearer view of internal anatomy of the heart and exact area of operation where various kinds of devices could be placed for plugging of various kinds of shunts with least discomfort.

In the diagnosis of various subsets of coronary artery disease with special reference to wall motion abnormalities and hemodynamic correlates both pharmacological and non-pharmacological approaches have been discussed.

Ultrasonic evaluation of coronary vasculature in comparison with coronary arteriography to study any luminal irregularity, atherosclerotic plaque and thrombotic lesions have been added so that an early management programme of CAD is planned with good index of sensitivity and specificity. An attempt has also been made to evaluate myocardial dysfunctions with the help of tissue Doppler, harmonic imaging and contrast technology.

Author has also tried to correlate various ECG diagnosed cardiac arrhythmias with its counterpart morphological features on echocardiography to consider later as one of the most reliable non-invasive modality in pre- and postoperative assessment of various types of cardiac arrhythmias.

Chapter on fetal and neonatal echocardiography gives an opportunity to peep deep into the fetal cardiac anatomy as early as 12 weeks of human gestation. Detection of fetal intracardiac malformations helps the fetal cardiac surgeons not only to manage various cardiac defects in their intrauterine life but also to follow these in their postnatal periods.

Chapter regarding age-related cardiovascular alterations occurring in human body and their assessment with echocardiography has been introduced to recognise fully the state of health and disease in elderly individuals. At the end of the book yet another chapter describing various systemic illnesses influencing the cardiac functions have been studied by the technique of echocardiography.

This book to my assessment satisfies all academic criteria being a very useful, cheap and a treasure-house of scientific knowledge gathered by the author over more than two decades in the field of diagnostic echocardiography.

I am sure, that this book is likely to act as a perfect guide to cardiac fellows, clinical cardiologists, physicians with interest in cardiovascular medicine, technical officers and those technicians in cardiology department who want to set up their echocardiographic laboratories in both private and governmental institutions.

K.C. Verma MD, DM
Sourabh Verma MD

Acknowledgements

More than two decades back when I started as a cardiology fellow, only a few echocardiographic machines were available in most of the premier institutions in India such as All India Institute of Medical Sciences (AIIMS), New Delhi; Command Hospital, New Delhi; and Institute of Cardiology, Chennai. Banaras Hindu University, where I was registered as a DM cardiology fellow, had acquired a new combined machine for conducting phonocardiogram, ECG, vectocardiogram and invasive intracardiac pressures, I was allotted a topic of echocardiographic incidence of tricuspid valvular disease in patients with combined/isolated rheumatic mitral stenosis. This machine was scanning the A-V valves in M-mode views only. But later on it was supplemented with 2-D echo machine, and I completed my project successfully. This study was presented by me during the world conference on open heart surgery and later published in the proceedings of the open heart surgery in Feb. 7-10-1985 by Drs K.R. Shetty and G.B. Parulkar. This encouraged me to have more practice and acquire more knowledge in the field of echocardiography and later it became my passion. During that period the first book on echocardiography in India was published by a group of doctors led by Dr. C. Lakshmikanthan from Institute of Cardiology, Chennai, in 1980 as an international edition. I read this book thoroughly and was greatly benefitted in basic understanding of the subject.

I later joined AIIMS, New Delhi, in 1981 for part-time training in investigative cardiology under the tutelage of Dr. M.L. Bhatia, Dr. U. Koul and Dr. Savitri Shrivastava who taught me the finer details of echocardiography and its correlationship with hemodynamics. After, finishing my training at AIIMS, I joined G.B. Pant Hospital, New Delhi, with Dr. M.P. Gupta, Dr. M. Khalilullah, Dr. K.K. Sethi and Dr. Romesh Arora, and acquired further skills in the field of non-invasive and invasive cardiology. During this period I was introduced to Col. S.K. Prasher working as graded specialist in medicine at Command Hospital, New Delhi, and learnt further as how to diagnose mild, moderate and severe pericardial effusion including echocardiograhic evaluation of cardiac tamponade. The teachings of these abovesaid doctors completely transformed me as a good investigator in the field of echocardiography and helped me as an independent worker for conducting echocardiograms with confidence for which I would ever remain indebted to them for the rest of my life. Thereafter, I published a few of my studies in national and international journals including paper presentation in many international conferences. I attended regularly national and international cardiological conferences and workshops in the field of echocardiography and clarified my doubts with national and international masters of the subjects.

I was also guided by Dr. Naveen C. Nanda, an international authority in echocardiography for establishing echocardiographic laboratory at Govt. Medical College, Jammu, for which I owe my respect and gratitude for his helpful gesture.

Attending international conferences organized by Dr. K.L. Chopra, Dr. H.K. Chopra and Dr. K.K. Aggarwal from Mool Chand Hospital, New Delhi, further enhanced my knowledge in clinical echocardiography for which I pay my respect to these fully deserving organizers. This book, therefore, is the outcome of continuing medical education in me contributed by various abovesaid national and international specialists in the field of clinical echocardiography.

Since it is difficult to communicate individually with various research workers of national and international fame and worthy masters in the field of clinical echocardiography whose direct and indirect help has been acquired to shape this book as a ready-reckoner and made easy educational guide suited to most of our postgraduate students in the field of general medicine and DM (Cardiology) fellows, I therefore take this opportunity through this book to thank them in person, acknowledge their contribution in absentia, and seek their blessings for the success of this project.

I am also very thankful to Dr. Manzoor Ahmed Malik as a model in Chapter 2 and Shri Devider Singh, my laboratory assistant, for helping me out in echocardiographic laboratory. Timely help extended by Shri V. Talwar, Yudhveer Sambyal, Sanjay Mengi and Ashu from Morex Computers and Leeward Graphics, Gandhi Nagar, Jammu, in DTP work and document setting is joyfully acknowledged.

K.C. Verma MD, DM

Contents

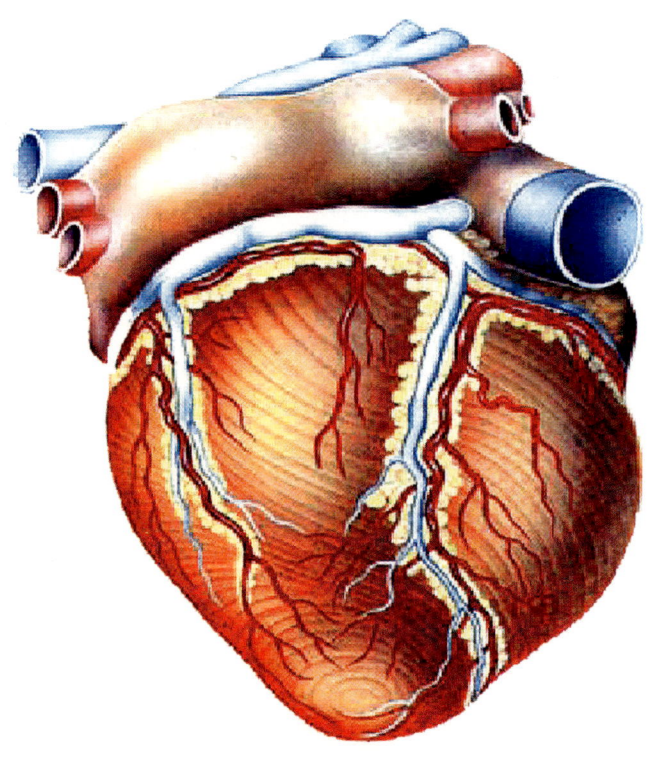

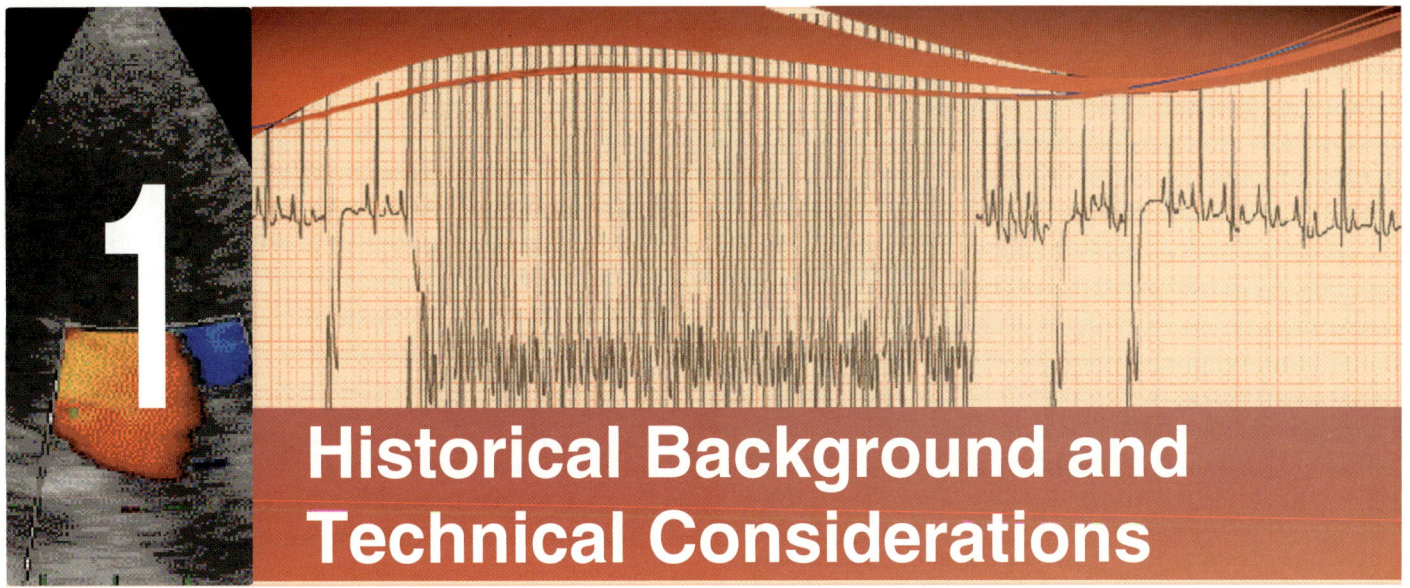

Historical Background and Technical Considerations

The first practical use of ultrasound was applied in sonar detection of submarines. This property was fully exploited for military objectives, mainly during the Second World War. Firestone published a study of flaw detection in metals, using an ex-military ultrasonoscope.

displaying the echoes on an oscilloscope with respect to time. In 1961, Edler after having modified the existing technique, visualised the various cardiac structures including the heart valves and myocardium. He also demonstrated various cardiac diseases such as mitral and aortic stenosis, left atrial tumors and pericardial effusion with the application of his technique. Echocardiography was introduced to the United States in 1963, by Reid. Since then the technique has been greatly refined, expanded and the number of medical publications on this subject have increased accordingly all over the world (Figs 1.1–1.3).

Fig. 1.1: Drs Edler and Feigenbaum demonstrating their M-mode echocardiographic machine during meeting of cardiac ultrasound Indianapolis in 1968

The first medical application of ultrasound was started as early as 1950 by Howry, Wild and Keidel. Later, two Swedish scientists, Edler and Hertz, in 1954 had the rare honour of visualising the cardiac structure in motion. This led to the beginning of M-mode echocardiography by simultaneously, recording and

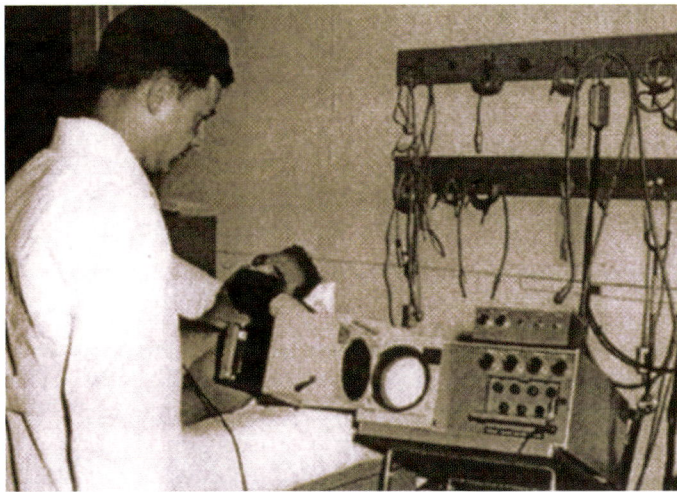

Fig. 1.2: Older model of M-mode echocardiograph using polaroid camera to record an echocardiogram

The supplementation of the Doppler technique to conventional M-mode and two-dimensional echocardiography represents a significant advance because it has provided the means for comprehensive, non-invasive evaluation of various cardiovascular diseases. Because Doppler echocardiography characterizes blood flow velocity patterns in various cardiac chambers and great vessels, it enables one to assess intracardiac flow disturbances produced by stenotic, regurgitant, and shunt lesions of both acquired and congenital cardiac defects. Neither M-mode nor the two-dimensional technique deals directly with intracardiac flow patterns, and hence they are of limited value in the assessment of regurgitant and stenotic lesions. The Doppler technique supplements information derived from cardiac catheterization and angiography, which are often required for definite determination of intracardiac flow dynamics. These invasive procedures are not practical for general screening and thus are not well suited for serial studies. Indeed, in selected cases, the Doppler technique may provide an alternative to cardiac catheterization in assessing cardiac surgical procedures (Table 1.2).

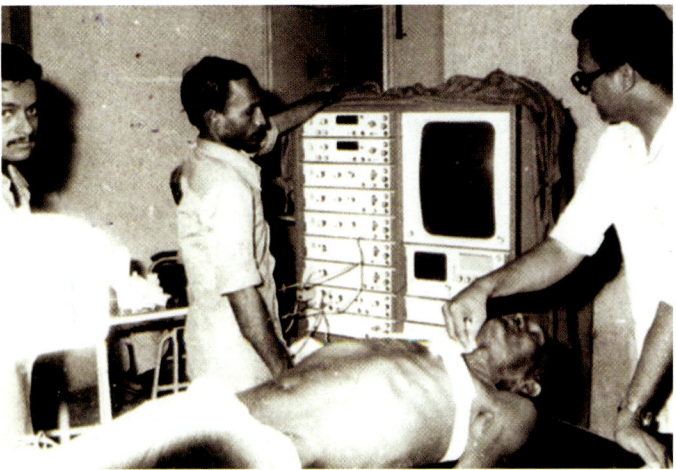

Fig. 1.3: The author performing simultaneous M-mode echocardiogram and phonogram during his postdoctoral study in cardiology in 1980 at Institute of Medical Sciences, Banaras Hindu University, Varanasi, India

Physical Properties of Ultrasound

Before putting echocardiography to its practical uses, certain knowledge of the physical properties of ultrasound is necessary to understand this technique fully.

Sound is the transmission of energy in the form of vibration (frequency) of particles in a particular medium. Frequency is the number of compressions or rarefactions per second. This is expressed in cycles per second or hertz (Hz). The audible range of human ear varies from 30–50 Hz to 15000 Hz (Fig. 1.17).

By definition, ultrasound has a frequency greater than 20,000 Hz, which means that it is above the range of human audibility. The frequencies used in cardiology range from one million Hz (MHz) to 7 MHz, with intensities of less than 100 milliwatts per cm^2.

The wavelength (λ) is the distance between two successive cycles. The velocity represents the speed with which the sound waves travel through a given medium. As all sound waves in a given beam have the same velocity, the distance by the ultrasound per unit of time is equal to the product of their frequency and wavelength.

$$C = \lambda f$$
C = velocity of sound in the medium
λ = wavelength
f = frequency in Hz

The soft tissues of t561he human body may behave like a homogenous conductor, such as normal saline, in which the propagation of ultrasound is relatively constant (1540 m/sec). On the other hand the velocity is much higher in bone (3380 m/sec), and much lower in air (330 m/sec). These media strongly absorb ultrasound, and are therefore very poor conductors (Table 1.4).

Acoustic Impedance

In technical terms, the acoustic impedance (Z) is the product of the density of the medium (P) and the velocity of sound in the medium (C): $Z = PC$.

The surface of separation between two media of different acoustic impedance is called an acoustic interface. At each acoustic interface, part of the ultrasound beam is reflected and part is refracted; the greater is the difference of acoustic impedance between two media (acoustic mismatch), the greater the amount of sound is reflected (Table 1.1).

Resolution and Penetration (Table 1.1)

When a frequency of 2.25 MHz is used, a wavelength of ultrasonic beam of 0.7 mm is obtained: $\lambda = C/f$. When the frequency is doubled (a value normally used in pediatric echocardiography), the wavelength is halved. Theoretically, the distance between two structures must be greater than a quarter of the wavelength for two separate echoes to be identified (resolution). In practice, it is difficult to obtain a better resolution than wavelength: therefore, the higher the frequency, the higher the resolution is. However, at high frequencies greater amounts of ultrasound are reflected by proximal tissues with a rapid fall of energy. As a result, the depth of penetration of the ultrasound beam is reduced and the distal echoes are attenuated. In other words, the higher the frequency and the shorter the wavelength, the better is the resolution. However, the ultrasound beam loses its energy of penetration and deep lying structures cannot be recorded. Piezo-electric crystals play a key role in ultrasound transducers currently in

Table 1.1: *Interpretation of technical term used in echocardiography*

Term used	Interpretation
Absorption	The transfer of ultrasound energy to the tissue during propagation
Acoustic impedance	The product of the density of the medium and velocity of sound differences in media 1 and 2 determine the ratio of transmitted versus reflected sound at the interface
Amplitude	The magnitude of the pressure changes along the wave; also, the strength of the wave (in decibels)
Attenuation	The net loss of ultrasound energy as a wave propagates through a medium
Cycle	The combination or sum of 1 compression and 1 rarefaction of a propagating wave
Dead time	The time in-between pulses that the echograph is not emitting ultrasound
Decibel	A logarithmic measure of the intensity of sound, expressed as a ratio to a reference value (dB)
Duty factor	The fraction of time that the transducer is emitting ultrasound, a unitless number between 0 and 1
Far field	The diverging conical portion of the beam beyond the near field
Frequency	The number of cycles through a medium
Half-layer value	The distance an ultrasound beam penetrates into a medium before its intensity has attenuated to one-half the original value
Intensity	The concentration or distribution of power within an area, often the cross-sectional area of the ultrasound beam, analogous to loudness
Longitudinal wave	A cyclic disturbance in which the energy propagation is parallel to the direction of particle motion
Near field	The proximal cylindrical-shaped portion of the ultrasound beam before divergence begins to occur
Period	The time required to complete 1 cycle, usually expressed in microseconds (μ sec)
Piezoelectricity	The phenomenon of changing shape in response to an applied electric current, resulting in vibration and the production of sound waves; the ability to produce an electric impulse in response to a mechanical deformation; thus, the interconversion of electrical and sound energy
Power	The rate of transfer over time of the acoustic energy from the propagating wave to the medium, measured in Watts
Pulse	A burst or packet of emitted ultrasound of finite duration, containing a fixed number of cycles travelling together
Pulse length	The physical length or distance that a pulse occupies in space, usually expressed in millimeters (mm)
Pulse repetition	The rate at which pulses are emitted from the transducer, i.e. the number of pulses emitted within a period of frequency time, usually 1 second
Resolution	The smallest distance between 2 points that allows the points to be distinguished as separate
Sensitivity	The ability of the system to image small targets at a given depth
Ultrasound	A mechanical vibration in a physical medium, characterised by a frequency > 20,000 Hz
Velocity	The speed at which sound moves through a given medium
Wavelength	The length of a single cycle of the ultrasound

Table 1.2: *M-Mode and 2-dimensional echocardiography in altered hemodynamics*

Echo-characteristics	Hemodynamic applications
M-Mode	
Early closure of the mitral valve	Acute, severe aortic regurgitation
Delayed closure of the mitral valve (B bump)	Elevated LV end-diastolic pressure
RV free wall early diastolic collapse	Pericardial tamponade
Mid-systolic notching of the aortic valve	Dynamic subaortic outflow tract obstruction
Diastolic mitral valve fluttering	Aortic regurgitation
Mid systolic notching of the pulmonary valve	Pulmonary hypertension
Rounding of the opening /closing points of a disk-type	Mechanical restriction to disc motion prosthetic valve
Systolic anterior motion of the mitral valve	Dynamic subaortic outflow track obstruction

Table 1.2: *M-Mode and 2-dimensional echocardiography in altered hemodynamics* (Contd...)

Echo-characteristics	Hemodynamic applications
Early systolic downward motion (beaking) of the IVS	LBBB
Gradual closure of the aortic valve	Reduced left ventricular stroke volume
Absent pulmonary valve A-wave	Pulmonary hypertension
Two dimensional	
Diastolic flattening of the IVS	RV volume overload
Systolic flattening of the IVS	RV pressure overload (elevated RVSP)
Dilated IVC with abnormal respiratory variation	Elevated RA pressure
Exaggerated IVS bounce, with respiratory variation	Pericardial constriction

IVC, inferior vena cava; **IVS,** interventricular septum; **LBBB,** left bundle branch block; **RA,** right atrial; **RV,** right ventricular; **RVSP,** right ventricular systolic pressure.

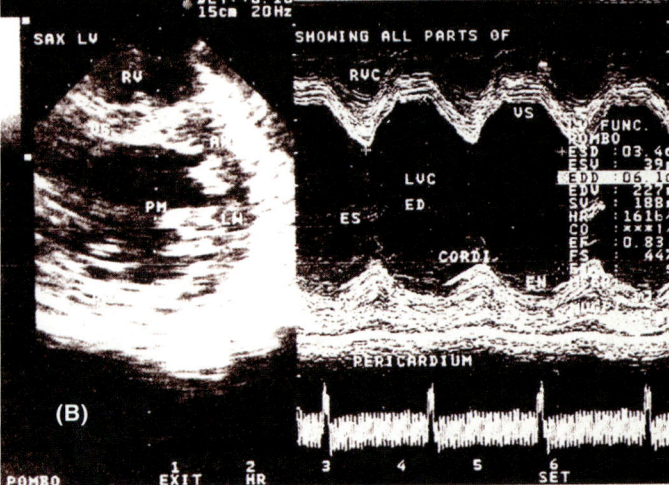

Fig. 1.4: Left panel color Doppler dual scan taken in apical 4C view showing mitral stenotic mosaic colored jet into LV and mitral regurgitation jet (blue) into LA. Right panel shows mainly blue colored jet mixed with yellow color in gross mitral regurgitation (MR)

Fig. 1.5A and B: Different structures of the heart as the ultrasond waves pass from chest through both the right and left ventricles. RVC = Right ventricular cavity, VS = Interventricular septum, LVC = Left ventricular cavity, ES = End systolic, ED = End diastolic cordi = Chordi tendine, EN = Endocardium, PLVW = Posterior left ventricular wall

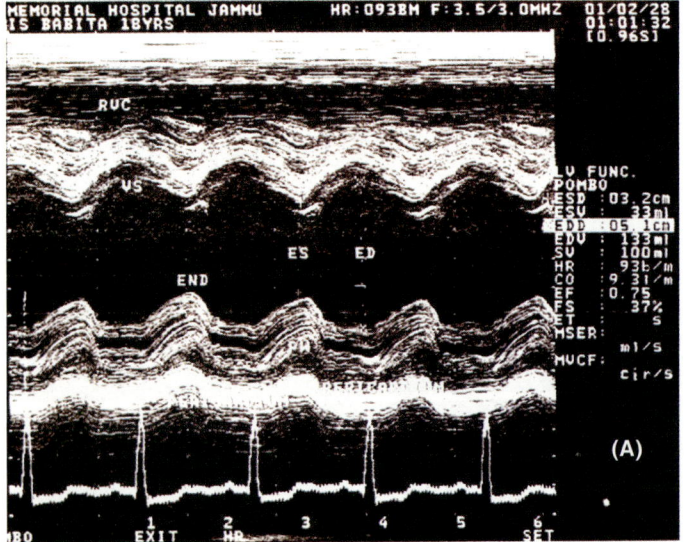

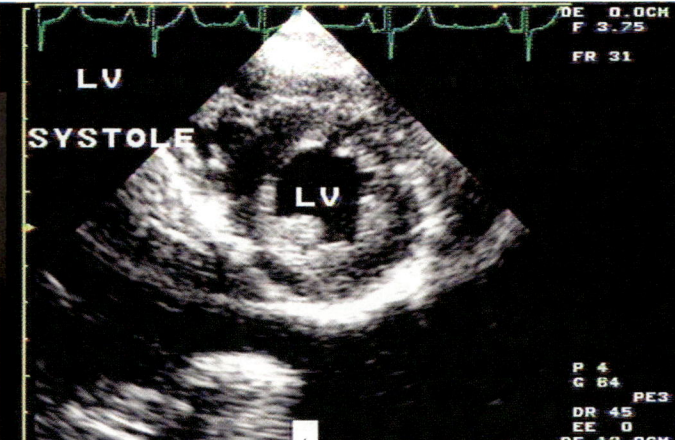

Fig. 1.6A: A short axis view of LV taken at high LPS region in 4th intercostal space showing LV size along with papillary muscles in systole

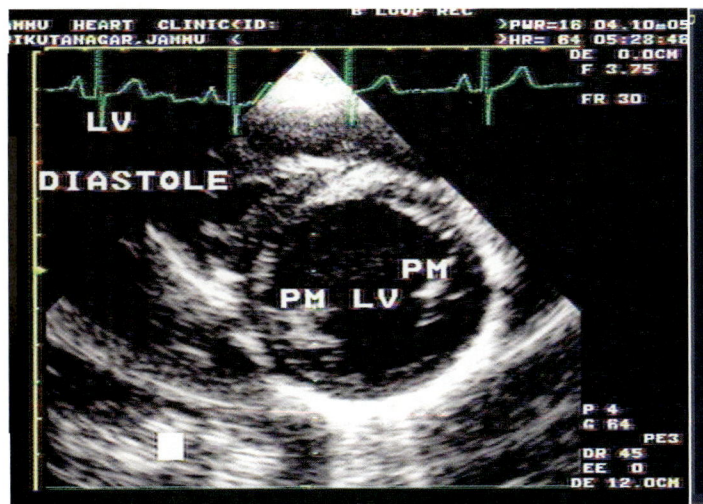

Fig. 1.6B: Short axis view of LV along with papillary muscles in diastole

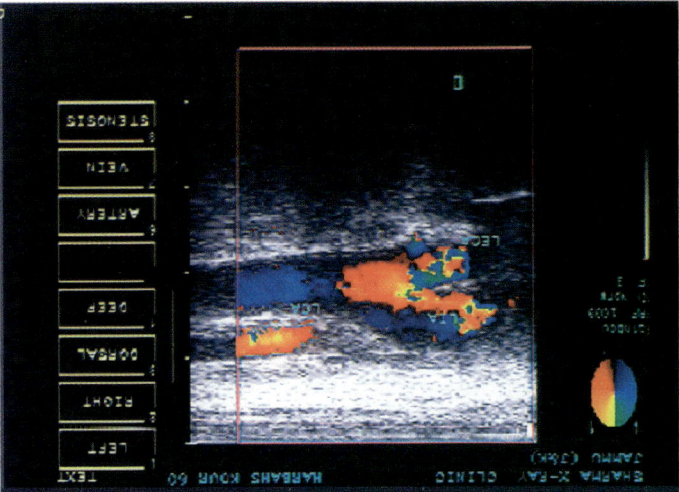

Fig. 1.9: Application of color bar in taking color flow velocity across the carotid arteries

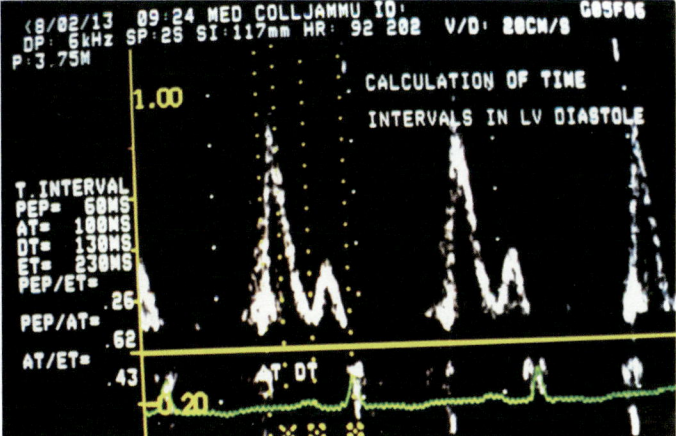

Fig. 1.7: Pulsed Doppler scan of mitral valve shows computer calculated various intervals as depicted on left hand panel of the scan used in hemodynamic correlates in various myocardial dysfunctions

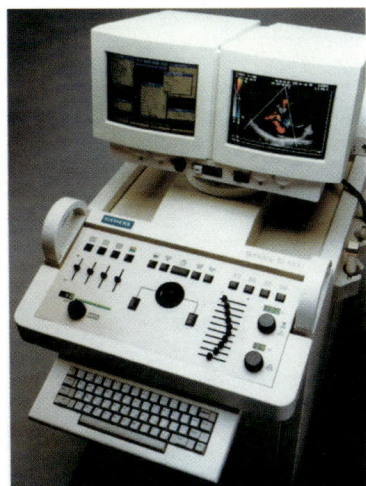

Fig. 1.8: Latest version of color Doppler echocardiographic machine used by the author to take various echocardiograms in this book

use. Piezo-electricity is the property of certain substances to change the mechanical energy of deformation into electric energy and vice versa.

Commercial transducers use ceramics as piezo-electric elements. The most commonly used are barium titanate and lead zinconate titanate. Behind the piezo-electric element is some backing material which absorbs the ultrasound directed backwards, and improves the shape of the forward beam. The echocardiography equipment acts both as transmitter and a receiver of ultrasound. It transmits for a very short time, and then "receives" the reflected echoes. The duration of the transmission is usually 1/1000 of the reception time and only lasts one microsecond. Therefore, there is an emission each millisecond. This method of acoustic imaging is called pulsed ultrasound (Fig. 1.27).

Reflection and Divergence

Light and sound are transmitted by similar physical laws. The ultrasound beam must be perpendicular to the structures under study to record the reflected echoes.

Certain properties of the ultrasonic beam must be appreciated. It remains essentially parallel for a given distance and then begins to diverge.

Lateral Resolution

The ultrasonic beam is as wide as the diameter of the transducer in the near field, but it undergoes divergence in the far field the beam is therefore not a point source, the diameter of the transducer usually being between 5 and 12 mm. This explains why two structures which are not in line with respect to the transducer, may appear artefactually aligned on the recording. This effect is more marked in the distal field. Acoustic lenses of known focal length (usually 5 to 10 cm), may be used to improve lateral resolution.

The Doppler Effect

Scientists have applied the Doppler effect in recording the velocities of normal and abnormal valvular structures of the heart. When a beam of ultrasound passes through a moving column of blood, there is some back-scattering of energy. The frequency of the reflected signal is modified by the velocity and direction of the blood flow with respect to the incidence of the ultrasonic beam. Movement towards the transducer increases the frequency and movement away decreases the frequency of the reflected signal. This change in frequency is proportional to the velocity of blood flow and the angle between the ultrasound beam and the moving target. When the direction of blood flow is perpendicular to the beam, its velocity cannot be measured. Using pulsed Doppler systems, the *Doppler effect* may be measured at a given distance from the transducer, so providing information on the velocity and direction of blood flow at a precise location within the thorax.

Instrumentation: (Uni-directional Echocardiography Display) (Fig. 1.15B)

The echocardiography functions both as a transmitter or pulsed ultrasound, and receiver of the reflected echoes. There are three modes of display of these echoes: A mode (A = amplitude), B mode (B = brightness) and M-mode (M = motion).

A-mode displays the reflected echoes as vertical spikes on a horizontal baseline. The amplitude of each spike varies with the intensity of each reflected echoes, the baseline being calibrated for distance. Although little used nowadays, it is very useful for adjusting the various echocardiographic controls.

B-mode retains the same horizontal baseline, but the reflected echoes are displayed as dots rather than spikes. The intensity or brightness of each spot is proportional to the amplitude of the spike. This mode is used for the display of two-dimensional echography, and also for the recording of M-mode echocardiograms on strip chart recorders.

M-mode is obtained by electronically tracking the B-mode on an oscilloscope. The B-mode echoes are therefore displayed with respect to time and their motion appears as a wavy line; in unidirectional echocardiography, M-mode is a method of presenting the different phases of the cardiac cycle, and of recording and analysing them. For conveniences, M-mode displayed from left to right on the oscilloscope, the top of the screen corresponding to the position of the transducer (Figs 1.16B and 1.21).

Controls

Most M-mode echographs have both A-mode and M-mode display, a fiberoptic strip chart recorder and various control knobs. The adjustments, which are made on the A-mode screen, are of two varieties:

Adjustment of the Position and Size of the Image: This depends on the size of the heart under study, the depth control having to be widened for children: this avoids reverberations and gives optimal visualisation of cardiac structures. The position control or delay allows the operator to change the position of the image without altering the depth control. This makes room for other physiological signals on the same recording.

Adjustment of the Quality and Intensity of the Image: This is performed by adjusting the emission and/or by processing the reflected echoes by a system of echo enhancement (A-mode). The gain-control allows enhancement of the reflected echoes without altering the intensity of the pulsed emission. Ultrasound is attenuated and decreases in intensity as it travels in the tissues, so that echoes reflected from deep lying structures are weaker than those reflected from proximal ones: to compensate for this effect, most echographs have a control which allows selective attenuation of near field echoes and/or enhancement or far field echoes (time-gain compensation) (Fig. 1.8).

The compensating mechanism is displayed as a "ramp", the start and slope of which may be adjusted. A separate adjustment (near gain) is used to control the intensity of near field echoes. Some echocardiographic machines have a programmable time-gain control which allows adjustment of the gain for each depth of examination.

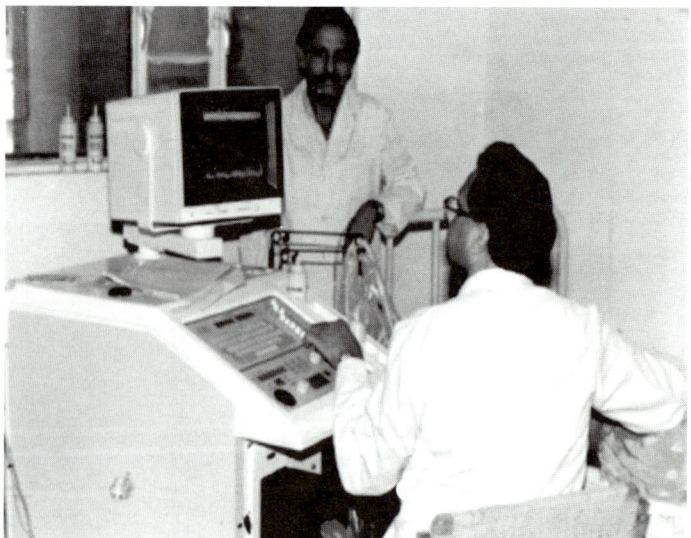

Fig. 1.10: Echocardiographic laboratory at Medical College Hospital, Jammu where part of work was done by the author as shown in this picture

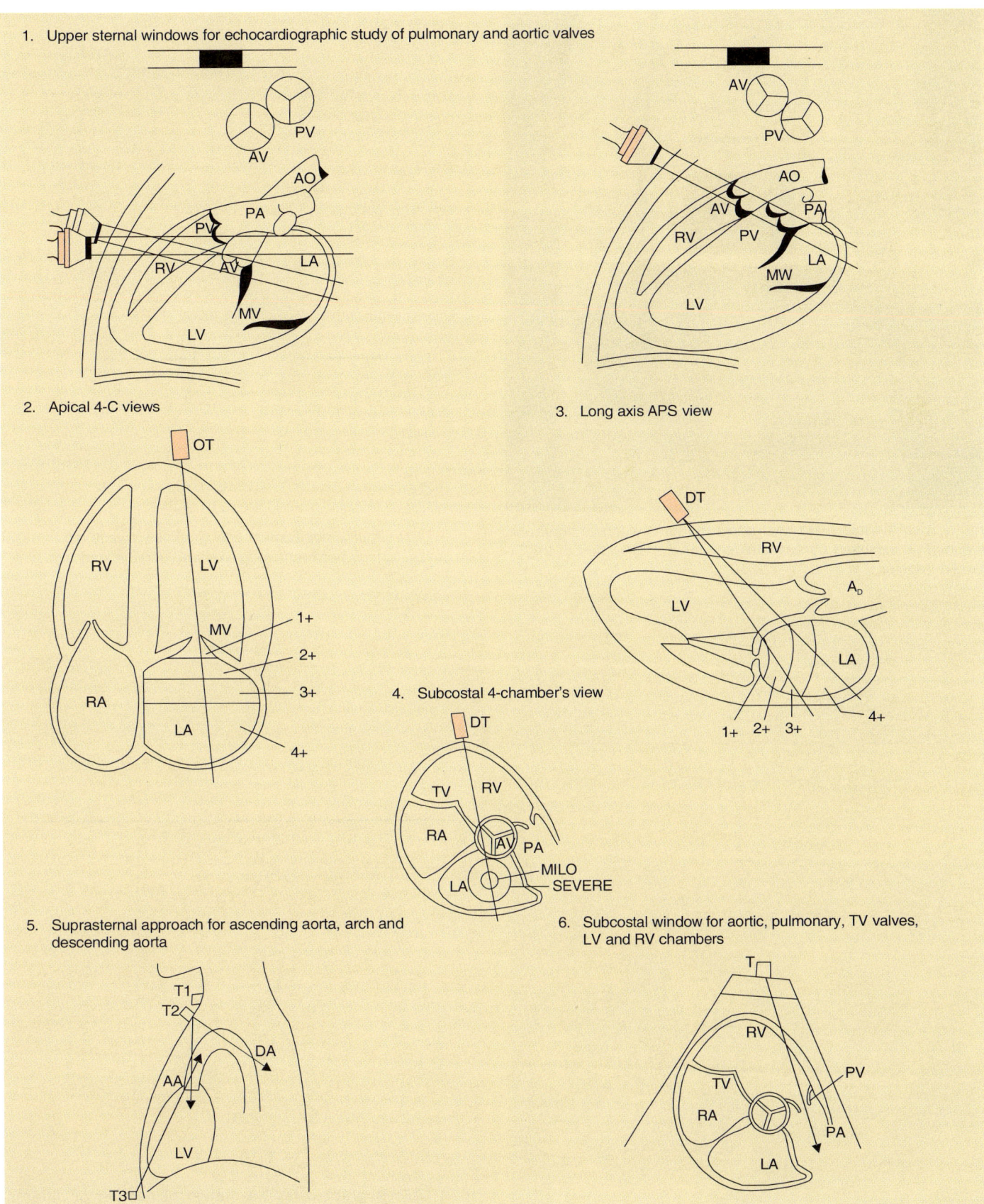

1. Upper sternal windows for echocardiographic study of pulmonary and aortic valves

2. Apical 4-C views

3. Long axis APS view

4. Subcostal 4-chamber's view

5. Suprasternal approach for ascending aorta, arch and descending aorta

6. Subcostal window for aortic, pulmonary, TV valves, LV and RV chambers

Fig. 1.11: Graphic representation of various views through different echocardiographic windows in taking M-mode, Doppler and color Doppler echocardiograms currently under use

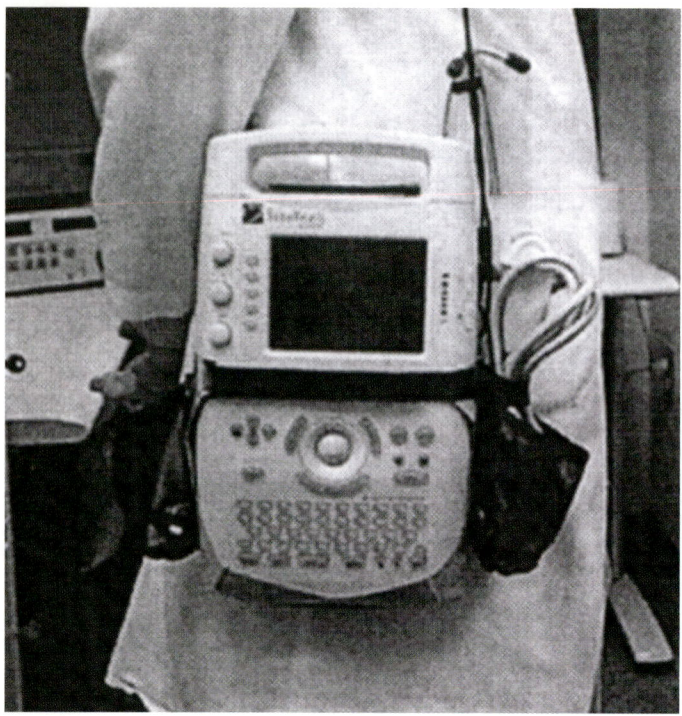

Fig. 1.12: Portable hand-held latest model of echocardiographic machine is exhibited by suspending over the shoulders of the attending doctor

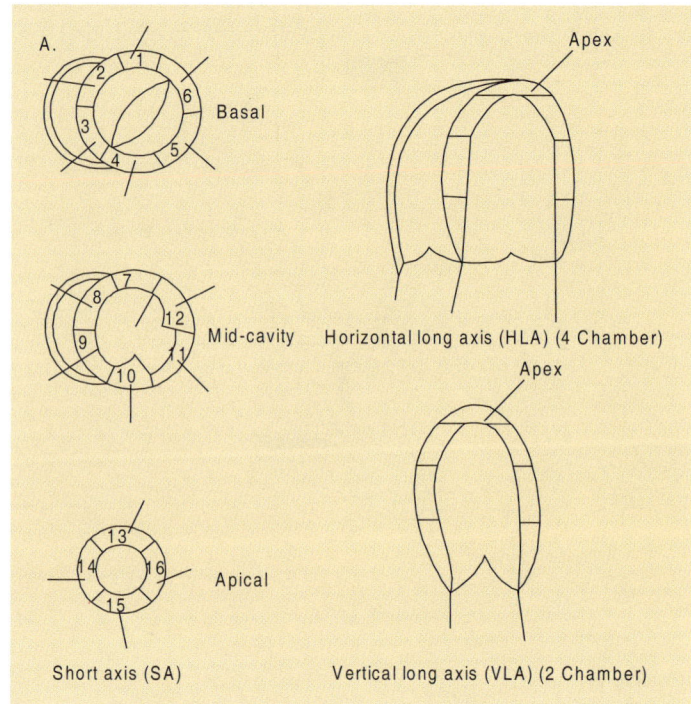

A.

Basal

Mid-cavity

Apical

Short axis (SA)

Apex

Horizontal long axis (HLA) (4 Chamber)

Apex

Vertical long axis (VLA) (2 Chamber)

Fig. 1.14A: Graphic depiction of echographic views taken at basal, mid cavity, apical, horizontal long axis and vertical long axis

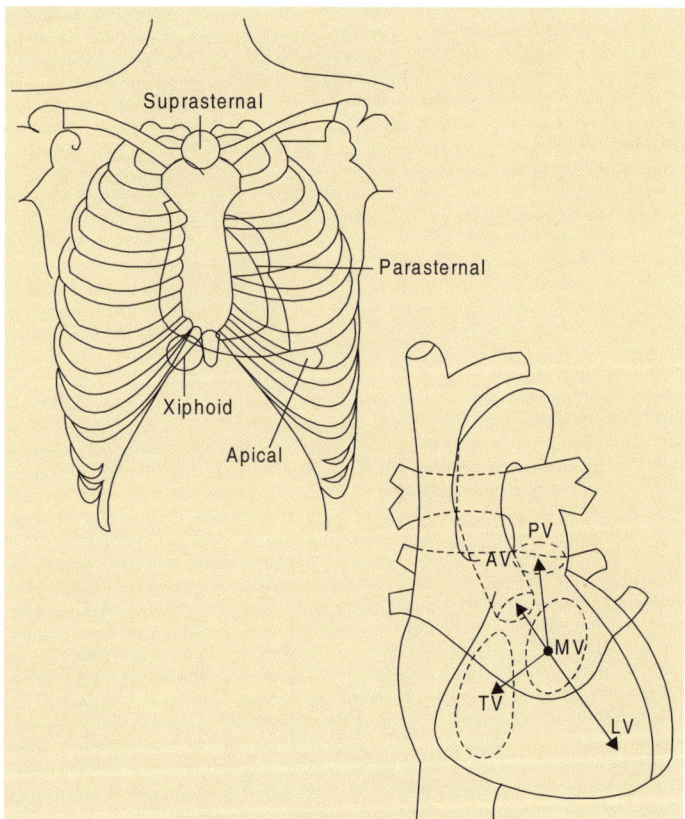

Suprasternal

Parasternal

Xiphoid

Apical

PV

AV

MV

TV

LV

Fig. 1.13: (left) Various echocardiographic windows on graphic cadaver and graphic visualisation of different cardiac valves by the application of these above depicted windows (right)

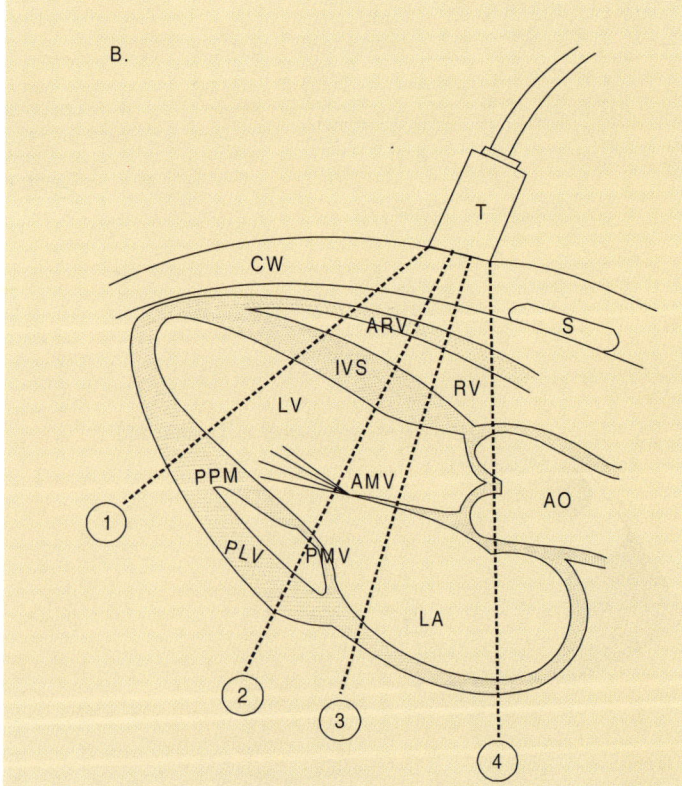

B.

CW

ARV

IVS

LV

RV

S

PPM

AMV

AO

PLV

PMV

LA

1

2

3

4

T

Fig. 1.14B: A graphic representation of number of different echocardiographic tracings of inner structures of the heart which can be obtained by moving the thoracic transducer at the sites of specified windows as shown in this diagram

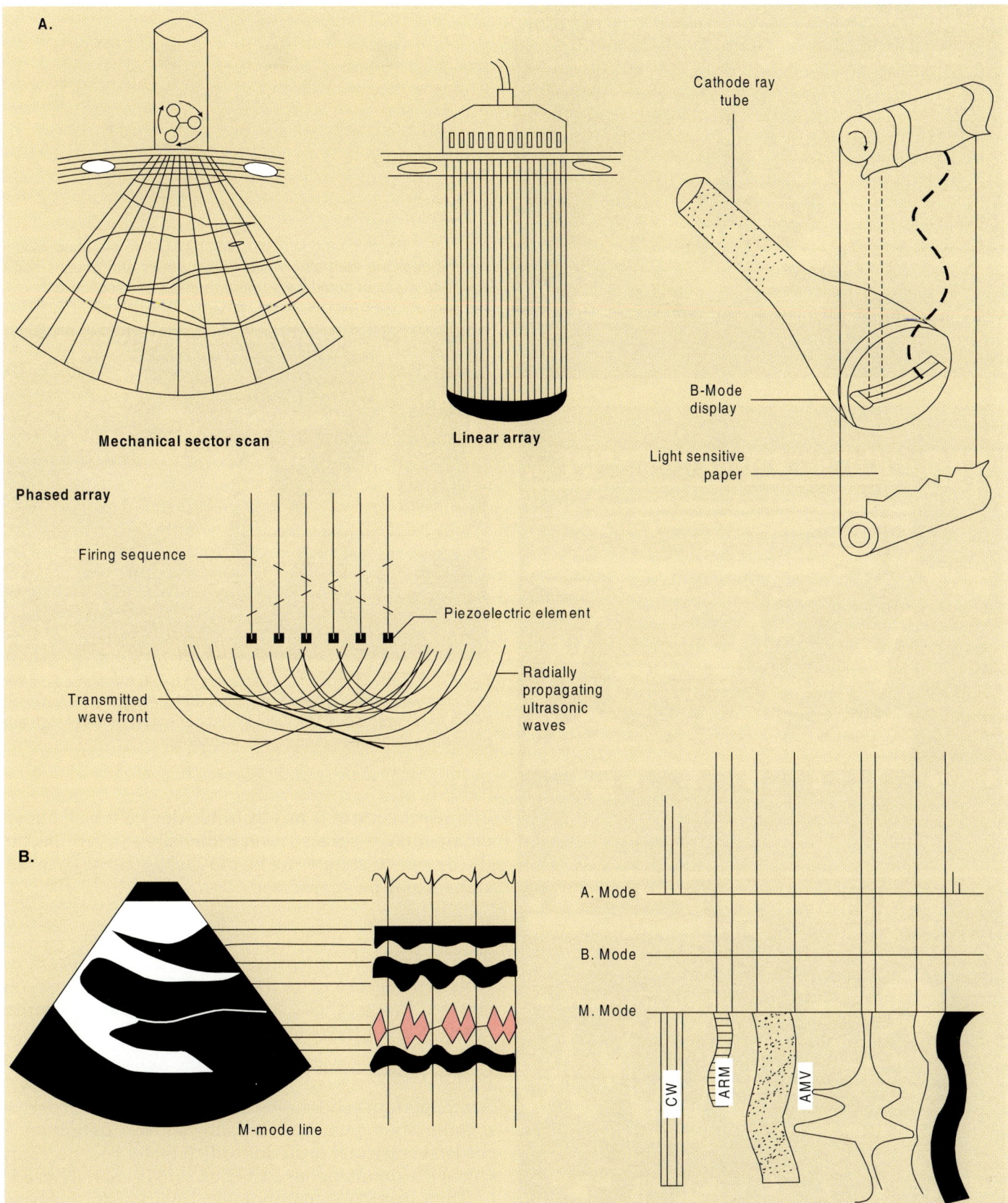

Fig. 1.15: (upper panel A) Showing different types of transducer, i.e. mechanical sector, linear array and phased array employed by the echographer and Lower panel B shows graphic representation of various modes used in obtaining live pictures for the evaluation of various diseases of the heart

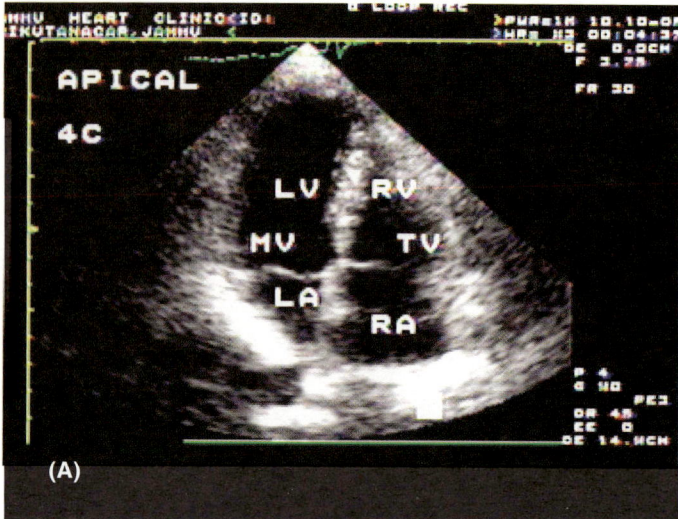

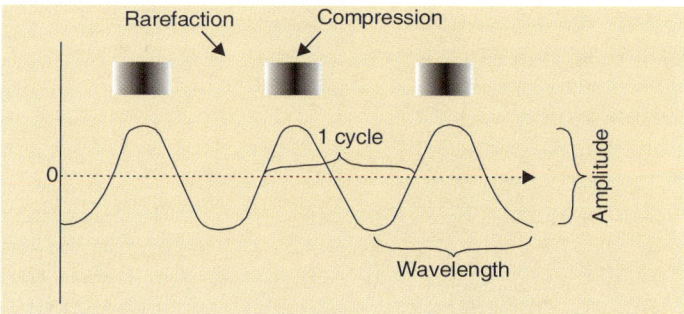

Fig. 1.17: Graphic representation of propagation of sound. Sound can be depicted as a sine wave whose peaks and troughs correspond to areas of compression and rarefaction, respectively

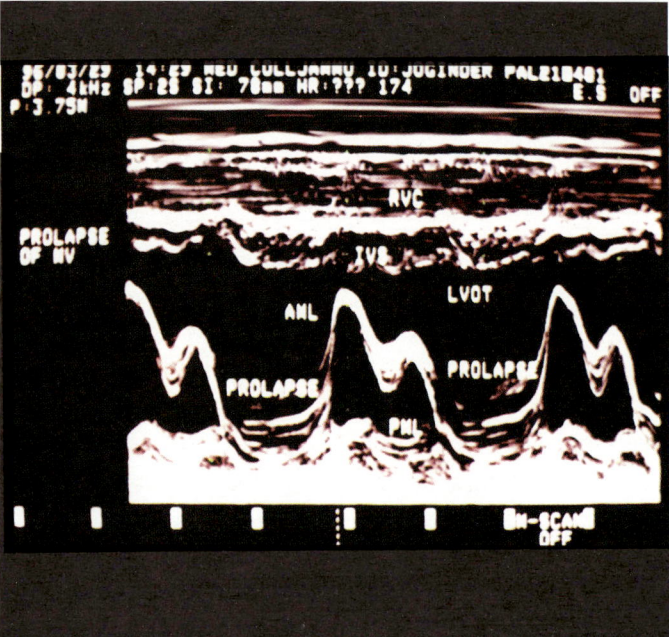

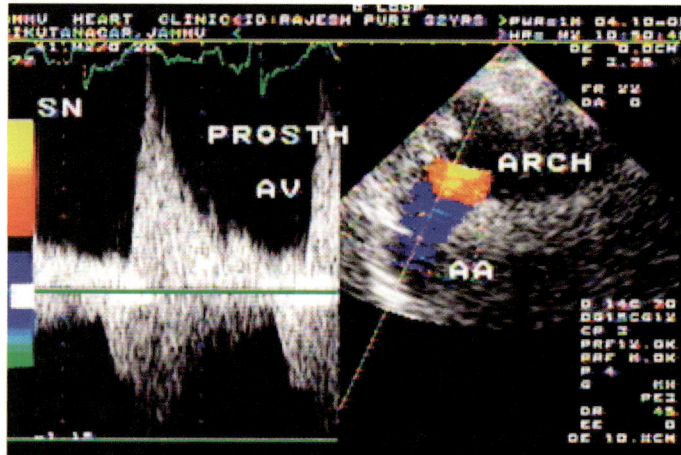

Fig. 1.18: Color Doppler echocardiogram taken through apical two chamber view showing near field clutter artifact at apical region simulating as an apical clot. This usually happens as a result of high amplitude oscillations emitted by the transducer

Reject

The reject control is an electronic device which allows elimination of signals of weak intensity at reception, but the threshold should not be too high, otherwise, useful signals may be suppressed.

Damping

This controls the intensity of the ultrasound beam on emission. It is useful for the identification of two closely situated strong echoes, such as the epicardio-pericardial complex from the neighbouring structures.

Switch Gain

Some modern echographs have a control which acts as a continuous damping and allows better definition of the left ventricular posterior wall. It is always a necessity to have a simultaneous ECG (lead II is generally used).

This serves as a chronological marker for echocardiographic events. In the early days of echocardiography, the only method of recording was by photographing the oscilloscope (usually by polaroid).

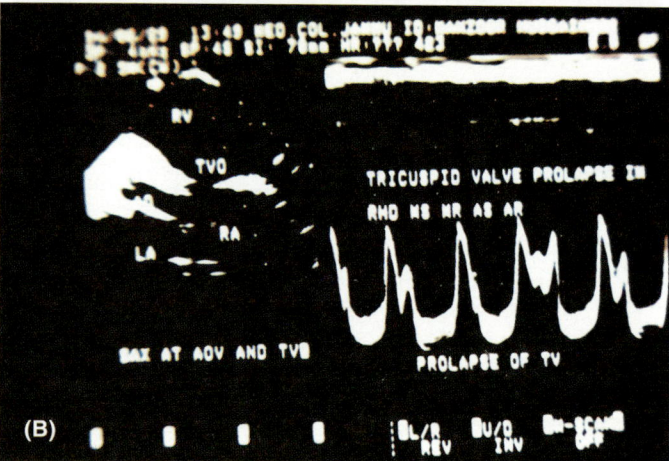

Fig. 1.16A and B: (A) 2-D apical four chamber view scan depicting all four chambers of the heart. **(B)** M-Mode scans of mitral (upper) and tricuspid (lower) valves

This was of limited value because of the relatively small number of cardiac cycles on each oscilloscopic sweep. Till recently it has become possible to record M-mode echocardiography on paper. The recording may be made at variable paper speeds of, 25 or 50 mm/sec for routine recording, 75 or 100 mm/sec for analysis of rapid events.

Several types of recording papers are commercially available; ultraviolet light sensitive and dry silver heart sensitive paper are the generally used, the essential feature being instantaneous development for immediate control of the quality of the recording (Fig. 1.15A).

Echocardiographic Laboratory (Fig. 1.10)

Echocardiography laboratory should have separate room for examination of patients and another for interpretation and filling of records; and it should be located as near to the intensive care unit and other wards as possible.

Two-Dimensional Echocardiography

Various systems have their own advantages and limitations. Mechanical sector scans have good proximal resolution, are more mobile and less costly than electronic systems; however, with phased array, simultaneous M-mode becomes possible, the transducer may be easier to use and dynamic focussing may be available (Figs 1.12, 1.15A and 1.31).

This comparison has been simplified, as the characteristics of each system may differ significantly from make-to-make. The recording is made on magnetic tape, and so the choice of recorder is critical; this may be influenced by the presence of a preexisting video system. The quality of image is related to the band width ¾ inch gives better image resolution than ½ inch tape.

A photographic system is a useful accessory; polaroid being the method offered by most manufacturers. More advanced equipment is necessary for better quality reproductions; for example, digital scan converters to freeze the image. Finally, it is essential to perform as many echocardiographs as possible, the machine offering the best value for money.

Organization of Echo Laboratory (Figs 1.10 and 1.27)

A set of transducers, each with a different frequency and focal length, is useful for 2-dimensional Doppler echocardiography. M-mode echocardiography transducers of 2.25 MHz frequency and focal length of 7/5 cm, are generally used to examine adults, whereas frequencies of 3.5 and 5.0 MHz are more appropriate for the examination of children and babies. These characteristics should be checked annually by the manufacturer.

Technicians may be employed to help position the patient and even to record the echocardiogram, under medical supervision, when a high patient turnover is expected. The echocardiogram may be reported on a standard printed sheet showing the normal values for the laboratory.

Three examinations a day is the minimum level of activity (American Heart Association) to maintain the quality of laboratory's results.

With the growth of computer industry, systems of automatic analysis have become available. These programs provide detailed analysis of left ventricular function (for research projects), but some systems may also be used for an automatic printout of results, and for administrative purposes.

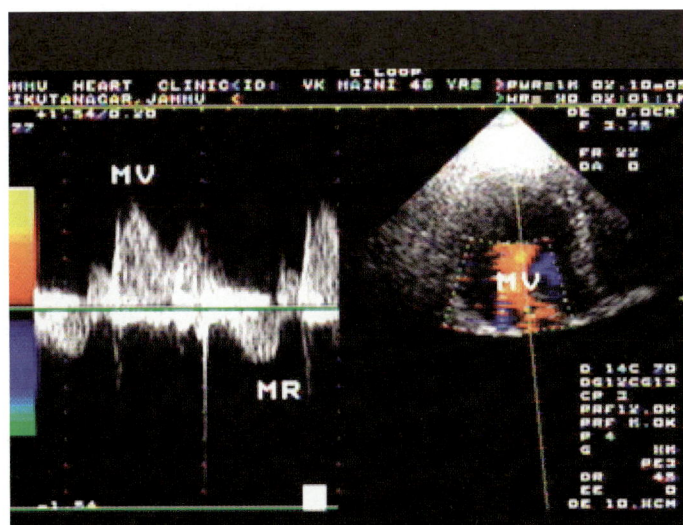

Fig. 1.19: Mild spectral widening of Doppler flow as blood passes through a roughened mitral valve

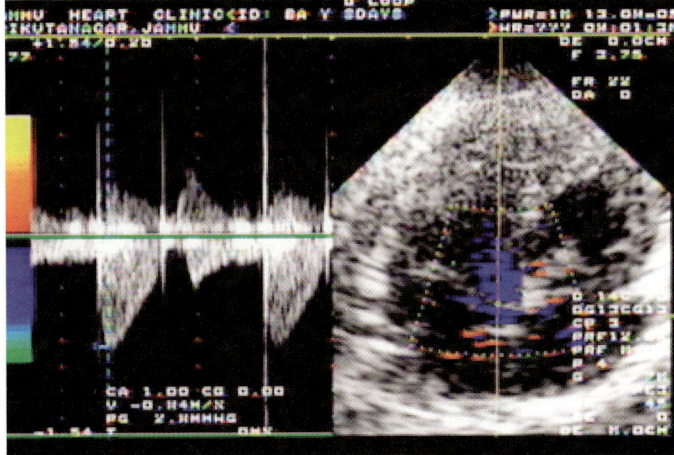

Fig. 1.20: Color Doppler blood flow velocity across ascending aorta through suprasternal notch window depicting mirror image backward velocity as an artifact. This can be mistaken as aortic regurgitation flow below the line

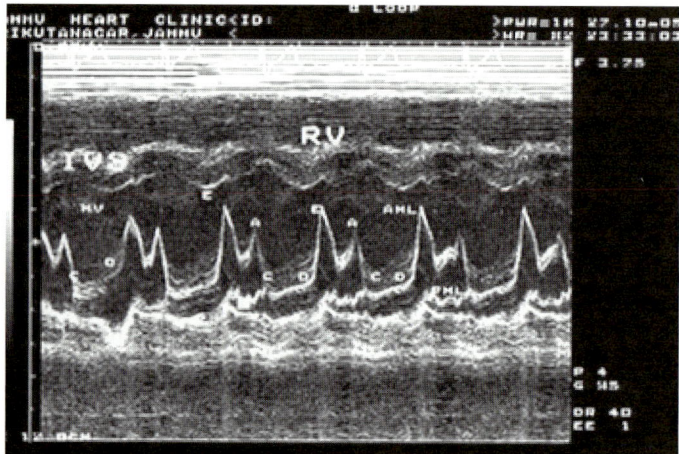

Fig. 1.21: M-mode echocardiogram showing morphology of normal mitral valve with various hemodynamic points as A, B, C, D, E, F and opening of anterior mitral and posterior mitral leaflets during diastole

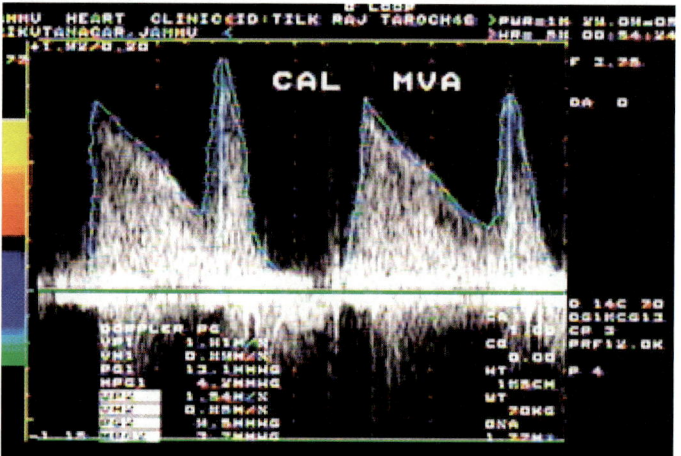

Fig. 1.22: 2-D Doppler flow across MV showing disturbed blood flow through inflow tract of LV with changing morphological features of all the hemodynamic points in patient with mild type of mitral stenosis

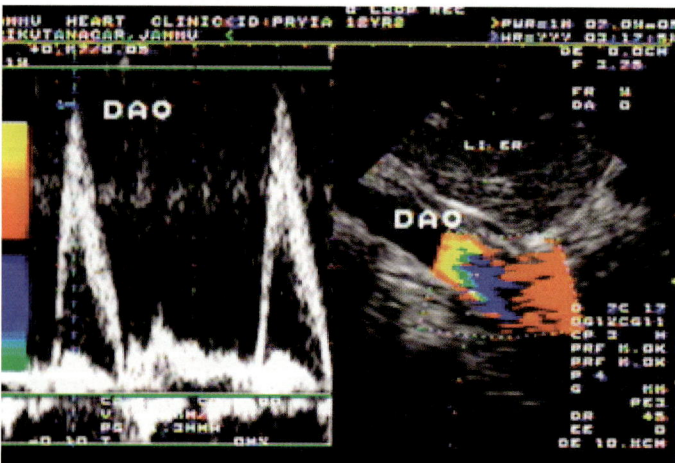

Fig. 1.23: Laminar, pulsatile flow in the abdominal aorta by the application of pulsed wave Doppler imaging. The signal depicts a narrow envelope during negotiating the Doppler flow

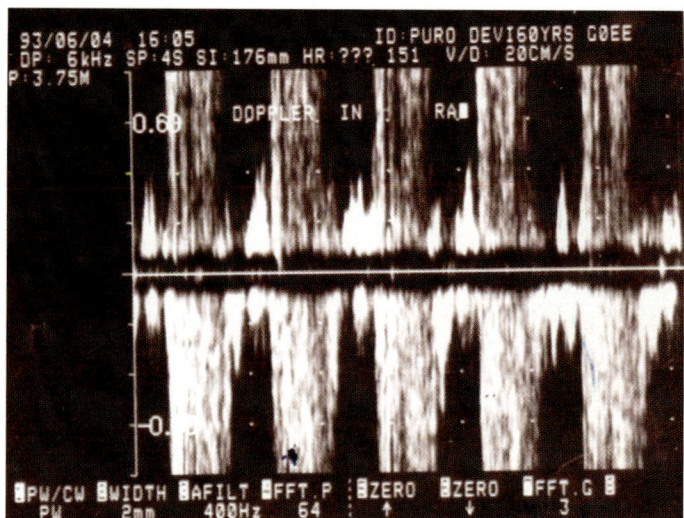

Fig. 1.24: An example of phenomenon of aliasing where velocity of flow can be seen above and down the line which can happen when velocity of flow crosses the prescribed limit of the pulsed Doppler technique. A case of severe tricuspid regurgitation when the sample volume was placed over the area of inflow tract of RV. In such situation, help of continuous wave Doppler can be acquired to record the true value of velocity flow

Table 1.3: *Echocardiographic windows used for records*
Transthoracic
Left parasternal
Apical
Subcostal
Right parasternal
Suprasternal
Transesophageal intravascular
Intracardiac
Intracoronary
Epicardial

Table 1.4: *Velocity of sound in air and other tissues of body*	
Medium velocity (m/sec)	
Air	330
Fat	1450
Water	1480
Soft tissue	1540
Kidney	1560
Blood	1570
Muscle	1580

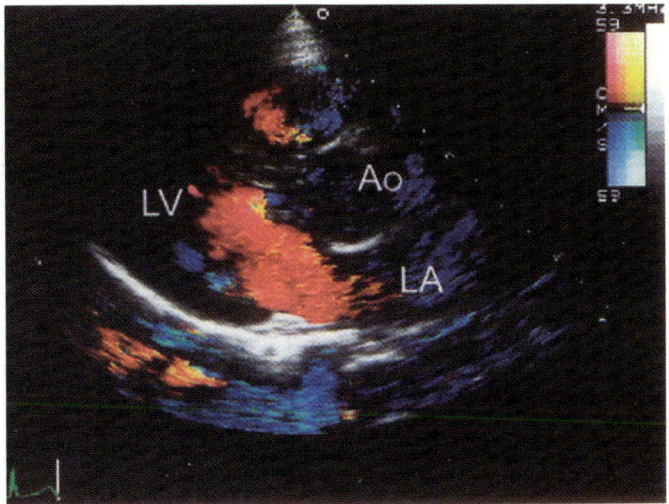

Fig. 1.25: Artifacts called Ghosts in color Doppler flow when color flow images are frozen to analyze or planimeter a jet of color flow

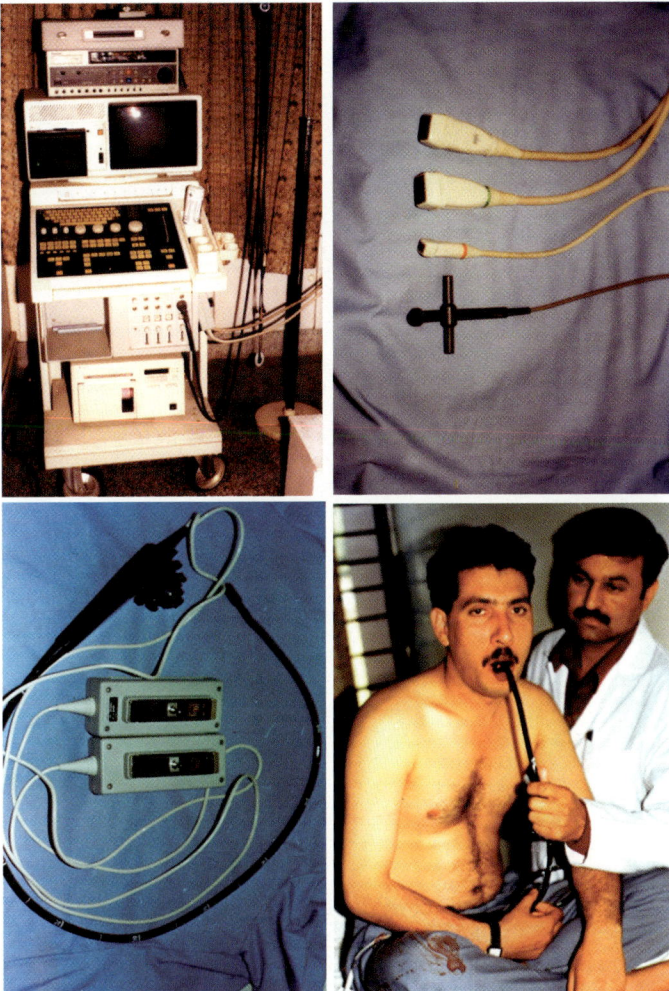

Fig. 1.27: Upper (left) panel shows echocardiography machine provided with ancillary tools used for obtaining graphs. Upper (right) panel showing mechanical, sector phased array and non-imaging or pedoff, continuous wave Doppler transducers being used for obtaining echoscans. Lower (left) panel shows the features of biplane transesophageal probe. Lower (right) panel showing laboratory assistant explaining the whole procedure to the patient prior to the performance of transesophageal echocardiography

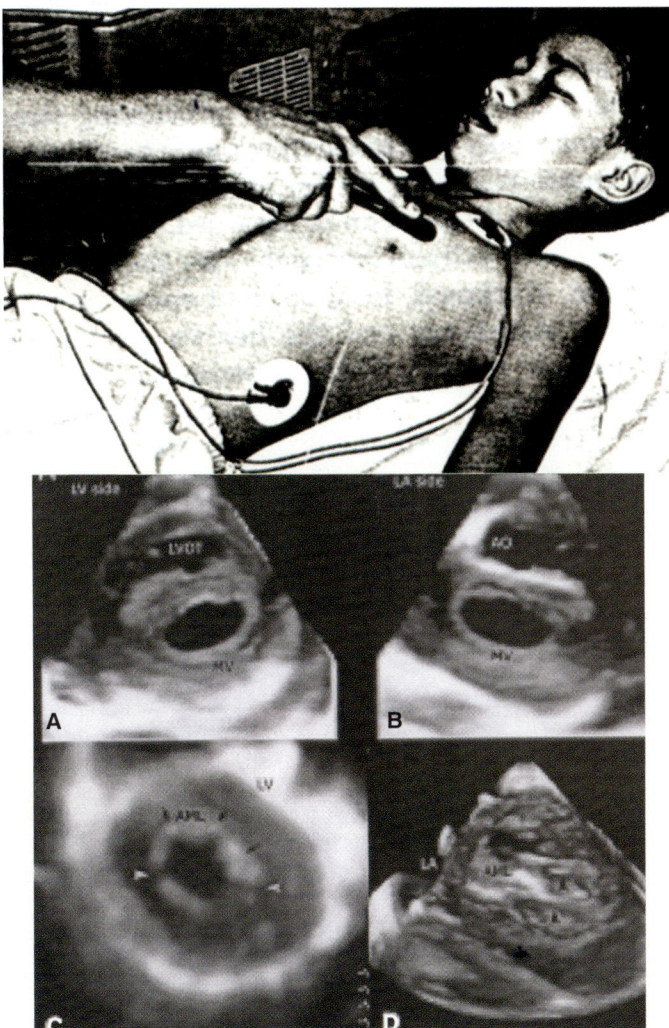

Fig. 1.26: Upper panel showing operator placing the specific transducer prior to obtaining transthoracic echoscans. Lower panel shows reconstruction of 3-Dimensional echoscan of MV

Digital Echocardiography (Figs 1.8, 1.9, 1.12, 1.22, 1.23, 1.26–1.29 and 1.33)

No doubt, videotape recordings of echocardiographic studies seems to be a versatile and cost-effective modality, but it does have certain limitations. It may record more informations than is required for use. A full study, including 2-dimensional, M-mode, spectral Doppler, and colour flow imaging may take 10 to 20 minutes of videotape. One of the major disadvantages of this approach is that the clinician frequently does not have the patience to view that much videotape. Furthermore, the tape may not be easily accessible to the referring clinician; it may still be in the instrument or it may be in shelf along with studies of 10 or 20

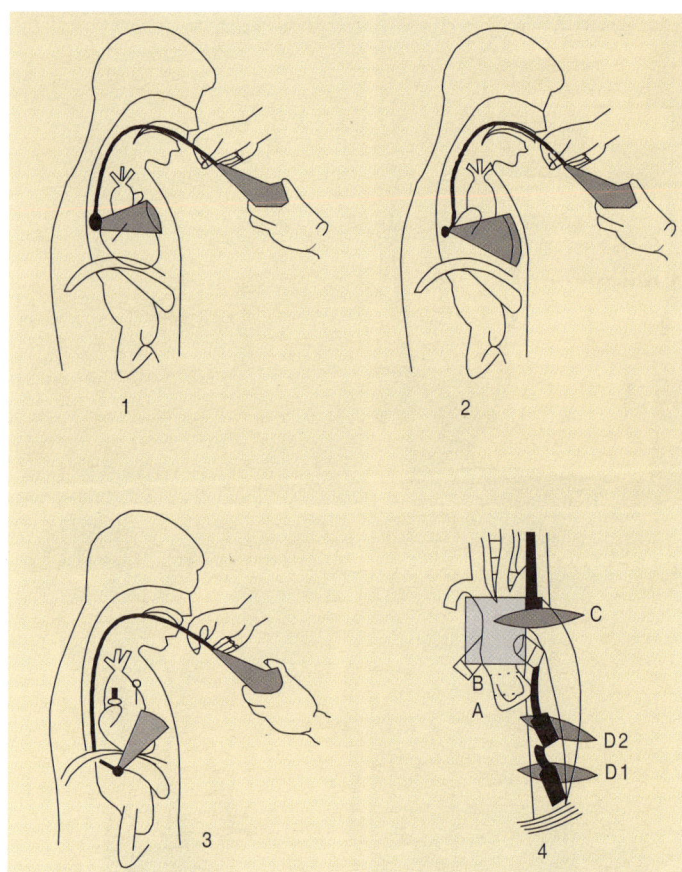

Fig. 1.28: Different types of windows and views employed in TEE. 1. Basal short axis, 2. Four chamber view, 3. Transgastric short axis, 4. At the level of thoracic aorta

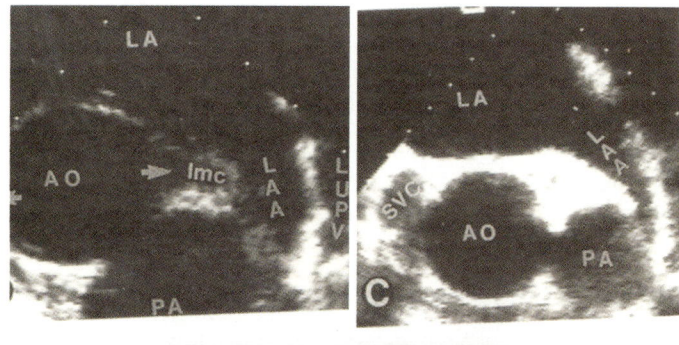

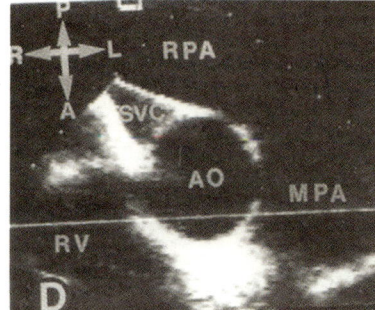

Fig. 1.29: Application of TEE in obtaining various structural scans in the study of anatomy of the heart

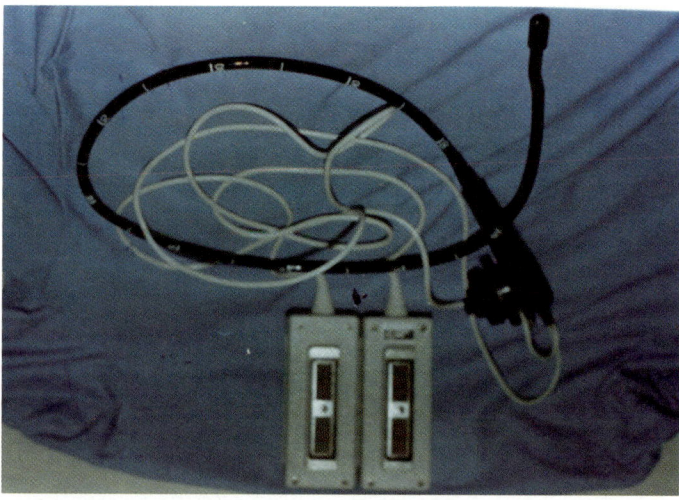

Fig. 1.30: Two connectors at the bottom of TEE probe which are to be fitted with the basic color Doppler echocardiographic machine to make it fully functional for obtaining TEE graphs

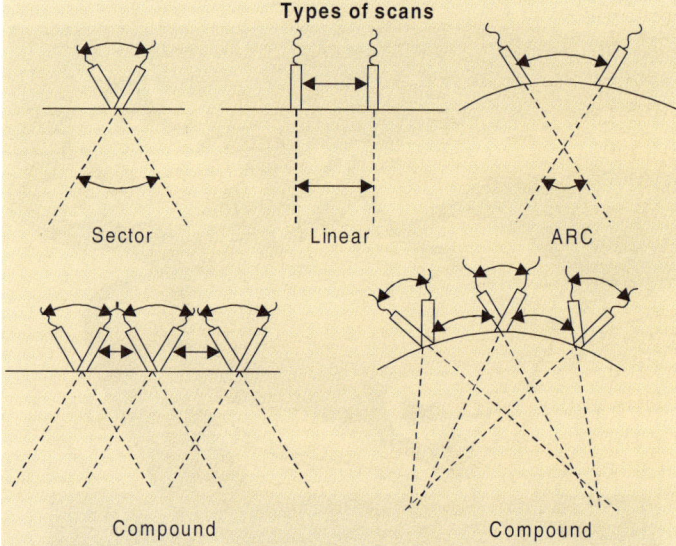

Fig. 1.31: Graphics depicting various types of scaners available for the study of echocardiographic imaging

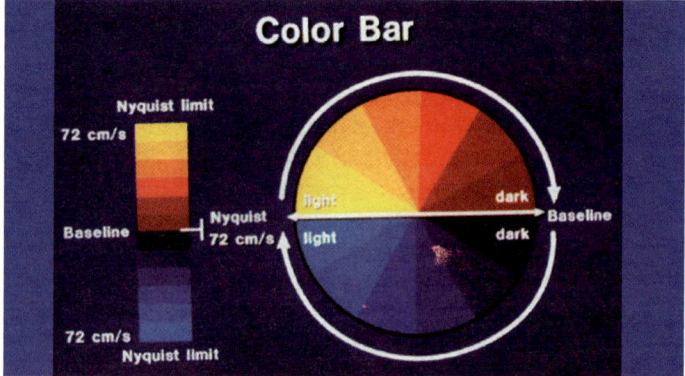

Fig. 1.32: Color bar and color aliasing. This concept is always kept in mind while working on color Doppler flow velocity recording. In this case the brightest step is shown the maximal measurable velocity or the nyquist limit and the lowest velocity or zero velocity is assigned to a color black or no color

patients on a 2-hour videotape. Merely finding a specific patient on a tape may be too time consuming for the average physician. As a result, relatively a few clinicians who have no special interest in echocardiography take the time to look at echocardiograms on videotape. It is also difficult to show videotape at conferences because an unedited videotape is lengthy.

Digital techniques with computer storage is an alternative means of assessing echocardiographic studies. One can use frame grabbers to digitally capture individual cardiac cycles and store them in a variety of different ways. A standard echocardiography with a commercially available frame grabber is inserted below the tape recorder and the computer monitor is mounted on its top. One can digitize and display a single full image, two views as a split image, or four examinations as a quad screen. Four views can be displayed simultaneously. Newer digital systems can display as many as 16 images on one screen. Digital recordings overcome many of the deficiencies of videotape. They make the examination readily accessible for the clinician to review. Individual studies which can be retrieved in 10 to 30 seconds. One can look at the study as long as is necessary without rewinding the videotape. This approach is ideal for analyzing serial studies. One can easily compare two, three, or four studies simultaneously to see whether or not any changes have occurred. Additionally with the study in the digital form, all of the versatility of digital technology including quantitation becomes easier. Automatic quantitation is feasible.

This method of digital recording facilitates the attending physician to have a brief review or abstract of the total case. The digital approach does not have sufficient information to replace videotape at this time. With the rapid advances in digital technology, however, this situation may change in the near future.

Tissue Doppler Imaging (Fig. 1.33)

Comparatively a recent application of the Doppler principle is tissue Doppler imaging. By adjusting gain and reject settings, the Doppler technique can be employed for recording the motion of the myocardium rather than the blood within it. To apply Doppler imaging to tissue, two important differences must be recognised.

First, because the velocity of the tissue is much lower than blood flow, the machine must be adjusted to record a much lower range of velocities. **Second**, because the tissue is a much stronger reflector of the Doppler signal compared with blood, additional adjustments are required to avoid oversaturation. When these factors are taken into account, a semiquantitative approach to myocardial velocity analysis is possible. Note how this early systolic frame displays the direction and relative velocity of the different myocardial segments.

One obvious limitation is that the incident angle between the beam and the direction of target motion varies from region to region. This limits the ability of the technique to provide absolute velocity information, although direction and relative changes in tissue velocity are displayed.

One potentially important derivation of this technique involves strain rate imaging. Strain is a measure of the deformation that occurs when force is applied to tissue. Strain rate is simply its temporal derivative. By measuring instantaneous velocity at two closely positioned points within the myocardium and knowing the initial distance between two points, both strain and strain rate can be determined. The Doppler tissue imaging technique has been used successfully to derive the velocity information needed to calculate strain rate accurately.

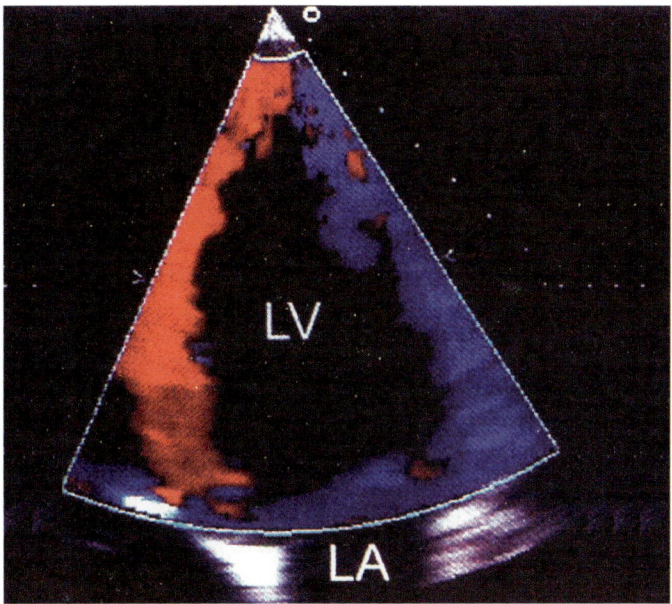

Fig. 1.33: Tissue Doppler scan depicting direction and relative velocity of different myocardial segments during early systole

Limitations of Echocardiography

As previously mentioned, ultrasound is absorbed by air and bone. Echocardiography is often difficult to perform in obese and emphysematous patients, and in those with deformities of the chest wall. However, by multiplying the number of M-mode and 2-dimensional examination, interpretable recordings may be obtained from almost all patients. Even when the recording is of poor quality, some simple problems may be resolved in most cases. The experience, skill and application of the operator play an important role. However, currently available technique of trans-esophageal echocardiography can be employed safely to overcome the difficulty of obtaining clear views particular in obese and emphysematous patients (Figs 1.28–1.30).

Bibliography

1. Aggarwal KK, Moos S, Philpot EF, Jain SP, Helmucke F, Nanda NC: Colour velocity determination using pixel colour intensity in Doppler colour flow mapping. *Echocardiography* 1989; 6:473.

2. Asberg A: Ultrasonic cinematography of the living heart. *Ultrasonics*, 1967; 6:113.

3. Burns PN: The physical principles of Doppler and spectral analysis. *JCU* 1987; 15:567.

4. Collins M, Hsieh A, Ohazama CJ, *et al*. Assessment of regional wall motion abnormalities; with real-time 3 dimensional echocardiography. *J. Am Soc Echocardiography* 1999; 12:7–14.

5. Chwartz MD, Decristofaro D: Review and evaluation of range gated, pulsed, echo-Doppler. *J Clin Eng* 1978; 3:153.

6. Dussik KT. Uber die Moglichkeit Hochfrequente Mechan-ischescbwingungen als Diagnostisches Hilfsmittel zu Venverten. *Z Neurol* 1941;174:153.

7. Edler I, Hertz CH. Use of ultrasonic reflectoscope for the continuous recording of movements of heart walls. *Kungl Fysiogr Sallsk Lung Forth* 1954; 24:40.

8. Edler I. The diagnostic use of ultrasound in heart disease. *Acta MedScand Suppl* 1955; 308:32.

9. Edler I. Ultrasound cardiogram in mitral valve disease. *Acta Chir Scand* 111:1956; 230.

10. Eggleton RC, *et al*: Visualization of cardiac dynamics with real-time B-mode ultrasonic scanner. In *Ultrasound in Medicine*. Edited by D. White. New York, Plenum Press, 1975.

11. Eyer MK, Brandestini MA, Phillips DJ, Baker DW: Colour digital echo/Doppler image presentation. *Ultrasound Med Biol*, 1981; 7:21.

12. Edler I, Gustafson A, Karlefors I: *et al*. The movements of aortic and mitral valves recorded with ultrasonic echo techniques (motion picture). Presented at the III European Congress of Cardiology, Rome, Italy, 1960.

13. Feigenbaum H, Zaky A: Use of diagnostic ultrasound in clinical cardiology. *J Indiana State Med Assoc* 1996; 59:140.

14. Flinn GS: Colour encoded display of M-Mode echocardio-grams. *J.Clin. Ultrasound* 1976; 4:339.

15. Feigenbaum H. Evolution of echocardiography. *Circulation* 1996; 93:1321.

16. Feigenbaum H. *Echocardiography*. 1st Ed. Philadelphia: LeaFebiger, 1972.

17. Firestone FA: Flaw detecting device and measuring instrument. *U.S. Patent* 1.1942; 280:226.

18. Feldman A, Ford P. *Scientists and Inventors*. New York: Facts on File, 1979.

19. Gramiak R, Waag R, Simon W. Cine ultrasound cardio-graphy, *Radiology* 1973; 107:175.

20. Griffith JM, Henry WL: A sector scanner for real time two-dimensional echocardiography *Circulation*, 1974;49:1147.

21. Goldberg P, Kimmelman BA. *Medical Diagnostic Ultrasound: A Retrospective* on its 40th Anniversary. Rochester, NY: Eastman Kodak Co., 1988.

22. Holmes JH. Diagnostic ultrasound during the early years of A.I.U.M. *J Clin Ultrasound*, 1980, 8:299–308.

23. Hatle L, Angelsen B: *Doppler Ultrasound in Cardiology: Physical Principles and Clinical Applications*, 2nd ed. Philadelphia, Lea and Fibger, 1984.

24. Hertz CH, Lundstrom K: A fast ultrasonic scanning system for heart investigation, 3rd International Conference on Medical Physics. Gotenburg, Sweden, August, 1972.

25. Hertz CH: Ultrasonic engineering in heart diagnosis. *Am J Cardiol*, 1976; 19:6.

26. King DL: Cardiac Ultrasonography: Cross-sectional ultrasonic imaging of the heart, *Circulation*. 1973; 47:843.

27. Kisslo JA, VonRamm OT, Thurstone FL: Dynamic cardiac imaging using a focused, phased-array ultrasound system. *Am J Med*, 1977; 63:61.

28. Kossoff G: Diagnostic applications of ultrasound in cardiology. *Australas Radiol* 1966; 63:101.

29. Kratochwil A, Jantsch C, Mosslacher H, Slany J, Wenger R: Ultrasonic tomography of the heart. *Ultrasound Med. Biol.*, 1974; 1:275.

30. Kuecherer HF, Abbott JA, Botvinick EH, Scheinman ED, O'Connell JW, Scheinman MM, Foster E, Schiller NB: Two-dimensional echocardiographic phase analysis. *Circulation*, 1992; 85:130.

31. Keidel WD: Uber cine Methode zur Registrierung del' Volumanderungen des Herzens am Menschen. *Z Kreislauf-forsch* 1950; 39:257.

32. Latson LA, Cheatham JP, Gutgesell HP: Resolution and accuracy in two-dimensional echocardiography. *Am J Cardiol*, 1981; 48:106.

33. Matsumoto M, Matsuo H, Ohara T, AbeH.: Use of kymo-two-dimensional echocardiography for the diagnosis of aortic root dissection and my cotic aneurysm of the aortic root. *Ultrasound Med. Biol.*, 1977; 3:153.

34. Millery DC. *Anecdotal History of the Science of Sound.* New York, Macmillan, 1935.

35. Morgan CL, Trought WS, Clark WM, Von-Ramm OT, Thurstone FL: Principles and applications of a dynamically focused scanners *JCU*, 1978; 6:385.

36. Nanda NC: *Textbook of Colour Doppler Echocardiography.* Edited by NC Nanda, Philadelphia, Lea and Febiger, 1989.

37. Omoto R: *Colour Atlas of Real-Time Two-dimensional Doppler Echocardiography*. Tokyo, Shindan-To-Chiryo Co., Ltd., 1984.

38. Phased array real time ultrasound system. *JCU*, 1978;6:385.

39. Ryan T, Armstrong WF, Feigenbaum H: Annular Array Technology: Application to Cardiac Imaging, *Echocardio-graphy*, 1987; 4:203.

40. Roelandt, JRTC. Seeing the invisible: A short history of cardiac ultrasound. *Eui' J Echocardiography* 2000;1.

41. Sokolov SY. Means for indicating/laws in materials. *U.S. Patent* 2.1937; 164:1125.

42. Schmidt W, Braun H. Ultrasonic mitral defect and in non-pathological Kreislauffol'sch 1958; 47:291.

43. Talbott JH. *A Biographical History of Medicine,* New York, Grune & Stratton, 1935, 290.

44. Wells PNT: Physics: *An Introduction to Echocardiography.* edited by G. Leech and G. Sutton, London, Medicine Ltd. 1978.

45. Yeh E: Reverberations in echocardiograms. *J Clin Ultrasound,* 1977, 5:84.

46. Wells PNT: Absorption and dispersion of ultrasound in biological tissue. *Ultrasound Med. Biol.,* 1:1975;3 69.

47. Wild PW. Early history of echocardiography. *J Cardiovascular Ultrasonography* 1996; 5:2.

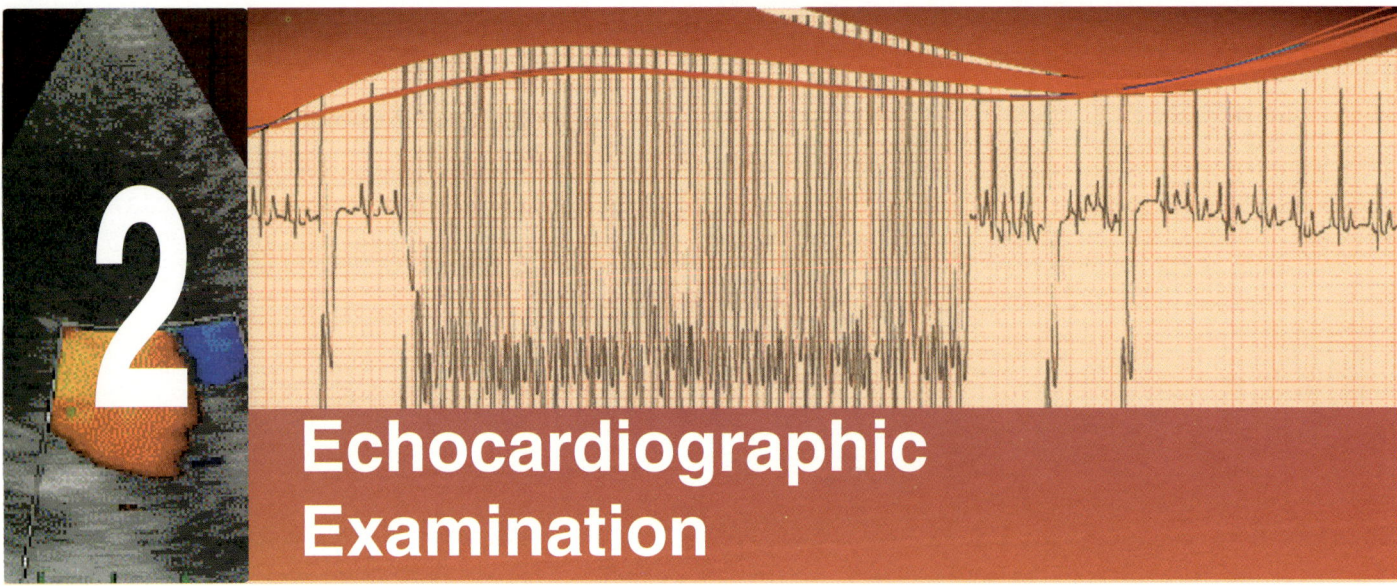

Echocardiographic Examination

The heart is situated within the thoracic cavity with an oblique long axis running from its apex to the base. This axis therefore, passes through the left ventricle and outflow tract and is partially surrounded by the right ventricle. Its obliquity changes from patient to patient. This long axis forms the echocardiographic landmark for the rest of the examination. The left heart cavities being scanned from the apex of the left ventricle to the aorta, and the other structures being studied in transverse view at various levels perpendicular to the long axis (Table 2.1).

In order to avoid interference due to lung intersecting the ultrasonic beam, the transducer has to be positioned over "acoustic windows", usually located in an intercostal space in the left parasternal region at the apex and subcostal area.

Table 2.1: *Echocardiography in the evaluation of heart murmurs*	
Category	Class
1. A murmur in a patient with cardiorespiratory symptoms	I
2. A murmur in an asymptomatic patient if the clinical features indicate at least a moderate probability that the murmur is reflective of structural heart disease	II
3. A murmur in an asymptomatic patient in whom there is a low probability of heart disease but in whom the diagnosis of heart disease cannot be reasonably excluded by the standard cardiovascular clinical evaluation	II
4. In an adult, an asymptomatic heart murmur that has been identified by an experienced observer as functional or innocent.	III

Positioning of the Patient

The patient is placed on a bed of convenient height for the operator to be able to examine/him or her comfortably. An ECG is connected. The examination is started in the supine position, but the patient may have to be turned into his/her left side, which brings the heart closer to the chest wall in order to record good quality M-mode tracings and to facilitate the location of the apex for apical views. The examination is easier with the operator on the patient's left side, holding the transducer in his left hand and adjusting the echocardiographic controls with his right hand. The different oscilloscopes are best viewed under dimmed light. A water soluble ultrasonic gel is used to obtain an airless contact between the transducer and the skin.

Recording Technique (Fig. 2.1A to F)

The "acoustic window" especially for M-mode recordings, is usually located in the third or fourth left intercostal space; this is where the investigation is started. The examination should be completed with routine apical and subcostal recordings.

Parasternal Views

Long Axis

This view allows the study of the aorta, mitral valve, left ventricle and left atrium. These structures may be recorded by M-mode scanning. The transducer is placed perpendicular to the chest wall to visualise the mitral valve, and then gradually angled towards the right shoulder to bring the aorta into view, and towards the apex to record the left ventricle.

Short Axis

The views are perpendicular (the transducer is rotated through 90°) to the long axis. They are recorded at different levels from the base to the apex of the heart by gradually changing the angle of the sector scan.

Apical Views

These views are mainly confined to two-dimensional echocardiography as they are very difficult to interpret in M-mode. They are as important as the parasternal views as all four chambers and the two atrioventricular valves may be visualised simultaneously. The aorta may also be recorded. With the patient in the left lateral position, the transducer is placed over the apex beat, and the examining plane directed upwards, towards the right shoulder.

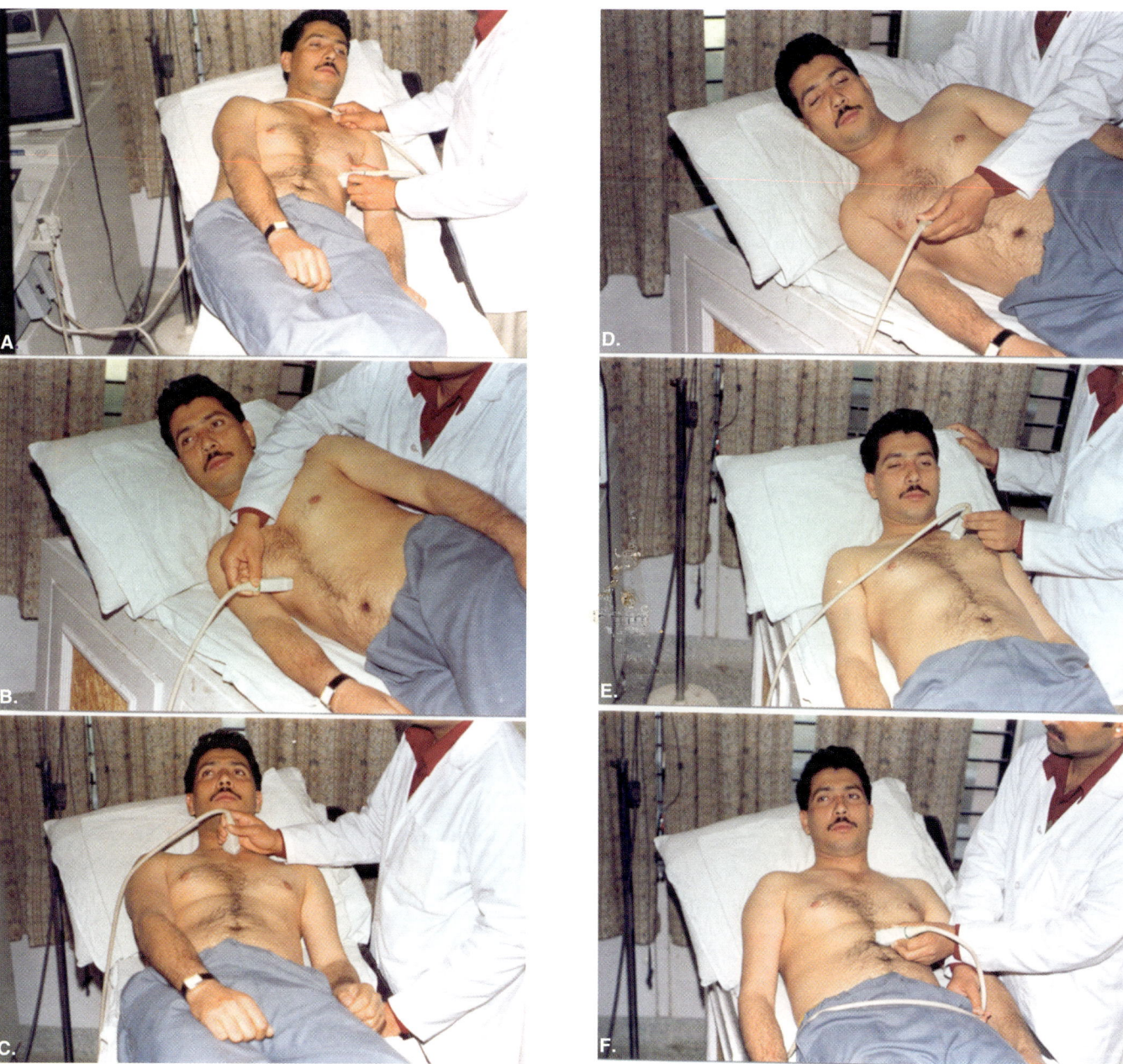

Fig. 2.1A to F: **(A)** Demonstrating bedside left lateral position of the model and hand held transducer, this is an ideal posture for obtaining apical 4.5 and 2 chambers view in M-mode, 2-D B/W and color Doppler scans. **(B)** Right lateral posture for aortic valve and ascending aorta. **(C)** Supine position with head and neck tilted backward in suprasternal notch for obtaining scans of ascending aorta and its valve, arch of aorta, descending aorta, right pulmonary artery, LA and carotid vessels including superior vena cava. **(D)** Demonstrating right lateral position for Doppler recording of velocity of aortic valve and ascending aorta, orientation between ascending aorta and LA, placement of aorta and pulmonary artery in the classification of cyanotic congenital heart defects. **(E)** Position for obtaining scans of descending aorta, right pulmonary artery, descending arch and its branches including left sided persistent superior vena cava. **(F)** Subcostal position for obtaining 2-D and 2-D color Doppler scans for 4, 5 chambers of the heart, RA, LA, TV, MV, AOV, PV and orientation between right and left ventricles. This window is an ideal for diagnosis of atrial septal defect (ASD). However, this position can also be used for IVC, portal vein and its various branches, abdominal aorta superior mesenteric artery and splenic vein

This is, in fact, another long axis view from the apex to the base of the heart. Two perpendicular planes may be defined, one taking in the four chambers and the other, at 90°, the left atrium and left ventricle views on echocardiography is considered as equivalent to right anterior oblique view in cardiac catheterization of left heart study. Apical views are essential for the assessment of left ventricular performance. They are easier to record in patients with easily palpable apex irrespective of the shape of the chest wall. In M-mode, they are mainly used to determine the maximum amplitude of prosthetic heart valves motion.

Table 2.2: *Transthoracic echocardiographic views*	
Two-dimensional imaging	**Doppler imaging**
Parasternal	*Parasternal*
Long axis	MR, AR, VSD
Medially angulated long axis	RV inflow, TR
Short-axis (multiple levels)	AR, TR, PS, PR, VSD
Basal	MR
MV level	
Papillary muscle level	
Apical	
Apical	*Apical*
Four-chamber	Mitral, tricuspid inflow; MR, TR
Two-chamber	Mitral inflow, MR
Long axis	MR, AR, AS, LVOT
Five-chamber	LV outflow, AR, AS, IVRT
Subcostal	*Subcostal*
Four-chamber	RV inflow, TR, ASD
Short-axis	TR, PS, PR
Basal	IVC, hepatic veins
Mid-ventricular	
Suprasternal	*Suprasternal*
Aortic arch in long-axis	Ascending/descending aortic flow,
Aortic arch in short-axis	AR, PDA, SVC
Right parasternal	*Right parasternal*
Ascending aorta	AS

AR, aortic regurgitation; AS, aortic stenosis; ASD, atrial septal defect; IVC, inferior vena cava; IVRT, isovolumic relaxation time; IV, left ventricle; lVOT, left ventricular outflow tract; MR, mitral regurgitation; MV, mitral valve; PDA, patent ductus arteriosus; PR, pulmonic regurgitation; PS, pulmonic stenosis; RV, right ventricle; SVC, superior vena cava; TR, tricuspid regurgitation; VSD, ventricular septal defect.

Subcostal Views

The patient is placed on his back with his legs flexed to relax the abdominal muscles (deep inspiration is sometimes useful), and the transducer placed in the subcostal area. Scanning through a horizontal plane, visualises the heart along its long axis, and the four cardiac chambers may be recorded. Rotation through 90° gives the various transverse views, extending as far

as the right atrium and the inferior vena cava. Increased angulation of the transducer towards the right side is required. This position is also used for M-mode and is very useful when the parasternal views are not obtainable.

A long axis view, morphologically comparable to the usual M-mode scan, may be recorded; but it must be appreciated that other myocardial zones are being visualised (interior portion of the interventricular septum, and lateral wall of the left ventricle).

The motion of the interatrial septum may also be recorded by two-dimensional imaging with simultaneous M-mode tracings.

Accessory Views (Fig. 2.9)

Other echocardiographic view may be obtained by positioning the transducer in the suprasternal notch, to visualise the aortic arch, right pulmonary artery and the left atrium; the right supraclavicular fossa, for analysis of the amplitude of aortic valve prostheses motion; the right parasternal area for the recording of the interatrial septum; and the left precordial area for the M-mode study of the left ventricular anterior wall.

Two-dimensional Echocardiography (Fig. 2.2)

As M-mode echocardiography only gives an image of the heart along a single line with respect to time, many techniques were suggested to visualise dynamic anatomical planes of the heart. Different terms have been proposed to describe these techniques. Cross-sectional echocardiography, real time two-dimensional, multi-scan and echotomocardiography. The principal technique used in two-dimensional echocardiographic recording is compound B scanning. A certain number of lines of B-mode are recorded simultaneously on the oscilloscope screen. When viewed together, they produce an image of a section of the heart which varies with the position and angle of the transducer. These images are reproduced at a rate of about 30 per sec, to give a dynamic, real-time scan.

Three different systems are available for two-dimensional echocardiography, but all use video systems for its recording (Fig. 2.3).

Mechanical Transducer: This is probably the simplest system. The image is obtained by a rapid rotation of one or several transducers by an electric motor. The resulting image is displayed as a sector of a circle, with each line of B-mode originating at the centre.

Linear Arrary Multiscan: This system comprises a linear array of a number of small ultrasonic elements on the transducer. The elements are activated rapidly in sequence each giving a line of B-mode echo. These systems require quite large transducers, which have two practical disadvantages; the transducer crosses the ribs and certain anatomical planes cannot be examined.

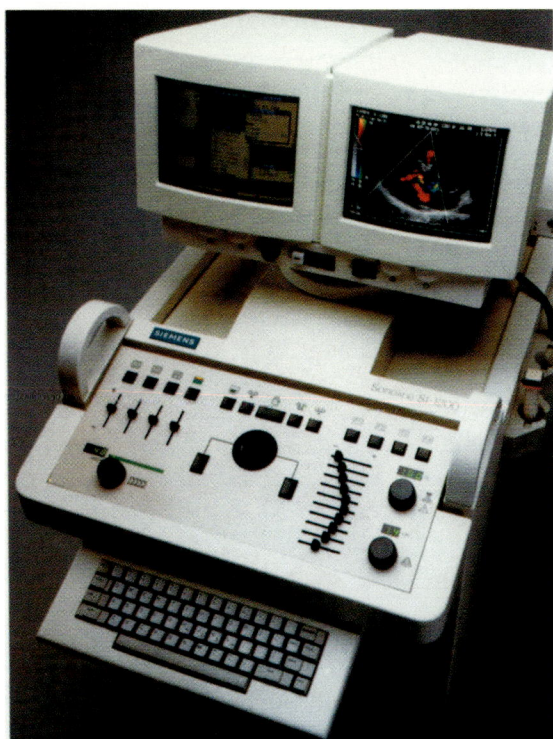

Fig. 2.2: Dedicated color Doppler echocardiography machine which is currently in use for obtaining M-mode, 2-D color Doppler scans for investigation in a heart patient

Phased Array Sector Scan: This is probably the most sophisticated technique for obtaining two-dimensional images of the heart. The transducer is about 2 cm wide allowing positioning between the ribs; it also employs multiple elements, usually about thirty, which are activated in sequence with an electronically timed delay so that the ultrasonic wavefront is at an angle with the transducer.

By changing the sequence or activation, it is possible to sweep the beam through a sector of 80° to 90°. These systems may also be equipped with a variable acoustic, focus.

These echocardiographs are costly but provide high quality echocardiograms. They are continually being perfected, and are probably, the future of echo-cardiography.

Simultaneous M-Mode: Phased array sector scans have the option of one or two line of M-mode which may be recorded at the same time as the two-dimensional image.

M-mode coupled with 2-D allows the recording of structures which are often difficult to visualise such as the pulmonary valve; it also offers a method for analysis of echocardiographic events which are too rapid to be studied by 2-D (Fig. 2.8).

It is also possible to integrate the sample volume of pulsed Doppler echocardiography on this line of M-mode.

Complementary System

Phono and Pulse Recording

This is recorded simultaneously with M-mode, and is useful in the study of the timing of heart sounds with respect to the valvular motion on echo, and also helps in the analysis of the function of prosthetic heart valves. It is essential that these cases are recorded at rapid paper speeds.

Dual Echo

This is the simultaneous recording of two modes of echocardiograms, a useful technique for measuring the isovolumetric periods.

Pharmacodynamic and Physiological Tests

Valsalva manoeuver, isometric or isotonic exercise tests, changing position, amyl nitrite, glyceryl trinitrate Dobutamine/Dipyridamole stress tests.

Other Parameters

Respiration, pressure curves, Doppler, etc.

Colour Doppler Flow Mapping (Fig. 2.18 A and B)

This technique employs two signal-processing termed as "moving of target indicators and autocorrelation." These are considered unique for medical ultrasonic systems. Flow patterns in various cardiac chambers and great vessels can be displayed simultaneously with real-time two dimensional imaging; colour coding helps to evaluate the directionality of flow: flow towards the transducer is shown in red, and flow moving away from the transducer is displayed in blue. Turbulent or variant flow, such as observed in the presence of regurgitant flow is denoted by mixed colour, mosaic patterns produced by adding green to the blue or red. This technique is quite useful in the assessment of all types of valvular regurgitation and shunt defects. It may also contribute significantly in the diagnosis of prosthetic malfunctioning with special reference to the para-prosthetic leaks.

The Normal Echocardiogram (Tables 2.1 and 2.2)

The Heart Valves

Mitral Valve

The echoes of the mitral valve usually act as a model guide for the rest of the echocardiographic examination, are the easiest to record and were among the first to be described.

Long Axis View (2-D) (Fig. 2.4)

The whole of the mitral apparatus from the papillary muscles to the left atrium may be visualised. Long axis may be recorded from the three routine transducer positions, but the best images are generally obtained with the transducer in the left parasternal region.

Valvular motion is difficult to study from still frames. The extreme positions of the mitral leaflets in systole and diastole and their precise motion on M-mode recording will be analysed. This method will also be used for the other heart valves.

Diastole (Fig. 2.7)

This is period of left ventricular filling when the mitral valve is opened and the aortic valve is closed.

In early diastole, the anterior mitral leaflet has a rapid anterior motion towards the inter-ventricular septum. The posterior leaflet moves in the opposite direction but with less amplitude. The mitral ring also has a slight posterior motion. During this phase the maximum separation of the two valves is attained. It is usually about 30 mm. The echoes of the anterior leaflet are in continuity with the posterior wall of the aorta which forms the anterior wall of the left atrium; the posterior leaflet is in echocardiographic continuity with the posterior wall of the left atrium. As they open, the two leaflets move down into the left ventricular cavity, defining the left ventricular inflow tract between the two leaflets and the outflow tract above the anterior mitral leaflet.

Systole (Fig. 2.6)

It is the onset of the ventricular contraction, when the mitral valve closes and the two leaflets come together.

The angle between the axis of the posterior wall of the aorta and the anterior mitral leaflet should not exceed 30°. The mitral ring has a slight anterior motion. The echocardiographic continuity of the posterior leaflet with the chordae and the posterior median papillary muscle is often well visualised. The distance between the free edge of the mitral valve and the papillary muscle may, therefore, be measured in systole.

The thickness of the valves and chordae may also be assessed.

Approximately, the same appearances are obtained by recording from the subcostal area; the apical view, however, visualises these structures from one of the extremities of the long axis.

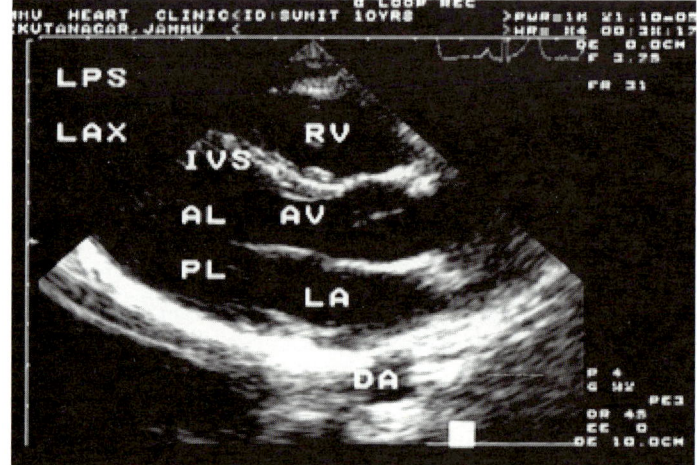

Fig. 2.4: 2D Scan taken at LPS long axis showing various structures as indicated including descending aorta (DA)

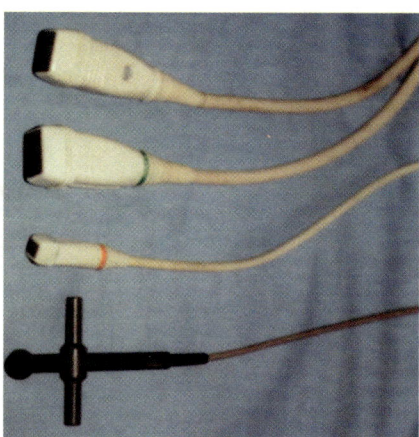

Fig. 2.3: (From top to bottom) Mechanical sector, phased array and non-imaging or pedoff continuous wave Doppler transducers being used for obtaining various types of echoscans

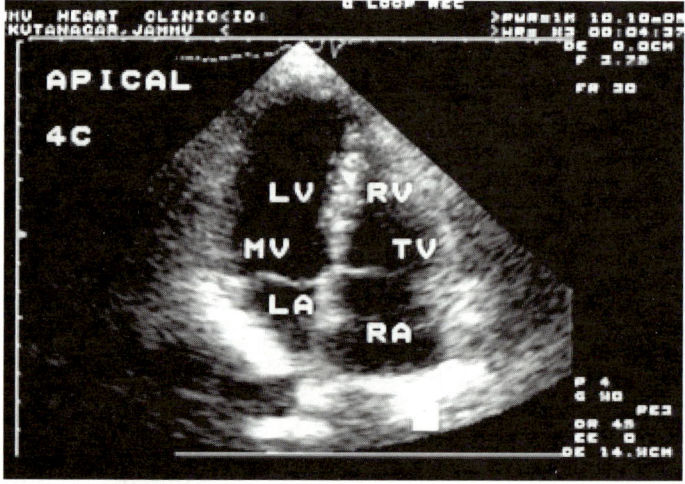

Fig. 2.5: Apical 4C view depicting all four chambers of the heart as indicated on the scan

Table 2.3: A comparison of 2-D and Doppler modes of echocardiography		
Objective	Two-dimensional echocardiography	Doppler
Ultrasound target	Tissue	Blood
Goal of diagnosis	Anatomy	Physiology
Type of information	Structural	Functional
Optimal alignment between beam and target	Perpendicular	Parallel
Prefer transducer frequency	High	Low

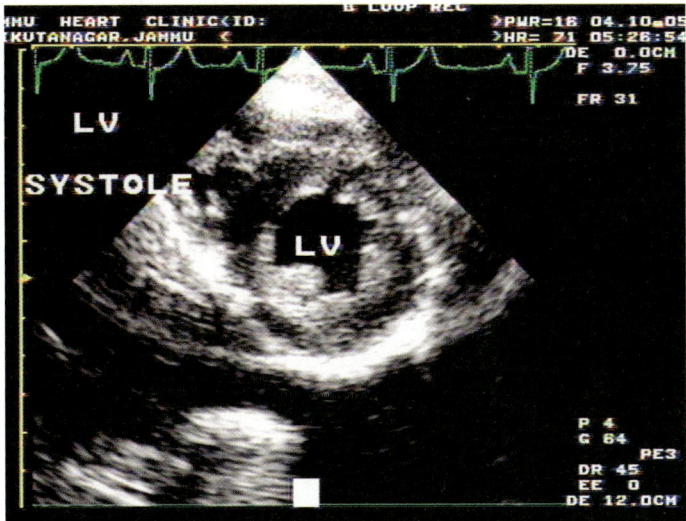

Fig. 2.6: Short axis view of LV taken at high LPS showing LV cavity, endocardium and papillary muscles during systole of the heart

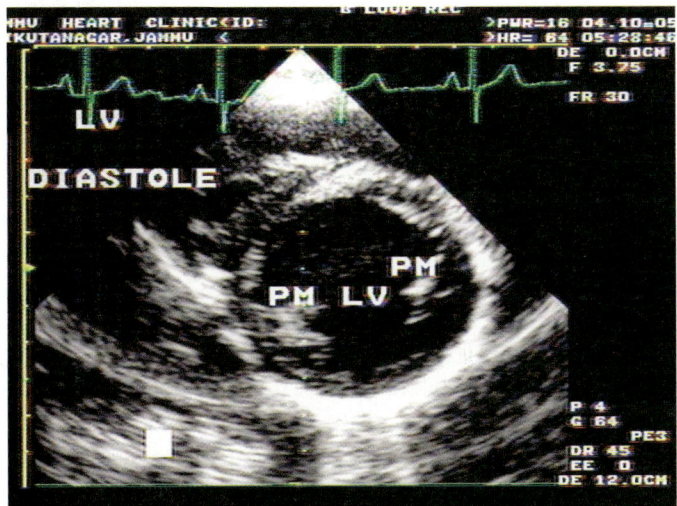

Fig. 2.7: Short axis view of LV taken at high LPS showing LV cavity, endocardium and papillary muscles during diastole of the heart

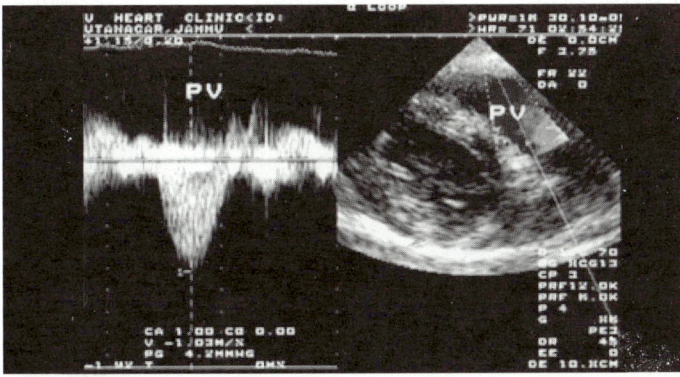

Fig. 2.8: Doppler flow velocity across PV taken at right 2nd-intercostal space directed towards right shoulder

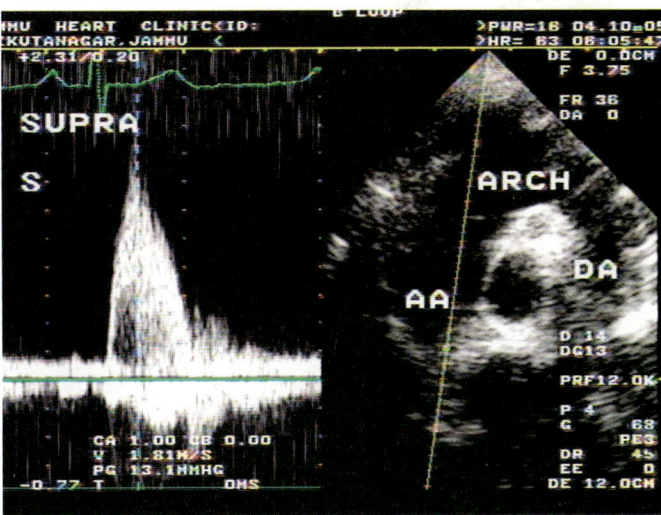

Fig. 2.9: Doppler flow velocity across ascending aorta in suprasternal notch(s)

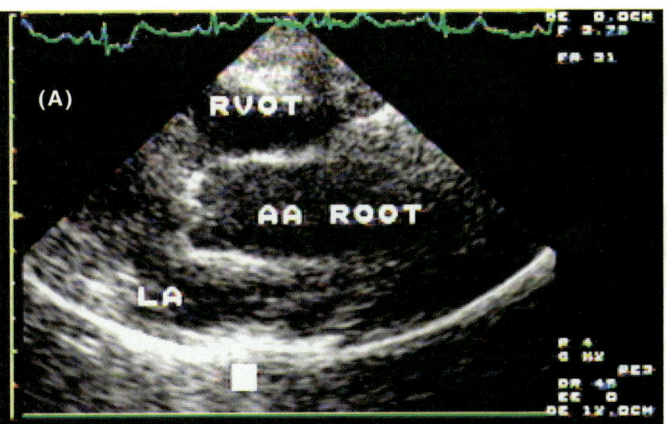

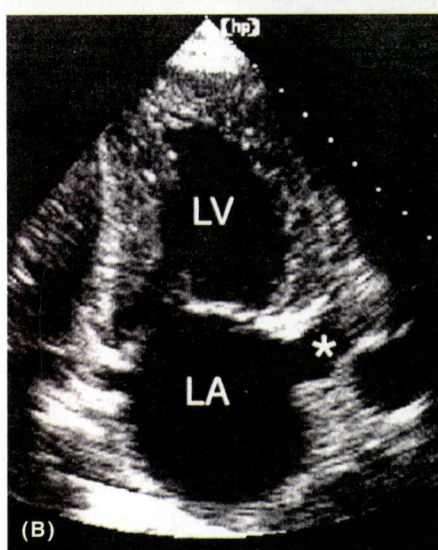

Figs. 2.10A and B: (A) LAX Upper LPS view showing both walls of ascending aorta which is useful view for determining size of aorta as in aneurysm seen frequently in Marfans syndrome and dissection of aorta. **(B)** Two chambers view especially for appendage of LA for any clot

Short Axis (2-D)

This view is recorded from the left parasternal area, in a plane perpendicular to the long axis (alternatively, the subcostal position may be used). Its principal advantage is that a good view of the mitral orifice is obtained in diastole, as the plane passes through the free border of the mitral leaflets. The orifice is oval in shape and has a shape of a fish's mouth; the surface area of the valve may be obtained by planimetry. It should be performed on a view in early diastole, when the mitral leaflets are furthest apart, and care must be taken to adjust the gain control so that the leaflets do not appear artifactually thickened. The anterolateral and posterior commissures form the two extremities of this ellipsoid.

In systole, the closure of the mitral valve with apposition of the two leaflets all along the width of the mitral orifice, should be verified. The same echocardiographic continuity is observed on mitral-aortic scanning.

M-Mode Measurements (Fig. 2.11)

Normal Appearance: The anterior and posterior leaflets of the mitral valve are assigned specific letters corresponding to their systolic and diastolic components as timed on the ECG. The systolic components are designated as C and D points. The diastolic components has E, F, A and B points. Each letter point coincides with a specific ECG function. The QRS on the ECG marks the onset of systole and coincides with the C point on the mitral leaflet. The T wave on the ECG coincides with the D point, signifying the end of systole. Shortly thereafter, the onset of diastole corresponds with the E point and the ventricle starts to relax at the F point. The P wave on the ECG triggers atrial contraction and the A "Kick" is then seen on the mitral valve. Normally the B point is not identified in patients without elevated end diastolic pressure and occurs just before the QRS.

C-D Amplitude: The C-D amplitude is a measurement from the C point to the D point. It is the closed systolic position during which the valve leaflets move with the mitral annulus. It normally has little to do with the valve itself and relates to the heart movement. These structures may be an important indicator of a systolic anterior motion (SAM) or mitral valve prolapse (posterior bulging into the atrial cavity). The normal value is 20 to 30 mm.

C-D Slope: The C-D slope measurement depicts the rate of movement of the valve leaflets as the annulus moves anteriorly in systole. The slope is measured by extending the line through points C and D and is a time-distance measurement. The normal valve is 35 mm/sec.

C-E Amplitude: The C-E amplitude is a measurement from the C point to the E point. It denotes the amplitude at which the mitral valve is opening. The E point is the most anterior excursion. The normal value is 20 to 33 mm (Fig. 2.12).

Left Ventricular Outflow Tract at the C Point: Measured from the left ventricular outflow tract from the left side of the septum to the C point on the mitral valve. The normal value is 20 to 33 mm.

Left Ventricular Out Flow Tract at D Point: It should be measured from the left side of the septum to the D point on the mitral valve. Its normal value varies from 12 to 33 mm.

D-E Slope: The D-E slope measurement signifies the opening movement of the mitral valve in early diastole. The slope is measured by extending the line through points D and E. This may be an indicator of left ventricular failure and elevated end systolic volume with a decreased D-E slope. The normal value is 240 to 380 mm/sec (Fig. 2.13).

D-E Amplitude: The D-E amplitude is a measurement of the maximum excursion of the anterior mitral valve after an early diastolic opening. The measurement is taken from the D point to the E point. It may be an important indicator of mitral regurgitation. The normal value is 17–30 mm.

E-F Slope: The E-F slope measures the rate of motion of the cusp in early diastole and expresses the rate of left atrial emptying. Since a slope is being measured, extend the line connecting the E and F points through 1 second in time. Draw a line from the bottom of the time line (at the point of intersection) and measure the distance along the vertical axis from the end of the completed line to the beginning of the time line. The normal value is 50 to 180 mm/sec (Figs 2.11A and B and 2.15).

A-C Slope: The A-C slope depicts the rate of systolic closure of the mitral valve. The measurement is made by extending a slope line through points A and C. A decreased rate of closure may indicate elevated left ventricular end-diastolic pressure or poor ventricular performance. The normal value is 350 to 360 mm/sec.

PR-AC Interval: The PR–AC interval is a measurement to detect premature closure of the mitral valve (Acute aortic insufficiency). It is taken from the beginning of the P wave on the ECG to the beginning of the Q wave on the ECG (for the PR component); the AC component is from the A point to the C point on the mitral valve. The interval is then determined by subtracting the AC from the PR interval. A time line of 0.04 sec is used for this calibration; normal values are less than 0.06 sec.

Fluttering of the Leaflet: Flutter may be seen as a fine oscillation of the anterior leaflet of the mitral valve in diastole. It may be secondary to aortic insufficiency, vegetations, coarse flutter and atrial fibrillation (Fig. 2.29A and B).

Table 2.4: *Normal measurements in adults*

RV dimension, supine (R)	0.7–2.3 cm
RV dimension, left lateral (R)	0.9–2.6 cm
LV dimension, supine (R)	3.7–5.6 cm
LV dimension, left lateral (R)	3.5–5.7 cm
LV posterior wall thickness (R)	0.6–1.1 cm
LV posterior wall excursion	0.7–1.7 cm
Ventricular septal thickness (R)	0.6–1.1 cm
Ventricular septal excursion	0.3–0.8 cm
LV outflow tract dimension (beginning S)	2.0–3.5 cm
Left atrial dimension (end-S)	1.9–4.0 cm
Aortic root diameter (R)	2.0–3.7 cm
Aortic cusp separation (early S)	1.5–2.6 cm
LV fractional shortening or % DMD	0.25–0.42
LV ejection fraction	45%–84%
Mean Vcf (LV)	1.02–1.94 circ/sec.
Ventricular septal thickening	0.30–0.65
Ventricular septal velocity (S)	3.3–7.0 cm/sec.
LV posterior wall thickening	0.36–0.95
Mean LV posterior wall velocity (S)	3.0–7.1 cm/sec.
Max. LV posterior wall velocity (S)	3.0–8.3 cm/sec.
Max. LV posterior wall velocity (D)	9.1–28 cm/sec.

Table 2.5: *Normal measurements from the suprasternal transducer position*

Aortic arch lumen diameter	24 ±1.1 mm
Right pulmonary artery lumen diameter	20 ±1.2 mm
Left atrial cephalocaudal diameter	52 ±12.7 mm
Left atrial anteroposterior diameter	42 ±7.3 mm

EF slope of MV

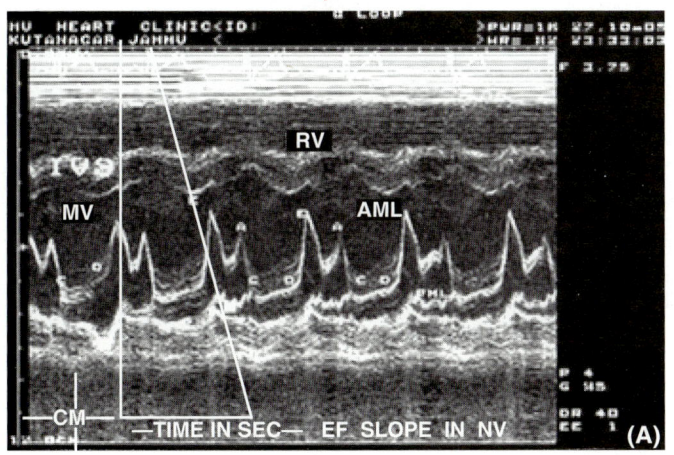

EF slope of TV

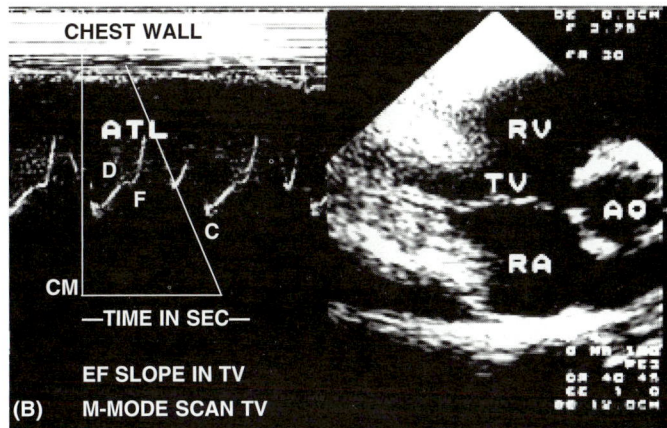

Fig. 2.11A and B: M-mode echocardiograms demonstrating calculation of EF slopes in MV and TV as shown with line diagrams on their respective scan

CE amplitude

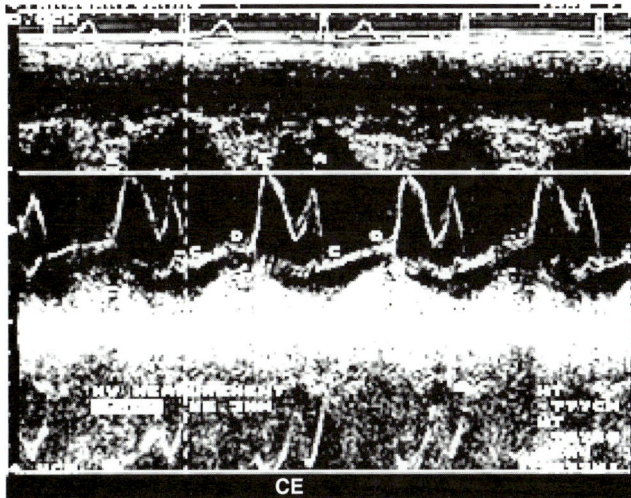

Fig. 2.12: It is the vertical distance between the C point and E of the anterior mitral leaflet

DE slope

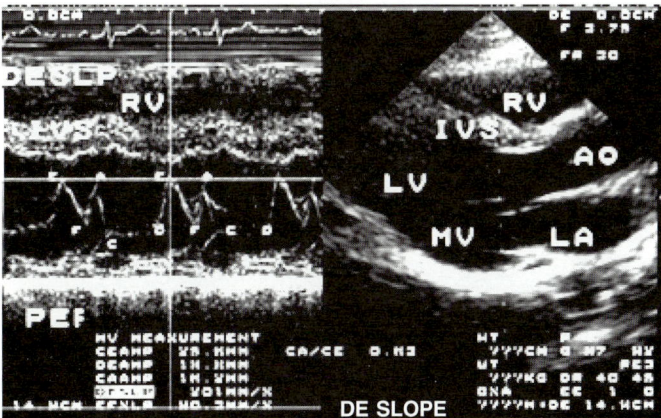

Fig. 2.13: It is opening slope of mitral valve and is measured by constructing a triangle with the diagonal over the DE slope as shown in the scan

CA amplitude

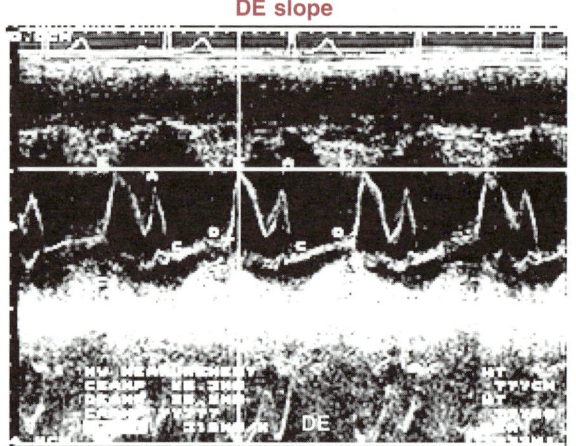

Fig. 2.14: It is measured from C point to meet the vertical line upto A point of the anterior mitral leaflet

DE slope

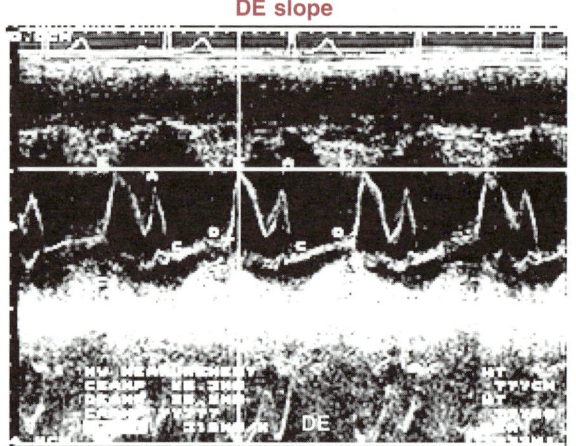

Fig. 2.15: It is the opening slope of the mitral valve and is measured by constructing a triangle with the diagonal over the DE slope as shown in the scan

EF slope

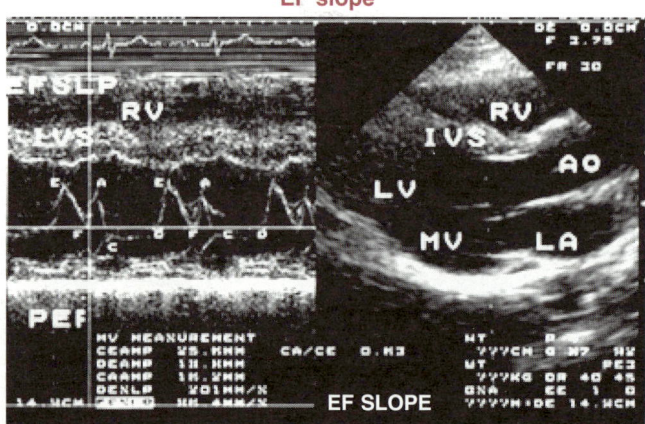

Fig. 2.16: It is the early diastolic closing slope of the anterior leaflet of the mitral valve. This is measured as the vertical distance in mm/sec. of a triangle constructed with the diagonal over the EF slope and the horizontal line to intersect 1 sec line as shown in the scan

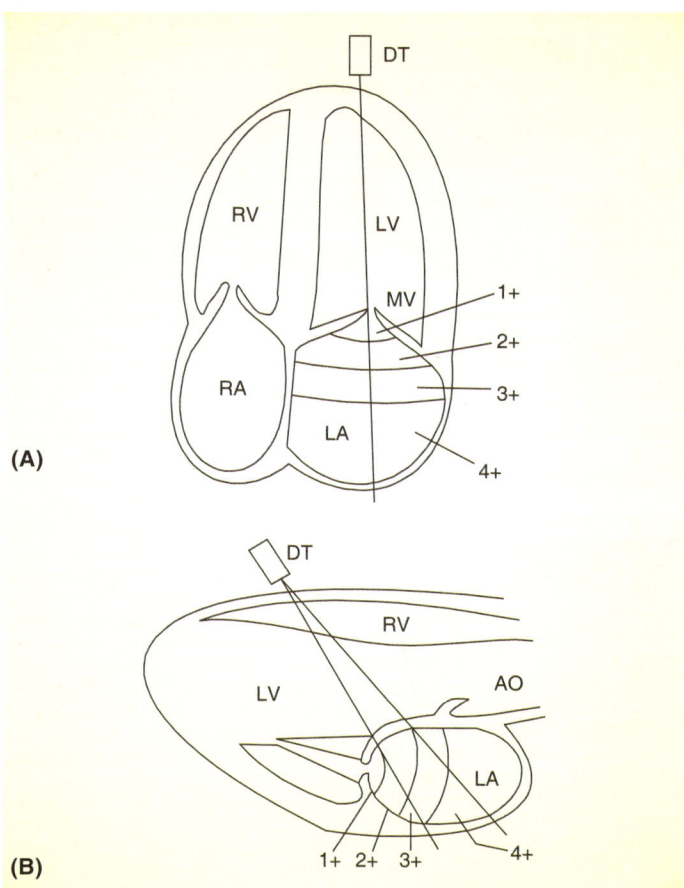

Fig. 2.17: A and B: Graphic representation of apical 4C and long axis views for demonstrating grades of MR focusing on the LA and LV cavities

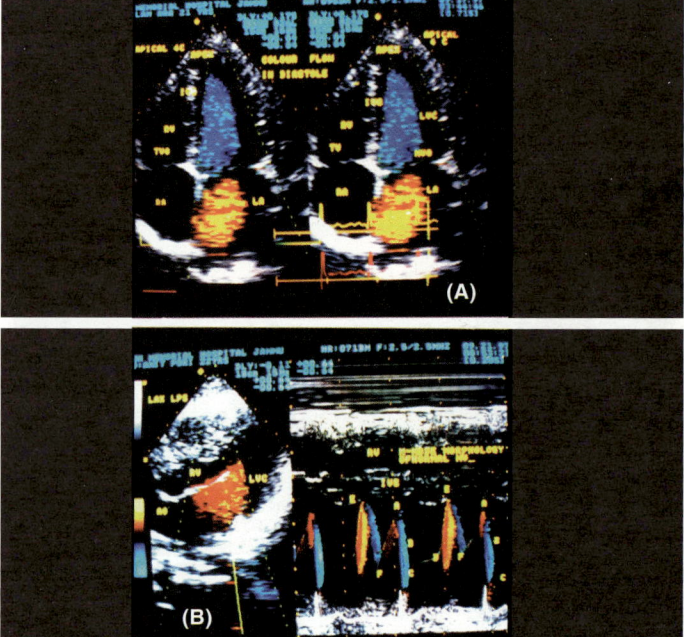

Fig. 2.18A and B: (A) Color flow in left atrium (red) and in aorta (blue) in a dual scan taken at LPS region in apical 4C view. **(B)** Normal color flow velocities of MV in both M-mode and 2-D echo scans

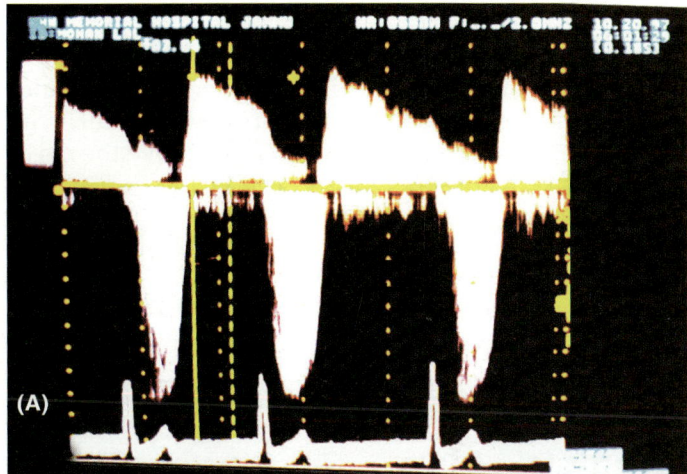

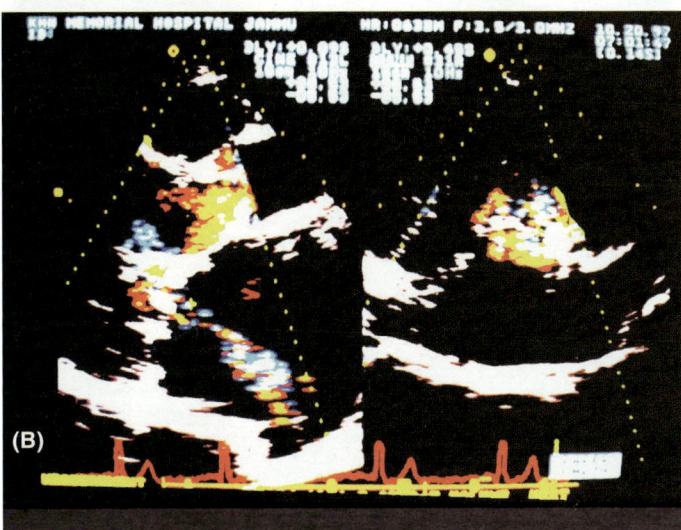

Fig. 2.19A and B: **(A)** Continuous wave Doppler in a patient suffering from mitral stenosis with grade 4 MR. **(B)** Color Doppler dual scan showing grade 4 MR as shown in the 2-D oblique 4C scan

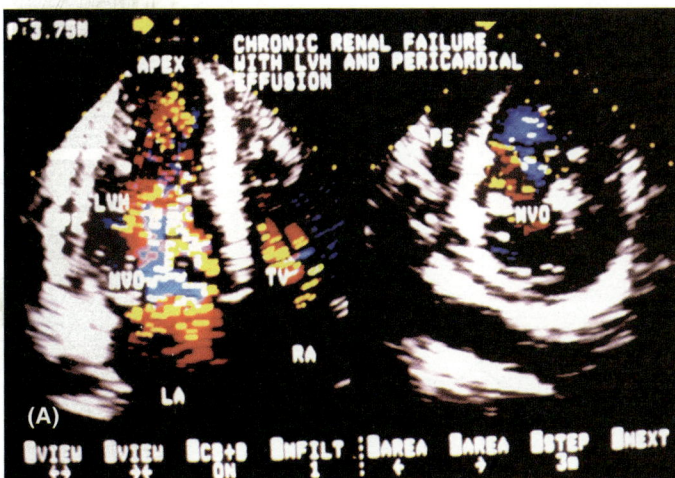

Fig. 2.20A: Color flows in apical 4C in dual scans show mosaic color jet approaching right up to apex of LV and down into LA in moderate pericardial effusion

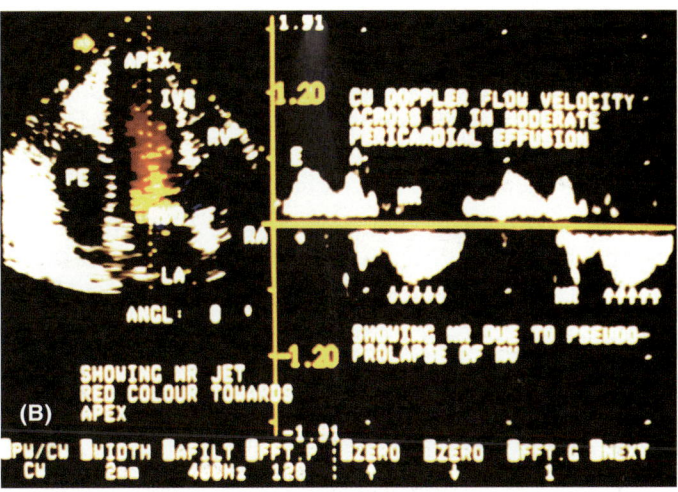

Fig. 2.20B: Color Doppler flow velocity of MV and mitral regurgitation as a result of pseudo prolapse of the valve(arrows) in patient with moderate pericardial effusion

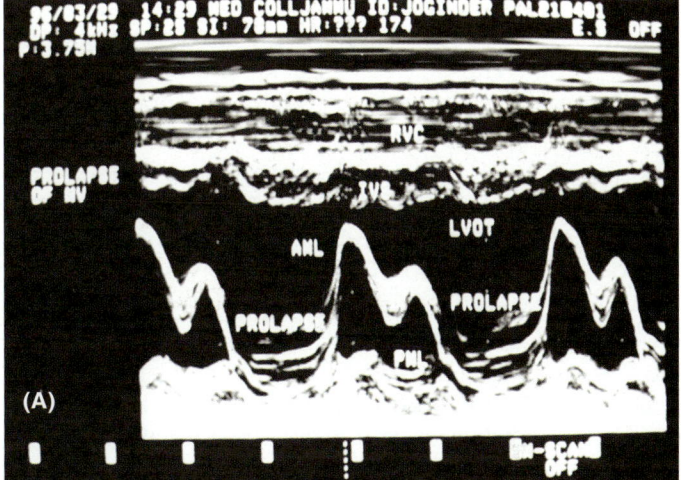

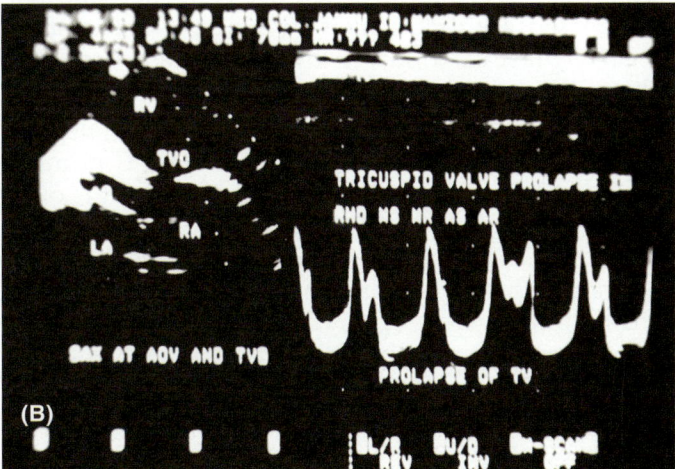

Fig. 2.21A and B: **(A)** M-Mode echoscan of mitral valve showing bowing of C-D line with multilayering echos as seen in mitral valve prolapse. **(B)** M-Mode echoscan of TV showing prolapse similar to the abnormalities as seen in MV prolapse

Systolic Anterior Motion: With systolic anterior motion, the anterior leaflet moves anteriorly after the onset of systole and then returns to its normal position just before diastole. Often it is seen with obstructive hypertrophic cardiomyopathy, and the degree of obstruction is directly related to the size of the systolic motion.

Pseudosystolic Anterior Motion (Figs 2.110 and 2.111): It may be seen when the chordal structures move anteriorly in systole and mimic the motion of SAM as seen with obstructive disorder. One can distinguish pseudo-SAM from obstructive SAM by following the systolic segment of the mitral leaflet. In pseudo-SAM, this segment remains in its normal position, and the chordal reflections move "over" the systolic segment. In obstructive SAM the motion is actually caused by the systolic segment of the mitral C-D portion of the leaflet (Fig. 2.110).

Multiple Echoes: In the absence of calcification the mitral complex is a thin, single reflection.

Multiple bright echoes resulting from fibrosis or calcification may be seen on either the anterior or the posterior leaflet. The degree of thickening or calcification is a function of the number of multiple echoes seen and may indicate a rheumatic process.

Posterior Leaflet of Mitral Valve: Observe whether the posterior leaflet moves posterior in diastole (Normal) or anterior (as seen in rheumatic disease such as mitral stenosis).

Posterior Bulging: Posterior bulging is indicated when the anterior or posterior leaflets or both are displaced posteriorly in systole. The normal C-D slope is interrupted by a posterior movement, usually 3 to 5 mm and usually indicates prolapse of mitral valve.

Space Beneath the Mitral Valve: Echoes posterior to the mitral valve in diastole that do not disappear as the gain is decreased, are abnormal. If there is an echo-free space in early diastole followed by an increased mass of echoes, this probably represents a myxoma or tumor.

Amputated E, Prominent A: It occurs with elevated left ventricular end diastolic pressure. The E point is diminished, and the A point is accentuated. (It is often seen in gross aortic insufficiency).

By tilting the transducer caudally towards the mitral valve and left ventricle, the same aorta-septal and aorto-mitral continuity is observed. Normally, the interventricular septum is located at the same level as the anterior aortic wall, but if the position of the transducer on the chest wall is nearer the aorta than the septum, a false image of overriding aorta may be obtained.

Aorta and Aortic Valve (Fig. 2.28A and B)

The aortic root and aortic cusps are normally recorded in routine examinations.

Long Axis View (2-D) (Fig. 2.22 A and B)

This view is obtained with the transducer positioned in the left parasternal area; the proximal aorta and the sinus of Valsalva, the anterior and posterior aortic walls with their parallel motion, and the 2 to 3 cm above the aortic valve may be recorded. During systole, these structures have an anterior motion.

Two of the aortic cusps are visualised in this plane (the right coronary and the posterior or non-coronary cusp). During diastole, the valves are closed giving rise

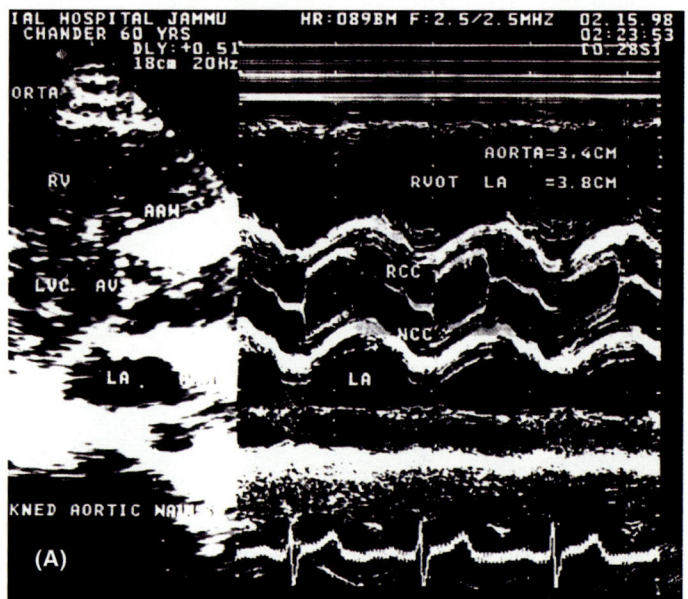

(A)

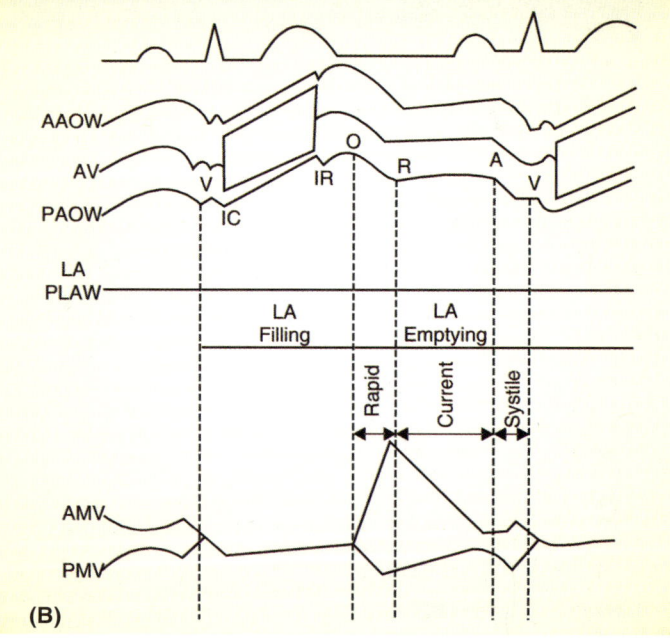

(B)

Fig. 2.22A and B: (A) 2-D and M-mode echocardiogram depicting normal morphology of Aortic valve including its cusps. (B) Graphic diagram showing various hemodynamic events of aortic valve in relation to mitral valve

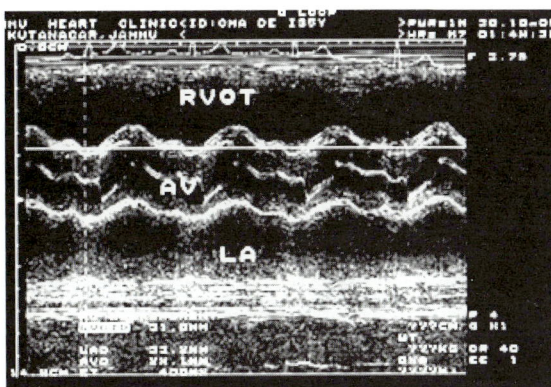

Fig. 2.23: RVOT—It is measured from the anterior heart wall to the anterior margin of the anterior aortic wall Normal value is variable. However,

$$\frac{RVOT}{LAD} = 1.5$$

It is diagnostic of RVOT stenosis in TOF when its value reaches up to 0.9.

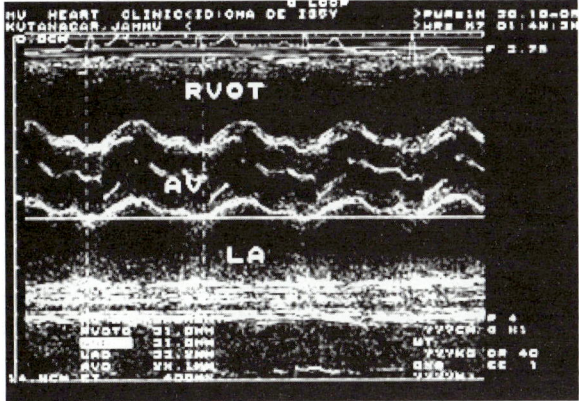

Fig. 2.24: AOD—Aortic root diameter at end diastole. This is measured from the anterior margin of the anterior aortic wall to the anterior margin of posterior aortic wall at the R wave of ECG
Normal values = 20–37 mm

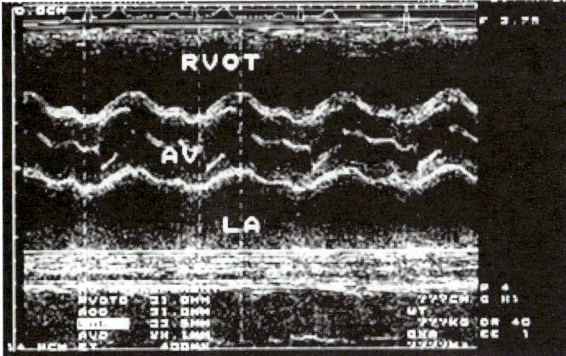

Fig. 2.25: LAD—Left atrial dimension. It is measured from the anterior margin of the posterior aortic wall to the leading edge of the left atrial posterior wall at end systole
Normal values = 15–40 mm
Rate of aortic cusp opening movement normal = 369 mm/sec
Rate of aortic cusp closing movement normal = 293 mm/sec

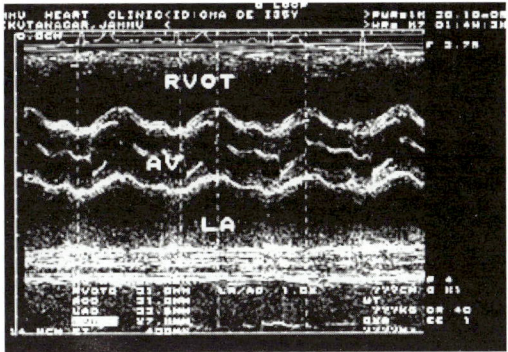

Fig. 2.26: AVD—It is the distance between the right coronary cusp and non-coronary cusp taken at early systole
Normal values = 15–26 mm
Left atrial posterior wall amplitude;
Normal values = <10 mm

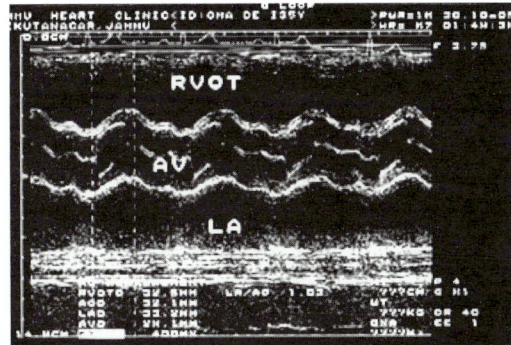

Fig. 2.27: LVET—It is measured between the opening and closing of aortic cusps.These measurements should be taken at a ECG paper speed of 100 mmsec
Eccentricity index: This is derived by dividing half of the aortic root diameter by the shortest distance between the aortic cusps position in diastole to the nearest aortic wall. It is diagnostic of bicuspid aortic valve

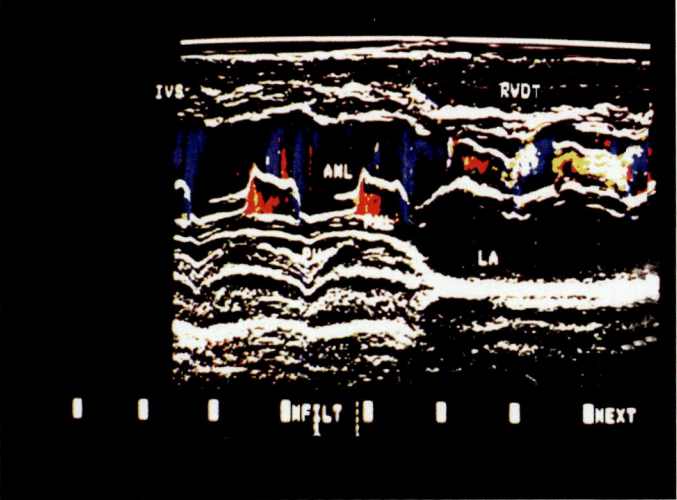

Fig. 2.28A: Color M-mode echoscan showing sweep from mitral valve to stenosed aortic valve

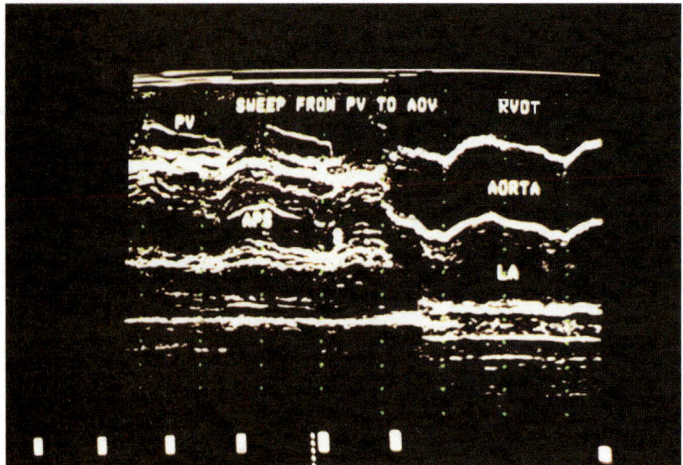

Fig. 2.28B: M-Mode echo scan showing sweep from pulmonary valve to aorta in normally positioned great vessels

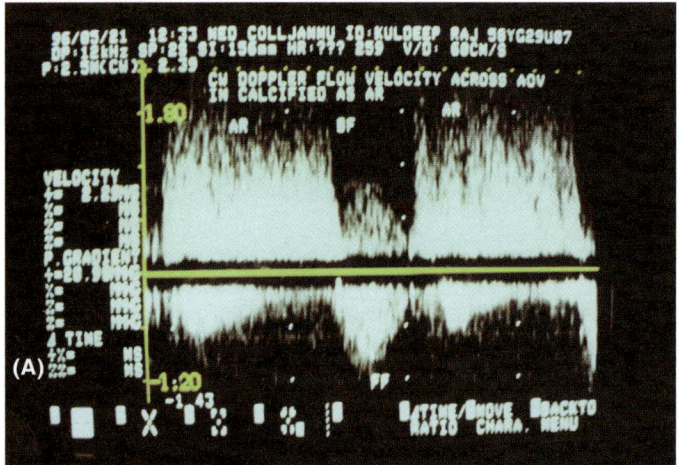

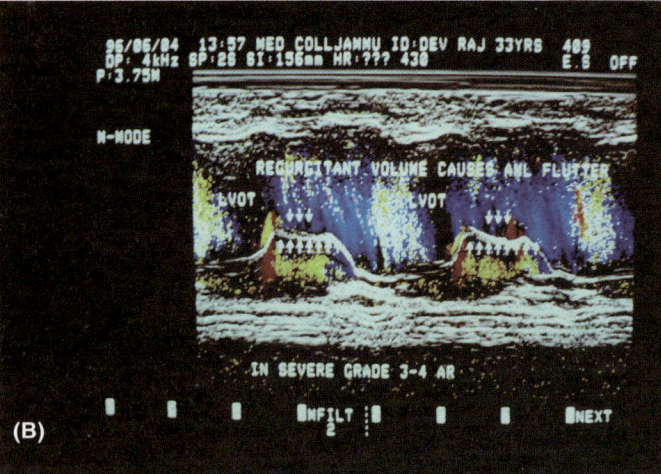

Fig. 2.29A and B: (A) Doppler flow velocity across AOV depicting gross AR in a patient suffering from moderate aortic stenosis and AR. **(B)** M-Mode echoscan depicting flutter of anterior mitral leaflet as shown in arrows caused by falling of aortic regurgitation jet on the valve during diastolic period of cardiac cycle

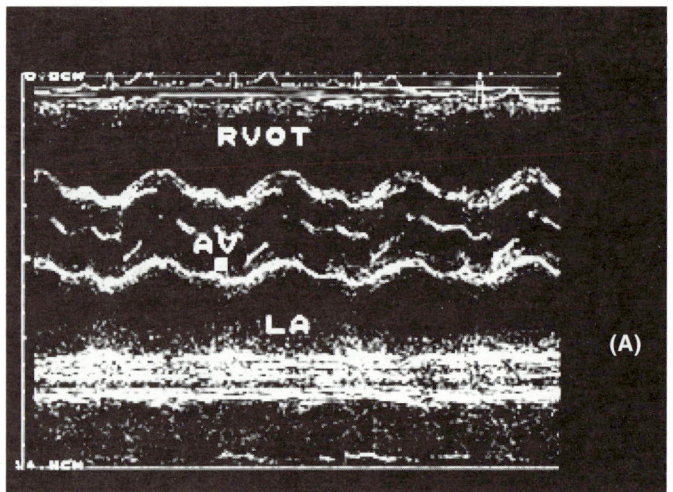

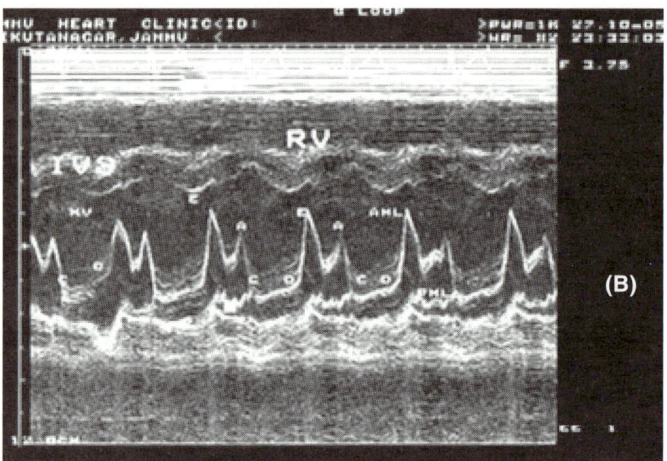

Fig. 2.30A and B: (A) M-Mode echocardiogram showing normal morphology of aortic valve and walls along with its relationship between LA and aorta. **(B)** M-Mode echoscan showing normal morphology of mitral valve in comparison to aortic valve

to a single echo equidistant from the two walls of the aorta. In systole, the valve opens and the echoes of the two cusps separate, the anterior cusps moving anteriorly to the anterior wall and the posterior cusp moving posteriorly to the posterior wall, each leaving a slight gap corresponding to the sinus of Valsalva. The continuity of the anterior wall of the aorta and the interventricular septum, and of the posterior wall of the aorta and the anterior mitral leaflet, is particularly well seen in long axis views (Fig. 2.28A).

The descending thoracic aorta is visualised as an oval echo-free space behind the heart. It may be followed down to the abdominal aorta by angling the transducer in the sagittal plane; this maneuver differentiates it from other causes of a retrocardiac echo-free space (Fig. 2.4).

It is possible, especially in children, to record the origin of the aorta and the aortic arch from the subcostal position by orientating the transducer obliquely upwards.

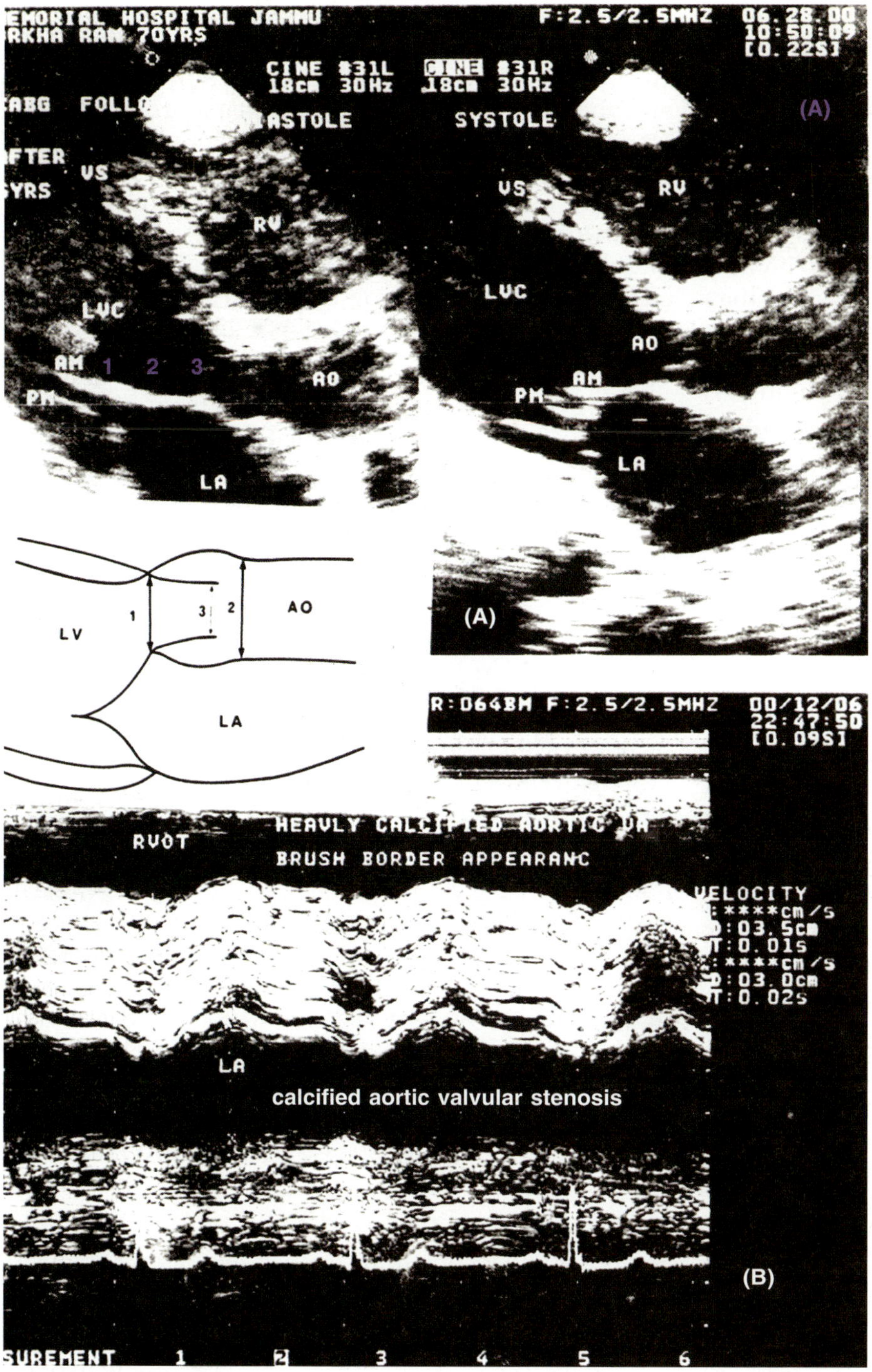

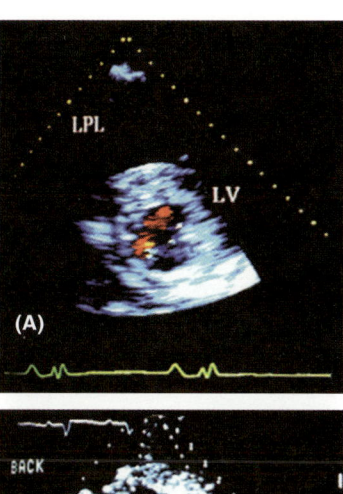

(A)

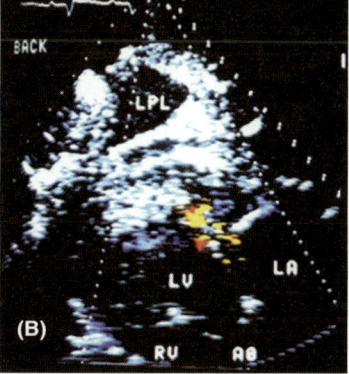

(B)

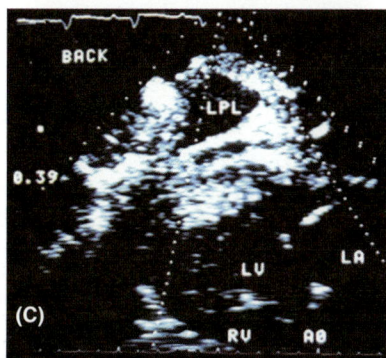

(C)

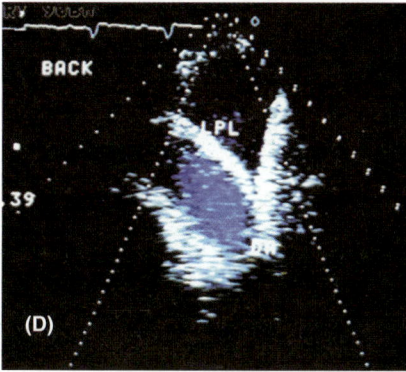

(D)

Fig. 2.31A and B: **(A)** 2-D, Long axis LPS view of aorta and LV showing how to determine the various diameters at aortic valve to calculate aortic valve area, flow and finally the stroke volume **(B)** M-Mode echoscan shows heavily calcified aortic valve typically called as *brush border appearance* leading to marked reduction in aortic valve area and aortic flow

Fig. 2.32A to D: Prominent flow signals are seen in the LV viewed in short axis **(A)** and long axis **(B, C)** by placing the transducer in left posterior intercostal space and viewing the heart through the large left pleural effusion (LPL). The Descending Aorta can also be viewed through the effusion **(D)**

The aortic arch, the origin of the cerebral vessels and the right pulmonary artery may be visualised from the suprasternal notch (Fig. 2.9).

The aortic cusps are recorded with transducer positioned in the left parasternal or subcostal area, with the sector plane at 90° to the long axis (Fig. 2.81).

In diastole, the aortic valve is closed and the three commissures resemble the Mercedes-Benz sign upside down. They are of equal length and the central point is located at the centre of the aortic ring. In systole, they separate and flatten against the aortic wall, and are difficult to visualise unless thickened by disease; the valvular surface area may be measured by planimetry.

Tilting the transducer obliquely upwards, sometimes brings the left main coronary artery into view at the centre of the left coronary cusp. The right coronary artery is more difficult to record as it lies anterior to the aorta. Only its ostium at the centre of the right coronary cusp is visible.

M-Mode Measurements

Aortic Root

Dimension: This is measured at the end of diastole at the onset of the first rapid deflection of the QRS complex from the leading edge of the anterior aortic root to the leading edge of the posterior aortic root. The normal value is 20 to 37 mm (Fig. 2.10A).

Thickening: Abnormal thickness with an increase in the amount of echoes or brightness of the aortic walls is usually caused by calcification. A decrease in wall motility may be noted (Fig. 2.31B).

Wall Amplitude: Wall amplitude is a measurement of the anterior motion of the posterior aortic wall during ventricular systole. It is obtained by drawing a horizontal line between the external boundaries of the posterior aortic wall in diastole and then measuring the maximal vertical distance from this line to the external boundary of the aortic wall during ventricular systole. Decreased values indicate low cardiac output and a reduced stroke volume.

Aortic Valve

Normal Appearance: The characteristic feature of the normal valve is the box-like configuration that presents as linear echo pattern formed by the right and non-coronary aortic cusps as they open in ventricular systole. The closed position in diastole presents as a dominant echo pattern in the middle of the aortic root.

The echoes of the aortic valve are recorded between the echoes of the two aortic walls. They have a characteristic box-like appearance in systole, with a linear median echo in diastole. The maximum separation of the anterior and posterior cusps is measured in early systole (normal = 16 to 25 mm). During systole, fine fluttering of the aortic cusps may be observed. The two cusps which are visualised, in 2-D, are the right coronary and the posterior non-coronary cusps. In recordings, when the aortic valve echoes are registered over several cardiac cycles, the systolic time intervals of the left ventricle may be measured. They correlate well with the values obtained by the traditional phonocardiographic methods with external pulse tracings. The pre-ejection (PEP) and ejection periods (EP) and their ratio may therefore, be measured (Fig. 2.22A and B).

Systolic Separation: Systolic separation is the maximum opening of the coronary cusps during the initial part of ventricular systole. A perpendicular line is drawn from the right coronary cusp to the non-coronary cusp at the opening movement, to leading edge at the onset of systole. The normal valve is 16–26 mm (Fig. 2.26).

Opening and Closing Rates: Opening and closing rates should be noted, as gradual closure of the cusps in systole may indicate low cardiac output, (i.e. congestive heart failure, cardiomyopathy, or mitral regurgitation).

Flutter: Flutter may be seen as fine oscillations of either or both of the coronary cusps during opening of the valve in ventricular systole. This is a normal variant of blood flowing through the cusps.

Interrupted Opening: Interrupted opening is seen as a midsystolic closure and reopening of the aortic valve in systole. It results from midsystolic obstruction of blood flow as seen in severe obstructive cardiomyopathy. An abrupt early systolic closure is seen in patients with discrete sub-aortic stenosis (Fig. 2.112A and B).

Thickening: Thickening of the cusps is seen with calcification or vegetations on the cusps. Vegetations may not hamper the cusp opening as is seen with aortic calcifications or stenosis (Fig. 2.117A and B).

Tricuspid Valve

The possibility of obtaining good views of the right heart chambers with 2-D echocardiography allows detailed study of the tricuspid valve; only two of its leaflets are recorded at any one time.

Long Axis View (2-D)

The tricuspid valve is usually recorded with the transducer in the left parasternal area tilted medially and sagittally. In practice, the apical and subcostal views give better images.

The apical or four-chamber view visualises the anterior and septal leaflets and their insertion, located slightly closer to the apex than the mitral leaflets. The portion of the septum between the septal leaflets of the mitral and tricuspid valves defines the anatomical

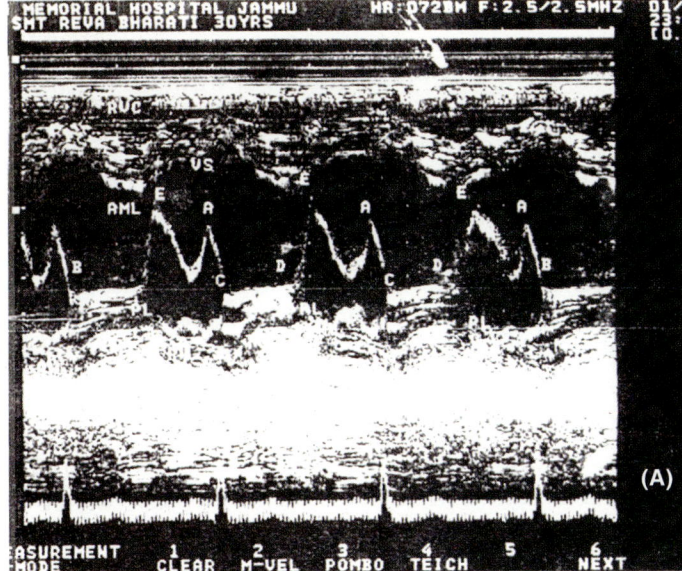

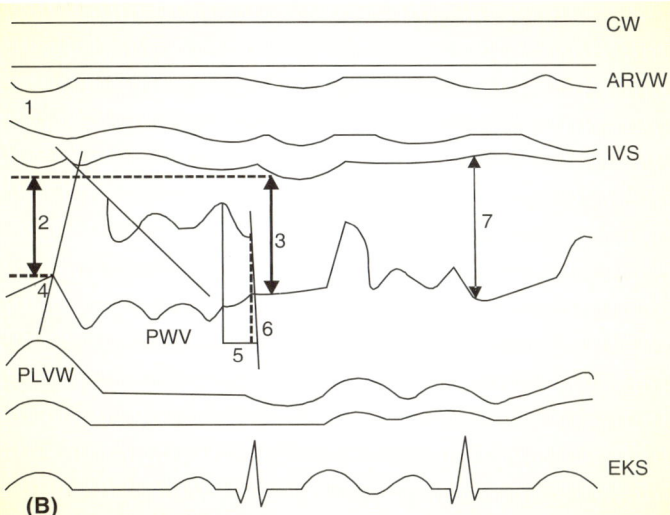

Fig. 2.33A and B: M-mode echocardiographic intervals and slopes in LV and mitral valve

Table 2.6: *M-Mode measurements of various slopes and intervals*

Item	Normal values	Significance
1. EF slope	75–120 mm/sec	Severity of mitral stenosis
2. DE Amplitude	>20 mm	Severity of mitral stenosis
3. CE Amplitude	20–32 mm	Movement of mitral annulus
4. DE Slope	240–380 mm/sec	Opening slope of AML
5. AC Slope	125–250 mm/sec	Prolonged by raised end-diastolic P
6. AC Interval	60 msec	Prolonged by raised end-diastolic P
7. Left ventricular out flow tract	20–34 mm	Diseases of IVS and MV

relationship of the left ventricle and the right atrium (membranous septum).

The subcostal view brings better visualisation of the tricuspid ring and its choradae tendinae (Figs 2.49B and 2.76).

Short Axis View (2-D)

This is usually recorded near the base of the heart, where the septal and anterior tricuspid leaflets are visualised to the left of the aorta. They have an anterior diastolic motion (Fig. 2.78).

M-Mode Measurements

Normal Appearance: The anterior leaflet can usually be visualised, at least in part, and moves like the mitral valve. The posterior and septal leaflets are not usually seen.

PR-AC Interval: The PR-AC interval is a measurement to detect premature closure of the tricuspid valve. A prolonged AC interval often indicates elevated right ventricular end diastolic pressure. The normal value is under 0.06 sec.

E-F Slope: The E-F slope is similar to that of the mitral valve. A significant decrease in E-F slope may indicate stenosis. The normal value is 60 to 125 mm/sec (Fig. 2.11B).

Posterior Echoes: Organised echoes posterior to the anterior leaflet may indicate a tumor mass, vegetation, or a ruptured sinus of a Valsalva aneurysm.

Fluttering: Fluttering is caused by fine oscillation of the anterior leaflet in diastole secondary to pulmonary insufficiency.

Thickening: Multiple bright echoes resulting from fibrosis or calcification or both may be seen on the anterior leaflet and may represent stenosis or vegetation.

Pulmonary Valve

This is one of the most difficult structures to record in M-mode. However, it is easier to locate in 2-D and its motion may be analysed by simultaneous M-mode recording. It is only visualised in the transverse view.

Usually, only the posterior cusp is recorded. It is a fine, mobile echo situated anteriorly and to the right of the aorta. It may also be recorded from the subcostal area (Figs. 2.8, 2.28B and 2.49A).

Normal Appearance: Part of the posterior leaflet of the pulmonary valve is visible on the M-mode tracing. The anterior wall of the right ventricle is seen anterior, and a characteristic thick mass of echoes (from the pulmonary root) is seen below the leaflet.

A Dip: The A dip is a pre-systolic downward motion of the posterior leaflet that coincides with the A point of the mitral valve and follows atrial contraction. The measurement is made by drawing a line from the F point to the B point and measuring the distance from the lowest point on the A dip to this line.

An absence of the A dip may indicate pulmonary hypertension or atrial fibrillation. An increase in the depth indicate pulmonary stenosis. This measurement fluctuates with normal respiration. The normal value is 1 to 8 mm.

E-F Slope: The E-F slope is similar to the E-F slope of the mitral valve and is measured in the same manner. A flattened or negative slope may indicate pulmonary hypertension. The normal value is 6 to 115 mm/sec.

Fluttering: Fluttering results from coarse oscillations of the posterior leaflet occurring with the onset of ventricular systole and often into early diastole. It indicates subpulmonic or infundibular stenosis.

Flying W Sign: The flying W sign is seen as a W-shaped wave during systole. It is caused by the midsystolic closure of the valve and is often a sign of pulmonary hypertension (Fig. 2.73A).

Premature Opening: Premature opening is detected by correlating the opening movement of the posterior leaflet with the P wave on the ECG. It occurs with increased pressure from the right ventricle against the pulmonary valve and may be caused by a ruptured sinus of Valsalva aneurysm, constrictive pericarditis, or tricuspid insufficiency.

The right ventricular systolic time intervals may be measured. The ratio of the pre-ejection period (PEP) to the right ventricular ejection time (RVET) is a good index of right ventricular function.

The Echocardiographic assessment of these indices gives useful information which can otherwise only be obtained by invasive haemodynamic investigations.

Cardiac Cavities

A series of dense linear echos 2–4 cm wide, anterior to the heart are recorded with the transducer in the left parasternal region. They correspond to the chest wall, a structure which is in direct contact with the anterior wall of the right ventricle.

Right Ventricle

Anatomical structure of the right ventricle (RV) is complex. It partially surrounds the left ventricle and, only by examination in a number of planes, its geometry can be studied with 2-dimensional echocardiography. The right heart is more completely visualised, especially the right atrium (RA), which can only be definitely visualised by this technique.

Long Axis (2-D)

In the usual parasternal position, only the anterior portion of the RV and the pulmonary infundibulum are visible. Angling the transducer medially in the true sagittal plane a view of the RV, tricuspid valve and RA may be obtained together with the anterior wall of the RV (Fig. 2.4).

In the apical 4 chamber view the two ventricles are recorded simultaneously along with their long axis, separated by the interventricular septum. The two atria and the interatrial septum are visualised posteriorly.

The apical and lateral wall of the RV may also be identified (Fig. 2.17A and B).

The 4 chamber view may also be obtained from the subcostal area but in this case the inferodiaphragmatic wall of the RV is visualised.

Short Axis View (2-D)

In the parasternal area, the short axis view at aortic level shows the pulmonary infundibulum circling around the aorta and continuing as the main pulmonary artery by angling the transducer, the pulmonary artery may be followed to its bifurcation. The RA is situated behind the tricuspid valve. Apical scanning gives a series of sections through the RV and shows its "crescent-like" shape around the LV. The same appearances may be recorded from the subcostal position by rotating the transducer 90° with respect to the 4 chamber view. Scanning towards the base of the heart shows the pulmonary infundibulum encircling the aorta and the RA. By orientating the beam towards the abdomen, the inferior vena cava (IVC) and its appearance in the RA with the Eustachian valve and the hepatic veins may be recorded. The internal dimension of the IVC varies with the respiratory cycle, decreasing during inspiration. This distinguishes it from the abdominal aorta (Figs 2.76–2.78).

M-Mode Measurement

Dimension: The dimension measurement should be made when the right side of the septum and the endocardium of the right ventricular anterior wall are clearly seen (and in the usual plane passing through the left ventricle at the chordal or the mitral valve level depending on the age of the patient). It should be measured at the onset of the QRS (end diastole). The normal value is 7 to 23 mm; in the left decubitus position, it measures slightly larger, 9 to 26 mm. If the right ventricular wall echo cannot be visualised, an estimate of 5 mm posterior to the last non-moving chest wall echo can be made as the relative location of the right ventricular wall.

Left Ventricle

One should always keep in mind that the inter-ventricular septum should be treated as a part of left ventricle (LV) as, it participates in left ventricular ejection and the interatrial septum with the left atrium.

Long Axis (2-D)

In the parasternal position, the anterior portion of the inter ventricular septum is visualised all along its length from its origin at the anterior wall of the aorta. These two structures are usually in the same plane, but when the heart lies horizontally, the septum bulges anteriorly and forms an obtuse angle with the aorta (Figs 2.46B, 2.47A and 2.48A).

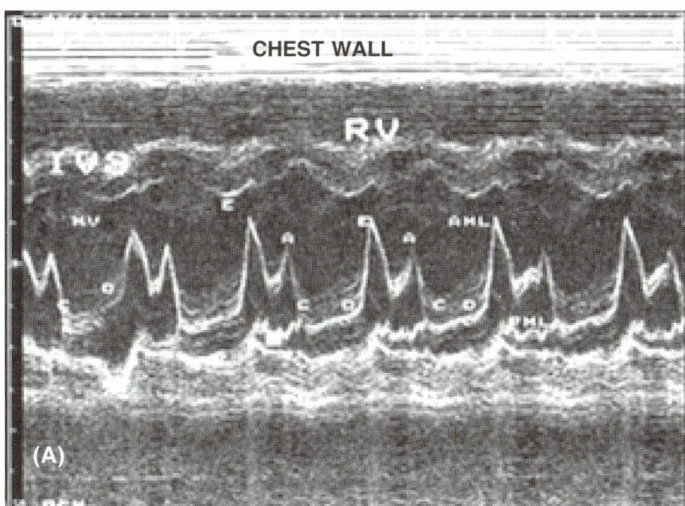

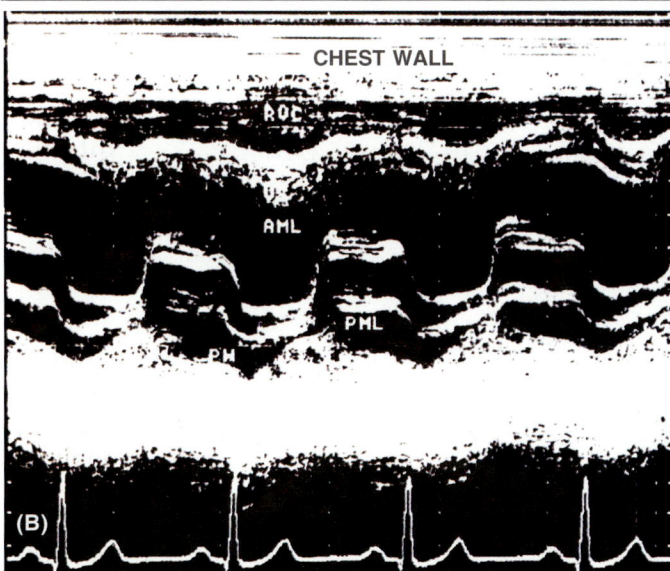

Fig. 2.34 A and B: **(A)** M-Mode echocardiogram of a normal mitral valve showing M shaped configuration along with different letters such as A, B, C, D, E and F used for opening and closing velocities of MV and hemodynamic derivatives. **(B)** Thickened anterior mitral leaflet with paradoxical movement of posterior leaflet in mild to moderate type of mitral stenosis

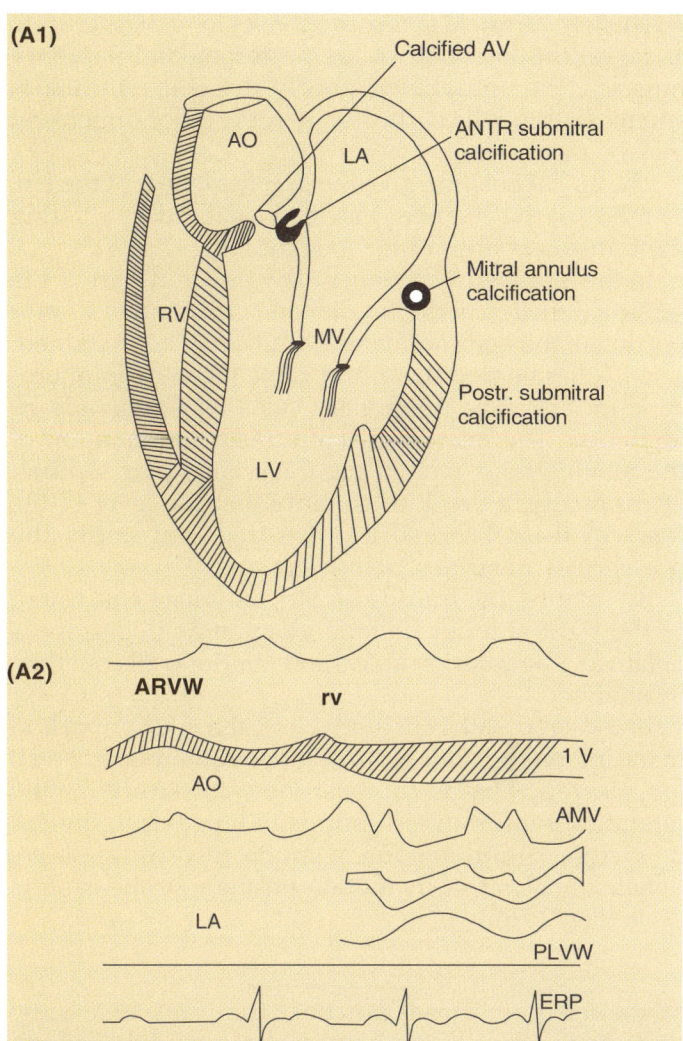

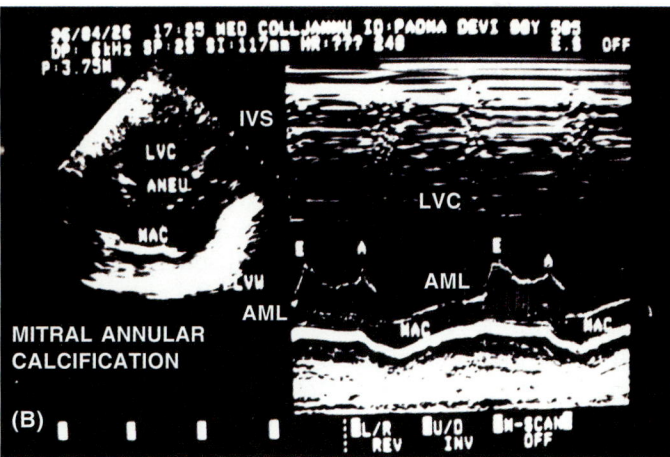

Fig. 2.35A and B: **(A1)** 2-D Graphic figure depicting calcification process over different parts of the heart as indicated including mitral and aortic annular calcification. **(A2)** Mitral annular calcification in a sweep from aorta to mitral valve. Black shaded area in the region of posterior mitral leaflet is indicated as MAC. **(B)** 2-D and M-mode echoscans show MAC with normal anterior and posterior mitral leaflets as shown in this scan

The left ventricle is recorded in its long axis, at least as far as the insertion of the posteromedial papillary muscles, the apex being poorly defined. The LA is situated behind the aorta; its anteroposterior dimension may be measured.

The apical position gives an excellent view of the LV, as much of the chamber may be visualised by rotating the transducer around the long axis (Fig. 2.54A).

In the so-called 4-chamber view, the mid-part of the septum (junction of the anterior and posterior or inferior portions), the apex and lateral walls may be examined. The LA lies behind the mitral valve taken in an infero-superior axis. The pulmonary veins may generally be identified. The interatrial septum is a continuation of the membranous part of the interventricular septum. Occasionally, a break in continuity at the level of the fossa oval is observed but this does not imply the presence of an atrial septal defect.

By rotating the transducer 90°, an image equivalent of the right anterior oblique view on angiography is obtained. The anterior, apical and inferior walls can then be studied.

In the subcostal 4 chamber view, the inferior portion of the interventricular septum and the anterolateral wall are viewed. This is the best view for studying the interatrial septum which normally bulges into the RA in systole. Simultaneous M-mode recording allows detailed analysis of its motion throughout the cardiac cycle (Fig. 2.76).

Short Axis View (2-D)

In the left parasternal position, the transverse view through the base of the heart sections the LA through its short axis posterior to the aorta.

The left ventricle may be studied in detail by scanning down towards the apex; the left ventricular outflow tract, and the papillary muscles may be considered the equivalent of the left anterior oblique angiographic view of the ventricle.

In short axis view, the length of the interventricular septum, which is concave towards the left ventricle and the inferior, anterior and lateral walls are very well visualised. Towards the apex, two muscular projections corresponding to the posterio-medial and antero-lateral papillary muscles of the mitral valve are observed. The same short axis views of the LV may sometimes be recorded from the subcostal position (Figs 2.53A, 2.67A, 2.79A and B, 2.82, 2.89, 2.106A and B and 2.121).

M-Mode Measurement

The left ventricle measurements should be made on M-mode tracing recorded just inferior to the tip of the mitral leaflet that includes a portion to the chordae tendineae. The interventricular septum and three layers of the posterior heart wall should be distinct and continuous throughout the cardiac cycle. The technique should involve a sweep with a decrease in gain to visualise the dense chordae from the endocardial surface of the posterior heart wall and the bright reflector of the pericardium from the posterior heart wall.

End Diastolic Dimension: End diastolic dimension (EDD) is a measure of the maximal left ventricular size in diastole. The vertical distance is measured from the left side of the septum to the endocardial surface of the posterior heart wall at the QRS (end diastole). The normal value is 3.5 to 5.7 cm (Fig. 2.36A and B).

End Systolic Dimension: End systolic dimension (ESD) is a measure of the minimal left ventricular size in systole. The vertical distance is measured from the endocardium to the left side of the septum. The dimension should be measured at the lowest point of septal motion in patients whose septal motion is normal. In patients whose septal motion is abnormal or paradoxical, the measurement should be made at the peak of the posterior wall motion. The normal value is 2.2 to 4.0 cm (Figs. 2.37B and 2.38A and B).

Wall Thickness: Wall thickness is a measure of the vertical distance from the epicardium of the posterior wall to the endocardium in end diastole at a point just before the pre-systolic "thinning" of the posterior wall (onset of the QRS). The normal value is 6 to 11 mm.

Wall Amplitude: Wall amplitude is a measure of the anterior motion of the posterior wall during systole. It is made by first drawing a horizontal line between the most anterior points of the endocardium in systole and then measuring the maximal vertical distance from this line to the endocardium of the posterior wall at a point just before the free wall begins to move anteriorly in systole (Fig. 2.38A).

A reduced wall amplitude may indicate myopathy, coronary artery disease, congestive heart failure, low cardiac output, or technical problems. Exaggerated wall motion may indicate left ventricular volume overload or coronary artery disease. The normal value is 5 to 14 mm.

Endocardial Velocity: Endocardial velocity is a measure of the velocity at which the endocardium of the posterior wall moves. It is made by extending a line from the endocardium in systole to the endocardium in diastole. The normal value is 20 to 35 mm/sec (Fig. 2.37B).

Septal/Posterior Wall Ratio: The septal/posterior wall ratio is calculated by the septal thickness in diastole to the posterior wall thickness in diastole. The normal value is 0.87 to 12 mm (Fig. 2.50A and 2.50B).

Stroke Volume: Stroke volume (SV) is an estimated measure of the amount of blood ejected from the left ventricle per cardiac cycle. It may be obtained from this formula (Fig. 2.38B):

$$SV = EDD^3 - ESD^3$$

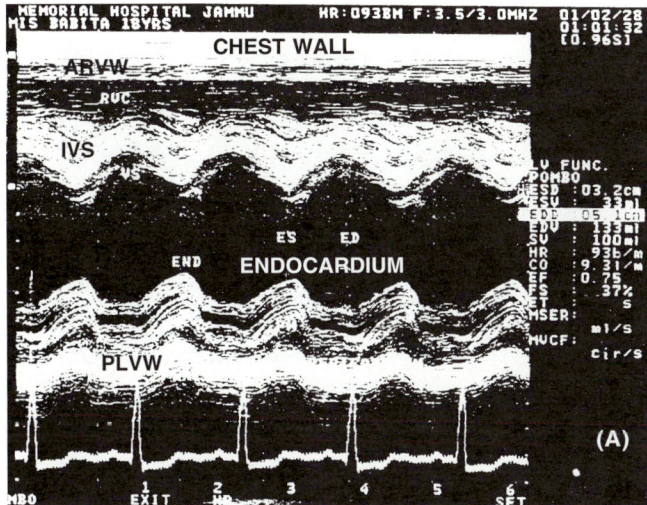

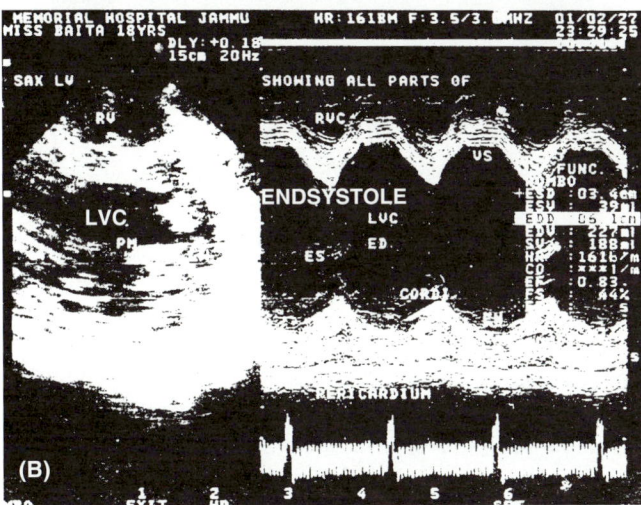

Fig. 2.36A and B: (A) M-Mode echocardiography shows different parts of the heart as indicated on the scan for measurements to classify a particular part is either normal or hypertrophied. **(B)** Measurements in end-systole and end-diastole to convert measurements from cm to volumes by cubic method as shown in this graph

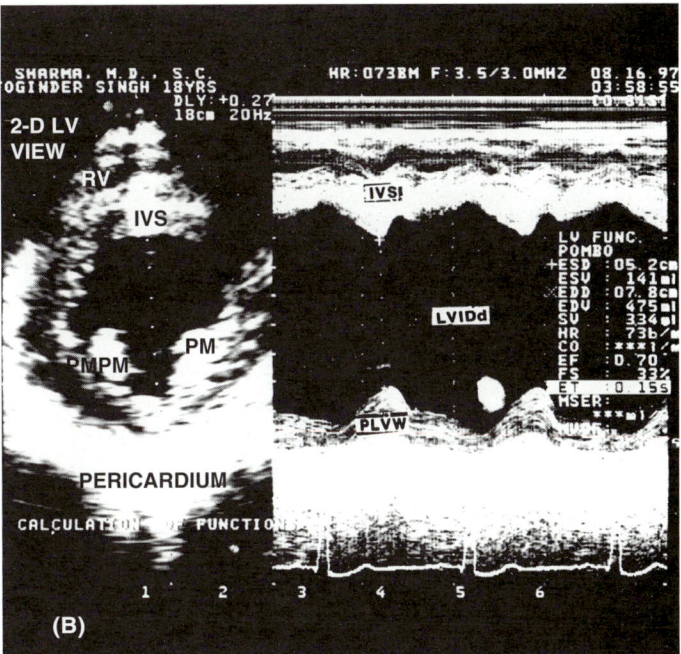

Fig. 2.37A and B: (A) M-Mode echocardiogram showing flat movements of IVS or marked hypokinesia of IVS, hypertrophy of posterior LV wall alongwith increased distance between E point of mitral valve and systolic contraction of IVS (EPSS) in patient with hypertension with ischemic heart disease. **(B)** 2-D and M-mode scan showing normal cardiac parameters with depiction of papillary muscles(PM) in 2-D scan on the left side and calculation of LV functions by POMBO method as shown on the scan on the right

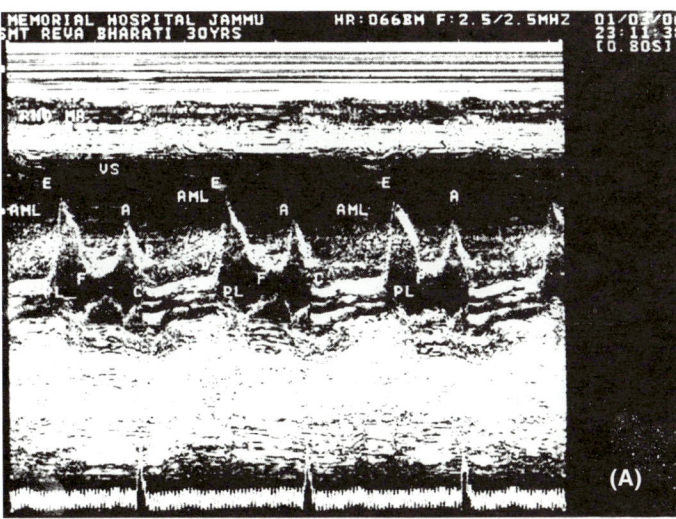

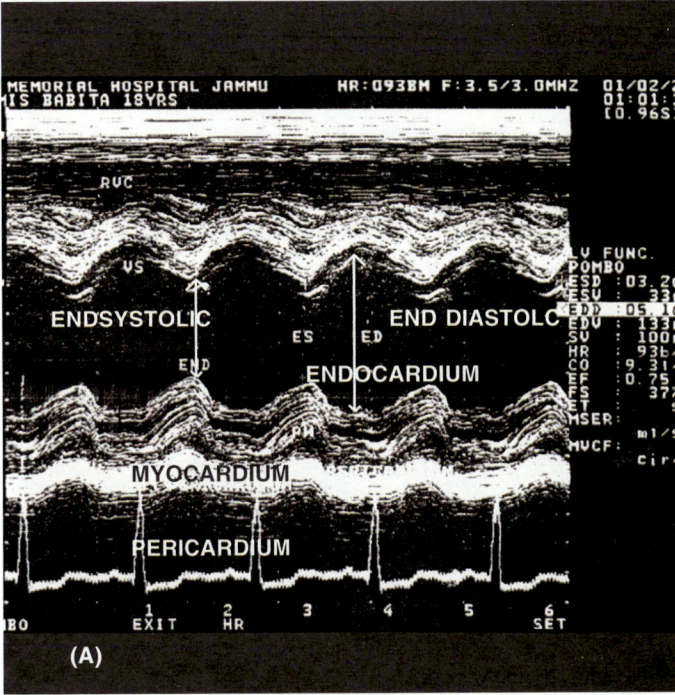

Fig. 2.38A: M-Mode echocardiogram showing relationship of different walls and cavities of the heart. It also helps in the measurements of various internal cardiac structures and cardiac volumes necessary for determining of cardiac functions

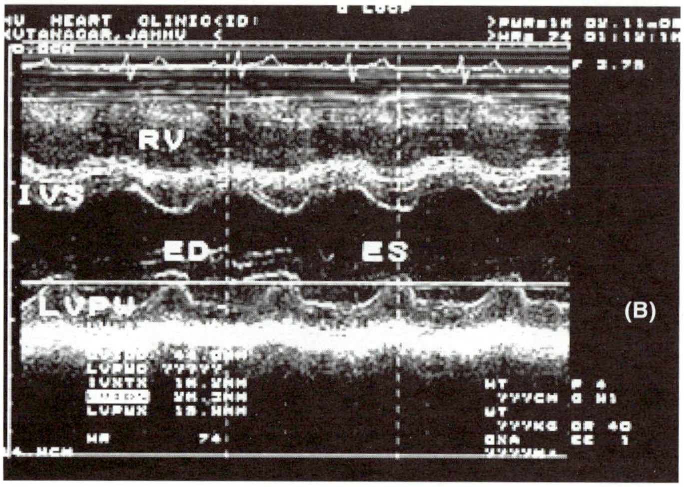

Fig. 2.38B: M-Mode echocardiogram showing as how to take end systolic and end diastolic measurements which in turn are automatically converted to respective volumes by the computer as marked on the scan

Measurements of Various Internal Cardiac Structures and Volumes

IVSTD

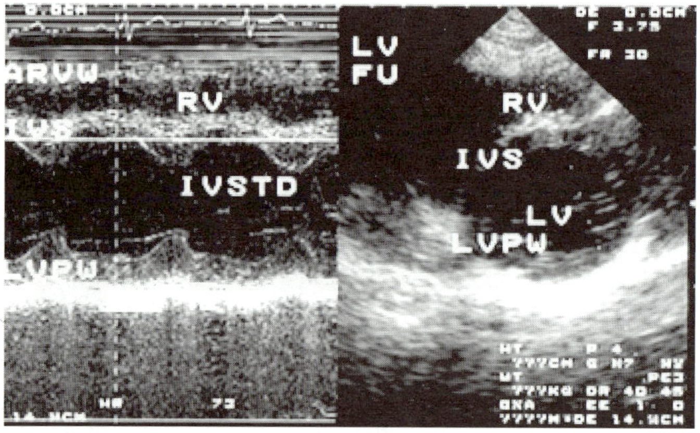

Fig. 2.39: Measurement of interventricular septum during diastole

IVSTS

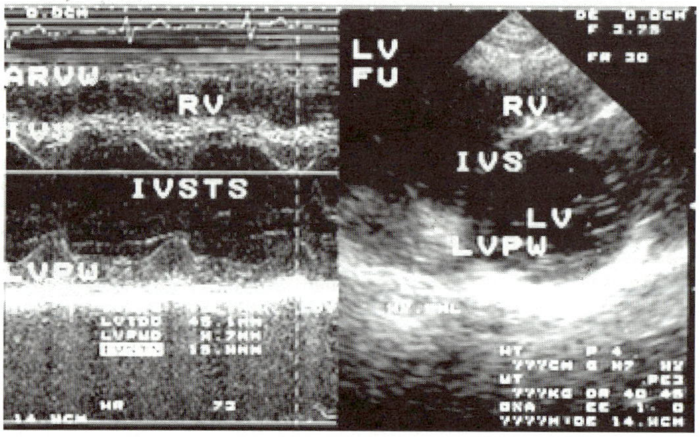

Fig. 2.40: Measurement of interventricular septum during systole

LVIDD

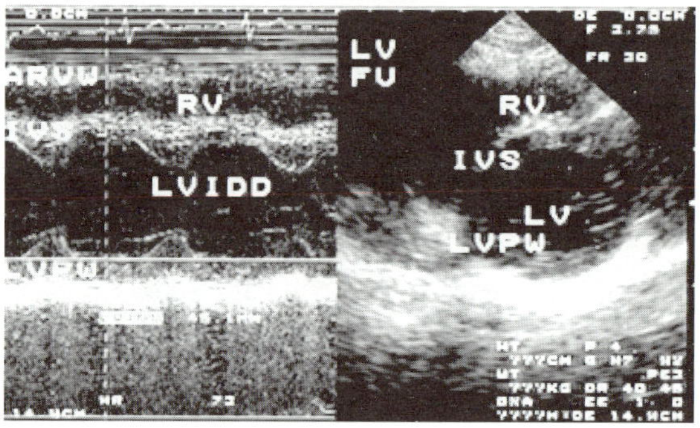

Fig. 2.41: LV internal diameter during end-diastole

LVIDS

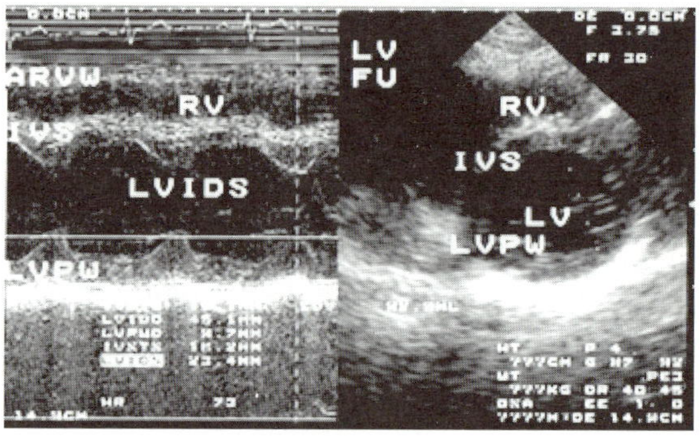

Fig. 2.42: LV internal diameter during end-systole

LVPWD

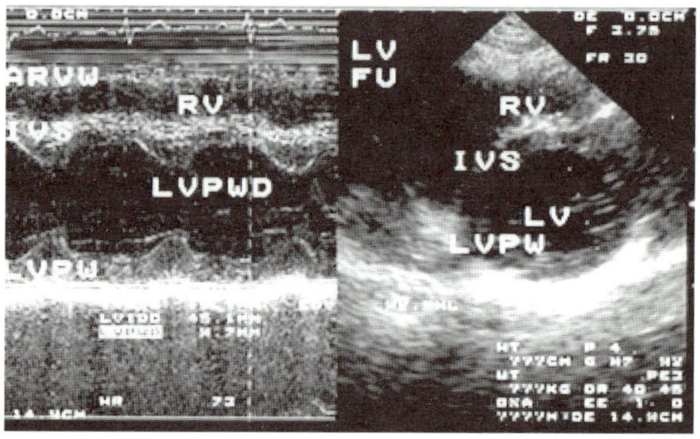

Fig. 2.43: LV posterior wall in end-diastole

LVPWS

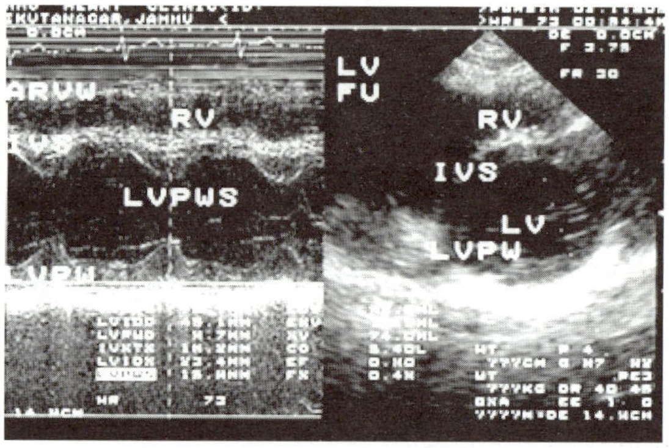

Fig. 2.44: LV posterior wall in end-systole

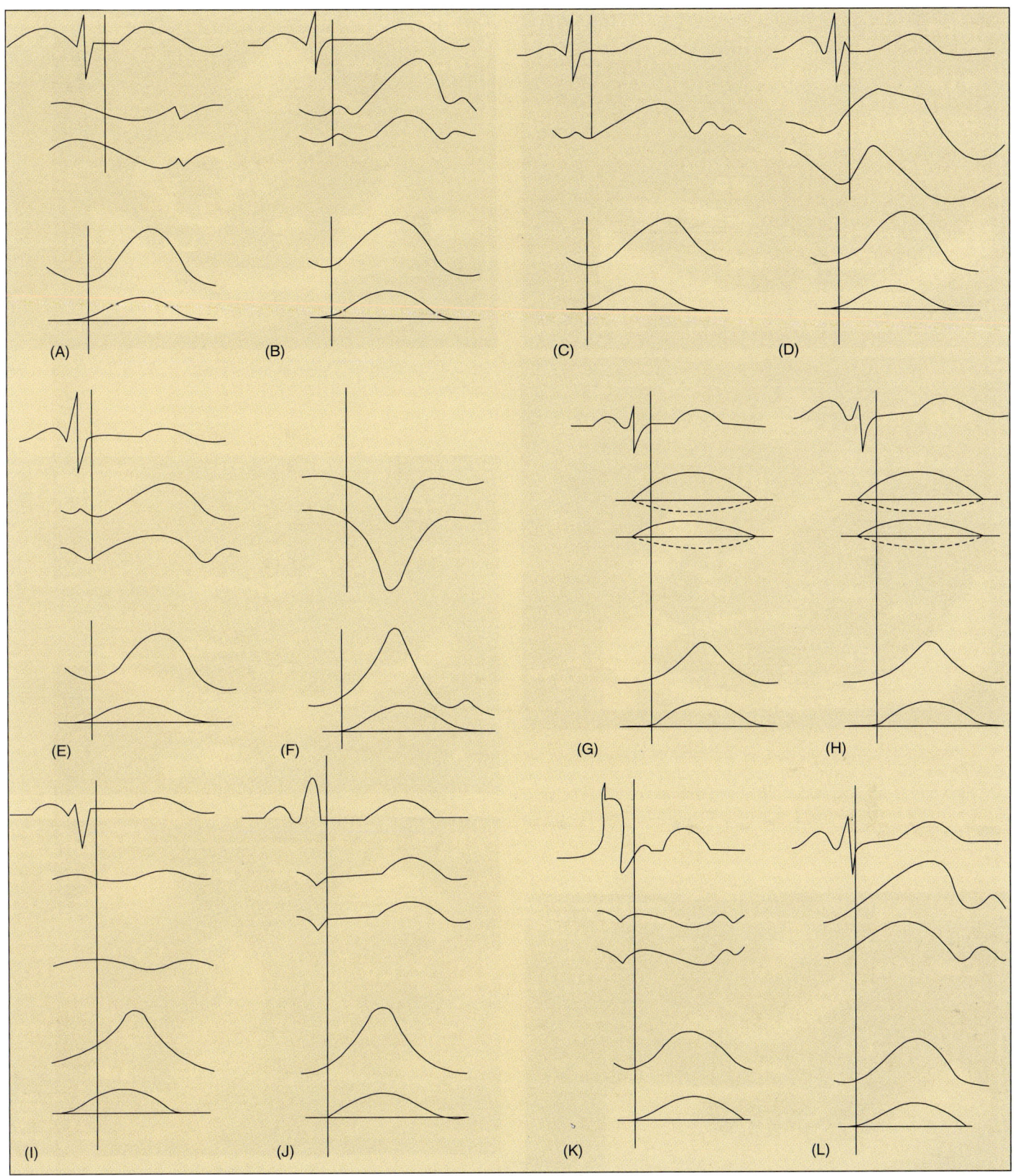

Fig. 2.45A to L: (A) Normal interventricular septal motion. (B) Paradoxical septal motion (Type A). (C) Flat septal motion (Type B). (D) Paradoxical septal motion of interventricular septum in pulmonary hypertension with right ventricular volume overload. (E) Rupture of aneurysm of sinus of valsalva into right atrium (Acute right ventricular volume overload). (F) Left ventricular volume overload. (G) Septal motion in coronary atherosclerotic heart disease. (H) Septal motion in congestive cardiomyopathy. (I) Hypertrophic obstructive cardiomyopathy. (J) Left bundle branch block. (K) Right ventricular endocardial pacing. (L) Constrictive pericarditis

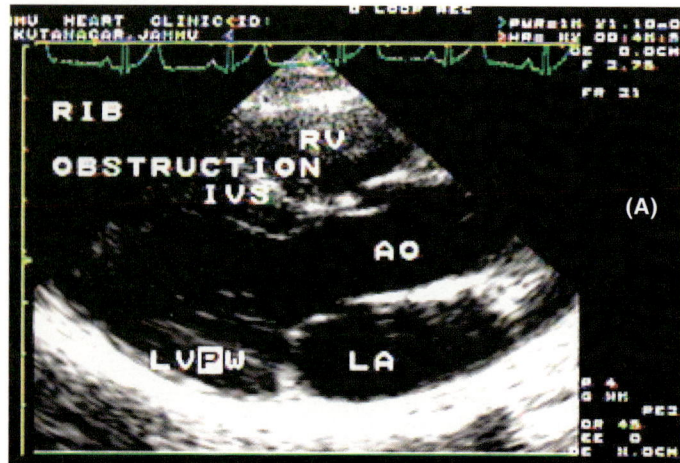

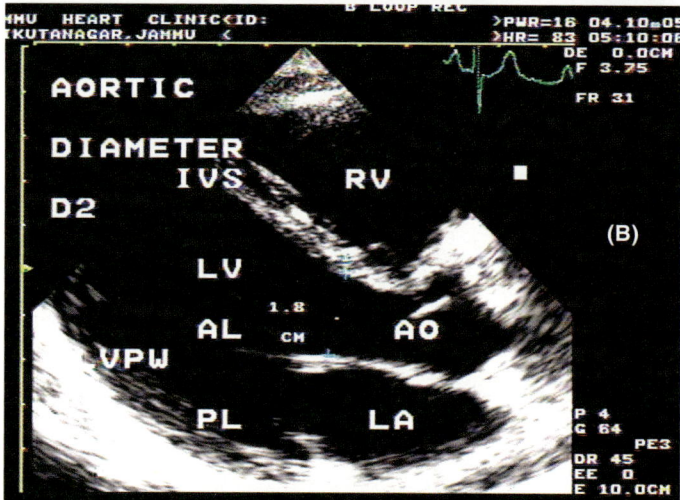

Fig. 2.46A and B: **(A)** Long axis left parasternal echo-scan of LV showing as how left ventricular apex and subapical areas can be truncated due to rib obstruction. **(B)** Long axis left parasternal view of the left ventricular showing various intracardiac structures as labelled on the scan

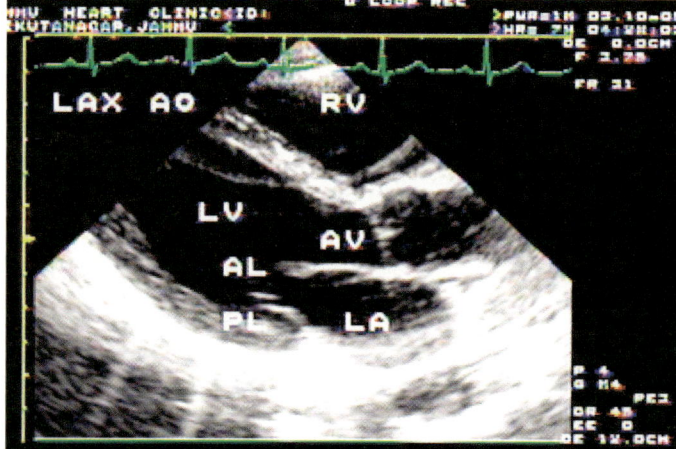

Fig. 2.47A: Shows how to determine diameter of aorta as indicated on scan for utilization in the calculation of hemodynamic data

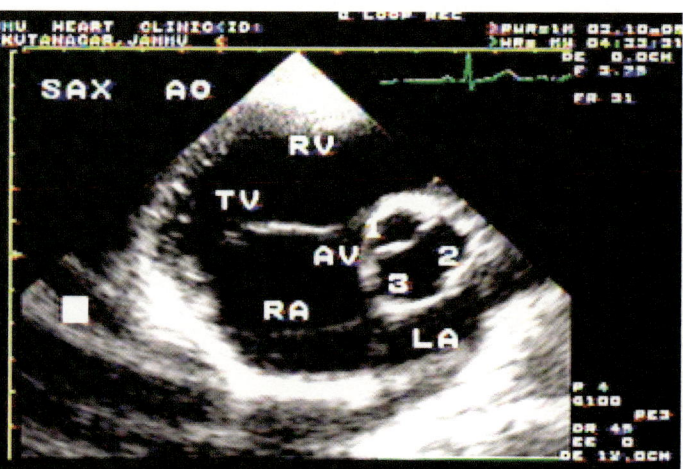

Fig. 2.47B: Short axis view at aortic cusps (1, 2, 3), LA RV and RA chambers

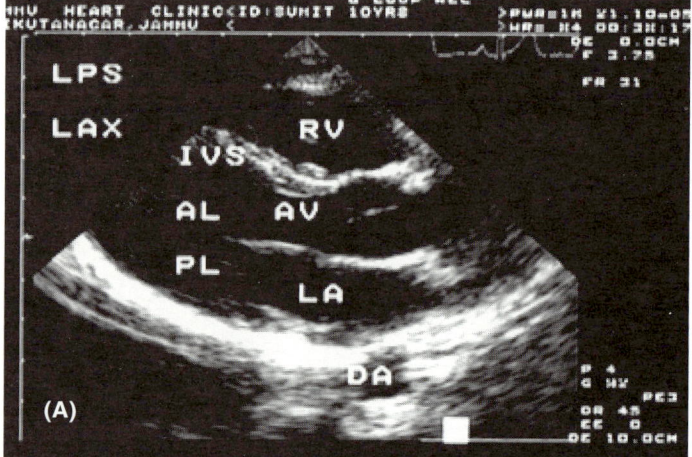

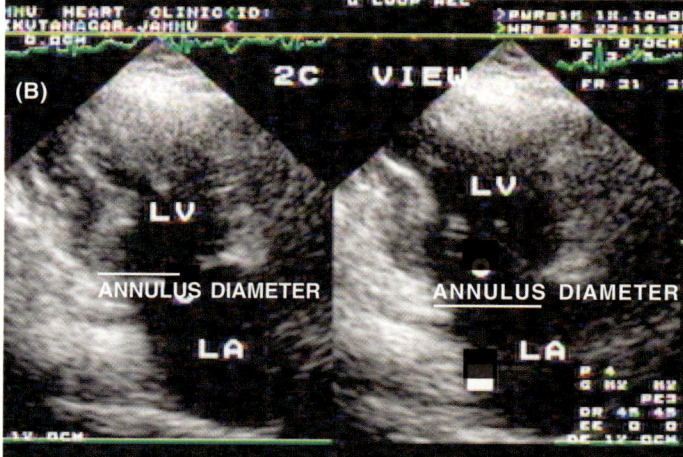

Fig. 2.48A and B: **(A)** LPS LAX view of LV showing intracardiac structures as indicated on scan along with depiction of descending aorta (DA) below the posterio-inferior LV wall. **(B)** Scan taken in oblique left parasternal position for acquiring 2-C view of intracardiac structures as indicated on scan of LV which is useful for obtaining mitral annulus diameter for calculating mitral flow

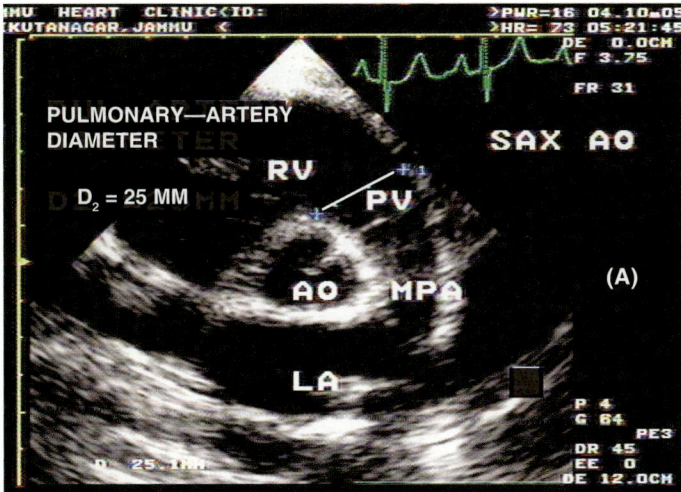

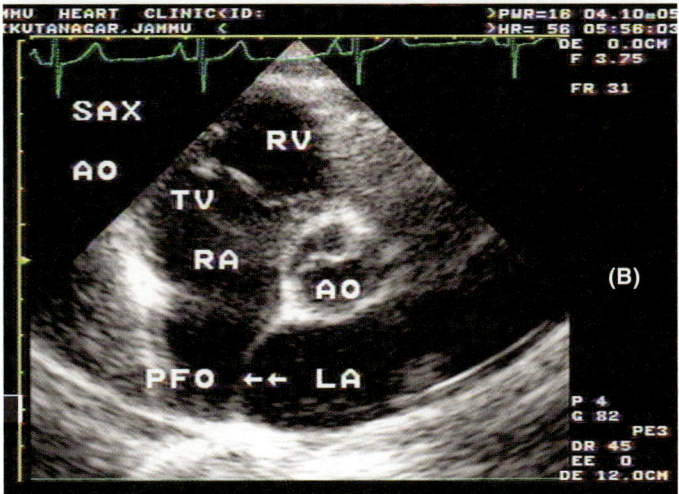

Fig. 2.49A and B: (A) short axis view at aorta taken at right upper parasternal area showing both aorta (AO) and main pulmonary artery (MPA). This view is useful for determining diameter of MPA for hemodynamic calculation of PA blood flow besides, it helps us to record the velocities of both the semilunar valves and their respective stenosis, regurgitation and vegetations. **(B)** Shot axis view at aorta which is helpful in profiling Interatrial septum, L-R shunt (ASD) R-L shunt and diseases of TV such as stenosis regurgitation and vegetations

Cardiac Output: Cardiac output (CO) is an estimated measure of the amount of blood ejected from the left ventricle per minute in litres: (Fig. 2.36A and B)

$$CO = (HR \times SV)/1000$$

where

HR = Heart Rate
SV = Stroke Volume

Ejection Fraction: The ejection fraction (EF) is the estimated percentage of blood filling the left ventricle in diastole that is ejected in systole (Fig. 2.37A and B)

$$EF = \frac{EDD^3 - ESD^3}{EDD^3} \times 100$$

Left Ventricular Mass: The left ventricular mass is the weight of the left ventricle and can be determined by: LV mass = (EDD + Septal thickness + Posterior wall thickness)^3 – EDD^3.

Note: These measurements are made in diastole and are invalid when asymmetric hypertrophy is present.

Left Atrium (LA) (Fig. 2.49A and B)

Dimension: The left atrium should be measured at the end of systole from the posterior wall of the aorta (leading edge) to the leading edge of the left atrial wall. The normal value is 19 to 40 mm (Fig. 2.57B).

Left Atrium/Aortic Root Ratio: The left atrium/aortic root ratio is the ratio of the atrial dimension taken at end systole to the aortic root dimension taken at end diastole. The normal value is 0.87 to 1.11 (Fig. 2.22A and B).

Left Atrial Index: The left atrial index is obtained by dividing the left atrial size by patient's body surface area. The normal value is 12 to 21 mm/m^2.

Interventricular Septum (IVS) (Figs 2.66A and B, 2.105A and B)

Wall Thickness: Wall thickness is a measure of the vertical distance from the right to the left ventricular wall at the onset of the QRS. Abnormal thickening may be seen in patients with obstructive or concentric hypertrophy. The normal value is 6 to 11 mm.

Wall Amplitude (Figs. 2.107A, 2.108A, 2.110, 2.111): Wall amplitude is a measure of the posterior motion of the left ventricular side of septum. It is obtained by drawing a horizontal line between the most posterior point of the septum during systole and then measuring the maximal vertical distance from this line to the septum just before the septum moves posteriorly in systole. The normal value is 5 to 12 mm.

Wall Motion (Figs 2.61–2.63): Normally the septum moves posteriorly after the onset of systole (as the posterior wall moves anteriorly). Following are the common septal abnormalities which can be observed in different situations:

1. Exaggerated septal motion may indicate hyperdynamic contractility—as seen in aortic or mitral insufficiency, ventricular septal defect, patent ductus arteriosus, increased cardiac output, or coronary artery disease- and implies left ventricular volume overload (Fig. 2.45A–L).

2. Paradoxical septal motion (the septum and posterior wall move anteriorly after the onset of systole) may be caused by left bundle branch block, ventricular aneurysm, atrial septal defect, or pulmonary or tricuspid insufficiency. It is indicative of right ventricular volume overload (Fig. 2.107B).

3. Flattened septal motion is observed when the left side of the septum moves poorly or not at all in systole. This indicates possible left anterior descending coronary artery disease, or it may result from technical problems connected with patient positioning.

Posterior Left Ventricular Wall (PLVW)

Definition of the limits of the left ventricular posterior wall is often difficult. The endocardium which is a fine structure must not be confused with echoes arising from chordae which are situated more anteriorly. They may be distinguished by their continuity with the echoes of the mitral leaflets and by the absence of a posterior end-diastolic motion (Fig. 2.36A).

The epicardium is recognised by the use of damping or switch gain controls. It may be distinguished from the pericardium, a denser echo-from which it may be separated by a small echo-free space in systole. The posterior walls moves anteriorly in systole with an amplitude of about 10 mm for about 0.36 sec. This motion is preceded by a small posterior movement (atrial contraction). At the end of systole it has a rapid posterior motion (lasting 0.08 to 0.10 sec) during rapid early diastolic filling; during the slow left ventricular filling phase, slight posterior motion is observed. The diastolic thickness of the posterior wall is measured from the most anterior endocardial echo to the most anterior epicardial echo; it is usually the same thickness as the interventricular septum. The systolic thickness is measured at its maximal thickness.

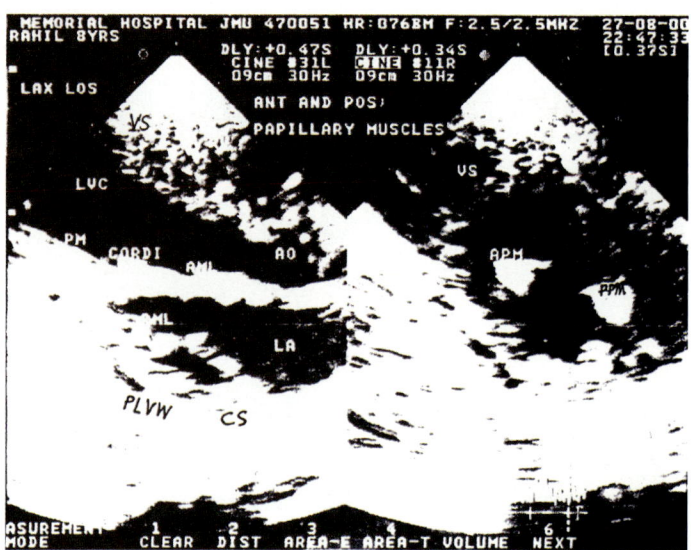

Fig. 2.50B: 2-D Scan in long axis and taken at LPS region depicts chordiae tendinae (left) and papillary muscles as shown in the scan (right)

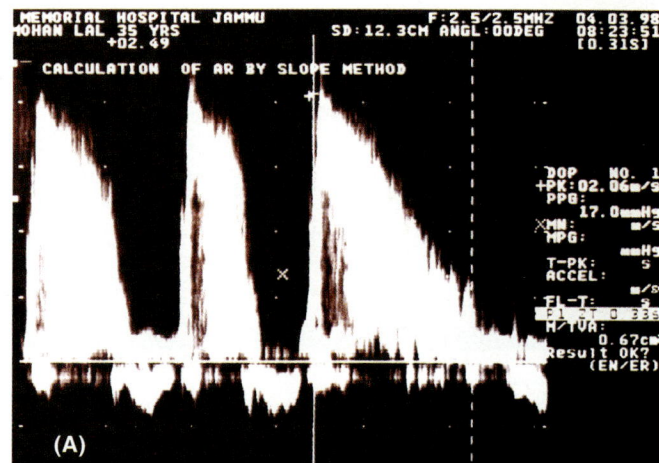

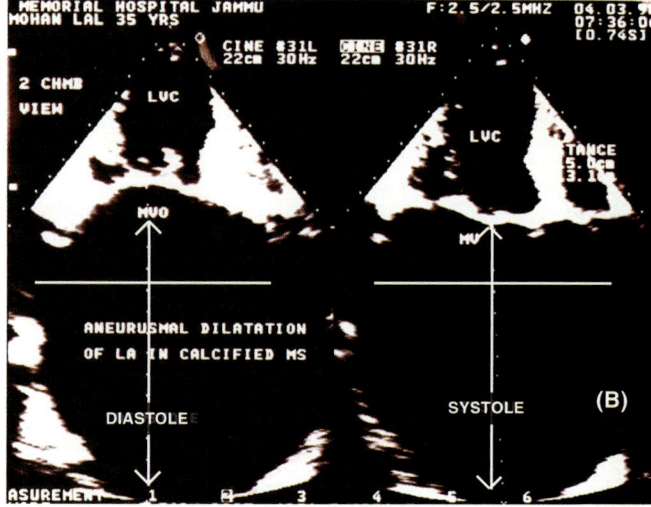

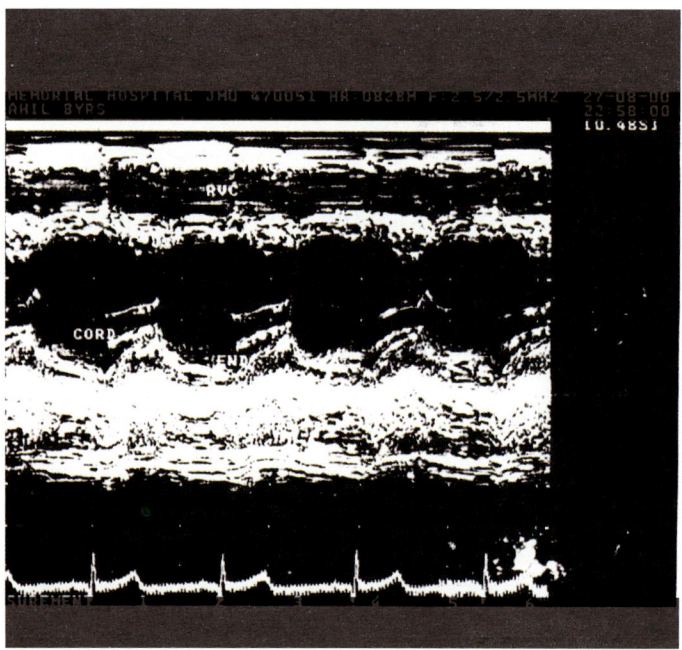

Fig. 2.50A: M-Mode echocardiogram showing RV, IVS, LV cavity, chordae tendinae and posterior left ventricular wall

Fig. 2.51A and B: (A) 2-D Scan of aortic regurgitation for determining severity of AR by the application of slope method. (B) 2-D Dual scan showing aneurysmal dilatation of LA in severe type of mitral stenosis

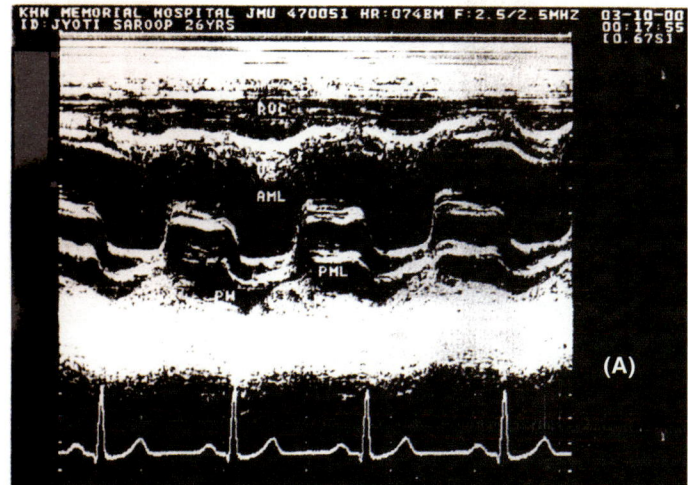

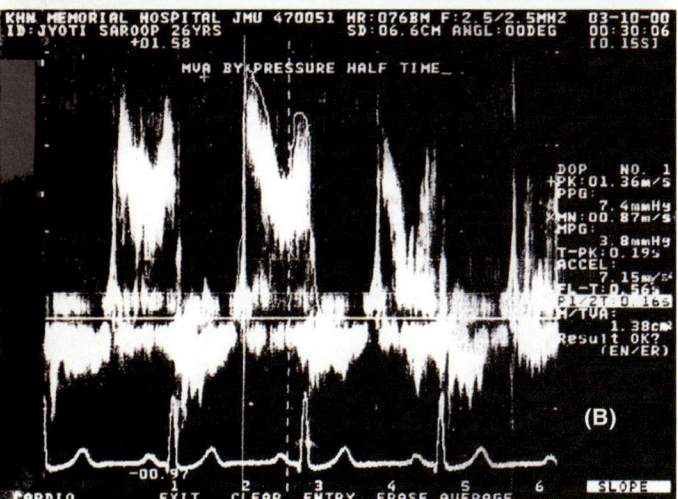

Fig. 2.52A and B: **(A)** M-Mode echocardiogram showing thickening of AML, reduction in EF slope, thichening and paradoxical movement of posterior mitral leaflet (PML) in moderate type of mitral stenosis. **(B)** Doppler flow across mitral valve for calculation of peak opening velocity, pressure half time, pressure gradient and finally determining the severity of mitral stenosis

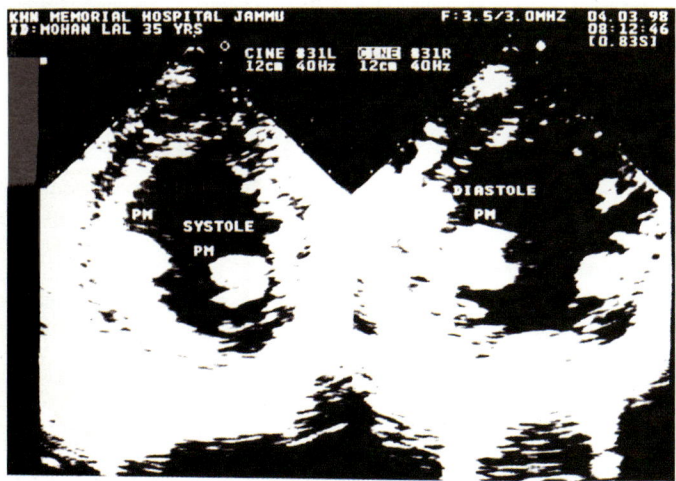

Fig. 2.53A: 2-D Short axis echogram showing hypertrophic papillary muscles during systole and diastole

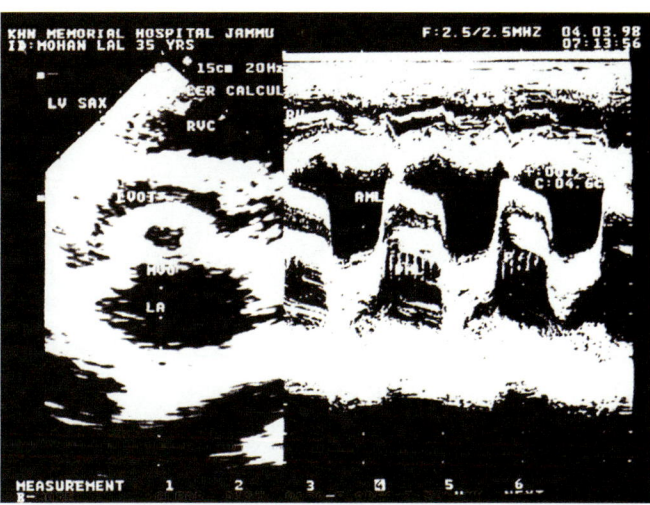

Fig. 2.53B: M-Mode echocardiogram depicts heavily calcified mitral valve with paradoxical movements of the posterior mitral leaflet (right) and reduced MVA with dilated LA (left)

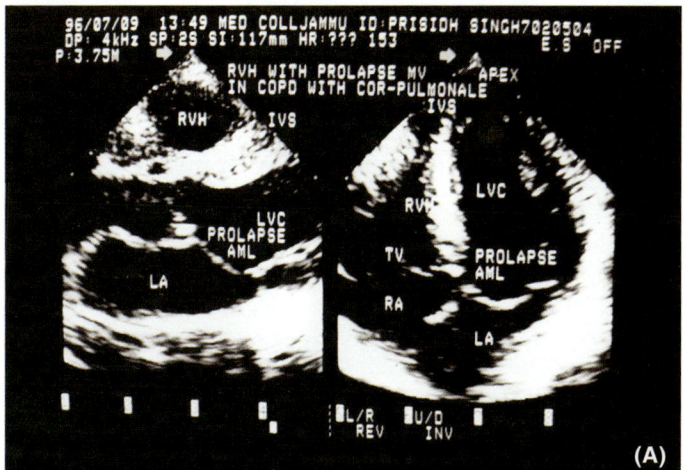

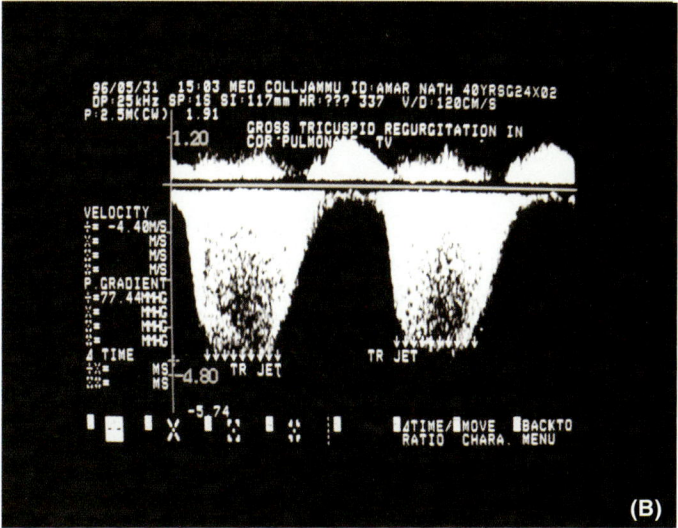

Fig. 2.54A and B: **(A)** M-Mode and 2-D apical 4C views showing significant mitral valve prolapse. **(B)** Doppler flow velocity across TV depicts gross TR in a patient suffering from chronic cor-pulmonale

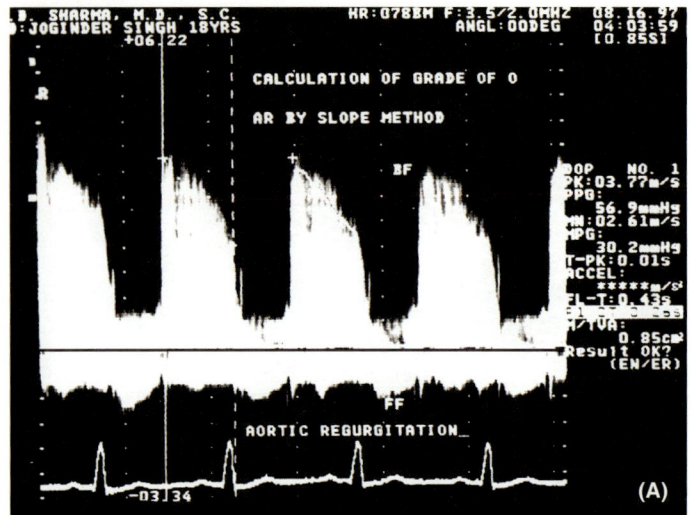

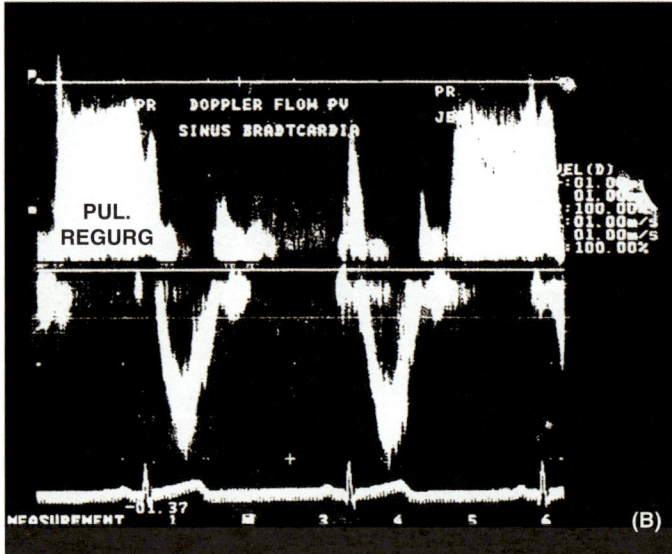

Fig. 2.55A and B: (A) Doppler flow velocity across aortic valve showing slope in aortic regurgitation to utilise it as a measure to determine the clinical grading and severity of aortic regurgitation. **(B)** Doppler flow velocity across pulmonary valve depicting gross pulmonary regurgitation in severe form of bradyarrhythmia in a patient with sick sinus syndrome

Study of the Left Ventricular Performance

The ability to record the left ventricle in diastole and systole provides a means of evaluating left ventricular performance.

Although M-mode echo only gives a unidimensional view, it does give good definition of the left ventricular wall and their motion throughout the cardiac cycle. 2-D studies give a global appreciation of the geometry of the cavity, but the definition of the endocardium is not as good. There is a source of error in the measurement of the left ventricular dimensions by this method.

In practice, M-mode studies remain valuable in the assessment of the quality of myocardial contractility.

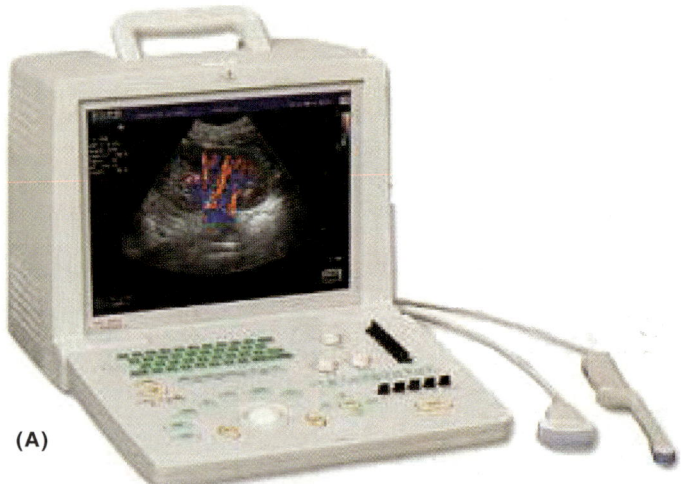

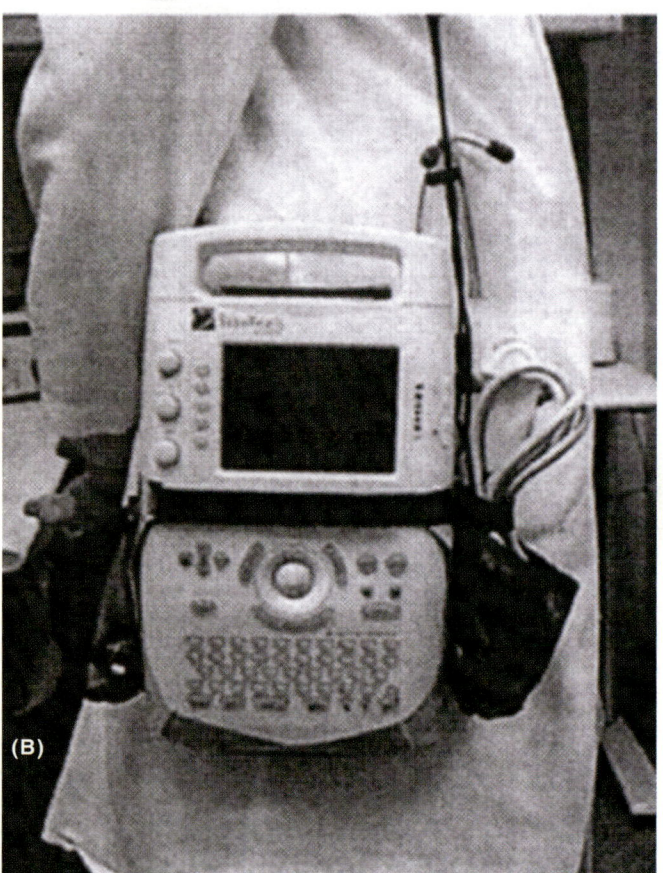

Fig. 2.56A and B: (A) Portable color Doppler echocardiography machine for instantaneous visualisation of cardiac structures right in the consulting chamber of the cardiologist. **(B)** Latest version of hand held echocardiographic machine which can be used for obtaining infomation even during routine or in emergency situation at the bedside of the patient. This is being depicted here around the shoulder of the doctor

Ventricular Volumes (Figs 2.36A, B, 2.37A and B)

Assuming that the left ventricle may be described as a prolate ellipse with a long axis twice the length of its short axis, and knowing the value of one of the short axis, it becomes possible to calculate the ventricular volume. Cardiac volumes can be obtained directly by either ellipse method or by trace method. This type of computer generated volumes can be obtained out of most of the currently available machines.

Portable Ultrasound Machines

During the past few decades, cardiologists were taught to perform physical examination by using their senses; indeed, most clinical diagnoses are still based on auscultation which requires the best skill to recognise abnormal sounds and different types of heart murmurs. However, awareness that abnormal physical findings are not always specific nor always sensitive has led to the development of an armamentarium of diagnostic procedures during the last few decades. In particular, ultrasound imaging allows the cardiac structures to be viewed dynamically, undoubtedly providing a new window on the heart. Currently, echocardiography is the most widely used and cost effective diagnostic imaging tool in cardiology and has largely replaced

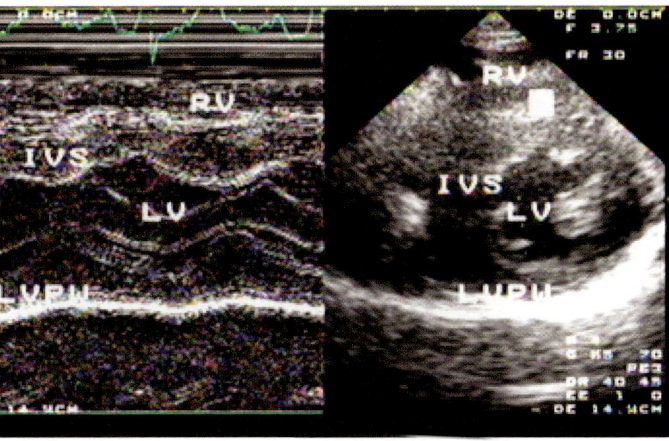

Apex

Fig. 2.58: Graphic tracing of various cardiac structures being scanned at different angulations of ultrasound beams

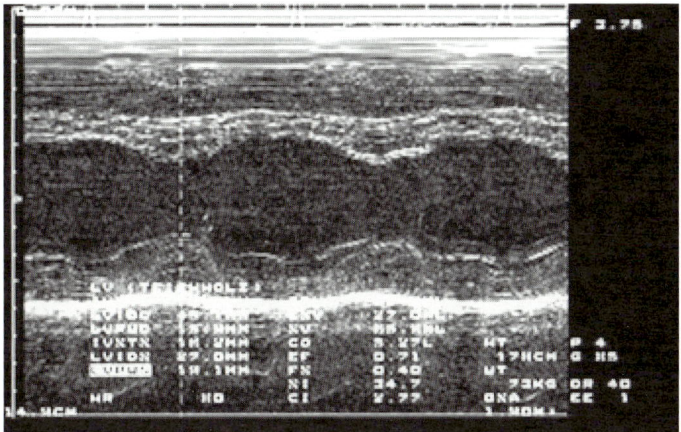

Fig. 2.59: Mid cavity

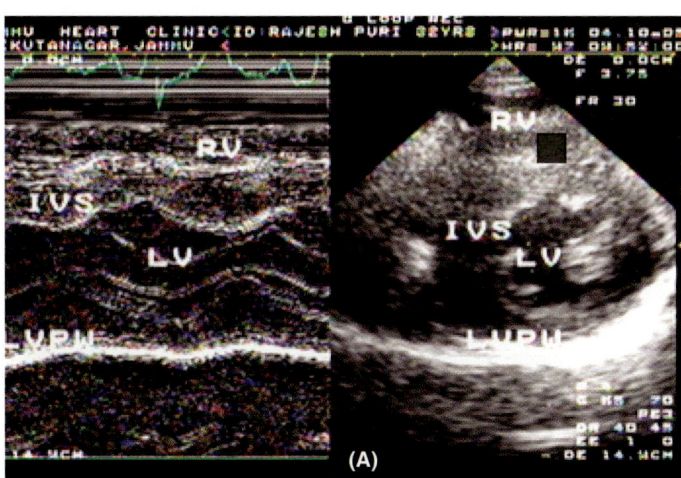

(A)

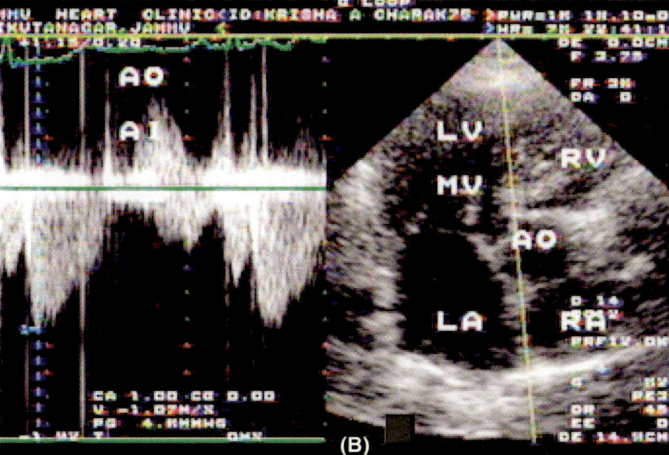

(B)

Fig. 2.57A and B: (A) M-Mode and 2-D view taken at high LPS shows concenteric LVH. **(B)** Doppler flow velocity of aorta in apical five chambers view

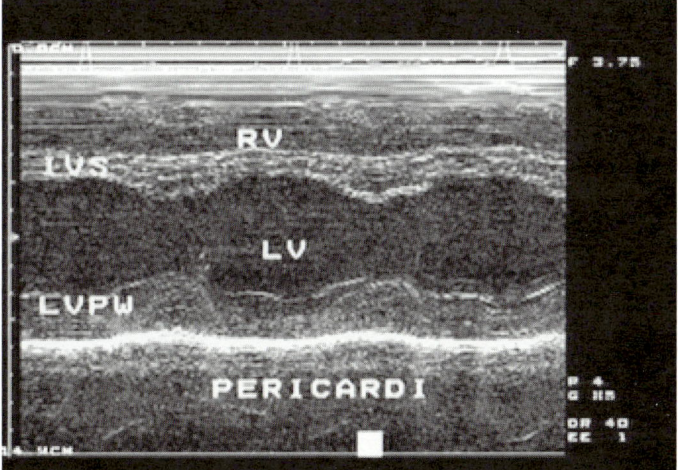

Fig. 2.60: Basal

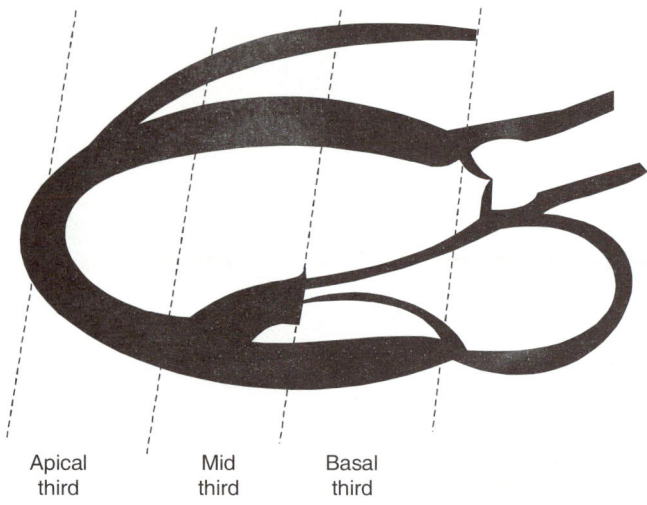

Apical   Mid   Basal
third   third   third

Fig. 2.61: Graphic representation

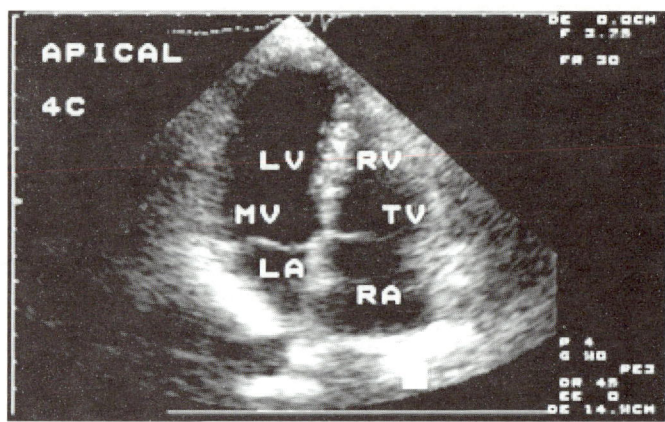

Fig. 2.64: 2-D Apical 4C scan for all the four chambers of the heart along with concordantly placed mitral and tricuspid valves in left-sided orientation

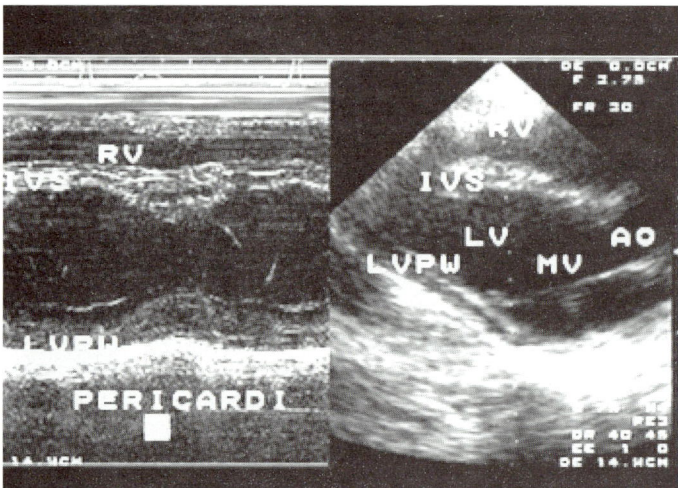

Fig. 2.62

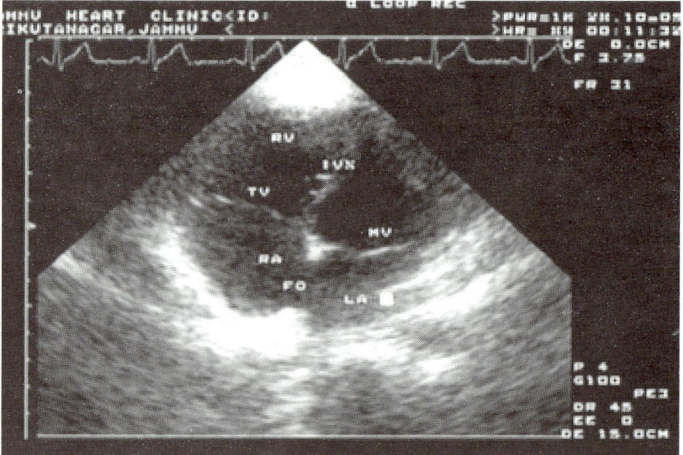

Fig. 2.65: 2-D Apical 4C scan for all the four chambers of the heart along with concordantly placed mitral and tricuspid valves in right sided orientation

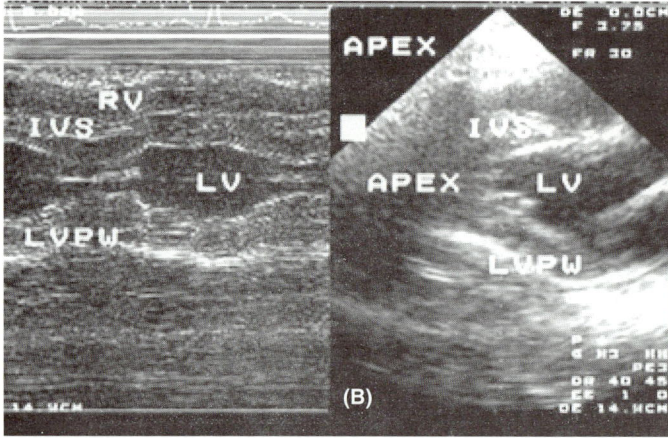

Fig. 2.63: Sub-apical

Figs 2.59 to 2.63: M-mode scans taken at LPS mid and upper regions to show that how LV cavity is oriented in these views and useful for diagnosing hypokinesia, dyskinesia paradoxical movements of IVS, cardiomyopathies and volume overload of LV and RV

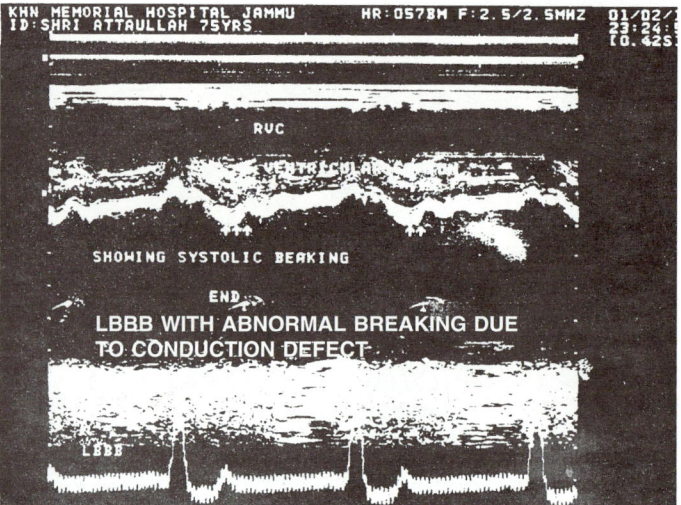

Fig. 2.66A: M-Mode echocardiogram showing abnormal beaking of IVS during systole as a result of conduction defect of LBBB

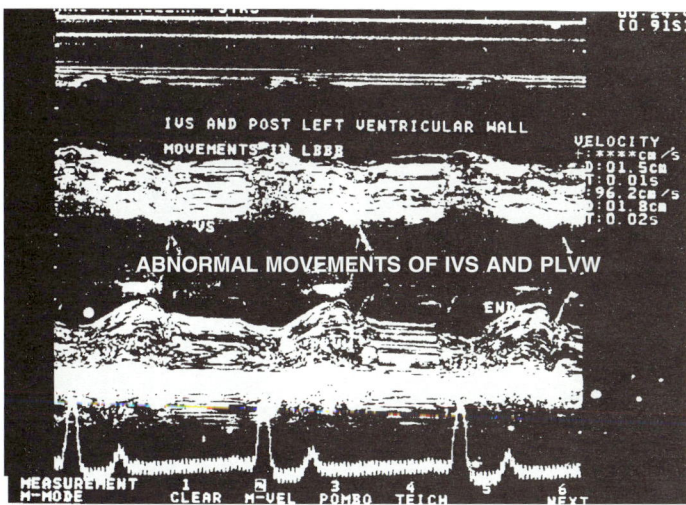

Fig. 2.66B: M-Mode echocardiogram shows abnormal contraction of posterior left ventricular wall with less thickening of IVS as compared to PLVW

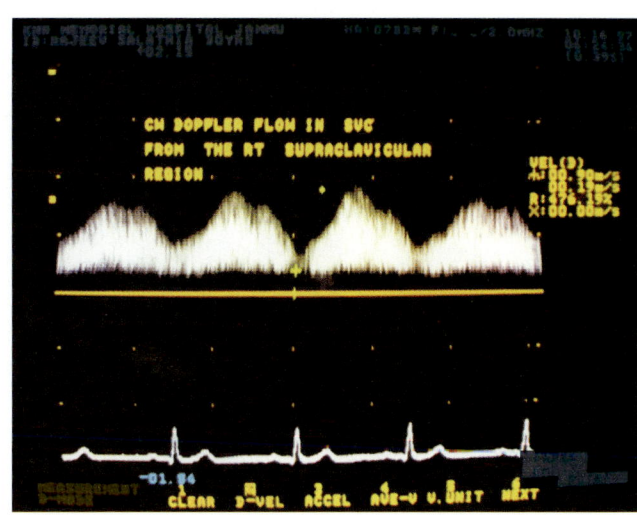

Fig. 2.68: Visualization of superior vena cava by the application of continuous wave Doppler probe placed at right supraclavicular region

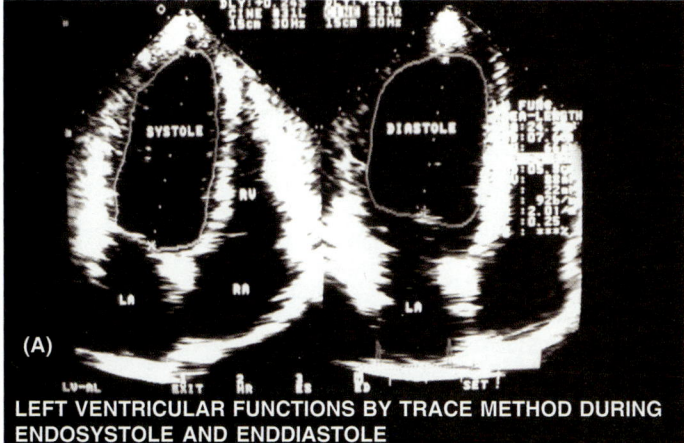

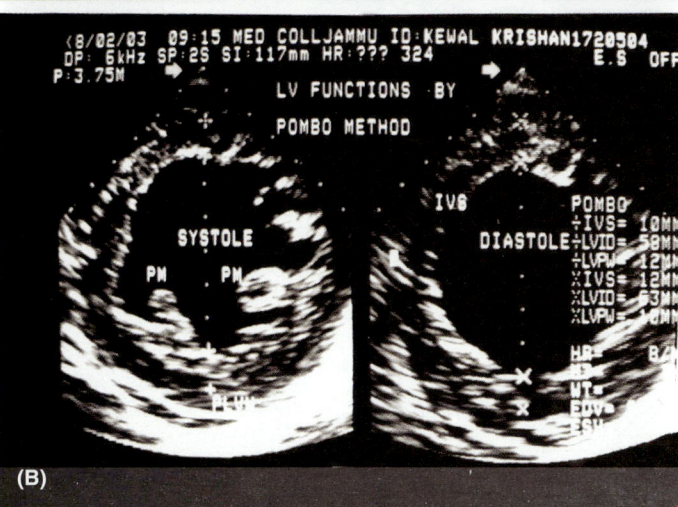

Fig. 2.67A and B: (A) 2-D Dual scan during systole and diastole in apical 4C views for calculation of LV functions by trace method as shown on the scan. **(B)** 2-D Dual scan taken both during systole and diastole for calculation of DLV functions by Pombo method as depicted on the scans

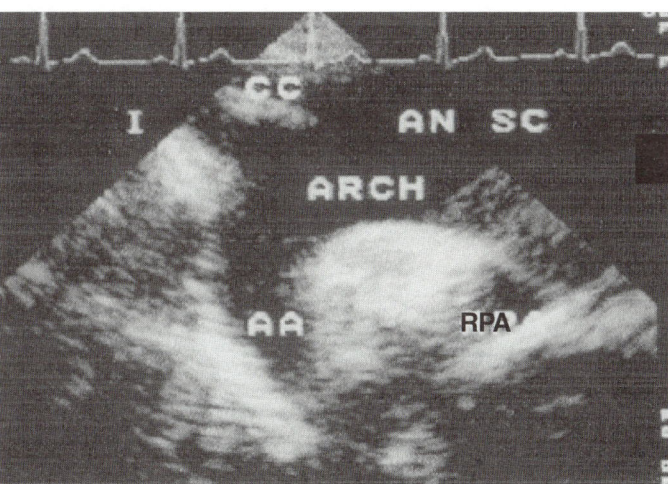

Fig. 2.69A: Suprasternal approach showing dilated left subclavian artery (AN–SC)

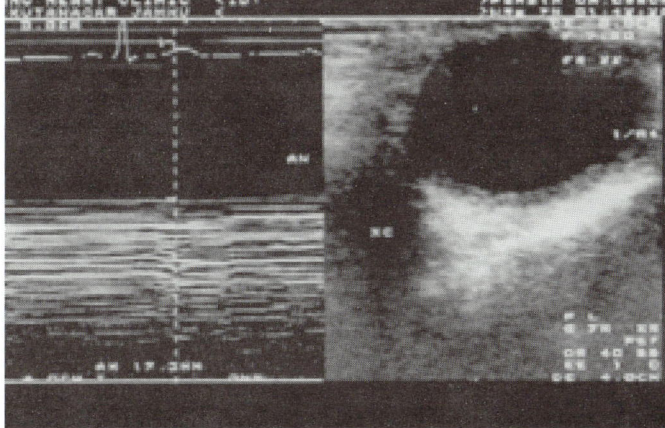

Fig. 2.69B: Short Axis Duplex scan at left subclavian artery showing aneurysmal dilatation of the vessel (AN)

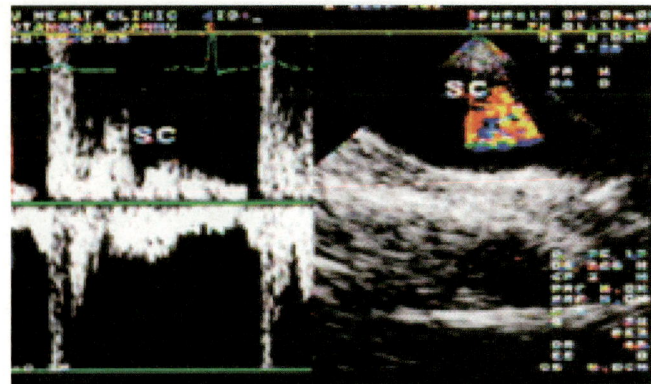

Fig. 2.69C: Color Doppler flow velocity across aneurysm of left sub-clavian artery

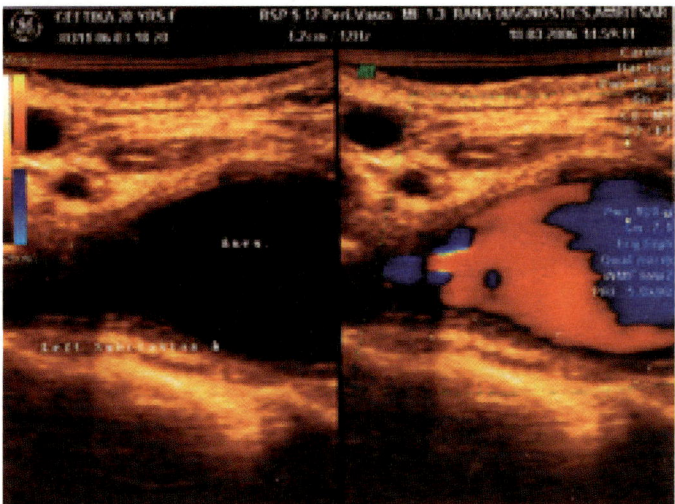

Fig. 2.69D: Color Duplex scan of left subclavian artery showing hugely dilated vessel with disturbed intraluminal blood flow

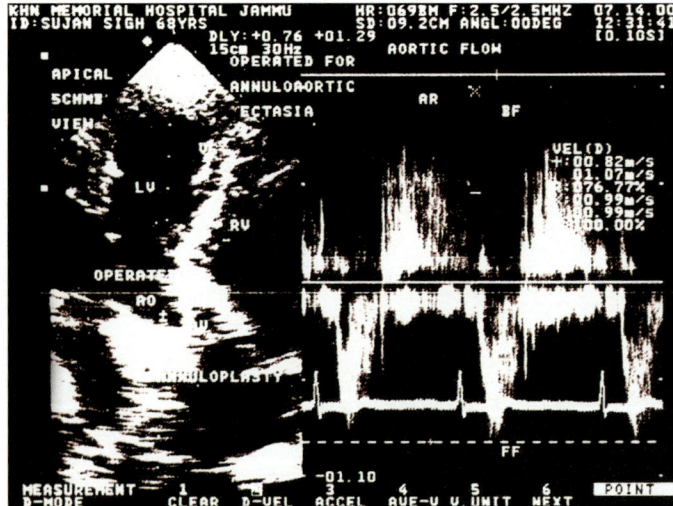

Fig. 2.70A: Apical 5C view of LV showing *annuloplasty* graft operation for the patient with annulo-aortic ectasia in Marfanoid syndrome

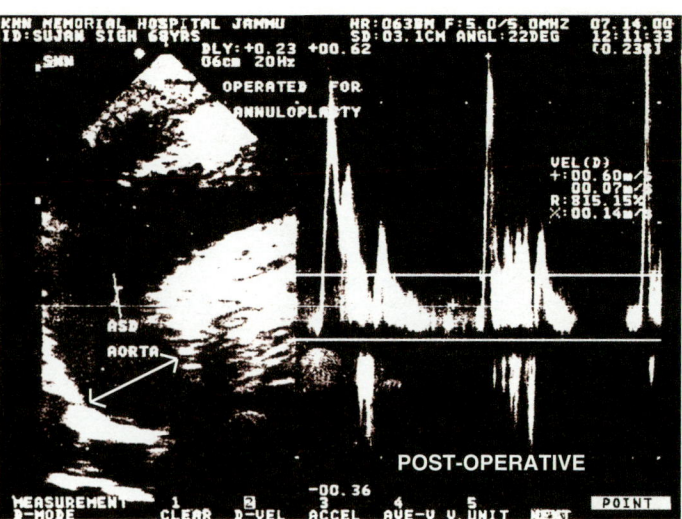

Fig. 2.70B: Suprasternal notch approach for ascending aorta showing aneurysmal dilatation of aorta with widened aortic annulus, clinically presenting as grade II-III. In the same patient AR disappeared after operation as shown in scan A

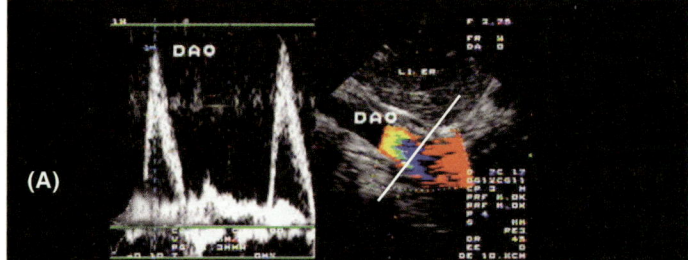
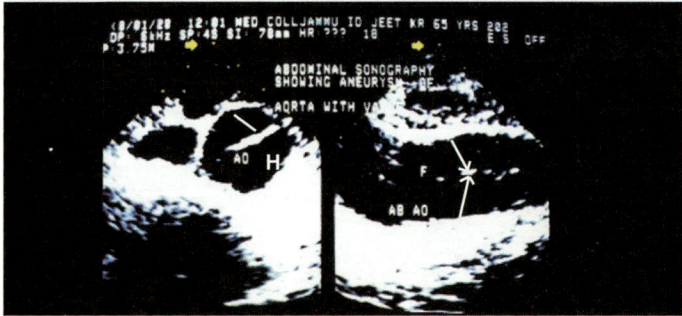
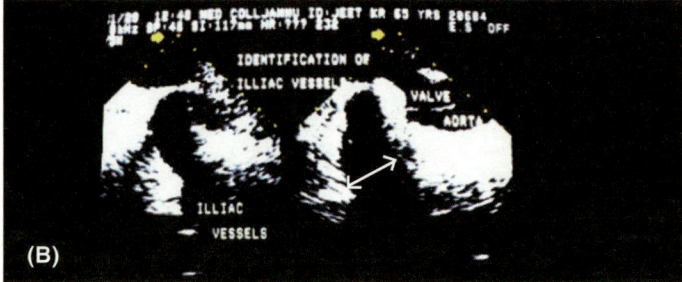

Fig. 2.71A and B: (A) Color Doppler flow across abdominal aorta taken at subcostal paraaortic window reveals normal laminar flow. **(B)** (upper) Subcostal approach for lower abdominal aorta revealed aortic band/valve as shown in graph, lower scan for illiac vessel shows irregular and fusiform configuration of illiac arteries due to atherosclerosis in an older person

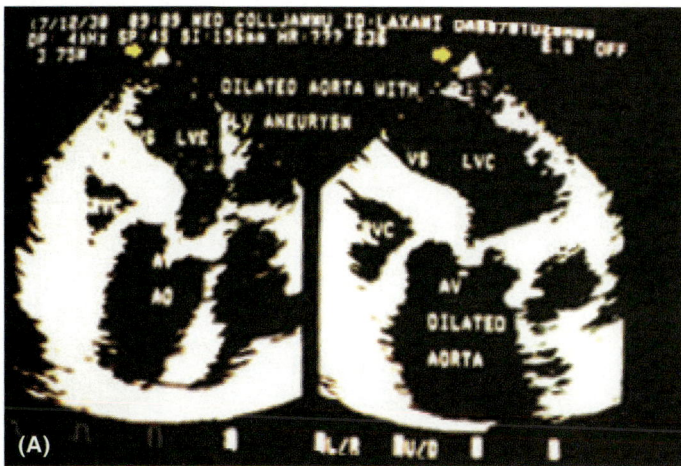

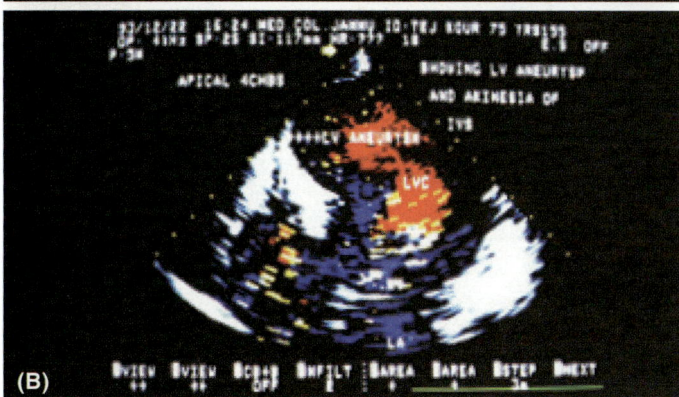

Fig. 2.72A and B: **(A)** Dual 4C Apical scans of LV showing aneurysmal enlargement of aorta, compressed LA, and thickened AOV. **(B)** Apical 4C view showing disturbed color flow patterns in LV aneurysm as indicated on the scan

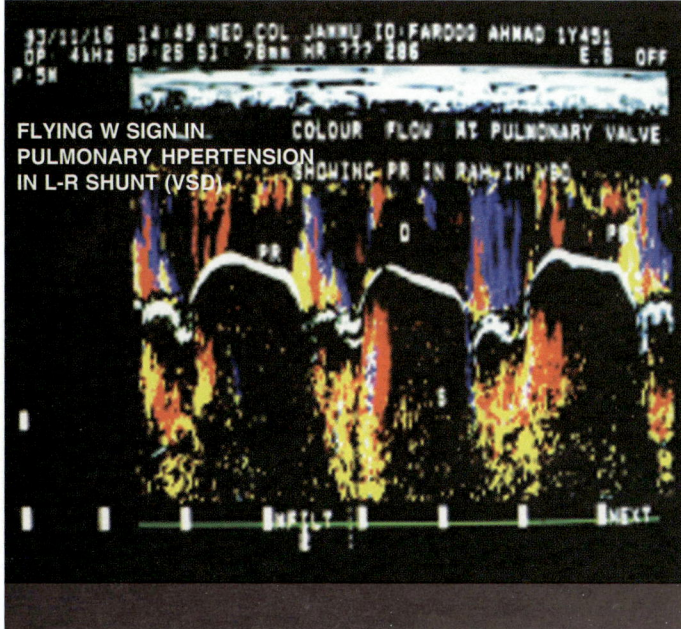

Fig. 2.73A: M-Mode echocardiogram shows flying w sign in pulmonary arterial hypertension and color flow shows pulmonary regurgitation jet

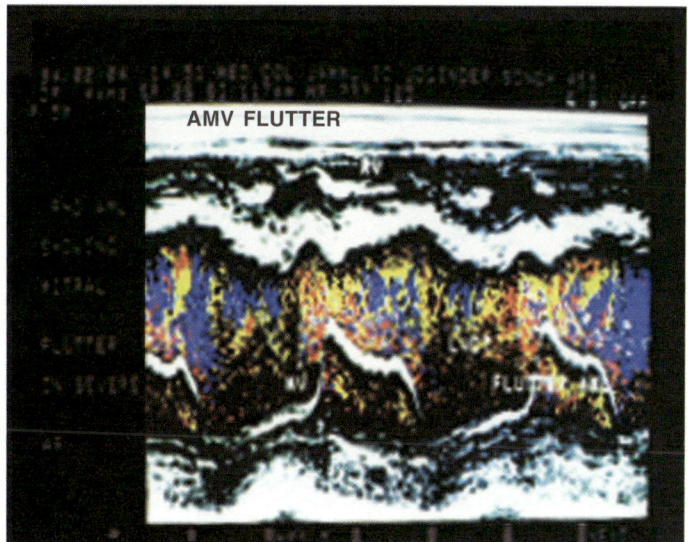

Fig. 2.73B: Color flow M-mode echocardiogram shows mitral valve flutter due to aortic regurgitant jet falling on the AML and causing restriction of movement of AML. This restriction gives rise to clinically detectable Austin Flint murmur goes after the name of the person who detected it for the first time. This has nothing to do with the organic disease of the mitral valve

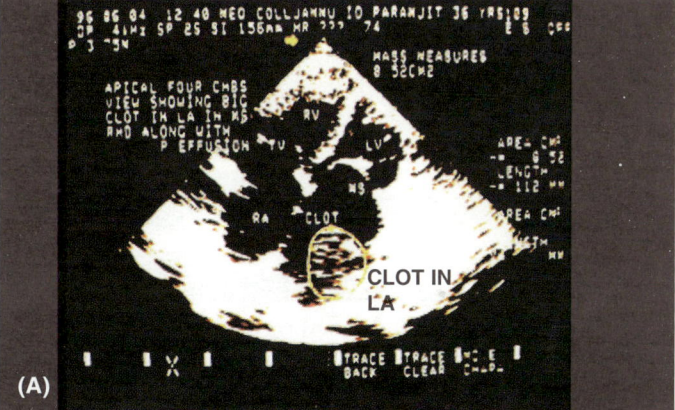

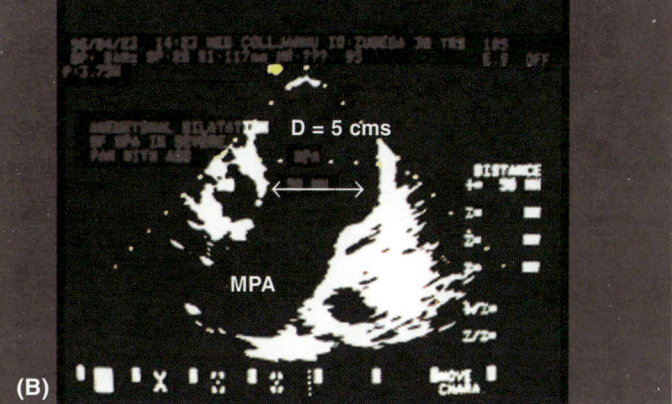

Fig. 2.74A and B: **(A)** Apical 4C view showing thickening of mitral valve in mitral stenosis and clot seen in left atrium (encircled). **(B)** 2-D short axis great vessel view showing aneurysmal dilatation of main pulmonary artery in patient with multivalvular dysfunctions in rheumatic heart disease

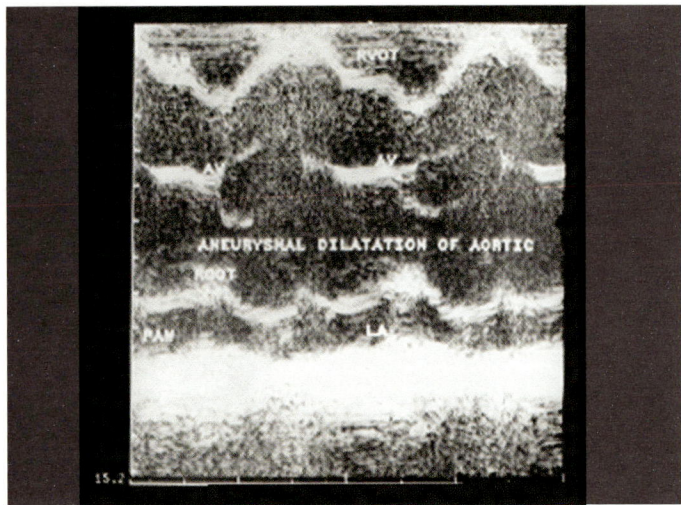

Fig. 2.75: M-Mode echo scan of aorta showing hugely dilated aorta with thinning of both aortic walls and compressed LA posteriorly

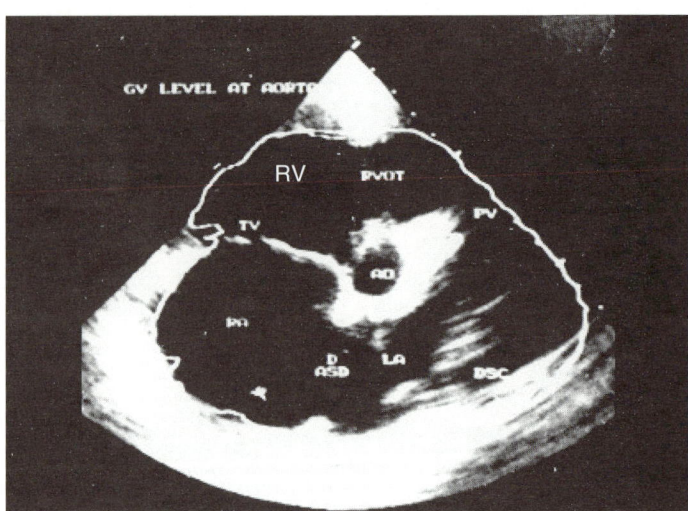

Fig. 2.78: Lower panel (short axis AO) showing large ASD

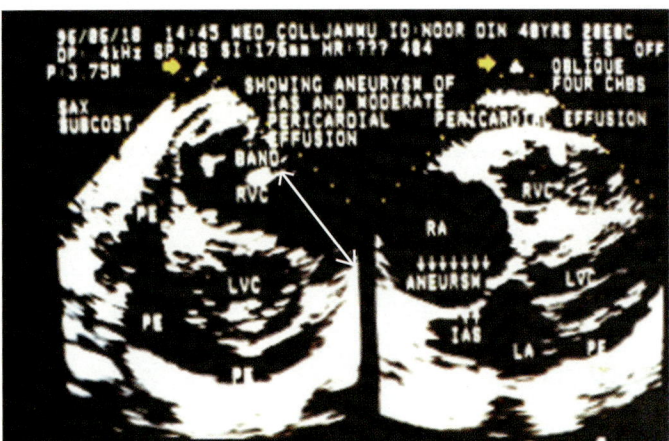

Fig. 2.76: Subcostal 4C view showing hugely distended RA and greatly stretched IAS creating a aneurysmal type of deformity of IAS

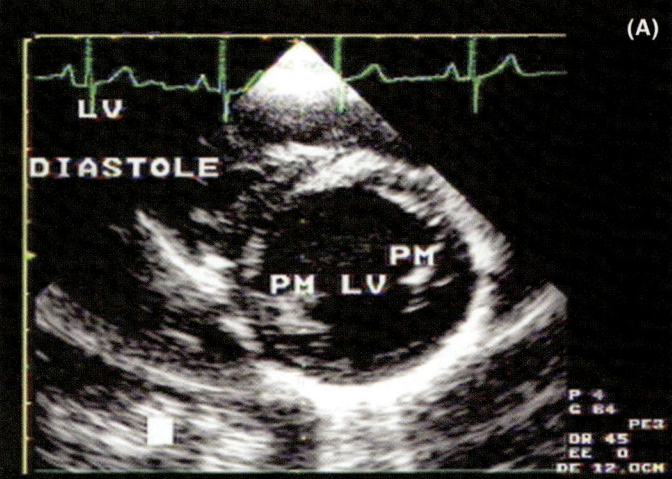

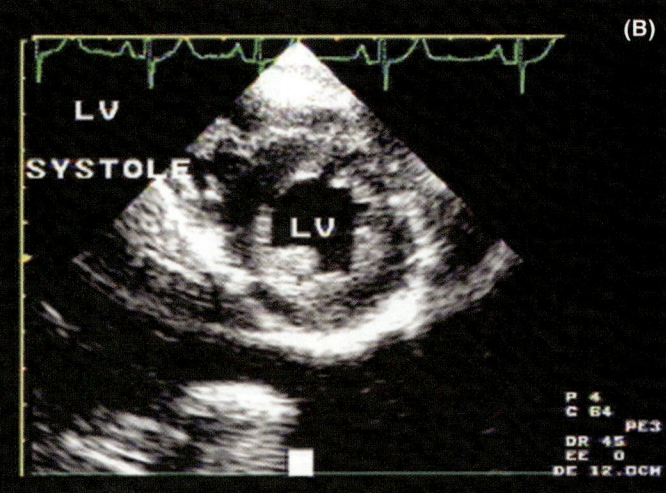

Fig. 2.79A and B: (A) Short axis view of LV taken at high LPS region in 4th intercostal space showing LV size along with papillary muscles in diastole. **(B)** Short axis view of LV along with papillary muscles in systole

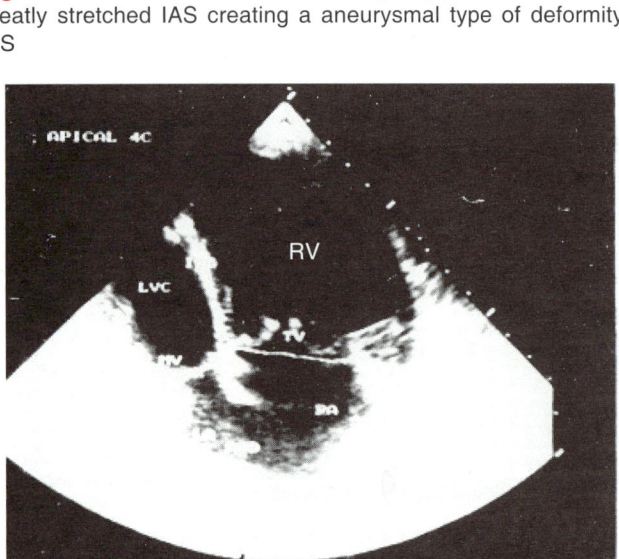

Fig. 2.77: Upper panel (4C view) showing absence of mid IAS as seen in ASD

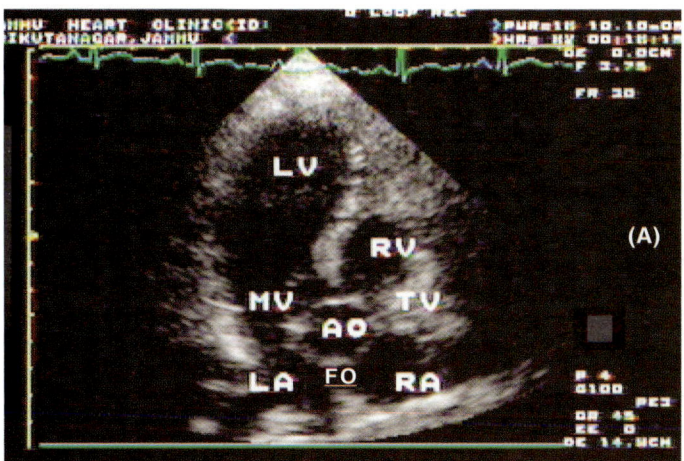

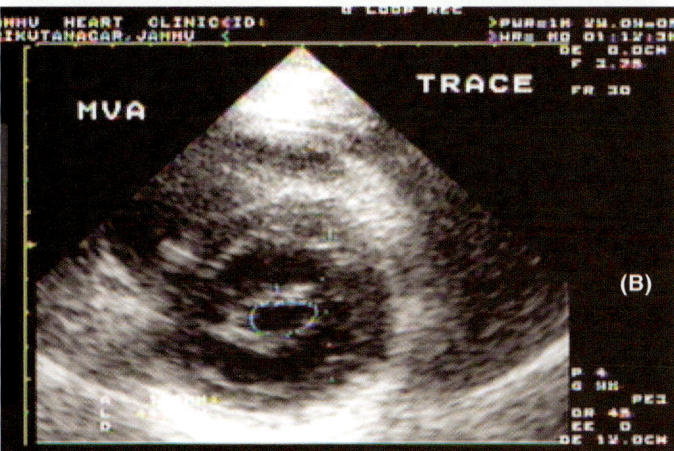

Fig. 2.80A and B: (A) LPS, Apical five chambers view showing all the four chambers, AV valves and aorta along with its valve. This view is useful to identify any intracavity mass / valvular vegetation and regurgitation when assisted by color Doppler technique. **(B)** Short axis of LV at upper LPS region for profiling of MV and trace method for determinig valvular stenosis

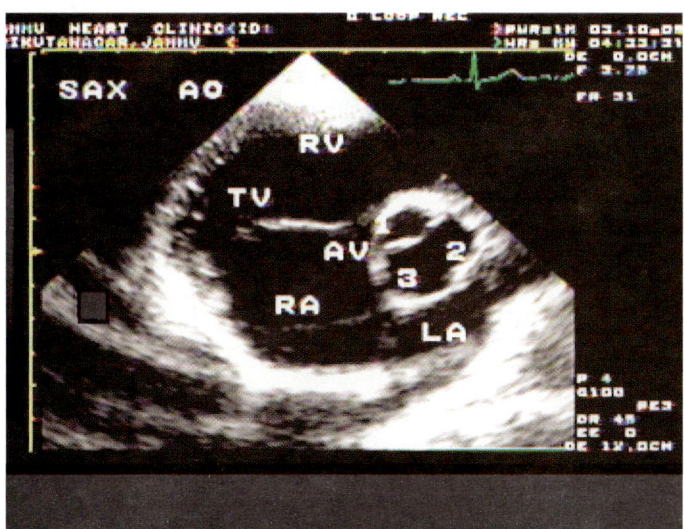

Fig. 2.81: Short axis view at aorta at high LPS region showing all the three cusps of aorta, TV, RA, LA, and RV

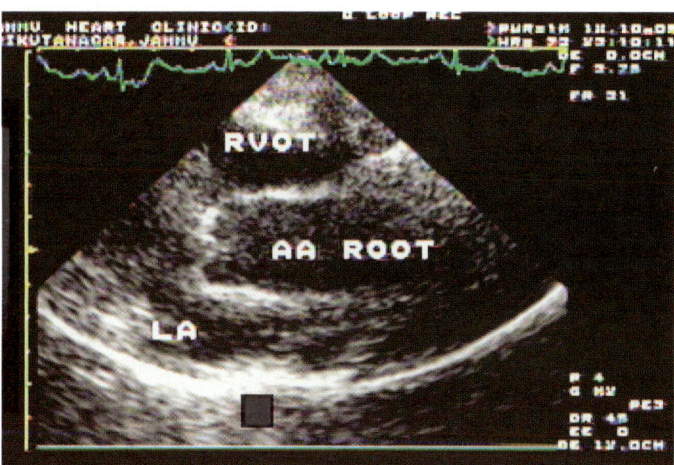

Fig. 2.82: Short axis view of root of aorta taken at high right parasternal area

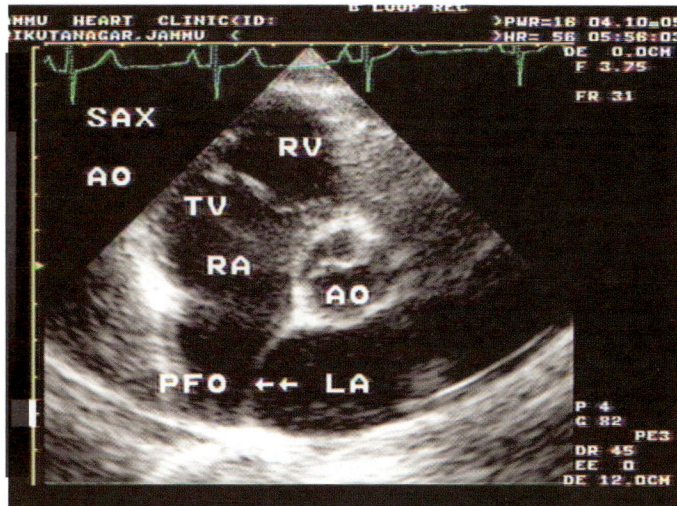

Fig. 2.83: Short axis view at aorta showing patent foramen ovale (PFO) besides other structures as shown on the scan

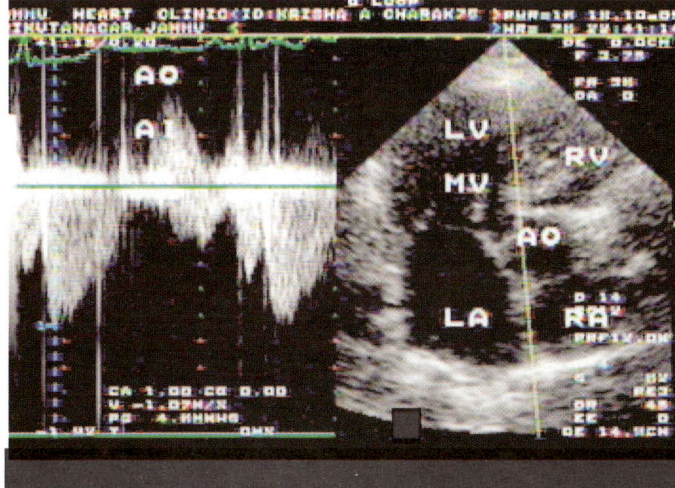

Fig. 2.84: Apical 5 C view of LV taken at low LPS region showing aortic valve velocity besides other structures as depicted on the scan

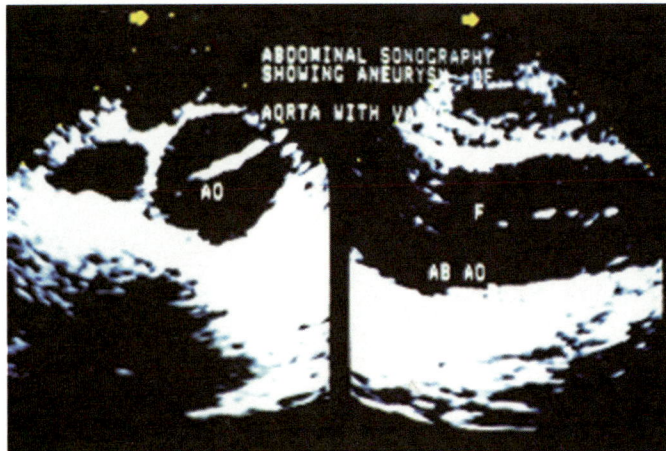

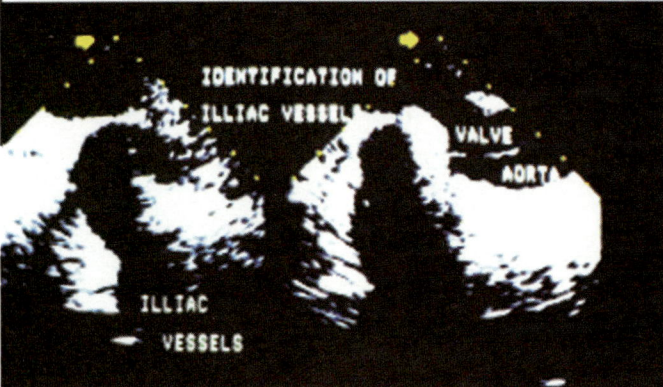

Fig. 2.85: Scan of abdominal aorta (upper) taken through subcostal window showing dilated aorta with valve and scan of illiac arteries showing variable fusiform dilatation and constriction (lower)

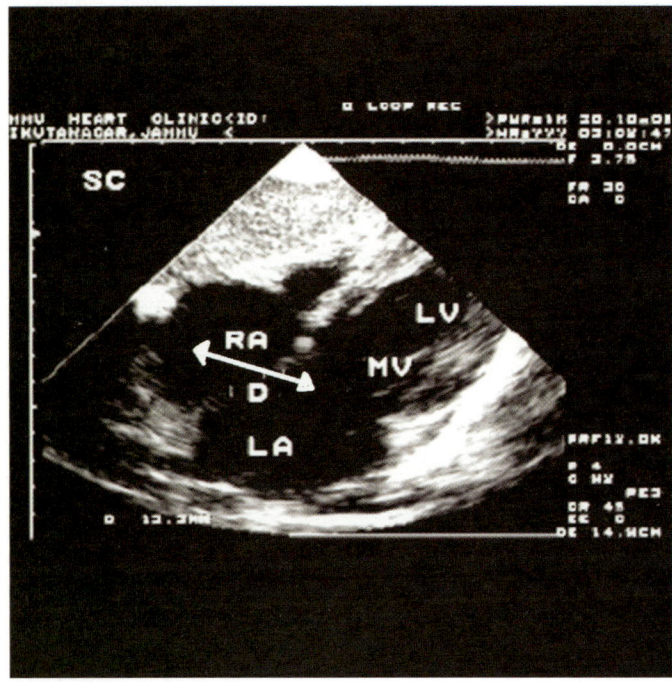

Fig. 2.86: Subcostal four chamber view taken at subxiphoid region showing small ASD(D)

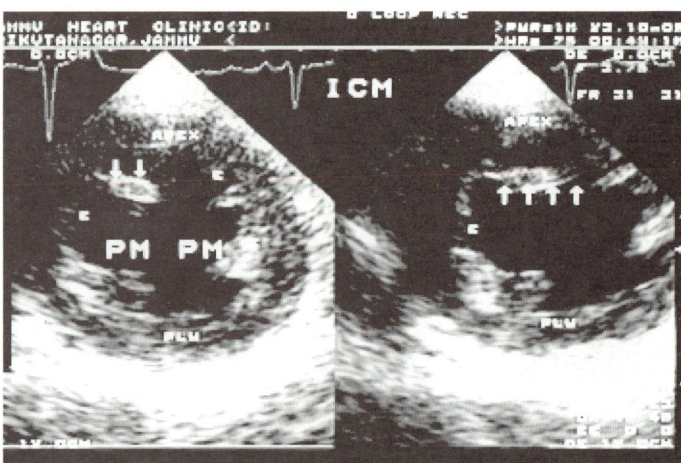

Fig. 2.87: Short axis dual scan taken at LPS apical region shows endocardium, papillary muscles and LV band (arrows)

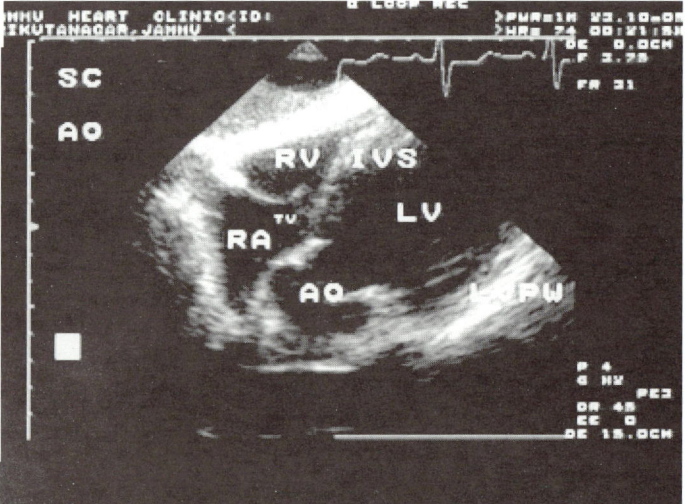

Fig. 2.88: Subcostal oblique view shows IAS TV/RA/AOV/V AND IAS RV

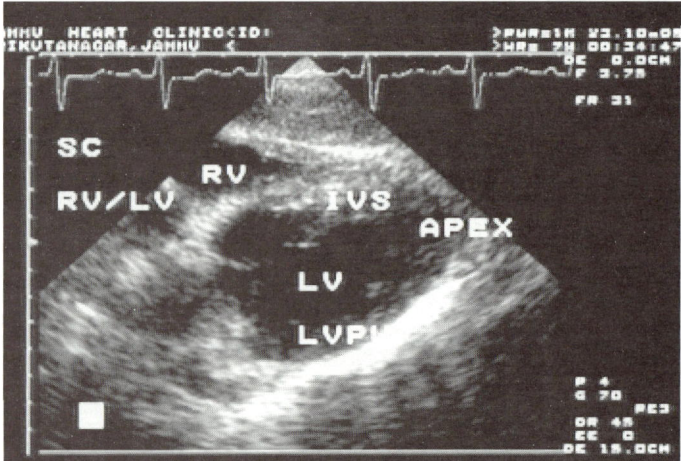

Fig. 2.89: Oblique SAX Subcostal view shows LV cavity for calculation of LV functions and its movements

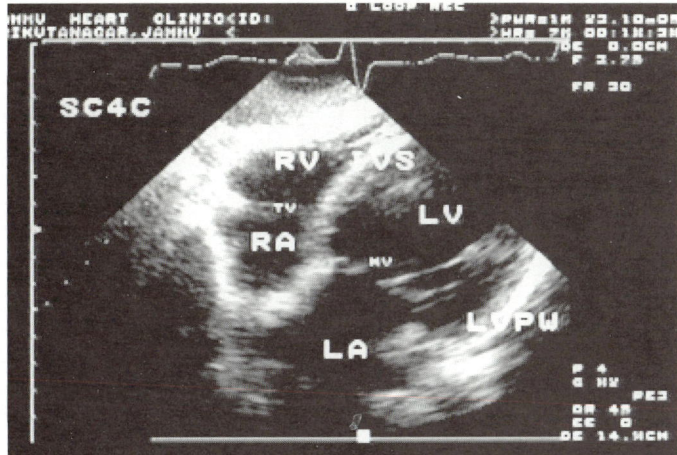

Fig. 2.90: Subcostal 4C view show all four chambers of heart along with AV valve

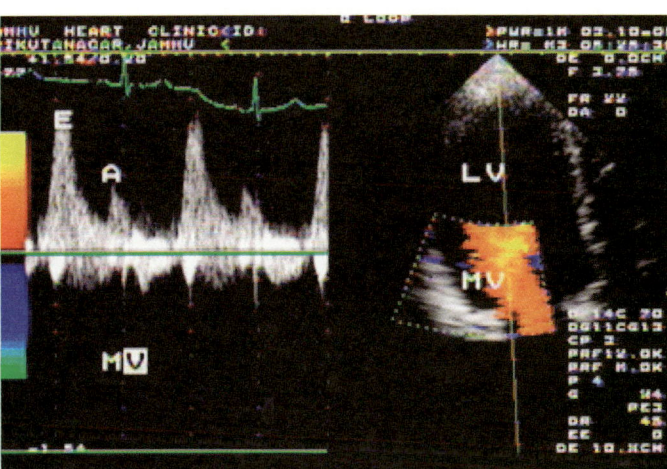

Fig. 2.93: Color Doppler flow velocity across MV at LPS apical 4C view

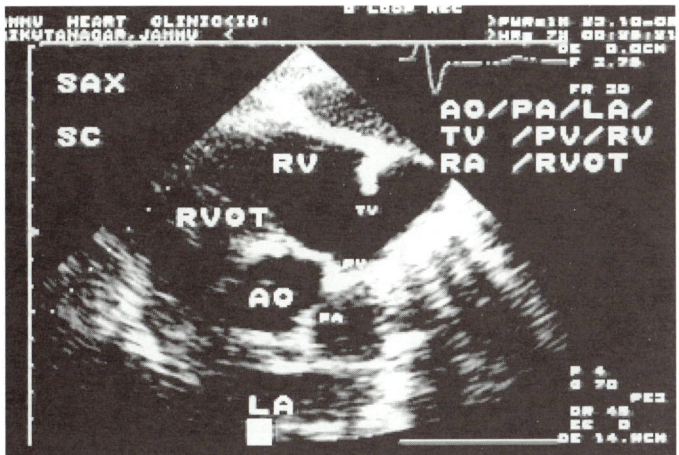

Fig. 2.91: Subcostal short axis view showing RV/TV/PV/RVOT/ RA/LA

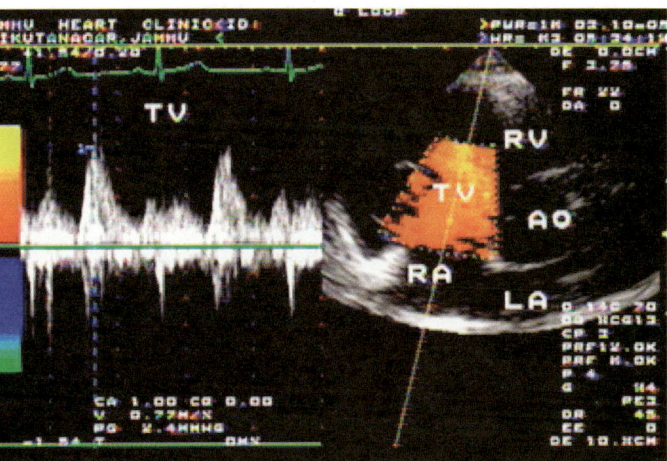

Fig. 2.94: Color Doppler flow velocity acrossTV taken at LPS short axis of aorta

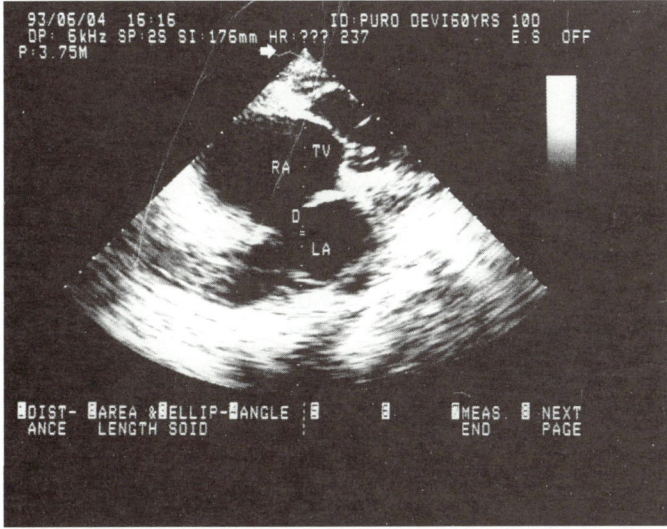

Fig. 2.92: Subcostal two chamber view show deficiency of mid IAS as seen in ASD (D)

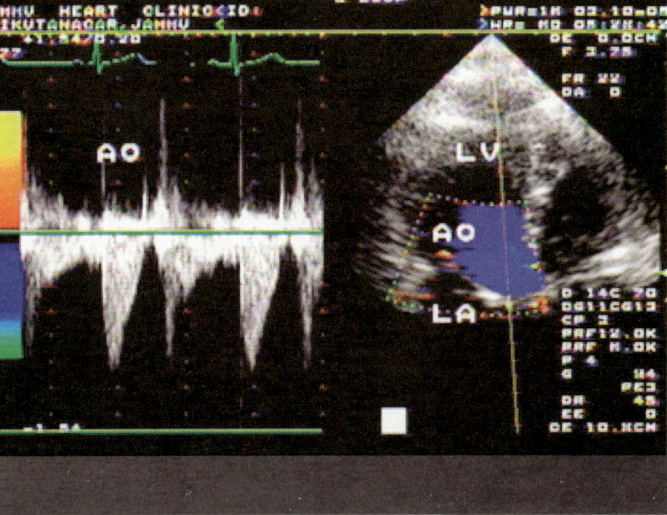

Fig. 2.95: Color Doppler flow velocity across aortic valve taken at apical 5C view

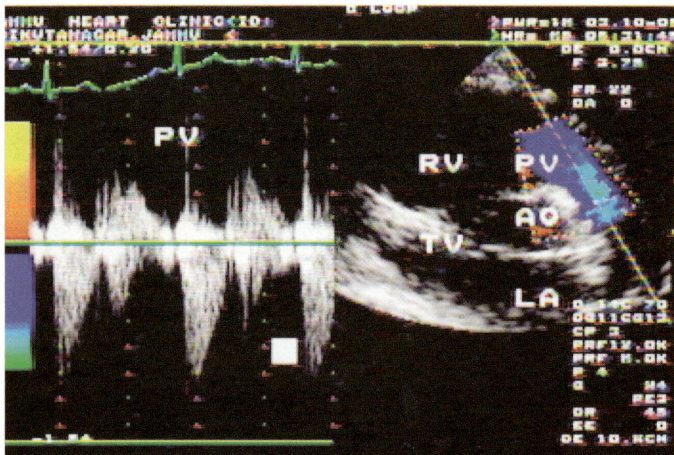

Fig. 2.96: Color Doppler flow velocity across pulmonary valve taken at short axis aorta

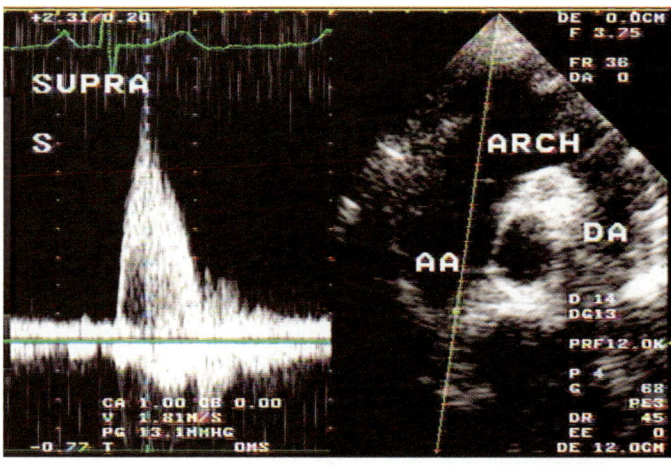

Fig. 2.99: Doppler flow velocity across ascending aorta showing laminar blood flow in normal individual (left) and visualising anatomic placement of ascending arch and descending aorta (right)

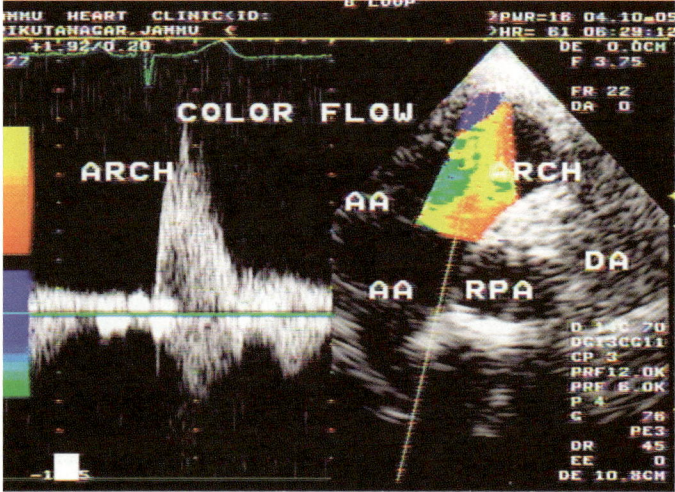

Fig. 2.97: Color Doppler flow velocity across ascending aorta at suprasternal notch window visualising ascending aorta, arch of aorta, descending aorta and right pulmonary artery in the centre

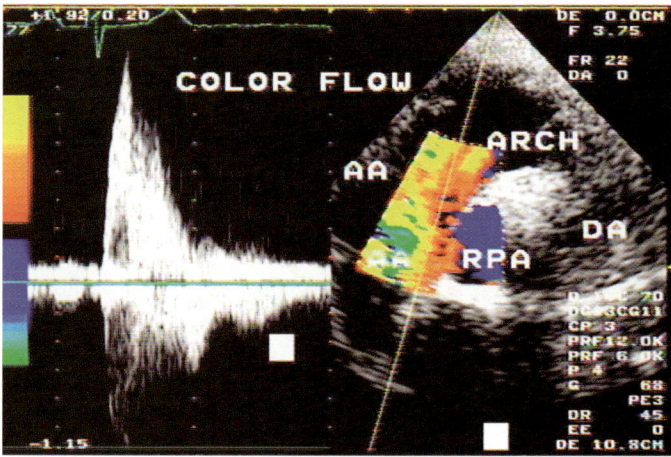

Fig. 2.100: Color Doppler flow velocity across ascending aorta (left) visualising ascending aorta (AA) in mosaic color and right pulmonary artery (RPA) in blue color (centre)

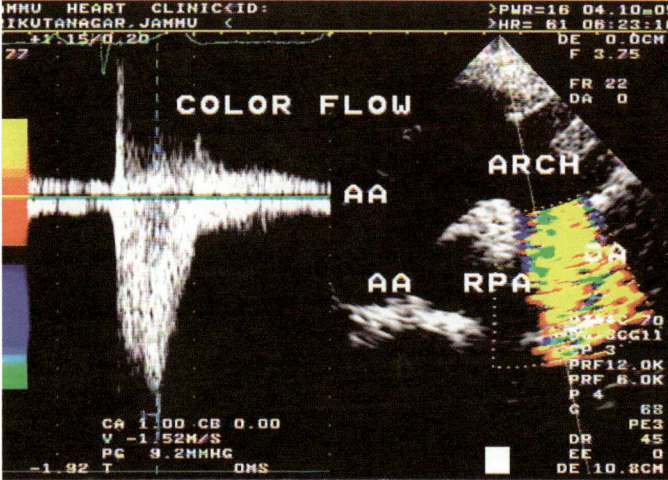

Fig. 2.98: Color Doppler flow velocity across descending aorta taken at suprasternal notch window

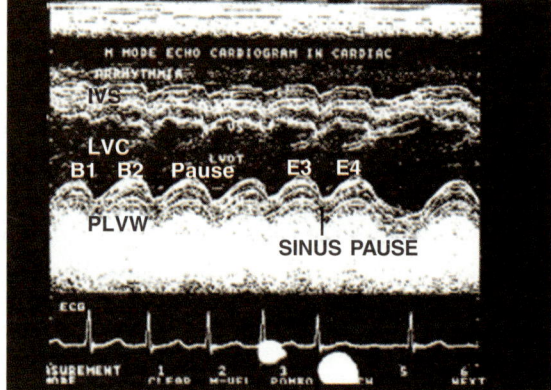

Fig. 2.101A: M-Mode echocardiograms showing IVS and PLVW contractions during both systole and diastole in atrial fibrillation with sinus pause . Note that after sinus pause the contraction of PLVW becomes more vigorous (B1, B2/ B3 and B4) and movements of IVS becomes almost flat as seen in figure

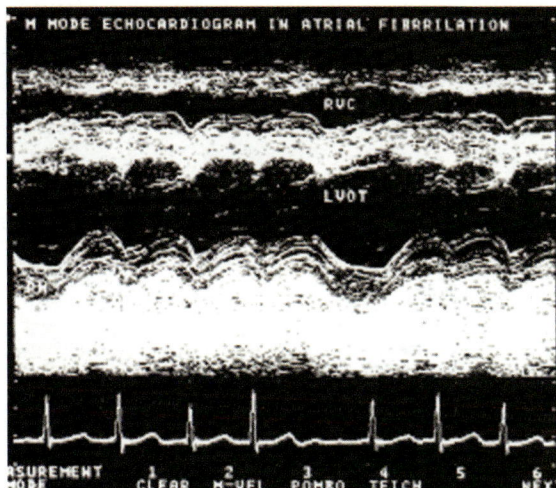

Fig. 2.101B: M-Mode echocardiograms showing IVS and PLVW contractions during both systole and diastole in atrial fibrillation with sinus pause. Note that after sinus pause the contraction of PLVW becomes more vigorous (B1,B2/ B3 and B4) and movements of IVS becomes almost flat as seen in figure

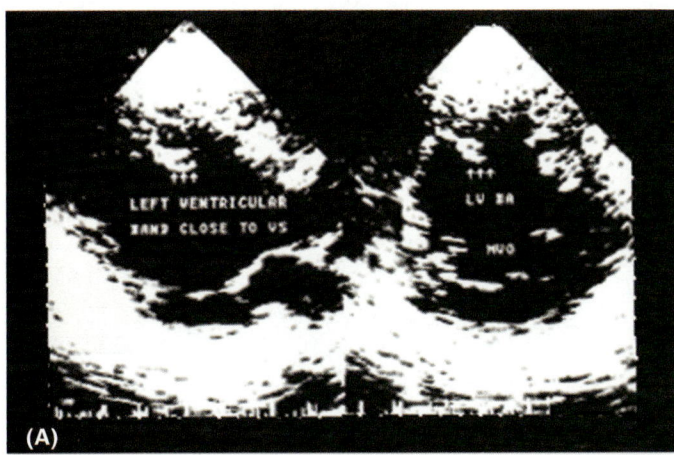

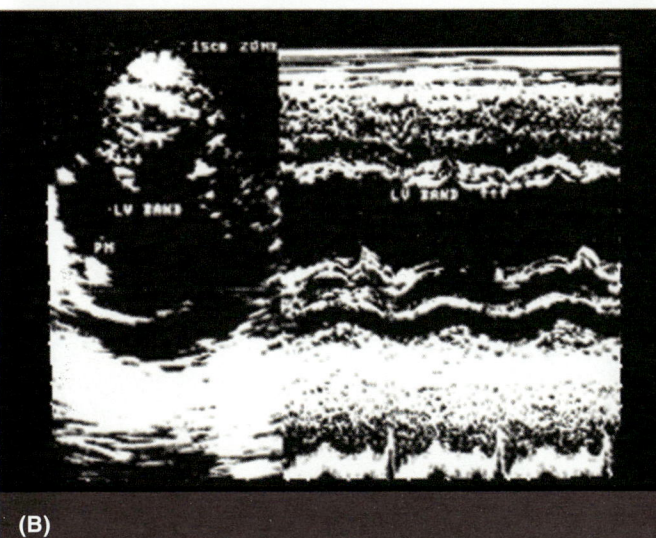

Fig. 2.102A and B: M-Mode and 2-D echocardiograms show left ventricular band as seen and marked in LVC

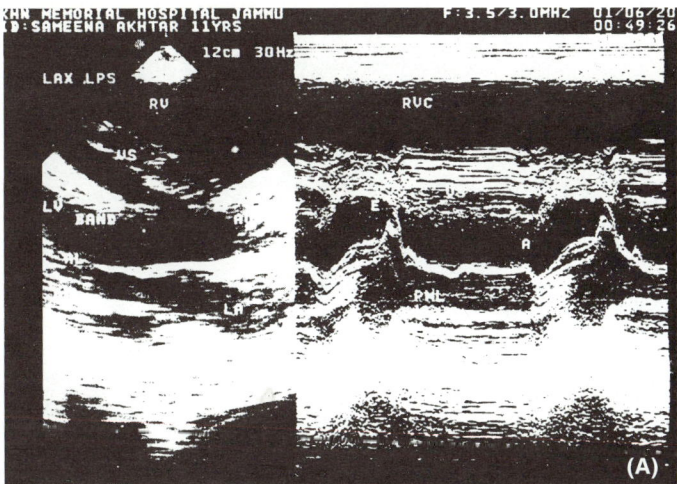

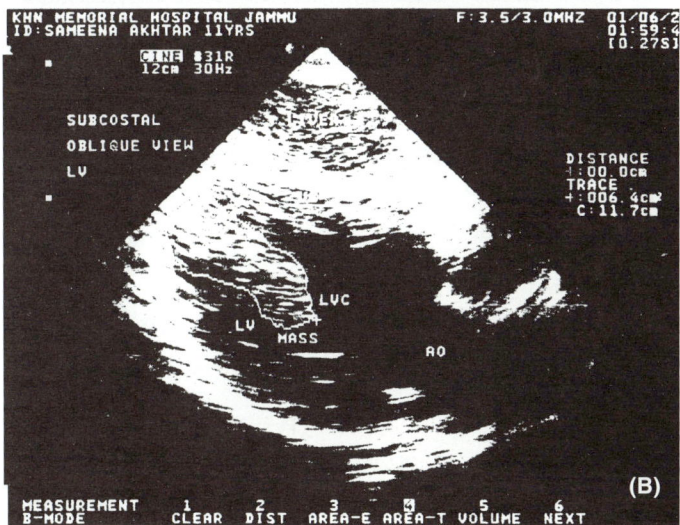

Fig. 2.103A and B: Hypertrophied LV band mimicking like a mass in 2-D long axis, M-mode (A) and oblique two chambers views through subcostal window

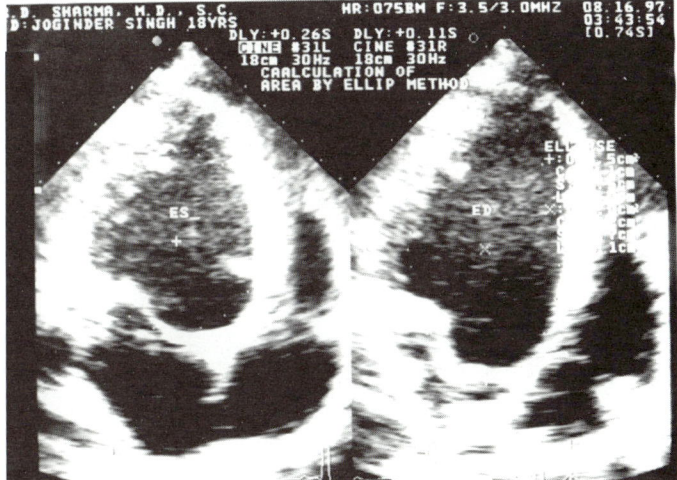

Fig. 2.104A: Apical 4C view during systole and diastole show spontaneous contrast as seen in a patient with dilated cardiomyopathy

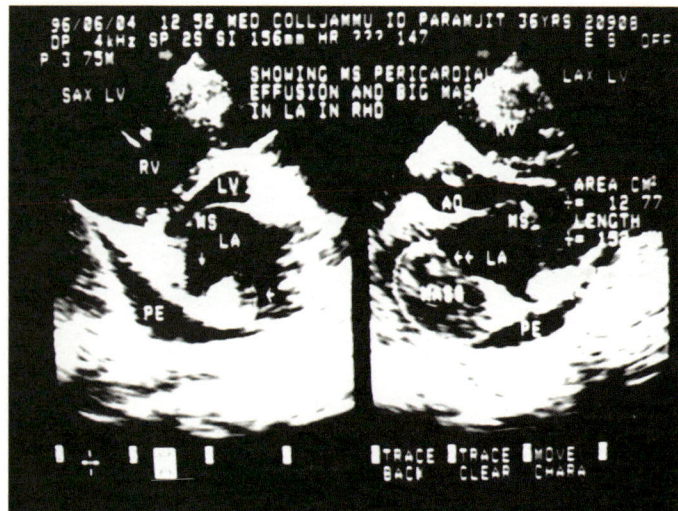

Fig. 2.104B: Dual scans in both long axis (right) and short axis (left) show a mass/clot with mild posteriorly located pericardial effusion (PE)

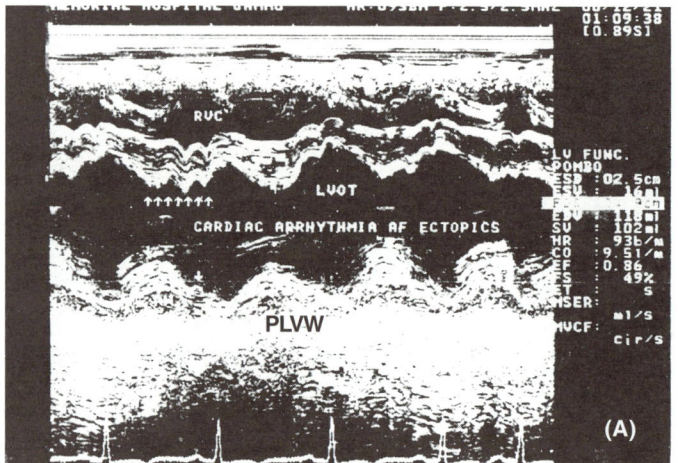

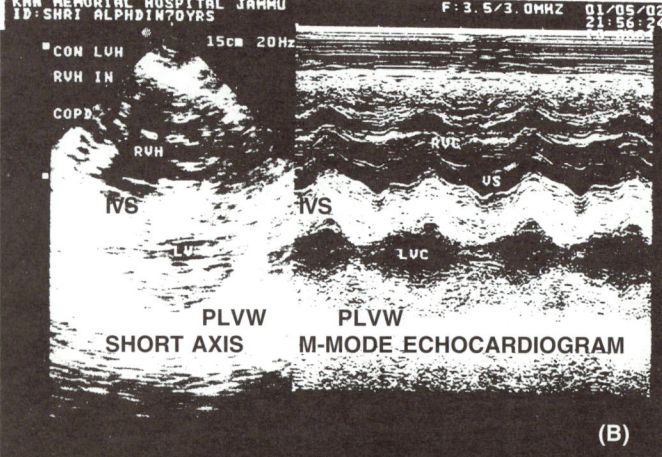

Fig. 2.105A and B: (A) M-Mode echoscan shows abnormal beaking of IVS in conduction defect in cardiac arrhythmia as shown on the scan. **(B)** 2-D and M-mode echoscans show RV moderator band in a patient with cor-pulmonale. It also reveals hypertrophy and dilatation of RV with compression of LV

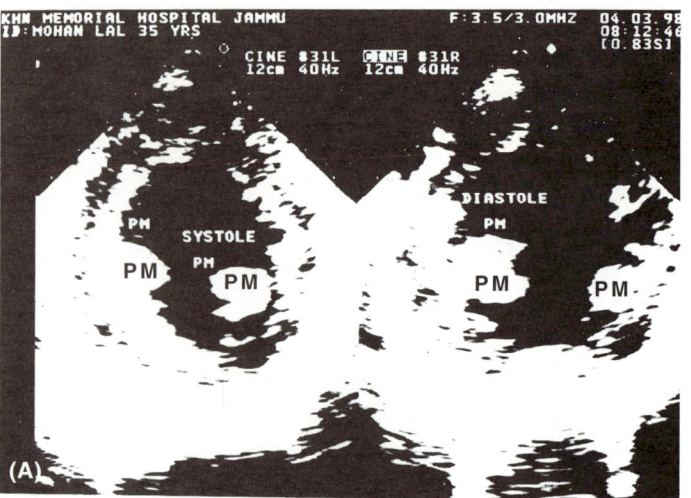

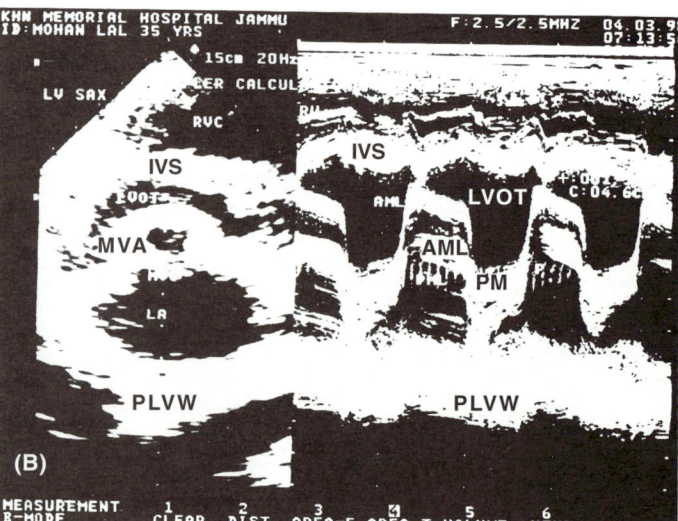

Fig. 2.106A and B: (A) Short axis 2-D echocardiogram showing both anterior and posterior papillary muscles to which respective chordi tendinae are attached. **(B)** M-mode and 2-D short axis echoscans showing mitral valve area (MVA) and thickening of both Anterior and posterior mitral leaflets (AML and PML) with paradoxical movemnt of PML as seen in mitral stenosis

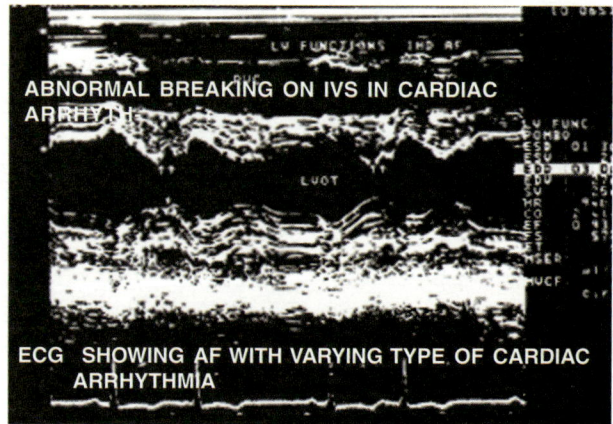

Fig. 2.107A: M-Mode echocardiogram showing abnormal thickening and beaking of IVS in varying grades of cardiac arrhythmia

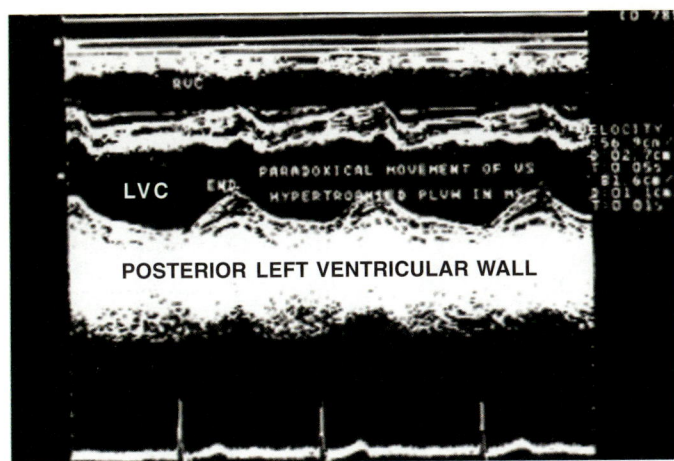

Fig. 2.107B: M-Mode echoscan shows paradoxical movements of IVS in relation to posterior LV wall movements in a patient with chronic obstructive lung disease

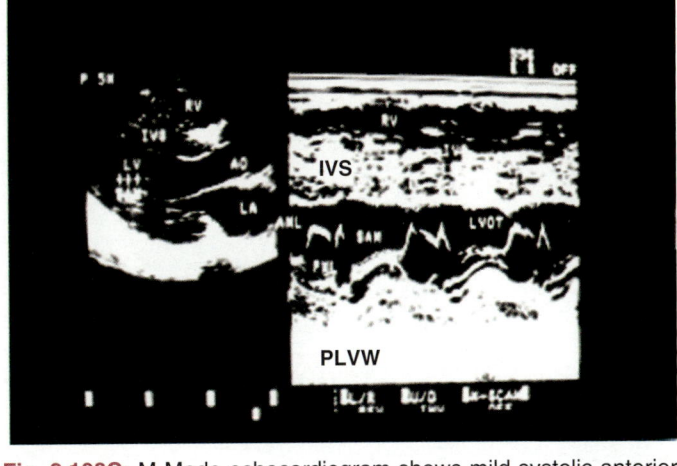

Fig. 2.108C: M-Mode echocardiogram shows mild systolic anterior motion of AML(SAM) of mitral valve in patient with hypertrophic cardiomyopathy

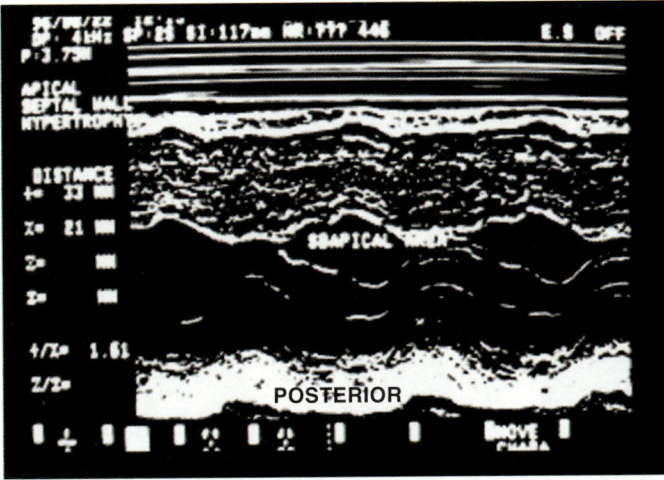

Fig. 2.108A: M-Mode echocardiogram showing marked hypertrophy of IVS as compared to PLVW in a patient with asymmetrical septal wall hypertrophy

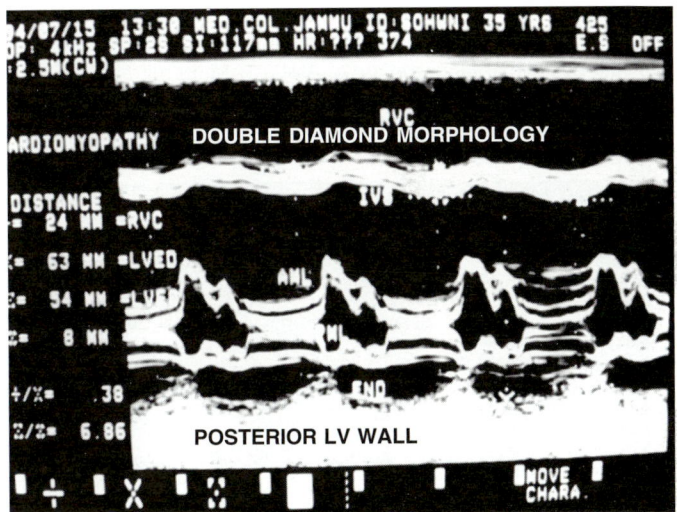

Fig. 2.109: Hypokinesia of IVS, dilated both RV and LV with thinning of IVS/PLVW. There is also increased distance of E point of AML to systolic thickening of (S) IVS as also called EPSS point distance due to poor contraction of LV. This scan also shows altered morphology of MV called double diamond appearance as shown in the scan which is frequently found in typical dilated cardiomyopathy

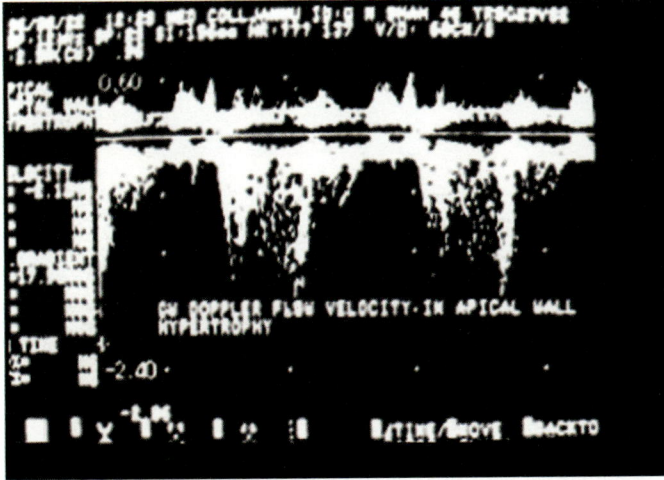

Fig. 2.108B: Doppler velocity at LVOT shows enhanced flow velocity in dynamic obstruction as seen in hypertrophic cardiomyopathy

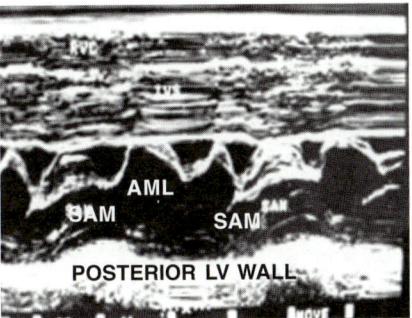

Fig. 2.110: M-Mode echocardiogram shows marked hypertrophy of IVS with systolic anterior motion of AML (SAM) of mitral valve seen in hypertrophic cardiomyopathy

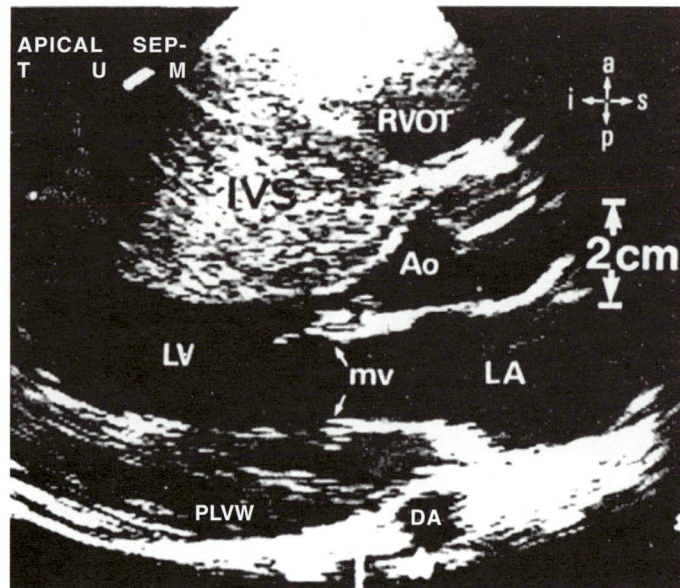

Fig. 2.111: M-Mode echocardiogram shows marked hypertrophy of IVS with systolic anterior motion of AML (SAM) of mitral valve seen in hypertrophic cardiomyopathy

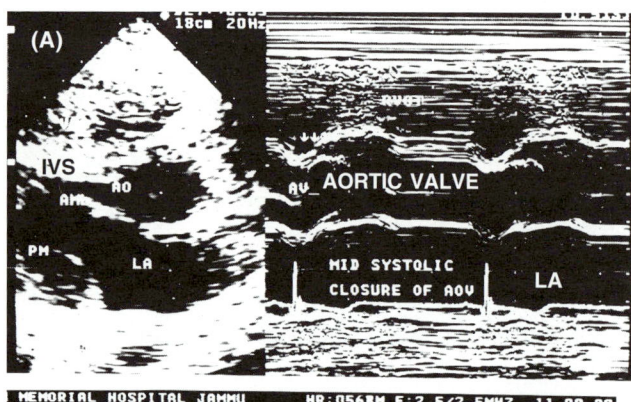

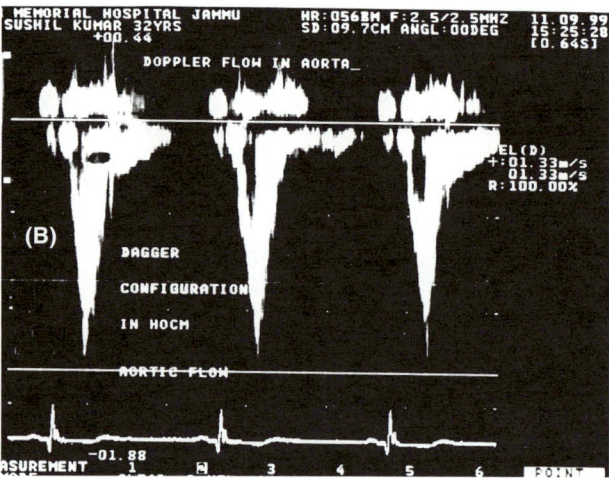

Fig. 2.112A and B: (A) 2-D and M-mode echoscans of aortic valve showing mid-systolic closure of mitral valve in hypertrophic cardiomyopathy as depicted on M-mode scan. **(B)** Doppler velocity taken at LVOT shows tappering of peak velocity waveform also called as dagger drawn appearance as seen in hypertrophic cardiomyopathy

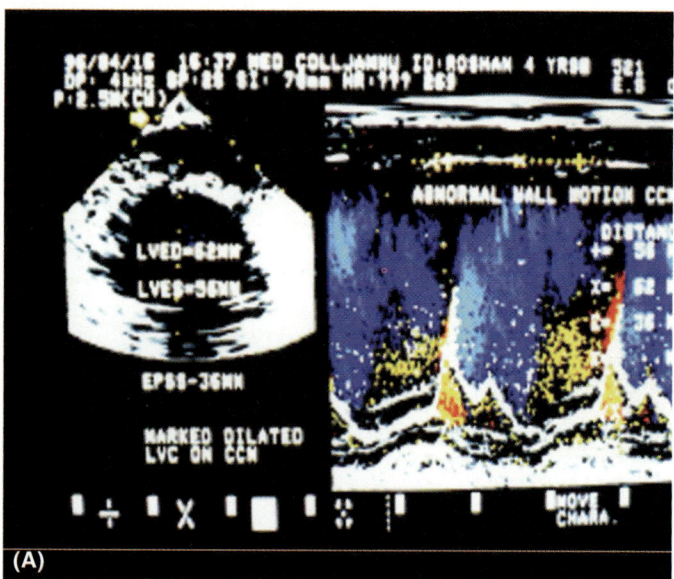

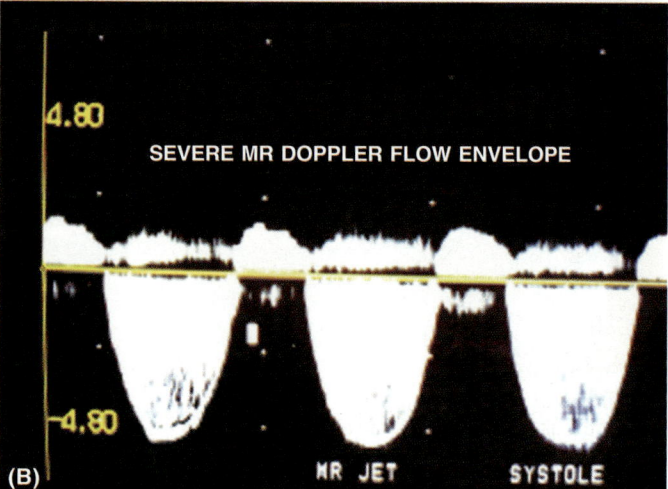

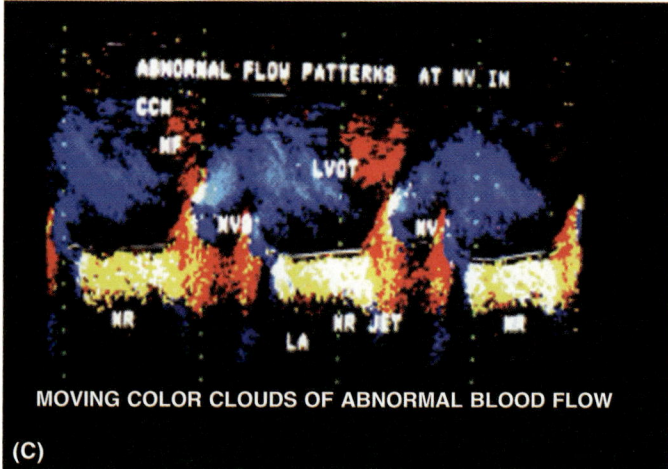

Fig. 2.113A to C: (A) 2-D and M-mode echocardiogram shows abnomal color flows through MV in dilated cardiomyopathy. **(B)** Doppler flow velocity showing typical envelope of severe MR in a patient with congestive cardiomyopathy. **(C)** Color M-mode echoscan in LV cavity showing moving cloud appearance of abnormal blood flows in dilated cardiomyopathy

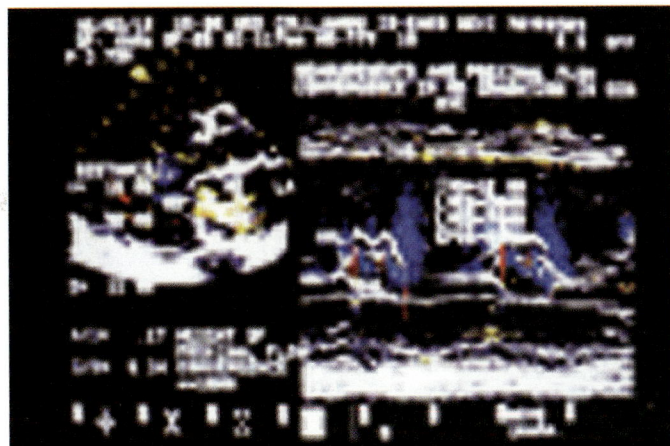

Fig. 2.114: Color M-mode and 2-D echo scans showing method of calculating LVEF and cardiac volumes

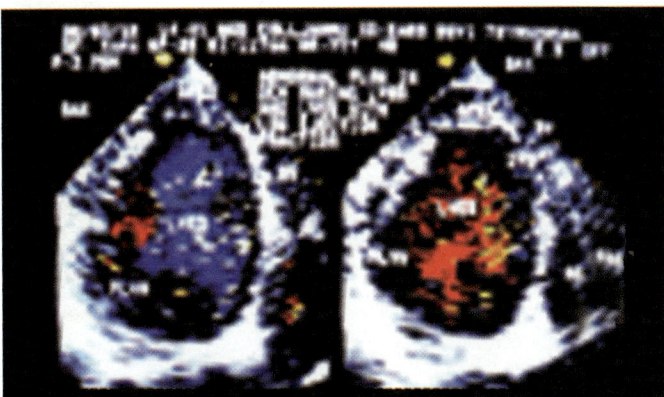

Fig. 2.115: 2-D Color flow dual scan taken at left parasternal region in short axis view showing mixture of red and blue color in both during systole and diastole as usually seen in dilated cardiomyopathy. There is hardly any difference in cardiac size during both phases of cardiac cycle as found in severe contractile dysfunctions of heart as in dilated cardiomyopathy

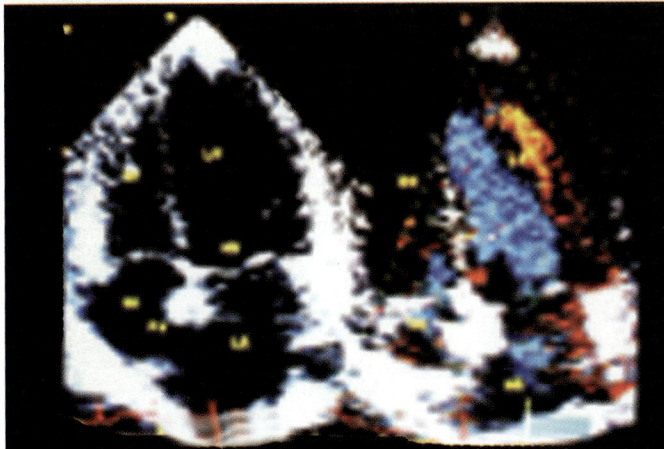

Fig. 2.116: Color dual 2-D scans showing dilated all four chambers of the heart (left) and abnormal mixture of blue and red color in LV cavity (right) as it happens in severely decreased contractile power of LV

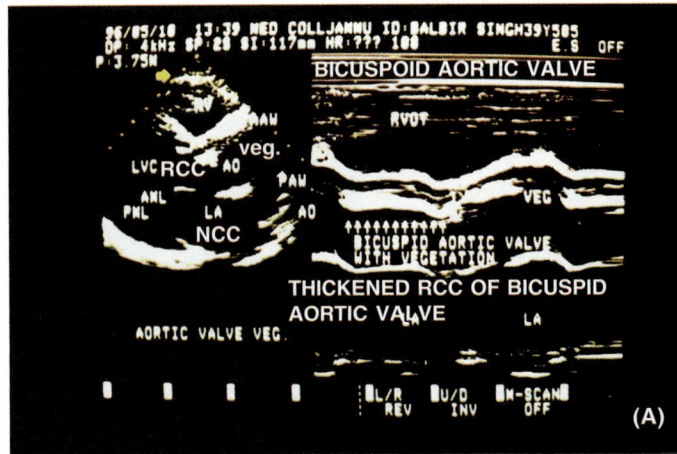

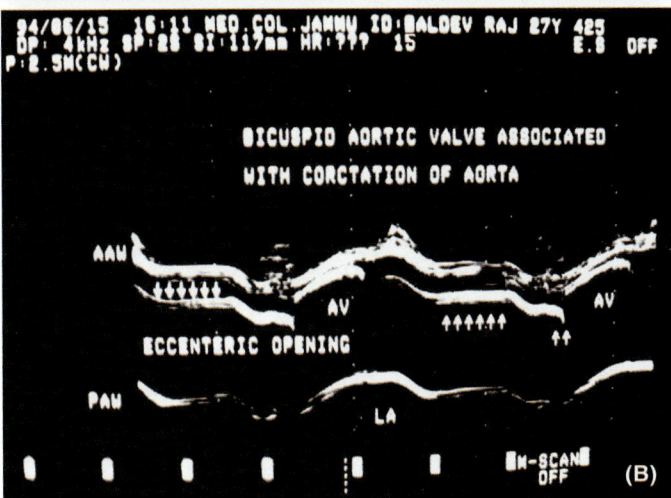

Fig. 2.117A and B: **(A)** M-Mode echoscan showing eccenteric opening of aortic valve with markedly thickened right coronary cusp (RCC) with vegetation as shown on scan in bicuspid aortic valve abnormality. **(B)** M-Mode echocardiogram showing eccenteric opening of native aortic valve with thickening of RCC in patient with bicuspid aortic valve associated with coarctation of aorta

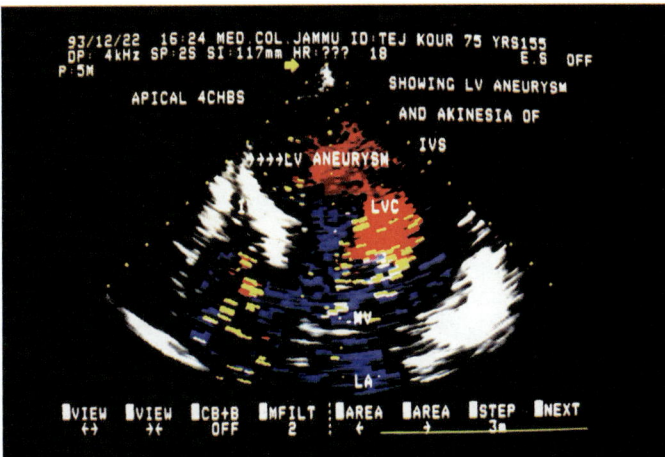

Fig. 2.118A: Apical 4C view of LV showing marked hypokinesia of IVS very low LVEF with abnormal color flows and LV aneurysm in a patient with CAD IHD and effort dyspnoea

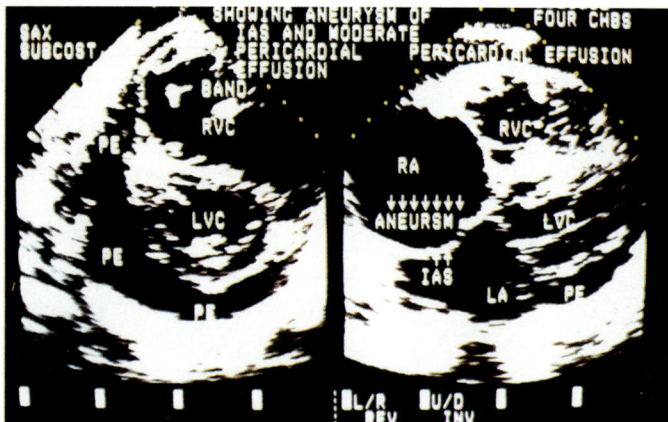

Fig. 2.118B: Subcostal dual scan approach in short axis and four chamber views shows distended interatrial septum giving the appearance of aneurysm in patient with moderate pericardial effusion (PE) with raised RA pressure as marked on the scan

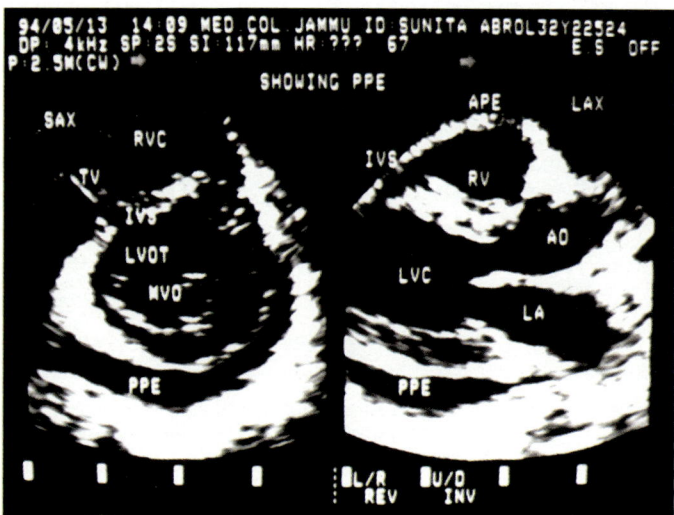

Fig. 2.119: Short axis and long axis left parasternal approach of LV showing mild pericardial effusion localised to posterior sac (PPE) only

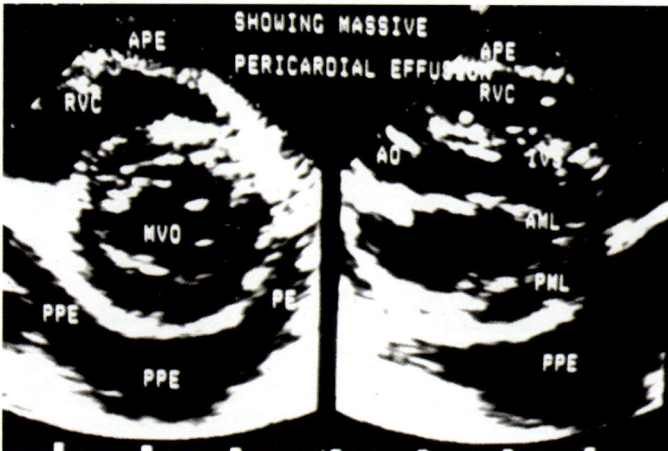

Fig. 2.120: Short axis and long axis left parasternal approach of LV showing moderate pericardial effusion localised to both anterior (APE) and posterior (PPE) sacs

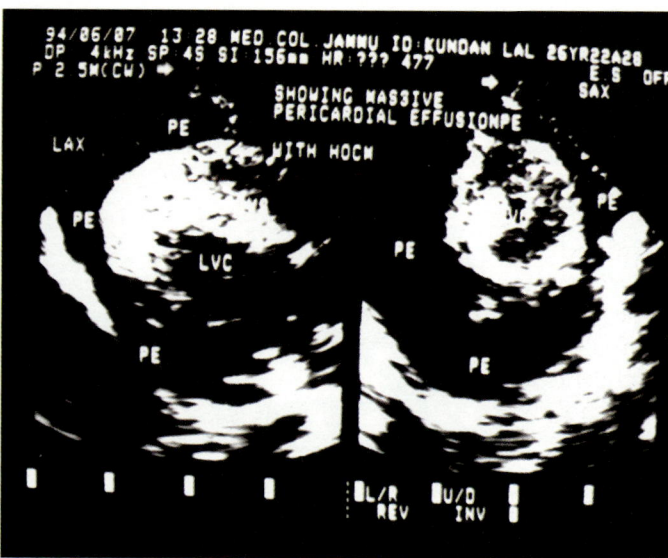

Fig. 2.121: Short axis and long axis left parasternal approach of LV showing moderately severe pericardial effusion localised to both anterior (APE) and posterior (PPE) sacs

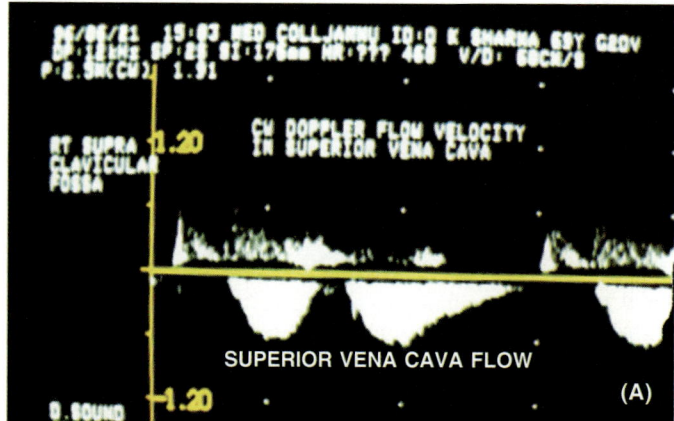

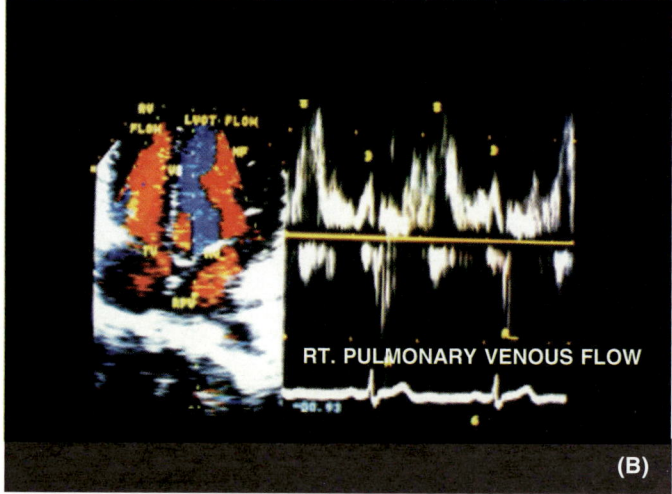

Fig. 2.122A and B: (A) Supraclavicular approach showing normal Doppler waveforms. **(B)** Color flow in apical 4C view (left) showing normal flows in MV, TV and LVOT and Doppler flow velocity across right pulmonary vein (right)

other imaging modalities in a wide variety of health care environments. Generally, a standard echocardiogram is requested whenever the physical examination is inconclusive or doubtful, or for evaluation of the severity of a known disease. However, echocardiography is becoming more and more complex and the significant equipment costs, standardised examinations, and required specialised personnel make standard echocardiography time consuming and expensive. The same factors limit access to echocardiography and create delays in getting important results to the bedside. Furthermore, it is generally assumed that to perform any echocardiographic examination an examiner must be completely trained, certified, and experienced.

Recent advances in ultrasound technology have led to the development of fully portable ultrasound machines, which can provide immediate assessment of heart morphology and physiology at the time of the first examination of the patient. Now we can add sonography to the examination encounter. These personal imagers are appropriately named "ultrasonic stethoscopes" since they allow us to look into the chest and see the heart and its pathology during the physical examination. Visualising the heart with the ultrasound stethoscope as part of the physical examination provides additional information beyond what we can perceive with palpation and auscultation, and allows us to confirm rapidly a cardiac abnormality and often to make a specific diagnosis in any clinical setting (Fig. 2.56 A and B).

Bibliography

1. Ahmadpour H, Shah AA, Allen JW, Edmiston WA, Kim SJ, Haywood LJ: Mitral E Point septal separation: A reliable index of left ventricular performance in coronary artery disease. *Am Heart J*, 1983; 106:21.
2. Albin G, Rahko PS: Comparison of echo-cardiographic quantitation of left ventricular ejection fraction to radionuclide angiography in patients with regional wall motion abnormalities. *Am J Cardiol*, 1991; 67:901.
3. Allen HD, Goldberg SJ, Shan DJ, Ovitt TW, Goldberg BB: Suprasternal notch. Echocardiography: Assessment of its clinical utility in pediatric cardiology. *Circulation*, 1977; 55:605.
4. Appleton CP, Hatle LK, Popp RL: Superior vena cava and hepatic vein Doppler echocardiography in healthy adults. *J Am Coll Cardiol*, 1987; 10:1032.
5. Bahler, RC, Trobel, TR, and Martin, P: The relation of heart rate and shortening fraction of echocardiographic indexes of left ventricular relaxation in normal subjects. *J Am Coll Cardiol*, 1984; 2:926.
6. Baker BJ, Scovil JA, Kane JJ, Murphy ML: Echocardiographic detection of right ventricular hypertrophy. *Am Heart J*, 1983; 105:611.
7. Bartzokis T, Lee R, Yeoh TK, Grogin H, Schnitthger I: Transesophageal echo-Doppler echocardiographic assessment of pulmonary venous flow patterns. *J Am Soc Echocardiogr*, 1991; 4:457.
8. Basnight MA, Gonzalez MS, Kershenovich, SC, Appleton CP: Pulmonary venous flow velocity: Relation to hemodynamics, mitral flow velocity and left atrial volume, and ejection fraction. *J Am Soc Echocardiogr*, 1991; 4:547.
9. Baumgartner H, Schima H, Kuhn P: Importance of technical variables for quantitative measurements by colour Doppler imaging. *Am J Cardiol*, 1990; 65:1026.
10. Benzing G, Stockert J, Nave E, Kaplan S: Evaluation of left ventricular performance: Circumferential fiber shortening rate in man. *Circulation* 1974; 49:925.
11. Berning J, Rokkedal-Nielsen J, Launbjerg J, Fogh J, Mickely H, Andersen PE: Rapid estimation of left ventricular ejection fraction in acute myocardial infarction by echocardiographic wall motion analysis. *Cardiology*, 1992; 80: 257.
12. Bhatt DR, Isabal-Jones JB, Villoria GJ, Nakazawa M, Yabek SM, Marks RA, Jarmakani JM: Accuracy of echocardiography in assessing left ventricular dimensions and volume. *Circulation*, 1978; 57:699.
13. Bierman FZ, Williams RG: Subxiphoid two-dimensional imaging of the interatrial septum in infants and neonates with congenital heart disease. *Circulation*, 1979; 60:80.
14. Bommer W, Weinert L, Neumann A, Neef J, Mason DT, DeMaria A: Determination of right atrial and right ventricular size by two-dimensional echocardiography. *Circulation*, 1979; 60:91.
15. Bommer W, Weinert L, Neumann A, Neef J, Mason DT, DeMaria A: Determination of right ventricular size by two-dimensional echocardiography. *Circulation*, 1979; 60:91.
16. Bruce CJ, Spittell PC, Montgoery SC, *et al*. Personal ultra sound imager: abdominal aortic aneurysm screening. *Echocardiogr* 2000; 13:674–9.
17. Buda AJ, Delop EJ, Meyer CR, Jenkins JM, Smith DN, Bookstein FL, Pitt B: Automatic computer processing of digital two-dimensional echocardiograms. *Am J Cardiol*, 1983; 52:384.
18. Cacho A, Prakash R, Sarma R, Kaushik S: Usefulness of two-dimensional echocardiography in diagnosing right ventricular hypertrophy. *Chest*, 1983; 84:154.
19. Engle SJ, Disessa TG, Perloff JK, Isabel Jones, J, Leighton J, Gross K, Friedman WF: Mitral valve E point to ventricular septal separation in infants and children. *Am J Cardiol*, 1983; 52:1084.
20. Feigenbaum H *et al*: Ultrasound measurements of the left ventricle. A correlative study with angiocardiography. *Arch Intern Med.*, 1972 129:461.
21. Feigenbaum H: Digital recording , display, and storage of echocardiograms, *J Am Soc Echocardiogr*, 1988; 1:378.
22. Felner JM, Blumenstein BA, Schlant RC, Carter AD, Alimurung BN, Johnson MJ, Sherman SW, Klicpera MW, Kutnerr MH, and Drucker LW: Sources of variability in echocardiographic measurements. *Am J Cardiol*, 1980; 45:995.
23. Feneley MP, Hickie JB: Validity of echocardiographic determination of left ventricular systolic wall thickening, *Circulation* 1984; 70:226.
24. Fneley M, Cavaghan T: Paradoxical and pseudoparadoxical interventricular septal motion in patients with right ventricular volume overload. *Circulation* 1986; 74:230.
25. Foale R, Nihoyannopoulos P, McKenna W, Klienebenne A, Nadazin A, Rowland E, Smith G: Echocardiographic measurement of the normal adult right ventricle. *Br. Heart J*, 1986; 56:33.

26. Fowles RE, Martin RP, Popp RL: Apparent asymmetric septal hypertrophy due to angled interventricular septum. *Am J Cardiol,* 1980; 46:386.

27. Germain P, Roul G, Kastler B, Mossard JM, Bareiss P, Sacrez A: Inter-study variability in left ventricular mass measurement. Comparison between M-mode echography and MRI. *Eur Heart J,* 1992;13:1011.

28. Gibson DG: Measurement of left ventricular volumes by echocardiography—comparison with biplane angiography. *Br Heart J,* 1971;33:614.

29. Goldberg BB: suprasternal ultrasonography, *JAMA,* 1971; 215:245.

30. Haendchen RV, Povzhitkov M, Meerbaum S, Maurer G, Corday E: Evaluation of changes in left ventricular end-diastolic pressure by left atrial two-dimensional echocardiography. *Am Heart J,* 1982;104:740.

31. Hammarstrom E, Wranne B, Pinto FJ, Puryear J, Popp RL: Tricuspid annular motion. *J Am Soc Echocardiogr.* 1991; 4:131.

32. Hatle L, Angelsen B: *Doppler Ultrasound in Cardiology: Physical Principles and Clinical Application.* 2nd Ed. Philadelphia, Lea & Febiger, 1985.

33. Henry WL, *et al.* Report of the American Society of Echocardiography Committee on Nomenclature and Standards in Two-dimensional Echocardiography. *Circulation,* 1980; 62:212.

34. Hiraishi S, DiSessa TG, Jarmakani JM, Nakanishi T, Isabel-Jones J, Friedman WF: Two-dimensional echocardiographic assessment of left atrial size in children. *Am J Cardiol,* 1983; 52:1249.

35. Hirata T, Wolfe SB, Popp RL, Helmen CH, Feigenbaum H: Estimation of left atrial size using ultrasound. *Am Heart J,* 1969; 78:43.

36. Hofstetter R, Bartz-Bazzanella P, Kentrup H, and Von Bernuth, G: Determination of left atrial area and volume by cross-sectional echocardiography in healthy infants and children. *Am J Cardiol,* 1991; 68:1073.

37. Iwase M, Hurui H, Miyaguchi K, Hayashi H, Yokota M, Takeuchi J, Ishiguro T, Sakuma S: Two-dimensional echocardiography and magnetic resonance imaging in diagnosis of idiopathic dilation of the right atrium. *Am Heart J,* 1990; 120:1231.

38. Jaffe WM, Dewhrust TA, Otto CM, Pearlman AS: Influence of Doppler sample volume location on ventricular filling velocities. *Am J Cardiol,* 1991; 68:550.

39. Kan G, Visser CA, Lie KI, Durrer D: Left ventricular volumes and ejection fraction by single plane two-dimensional apex echocardiography. *Eur Heart J,* 1981; 2:339.

40. King ME, Braun H, Goldblatt A, Liberthson R, and Weyman AE: Interventricular septal configuration as a predictor of right ventricular systolic hypertension in children: A cross-sectional echocardiographic study. *Circulation,* 1983; 68:68.

41. Klein AL, Stewart WC, Cosgrove DM, Salcedo EE: Intraoperative epicardial echocardiography: Technique and imaging planes. *Echocardiography,* 1990; 7:241.

42. Klein AL, Tajik AJ: Doppler assessment of pulmonary venous flow in healthy subjects and in patients with heart disease. *J Am Soc Echocardiogr,* 1991; 4:379.

43. Kronzon I, Mehta SS: Giant left atrium. *Chest,* 1974, 65:677.

44. LaBarre TR, Stamto NJ, Hwang MH, Jacobs WR, Stephanides L, Scanlon PJ: Left atrial apendage aneurysm with associated anomalous pulmonary venous drainage. *Am Heart J,* 1987; 114:1243.

45. Lambertz H, Braun C, Krebs W: Determination of the size of the right atrium using two-dimensional echocardiography, *Z. Kardiol* 1984; 73:393.

46. Lange LW, Sahn DJ, Allen HD, Goldberg SJ: Subxiphoid cross-sectional echocardiography in infants and children with congenital heart disease. *Circulation,* 1979; 59:513.

47. Lehmann KG, Lee FA, McKenzie WB, Barash PG, Prokop EK, Durkin MA, Ezekowitz MD: Onset of altered interventricular septal motion during cardiac surgery. *Circulation,* 1990; 82:1325.

48. Levine RA, Gibson TC, Aretz T, Gillam LD, Guyer DE, King ME, Weyman AE: Echocardiographic measurement of right ventricular volume. *Circulation,* 1984; 69:497.

49. Lin S L, Tak T, Kawanishi DT, Rahimtoola SH, Chandaratna PAN: Accuracy of Doppler ultrasound in evaluating changes of left ventricular diastolic properties. *Echocardiography,* 1990; 7:515.

50. Massie BM, Schiller NB, Ratshin RA, Parmley WW: Mitralseptal separation: New echocardiographic index of left ventricular function. *Am J Cardiol,* 1977; 39:1008.

51. Masuyama T, Lee JM, Tamai M, Tanouchi J, Kitabatake A, Kamada T: Pulmonary venous flow velocity pattern as assessed with trans-thoracic pulsed Doppler echocardiography in subjects without cardiac disease. *Am J Cardiol,* 1991; 67:1396.

52. Meyer RA, Schwartz DC, Benzing G, Kaplan S; Ventricular septum in right ventricular volume overload: An echocardiographic study. *Am J Cardiol,* 1972; 30:349.

53. Miki S, Murakami T, Iwase T, Tomita T, Suzuki Y, Kawai C: Dependence of Doppler echocardiographic transmitral early peak velocity on left ventricular systolic function in coronary artery disease. *Am J Cardiol,* 1991; 67:470.

54. Mueller TN, Kerber RE, Marcus ML: Comparison of interventricular septal motion studied by ventriculography and echocardiography in patients with atrial septal defect. *Br. Heart J,* 1978; 40:984.

55. Mueller X, Stauffer JC, Jaussi A, Goy JJ, Kappenberger L: Subjective visual echocardiographic estimate of left ventricular ejection fraction as an alternative of conventional echocardiographic methods: Comparison with contrast angiography. *Clin Cardiol,* 1991; 14:898.

56. Myreng Y, Smiseth OA, Risoe C: Left ventricular filling at elevated diastolic pressures: Relationship between transmitral Doppler flow velocities and atrial contribution. *Am Heart J,* 1990; 119:620.

57. Okamoto M, Beppu S, Nagata S, Park YD, Masuda Y, Sakakibara H, Nimura Y Echocardiographic features of the eustachian valve and its clinical significance (author's translation). *J Cardiogr,* 1981; 11:271.

58. Okamoto M, Nagata S, Park YD, sure of contractility. *Am J Cardiol,* 1992; 69:403.

59. Pai RG, Bodenheimer MM, Pai SM, Koss JH, Adamick RD: Usefulness of systolic excursion of the mitral annulus as an index of left ventricular systolic function. *Am J Cardiol,* 1991; 67:222.

60. Pandian NG Ultrasound stethoscopy: adding another sense art and scien physical examination. *Thoraxcentre J* 2001; 4:91–2.

61. Petrovic O, Feigenbaum H, Armstrong WF, Ryan T, West SR, Green-Hess D, Stewart J, Mattson JL, Fineberg NS: Digital averaging to facilitate two-dimensional echocardiographic measurements. *JCU*, 1986; 14:367.

62. Pinheiro L, Nanda NC , Jain H, Sanyal R: Transesophageal echocardiographic imaging of the pulmonary veins. *Echocardiography*, 1991; 8:741.

63. Pinto FJ, Wranne B, St. Goar FG, Schinttger I, Popp RL: Hepatic venous flow assessed by transesophageal echocardiography. *J Am Coll Cardiol*, 1991; 17:1493.

64. Pombo JF, Troy BL, Russel RO, Jr: Left Ventricular volumes and ejection fraction by echocardiography. Circulation, 1971; 43: 480.

65. Popp RL and Harrison DC: Ultrasonic cardiac echography for determining stroke volume and valvular regurgitation. *Circulation*, 1970; 41:493.

66. Report of the American Society of Echocardiography Committee on Nomenclature and Standards: Identification of Myocardial Wall Segments. November, 1982.

67. Reynolds T, Appleton CP: Doppler flow velocity patterns of the superior vena cava, inferior vena cava, hepatic vein, coronary sinus, and atrial septal defect: A guide for the echocardiographer. *J Am Coll Cardiol*, 1991; 17:1493.

68. Reynolds T, Szymanski K, Langenfled K, Appleton CP: Visualization of the hepatic veins: New approaches for the echocardiographer. *J Am Soc Echocardiogr* 1991; 4:93.

69. Sahn DJ, DeMaria A, Kisslo J, Weyman A: Recommendations regarding quantitation in M-mode echocardiography; Results of a survey of echocardiographic measurements. *Circulation*, 1978; 58:1072.

70. Salustri A, Trambaiolo Point of care echocardiography: small, smart and quick. *Eur Heart J* 2002; 23: 1484–7.

71. Sasse L: Echocardiography of left atrial wall. *JAMA*, 1974; 228:1667.

72. Schiller NB, Shah PM, Crawford M, DeMaria A, Devereux R, Feigenbaum H, Gutfesell H, Reichek N, Sahn D, Schnittger I, Silverman NH, Tajik AJ: Recommendations for quantitation of the left ventricle by two-dimensional echocardiography. *J Am Soc Echocardiogr*. 1989; 2:358.

73. Schiller NB, Shah PM, Crawford M, DeMaria A, Devereux R, Feigenbaum H, Gutgesell H, Reichek N, Sahn D, Schnittger I, Silverman N, Tijik A: Recommendations for Quantitation of the Left Ventricle by Two-Dimensional Echocardiography. *J Am Soc Echocardiogr*, 1989; 5:362.

74. Schnittger I, Gordon EP, Fitzgerald PJ, Popp RL: Standardized intracardiac measurements of two-dimensional echocardiography. *J Am Coll Cardiol*, 1983; 2:934.

75. Silverman NH, Hudson S: Evaluation of right ventricular volume and ejection fraction in children by two-dimensional echocardiography. *Pediatr Cardiol*, 1983; 4:197.

76. Skorton DH, McNary CA, Child JS, Newton FC, Shah PM: Digital image processing of two-dimensional echocardiograms: Identification of the endocardium. *Am J Cardiol*, 1981; 48:479.

77. Slovis TL, Clapp SK, Farooki ZQ: Non-invasive evaluation of the inferior vena cava. The value of sonography. *Am J Dis Child*, 1984; 138:277.

78. Spencer KT, Anderson AS, Bhargava A, *et al*. Physician performed point of care echocardiography using a laptop platform compared with physical examination in the cardiovascular patients. *J Am Coli Cardiol*, 2001; 37: 2013–8.

79. Starling MR, Crawford MH, Soreson SG, O'Rourke RA: A new two-dimensional echocardiographic technique for evaluating right ventricular size and performance in patients with obstructive lung disease. *Circulation*, 1984; 66:497.

80. Strunk BL, Fitzgerald JW, Lipton M, Popp RL, Barry WH: The posterior aortic wall echocardiogram: Its relationship of left atrial volume change. *Circulation*, 1976; 54:744.

81. Tajik AJ, Seward JB, Hagler DJ, Mair DD, Lie JT: Two-dimensional real-time ultrasonic imaging of the heart and great vessels: Technique, image orientation, structure identification, and validation. *Mayo Clin Proc*, 1978; 53:271.

82. Vourvouri EC, Koroleva LY, Ten Cate FJ, *et al*. Clinical utility and cost effectiveness of a personal ultrasound imager for cardiac evaluation during consultation rounds in patients with suspected, 2003; 89:727–30.

83. Vourvouri EC, Poldermans D, Schinkel AFL, *et al*. Left ventricular hypertrophy screening using a hand-held ultra sodevi. *Eur Heart J*, 2002; 23:1516–21.

84. Weyman AE, Dillion JC, Feigenbaum H, Chang S: Echocardiographic patterns of pulmonic valve motion in pulmonic stenosis. *Am J Cardiol*, 34:644, 1974.

85. Yoshikawa J, Kato H, Owaki T, Tanaka K: Study of posterior left atrial wall motion by echocardiography and its clinical application. *Jpn: Heart J*, 1975; 16:683.

86. Zile MR, Tanaka R, Lindroth JR, Spinale F, Cardabello BA, Mirsky I: Left ventricular volume determined echocardiographically assuming a constant left ventricular epicardial long-axis/short-axis dimension ratio throughout the cardiac cycle. *J Am Cardiol*, 1992; 20:986.

87. Zwehl, W, Levy, R, Garcia, E, Haendchen, RV, Childs, W, Corday, SR, Meerbaum, S, and Corday, E: Validation of a computerized edge detection algorithm for quantitative two-dimensional echocardiography. *Circulation*, 68: 1127, 198

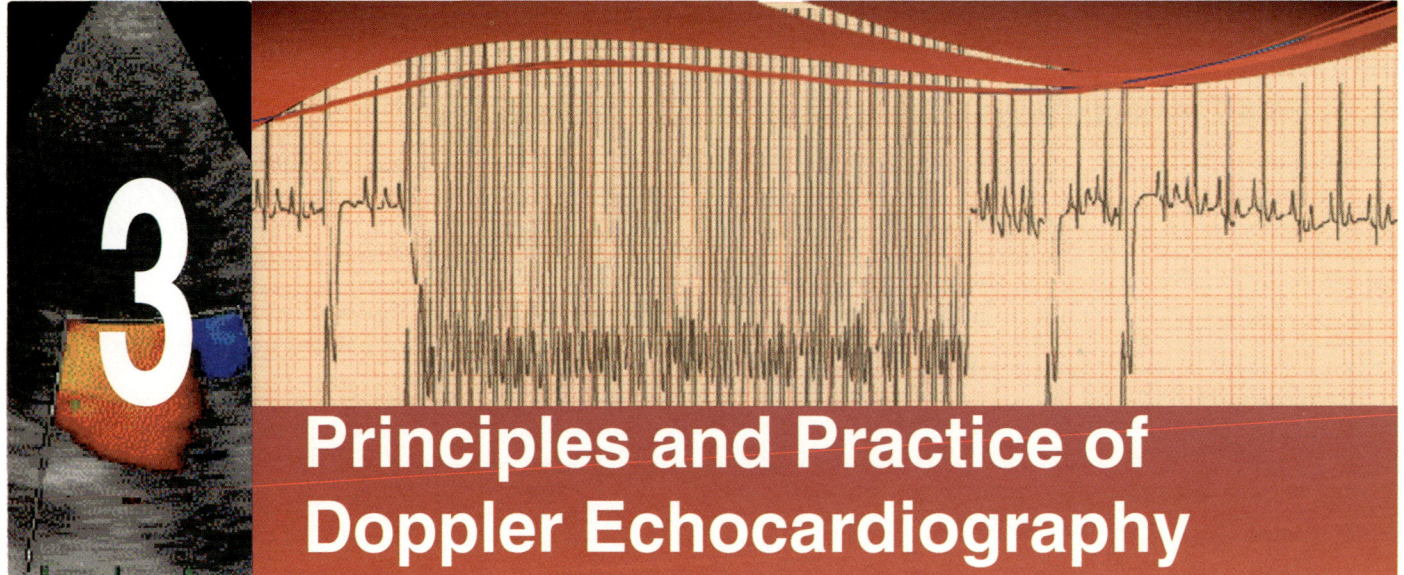

Principles and Practice of Doppler Echocardiography

Since both M-mode and 2-dimensional echocardiographic techniques do not directly deal with intracardiac flow patterns, hence they are found to be of very limited value in the evaluation of most stenotic and regurgitant cardiac defects. Pulsed Doppler and colour Doppler echocardiography, therefore, supplements hemodynamic information derived from the cardiac catheterisation and angiography which are frequently needed for specific determination of intracardiac flow dynamics. Doppler technique thus, may provide an alternative to cardiac catheterisation in the evaluation of preoperative and postoperative follow up cases of cardiac surgical interventions in both congenital and acquired heart ailments.

Basic principle of Doppler echocardiography is dependent upon the fact that ultrasonic waves generated by the transducer and directed at cardiac chambers are reflected by the moving blood cells in such a manner that the reflected waves have a frequency different from that of the incident beam, which is further based upon the direction and velocity of blood flow relative to the incident beam. When the flow is directed towards the transducer, the frequency of the returning signals is higher than the transmitted frequency, when compared to the motion of the red blood cells away from the transducer resulting in lower frequency of the reflected ultrasonic beam. This change in the frequency of the ultrasonic beam produced by moving targets is called the Doppler frequency shift, is named after the Austrian physicist Johann Doppler, Professor of Mathematics and Geometry who first described this phenomenon in relation to reflection of light waves from planets and other celestial bodies in 1842. The Doppler equipment measures this Doppler shift (Δf), which is proportional to the velocity of blood flow and is incorporated in the Doppler equation (Tables 3.1 and 3.2).

$$\Delta f = \frac{v \times 2 f_o \times \cos \theta}{C}$$

where v represents the velocity of moving targets blood cells, f_0 is the frequency of the incident ultrasonic beam, C is the speed of sound in tissue, which averages 1,540 m/sec and θ is the angle subtended by the incident ultrasonic beam with the direction of blood flow. Cosine (cos) θ equals 1 if the ultrasonic beam is kept parallel to the direction of blood flow, and in this setting, the magnitude of Doppler frequency shift becomes proportional to the velocity of blood flow. If the cross-sectional area of a given vessel or cardiac chamber is known from two-dimensional echocardiography, stroke volume can be derived by multiplying the cross-sectional area with the area under the Doppler flow-velocity curve. In selected patients, both left and right ventricular outputs can be measured separately by sampling in the pulmonary and systemic circulations, respectively. This procedure makes it feasible to calculate the degree of shunting in patient with systemic-pulmonary communications such as atrial and ventricular septal defects.

All the cardiac chambers and blood vessels can be interrogated for obtaining various patterns of blood flow by Doppler echocardiography. Normal flow is characterised by velocities that are generally in the same direction and magnitude at a given time in the cardiac cycle. The resultant Doppler signals, nearly, at the same frequency are often referred to as the "narrow band". On the other hand, flow through a stenotic valve produces, downstream from the narrowed orifice, velocities of multiple magnitudes and directions. A regurgitant jet also produces similar findings (Table 3.3).

A higher velocity flow can always be isolated from that of normal or laminar flow by the help of the Doppler signals recorded on strip chart papers or videotape using

Table 3.1: *Doppler echocardiography pressure drop or gradient measurement*

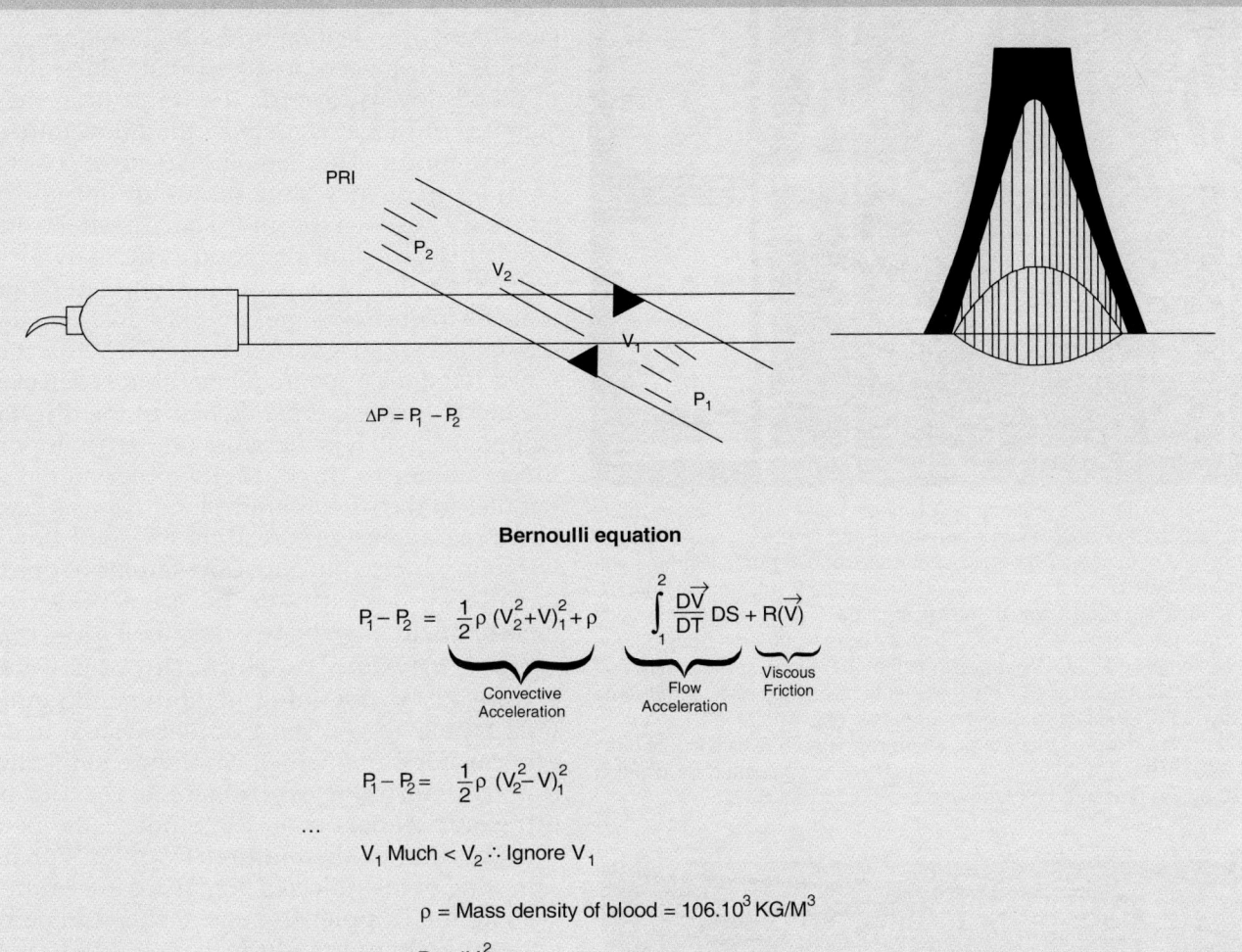

Bernoulli equation

$$P_1 - P_2 = \underbrace{\frac{1}{2}\rho\,(V_2^2 + V)_1^2}_{\substack{\text{Convective}\\\text{Acceleration}}} + \rho \underbrace{\int_1^2 \frac{D\vec{V}}{DT}\,DS}_{\substack{\text{Flow}\\\text{Acceleration}}} + \underbrace{R(\vec{V})}_{\substack{\text{Viscous}\\\text{Friction}}}$$

$$P_1 - P_2 = \frac{1}{2}\rho\,(V_2^2 - V)_1^2$$

...

V_1 Much $< V_2$ ∴ Ignore V_1

ρ = Mass density of blood = 106.10^3 KG/M^3

∴ $\Delta P = 4V_2^2$

Table 3.2: *Clinical application of the Bernoulli equation*

Application	Clinical utility
Peak velocity through a stenotic valve	Aortic stenosis maximal gradient
TR jet velocity	RV systolic pressure
LV outflow tract contour and velocity	HOCM gradient
Peak velocity across VSD	RV systolic pressure
End-diastolic velocity of PR jet	Pulmonary artery diastolic pressure
Velocity through a PDA	Pulmonary artery systolic pressure
MR contour and velocity	Left ventricular dp/dt

HOCM, hypertrophic obstructive cardiomyopathy; LV, left ventricle; MR, mitral regurgitation; PDA, patent ductus arteriosus; PR, pulmonic regurgitation; RV, right ventricular; VSD, ventricular septal defect; TR, tricuspid regurgitation.

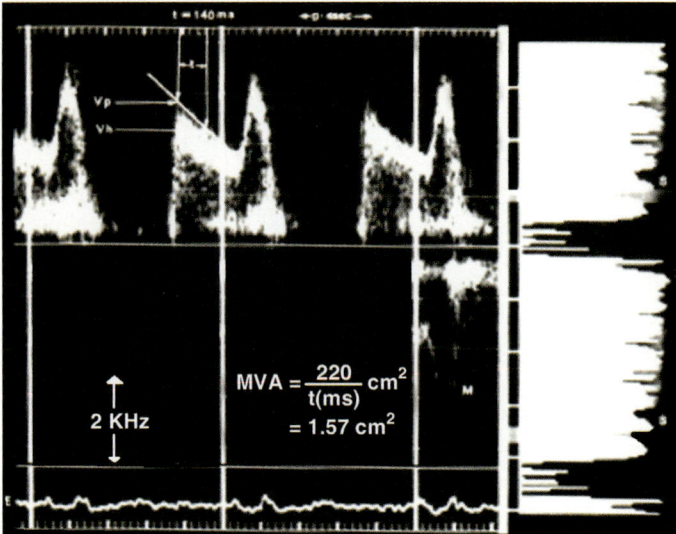

Fig. 3.1: In Doppler estimation of mitral valve orifice size in mitral stenosis by the application of pressure half time technique Doppler tracing is obtained by the help of pulsed Doppler probe. Sample volume is placed over the inflow tract of LV at the level of mitral annulus and angled in such a way that a the maximal Doppler frequency shifts is obtained and perfect morphology of MV is recorded as depicted in this exemplified case. Vp represents the peak Doppler frequency shift in early diastole,whereas Vh represents frequency shift at half time obtained by dividing Vp by the square root of 2. The time taken by Vp to drop to Vh represents the pressure half time (t), which in this case is 140 msec. The mitral valve area (MVA) is calculated by dividing 220 by the pressure half time and measured as 1.57 cm^2

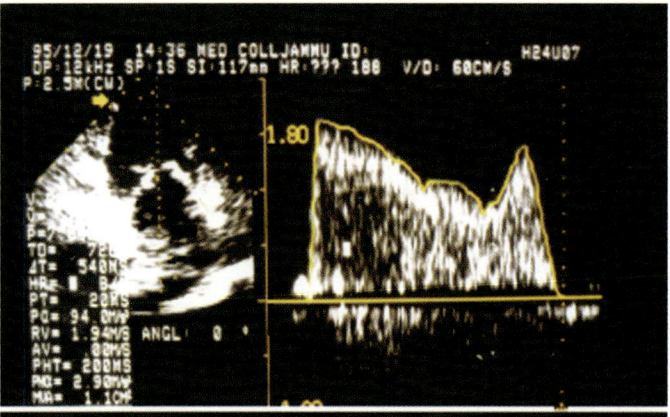

Fig. 3.2: Computer generated pressure half time and mitral value area (left panel) by just tracing the Doppler velocity spectrum of stenosed mitral valve (right panel)

a fast Fourier transform or Chrip-Z process. Unlike the frequency of the transmitted ultrasonic beam, the Doppler frequency shifts are of small magnitude and hence are in the audible range. These Doppler audio signals can also be used to distinguish normal from disturbed or turbulent flow. Because normal blood flow is organised and adjacent red blood cells cause similar Doppler shifts, the corresponding audio signals have a smooth, audio quality. On the other hand, flow

disturbances produce audible signals that are dissonant and harsh. High velocity flows unaccompanied by significant turbulence produce high-frequency whistling sounds. It has been observed that, when the direction of blood flow is towards the transducer, the reflected signal is of higher frequency than the emitted signals. On the monitor screen, the spectral display of the Doppler frequency shift shows an upright deflection above the baseline (positive signal). On the other hand, when the direction of blood flow is away from the transducer, the frequency of the reflected signal is lower than the frequency of the emitted signal, and the spectral display shows an inverted deflection below the baseline (negative singal). No frequency shift is detectable when the blood flow is perpendicular to the direction of the Doppler signal. It is therefore of utmost importance for the examiner to direct the Doppler signal as nearly parallel to the direction of blood flow as possible, for obtaining an accurate reading of blood flow velocity. For more clinical purposes, deviations of upto 20° from parallel are acceptable because the error in the measurement of velocity is less than 6%.

Currently two types of Doppler systems are employed for obtaining hemodynamic information. First type is the pulsed Doppler system like M-mode echocardiography which employs a single transducer that transmits as well as receives the reflected ultrasonic signals from the blood cells. Because the transmission of the emitted Doppler signal and the sampling of the reflected signal are intermittent in this system, the Doppler frequency shift can be measured without ambiguity only if its magnitude is less than half the pulse repetition frequency (PRF). Doppler frequency shifts greater than half the samplings frequency (called the Nyquist limit) create artifacts in the display of the Doppler signal. This phenomenon is called aliasing and results in truncation and displacement of the top portion of a high-velocity signal into the opposite frequency range. The presence of aliasing makes it difficult or impossible to measure the velocity of blood flow or to determine accurately the direction of blood flow signals. Aliased signals point towards the disturbed flow, and it is not generally noted in patients with normal laminar low-velocity flows.

Facility of range resolution as found in pulsed mode allows the echographer to record the given flow at any selected location in a given cardiac chamber or great vessel. This range resolution is accomplished by introducing a gate delay interval, which permits the receiver to analyse only those signals returning to the transducer during a pre-selected time window corresponding to a delay of 30 μsec/cm depth. The Doppler signal thus derived from a small localised region is called the **sample volume** and it has the shape

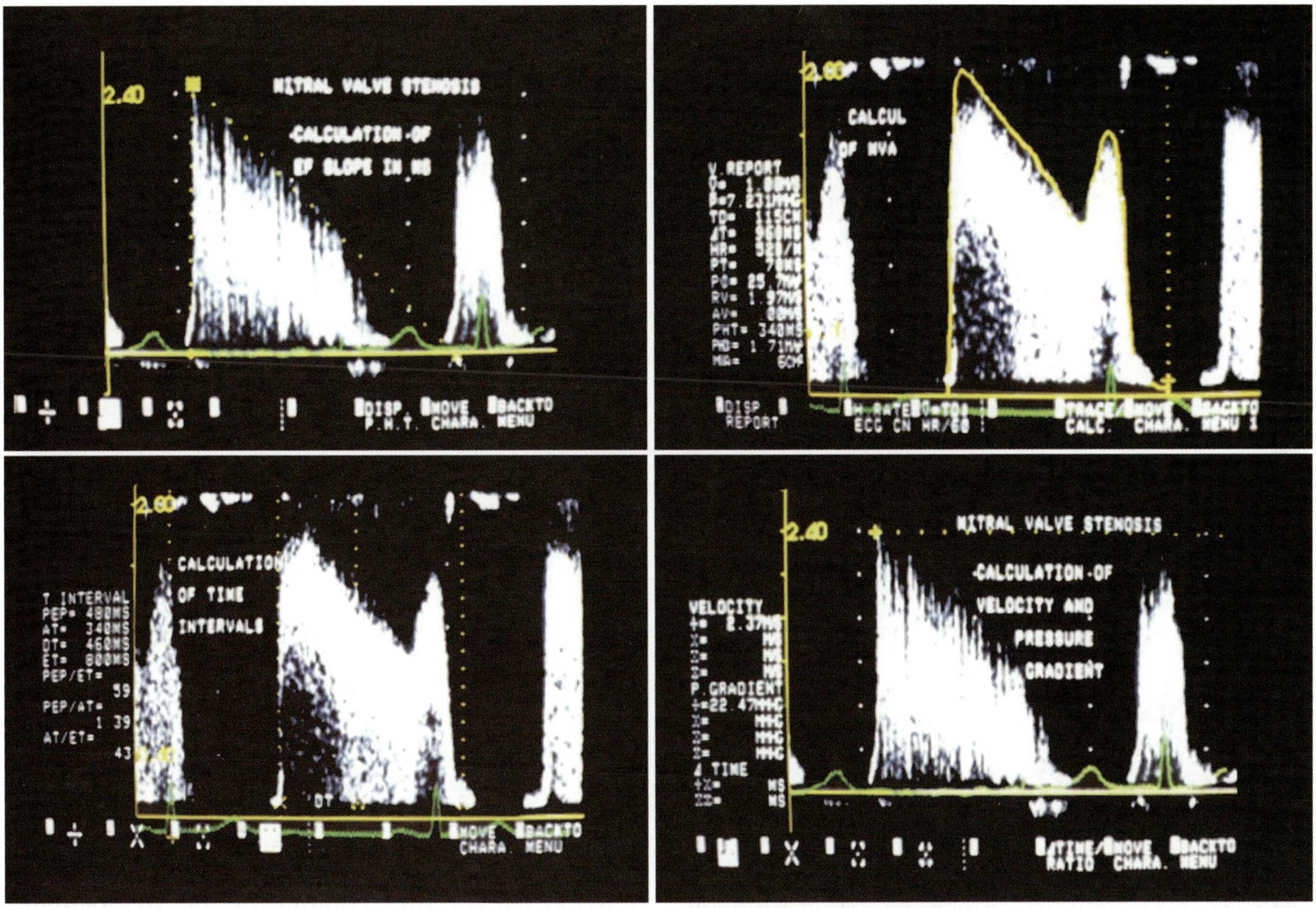

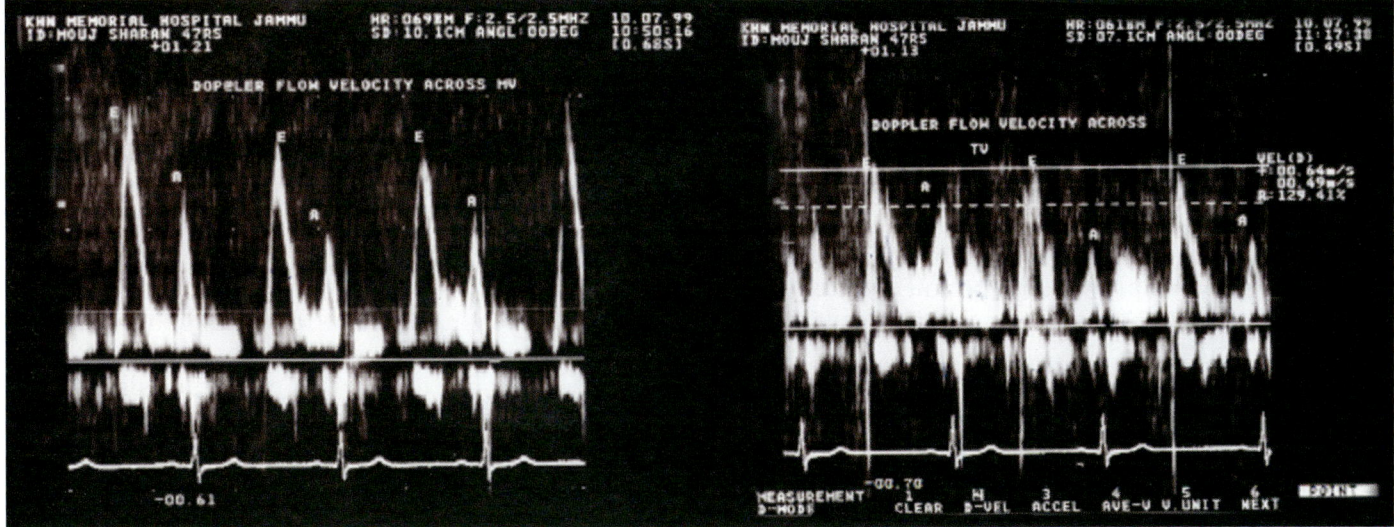

Fig. 3.3: Calculation of EF slope of MV (upper left), MVA by trace method (upper right), determination of various time intervals used in hemodynamic calculations (lower left), and calculation of MVA by the application of velocity and pressure gradient (lower right)

Fig. 3.4: Pulsed Doppler flow velocities across mitral (left) and tricuspid valve (right) in the absence of their respective valvular regurgitation

NOTE: In the absence of valvular regurgitation or intracardiac shunts, the stroke volume through each of the four valves should be equal.

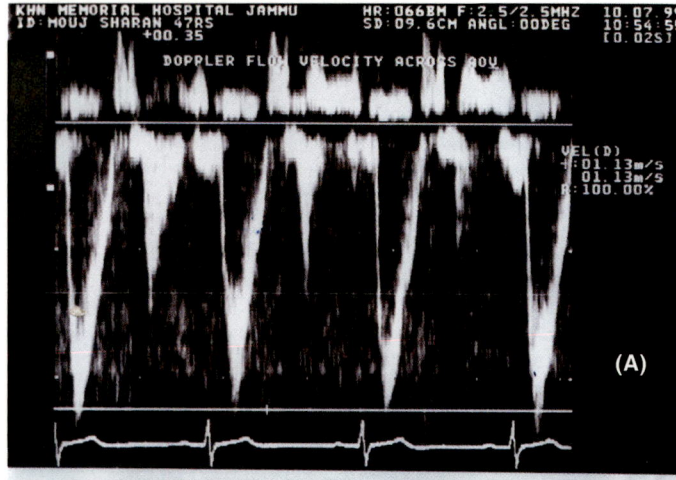

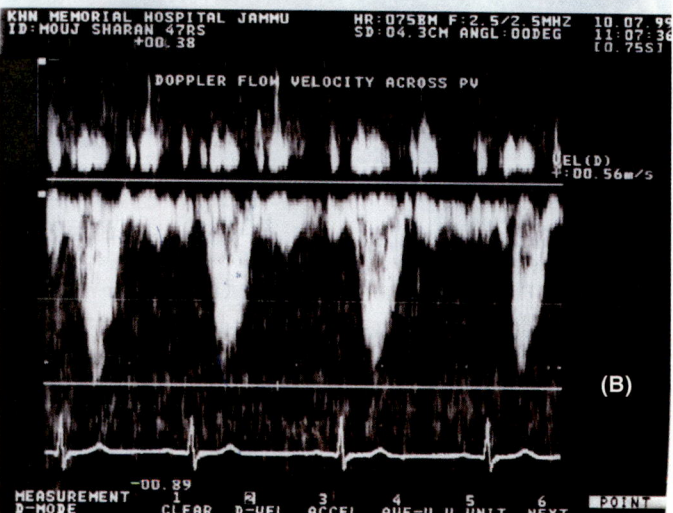

Fig. 3.5A and B: Pulsed Doppler flow velocities across aortic valve **(A)** and pulmonary valve **(B)** in the abscence of their respective valvular regurgitation

of a tear drop and measures approximately 2 by 3.8 mm for a 3.0 MHz transducer. In some newer equipment, the axial size of the sample volume is variable and can be modified by the examiner, whereas in other Doppler apparatus, the size of the sample volume is fixed because an overly large sample volume permits admixture of signals from adjacent chambers or vessels resulting into erroneous calculations.

Second type of Doppler mode is the **continuous-wave Doppler system** which employs a transducer with two piezoelectric crystals, one continuously broadcasting ultrasound and the other continuously receiving signals reflected from the blood cells and the tissues. A great advantage of this system is that the maximum measurable velocity is unlimited, because of continuous wave Doppler samples. By observing Doppler shifts all along the entire ultrasonic beam one may encounter certain drawback in this type of Doppler system for the exact location of flow disturbance. It is just to exemplify that in patients with a high-velocity jet in the vicinity of the aortic valve, it is not possible to determine, whether the abnormal jet originates from valvular or from supra-valvular aortic stenosis. Similarly, from the apical transducer position, it may not be possible to differentiate normal aortic systolic flow from that produced by mitral regurgitation.

It would be much easier to use simultaneous recording of Doppler and real time 2-dimensional echocardiography to assess cardiac lesions. It would be advantageous to acquire equipment which combines two-dimensional imaging with both pulse and continuous-wave Doppler techniques. The pulsed-wave system, with its ability to provide range-specific velocity information, permits systematic investigation of various cardiac chambers and vessels, for detection and mapping of flow disturbances. On the other hand, the continuous-wave Doppler system has its great strength and its ability to measure accurately the velocity of abnormal jets. In situations where one may find higher velocities the instrument can be switched to the continuous mode, which has no limit on maximum velocity that can be measured.

Although such a procedure also results in the loss of range resolution, such high velocities are generally found only in localised areas, so range resolution is unnecessary. In patients with cardiac lesion giving higher velocities one may take the help of third system called **extended-range Doppler** or **adaptive Doppler**, in an attempt to solve the problem of aliasing that occurs in conventional pulsed Doppler equipment. This approach is based on the concept that although some of the ultrasonic energy in the area of the Doppler sample volume is reflected back towards the transducer, another component of this ultrasonic energy is transmitted beyond the region of the Doppler sample volume. This transmitted energy can be used to examine a patient for Doppler shift signals arising from deeper areas. As this method of extended range Doppler effectively increase the pulse repetition frequency, hence high flow velocities can be recorded without interference from aliasing.

Since this system picks up Doppler signals from two or more sampling regions at different depth, it is therefore, potential to have an ambiguous recording though to a very smaller range of values.

Finding out an adequate acoustic window in Doppler examination is of utmost importance, as poor acoustic window may result into low quality two dimensional Doppler signal and in turn print out poor quality Doppler graph.

It is just to give an example that in an emphysematous patient one may not be able to obtain adequate Doppler signals due to non availability of an adequate acoustic

Table 3.3: *M-mode and 2-dimensional echocardiography in altered hemodynamics*

Echo-characteristics	Hemodynamic applications
M-mode	
Early closure of the mitral valve	Acute, severe aortic regurgitation
Delayed closure of the mitral valve (B bump)	Elevated LV end-diastolic pressure
RV free wall early diastolic collapse	Pericardial tamponade
Mid systolic notching of the aortic valve	Dynamic subaortic outflow tract obstruction
Diastolic mitral valve fluttering	Aortic regurgitation
Mid systolic notching of the pulmonary valve	Pulmonary hypertension
Rounding of the opening/closing points of a disk-type prosthetic valve	Mechanical restriction to disc motion
Systolic anterior motion of the mitral valve	Dynamic subaortic outflow track obstruction
Early systolic downward motion (beaking) of the IVS	LBBB
Gradual closure of the aortic valve	Reduced left ventricular stroke volume
Absent pulmonary valve A-wave	Pulmonary hypertension
Two-dimensional	
Diastolic flattening of the IVS	RV volume overload Systolic flattening of the
Systolic flattening of the IVS	RV pressure overload (elevated RVSP)
Dilated IVC with abnormal respiratory variation	Elevated RA pressure
Exaggerated IVS bounce, with respiratory variation	Pericardial constriction

IVC, inferior vena cava; IVS, interventricular septum; LBBB, Left bundle branch block; RA, right atrial,

RV, right ventricular; RVSP, right ventricular systolic pressure.

window and therefore, one may fail to demonstrate significant mitral regurgitation by transthoracic 2-D Doppler echocardiography.

Doppler Technique in the Assessment of Individual Cardiac Structure

Given below is the description of individual area examination with respect to plane, sample volume position, particular technique employed and details of morphology obtained from a scanned structure.

Superior Vena Cava (SVC)

Plane: Preferred plane—suprasternal notch, short axis; in some individuals subcostal plane can also be used.

Sample Volume Position: In SVC, which is found to the right of the ascending aorta, and right pulmonary artery. The sample volume is placed centrally and parallel to the walls of the SVC. In the subcostal position, the SVC is visualised from the sagittal four-chamber plane with the transducer angled anteriorly. The SVC is located as it enters the right atrium (RA) and the sample volume is placed in the centre of the SVC parallel to the SVC walls.

Description of Waveform (Fig. 3.54B)

A biphasic waveform is usually found. The larger peak occurs in systole and the second and smaller peak occurs in early and mid-diastole. It does show respiratory variation in peak velocity.

Velocity Findings: Directional Findings

Systole: Suprasternal negative; subcostal positive.
Diastole: Suprasternal negative; subcostal positive.

Abnormal Flow: Causes of Flow Disturbance

1. Anomalous pulmonary venous return into SVC.
2. Arteriovenous malformation with increased flow into SVC.
3. Tricuspid regurgitation may cause a flow disturbance.

Causes of Jets

Stenosis superior to sampling site in SVC, most commonly seen in Mustard baffles for transposition of the great vessels.

Right Atrium (RA)

Plane: Apical four-chamber plane is preferred. The RA can also be evaluated easily from subcostal positions. Short axis precordial position can be used to image the RA, but very little information can be gathered in this plane.

Sample Volume Position: The usual method for study of the RA is to place the sample volume superior to the tricuspid valve ring. When searching for a jet of flow disturbance the entire atrium should be studied.

Technique: The transducer is positioned in the standard apex or subcostal four-chamber plane. For Doppler interrogation, the septum should be parallel to the course. When a predetermined velocity signatures are traced, the transducer can be moved in the elevation plane within the RA to obtain peak velocity. Measurable velocity are not usually found in most other locations within the right atrium.

Description of Waveform

The first peak occurs early during the rapid ventricular filling phase. A second peak occurs with atrial contraction. The configuration has the appearance of motion of the tricuspid valve as imaged by M-mode technique.

Directional Velocity Findings

Systole: Not much signal in normal
Diastole: Positive

Abnormal Flow:

Causes of Flow Disturbance

1. Any cause for a left-to-right shunt at the atrial level
2. Tricuspid insufficiency
3. Superior vena cava stenosis.

Causes of a Jet

1. Systolic negative directional high velocity:
   a. Tricuspid insufficiency
   b. Mitral regurgitation with atrial septal defect
   c. Left ventricle/right atrial shunt
   d. Endocardial cushion valve regurgitation
2. Positive directional shunt—SVC obstruction

Atrial Septum

It is essential to scan atrial septal defects (ASD).
Plane: Subcostal plane 90° to the four-chamber plane. (Figs 3.9 and 3.23)
Sample Volume Position: On both sides of the interatrial septum in the area of an imaged or presumed ASD.
Technique: The whole atrium can be scanned. The sample volume should be as perpendicular as possible to the atrial septum. When a velocity is found, the transducer must be moved in the elevational plane to maximize the velocity and reduce spectral broadening.

Description of Waveform

In the normal recordings, few velocities are found. In patients with ASD, two or three peaks are usually found. The largest peak occurs in systole and is followed by

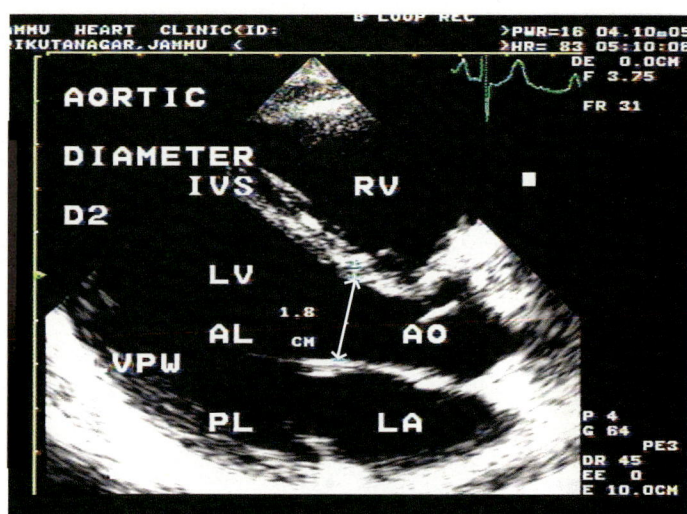

Fig. 3.6: An example of stroke volume calculation is shown. The cross sectional area of the outflow tract of aorta or pulmonary artery is measured. The time velocity integral is determined by planimetry. The calculation for stroke volume (SV) is shown

$$SV = D^2 \times 0.785 \times TVI$$
$$SV = 2.42 \times 0.785 \times 19$$
$$= 86CC$$

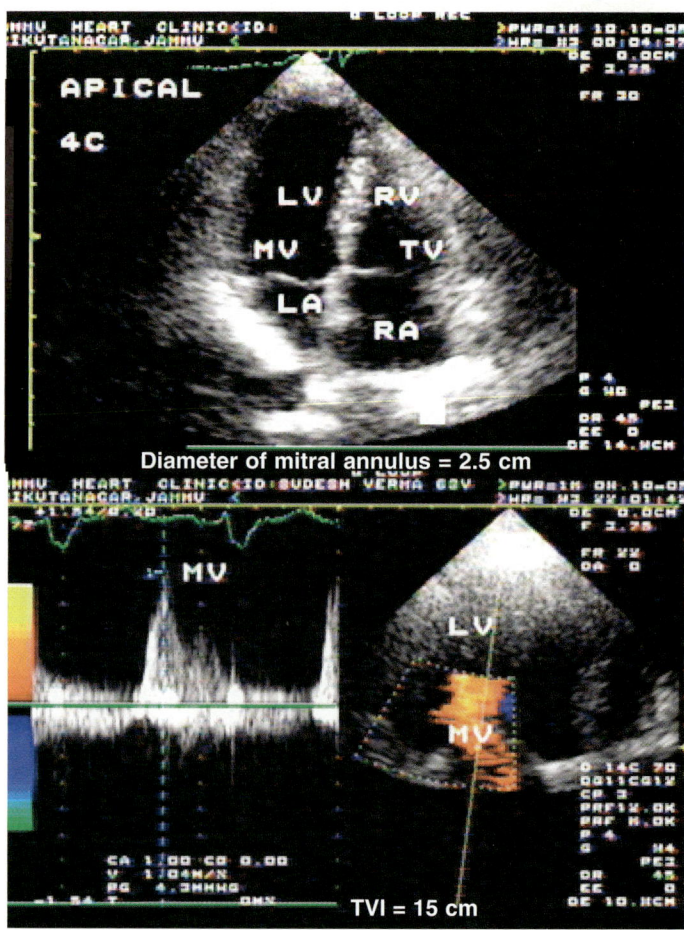

Fig. 3.7: Apical four chambers view for calculation of mitral annulus diameter (D) and stroke volume

$$SV = 2.52 \times 0.785 \times 15 = 74 \ CC$$

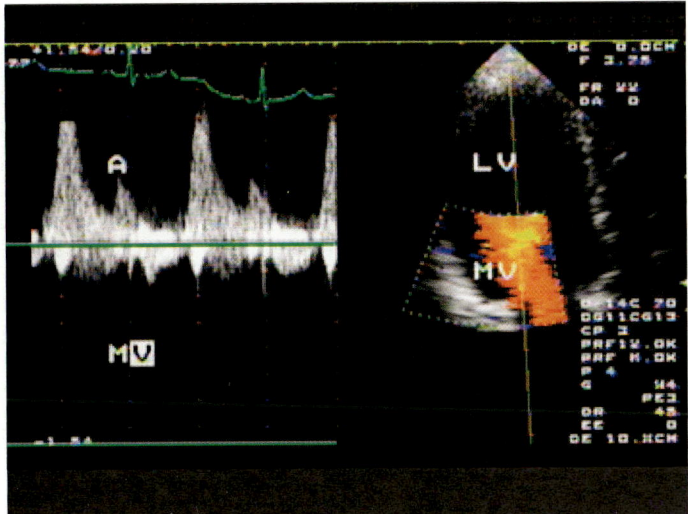
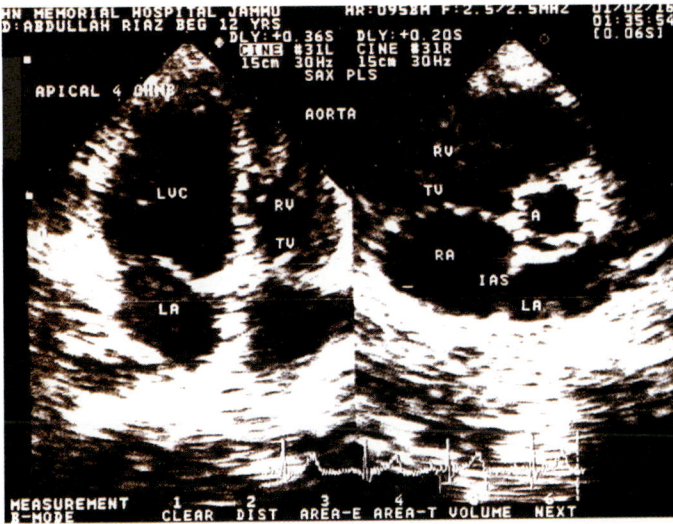
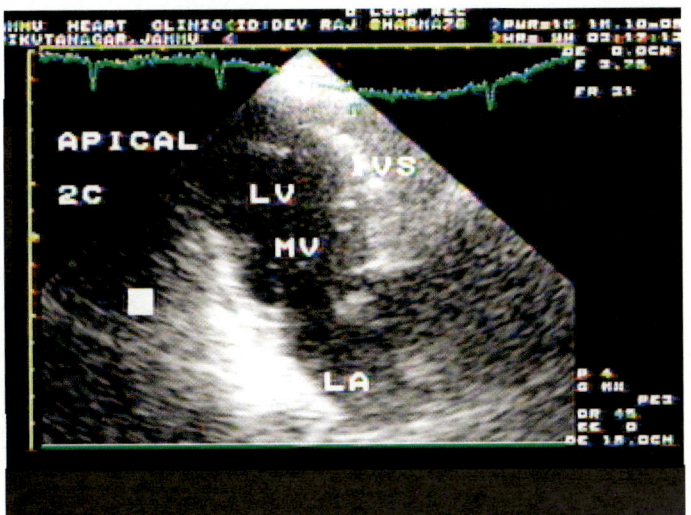
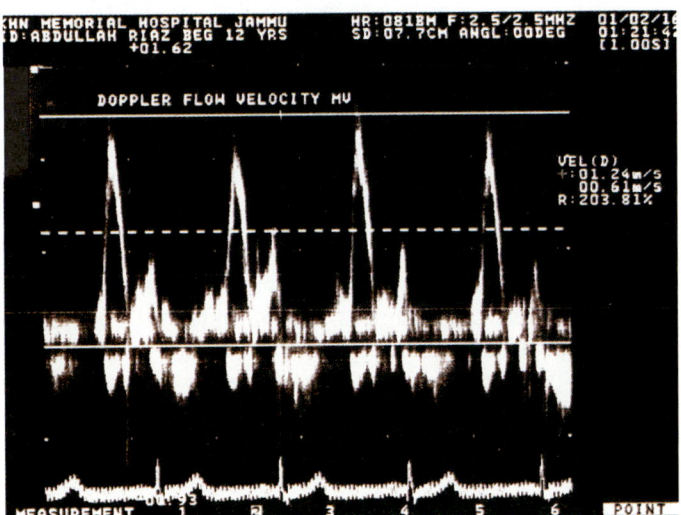

Fig. 3.8: Alternatively the diameter is measured from the four chamber (right upper) and two chambers view (left lower). The Doppler recording of mitral inflow is depicted at (right lower)

$$SV = (\pi \times r^1 \times r^2) \times 22$$
$$= 152cc$$

one smaller, broad peak in diastole or two distinct, small peaks; one in early diastole and the second following the P wave on EKG. Respiratory variation in velocity magnitude frequently occurs in this area.

Directional Velocity Findings

Systole: Positive in right atrium with left-to-right shunt; negative in left atrium with right-to-left shunting as in ASD.
Diastole: Same as systole.

Abnormal Flow

Few velocities are found in the area except in the area of an ASD. When the sample volume enters the area of the ASD, velocities are more pronounced.

Causes of a Jet

It is usually not found in normal circumstances but in some instances one may encounter a jet due to mitral regurgitation associated with ASD.

Right Ventricular Inflow

Plane: Apical four-chamber plane (preferred).

Other Possible Planes: Precordial Short Axis.

Sample volume position: Just distal to tricuspid valve.

Technique: Similar to the method described for the apical four-chamber plane for right atrium but the sample volume is moved to the inflow of the tricuspid valve.

Description of Waveform (Fig. 3.4B)

The first peak represents diastolic rapid filling and the second peak is due to atrial contraction. Higher velocities can occur with inspiration and lower ones with expiration.

Directional Velocity Findings

Systole: Velocities are not usually recorded.
Diastole: Positive velocity

Abnormal Flow

Cause of flow disturbance: Those defects which increase tricuspid flow. Examples include ASD, anomalous pulmonary venous return and tricuspid insufficiency.

Causes of a Jet

1. Systolic negative velocity-tricuspid insufficiency, ventricular septal defect (VSD)
2. Diastolic positive velocity-tricuspid stenosis, VSD

Right Ventricular Outflow Tract (RVOT)

Plane: Short axis, sagittal subcostal.
Sample Volume Position: In RVOT proximal to the pulmonary valve.
Technique: The patient is positioned in the left decubitus and examined by imaging the parasternal short-axis plane. For subcostal imaging, the patient is placed in supine position and the transducer is placed in the sagittal plane and angled leftward and anteriorly.

Description of Waveform (Fig. 3.10)

The waveform looks like a pulmonary artery waveform. In some patients, however, it will be of lower apparent magnitude because the interception angle may not be as favourable as for the pulmonary artery.

Velocity Findings:

Directional Findings

Systole: Negative
Diastole: None in normal circumstances

Abnormal Flow:

Causes of flow disturbance

Right ventricular muscle bundles. VSD, tricuspid stenosis, and pulmonary insufficiency.

Causes of Jet

1. Tricuspid stenosis (either direction)
2. VSD (variable direction dependent upon relative location of the sample volume and the VSD
3. Pulmonary insufficiency (positive direction)
4. Infundibular stenosis

Potential Problems

The subcostal plane provides excellent beam alignment but the examination causes patient discomfort. Further, the sample volume is far from the transducer and the maximal velocity that can be recorded by pulse. Doppler is thus reduced. This plane is more useful for infants and small children. The precordial short-axis plane can be difficult to image in some larger and older individuals.

Interventricular Septum (IVS)

Plane: Precordial long axis, precordial short axis at mitral-chordal plane, subcostal four chamber, subcostal sagittal (all preferred); apex four-chamber short axis and apex two chamber planes (possible).
Sample Volume Position: Search in both ventricles and the septum itself for a jet by scanning the entire area.
Technique: The sample volume can be placed beneath aorta in the long axis plane and moved through the septum to the right ventricle just under the tricuspid valve. The transducer is often angled slightly inferiomedially to allow better interrogation of the membranous area of the septum. The remaining length of the septum should be interrogated for muscular ventricular septal defects. In the short axis plane, the ventricles are each interrogated along the breadth of the septum. Several areas should be studied from the apex, including the area of the papillary muscles and the area at the level of the mitral valve. The same technique should be applied to the subcostal four-chamber plane. A sagittal plane can be obtained by 90° transducer rotation with anterior leftward angulation, which allows interrogation of the septum by the right ventricular outflow tract. If the apical views are used, a ventricular septal defect jet may be perpendicular and not appreciated by the Doppler technique. Apical view are helpful in detecting muscular ventricular septal defects (Figs 3.11 and 3.15).

Description of the Waveform

In normal recordings waveforms are usually nondescript since planes perpendicular to the interventricular septum are not compatible with Doppler interrogation.

Directional Velocity Findings

Systole: Usually none.

Diastole: Not established; usually low in magnitude; perpendicular to the septum.

Abnormal Flow:

Causes of Flow Disturbance

Ventricular septal defect

Causes of a Jet: Restrictive ventricular septal defect.

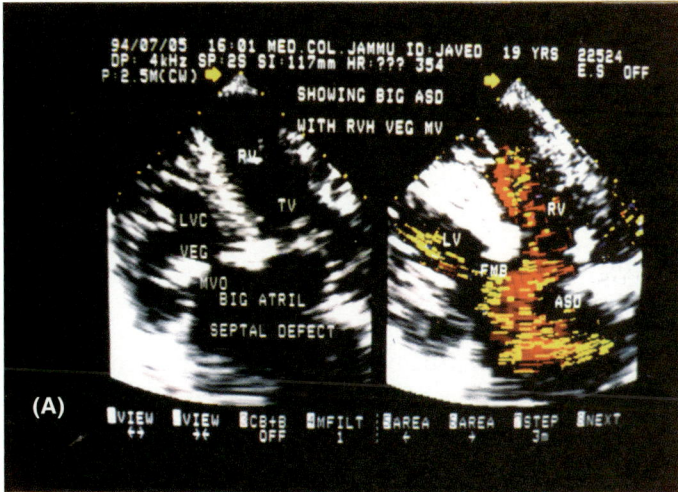

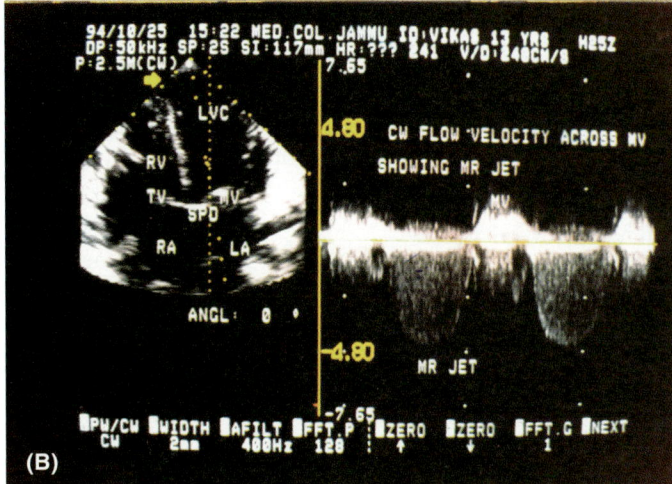

Fig. 3.9A and B: Large secundum atrial septal defect in dual 2-D scan both b/w and color (upper) and septum primum defect with large L-R shunt with gross MR (lower panel)

> In the presence of an intracardiac shunt, Qp/QS provides a mean to quantify the magnitude of shunting. In this example from a patient with a large secundum atrial septal defect, stroke volume (SV) through the pulmonary (right lower) and aortic (right upper) valves are measured and the Qp/Qs is estimated.

Fig. 3.10A and B: In the presence of an intracardiac shunt, Qp/QS provides a mean to quantify the magnitude of shunting. In this example from a patient with a large secundum atrial septal defect, stroke volume (SV) through the pulmonary (B) and aortic (A) valves are measured and the Qp/Qs is estimated, noted below.

An example;

$$QpSV = D^2 \times 0.785 \times TV1$$
$$= 1.62 \times 0.785 \times 56 = 113 \text{ CC}$$
$$QsSV = D^2 \times 0.785 \times TV1$$
$$= 1.52 \times 0.785 \times 25 = 44 \text{ CC}$$

Hence $\quad Qp/Qs = 113/44 = 2.5$

Potential Problems

Localisation of tiny jets is sometime difficult but one should try hard to find by placing sample volume in different angles and planes.

Main Pulmonary Artery

Plane: Parasternal short axis (preferred); sagittal subcostal suprasternal.

Sample Volume Position: Distal to the valve in the main pulmonary artery.

Technique: The patient is positioned in the left lateral decubitus for the parasternal short-axis. Both the aorta and pulmonary artery are visualised. In cases where it is difficult to locate it can be traced by rotating the patient further to the left. For subcostal imaging, the transducer is aligned as for to the right of ventricular outflow tract.

Description of Waveform (Fig. 3.7)

The initial systolic deflection is narrow in spectral widths and broadens after the peak. Usually relatively wide spectral broadening occurs during deceleration phase in some patients, the broadened spectrum continues until the trace again reaches baseline. In late diastole, small negative deflection occurs in patients with normal pulmonary artery pressure. This wave is due to increased right ventricular pressure sufficient to cause diastolic opening of the pulmonary value.

Directional Velocity Findings

Systole: Negative.
Diastole: A small positive peak may occur in early diastole. This probably results from filling the sinus of Valsalva. A negative presystolic velocity is encountered in normal persons.

Abnormal Flow:
Causes of Flow Disturbance

VSD, pulmonary stenosis of any kind, shunts into the pulmonary artery of any kind.

Causes of a Jet

1. Pulmonary stenosis of any kind (negative direction).
2. A pulmonary insufficiency jet may be detected close to the valve as a positive directional high velocity.
3. Patent ductus arteriosus (PDA), aortico-pulmonary window, and shunts created at operation.

Potential Problems

It may be difficult to obtain signatures of the pulmonary artery in short axis due to over shadowing of lung tissue. The patient can then be turned greater than 90° in the left decubitus. The sagittal subcostal approach may be tried but the distance to the pulmonary artery is significant, thus limiting the maximal pulsed Doppler velocity. From this latter location, the elevational angle is difficult to determine. The sagittal subcostal scanning is also reported to be uncomfortable and cannot usually be performed successfully in larger children and adults.

Left Atrium (LA)

Plane: Preferred apical four-chamber. Short axis precordial and apical two chamber possible.
Sample Volume Position: Superior to mitral valve ring (when searching for a jet or a flow disturbance, the entire atrium should be studied).
Technique: It can be visualised through an apical four chamber view. For Doppler interrogation, the septum should be parallel to the cursor. When a velocity of interest is found, the transducer should be moved in the elevational plane to obtain peak velocities in normal patients. Most other locations in the left atrium do not produce measurable velocities.

Description of Waveform (Fig. 3.29)

The first peak occurs in early diastole and corresponds to the rapid ventricular filling phase. A second presystolic peak is associated with atrial contraction. The configuration has the appearance of the mitral valve image on an M-mode echocardiogram.

Directional Velocity Findings

Systole: Minimal detectable velocities.
Diastole: Positive.

Abnormal Flow:
Causes of a Flow Disturbance

1. Right-to-left shunts at atrial level may produce a flow disturbance.
2. Increased transmitral flow;
   a. Mitral regurgitation
   b. Increased pulmonary venous return for any reason.

Causes of a Jet

1. Mitral insufficiency; Systolic negative velocity.
2. Possible causes—supravalvular stenosing ring, cor triatriatum, and pulmonary venous stenosis.

Potential Problems

The left atrium can be distant to the transducer, thus limiting the maximal pulsed Doppler velocity.

Left Ventricular Inflow

Plane: Apical four-chamber (preferred); apex long-axis plane (also possible).

Sample Volume Position: In the left ventricle just distal to the mitral ring.

Technique: Same as for left atrium in apical four-chamber plane. The sample volume should be advanced into the mitral valve and located near the leaflet tips. If the sample volume is placed more medially, left ventricular outflow tract velocity will be recorded. This negative systolic velocity from the outflow tract could be mistaken for mitral regurgitation.

Description of Waveform (Fig. 3.4A)

The initial peak occurs during the rapid filling phase in early diastole. A second and usually smaller peak occurs in later diastole as a result of atrial contraction. In atrial fibrillation, the second peak is missing and with other atrial arrhythmias several peaks can be seen (one with each contraction). Little respiratory variation occurs in mitral velocities as compared to that which occurs in tricuspid velocities. Normal peak mitral velocity is generally higher than normal peak tricuspid velocity. A negative systolic deflection after the aortic valve opens usually represents left ventricular outflow velocity.

Velocity Findings:
Directional Findings

Systole: Normally no velocity is recorded.
Diastole: Positive.

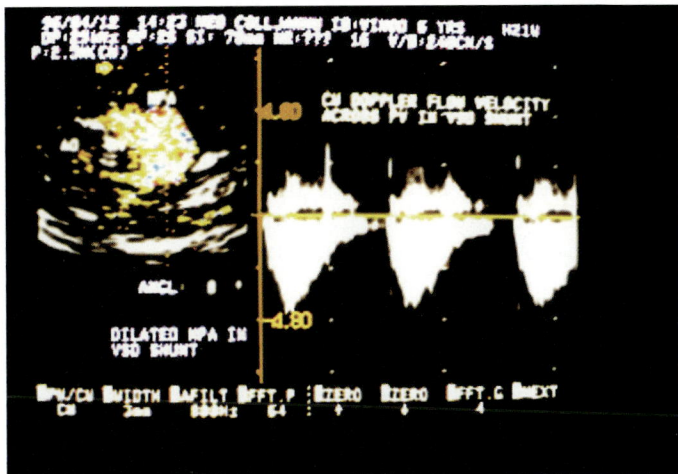

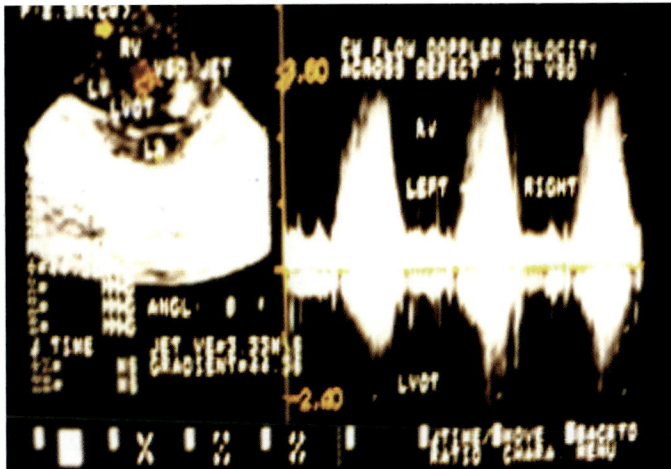

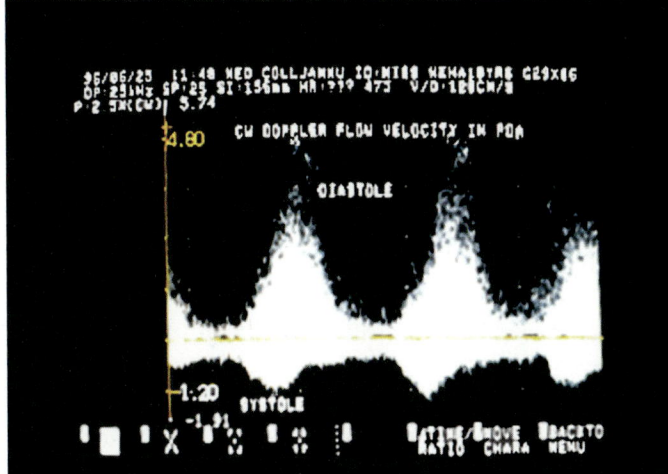

Fig. 3.11: Both in upper and lower panels show two cases of (L–R). Upper panel shows continuous wave Doppler determining the velocity across PV in VSD. In lower panel a case of PDA in which CW Doppler has been employed to record the peak velocity. In both the cases ratio of Qp/Qs was calculated and severity of shunt was identified in their preoperative period

Abnormal Flow:

Causes of Flow Disturbance

Increased mitral flow for any reason (ventricular septal defect, patent ductus arteriosus, mitral regurgitation).

Causes of a Jet

1. Mitral stenosis—diastolic positive high velocity
2. Mitral regurgitation—systolic negative high velocity.

Potential Problems

Placing the sample volume parallel to flow may be difficult because flow passes leftward to the usual cursor location. Elevational beam adjustment requires care. Correct placement of the sample volume is essential as erratic location of sample volume may overlap the LVOT velocity.

Left Ventricular Outflow Tract (LVOT)

Plane: Apex five chamber, apex two chamber, subcostal five chamber and subcostal sagittal (apical and suprasternal views are preferred).

Sample Volume Position: Left ventricular outflow tract below aortic valve and away from mitral leaflets.

Technique: The patient is usually positioned in the left decubitus. The transducer is placed on the point of maximal impulse and oriented in such a way that a short-axis four-chamber view is obtained. It is then angled superiorly so that the aortic valve is imaged.

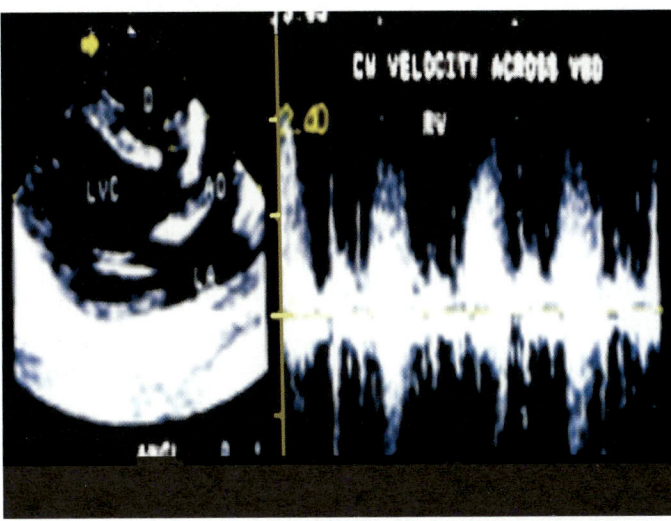

Fig. 13. 12A

Alternatively, the transducer can be placed in the apex long-axis (two chamber) plane to image the LVOT. The sample volume is then directed parallel to the interventricular septum and positioned just below the aortic valve. Elevation adjustments are then made to achieve maximal velocities.

Description of Waveform (Fig. 3.36)

The velocity profile almost closely resembles with that of the ascending aorta with an abrupt systolic stroke away from the baseline. Spectral dispersion occurs at peak velocity and some spectral scattering remains as the curve again reaches baseline. Little waveform is seen in diastole unless mitral inflow velocities are mixed with that of the LVOT waveform.

Velocity Findings:
Directional Findings

Systole: Negative.
Diastole: No waveform.

Abnormal Flow:
Causes of Flow Disturbance

Aortic insufficiency, subaortic stenosis.

Causes of a Jet

Systole: Subaortic stenosis (discrete membranous fibromuscular subaortic stenosis. Also in idiopathic hypertrophic subaortic stenosis (IHSS), although an additional jet of mitral regurgitation is often present in IHSS (Fig. 1.13).
Diastole: Aortic insufficiency, subaortic tunnel.

Potential Problems

Mitral signals, especially in children and when distant sample volume placement is necessary, can contaminate left ventricular outflow tract signals. The left ventricular outflow tract is difficult to image parallel to flow.

Ascending Aorta (AAO)

Plane: Suprasternal notch, short axis (preferred): right upper sternal border, apex and subcostal planes are also possible.
Sample Volume Position: In mid-ascending aorta.
Technique: Suprasternal notch transducer that allows the sample volume to be centred in the ascending aorta and placed parallel to blood flow. Once the sample volume is positioned in the two visualised planes, the transducer is moved in the elevational plane until maximal velocity is recorded. Other transducer locations usually record submaximal aortic velocities as uncertain beam intercept angles. From the apex and subcostal positions, velocity will be reversed in direction.

Description of Waveform (Figs. 3.20 and 3.21)

The initial systolic deflection has a rapid, narrow upstroke. Spectral broadening occurs at the peak. The down slope usually has a wider spectrum than the upstroke. During early diastole a slight reversal of velocity is usually noted. The upstroke of the velocity curve is more rapid than in the pulmonary artery, so peak velocity is reached earlier in systole.

Velocity Findings:
Directional Findings

Systole: Positive from the suprasternal notch and upper right sternal border positions. Negative from the apex and subcostal position.
Diastole: Small negative deflection in early diastole in the suprasternal plane.

Abnormal Flow:
Causes of Flow Disturbance

Any type of aortic stenosis. Any lesion that causes a pulmonary disturbance can cause aortic disturbance by induction.

Causes of a Jet

1. A positive directional jet is usually evidence of aortic stenosis.
2. A large negative directional jet close to the aortic valve is usually evidence of aortic insufficiency.

Potential Problems

Sampling at the junction of the transverse arch and ascending aorta with a standard imaging transducer does not allow detection of maximal velocities because of an unfavourable intercept angle. Some patients, especially when intubated, do not tolerate the pressure of a transducer in the suprasternal notch.

Descending Aorta (DAO)

Plane: Suprasternal notch short-axis plane.
Sample Volume Position: At the junction of the transverse aortic arch and descending aorta. In a few patients, the sample volume can be placed more distally in descending aorta and still be reasonably aligned with flow.
Technique: The same as for the suprasternal notch velocity in the ascending aorta but the transducer is angled to the left and posteriorly to bring the descending aorta into view. The sample volume is usually placed in the location most parallel to flow. This location is usually the junction of the transverse and descending aorta.

Table 3.4: *Doppler velocity measurements in normal individuals*

	Children		Adults	
	Mean	*Range*	*Mean*	*Range*
Mitral flow	1.00 m/s	0.8–1.3 m/s	0.90 m/s	0.6–1.3 m/s
Tricuspid flow	0.60 m/s	0.5–0.8 m/s	0.50 m/s	0.3–0.7 m/s
Pulmonary artery	0.90 m/s	0.7–1.1 m/s	0.75 m/s	0.6–0.9 m/s
Left ventricle	1.00 m/s	0.7–1.2 m/s	0.90 m/s	0.7–1.1 m/s
Aorta	1.50 m/s	1.2–1.8 m/s	1.35 m/s	1.0–1.7 m/s

Description of Waveform

Same pattern as for the ascending aorta except the velocity is displayed with the opposite polarity and usually has more spectral broadening (Figs 3.12 and 3.26).

Directional Velocity Findings

Systole: Mainly a negative velocity.

Diastole: Reversed flow can occur in patent ductus arteriosus.

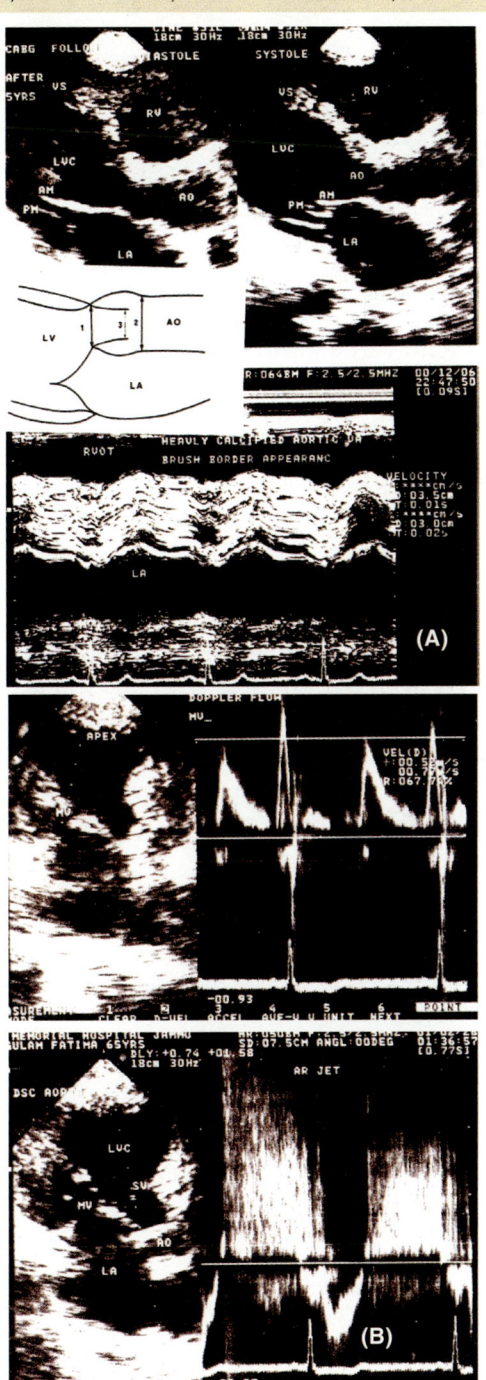

(A)

(B)

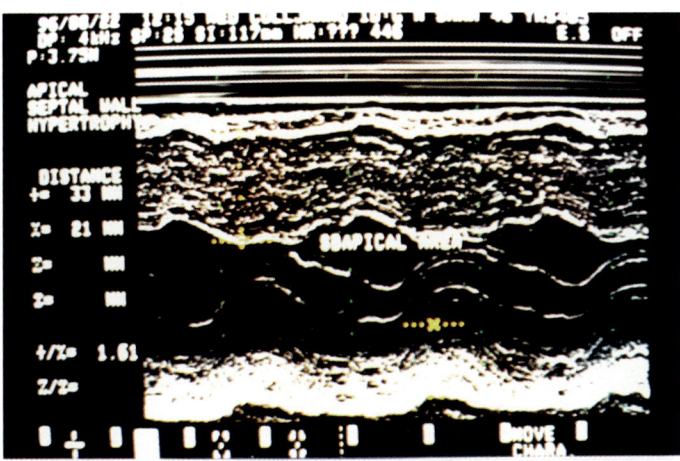

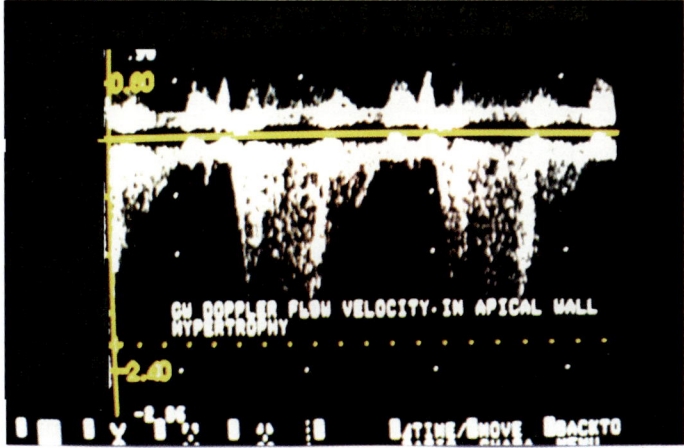

Fig. 3.13: Upper panel shows marked septal wall hypertrophy as a part of HOCM. In lower panel showing CW Doppler flow velocity in subaortic region for the calculation of LV pressure in the application of Bernoulli equation

Fig. 3.14A and B: (A) A case of calcified aortic stenosis (below) with two chamber oblique view (above) for measuring aortic diameter. (B) Mitral velocity (above) and severe aortic regurgitation in lower panel

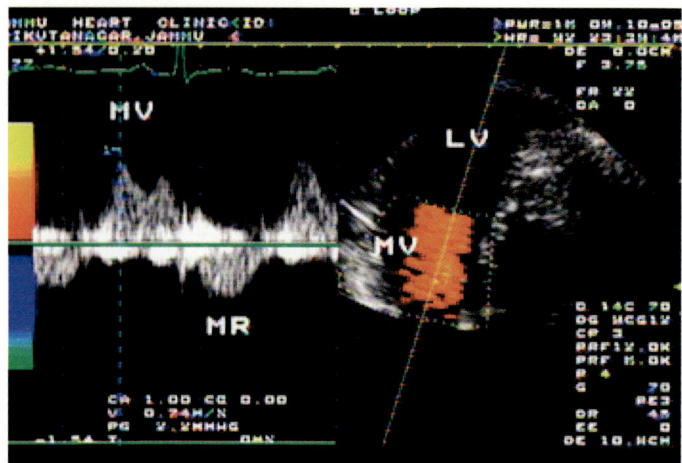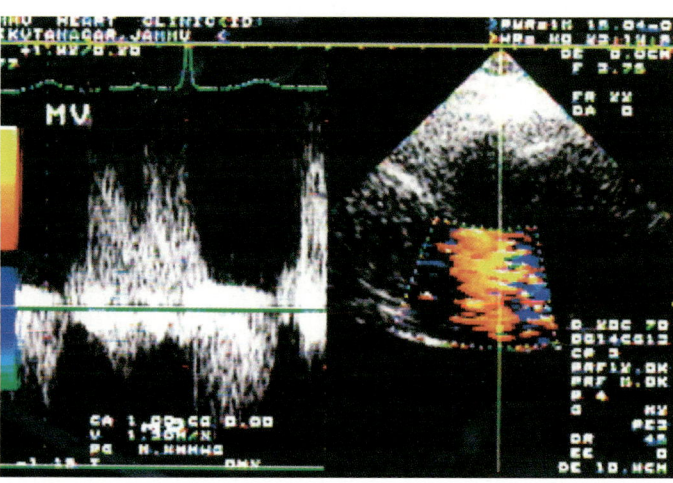

Fig. 3.15: An example of how regurgitant volume (RV) and regurgitant fraction (RF) can be measured has been cited from the formula and respective scans of MV and aortic valve. Showing mitral flow velocity in two chamber view of LV at the level of mitral annulus

Fig. 3.16: Apical 4C left parasternal view showing mosaic colored mitral obstructive flow (right) and wider spectral waveforms on continuous wave Doppler flow through roughened mitral valve (left) with MR in patient with mild degenerative mitral valve disease

In patients with valvular regurgitation, differences in stroke volume across different valves provides a quantitative assessment of severity.

$$SV_M = TV1_M \times CSAM$$
$$SV_A = TV1_A \times CSAA$$
$$RV_A = SV_A \times SV_M$$

SV_M = Stroke volume at mitral valve
SV_A = Stroke volume at aorta
RV_A = Regurgitant volume
TV_1 = Time velocity integral
CS_A = Cross sectional area

Differences in stroke volume (SV) across the aortic and mitral valves may reflect regurgitation at one of these sites. In a patient with aortic regurgitation, regurgitant volume (RVA) is simply the difference between the aortic stroke volume and the mitral stroke volume. For CSA calculation diameters at mitral anulus and aortic outflow tract can be measured from two to three scan taken one after the other to eliminate any error in calculation.

Regurgitation volume = aortic systolic flow – mitral diastolic flow

Regurgitation fraction in aortic regurgitation can also be calculated as:

$$Regurgitant\ fraction\ (\%) = \frac{Regurgitant\ volume}{Aortic\ outflow\ volume} \times 100\%$$

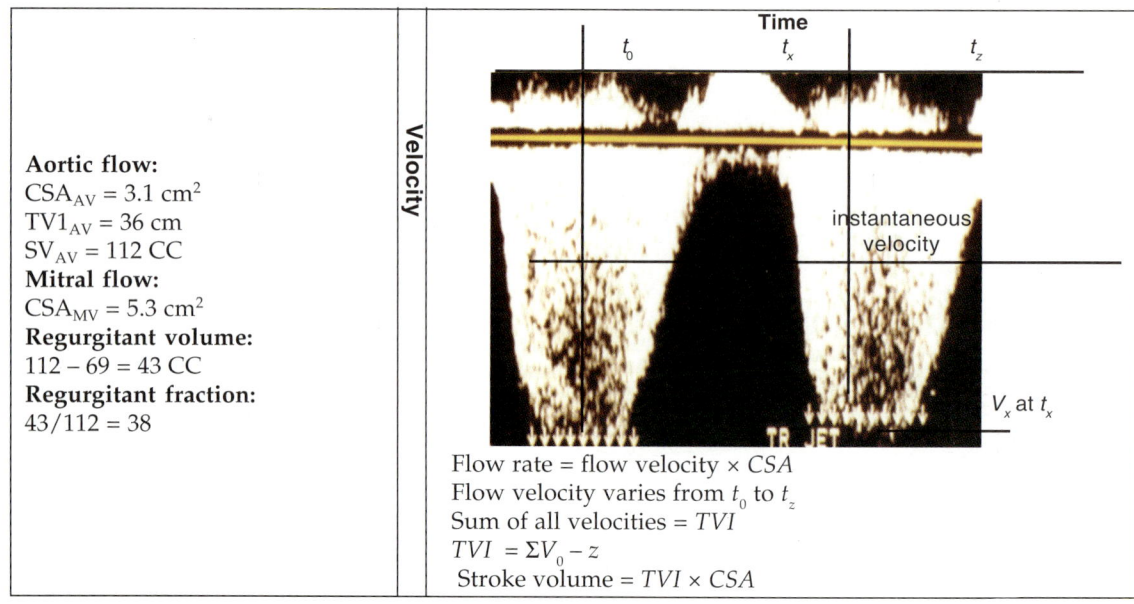

Aortic flow:
$CSA_{AV} = 3.1\ cm^2$
$TV1_{AV} = 36\ cm$
$SV_{AV} = 112\ CC$
Mitral flow:
$CSA_{MV} = 5.3\ cm^2$
Regurgitant volume:
$112 - 69 = 43\ CC$
Regurgitant fraction:
$43/112 = 38$

Flow rate = flow velocity × CSA
Flow velocity varies from t_0 to t_z
Sum of all velocities = TVI
$TVI = \Sigma V_0 - z$
Stroke volume = $TVI \times CSA$

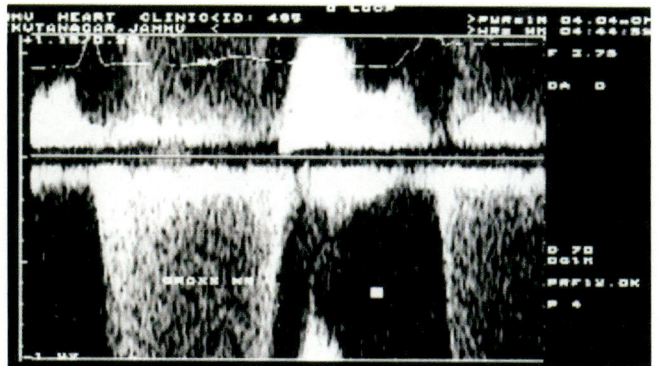

Fig. 3.17: Doppler flow across mildly stenosed mitral valve with grade III-IV type of mitral regurgitation

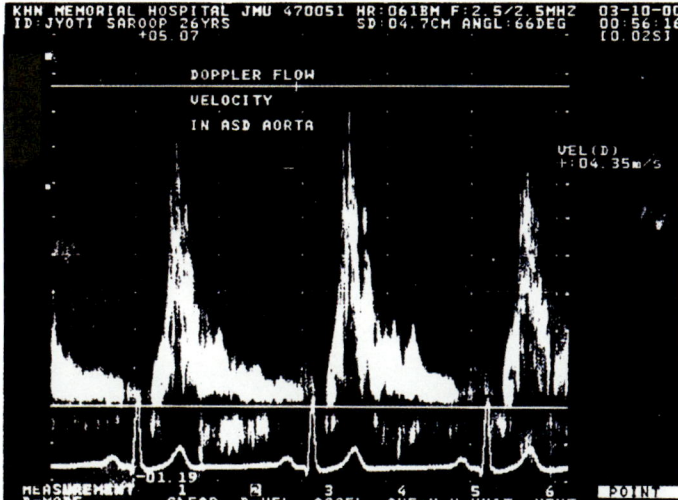

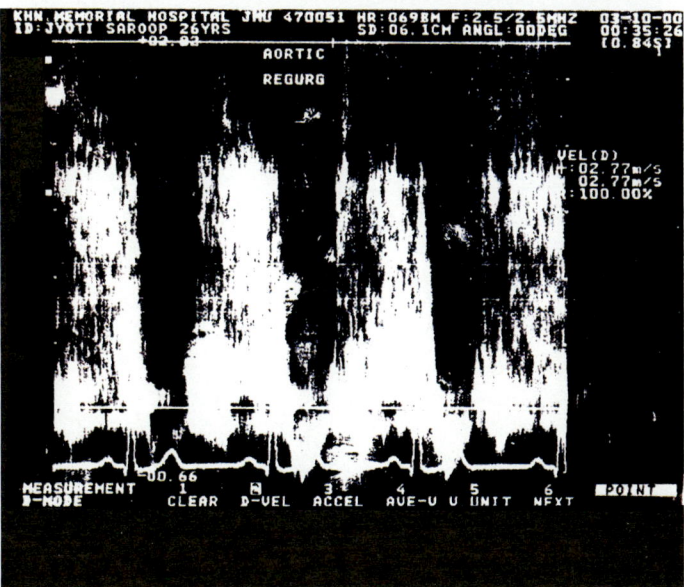

Fig. 3.18: Upper panel shows CW Doppler flow velocity in aortic stenosis. Pressure gradient across the valve was calculated according to the Bernoulli formula, i.e. Pressure gradient = 4 × V^2 = 4 × 4.35^2 mm of Hg. Similarily In the lower panel diastolic pressure gradient in case of severe aortic regurgitation was calculated

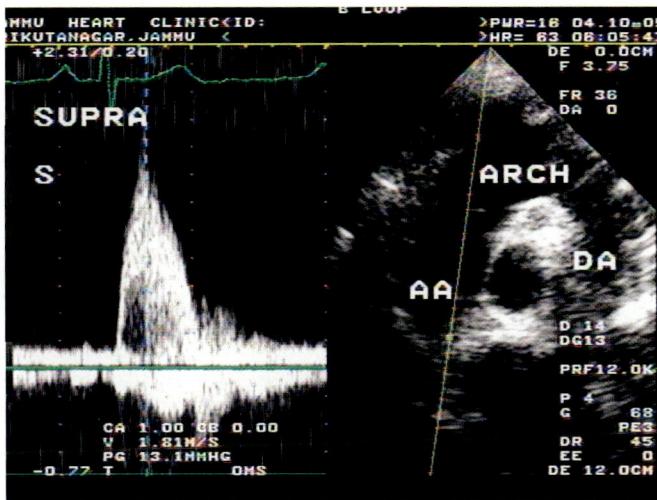

Fig. 3.19: Upper panel shows CW Doppler peak velocity of aortic valve in moderately severe aortic stenosis . Pressue gradient across the valve was calculated by the application of Bernoulli formula.

Abnormal Flow:

Causes of Flow Disturbance

Most velocities look somewhat disturbed in this position because flow is changing direction. Most flow disturbances found in the ascending aorta have relaminarised by the time they reach this location. Any lesion in the transverse aorta (a dissection, supravalver aortic stenosis or tubular hypoplasia) could cause a flow disturbance in the descending aorta.

Cause of a Jet

Coarctation of the aorta.

Potential Problems

Spectral Broadening: Causes a major problem in this location. Imaging is not usually a problem.

Summary of Various Hemodynamic Informations as Derived by Doppler Echocardiographic Equations

A. **L.V. volume** is best measured using the modified Simpson method (disk summation method). This involves tracing the LV area from two orthogonal views (typically A4C and A2C) and dividing the LV into a number of cylinders of equal height. Volume is calculated by adding up the totals of all combined cylinders. All modern machines and digital echo reading systems have integrated software to create and combine the volume data after simply tracing the LV areas in both apical views.

B. **Ejection fraction (EF)** is the standard measure of LV systolic function. It can be measured using two primary methods:

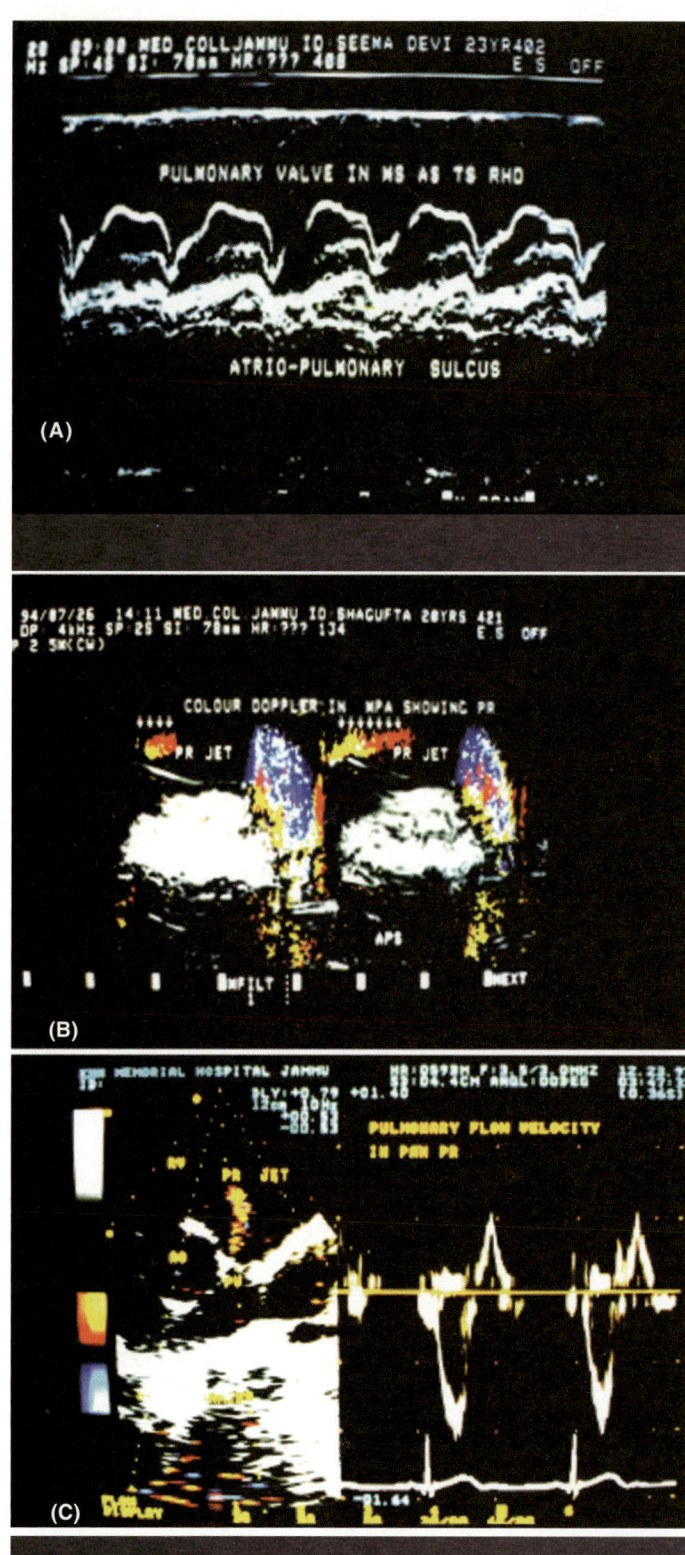

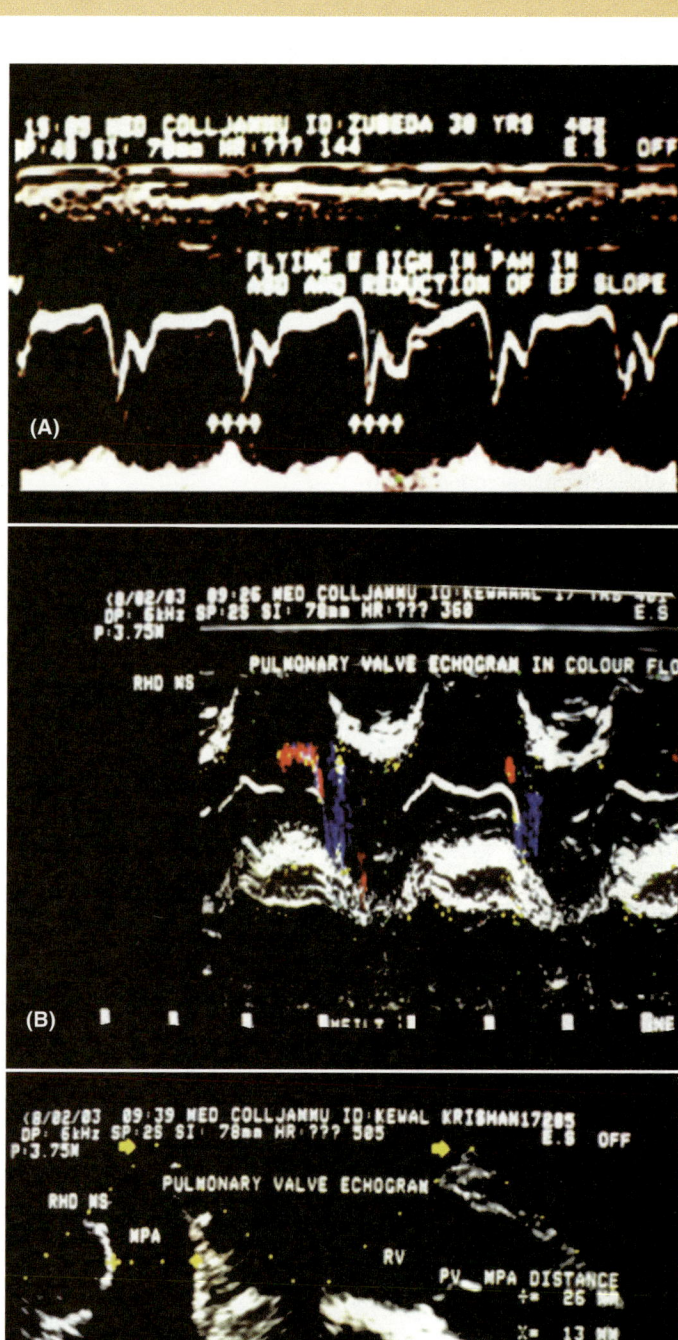

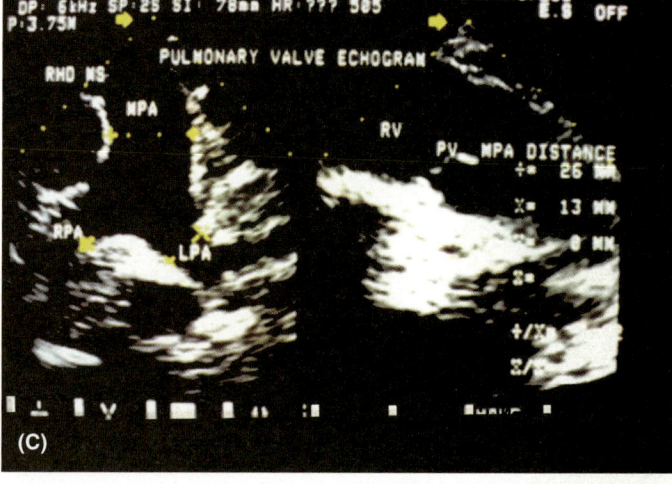

Fig. 3.20A to C: Upper panel shows M-mode pulmonary valve scan depicting reduced EF slope and thickening recorded at the level of atrio-pulmonary sulcus in PV stenosis. Middle panel shows color flow of pulmonary regurgitation jet in severe pulmonary arterial hypertension. In lower panel as in middle shows CW Doppler flow velocity as calculated by Bernoulli formula for grading the severity of pulmonary disease

Fig. 3.21A to C: Upper panel shows M-mode echo scan of pulmonary valve depicting typical flying W sign as observed in severe pulmonary arterial hypertension. In middle panel color PV M-mode scan shows reduction in EF slope and PR jet in moderate pulmonary arterial hypertension. The lower panel shows the measurement of diameters of MPA at the level of pulmonary valve for the determination of stroke volume by the application of formula; Area = 0.785*D2. Stroke volume = 0.785*D2*TVI = ml

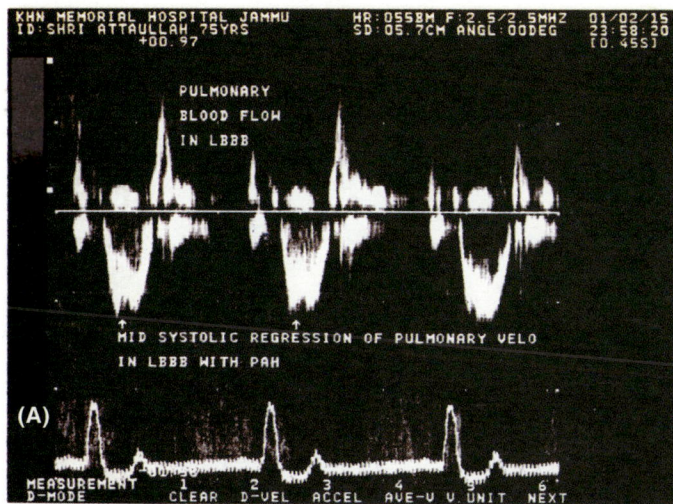

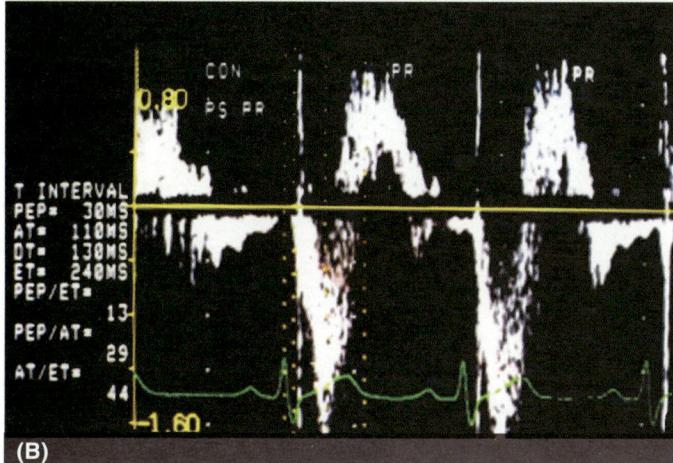

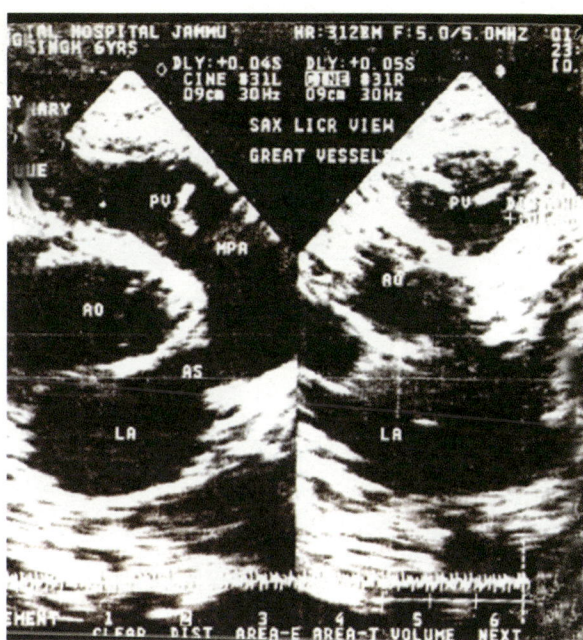

Fig. 3.23B: Reveals as how to calculate pulmonary and systemic blood flow with finding out of cross sectional area at pulmonary and aortic conduits

Fig. 3.22A and B: (A) Upper panel CW Doppler flow velocity across PV showing systolic regression of peak velocity in severe pulmonary arterial hypertension. **(B)** Lower panel shows calculation of various hemodynamic time intervals by pulsed Doppler particularly PEP/AT and AT/ET ratios for the determination of severity of pulmonary arterial hypertension

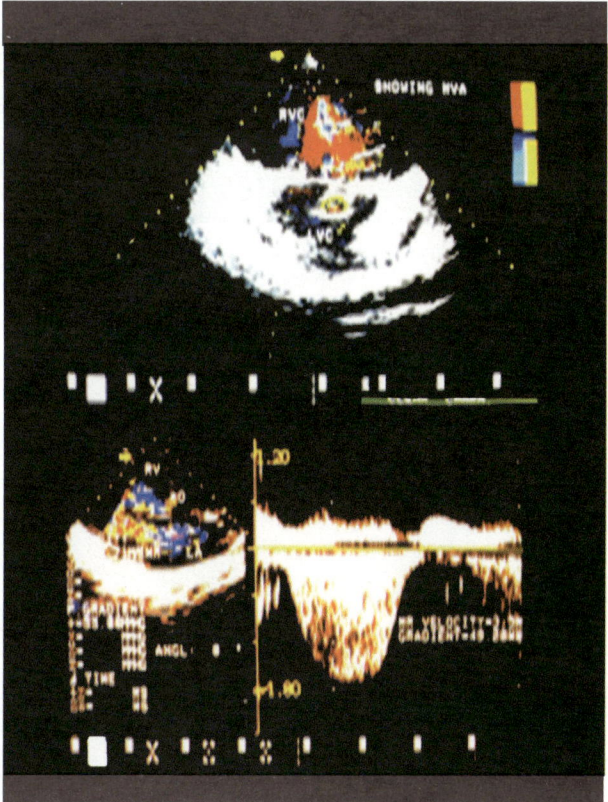

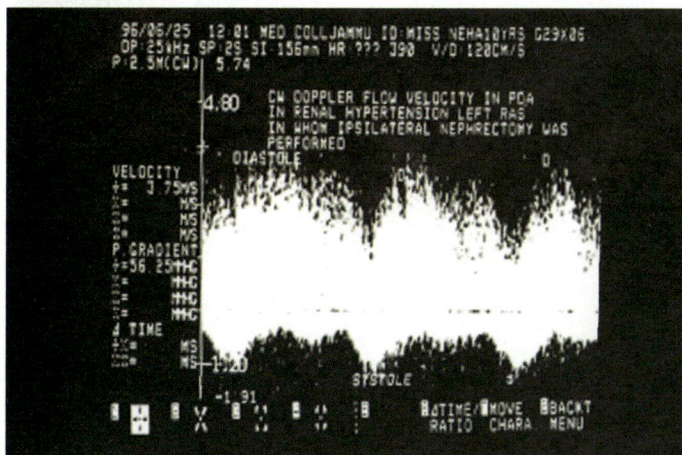

Fig. 3.23A: Continuous wave Doppler scan of PDA flow velocity for the calculation of Qp/Qs ratio for determination of preoperative severity of PDA shunt.

Fig. 3.24: Color flow scan at MV determining the severity of mitral stenosis by finding out MVA by trace method as shown in color scan

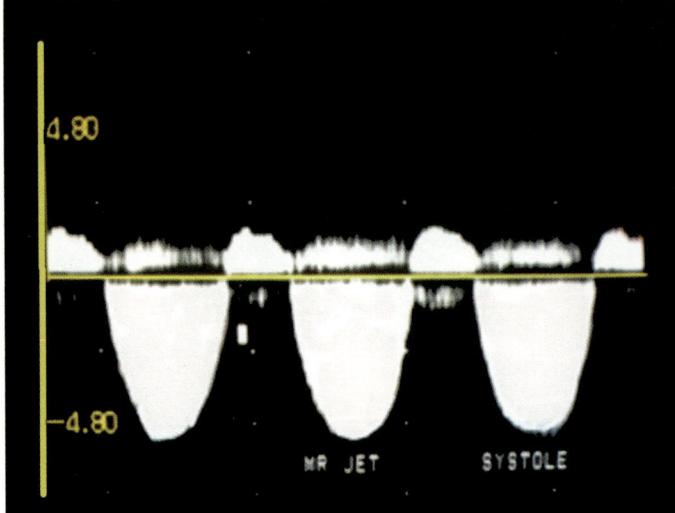

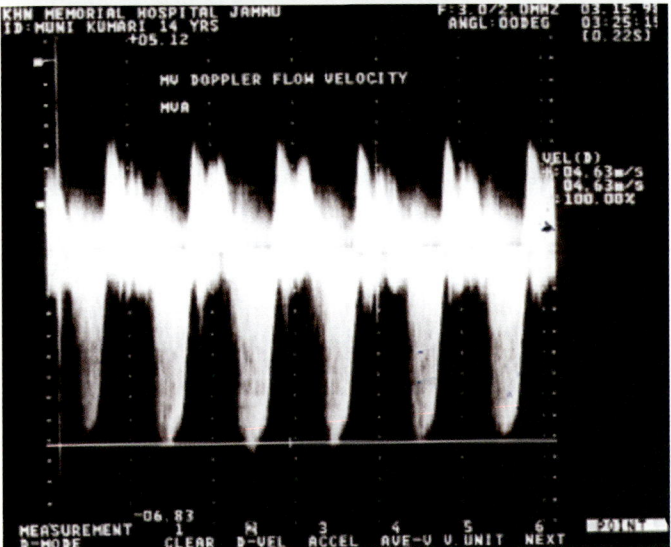

Fig. 3.25: Upper panel shows CW Doppler scan of MR jet envelope in dilated cardiomyopathy with diastolic gradient of 4×4.80^2 85 mmHg. Similarily lower panel shows a peak Doppler velocity of 4.63 m/sec preliminary to the calculation of pressure gradient by the application of Bernoulli formula

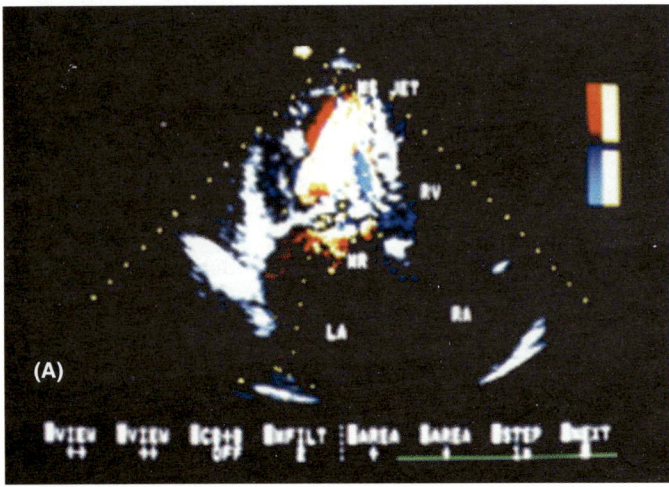

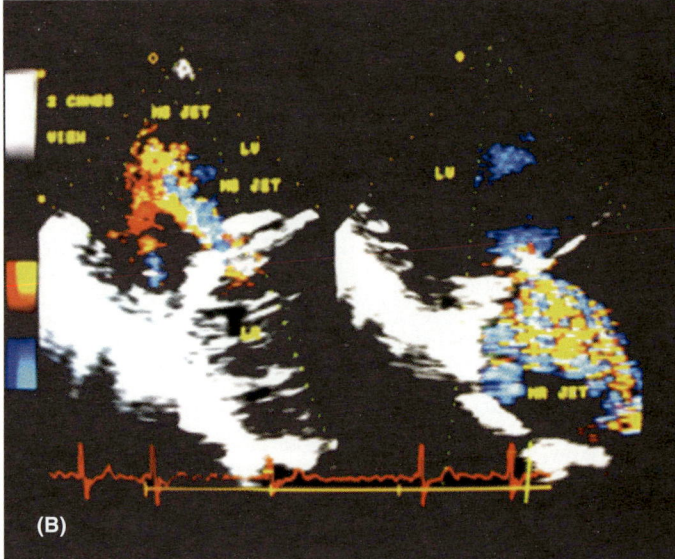

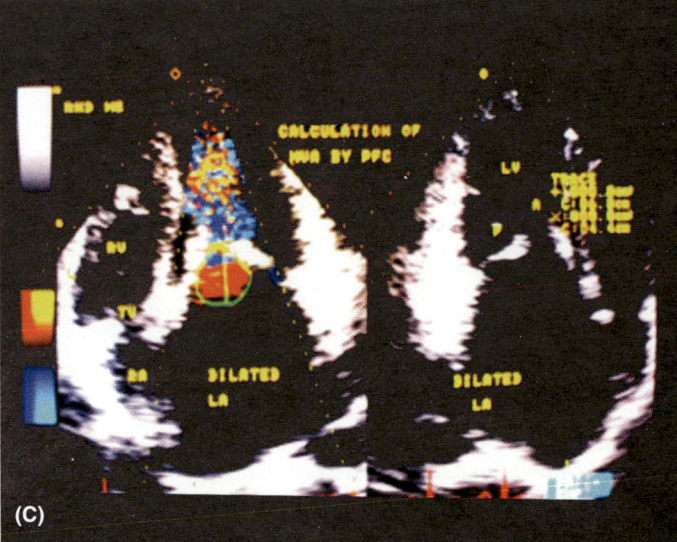

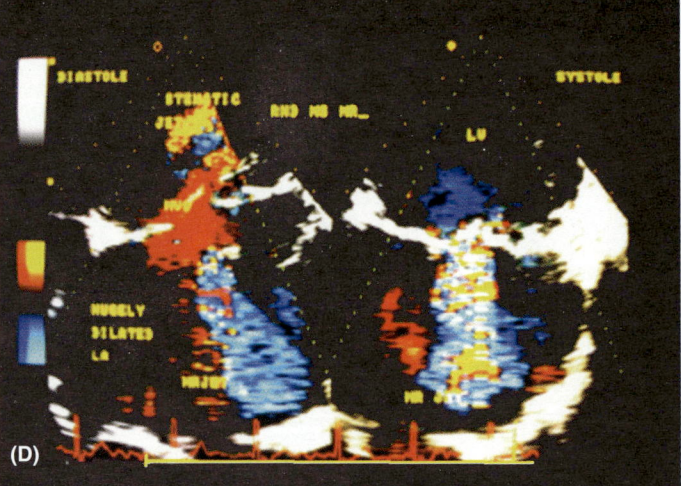

Fig. 3.26A to D: An example as how to determine the severity of mitral regurgitation by the application of proximal isovelocity surface area

$$\text{Flow} = 2\pi \times r^2 \times \text{Va}$$
$$\text{ERO} = \text{Flow} + V_{MR}$$
$$\text{RV} = \text{ERO} \times \text{TV}_{MR}$$

Table 3.5: *Measurement of flow rate, orifice area and regurgitant volume*

To measure regurgitant flow rate	*To measure effective regurgitant orifice area*	*To measure regurgitant volume*
Flow rate = $6.25 \times r^2 \times V_a$	ERO = Flow rate/V_{MR}	RV = ERO × TVI$_{MR}$
Flow rate = 6.28.682 × 30	ERO = 87/523	RV = 0.17 × 187
Flow rate = 87 cc	ERO = 0.17 cm^2	RV = 31 cc

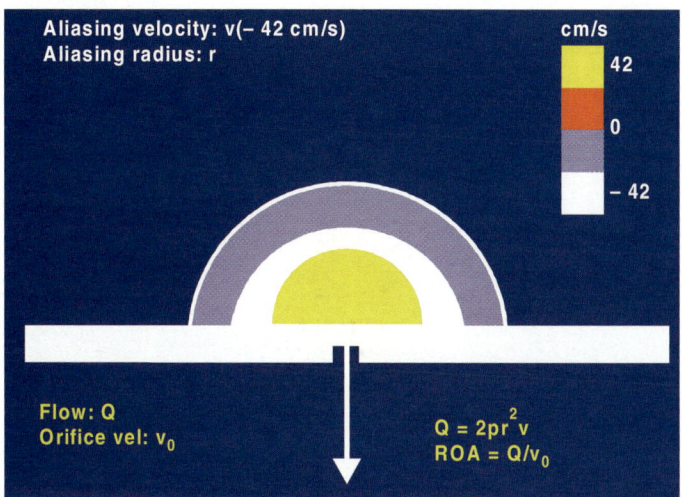

Fig. 3.27: The proximal convergence method uses the aliasing velocity of the color Doppler scan, it is possible to measure the radius to an isovelocity shell as blood converges on the regurgitant orifice, assuming a hemispheric shape to the shell, flow rate is given as Q = 2pr^2 × v dividing this flow rate by the maximal velocity through the orifice (given by CW Doppler) yields an estimation for the regurgitant orifice area (ROA)

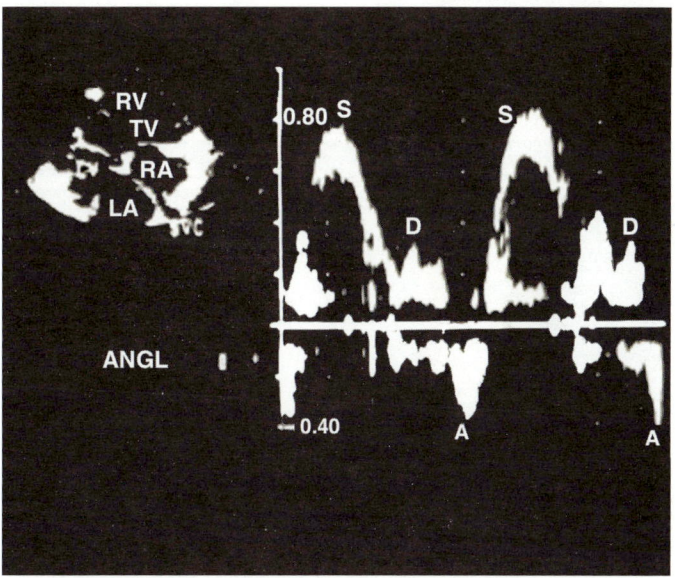

Fig. 3.29: Normal Doppler pulmonary venus waveforms

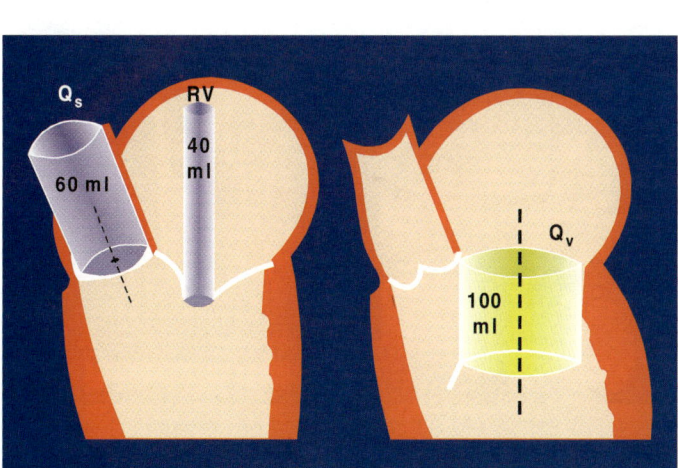

Fig. 3.28: The principle of the volumetric assessment of valvar regurgitation. By measuring stroke volume in two areas of the heart, it is possible to use the difference between these to estimate regurgitant volume. Q_s = systemic stroke volume, Q_v = stroke volume across regurgitant valve, RV = regurgitant volume

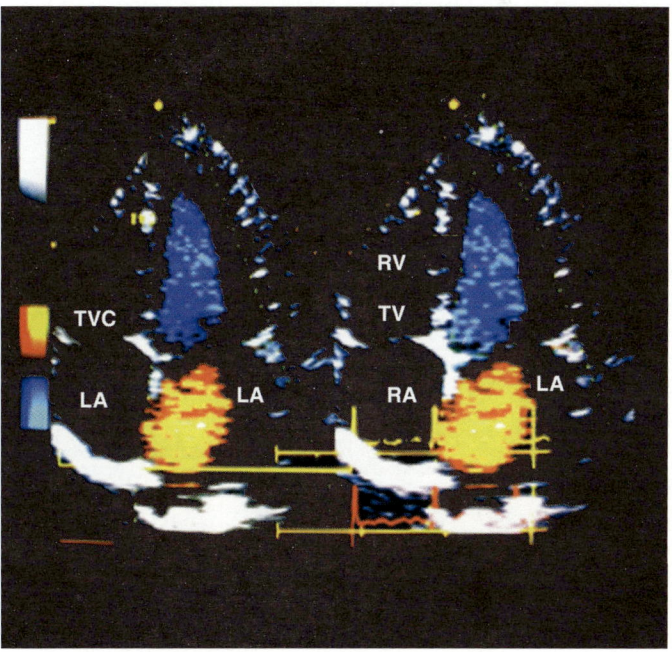

Fig. 3.30: Normal color flows in LA and pulmonary vein

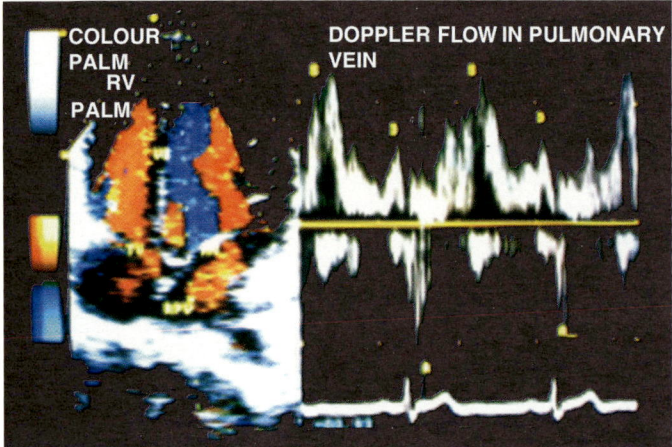

Fig. 3.31: Mild rise in pulmonary venous pressure

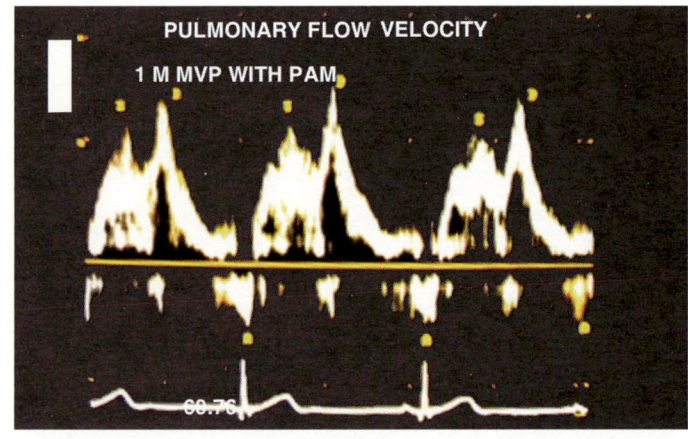

Fig. 3.34: Moderate rise in pulmonary venous pressure

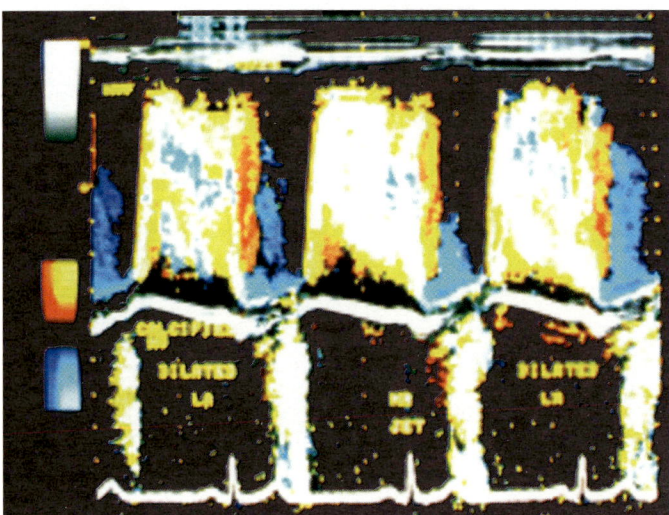

Fig. 3.32: A case of RHD, MS + MR with raised pulmonary venus presssure

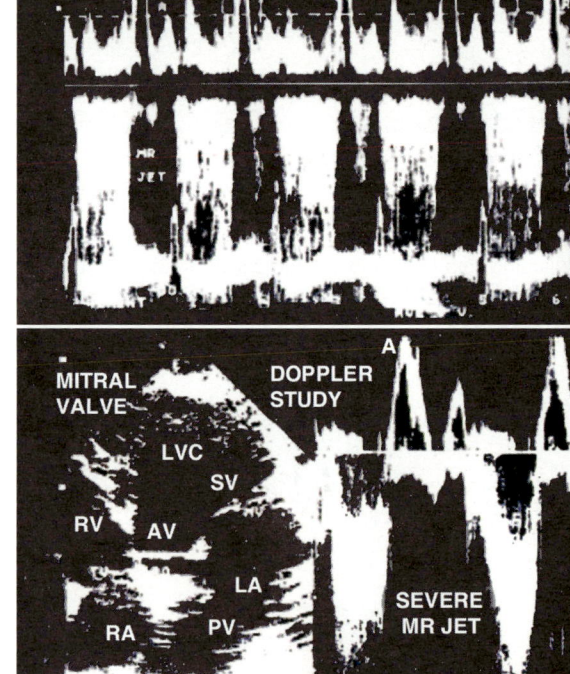

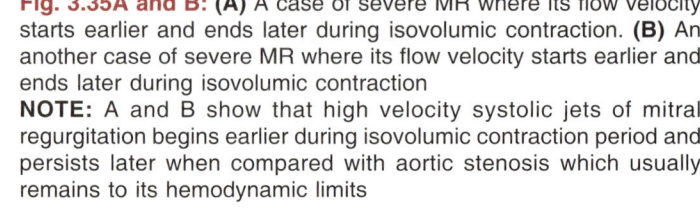

Fig. 3.35A and B: (A) A case of severe MR where its flow velocity starts earlier and ends later during isovolumic contraction. **(B)** An another case of severe MR where its flow velocity starts earlier and ends later during isovolumic contraction

NOTE: A and B show that high velocity systolic jets of mitral regurgitation begins earlier during isovolumic contraction period and persists later when compared with aortic stenosis which usually remains to its hemodynamic limits

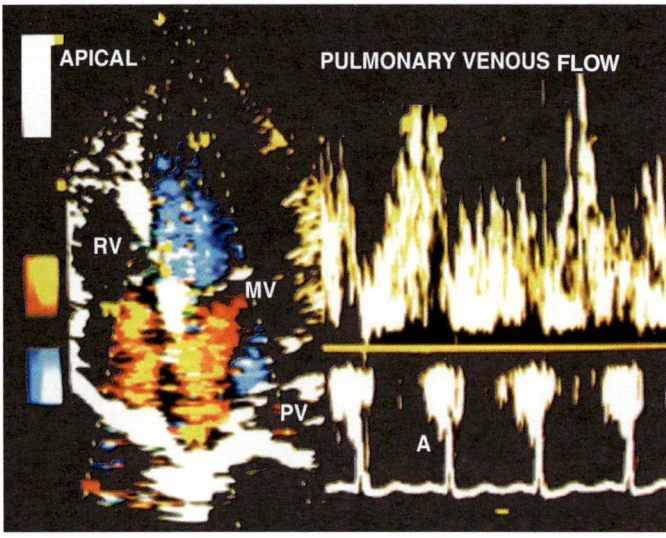

Fig. 3.33: Reversal of flow in severe MR

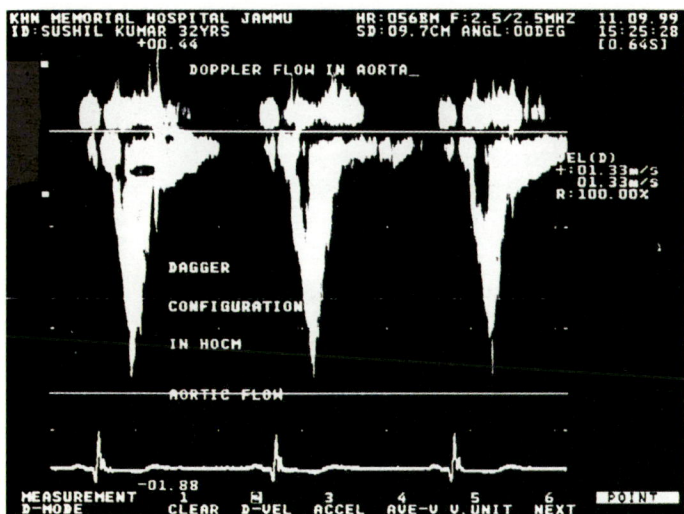

Fig. 3.36: A case of subaortic obstruction due to HOCM where its velocity flow restricts to its isovolumic phase of contraction

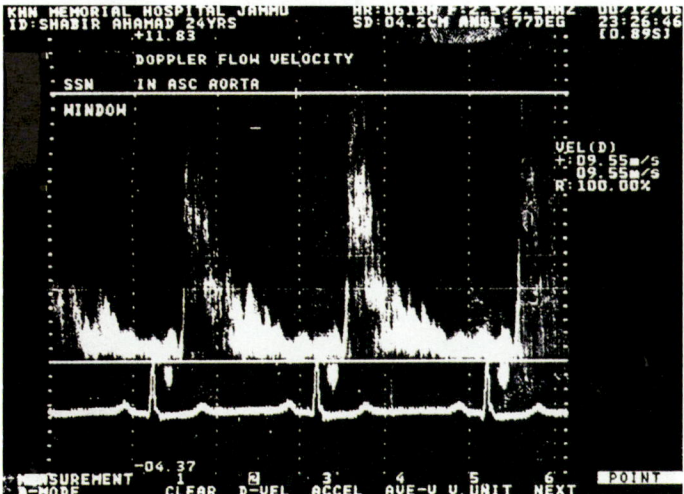

Fig. 3.37: A case of severe valvular aortic stenosis where its velocity flow restricts to its isovolumic phase of contraction

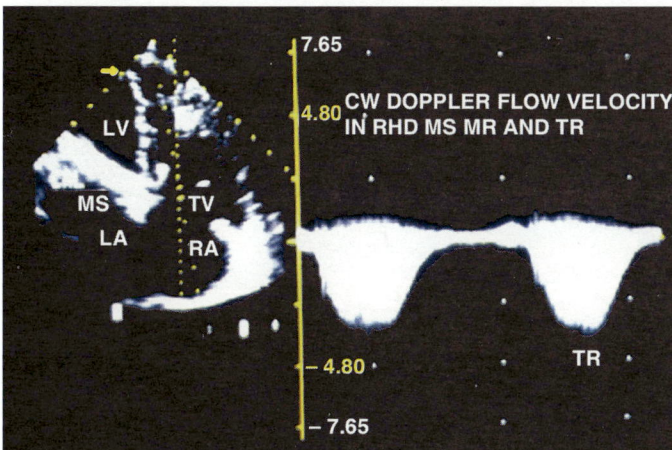

Fig. 3.38: 2-D and colour Doppler across tricuspid valve in patient with gross tricuspid regurgitation jet

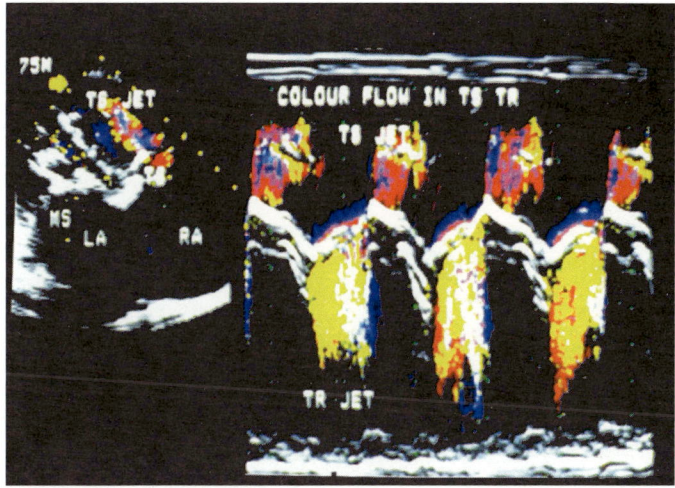

Fig. 3.39: 2-D and Doppler flow velocity across tricuspid valve in another patient with gross tricuspid regurgitation jet

An example;

$$PVR = TRV/TV1OT \times 10 + 0.16$$
$$= (4.17/9) \times 10 + 0.16$$
$$= 0.46 \times 10 + 0.16$$
$$= 4.8 \text{ Woods Units}$$

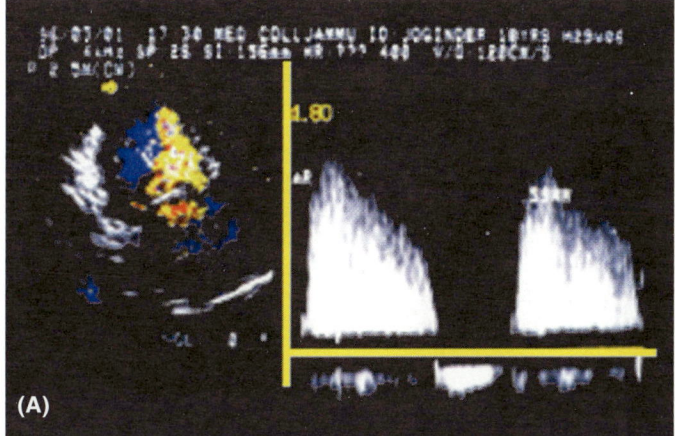

(A)

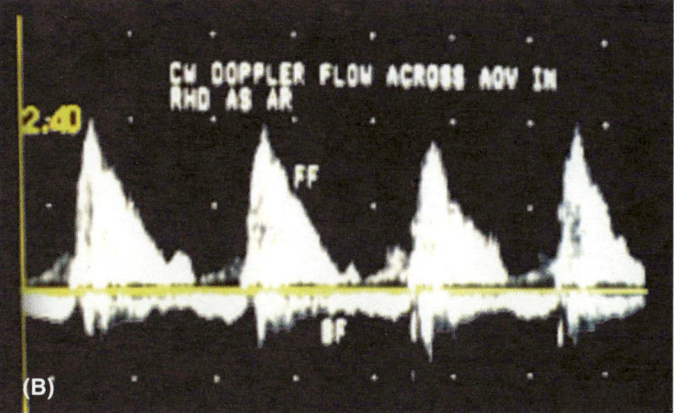

(B)

Fig. 3.40A and B: (A) CW Doppler flow velocity in calculation of diastolic gradient in severe aortic regurgitation. **(B)** CW Doppler flow velocity in aortic stenosis for determination of pressure gradient across the aortic valve by the application of Bernoulli equation

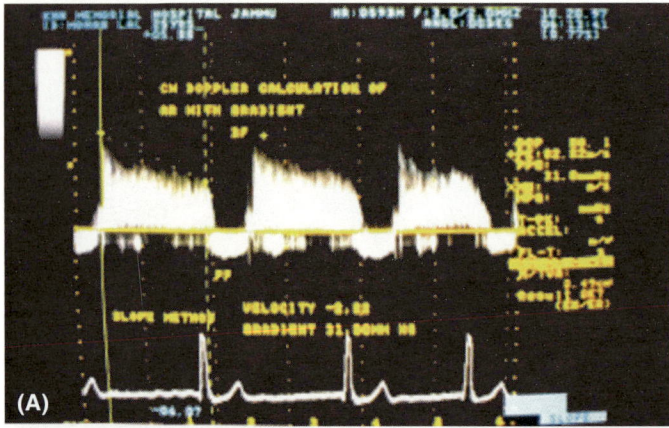

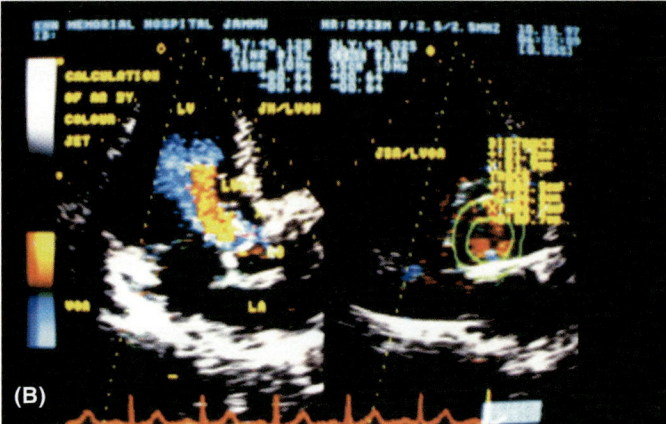

Fig. 3.41A and B: (A) Shows how to calculate gradient and severity of aortic valvar disease by slope method. **(B)** Application of Bernoulli equation to estimate left ventricular end diastolic pressure after determining the velocity of the aortic regurgitation (AR) at end-diastole, the aortic to left ventricular pressure gradient is calculated. By subtracting this value from the aortic diastolic pressure LVEDP is determined

Peak Flow Velocity of Tricuspid Regurgitation

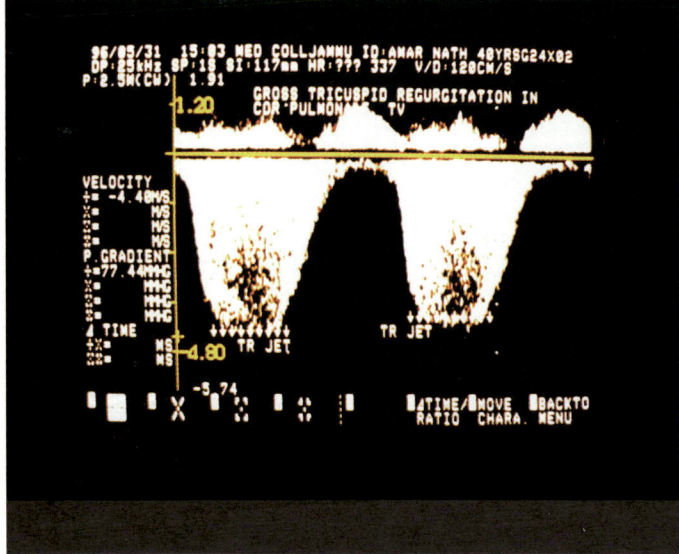

Fig. 3.42A

Time Velocity Integral (TVI) of the RVOT

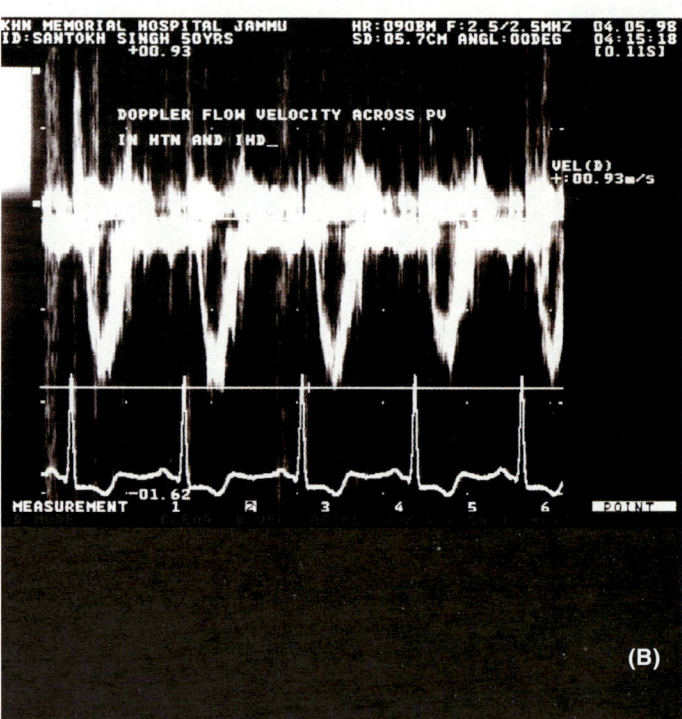

Fig. 3.42A and B: Pulmonary vascular resistance (PVR) = Peak velocity of tricuspid regurgitation (TR) jet and the time velocity integral (TV1) of the right ventricular outflow tract

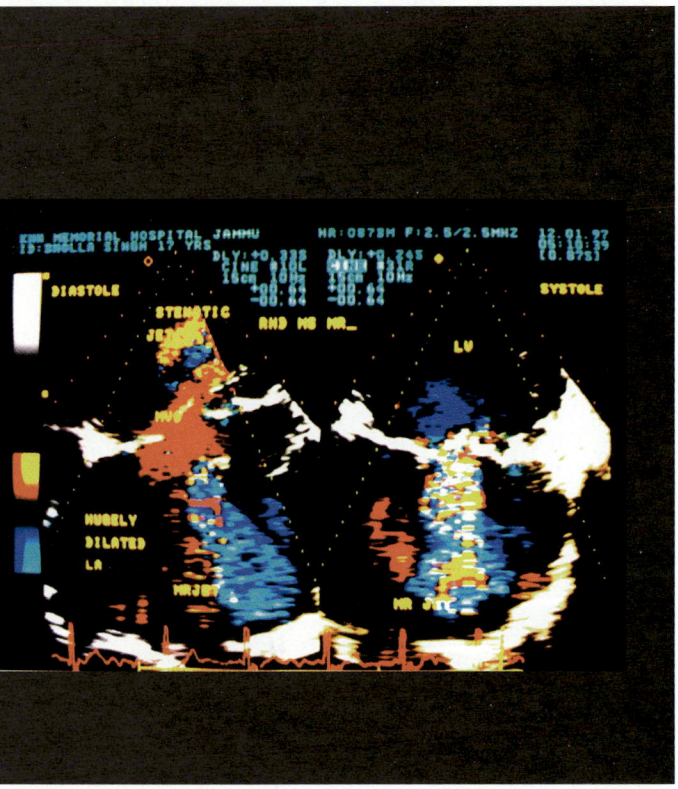

Fig. 3.43: 2-D Color flow showing severe MR jet in both in blue and yellowish red which becomes the baseline for application of proximal isovelocity surface area equation

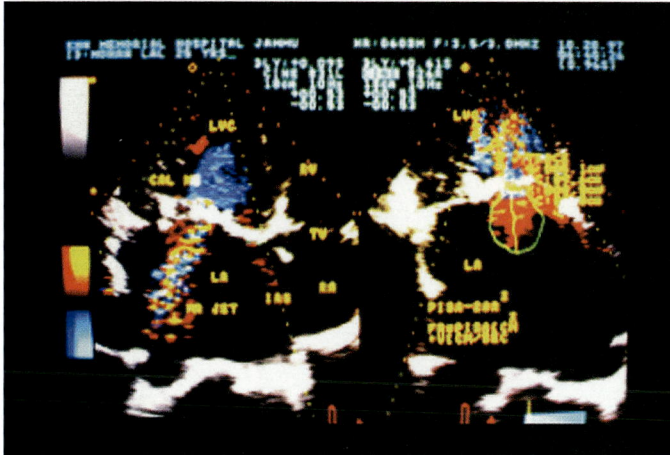

Fig. 3.44

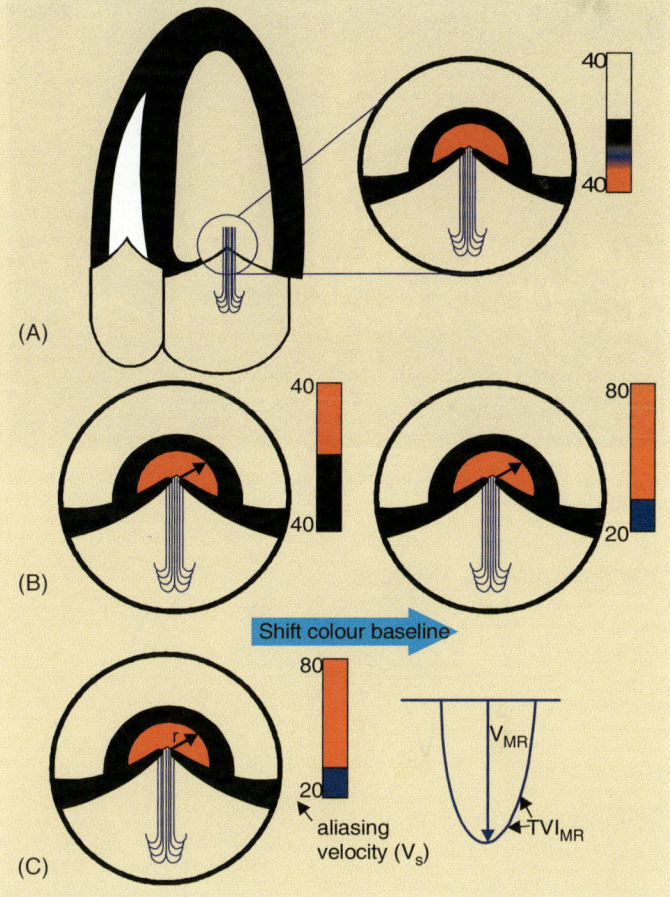

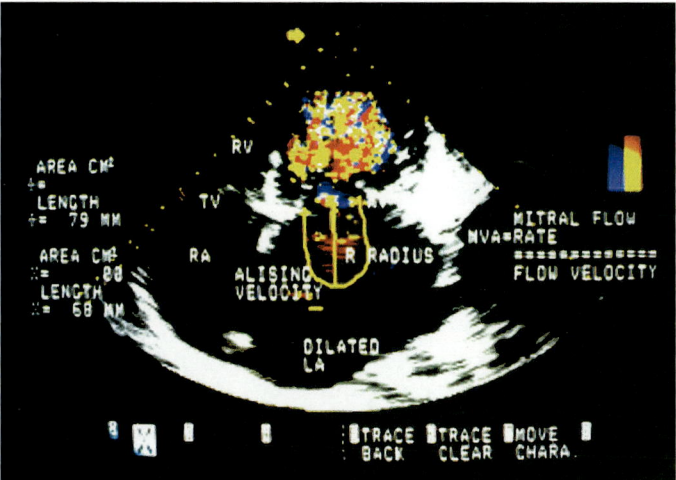

Fig. 3.44 and 3.45: 2-D Color Doppler MV showing an example of how MS grading is determined by application of proximal isovelocity surface area

Fig. 3.46: Estimation of severity of mitral regurgitation (MR) by the application of the proximal isovelocity surface area method. **(A)** The schematic demonstrates how regurgitant flow converges and accelerates in a series of isovelocity shells, indicated by the red and blue patterns. **(B)** The radius of the shell is measured, after the baseline has been shifted to maximize its size. From this, the surface area of the shell is determined. **(C)** Using the continuity equation, the calculations required to measure flow, effective regurgitant orifice (ERO) area and regurgitant volume(RV) are determined r = radius,Va aliasing velocity; VMR, maximal MR jet velocity

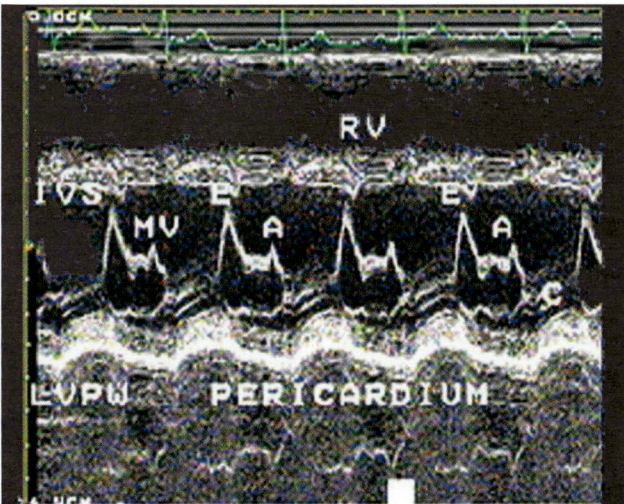

Fig. 3.47: Showing M-mode signatures of normal mitral valve depicting E wave

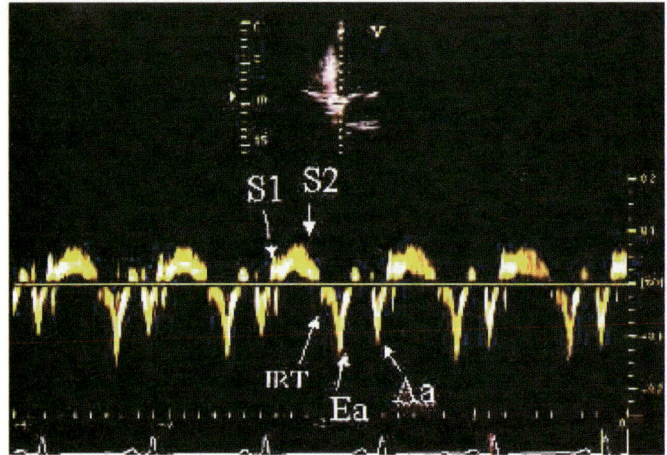

Fig. 3.48: Normal tissue Doppler flow velocity at mitral annulus depicting Ea wave

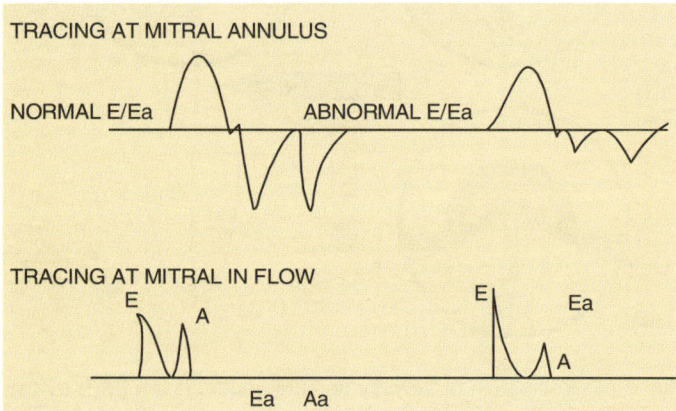

NOTE: In normal individual E/Ea = 5 – 10 whereas in elevated LV filling pressures it is 15–40

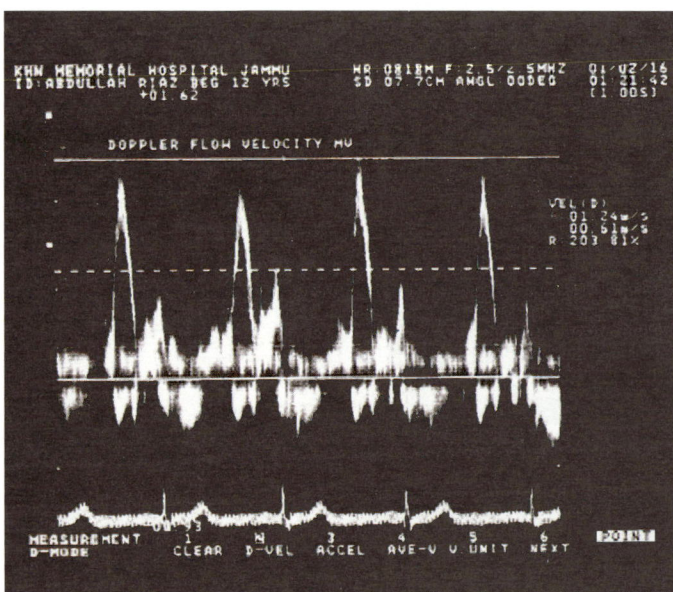

Fig. 3.49: Larger E wave indicating elevated left ventricular filling pressure

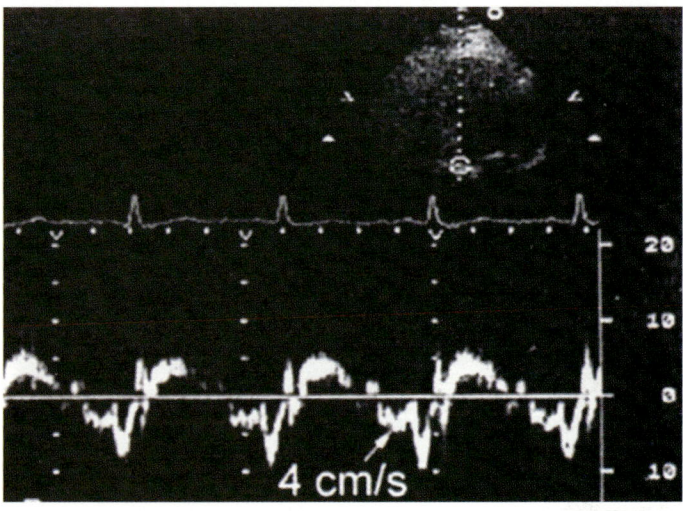

Fig. 3.50: Decrease in Ea wave in gross dysfunction of LV with increased filling pressures on tissue Doppler scan

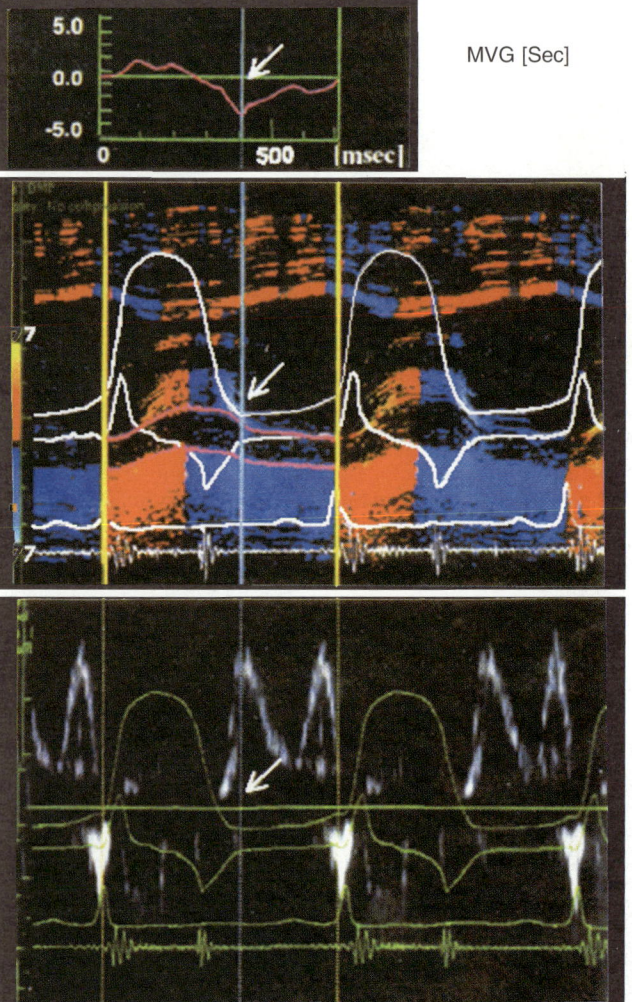

Fig. 3.51: Myocardial velocity gradient (MVG) (upper panel), tissue Doppler M-mode (middle panel), and transmitral velocity recording (lower panel) with LV pressure and phonocardiogram (PCG) in a patient with hypertrophic cardiomyopathy

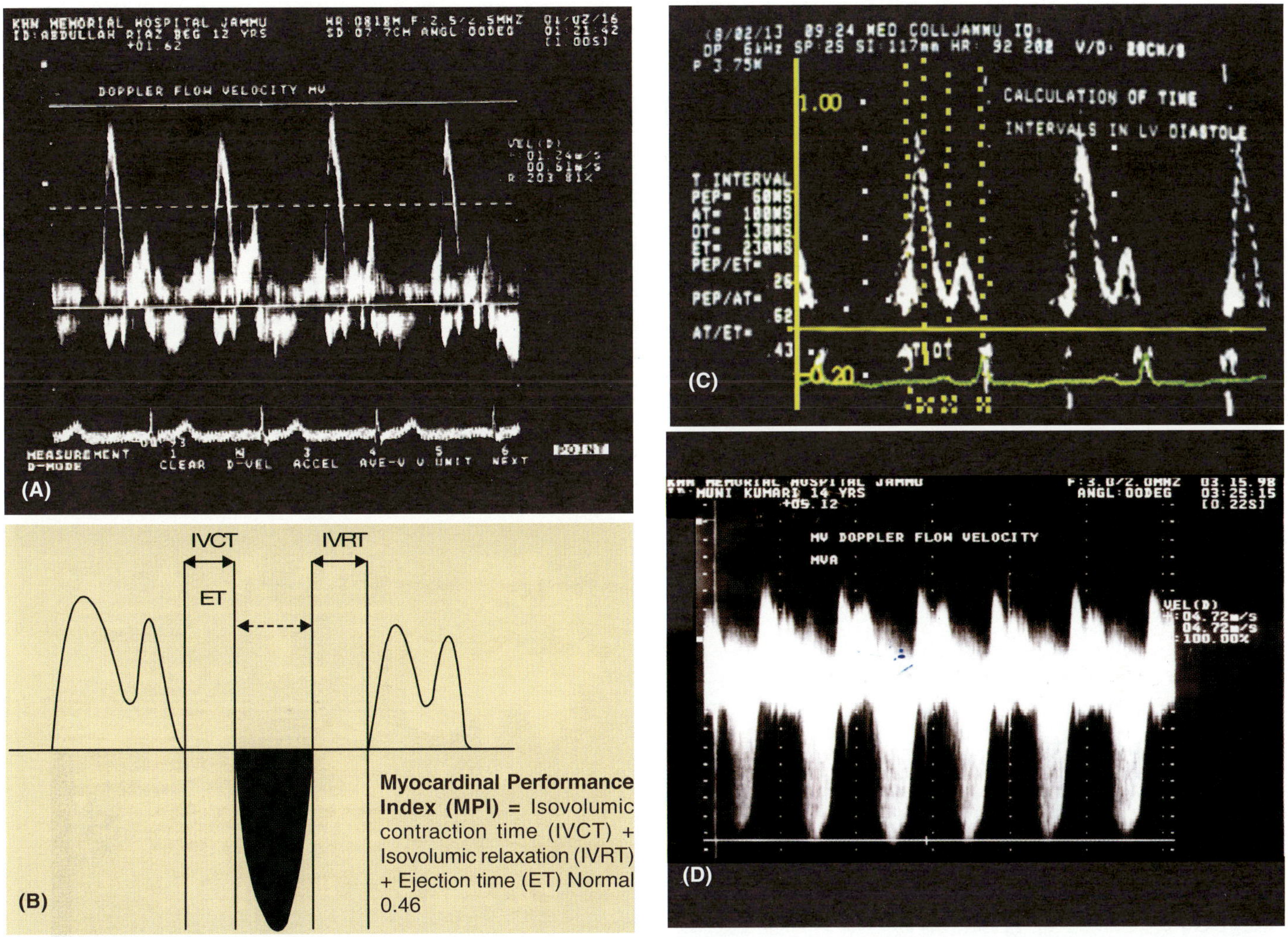

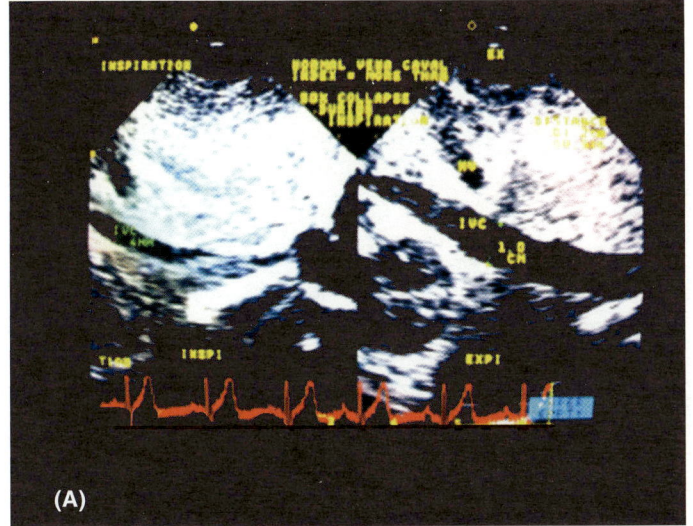

Fig. 3.52A to D: **(A)** Pulsed Doppler flow velocity of normal MV. **(B)** Graphic technique of calculation of myocardial performance index as shown in this figure. **(C)** Pulsed Doppler tracing from a normal MV with calculation of hemodynamic intervals. **(D)** Doppler flow velocity signatures from a patient suffering from MV disease with gross MR in calculation of MPI

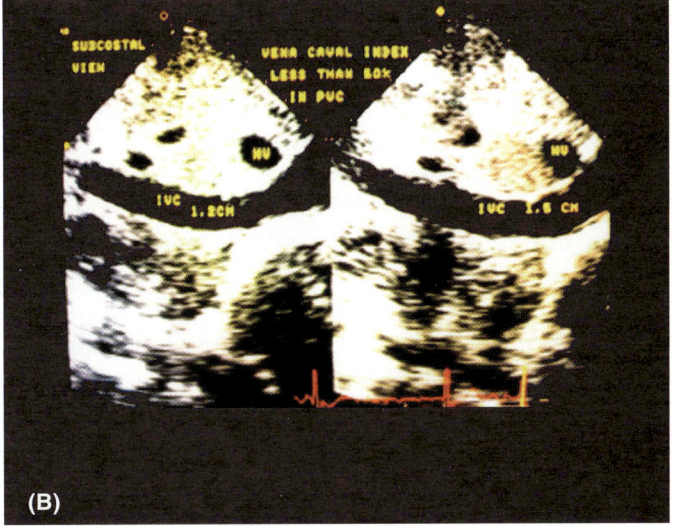

Fig. 3.53A and B: **(A)** Normal inspiratory collapse of IVC in a healthy normal person. **(B)** Failure of inspiratory collapse of IVC less than 50% in a patient with very high right atrial and ventricular pressure in cor-pulmonale

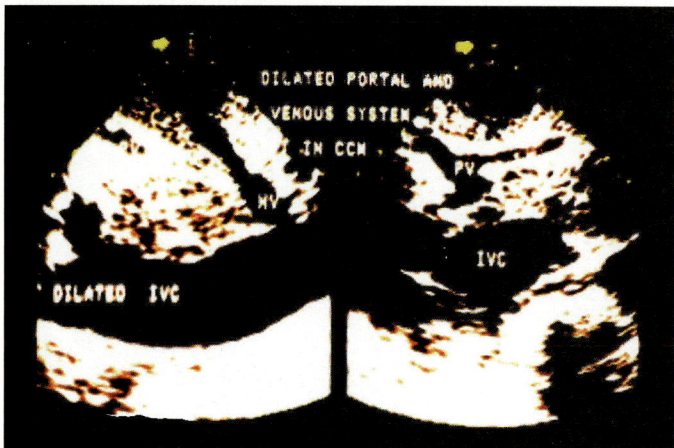

Fig. 3.54A: Dilated peripheral venous system particularly hepatic and IVC in case of dilated cardiomyopathy. It indicates raised RA and RV pressure

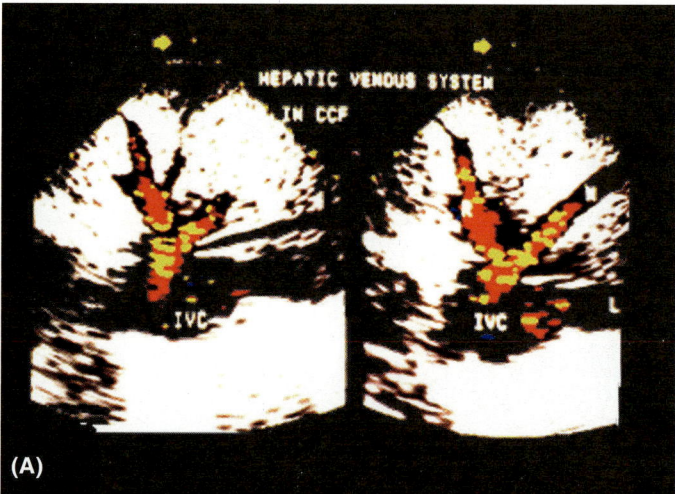

(A)

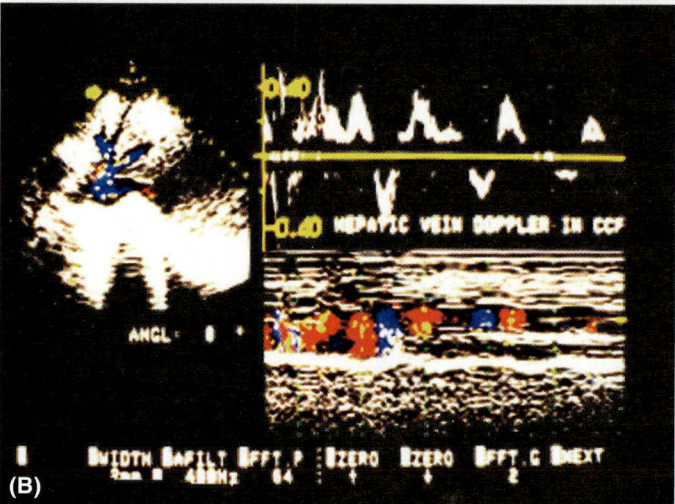

(B)

Fig 3.55A and B: (A) Color flow patterns in IVC and its branches due to raised venous pressure in right-sided heart failure. **(B)** Depicts reversal of flow on pulsed Doppler and mosaic pattern of color of blood flow in hepatic vein indicating raised peripheral venous pressure in congestive heart failure

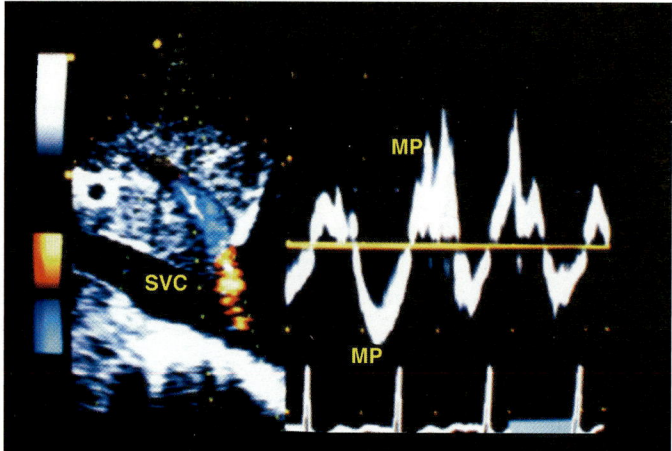

Fig. 3.54B: Pulsed color Doppler flow velocity showing reversal of flow in case of right-sided heart failure indicating raised peripheral venous pressure

1. EF from volume data obtained by **Simpson s method:**
   Stroke volume (SV) = end-diastolic volume (EDV) – end-systolic volume (ESV)

   $$EF = SV/EDV \times 100\%$$
   $$\textbf{EF = EDV}\ \check{}\ \textbf{ESV/EDV}\quad \textbf{100\%}$$

2. **Quinones method** is based on measurement of internal dimensions of the LV:

   $$EF = [(\%\Delta D^2) + (1 - \% D^2)]\ [\%\Delta L]$$

   $\%\Delta D^2$ = fractional shortening of the square of the minor axis
   $$= LVE\ \Delta d^2 - LVEDs^2/LVED^2$$

   $\%\Delta L^2$ = fractional shortening of the long axis, mainly related to apical contraction (15% for normal; 5% for hypokinetic; 0% for akinetic; – 5% for dyskinetic; – 10% for apical aneurysm)

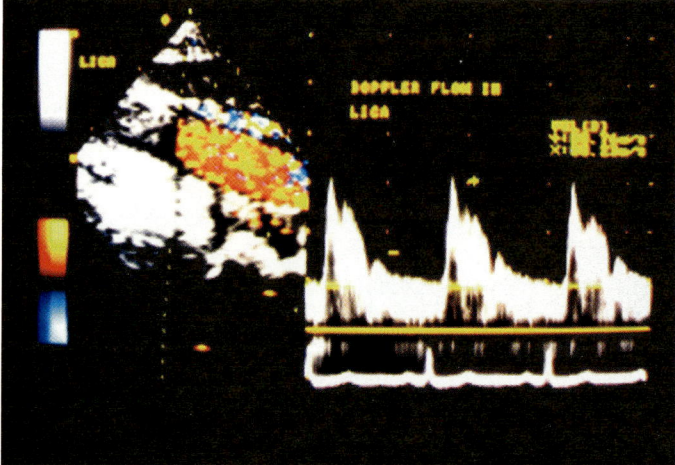

Fig. 3.56: Color Doppler flow velocity across left internal carotid artery shows mosaic pattern and enhanced flow velocity indicating thickened and irregular intimal lining

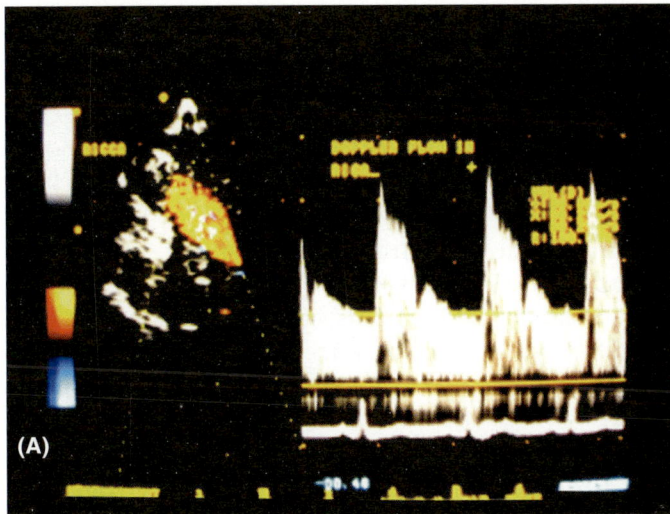

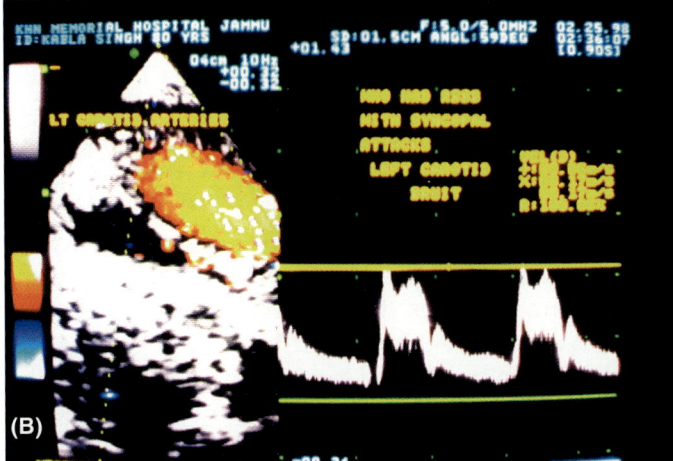

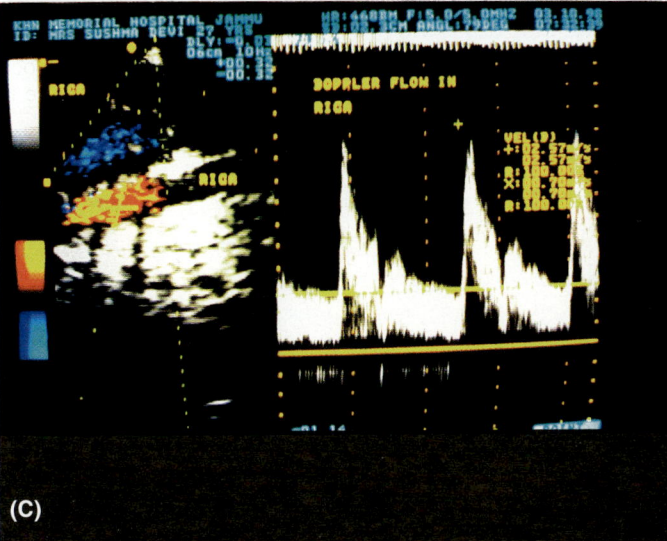

Fig. 3.57A to C: (A) Color Doppler flow velocity across right internal carotid artery with broadned spectral of flow indicating obstructive pathology in this vessel **(B)** Color Doppler scan of left internal carotid artery obstruction with post- stenotic dilatation of vessel with mosaic color in a patient with recurrent syncopal episodes. **(C)** Color Doppler flow velocity in the region of right internal carotid artery shows near normal flow pattern

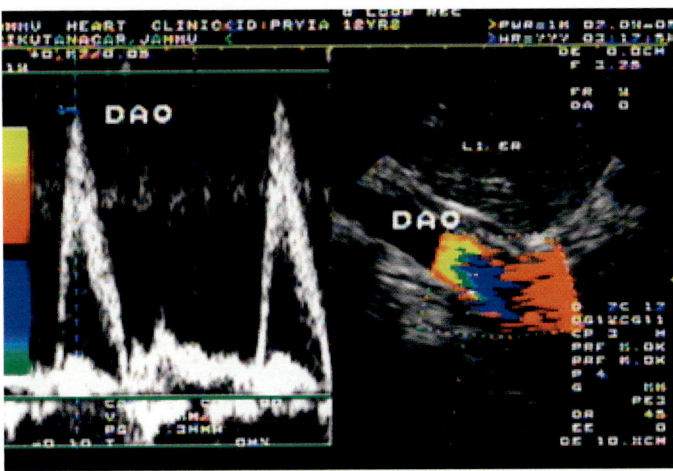

Fig. 3.58: Laminar flow through the abdominal aorta recorded from the subcostal window with pulsed Doppler transducer. The vertical velocity spike at endsystole indicates aortic valve flow

LVEDd = LV end-diastolic diameter
LVEDs = LV end-systolic diameter (PLAX view)

C. Transvalvular pressure gradient: The **Bernoulli equation** allows measurement of relative pressure differences across valves, shunts, or the LVOT. In its complete form, the Bernoulli equation is too complex for routine clinical use, as it incorporates three main components: convective acceleration; inertial term (flow acceleration); and viscous friction In many clinical situations, the latter two components can be ignored, leaving the flow gradient across an orifice to be derived from the convective acceleration term alone:

$$\Delta P = 4 \times (V_2^2 - V_1^2)$$

where V_2 is velocity distal to an obstruction and V_1 is velocity proximal to an obstruction.

Flow proximal to a narrowed orifice (V_1) is much lower than the peak flow velocity (V_2) and can frequently be ignored leaving a **simplified Bernoulli equation:**

$$\Delta P = 4V^2$$

The simplified Bernoulli equation is unreliable when:
1. V_1 is greater than 1.0 m/s, which occursin serial lesions (subvalvular and valvular stenosis) and mixed stenosis with regurgitation.
2. Viscous resistance becomes significant in the evaluation of long stenoses (e.g. coarctation or a tunnel-like ventricular septal defect).
3. When the inertial term (flow acceleration) is not negligible (flow through normal valves).

It is important to realize that the Bernoulli equation represents the **maximal instantaneous gradient** across a stenosis, which is always higher than the customary peak-to-peak gradient (they do not occursimultaneouslyless physiologic) measured in the catheterization laboratory.

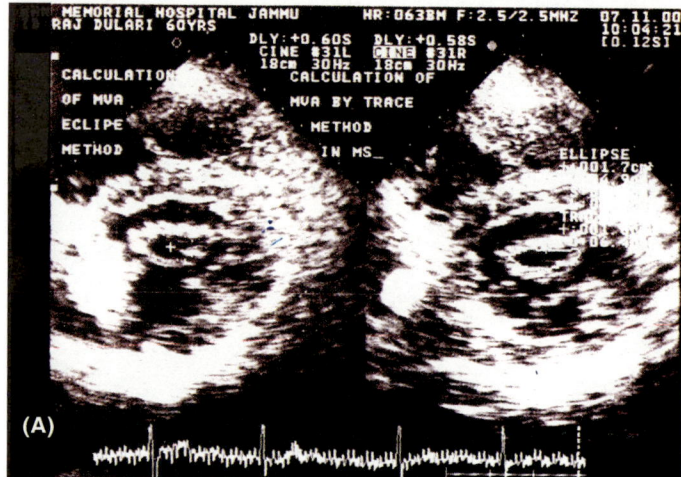

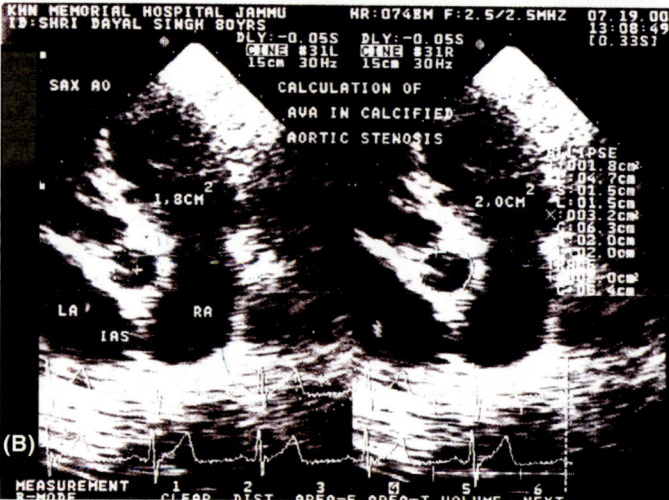

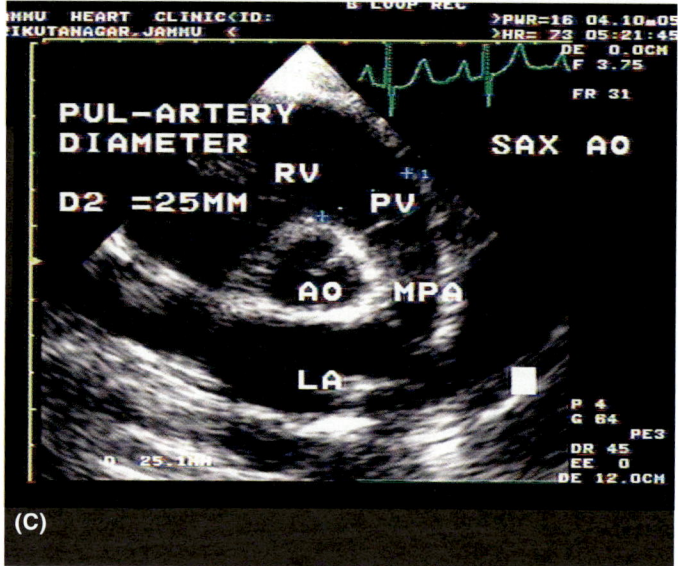

Fig. 3.59A to C: **(A)** and **(B)** Computer generated calculation of mitral and aortic valvular areas by trace method in short-axis planes of LV and Aorta. **(C)** Measurement of pulmonary area by determining the diameter of main pulmonary artery in short axis plane of great vessels. After measuring the diameter D², the area is calculated by formula area = MV², hence A = 0.785 × D²

Flow within the heart is pulsatile; hence, mean gradients are an important measure and are obtained by integrating the velocity profile over the ejection time. This can be obtained readily with software available on all modern echo machines by simply tracing the area of the velocity profile. The mean pressure gradient is then derived from the mean velocity data using the Bernoulli equation.

D. Intracardiac pressure measurement

1. **Pulmonary artery systolic pressure (PASP)** is estimated from the tricuspid regurgitation (TR) peak velocity. Provided there is no tricuspid valve obstruction, peak TR velocity will depend on the pressure gradient between the right ventricle and the right atrium (difference between peak right ventricular systolic pressure (RVSP) and right atrial (RA) pressure). Therefore, estimated RVSP is equal to this pressure difference (determined from the peak TR velocity using the Bernoulli equation) and the estimated RA pressure (Table 3.6). Provided there is no obstruction across the pulmonic valve, the RV systolic pressure will be similar to the PASP. PASP = 4 × (peak TR velocity)² + estimated RA pressure.

2. **Pulmonary artery diastolic pressure (PADP)** Pulmonary regurgitation represents the pressure difference between the pulmonary artery (PA) and the RV. Hence, the end pulmonary regurgitation velocity can be utilized to measure the end diastolic pressure difference between the PA and RV. The RV end diastolic pressure should be similar to the RA pressure, hence, addition of estimated RA pressure to the end diastolic pressure difference between PA and RV will estimate the PADP.

Table 3.6: *Estimation of RA pressure*

IVC	Change with respiration/sniff	Est. RA pressure
Normal (<2 cm)	Collapse or decrease >50%	5 mm Hg
Normal (<2 cm)	Decrease <50%	10 mm Hg
Dilated (>2 cm)	Decrease <50%	15 mm Hg
Dilated with dilated Hepatic Veins	No change	20 mm Hg

PADP = 4 × (end pulmonary regurgitant velocity)² + estimated RA pressure

3. **Estimated RA pressure** can be estimated from the size of the inferior vena cava and its response to changes in respiration or a sniff.

4. **Estimated left atrial pressure (LAP)/LV diastolic pressure (LVEDP):** Providing there is no mitral stenosis, LVEDP and LAP should be the same. This

important measure of LV diastolic function can be estimated by several methods.

(a) **Deceleration time of mitral inflow (DT):** A DT less than 150 milliseconds is strongly suggestive of an elevated LVEDP/LAP greater than 20 mm Hg.

(b) **Difference between pulmonary venous atrial duration and mitral atrial duration:** Normally mitral A-wave duration is greater than pulmonary venous atrial reversal (Ar) duration. When LVEDP is increased, the velocity and duration of the mitral A decreases, whereas pulmonary vein Ar velocity and duration increase. The difference between the duration of the Ar wave and the mitral A wave correlates with LVEDP. An Ar-A duration of more than 50 milliseconds is quite specific for an elevated LVEDP greater than 20 mm Hg. The primary limitation with this method is the difficult in accurately measuring the duration Ar.

(c) **Combined mitral inflow/CMM index (E/V_p):** This index has been demonstrated to correlate with LAP/LVEDP, especially when these filling pressures are elevated. A ratio greater than 2.0 is suggestive of elevated filling pressures.

(d) **Combined mitral inflow/DTI index (E/E_n):** This index has been shown as a semi-quantitative measure of LVEDP. A ratio (using the septal E_a) of less than 8 suggests filling pressures. However, values between 8 and 12 were nonspecific. Others have correlated E/E_n with LAP using the E_0 from the lateral annulus.

E. dp/dt: This index of LV contractility is the rate of pressure increase during iso-volumic contraction and is traditionally obtained using invasive pressure transducers. It can be estimated from the continuous wave Doppler mitral regurgitant jet. During isovolumic contraction there is no change in LAP; therefore; mitral regurgitant velocity changes reflect dp/dt, with more rapid increases in mitral regurgitant velocity being associated with increased contractility. The pressure change 1 m/s and 3 m/s = 4 ($V_2^2 \cdot V_1^2$) = 32 mm Hg. The time difference between 1 m/s and 3 m/s is measured from the mitral regurgitation jet, and dp/dt is calculated as follows:

$$dp/dt = 32 \text{ mm Hg/time}(s)$$

This has been demonstrated to correlate well with invasively measured dp/dt (normal is greater than 1200 mm Hg/s). Similarly, dp/dt can be calculated for the right ventricle, with the only difference being to measure the time difference between 1 m/s and 2 m/s. Hence, dp/dt = 12 mm Hg/time (s).

F. Continuity equation is an application of the principle of conservation of mass, which states that flow across a conduit of varying diameter is equal at all points. This equation is especialy useful in the quantifying of a stenotic aortic valve area that cannot be accurately planimetered from the transthoracic window. Flow at any point in the heart is the product of the cross-sectional area (CSA) by the flow velocity. As flow velocity varies during ejection in a pulsatile system, individual velocities must be integrated to measure total volume of flow (velocity time integral, VTI). This is determined by tracing the spectral Doppler profile, using standard measurement software built into all echocardiography machines.

Bibliography

1. Adhar GC, Abbasi AS, Nanda NC: Doppler echocardiography in the assessment of mitral regurgitation and mitral valve prolapse. In *Doppler Echocardiography* (Nanda, NC Ed.), p. 188. New York, Igaku-Shoin Medical Publishers, 1984.

2. Adhar GC, Nanda NC: Doppler echocardiography. *Echocardiography,* 1984; 1:219.

3. Angelsen BAJ, Brubakk AO: Transcutaneous measurement of blood flow velocity in the human aorta. *Cardiovasc Res* 10:368, 1976.

4. Bengur AR, Snider AR, Vermillion RP, Freeland JC: Left ventricular ejection fraction measured with Doppler colour flow mapping techniques. *Am J Cardiol* 1991;68: 669.

5. Bommeer WJ, *et al.* Quantitation of aortic regurgitation with two-dimensional Doppler echocardiography (Abstract). *Am J Cardiol* 1981;47:412.

6. Bouchard A, Blumelin S, Schiller NB, Schlitt S, Byrd II BF, Ports T, Chatterjee K: Measurement of left ventricular stroke volume using continuous wave Doppler echocardiography of the ascending aorta an dM-mode echocardiography of the aortic valve. *J Am Coll Cardiol* 1987;9:75.

7. Braubakk AO Angelsen BAJ, Hatle L: Diagnosis of valvular heart disease using transcutaneous Doppler ultrasound. *Cardiovasc Res* 1977;11:461.

8. Bruce CJ, Spittell PC, Montgomery SC, *et al.* Personal ultrasound imager: abdominal aortic aneurysm screening. *J Am Soc Echocardiogr* 2000; 13:674–9.

9. DeMaria AN, Smith MD: Quantitation of Doppler colour flow recordings: *J Am Coll Cardiol* 1992; 20:439.

10. Dubin J, Wallerson DC, Cody RJ, Devereux RB: Comparative accuracy of Doppler echocardiographic methods for clinical stroke volume determination. *Am Heart J* 1990;120:116.

11. Durell M, Nanda NC: Doppler colour flow mapping. In *Doppler Echocardiography* (Nanda, NC, Ed.) p. 515. New York, Igaku-Shoin Medical Publishers, 1984.

12. Elkayam U, *et al.* The use of Doppler flow velocity measurement to asses the hemo-dynamic response to vasodilators in patients with heart failure. *Circulation* 1983; 67:377.

13. Fisher DC, *et al.* The mitral valve orifice method for noninvasive determination of cardiac output by two-dimensional echo-Doppler: validation and initial clinical trials. (Abstract.) *Am J Cardiol* 1982; 49:932.

14. Fisher DC, Sahn DJ, Friedman MJ, Larson D, Valdes-Cruz LM, Horowitz S, Goldberg SJ, Aller HD: The mitral valve orifice method for noninvasive two-dimensional echo Doppler determinations of cardiac output. *Circulation* 1983; 67:872.

15. Goldberg SJ, *et al*. Range gated echo-Doppler velocity and turbulence mapping in patients with valvular aortic stenosis. *Am Heart J*, 1982; 103:858.

16. Goldberg SJ, Sahn DJ, Allen HD, Valldes-Cruz LM, Hoenecke H, Carnahan Y: Evaluation of pulmonary and systemic blood flow by two-dimensional Doppler echocardiography: Initial experience and review of the literature. *Mayo Clin Proc* 1984; 484:59.

17. Goodkin GM, Spevack DM, Tunick P A, *et al*. How useful is hand-carried bedside echocardiography in critically ill patients? *J Am Coll Cardiol* 2001; 37:2019–22.

18. Gross C, Wamm SL: Doppler echocardiography in the assessment of prosthetic cardiac valves. In *Doppler Echocardiography* (Nanda, NC, Ed.) , 22. New York, Igaku-Shoin Medical Publishers, 1984.

19. Habib GB, Zoghbi WA: Doppler assessment of right ventricular dynamics in systemic hypertension: Comparison with left ventricular filling. *Am Heart J* 1992; 124:1313–1320.

20. Harrison MR, Cliftom GD, Pennell AT, DeMaria AN, Cater A: Effect of heart rate on left ventricular diastolic transmitral flow velocity Atterns assessed by Doppler Echocardiography in normal subjects. *Am J Cardiol* 1991; 67:622.

21. Hatle J, *et al*: Noninvasive assessment of pressure drop in mitral stenosis by Doppler ultrasound. *Br Heart J* 1978; 40:131.

22. Hatle L, Angelsen B, Tromsdol A: Noninvasive assessment of atrioventricular pressure half time by *Doppler ultrasound. Circulation*, 1979; 60:1096.

23. Hatle L, Angelsen B: *Doppler Ultrasound in Cardiology-Physical Principles and Clinical Applications.* Philadelphia, Lea & Febiger, 1982.

24. Hatle L, Angelsen BA, Tromsdol A: Non-invasive assessment of aortic stenosis by Doppler ultrasound. *Br Heart J* 1980; 43:284.

25. Himura Y, Kumada T, Kambayashi M, Hayashida W, Ishikawa N, Nakamura Y, Kawai C: Importance of left ventricular systolic function in the assessment of left ventricular diastolic function with Doppler transmitral flow velocity recording. *J Am Coll Cardiol.*

26. Ihlen H, Amlie JP, Dale J, Forfang K, Nitter-Hauge S, Otterstad JE, Simonsen S, Myhre E: Determination of cardiac output by Doppler echocardiography. *Br Heart J* 1984; 51:54.

27. Isaaz K Ethevennot G, Admant P, Brembilla B, Pernot C: A simplified normalised ejection phase index measured by Doppler echocardiography for the assessment of left ventricular performance. *Am J Cardiol*, 1990; 65: 1246.

28. Kitabatake A, *et al*. Noninvasive estimation of pulmonary artery pressure from velocity pattern of right ventricular ejection flow by pulsed Doppler technique. *J Am Coll Cardiol*, 1983; 1:657.

29. Kitabatake A, Inoue M, Asao M, Ito H, Masuyama T, Tanouchi J, Morita T, Hori M, Yoshima H, Ohnishi K, Abe H: Noninvasive evaluation of the ratio of pulmonary systemic flow in atrial septal defect by Duplex Doppler echocardiography, *Circulation* 1984; 69:73.

30. Lbanoff A, Rodbard S: Atrioventricular pressure half time: measure of mitral valve orifice area. *Circulation*, 1968; 38:144.

31. Lightly GW, Garbiulo A, Kronzon I, Politzer F: Comparison of multiple views for the evaluation of pulmonary arterial blood flow by Doppler echocardiography. *Circulation* 1002; 1986;74.

32. Meijboom EJ, Rijsterbirgh H, Bot H, DeBoo JAJ, Roelandt JRTC, Bom N: Limits of reproducibility of blood flow measurements by Doppler echocardiography. *Am J Cardiol* 1987; 59:133.

33. Myreng Y, Smiseth OA: Assessment of Left ventricular relaxation by Doppler echocardiography. *Circulation* 1990; 81:260.

34. Nichol PM, Boughner DR, Persaud JA: Noninvasive assessment of mitral insufficiency by transcutaneous Doppler ultrasound. *Circulation* 1976; 54:656.

35. Omoto R (Ed.): Colour Atlas of Real-Time Two-dimensional Doppler Echocardiography. Tokyo, Shindan-To-Chiryo, 1984.

36. Omoto R, *et al*. The development of real-time two-dimensional Doppler echocardiography and its clinical significance in acquired valvular diseases with special reference to the evaluation of valvular regurgitation. *Jpn Heart J* 1984; 25:325.

37. Pandian NG. Ultrasound stethoscopy: adding another sense to the art and science of physical examination. *Thoraxcentre J* 2001; 4:91–2.

38. Panidis IP, Ross J, Mintz GS: Effect of sampling site on assessment of pulmonary artery blood flow by Doppler echocardiography. *Am J Cardiol* 1986; 58:1145.

39. Quinoes MA, *et al* Assessment of pulsed Doppler echocardiography in detection and quantification of aortic and mitral regurgitation. *Br Heart J* 1980; 44:612.

40. Roelandt JRTC. A personal ultrasound imager (ultrasound stethoscope). A revolution in the physical diagnosis. *Eur Heart J* 2002; 23:523–27.

41. Rugolotto M, Hu BS, Liang DH, *et al*. Rapid assessment of cardiac anatomy and function with a new hand-carried ultrasound device (OptiGo): a comparison with standard echocardiography. *Eur J Echocardiogr* 2001; 4:262–9.

42. Salustri A, Trambaiolo P Point-of care echocardiography: small, smart and quick. *Eur Heart J* 2002; 23: 1484–7.

43. Schuster AH, Nanda NC: Doppler echocardiographic features of mechanical alternans. *Am Heart J* 1984; 107:580.

44. Seward JB, Douglas PS, Erbel R, *et al*. Hand-carried cardiac ultrasound (HCU) device. A report from the echocardiography task force on new technology of the nomenclature and standard committee of the American Society of Echocardiography. *J Am Soc Echocardiogr* 2002; 15:369–73.

45. Shapiro SM, Bersohn MM, Laks MM: In search of the Holy Grail: The study of diastolic ventricular function by the use of Doppler echocardiography. *J Am Coll Cardiol* 1992; 70:1341.

46. Spencer KT, Anderson AS, Bhargava A, *et al*. Physician-performed point-of-care echocardiography using a laptop platform compared with physical examination in the cardiovascular patients. *J Am Coll Cardiol* 2001; 37:2013–8.

47. Stevenson JG, Kawabori I, Guntheroth WG: Detection of pulmonary insufficiency by pulse Doppler echocardio-

graphy: validation sensitivity, specificity and correlation with M-mode echocardiography. *Circulation* 1980; 62:251.

48. Stevenson JG, Kawabori I, Guntheroth WG: Validation of Doppler diagnosis of tricuspid regurgitation. *Circulation* 1981; 64:55.

49. Stewart RAH, Joshi J, Alexander N, Nihyo-yannopoulos P, Oakley CM: Adjustment for the influence of age and heart rate on Doppler measurement of left ventricular filling. *Br Heart J* 1992; 68:608.

50. Vourvouri EC, Koroleva LY, Ten Cate FJ, *et al.* Clinical utility and cost effectiveness of a personal ultrasound imager for cardiac evaluation during consultation rounds in patients with suspected cardiac disease. *Heart* 2003; 89:727–30.

51. Vourvouri EC, Poldermans D, Schinkel AFL, *et al.* Left ventricular hypertrophy screening using a hand-held ultrasound device. *Eur Heart J* 2002; 23:1516–21.

52. Vourvouri EC, Poldermans D, De Sutter J, *et al.* Experience with an ultrasound stethoscope. *J Am Soc Echocardiogr* 2002; 15:80–5.

53. Zoghbi WA, Habib GB, Quinones MA: Doppler assessment of right ventricular filling in a normal population. *Circulation*, 1990; 82:1316.

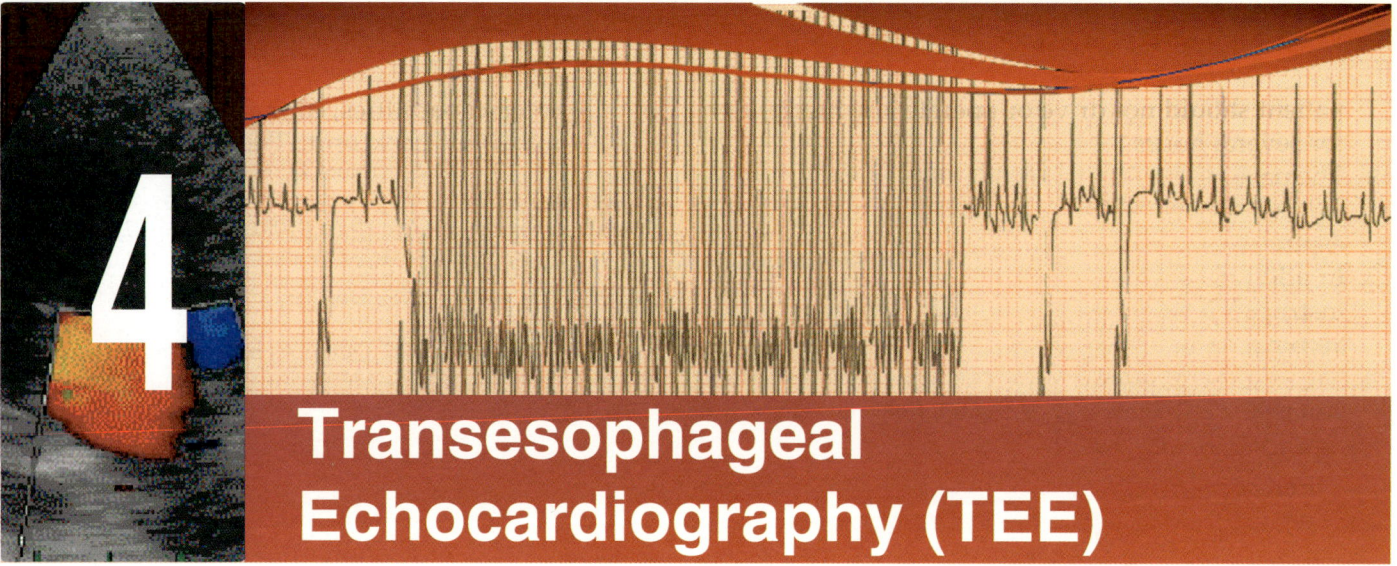

Transesophageal Echocardiography (TEE)

Transesophageal echocardiography is an extremely useful tool in diagnostic cardiology. The proximity of the heart to the oesophagus and the use of high-frequency transducers allows detailed visualisation of cardiac anatomy. Furthermore, Doppler techniques permit evaluation of cardiovascular flow velocities in a safe, semi-invasive manner.

Frazim and his associates were the first to perform transesophageal echocardiographic studies by M-mode recordings with certain limitations. In 1981, Souquet, Hanrath and colleagues developed and clinically evaluated transesophageal two-dimensional phased-array imaging systems, having employed a 2.5 MHz phased-array ultrasound transducers mounted at the tip of an endoscope. However, clinical interest in the technique remained limited as image quality was poor and only morphologic information could be obtained. In 1986 with the introduction of the second generation of single (transverse) plane transesophageal probes which provided the combination of high-resolution imaging (centred around 5.0 MHz) and colour flow mapping that this technique has become accepted globally as a major new diagnostic technique in the investigation of both congenital and acquired heart ailments and wider number of clinical applications in the field of clinical cardiology. Since then there has been tremendous progress in the development of endosonoscopic probes which have led to the finer views of the normal and altered anatomy of the heart with distinctive objective in the investigation of heart ailments such as:

1. Providing higher resolution imaging.
2. Development of smaller probes for studies in children.
3. The incorporation of additional imaging planes and Doppler facilities.

4. The development of ultrasound generated three-dimensional views.

Flow Chart in TEE

1. Obtain a careful history, particularly, history of dysphagia or esophageal disease.
2. Obtain informed consent.
3. Ensure that the patient has not eaten within at least 4 hours before the TEE procedure.
4. Obtain baseline vital signs, including blood pressure, heart rate, oxygen saturation, and continuous ECG. Vital signs are also monitored throughout the study.
5. Establish intravenous access to administer medications or a contrast agent.
6. Remove dentures and any loose objects in the patient's mouth.
7. Apply local pharyngeal anesthesia. Use of a drying agent and sedation depends on the physician.
8. Examine the TEE probe to ensure there are no visible signs of damage. Insert the TEE probe and secure a bite lock in place.
9. Obtain and record two-dimensional, Doppler, and colour-flow images according to institutional protocol.
10. When the study is completed, remove the TEE probe. Clean and soak the probe in glutaraldehyde-based disinfecting solution (e.g. Sporcidin) for at least 10 to 15 mins. or according to manufacturer's recommendation. Rinse the probe thoroughly. Examine the probe for any visible damage and then return it to storage.
11. If sedation has been used, continue to monitor the patient until the vital signs return to baseline. The

patient should not drive or operate any machinery for several hours.

12. The patient should not take anything by mouth for at least 1 hour after the procedure to avoid potential aspiration.

13. In addition to oral instructions, written discharge instructions are usually given to the patient or the accompanying person in outpatient settings.

Advantage of Transesophageal over Transthoracic Echocardiography (Table 4.1)

1. Different imaging approach allows the visualisation of structures not seen from the transthoracic windows.

2. Higher ultrasound frequencies can be used, providing higher image resolution.

3. No obstruction to ultrasound by chest wall structures, or lung tissue.

4. Improved signal-to-noise ratio allows better detection of poor echo-reflective structures (intracardiac tumor, thrombi).

5. Reduced target range for pulsed Doppler, and higher sensitivity of colour flow imaging, when studying posterior cardiac structures.

Requirements for Organisation of TEE Laboratory

Even though any facility which already has these diagnostic units in full function along with the supporting professional and technical staff can consider setting up TEE, it is preferable in those institutions where the facilities of both Cardiology and Cardio-vascular Surgical Services are already made available due to initial capital expenditure, number of patients and necessary requisite of highly trained multi-disciplinary staff. (Fig. 4.4A–C).

Site: TEE is usually carried out in the cardiac ultrasound laboratory after the cardiologists has gained confidence by watching and performing esophageal intubations in the UGIE unit even though it can be performed at the patients bed side, no matter where it is located. TEE hardware is portable enough that it can be carried to any location of the medical centre such as critical care units (ICU, CCU) and operating rooms. It can even be performed in the cardiologists office or even in the emergency room, if needed.

Equipment: Proper functioning of all equipment involved during TEE cannot be overemphasized. The mainstay of TEE is a nonfiberoptic echo scope which consists of a phased array mono (64 elements) or biplane (48 elements) 5 MHz transducer ($13 \times 7 \times 4$ mm) mounted at the tip of a 70 to 100 cm flexible tube (9–11 mm in diameter) interfaced with a two-dimensional ultrasound machine which contains pulse and colour

flow Doppler capabilities, along with video image recorder and play back unit. The echoscope can be anteflexed (120°), retroflexed (90°) and also has the capability to move laterally to the right or left (90°each) by steering knobs at its proximal end. A special size 6.7 mm pediatric probe is also now available at few centres for use in infants and young children. Besides TEE, other equipment for monitoring patients during procedures is needed. These are pulse oximeter for respiratory monitoring and electrocardiographic and blood pressure recording for cardiac monitoring. A portable or built in wall suction apparatus, O_2 supply and updated emergency resuscitation cart should also be available when and wherever TEE is being performed.

Training of Manpower

Technicians: Besides obtaining an informed consent under a cardiologist's instructions, he or she is responsible for inspecting the echoscope prior to its use and checking for any electrical current leakage by its accompanying leakage current testing kit. This requirement is very important, and the echoscope needs to be tested at least once every two weeks. As the image orientation and image recording differs, the technician's familiarization with the various levels of TEE imaging is also necessary. This can easily be learned from a cardiologist during the study and formal sit down interpretation. The next most important task of the technician is the proper aftercare of the echoscope. Thorough physical cleansing of the echoscope is an essential prerequisite to effective disinfection. The echoscope should first be rid of proteinaceous material with enzyme treatment (protozyme) and then immersed in aqueous 2% alkaline gluteraldehyde (Cidex) for at least 20 minutes. Gluteraldehyde provides rapid high level germicidal activity. An inconvenient side-effect of the gluteraldehyde disinfection is the risk of occasional dermatitis, conjunctivitis and sinusitis in the person handling it. The echoscope, after having been treated with gluteraldehyde, can be washed in sterile water and dried for 30 minutes before its next use.

Gas sterilization by ethylene dioxide has no practical utility in the routine disinfection of the echoscope between two procedures, because it is time-consuming; however, it remains the best available method for getting rid of infections, including hepatitis B, HIV, tuberculosis etc. Besides being time-consuming, this process of sterilization is also expensive. It requires at least 30 minutes exposure to ethylene dioxide followed by prolonged aeration of up to 24 hours to elute any retained disinfectant.

Nurse: The presence of a registered nurse during TEE is necessary to watch the patients respiratory rate, O_2 saturation by pulse oximeter, and blood pressure before,

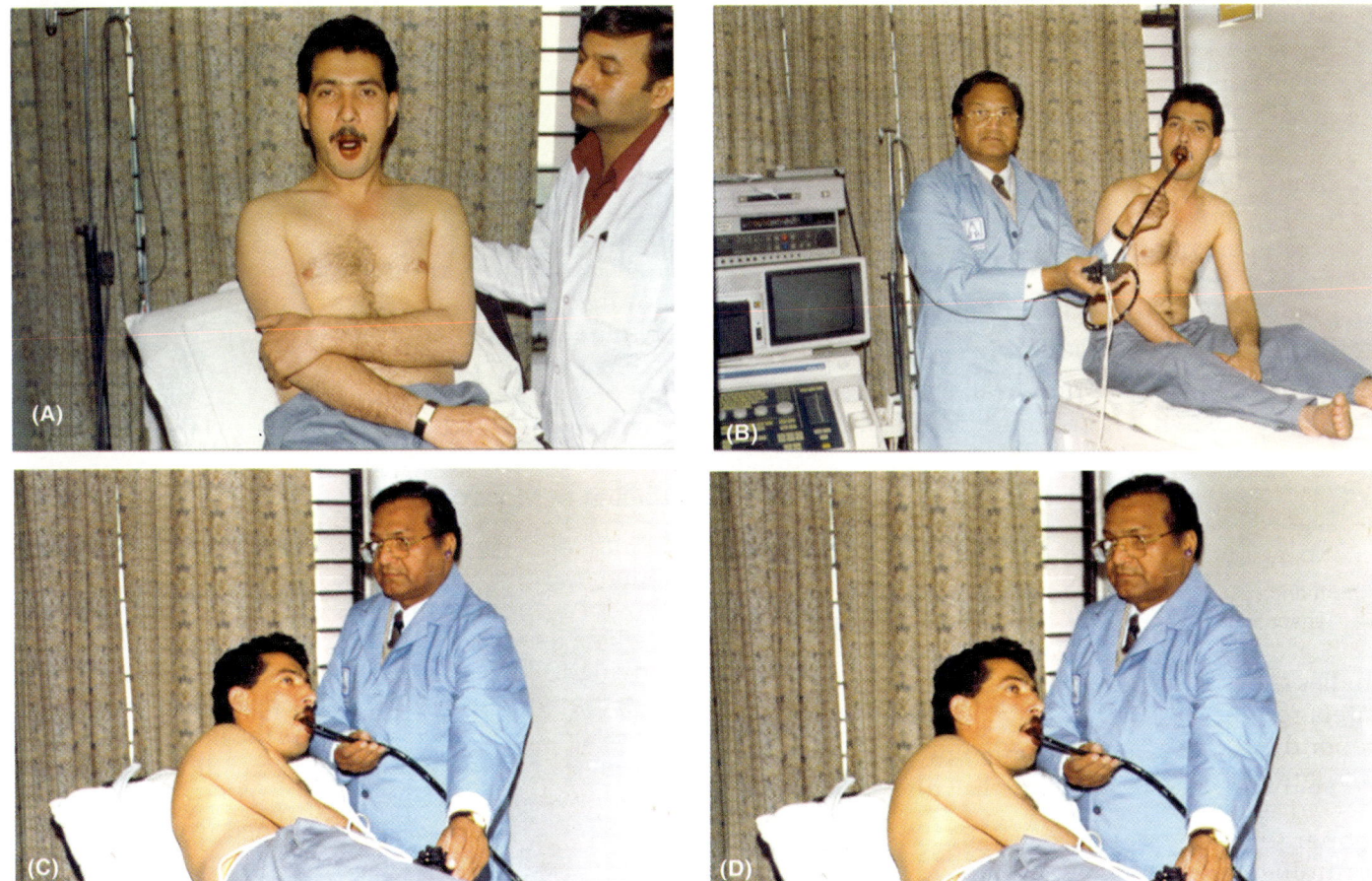

Fig. 4.1A to D: (A) Preparing for undertaking Trans-esophageal echocardiography test in hospital laboratory Jammu. **(B)** Introduction of esophageal probe in the mouth by the author. **(C)** The model is asked to turn to left lateral position to introduce the transducer further into the esophagus and finally into the gastric cavity for making various required views. **(D)** TEE probe has been finally placed into the gastric cavity

during and after the procedure. He/she can also administer supplemental IV medications and apply suction should they become necessary. His/her role is indispensable when IV prophylactic antibiotic needs to be administered one half to one hour prior to an 8–12 hours following the procedure in high risk patients. These responsibilities and their efficient and smooth carrying out can be easily and quickly learned by a nurse by observing the function of endoscopy unit.

Cardiologist: Because TEE requires the expertise of two different disciplines, i.e. cardiology and UGIE, it is universally agreed that initial training of cardiologists in TEE should be under the technical supervision of an experienced gastroenterologist. This should begin with a clear comprehension of the contraindications, risks and complications of esophageal intubation and end with a sufficient number of supervised echoscope insertions. A minimum of 30–50 esophageal intubations has been suggested for technical and safety considerations for a under training TEE operator. This threshold is quite

arbitrary and no doubt will vary from institution to institution. Observe the technique of esophageal insertion by the gastroenterologists in at least 10 patients before attempting intubations under their supervision (minimum 25–30). This step-up approach will increase the level of comfort by eliminating fear and anxiety due to unfamiliarity with esophageal insertions on the part of the cardiologists to be trained. Gastroenterologists have been very cordial and courteous to their cardiologist colleagues in preparing them to set up and perform TEE.

Anesthesiologist: As the anesthesiologists are already trained in nasotracheal, orotracheal, orogastric and esophageal intubation and deal with sedated or anesthetized patient, passing the echoscope under these conditions does not pose a problem for them. However, they do need tutelage in the assessment of tomographic anatomy, function, pulse Doppler and colour flow Doppler principles. These can be learned from their cardiologist colleagues who interpret echocardiographic

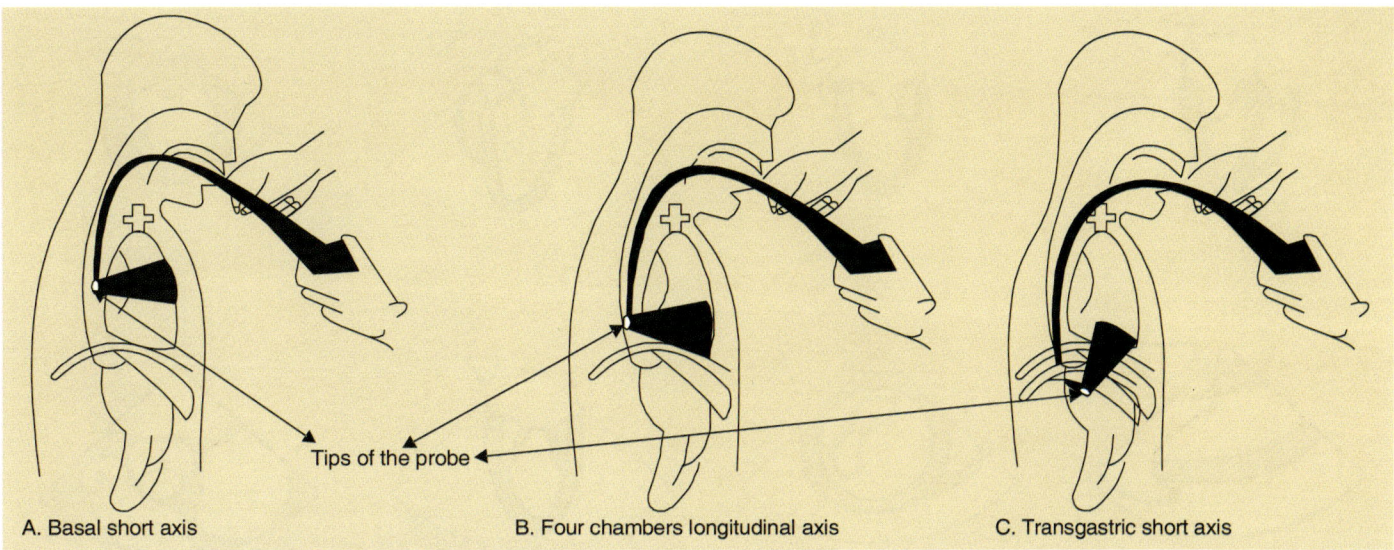

Fig. 4.2: Diagrammatic representation of the three axes around which various cross-sectional views of the heart are obtained in the performance of TEE. **(A)** Basal short axis (25–30 cm from the incisors). **(B)** Four chamber longitudinal axis (30–35 cm from incisors). **(C)** Transgastric short axis (40–45 cm from the incisors).

studies at their institution. The optimal duration of such tutelage will vary from individual to individual, depending upon the basic familiarity with echocardiographic techniques. It should be emphasized that, for optimal use of intraoperative TEE, a close cooperation is needed between anesthesiologist, cardiologist and cardiac surgeon, because multidisciplinary knowledge is often required.

Technique of Transesophageal Echocardiography (Figs 4.1–4.3)

Transesophageal echocardiography is performed using a two-dimensional Doppler colour-flow echocardiographic system, with a multicrystal phased-array of 5 MHz ultrasound transducer tip, attached to a conventional flexible endoscope. The transducer tip size is 10 to 13 mm in diameter, the shaft size is 9 mm in diameter, and the length is 60 to 10 cm. Inner and outer dials on the endoscope handle allow for posterior flexion and right and left lateral movement, respectively. Anterior and posterior flexion is used most commonly with monoplane imaging and right and left lateral movement is usually employed with biplane imaging, when converting from short to long range views.

Patient is usually kept on fast for 4 to 6 hours before endoscopy. Intravenous access and 12-lead electrocardiographic monitoring are established. Since endoscopy is unpleasant for most patients, short-acting intravenous benzodiazepines are commonly administered before the test. Some operators also use anticholinergic agent such as glycopyrrolate to lessen secretions. The pharynx is anaesthetised with topical local anaesthetics to suppress the gag reflex. As with any invasive procedure, verbal reassurance is an important means of reducing patient anxiety improving compliance and reduce the need for sedation.

Incubation is usually performed with the patient in the left lateral decubitus position, with the neck slightly flexed. However, in intubated patients or patients with chest-trauma, the test can be performed in supine posture. Dentures should be removed, or a bite guard should be used, so that the probe is not damaged. Once the transducer is positioned behind the heart, it can be advanced and withdrawn, rotated laterally and medially, and anteflexed and retroflexed, to obtain cardiac images. Biplane imaging provides longitudinal windows not available with monoplane imaging, thus facilitating visualisation of structures most anterior and posterior, as well as the left atrium, left ventricular inflow, right ventricular outflow, ascending aorta and venae cavae. The various views are undertaken by using a monoplane, a biplane and later multiplane transesophageal echocardiographic probes and the patient is continuously monitored with ECG, blood pressure, and pulse oximetry for oxygen saturation.

Intravenous antibiotics are usually administered prophylactically to all patients with prosthetic heart valves. All patients suffering from critical illness such as aortic dissection should receive an appropriate sedation and drugs to control their blood pressure.

Cardiac Imaging Planes in Transesophageal Echocardiography (Figs 4.3 and 4.5)

Single Plane Approach

The majority of current generation single-plane probes usually have an imaging frequency centred around 5 or 5.6 MHz and have a phased-array transducer containing

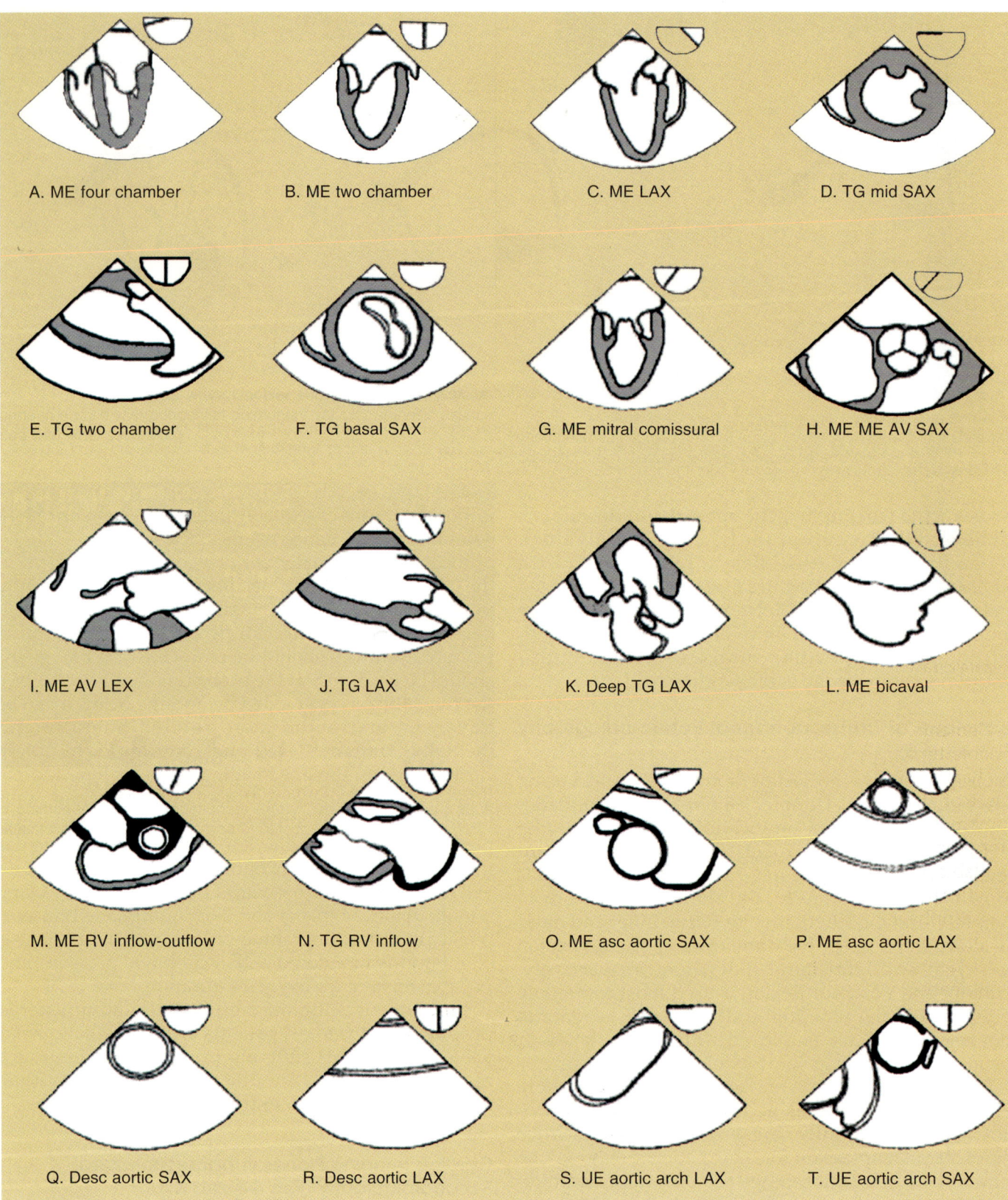

Fig. 4.3 A to T: Standard TOE views ME, mid oesophageal; LAX long axis, TG, transgastric, SAX, short axis, AV, aortic valve; RV, right ventricular

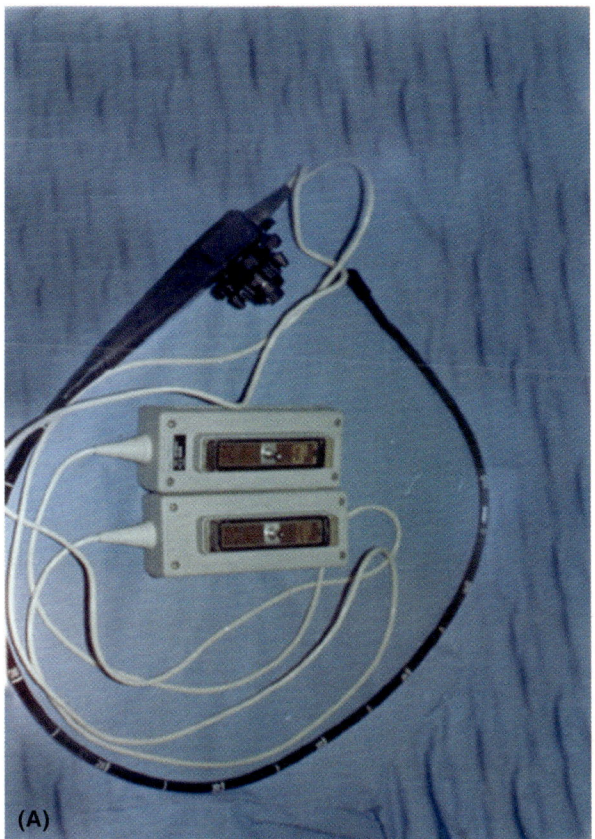

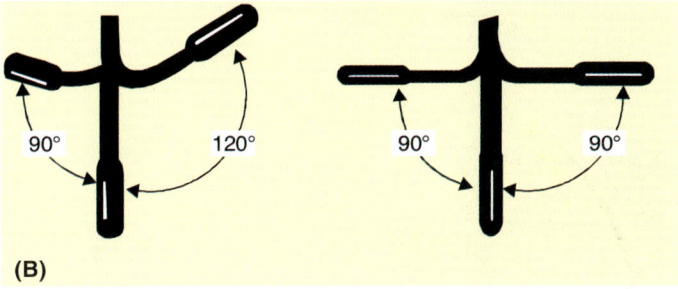

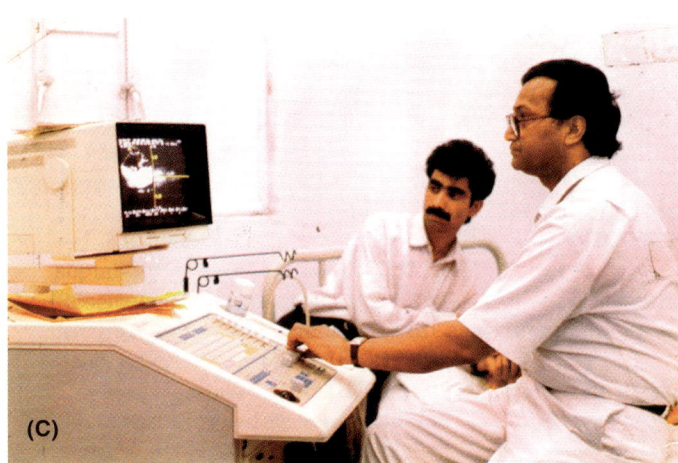

Fig. 4.4A to C: (A) Biplane TEE probe used frquently for study. **(B)** TEE probe being rotated at different angles to acquire the view under study. **(C)** Preparation and editing of TEE report for final diagnosis, here by the author himself

64 elements. The ultrasound elements are mounted at the flexible tip so as to provide transverse plane images of the heart; that is their scan plane is at right angles to the shaft of the endoscope. Cross-sectional imaging, in combination with colour flow mapping and pulsed wave Doppler interrogation, is provided on all currently available probes. More recently continuous wave Doppler facilities have become available on selected phased-array transesophageal probes. In addition, one annular array mechanical system is available, that allows a dynamic shift in imaging frequency from 5 to 7.5 MHz in combination with both high pulse repetition frequency Doppler and continuous wave Doppler.

Biplane Approach

Current generation biplane probe have two separate ultrasound transducer element arrays mounted at the tip of the endoscope so as to provide both transverse axis and longitudinal axis images of the heart and the great vessels. Conventionally, the more distal transducer provides the standard transverse axis images. By switching a button on the ultrasound system the more proximal transducer is activated and generates longitudinal plane images.

Advantages of (Biplane) Transesophageal Echocardiography

1. Facilitates three-dimensional conceptualization of the heart and complex structures (e.g. mitral valve apparatus).

2. Longitudinally aligned structures are better visualised than in the transverse planes (venae cavae, right ventricular apex, thoracic aorta).

3. Reduces probe manipulation.

Multiplane Approach

The ultimate goal in transesophageal probe design, however, remains the construction of high-resolution, multiplane imaging probes. In these probes, a 48 or 64-element phased-array transducer is mounted on a circular footprint, which can be rotated from 0 degrees (transverse plane) through 90 degree (longitudinal plane) to almost 180 degrees (reversed transverse plane). Since in clinical practice lateral angulation of an endoscope within the oesophagus beyond 30 degrees is rarely possible without causing considerable discomfort to the patient, this multiplane approach therefore can provide a number of additional imaging planes not

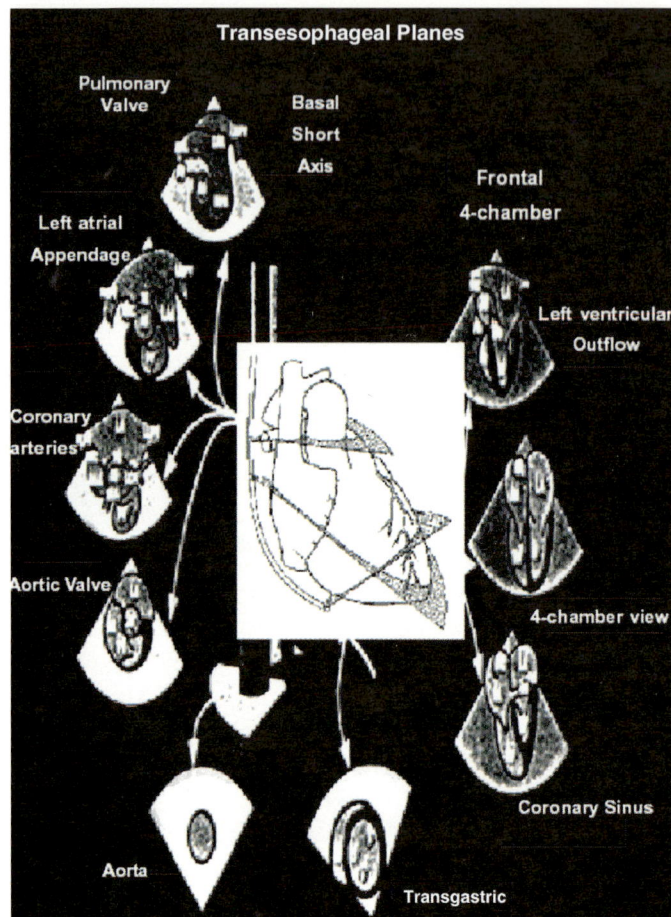

Fig. 4.5: Graphic representation of different types of TEE views at different levels as shown in this diagram

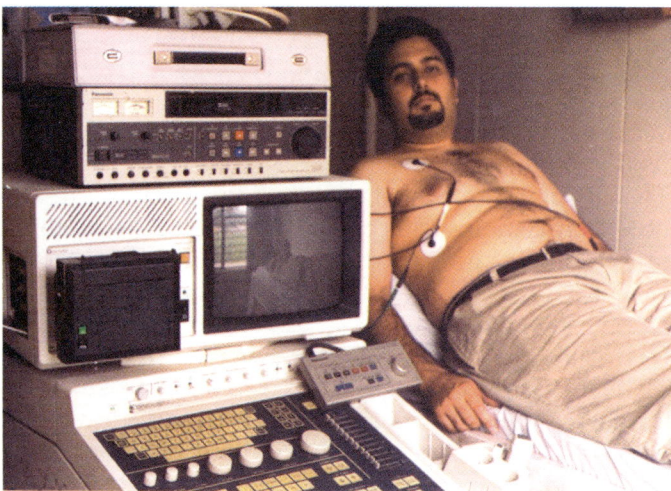

Fig. 4.6: ECG electrodes on the chest of model (right) and echocardiography machine (left)

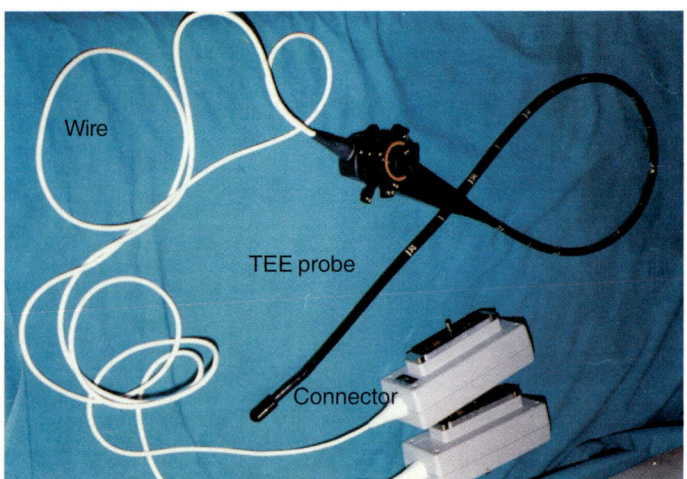

Fig. 4.7: Typical features of biplane TEE probe used in most of the patients studied

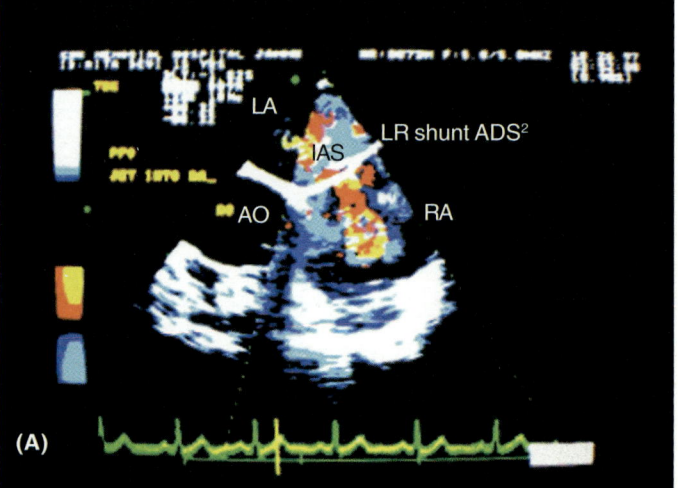

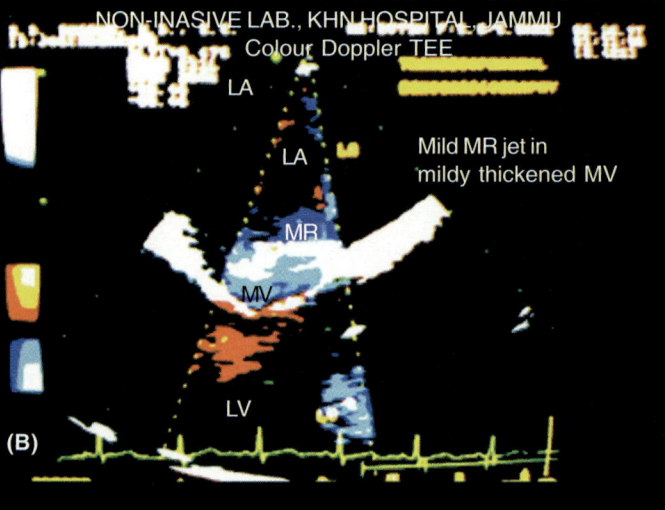

Fig. 4.8A and B: (A) L–R shunt across interatrial septum in ASD secundum in a biatrial basal plane TEE scan. **(B)** 2-Chamber view showing mild MR jet into LA in a patient with mildly thickened mitral valve

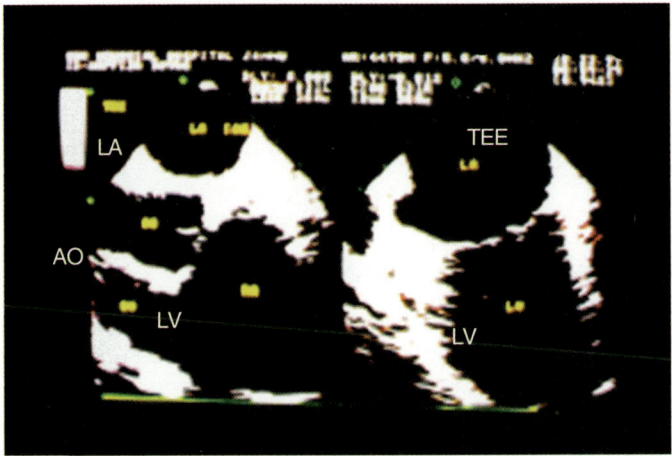

Fig. 4.9: Short axis plane view shows two chambers LA/LV and MV(right). LA/LV/AO/RVOT(left)

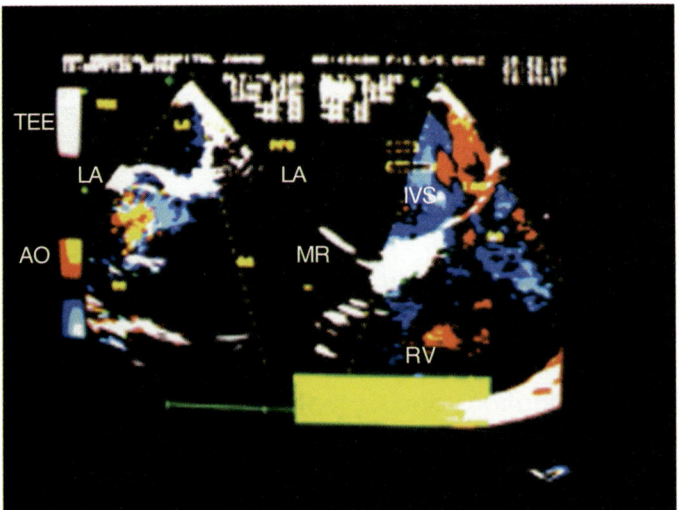

Fig. 4.10: Basal short axis view shows different cardiac structures as indicated on the scans

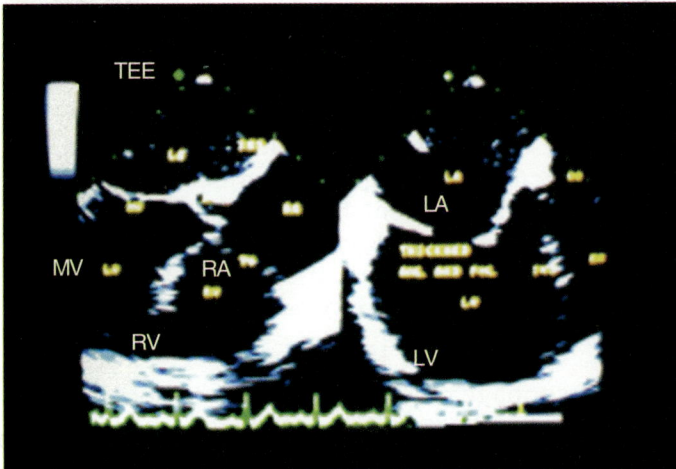

Fig. 4.11: TEE scans show different anatomical structures with thickening of both MV and aortic valves

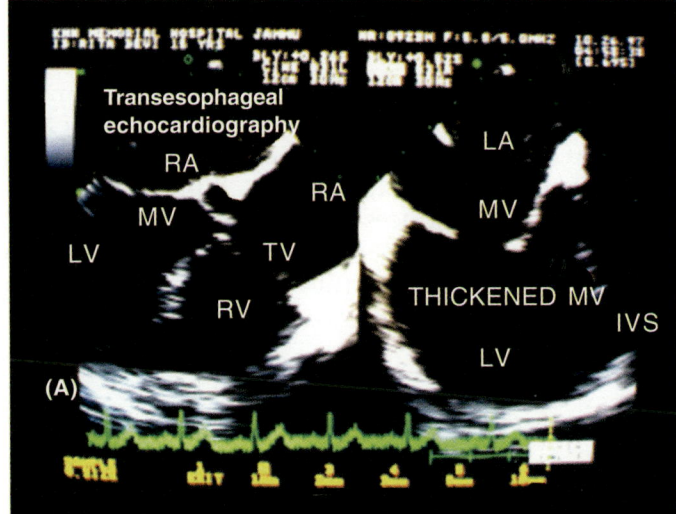

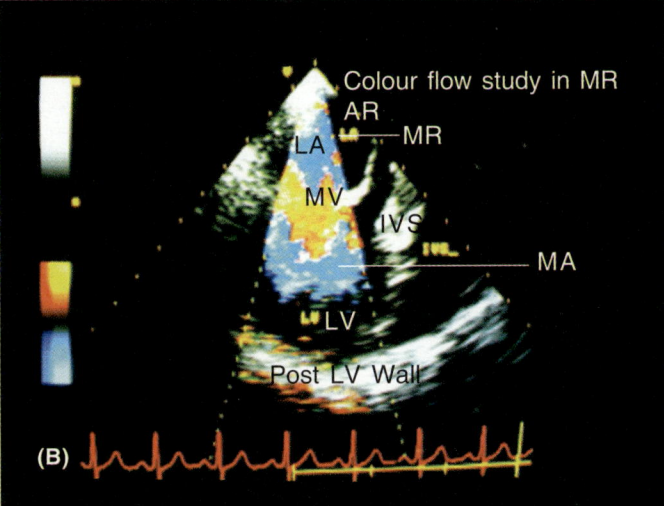

Fig. 4.12A and B: (A) Anatomical internal structures as seen through TEE windows. **(B)** Color flow 2D.TEE showing mainly biatrial view depicting LA/RA, intervening IAS and mitral valvular apparatus in one of the patients who had mitral valvular regurgitation as visualised by a blue jet entering into LA

normally available using standard biplane probes. A further advantage of this system is that the required imaging planes can normally be obtained from the one transducer position within the oesophagus.

Advantages of Multiplane Transesophageal Echocardiography (Table 4.1)

1. Optimisation of imaging and Doppler flow mapping.
2. Minimal repositioning facilitates and shortened examinations.
3. Transitional (oblique) planes reduce interpretation problems of both single and biplane TEE.
4. Best for three-dimensional reconstruction.

Cardiac Imaging Views in Transesophageal Echocardiography (Fig. 4.5)

Structures which are anatomically anterior are most distant from the oesophageal probe and therefore appear at the bottom of the video monitor screen with monoplane (horizontal) imaging. Biplane or longitudinal imaging produces anterior structures at the top, posterior structures at the bottom, basal structures to the right and apical structures to the left of the video monitor.

Transgastric (Short Axis View) (Fig. 4.2C)

The transducer is initially advanced 45 to 50 cm from the teeth yields a short axis view of both ventricles and the posteromedial and anterolateral papillary muscles. It gives information about papillary muscles, and wall thickness and contraction pattern of the ventricles. This view may be used to monitor intraoperative left ventricular functions. Biplane imaging at this level provides good visualisation of the cardiac apex, mitral apparatus and papillary muscles.

Supradiaphragmatic (Four-Chamber View)

Slight retroflexion of the endoscope at approximately 30 cm yields the 4 chamber view of the heart. This perspective gives the best views of the atrioventricular valves and subvalvular apparatus and the left ventricular outflow tract. Incompetent mitral, tricuspid and aortic valves are best examined at this level. The corresponding biplane view allows detailed inspection of the interatrial septum and detection of a patent foramen ovale (Figs 4.19 and 4.20).

Right Ventricular Inflow View (Fig. 4.3M)

This is obtained by rotating the endoscope to the patient's right at about 25 to 30 cm. The tricuspid valve, inferior vena cava, coronary sinus and interatrial septum are seen. The degree of tricuspid regurgitation is best evaluated by this view. Corresponding longitudinal biplane views allow evaluation of both atria, aorta and superior and inferior venae cavae.

Basal Four-Chamber View (Fig. 4.3A)

As the transducer is withdrawn, further images of the atrioventricular valves and support apparatus, the atria, ventricles and left ventricular outflow tract are obtained. Pulsed-wave Doppler and colour flow echocardiography can be used to assess the presence and severity of mitral and tricuspid regurgitation. Quantification of mitral regurgitation is determined by comparing the area and length of the mitral regurgitant jet with those of the left atrium and the ventricle.

Basal Short Axis (Fig. 4.2A)

The aortic valve, aortic root, proximal ascending aorta, proximal coronary and pulmonary arteries, atrial appendages, atrial septum, superior vena cava and pulmonary veins are viewed as the endoscope is withdrawn further up the oesophagus.

Thoracic and Aortic Imaging (Fig. 4.3Q–T)

Transesophageal combined with transthoracic echocardiography permits visualisation of almost the entire thoracic aorta. The descending aorta is visualised by counter-clockwise rotation of the transducer from the basal short axis view of the left ventricle. Although a small section of the ascending thoracic aorta is obscured from monoplane horizontal imaging by the airfilled trachea, this region can be seen on biplane longitudinal imaging (Table 4.1).

Contraindications and Complications of Transesophageal Echocardiography (Tables 4.2 and 4.3)

Morbidity and mortality rates after transesophageal echocardiography are extremely low. The most frequently reported complication of transesophageal echocardiography is a trauma to oesophagus. Oesophageal perforation has been reported in patients with undiagnosed oesophageal tumors, and bleeding from traumatic lesions caused by the endoscope in a patients receiving thrombolytic therapy immediately after completion of the procedure. Other rare complications include supraventricular and ventricular tachycardias, transient vocal cord paralysis, oesophageal burns. The later may be caused by electrical heat of the transesophageal probe. Newer probe have self-contained thermal sensors to monitor probe temperature and alert the operator for this mishap.

Transesophageal echocardiography should not be performed in patients with oesophageal abnormalities such as strictures, diverticuli, tumors or inflammation, and caution should be exercised in patients with bleeding disorders or coagulopathies.

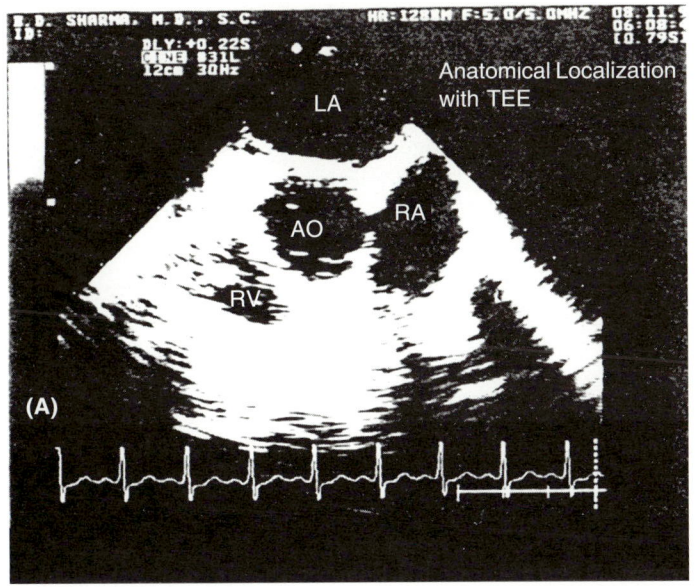
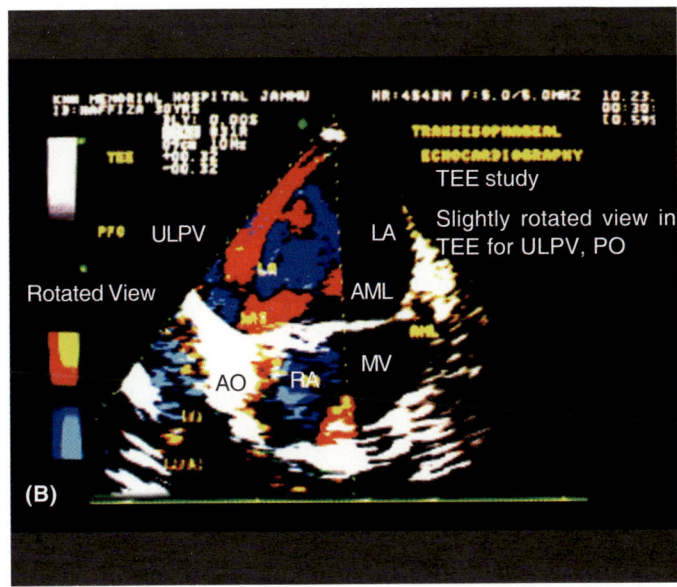

Fig. 4.13A and B: (A) Anatomical relationship of the internal structures as visualised by basal short axis plane through great vessels level on TEE technique. **(B)** Relationship of different internal structures as seen through color flow TEE scans

Table 4.1: *Indications for transesophageal echocardiography*

Diagnostic	*Intraoperative and perioperative monitoring*	*Adjunct of interventional cardiology*	*Postsurgical surveillance*
1. Inadequate transesophageal echocardiography study for any reason, e.g. obesity, thoracic cage deformity, emphysema, etc	1. Effect of anesthesia on cardiac function	1. Preceding elective cardioversion	1. Corrected congenital heart disease
2. Nondiagnostic or equivocal transesophageal echocardiography study	2. Left ventricular function	2. Preceding and during mitral valvuloplasty	2. Repaired aortic dissection
3. Left atrial appendage/thrombi	3. Intracardiac air and marrow emboli	3. Preceding and during aortic valvuloplasty	3. Cardiac valve repair
4. Other intracardiac thrombi and tumors	4. Adequacy of surgical valve repair	4. During transcatheter closure for ASD	4. Prosthetic valve function
5. Infective endocarditis and its complications, e.g. annular abscess	5. Adequacy of prosthetic valve function	5. During coronary angioplasty	5. Orthotopic cardiac transplantation
6. Assessing of severity of valvular regurgitations	6. Adequacy of congenital heart disease correction	6. During endomyocardial biopsy	
7. Prosthetic valve dysfunction			
8. Aortic dissection			
9. Carcinoid heart disease			
10. Congenital heart disease			
11. Coronary artery disease			

Table 4.2: *Contraindications to TEE*

Major (absolute)		*Minor (relative)*	
1.	Lack of informed consent	1.	Perforation
2.	Lack of expertise in inserting echoscope	2.	Oropharyngeal distortion
3.	Uncooperative patient	3.	Cervical spondylosis
4.	Esophageal obstruction	4.	Esophageal diverticulum (Zenker's)
5.	Gastric volvulus	5.	Esophageal varices
6.	Upper GI bleeding	6.	Paraesophageal Hernia of gastric cardia
7.	Cervical spine injury	7.	Postoperative esophageal surgery

Table 4.3: *Complications during and/or following TEE*

Major		*Minor*	
1.	Transient bacteremia	1.	Sore throat (common)
2.	Dysphagia	2.	Edema of uveola (occasional)
3.	Aspiration pneumonitis	3.	Nonsustained arrhythmias (occasional)
4.	Esophageal perforation (potential but rare)	4.	Parotid or submandibular gland swelling
5.	Esophageal mucosal tear (Mullory-Weiss Syndrome)		
6.	Hematemesis		
7.	Unilateral vocal cord paralysis		
8.	Glaucoma exacerbation		
9.	Hypoxia		
10.	Laryngospasm		
11.	Sustained cardiac arrhythmias		
12.	Embolization of left atrial wall thrombus		
13.	Buckling of tip of TE probe.		

Clinical Applications of Transesophageal Echocardiography

Transesophageal echocardiography is now being employed for number of clinical applications such as diagnostic, intraoperative and perioperative monitoring, supplement to interventional cardiology and inpost surgical surveillance. However following is the list of various common clinical situations where cardiologist is consulted for his expert opinion in his routine clinical hospital practice:

1. Valvular heart disease
2. Infective endocarditis
3. Coronary artery disease
4. Aortic dissection
5. Prosthetic valve dysfunction
6. Cardiac Mass lesions (Figs 4.34, 4.37, 4.43 and 4.45)
7. Congenital heart disease
8. TEE in critically ill patients
9. TEE in Interventional cardiology
10. Intraoperative and peri-operative monitoring.

Valvular Heart Disease (Figs 4.8–4.14 and 4.19)

Rheumatic fever is one of the leading causes of malfunctioning of both AV and semilunar valves in most of the developing countries of the world. Mitral valve is affected commonly followed by aortic, tricuspid and

rarely pulmonary valve. Most of the pathological lesions can be diagnosed with TTE but with certain limitations. TEE can overcome these limitations easily and in most of the cases an accurate diagnosis can be made with good index of sensitivity and specificity.

Organic lesion of the mitral apparatus is more easily visualised by transesophageal than by transthoracic echocardiography. The extent of valvular and sub-valvular calcification, leaflet mobility and the severity of mitral regurgitation can be accurately defined. Aortic, tricuspid and even pulmonary valves can also be inspected by the transesophageal approach.

Although transthoracic Doppler techniques can assess mitral transprosthetic gradients and provide data about the haemodynamic performance of prostheses, identification of the cause of malfunction is often difficult; nevertheless, in most cases, transesophageal echocardiography can accurately identify the malfunction. Thus, recently transthoracic and transesophageal echocardiography are used to evaluate recombinant tissue plasminogen activator therapy in prosthetic mitral valve thrombosis. Pretreatment transesophageal echocardiography identified thrombus formation on mitral prosthetic leaflets; and, post-thrombolytic echo showed complete resolution of the thrombi and resumption of normal bioprosthetic function.

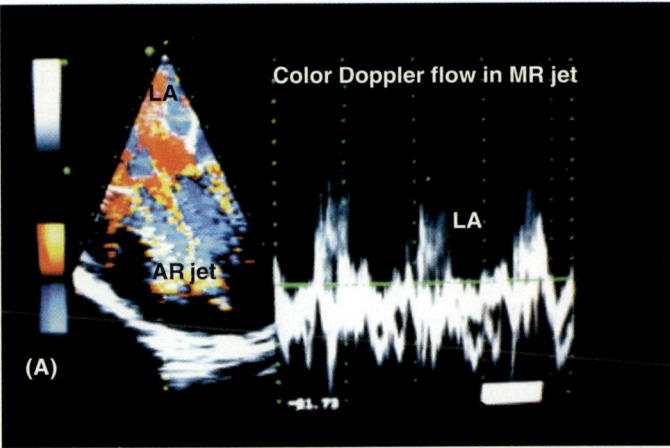

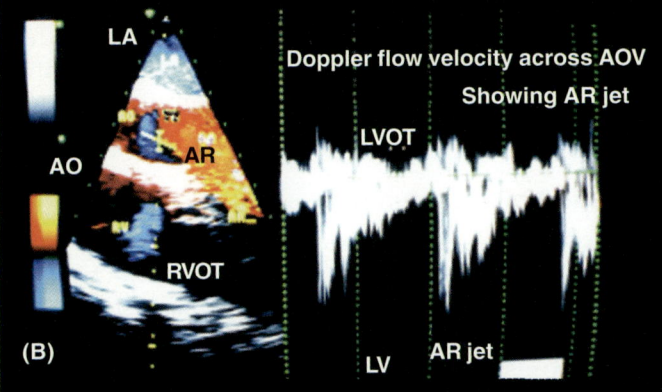

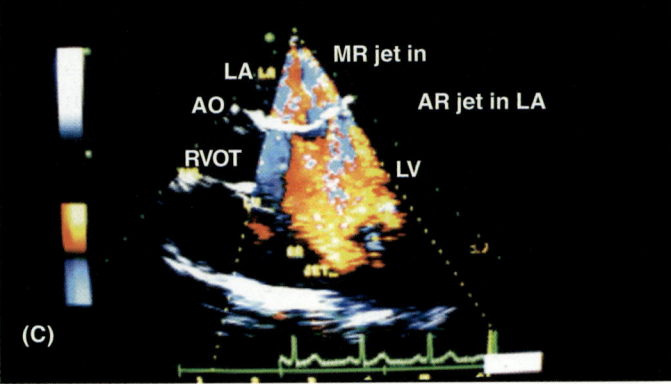

Fig. 4.14 A to C: Color flow and color Doppler flows in one of the patients suffering from RHD, MS, MR AR and pulmonary hypertension in different angles and planes as shown in these TEE scans

Balloon valvuloplasty of stenotic mitral valve may be contraindicated in the presence of left atrial or appendiceal thrombus. In this clinical setting, transesophageal echocardiography provides accurate data on the presence of atrial thrombi.

Infective Endocarditis (Figs 4.35, 4.41 and 4.45)

Knowledge of TEE has revolutionised the development of life saving antimicrobial and surgical therapies in infective endocarditis. TEE technique has proved useful for the visualisation of various valvular abnormalities leading to infective endocarditis; and urgency surgical intervention.

Transesophageal echocardiography has been shown in various studies—to have >90% sensitivity for detecting vegetation, compared with 60% sensitivity for transthoracic echocardiography. The transesophageal route also demonstrated high degree of specificity.

It is highly versatile and useful in delineating small vegetation (<5.0 cm), valve ring abscesses, mycotic aneurysms, chordal tears, flail leaflets and valve disruptions. Furthermore, it is probably superior to transthoracic echocardiography for visualisation of vegetations of mural infective endocarditis and particularly in bacteraemic patients with intracardiac shunts, intracardiac catheters or pacemakers.

Another important role of transesophageal echocardiography in infective endocarditis is in the ability of the procedure to assess valve function for purposes of surgical intervention. Evaluating whether single or multiple valves are involved and identification of ring abscesses, influences the nature and extent of subsequent surgery. Furthermore, Doppler techniques can identify dysfunctional valves before surgery. Transesophageal Doppler echocardiography has proved especially useful in patients with prosthetic valve endocarditis with congestive cardiac failure. Regurgitant jets on Doppler mode can indicate the exact site of lesion limiting either to a transvalvular, paravalvular areas or to intracardiac communication. In addition, intraoperative transesophageal echocardiography can also reliably assess the surgical outcome of a valvular repair.

Coronary Artery Disease (Figs 4.22 and 4.40)

Highly-frequency transesophageal transducers permit adequate non-invasive visualisation of the proximal areas of the coronary arteries, providing information on luminal narrowing and blood flow. The proximal left coronary arterial system is more frequently visualised (90% of patients) than the right (< 50% of patients).

In addition, the distances of stenotic lesions from vessel origins were accurately recorded by the transesophageal probe. Thus, the investigators concluded that transesophageal echocardiography accurately identified left main coronary artery stenosis in a large number of patients. The procedure was, however, less useful in identifying stenotic lesions in proximal portions of the left anterior descending left circumflex and right coronary arteries. Transesophageal Doppler studies have been performed in the assessment of coronary flow reserve, which is defined as the difference between baseline flow and maximal flow; the later being induced either by physiological stimuli, such as ischaemia, or by pharmacological agents, such as dipyridamole or

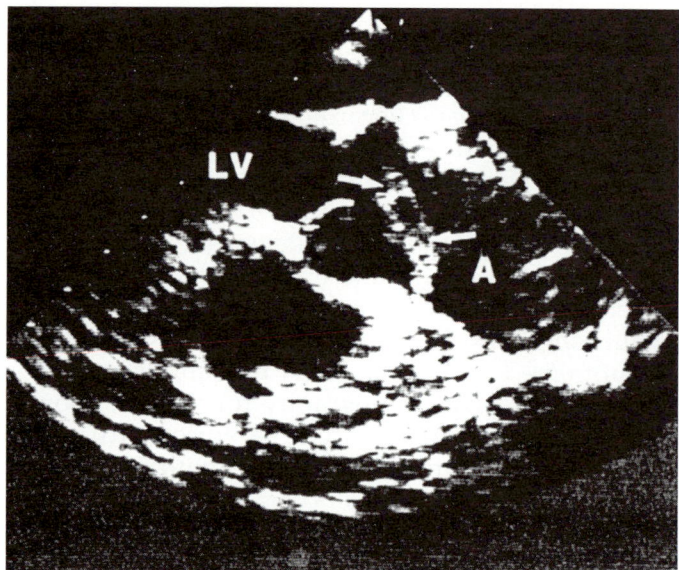

Fig. 4.15: TEE echoscan showing mobile mass in ascending aorta (arrow)

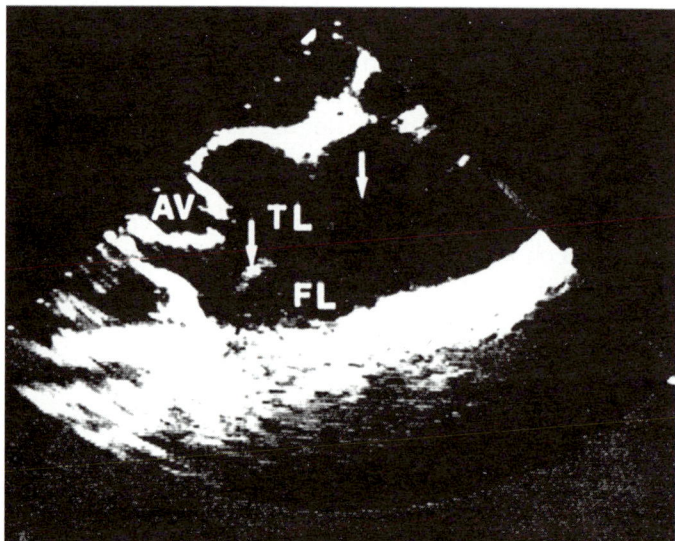

Fig. 4.16: Ascending aorta with dissection, bicuspid aortic valve with possible thrombosis. Seen also is the false lumen (FL) and true lumen (TL) of the dissection

adenosine. Coronary flow reserve is considered a meaningful indicator of the functional significance of coronary artery stenosis. Thus, a recent clinical series showed that transesophageal Doppler studies provided a safe and effective means of measuring coronary flow reserve ratio during adenosine infusion.

Furthermore, Doppler transesophageal echocardiographic assessment of coronary blood flow reserve during dobutamine infusion can be compared with transesophageal 2-dimensional analysis of left ventricular wall motion for the detection of left anterior

descending coronary artery disease. Both techniques are equally sensitive for diagnosing left anterior coronary artery disease, It has been seen that coronary flow reserve is a more sensitive detector of left anterior descending artery stenosis than 2-dimensional transesophageal left ventricular views for analysis of wall motion.

Aortic Dissection (Figs 4.16, 4.36 and 4.50)

One of the most useful applications of TEE is to detect aortic dissection in critically sick patients and demonstrate dissection in a quick and portable manner. It, therefore, makes the TEE procedure superior to other available methods. With the multiplane TEE transducer, demonstrating the presence of thrombus or flow in the false lumen can usually identify the site and extent of the dissection. This information is pertinent to the management of these patients.

Prosthetic Valve Dysfunction

On account of dense material used in the preparation of prosthetic valves which gives bright reflections on transthoracic 2-dimensional echocardiography, it, therefore, becomes much difficult for a echocardiographer to assess the valvular functions accurately. Evaluating the presence of thrombus or vegetation on prosthetic valves has been particularly challenging from the transthoracic approach. Transesophageal echo, approaching the prosthetic valves from a different angle, enables visualisation of the hidden area of the prosthesis, particularly the left atrial side of the prosthetic mitral valve. Moreover, its superior resolution, can detect small vegetations or thrombi on prosthetic valves (Figs 4.30 and 4.33).

Transesophageal Echocardiography in Critically Ill Patients

Postoperative patients and those who are on mechanical ventilators are at increased risk for developing critical complications. Two-dimensional echocardiography is quite unsatisfactory and of low diagnostic yield when compared to TEE which is considered as the best modality in the diagnosis of various complications in critical situations. Often, diagnosis can be obtained at the bedside in 15–20 min. Surprisingly, such patients tolerate TEE well with minimal risks and side effects. TEE can be safely performed in most critically ill-patients in critical care units and has a definitive role in the diagnosis and expeditious management of such patients, some of whom can be sent to surgical operations without further investigation. TEE is also very useful in various cardiopulmonary emergencies such as postoperative hypotensive states, localised cardiac temponade, acute

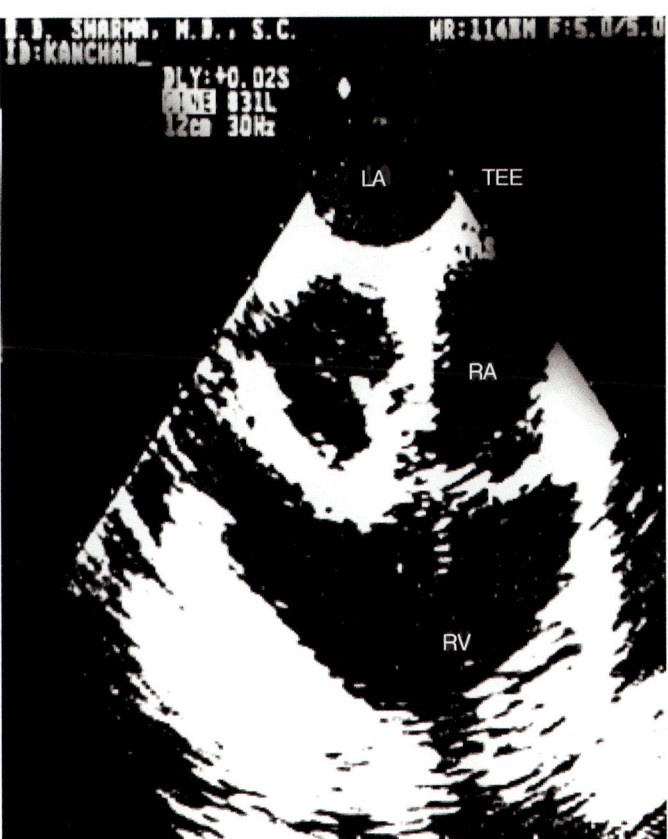

Fig. 4.17: Basal short axis plane showing anatomical relationship of the internal cardiac structures as indicated on the scan

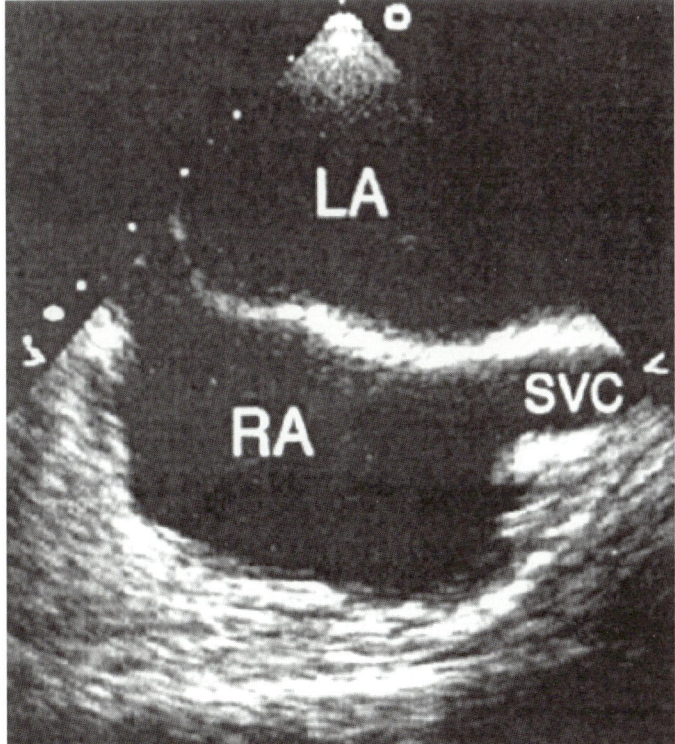

Fig. 4.18: Vertical plane in esophagus through bicaval view demonstrates LA/RA, IAS and entery of superior vena cava (SVC)

MR due to ruptured cardiae tendinae, papillary muscle, IVS rupture, pulmonary thrombo-embolism in the main pulmonary artery, its branches and acute dissecting hematoma (Figs 4.36, 4.38, 4.46 and 4.49).

Transesophageal Echocardiography in Interventional Cardiology (Table 4.1)

Transesophageal echocardiography has been proved very useful during certain interventional procedures, e.g. prior to cardioversion to exclude left atrial appendage thrombus, during valvoplasty (both aortic and mitral) transcatheter closure of ASD, assessing LV functions during angioplasty, removal of intracardiac catheter and insertion of pacemaker in early pregnancy to avoid radiation. With the help of TEE interventional cardiologists have been encouraged to perform interventional procedures more frequently with least post-procedural morbidity and mortality.

Intraoperative and Perioperative Monitoring (Table 4.1)

TEE is being increasingly used in the operative room during (intraoperative) and immediately to six hours postoperative (perioperative) by cardiac surgeons and anesthesiologists during operative intervention of various congenital and acquired heart diseases and major vascular surgery. There are three main indications for such monitoring. They are baseline preoperative (pre-bypass) diagnosis, monitoring of left ventricular function, and assessing efficacy of surgical intervention before discontinuation of cardiopulmonary bypass. Perioperative TEE monitoring is usually limited to continuation of monitoring of left ventricular function following surgery in unstable patients who have undergone revascularization. Segmental wall motion abnormalities are detectable much earlier by TEE than any other invasive or noninvasive cardiac monitoring methods currently employed. Other problems for which TEE has been used are the detection of venous air embolism, bone marrow embolism during insertion of hip prosthesis and intraoperative TEE monitoring for myocardial ischemia during major noncardiac vascular surgery in order to reduce the incidence of cerebral stroke. Displacement of a friable and, protruding atherosclerotic material by aortic arch cannulation or by high pressure jet emerging from the cannula tip may play an important role in the creation of embolization and stroke. TEE is not only found contributory in clarifying physiology of dynamic obstruction, in HOCM but also in planning the extent of resection, assessing the immediate result, and excluding important complications. Transesophageal echocardiography is very useful modality in the evaluation of a cardiac mass lesion. For patients who have unexplained strokes, TEE may demonstrate the potential source of emboli, such as the presence of thrombus in the left atrial appendage

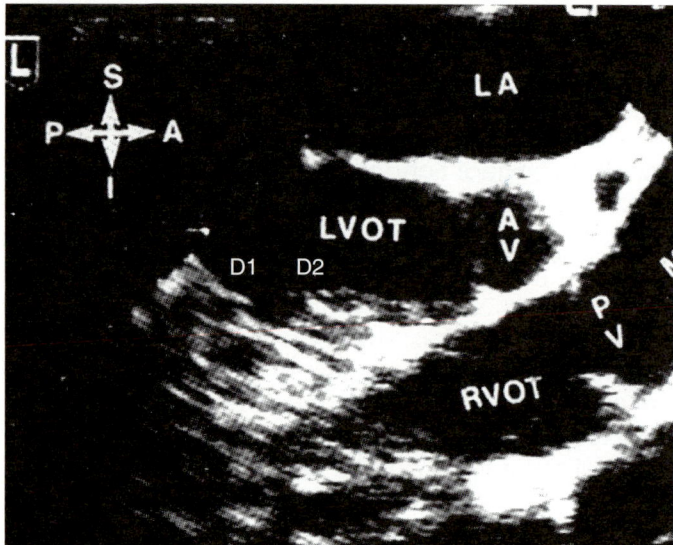

Fig. 4.19: Oblique basal short axis view demonstrating the exact location of aortic valve and LVOT. This can also help us determining the outflow area in the final calculation of stroke volume and cardiac output (D1 and D2)

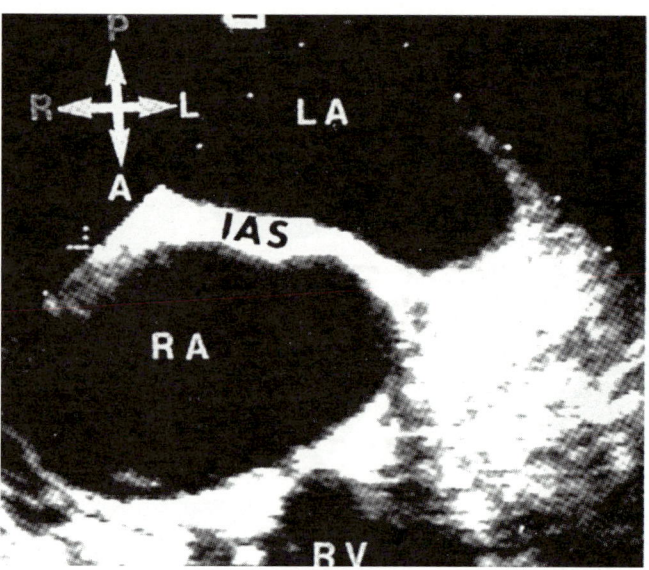

Fig. 4.20: Basal short axis view also called as biatrial view demonstrating the placement of two chambers(LA/RA) with intervening interatrial septum.This view is very helpful in the final diagnosis of secundum type of atrial septal defect, (ASD)

Table 4.4: *Showing various imaging planes in transesophageal echocardiography in the assessment of congenital heart disease*

	Standard examination planes	*Visualisation of cardiac structures*	*Pathology observed*
(i)	Transgastric planes	Ventricular morphology	Ventricular dominance
		Ventricular relations	Superio/inferior ventricles
		Ventricular function	Parachute MV
		Chordal apparatus MV	Interruption of
		Inferior atrioventricular vein	Individual drainage
		Hepatic veins	Common valve orifice
		Atrioventricular valves	
(ii)	Lower oesophagus	Coronary sinus (CS)	Unroofed CS
		Dilated CS	Muscular inlet VSD
		Muscular inlet septum	Ebstein's malformation
		Tricuspid valve	Offsetting atrioventricular valves
		4-chamber view	Atrio-ventricular septal defects
			Perimembranous VSD
(iii)	Left atrial views	Mitral valve	Valvular regurgitation
		Atrial septum	Patent oval foramen
		Atrial chambers	Deficiencies of the fossa ovalis
		Pulmonary veins	Anomalous connection

or the presence of pedunculated, mobile, atheroseclerotic plaque in the aorta. TEE may also demonstrate the presence of an atrial septal defect, patent foramen ovale, or atrial septal aneurysm. The latter is known to increase the chances of thrombo-embolic phenomenon in the absence of LA thrombosis (Fig. 4.16).

Transesophageal Echocardiography in Congenital Heart Diseases (Figs 4.8A and 4.48)

The first pediatric probe was developed in late 1980, and an initial clinical experience with its use was reported by Omoto and colleagues. The original design featured a 5 MHz 24-element phased-array transducer mounted at the tip of a pediatric gastroscope. The maximal shaft diameter measured just under 7 mm. This miniaturisation could only be accomplished by a reduction in the number of ultrasound crystals (and hence connecting wires), as well as by sacrificing the lateral steering mechanism. To cater to the need of children, the total shaft length measured upto 70 cm. The tip of the transducer measured roughly 7 mm in maximal width and 8 mm in maximal height. Thus transducer tip circumference was just under 30 mm.

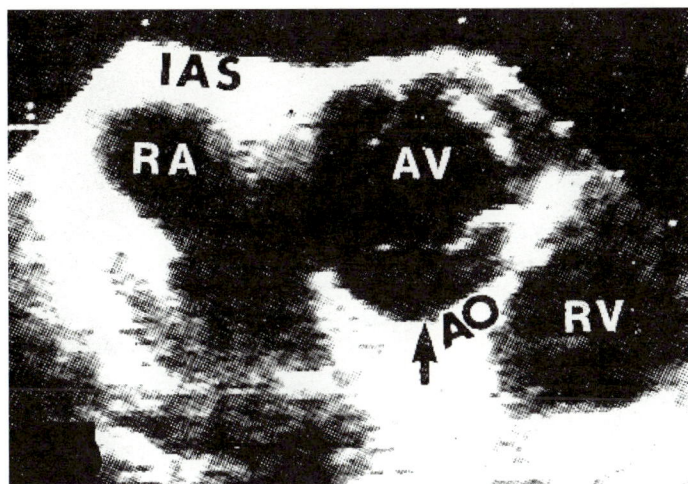

Fig. 4.21: Basal short axis view showing LV, IAS, RA, RV, AO and aortic valve

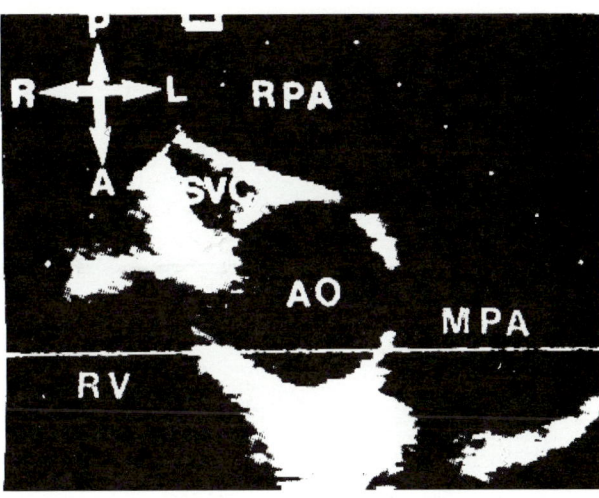

Fig. 4.24: Short axis basal plane passing through great vessels depicting aorta as a central structure and is surrounded by to its right SVC, to its left MPA, to its posterior RPA and to its anterior Aorta. It also visualises RV lying anterior to superior vena cava (SVC)

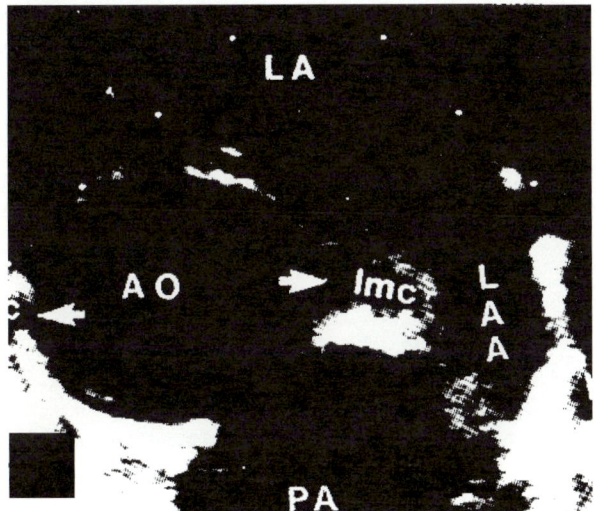

Fig. 4.22: Basal short axis plane showing relationship between aorta and emerging left main coronary artery (lmc). This view also depicts close association of left atrial appendage and left main coronary artery. Moreover, pulmonary artery (PA) is seen distal to aorta (AO)

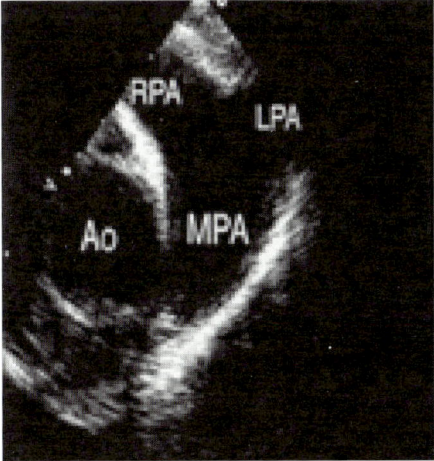

Fig. 4.25: Horizontal plane in high esophagus position TEE shows main pulmonary artery and its two branches LPA and RPA closely related with ascending aorta (AO)

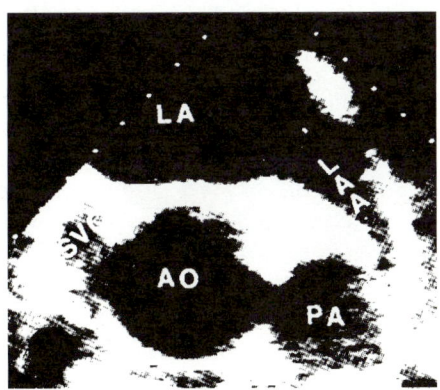

Fig. 4.23: Short axis plane through great vessels showing relationship between LA/AO/PA and left atrial appendage (LAA)

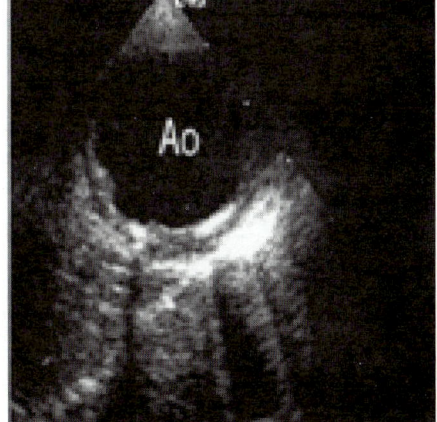

Fig. 4.26: TEE with slightly probe rotated upward it visualizes aorta (AO) to its entire thickness

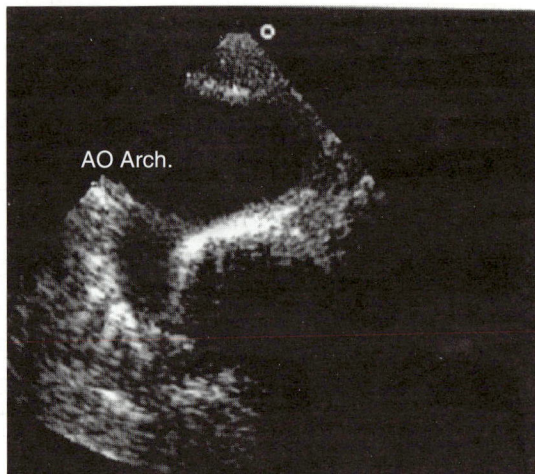

Fig. 4.27: TEE Distal aortic arch (AO arch) can be visualised comfortably positioning the probe in the vertical plane

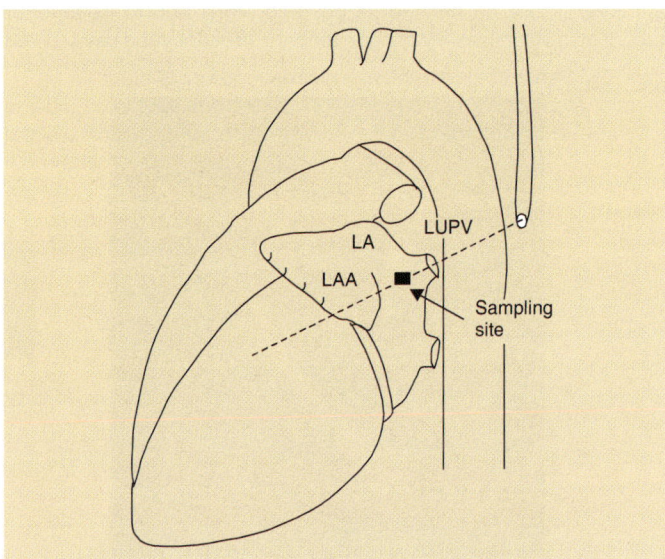

Fig. 4.28: Diagrammatic relationship between left upper pulmonary vein and left atrial appendage which is very close with descending aorta when two chamber view are constructed through positioning TEE probe in the short basal view in lower esophagus

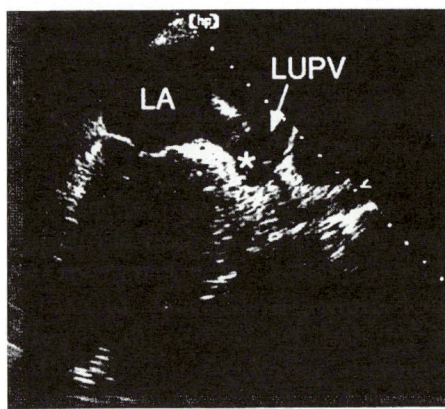

Fig. 4.29: Upper two chamber view visualising LA appendage and left upper pulmonary vein (LUPV)

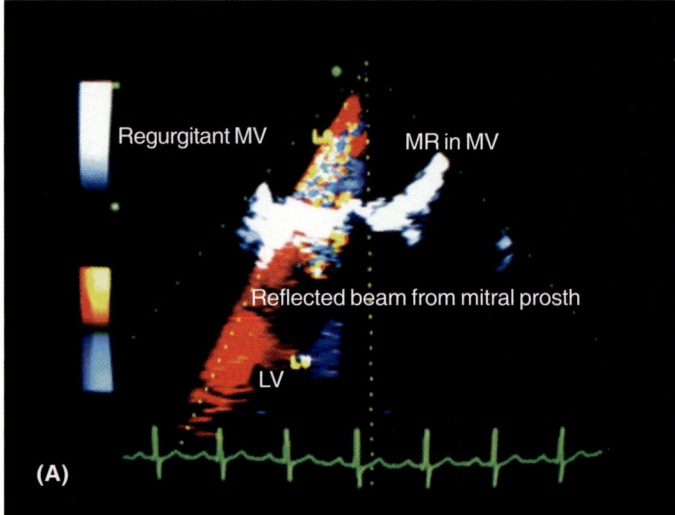

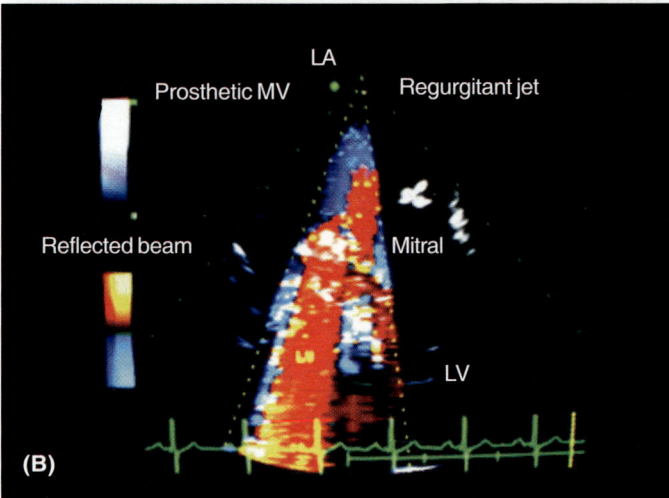

Fig. 4.30A and B: Color flow TEE showing mitral valve prosthetic MR jet entering into LA as blue stream and reflected ultrasound beam from the solid body of the prosthesis

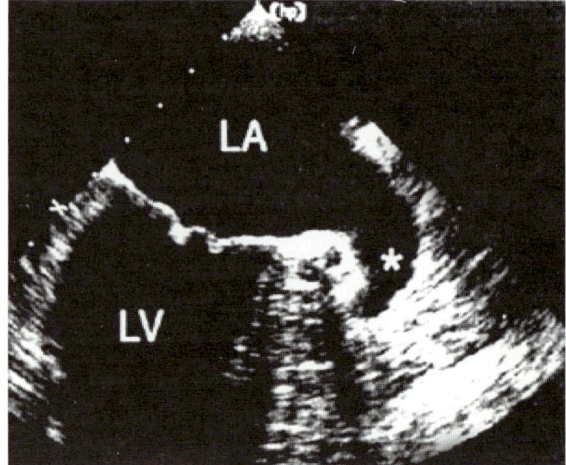

Fig. 4.31: Short axis basal plane for two chamber view for LA/LV with opening and closing excursion of MV during systole and diastole respectively

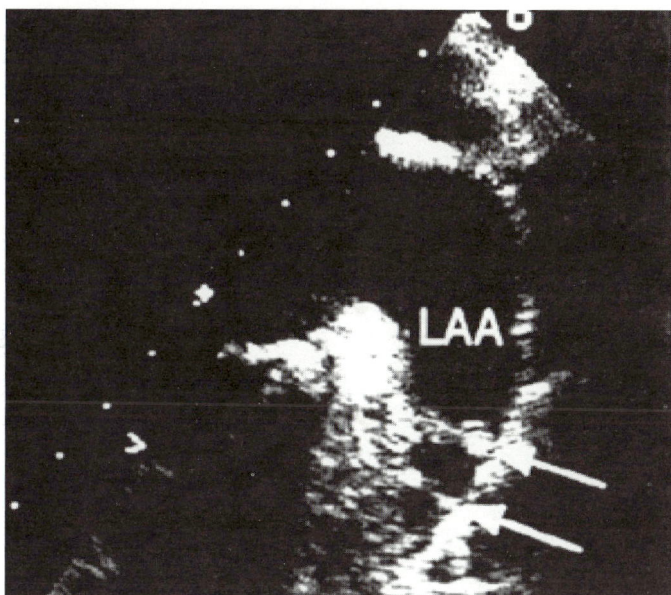

Fig. 4.32: Constructing vertical plane at mid esophagus reveals left atrial appendage with shaggy intraluminal structure some times mistaken as an organised thrombosis (arrow)

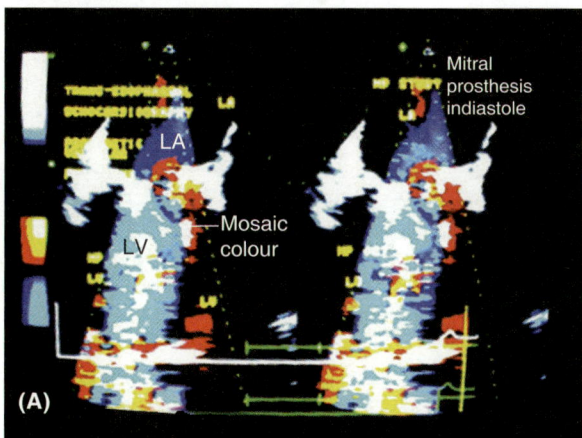

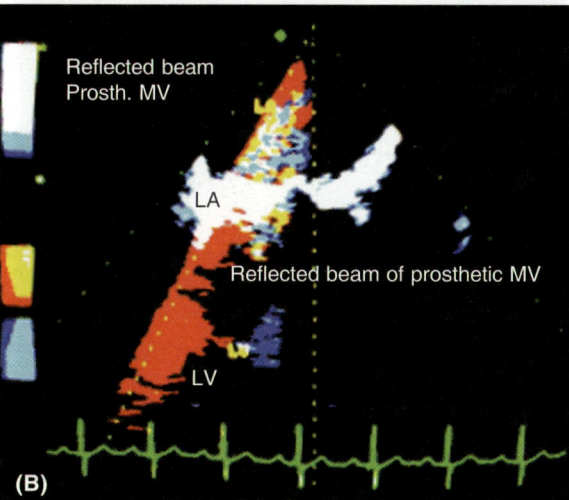

Fig. 4.33A and B: Mosaic color flow in a regurgitant prosthetic MV (A) and reflected ultrasound beam (B)

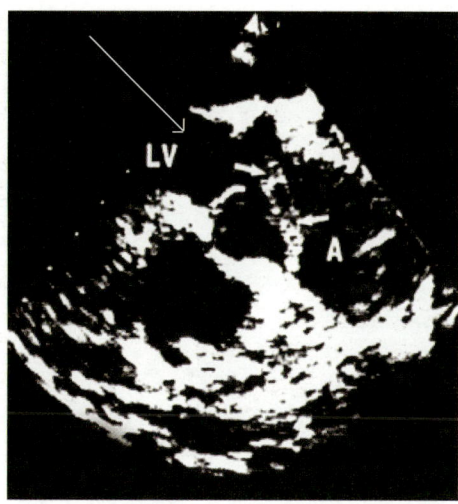

Fig 4.34: Mobile mass (arrow) in the ascending aorta (A) as visualised by TEE

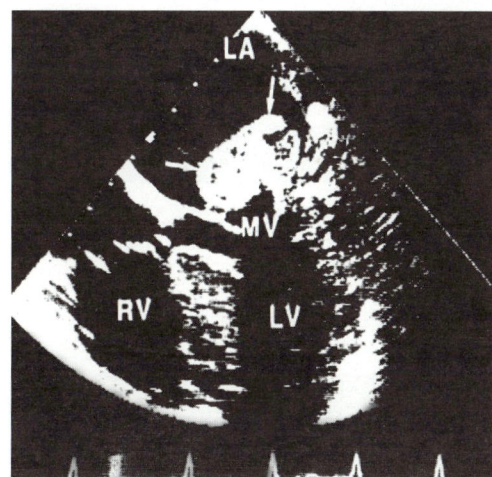

Fig. 4.35: 2-Chamber view showing mass echo on the mitral valve (MV) as a result of infective endocarditis (arrow)

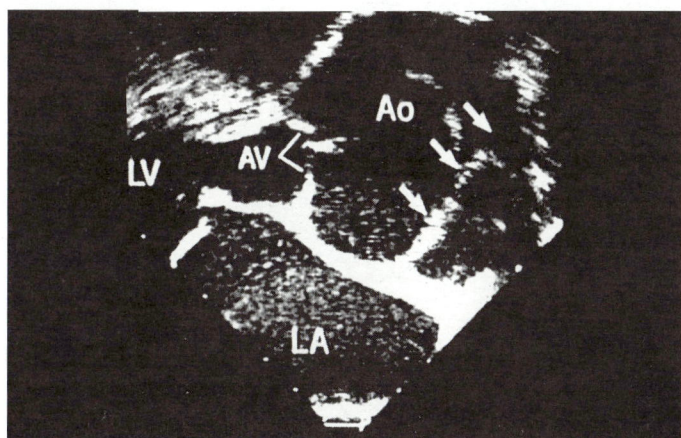

Fig. 4.36: Short axis upside down view shows dissection of aorta. False lumen and flap have been shown by arrows one can also see spontaneous contrast in LA

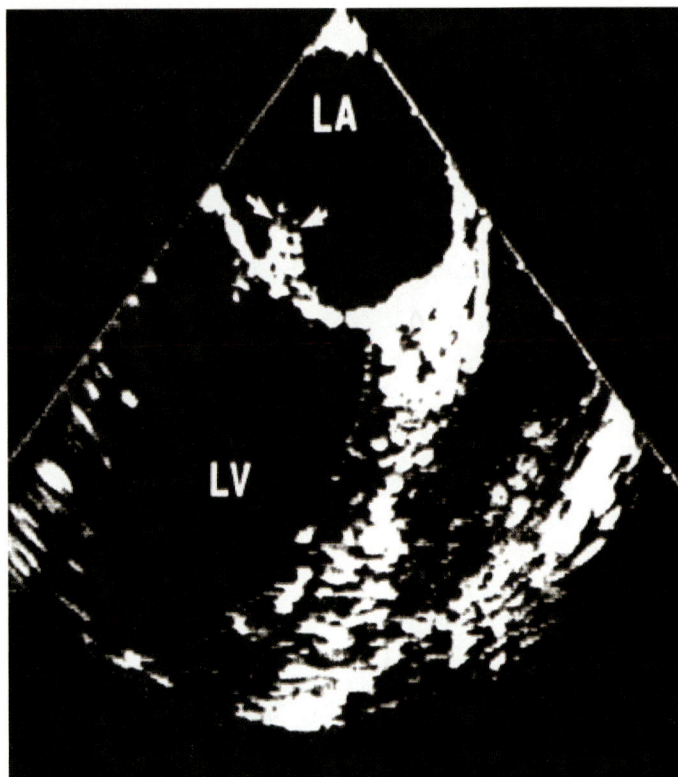

Fig. 4.37: 2-Chamber view visualising LA, LV and two leaflets of mitral valve which are affected by a fixed mass (arrow)

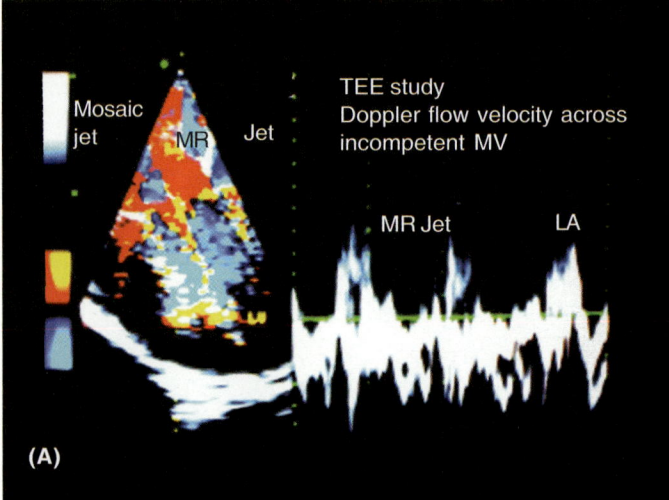

(A)

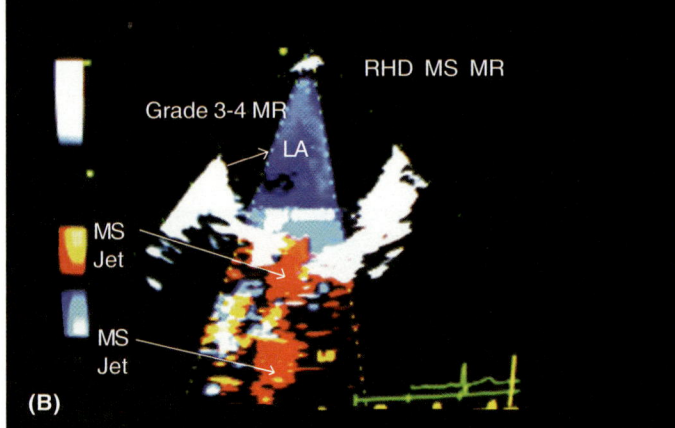

(B)

Fig. 4.39A and B: Color Doppler flow velocity across MV in a patient with RHD, MS, MR and AR (A) and color flow scan showing grade 3-4 MR as seen blue color jet spreading throughout the cavity of LA

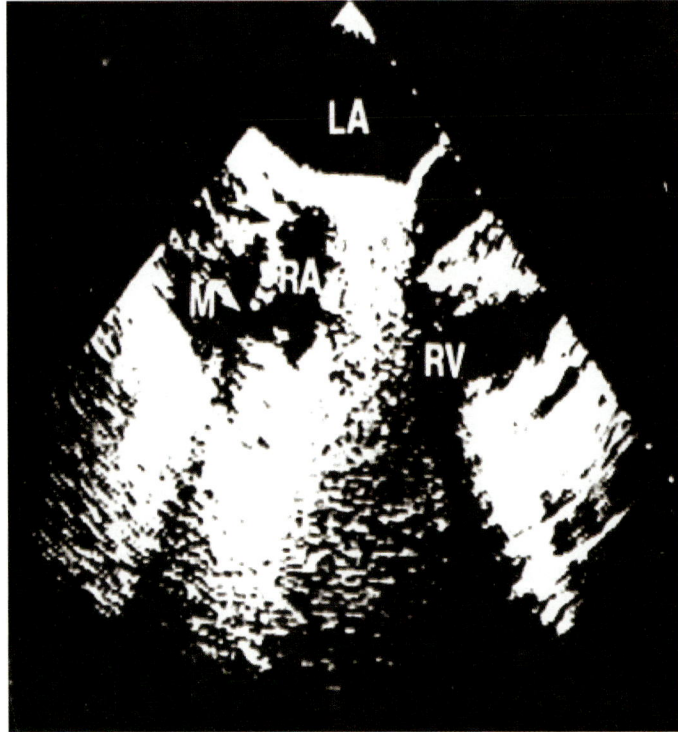

Fig. 4.38: A big pericardial hematoma (M) compressing right atrium (RA) in a patient with pericardial temponade visualised by TEE

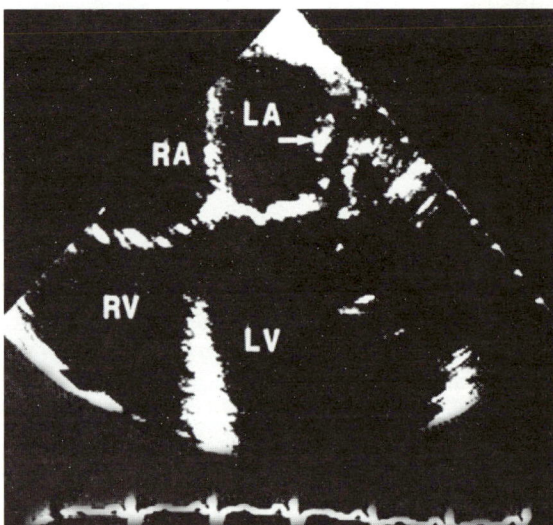

Fig. 4.40: Flail mitral valve (arrow) after rupture of papillary muscle following an acute myocardial infarction in four chamber TEE view

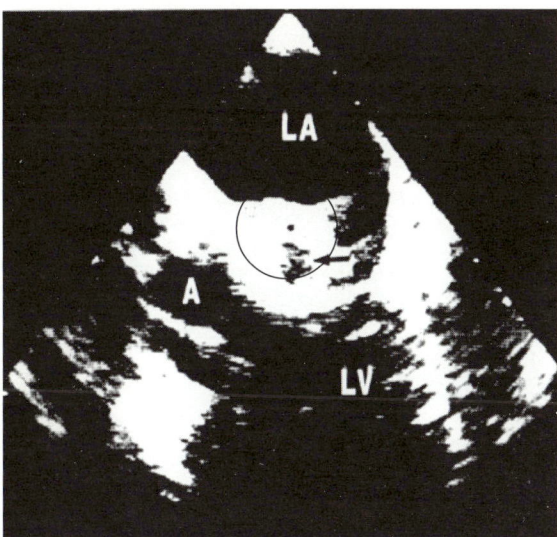

Fig. 4.41: Basal 2-chamber TTE view showing aortic root abscess (arrow) following aortic valve endocarditis

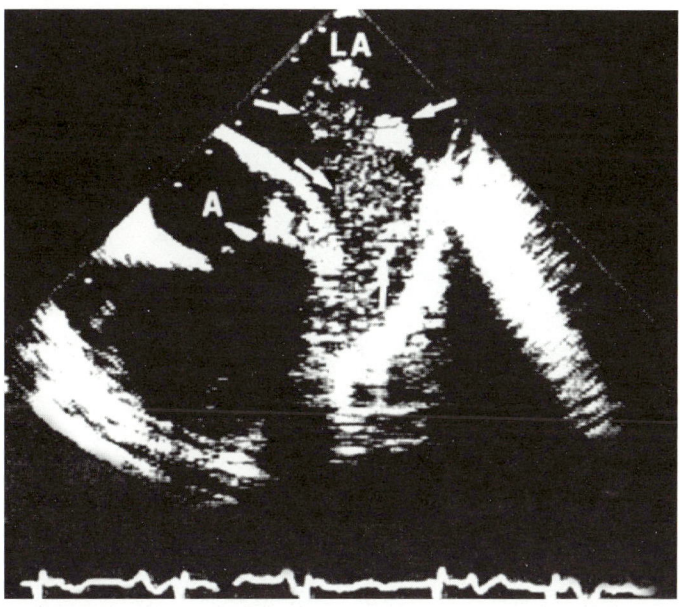

Fig. 4.43: Short axis plane showing thrombosis in the left atrial appendage (arrow)

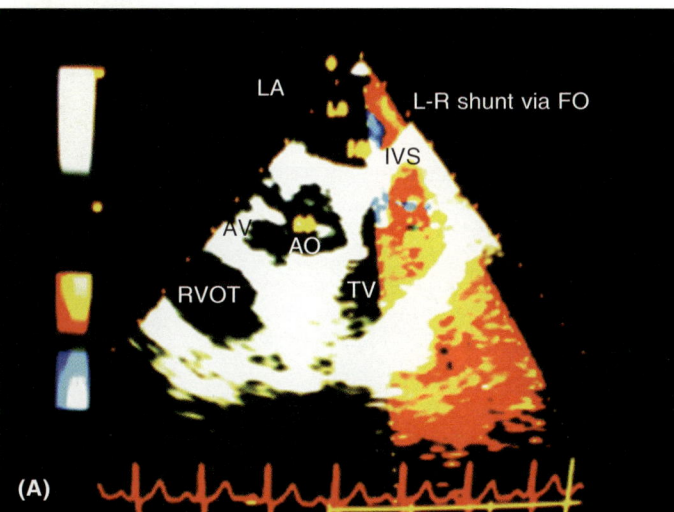

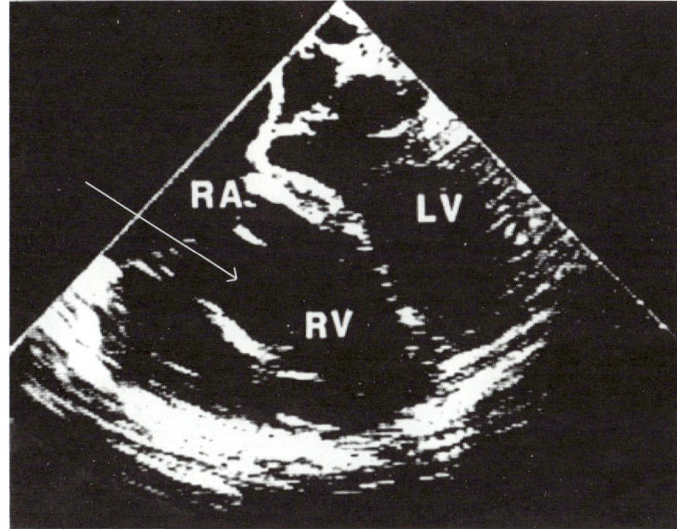

Fig. 4.44: Dilated right ventricle in a patient with chronic cor-pulmonale

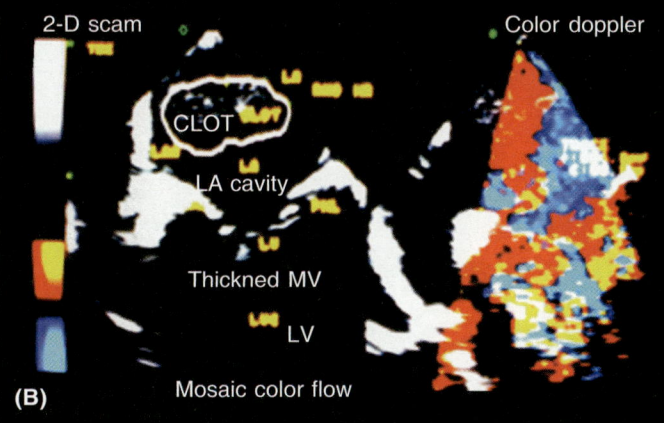

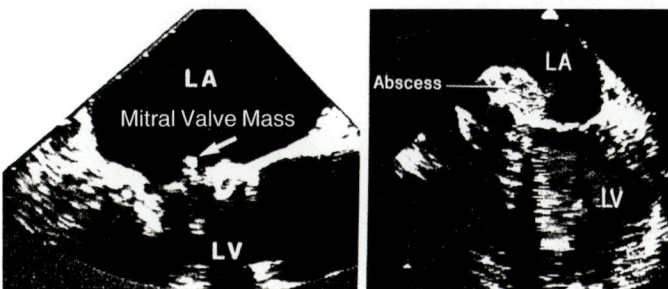

Fig. 4.42A and B: (A) Mild L-R shunt through persistent foramen ovale. **(B)** Dual 2-D scan showing marked thickened MV and clot (arrow, left) and gross MR with mosaic color as it happens in severe regurgitant flow with roughned valve (right)

Fig. 4.45A and B: (A) Basal 2-chamber plane view showing mitral valve mass mimicking like infective vegetation. **(B)** A large bacterial abscess localised in the region of aortic root. Clinically the patient presented with bacterial infection with gross aortic regurgitation

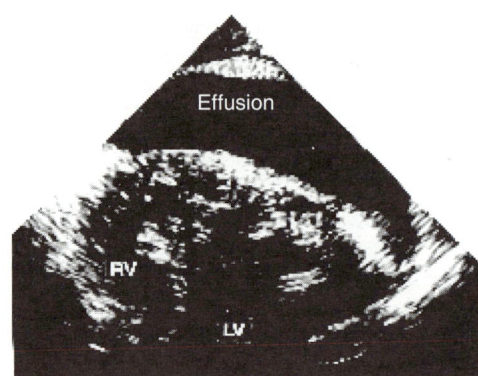

Fig. 4.46: Short axis plane demonstrating moderate type of pericardial effusion

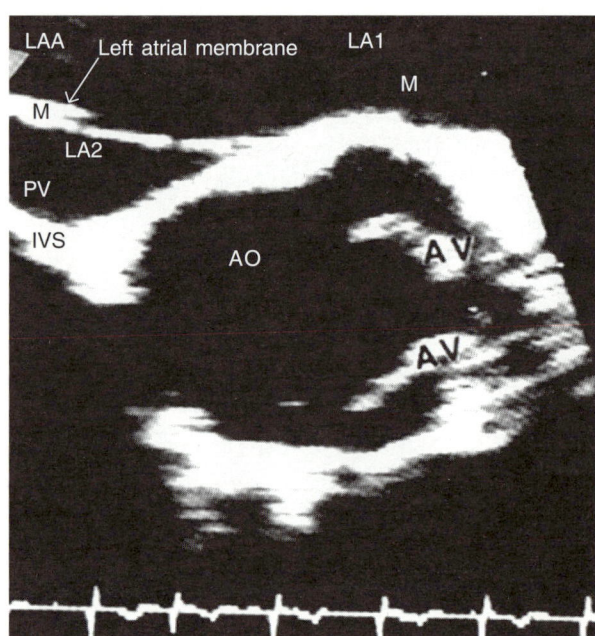

Fig. 4.48: TEE scan shows how left atrial membrane (M) divides LA cavity into upper (LA1) and lower (LA2). It is further clarified that upper larger division is connected with LA appendage (LAA) and lower smaller one receives low frequency pulmonary venus blood flow (pv) in patient with cor triatriatum

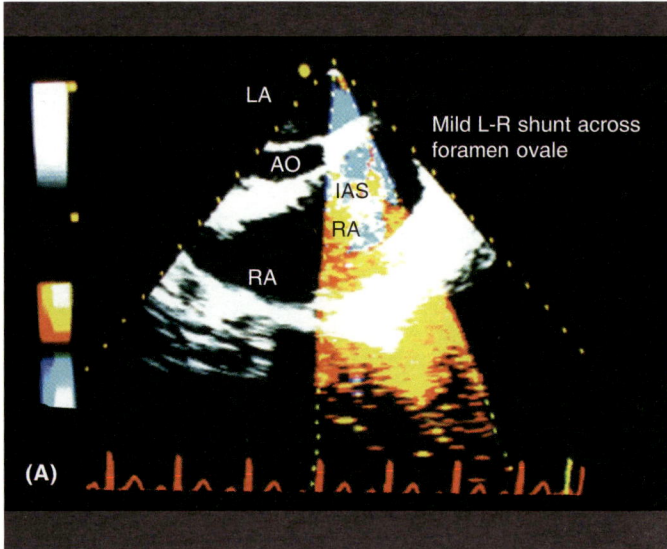

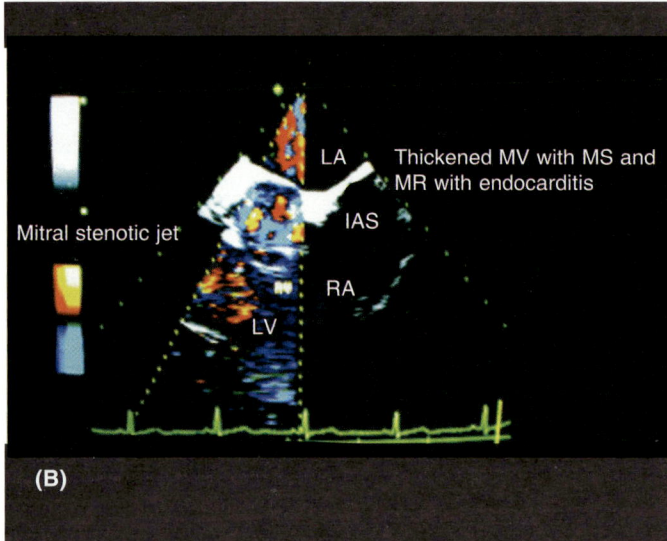

Fig. 4.47A and B: **(A)** Mild L-R shunt flow across IAS through foramen ovale as seen through TEE. **(B)** Thickened MV with stenotic jet and mild MR jet into LA cavity with infective endocarditis and complete closure of foramen ovale

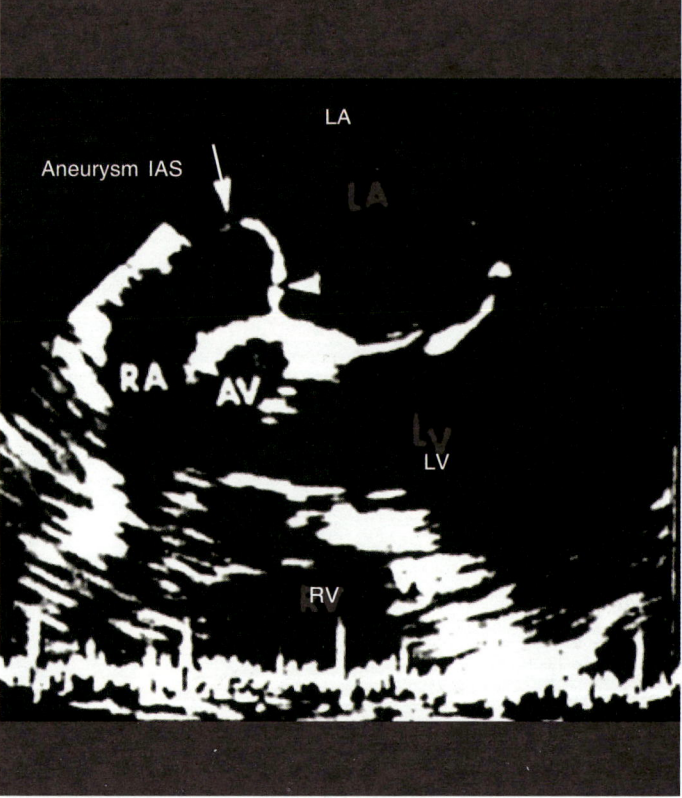

Fig. 4.49: TEE 4C view in horizontal plane, showing aneurysm (arrow) of interatrial septum which is considered as a site for developing thrombosis/clot and further may predispose to thrombo-embolic phenomenon

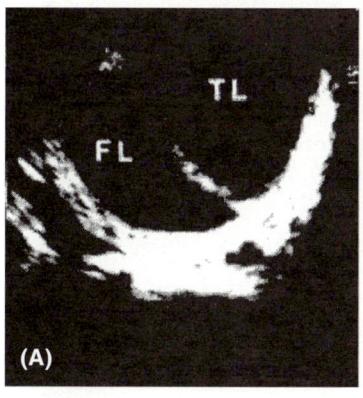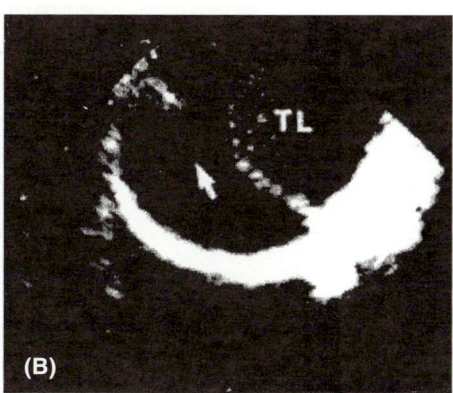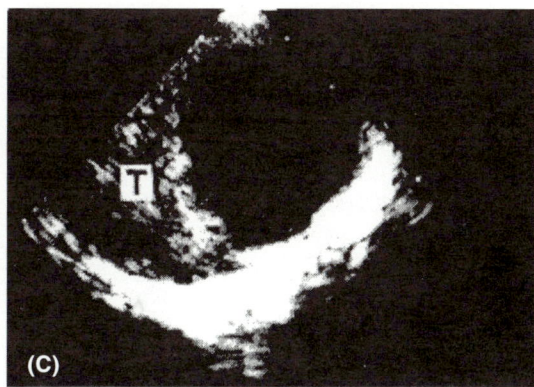

Fig. 4.50A to C: (A) TEE, scan depicts a double lumen with pulsatile flow in both the true (TL) and false (FL) lumens of the aorta. **(B)** After 4 days, the same patient revealed spontaneous contrast within the false lumen. **(C)** After 8 weeks, the spontaneous contrast previously noted in the false lumen is replaced by Thrombus (T) in an elderly patient with aortic dissection

Table 4.5: *Comparative evaluation between transthoracic (TTE) transophageal (TEE) and epicardial (EE), 2D-echocardiography*

	TTE	TEE	EE
Mitral stenosis	++++	++++	+++
Atrial myxoma	++++	++++	+++
Dissecting aorta	+	++++	—
Left atrial thrombus	+	++++	—
Prosthetic valve dysfunction	++	++++	+++
Quantitation of valvular regurgitation	++	++++	+++
Atrial septal defects	+	++++	+++
Valvular endocarditis	++	++++	+++

However, with the rapid evolution of paediatric transesophageal imaging as an adjunct to the diagnostic armamentarium in paediatric cardiology, several further probe designs have become available. These include a 48-element 5 MHz phased-array single-plane probe. Although this probe has slightly larger dimensions than the probe developed by Omoto et al, it allows safe studies in children down to 3.5 kilograms bodyweight. In this new probe, there was improvement in cross-sectional imaging resolution, the near field artifact reduced, and the depth at which both colour and pulsed wave Doppler studies could be carried out was found much improved.

Mechanical probes have been developed for paediatric imaging and array systems have become available in two sizes with an 11.5 and 9 mm transducer tip diameter. Both probes provide a dynamic shift in imaging frequency from 5 to 7.5 MHz and continuous wave Doppler facilities.

Neonatal transesophageal probe has also been developed which allows studies in premature infants. The maximal shaft diameter of this probe measures just 4 mm and the tip measured 4 × 5 mm. However, because of the considerable deduction of the total number of ultrasound elements to 17, this probe does not provide high-resolution cross-sectional imaging. Nonetheless, the probe allows for the acquisition of high-quality Doppler and colour flow mapping information in either the critically ill neonate or after neonatal cardiac surgery.

In order to overcome the shortcomings of single plane transverse axis imaging in the assessment of lesions involving the right ventricular outflow tract and the ventriculo-arterial junction, a single-plane longitudinal axis transducer has been developed for use in children. Although this approach offers several advantages in the evaluation of outflow tract lesions, the longitudinal imaging plane proved to be only an adjunct to transverse axis imaging rather than a viable alternative.

Bibliography

1. Acar J, Cormier B, Grimberg G, *et al*. Diagnosis of left atrial thrombi in mitral stenosis—Usefulness of ultrasound techniques compared with other method. *Eur Heart J* 1991; 12:70–76.
2. Burke RP, Wernovsky G, Van der Welde M, *et al*. Surgery for congenital heart disease. Video-assisted thoracoscopic surgery for congenital heart disease. *J Thorac Cardiovasc Surg* 1995; 109:499–508.
3. Feinberg MS, Hopkins WE, Davila-Roman VG, Barzilai B. Multiplane transesophageal echoardiographic Doppler imaging accurately determines cardiac output measurements in critically ill patients. *Chest* 1995; 107:769–773.
4. Fisher EA, Stahl JA, Budd JH, Goldman ME. Transesophageal echocardiography: procedures and clinical application. *J Am Coll Cardiol* 1991; 18:1333–1448.
5. Losi MA, Betocchi S, Briguori C, *et al*. Recombinant tissue-type plasminogen activator therapy in prosthetic mitral valve thrombosis: assessment by transthoracic and transesophageal echocardiography. *Int J Cardiol* 1995; 48:219–224.
6. Redberg RF, Sobol Y, Chou TM. Adenosine induced coronary vasodilatation during transesophageal Doppler echocardiography. *Circulation* 1995; 92:190–96.

7. Samadarshi TE, Nanda NC, Gatewood RP, *et al.* Usefulness and limitations of transesophageal echocardiography in the assessment of proximal coronary stenosis. *J Am Coll Cardiol* 1992; 19:572–580.

8. Shah PM. Shapiro J. Intraoperative transesophageal echocardiography: An anaesthesiologists perspective. *Acta Anaesthesiol Scand* 1991; 35:683–692.

9. Shapiro SM, Bayer AS. Transesophageal and Doppler echocardiography in the diagnosis and management of infective endocarditis. *Chest* 1991; 100:1125–1130.

10. Stoddard MF, Prince CR, Morris GT. Coronary flow reserve assessment by dobutamine transesophageal Doppler echocardiography. *J Am Coll Cardiol* 1995; 25:325–332.

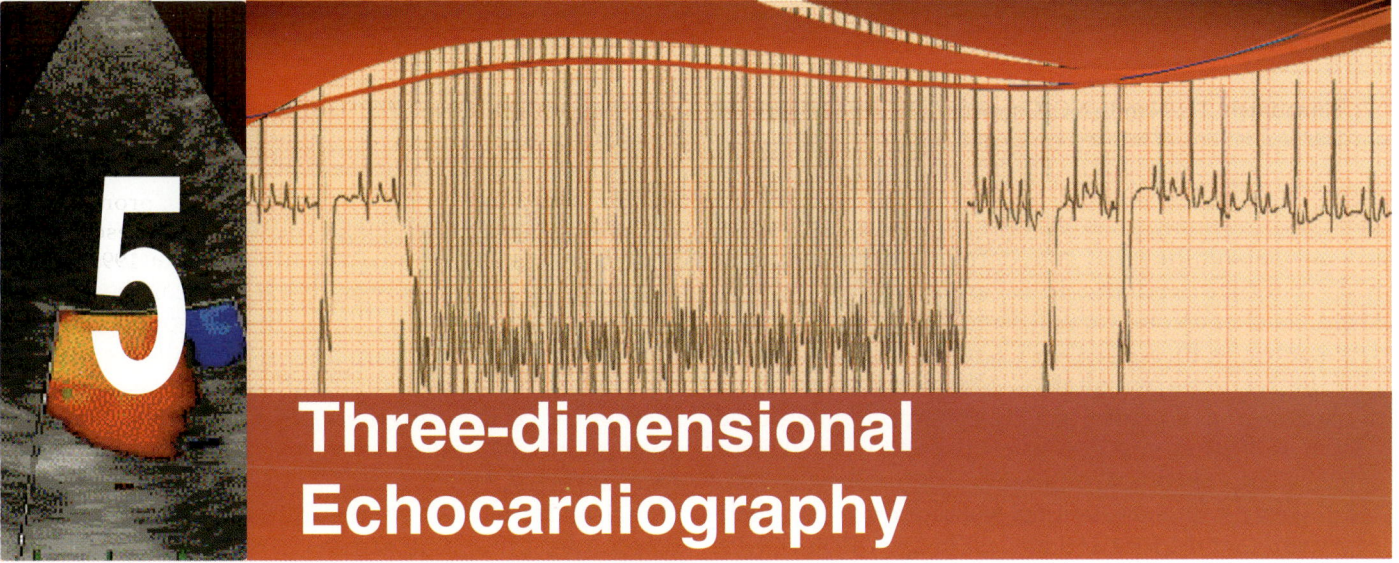

Three-dimensional Echocardiography

At times one may not be able to obtain an effective imaging through 2-D transthoracic and to some extent even with transesophageal echocardiography. But currently 3-D echocardiography with improved equipment and computer technology allows better and more effective imaging of the heart in multiple sequential planes by overcoming chest wall difficulties. The acquisition and display of images of the heart in three dimensional space has been attempted for more than a decade, but several technical limitations have hampered its clinical acceptance. In particular, the quality of precordial images has often been less than optimal and the time required for reconstruction of the images prohibitively long. The multiplane transesophageal probe represents the most technological innovation for reconstruction of better quality of cardiovascular imaging, transesophageal approach therefore, offers a relatively stable site for the imaging probe and, together with the superior quality of the tomographic images, it therefore, forms an ideal window to three dimensional reconstruction.

In order to get better view of intracardiac structures it needs spatial orientation in three dimensions for better understanding and best possible image interpretation. The scope and efficacy of the emerging 'real-time three-dimensional transthoracic echocardiography' technique for comprehensive assessment of cardiac anatomy, physiology, pathomorphology and pathophysiology in patients with structural heart disease have been thoroughly discussed in this chapter.

Conventional two-dimensional (2-D) echocardiography requires comprehensive knowledge of a series of multiple orthogonal planar or tomographic images into an imaginary multidimensional reconstruction for better understanding of complex intracardiac structures and their spatial relation with surroundings. The emerging three-dimensional (3-D) echocardiographic imaging technique is a major step ahead towards the final goal of complete visualisation and comprehensive assessment of cardiac anatomy, physiology, pathomorphology and pathophysiology in real-time, which could potentially facilitate image interpretation and reduce inter-observer variability. Three-dimensional echocardiography started in the early 90's and is based on serial acquisition of 2-D images but limitations like electrocardiographic (ECG) and respiratory gating, motion artifacts, time consuming off-line reconstruction and analysis restricted its use only as a research tool. Various workers, in recent past have demonstrated the potential clinical applicability of newer generation real time 3-D echocardiography with advances in technique for image acquisition and digital data processing in noninvasive evaluation of heart diseases. The real-time 3-D echocardiography is the only on-line 3-D method based on real time volumetric scanning, as compared with other 3-D imaging techniques such as magnetic orientation of image in three dimensions for better understanding and enhanced image interpretation.

Technique (Fig. 5.1)
Technique of Image Acquisition
To start with, basic cross sectional images are acquired with the help of the probe in its predetermined rotational movements in obtaining 3-D images. Besides acquiring these basic cross sectional images, one should always keep in mind, the position and orientation of the heart in relation to imaging planes. This may vary during the cardiac and respiratory cycles and hence the tomographic images must be timed according to cardiac cycle. Spatial registration is controlled by a computer algorithm logic which controls the image acquisition in a given plane at a predetermined time in the respiratory

cycle. Temporal information is obtained by measuring cardiac cycle variation by ECG gating.

Rotational Scanning

Rotational scanning gives the echographer an additional advantage over the other conventional scanning modes and is considered the ideal means of acquiring 3-dimensional reconstruction images gathering optimal data sampling through a very small acoustic window with better imaging quality. The imaging plane is rotated around its central axis by a computer monitored system and the data is generated usually with 20 steps with the help of conical volume.

However, with the rotational technique it is extremely important that the first and the last images acquired are mirror images to avoid a mismatch between images in the conical volume, which will result in artifacts in the final display. Thus the transducer position and its central axis of rotation must remain fixed during the full 180° arc sampling.

The Esophageal Probe

In this procedure multiplane transesophageal probes can be used provided the rotation of the transducer array can be controlled to obtain predetermined sequential images with spatial and temporal registration. This can be monitored by a computer controlled step motor externally interfaced to the control knob of the transducer array. Usually 5 MHz, 64 element rotational array transducer is employed for this purpose. After being positioned in the esophagus, the probe can be kept in a steady position by locking the antero-posterior flexion control in the anterior position. The scanning plane can be continuously, rotated through 180°, starting from a longitudinal imaging position, by a control knob on the handle of the echoscope. The control knob of the multiplane probe is mechanically rotated by a step motor through a custom built wheel-work interface which permits step progress of the imaging plane over a span of 180° to produce a conical data volume with its apex in the transducer (Fig. 5.2).

The Precordial Probe

Preselected transducer is mounted in a prototype housing with a cogwheel which fits into a cylindrical holder. The step motor is mounted on the holder and through a wheel-work interface, rotates the cogwheel and the transducer inside the holder. A micro switch controls the start at 0° and the end at 180° of the image acquisition.

Equipment and Reconstruction System (Fig. 5.1)

It has already chosen instrument and the video output is interfaced with the three dimensional reconstruction system. This technique consists of a steering system for the computer controlled image acquisition and the software for three dimensional reconstruction and display.

The Image Acquisition

A particular desirable image can be constructed by the step motor controlling transducer rotation (either oesophageally or precordially) which can be applied over the thorax or placed through the esophageus. It is activated by the steering logic which allows optimal temporal and spatial registration of a cardiac cross section by considering heart cycle variation by ECG gating and respiratory cycle variation by impedance measurement. When a cardiac cycle is selected by the steering logic and corresponds to a pre-selected respiratory phase, the cardiac cross section is sampled at 40 ms intervals during a complete heart cycle. The cross section is digitised and stored in the computer memory. The step motor is then activated and rotates the control knob of the esophageal multiplane probe, the precordial transducer 2° to the next cross section where the same logic is followed. To encompass the whole heart (or region), 90° sequential standardised cross section must be obtained each during a complete heart cycle.

The Image Processing

Once the acquisition of the image has been finished cross section images are resampled in the correct sequence according to their ECG phase in volumetric data sets ($256 \times 256 \times 256$ pixel/each 8 bit). After this stage, a mathematical interpolation is used to create pixel intensities to generate the three dimensional image elements to fill the gaps. In order to improve over all quality of a image of 3-D reconstruction several steps are initiated to reduce noise, enhance edges spatial artifacts and improvement in contrast background.

The Dimensional Reconstruction

Out of three-dimensional echocardiography one can expect various datasets such as:
1. A two dimensional display from individual selected cut planes (any plane echocardiography); or from parallel short axis cuts (along a defined long axis); or from long axis cuts (up to eight different views, at different angle increments).
2. A volume rendered technique from any defined cut plane, differential algorithms are applied to represent the information in space.

Concerning volume rendered display, a threshold value is used to identify the borders of the object of interest and to separate cardiac structures from the blood pool and background. Brightness and shading are used to give the perception of depth and different algorithms can be combined to obtain the best results according to the region of interest. The final acquired 3-dimensional image of a cardiac structure aptly resembled with the anatomy and carries close relationship with its neighboring ones, thereby differentiating the normal structure from that of a diseased one.

The Examination Technique

The main advantage of rotational approach is that it allows the acquisition of the images with same multiplane probe used for the standard examination, and is considered more comfortable to the patient than other acquisition techniques. The acquisition of the cross sectional images for three dimensional reconstruction is the part of the standard diagnostic study after having considered various precautions, proper preparation of the patient and insertional technique of TEE multiplane probe. The settings of the ECG and respiration gating are selected after two or three rotational scans to assure that the scanned volume encompasses the structures of interest. The rotation of the scan plane is switched to the step motor under control of the steering logic of sample of the cross sectional images.

In order to carry out transthoracic procedure a transducer has to be placed either in the left parasternal or apical regions. The transducer is mounted in the cylindrical holder connected to the computer algorithm. The operator has to find the central axis around which the imaging plane is rotated to include the structure of interest in the centre of the sector during the whole rotation. Since the spatial coordinate system changes with tranducer movement, the operator must be able to keep the transducer stationary during the procedure. The movements of the patient during the image acquisition must be kept to his minimal possible which is done by explaining the details of the procedure during pre-study period. Positioning the probes, the calibration process, and recording and storage of the cross sectional images requires approximately 7–10 minutes more than the time needed for a standard cross sectional examination.

Three-dimensional reconstruction is performed off line and processing times vary between 30 and 45 minutes, which is further dependent upon the various difficulties faced to select the optimal cut planes to visualise a given structure or region of interest, as there may be significant anatomical variability between patients and countless cut planes can be selected. Valve leaflets can be visualised from above or from below and the septa from the right or left side, almost identical cuts when observed during surgical procedure.

Any Plane Cross Sectional Imaging

The limitations of acoustic access and registration of individual cross sectional images can potentially be overcome by three-dimensional echocardiography.

From the original three dimensional dataset, new individually optimised and otherwise unobtainable image planes can be computed and displayed in motion (dynamic any plane echocardiography). A zoom facility allows visualisation of detailed structures. Slicing of a given structure can be performed with parallel scanning in a way similar to computed tomography or magnetic resonance imaging. Up to eight longitudinally cut planes with different angle interval spatial appreciation. Futhermore, the final assessment of cavity dimensions or the evaluation of a given structure will be more objective and less operator dependent.

Quantification and Volume Measurements (Fig. 5.12)

Various cross sectional approaches for measuring left ventricular volume have been proposed, but all make some assumptions about cavity shape. 2-D with standard cross-sectional echocardiography only a limited number of planes can be obtained; thus a theoretical geometrical model must be assumed which is often far from the reality. From the three dimensional dataset, orthogonal long axis cut planes can be automatically selected, which partially compensates the geometric assumptions involved in biplane methods.

The major advantage of three-dimensional echocardiography over standard cross sectional imaging relies on more objective assessment of ventricular shape and size, since it does not depend on any specific transducer location or orientation plane. Thus, three-dimensional echocardiography should be able to define chamber volume in an accurate and reproducible manner. Manual tracings of endocardial borders from a series of parallel short axis cut planes of the left ventricle at variable intervals allow computation of left ventricular volumes independent of theoretical models. Volumes of individual slices are calculated ($V = A \times h$, where A = area of the slice, and h = distance between adjacent cut planes) and summed to obtain the total volume. Serial studies with three dimensional echocardiography will provide more insight into the natural history of complex cardiac pathology and into the rate of progression of its severity (for example, ventricular remodeling).

Distance Measurements

The different surface points of a three-dimensional reconstruction are not in one plane. Thus a distance measurement must always take the depth into account. From the volume rendered display, the definition of a start and end point of the distance to be measured will result in the computation of the distance in the voxel space.

Area Measurements

Although area measurements can only be applied to cross-sectional images, three-dimensional echocardiography permits sectioning of the heart in any desired orientation. Thus cut planes can be selected which cross section the structure in the desired optimal orientation. This makes orifice area measurement more accurate (Figs 5.4 and 5.5).

Morphological Diagnosis

With an integrated system for three-dimensional reconstruction shows that the potential goal of the objective display of the anatomy and the complex relationships among the different structures of the heart can be achieved.

The possibility of obtaining unrestricted cross sectional images coupled with the volume rendered dynamic display allow us to explore fully the morphological features of a given structure for three dimensional reconstruction. With both the transesophageal and the transthoracic approach, rotational scanning can be performed with the mitral valve remaining in the centre of the sector during the whole acquisition, which allows adequate sampling of information and subsequent optimal reconstruction. The aortic valve can be observed from above or from below, which enhances evaluation of leaflet morphology.

Present Problems with Three-dimensional Echocardiography

1. Acquisition of processing time (storage space, computing power)
2. Transducer stability during acquisition
3. Limited resolution
4. Susceptibility to background noise artefacts
5. No on line three dimensional representations.

Three dimensional echocardiography is one of the few modalities which can offer a major potential role for the comprehensive evaluation of patients with congenital heart disease. Dynamic volume rendered reconstructions provide accurate spatial information, especially in complex congenital heart defects.

Images of acquired or congenital pathology can be displayed from views which simulate exposure of the affected structure. Thus, in patients who are candidates for cardiac surgery, three dimensional echocardiography can provide a dynamic view of the surgical anatomy of the heart. The surgeon can observe the affected structure in a way similar to that which you will find later in the operating room. Clearly this will facilitate the surgical planning of procedure.

Till date the limitations of the critical factors determining the results of three dimensional reconstruction, **firstly** is the quality of the original cross sections. No software can compensate for low standard cross sectional image quality and defective image acquisition. An appropriate gain setting and basic image quality are crucial for the accuracy of the reconstruction.

Secondly, there is critical factor which is related to the processing filter and segmentation. If these algorithms remove too many echoes, the viewer may interpret the gaps as septal defects. If the algorithm does not remove enough noise, confusing echoes will appear in the reconstruction and can be mistaken for vegetation or thrombus.

Thirdly, the resolution in the conical volume is non-uniform in two dimensions, worsening progressively from the central axis to the lateral field and from the top to the bottom. Thus when a tangential cut plane is computer reconstructed and displayed the resolution will be different in any given point of this cut plane and may affect the interpretation of the images.

Future Directions in 3-Dimensional Echocardiography

The development of new software will further improve the final image quality in three dimensional echocardiography. The possibility of color Doppler flow

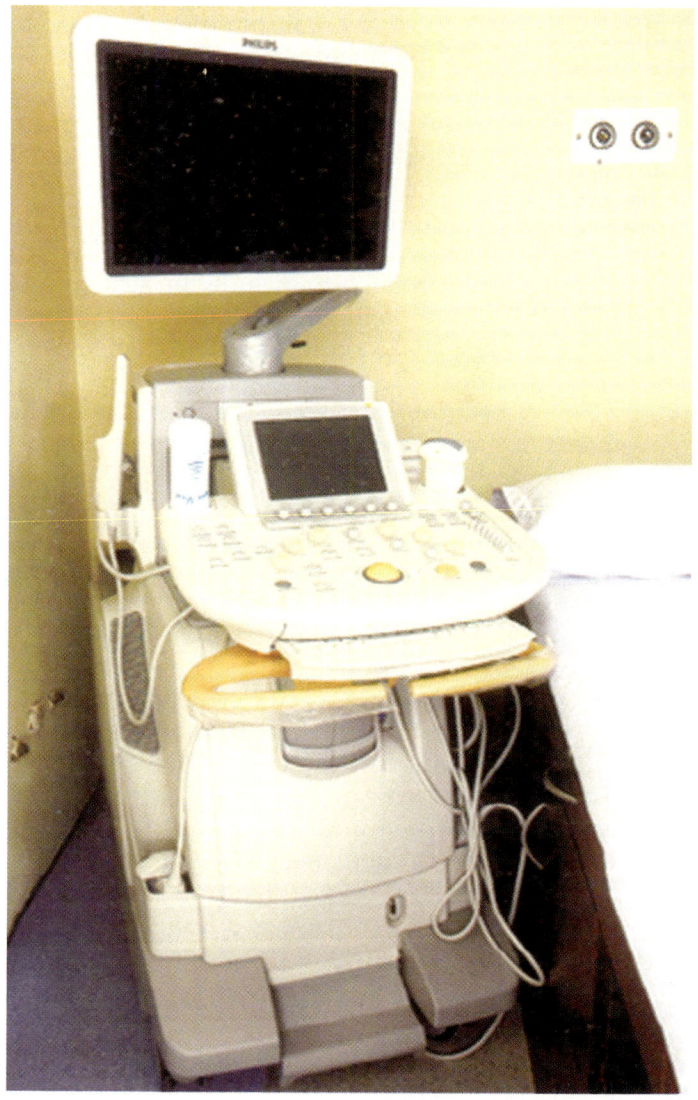

Fig. 5.1: 4D Ultrasound

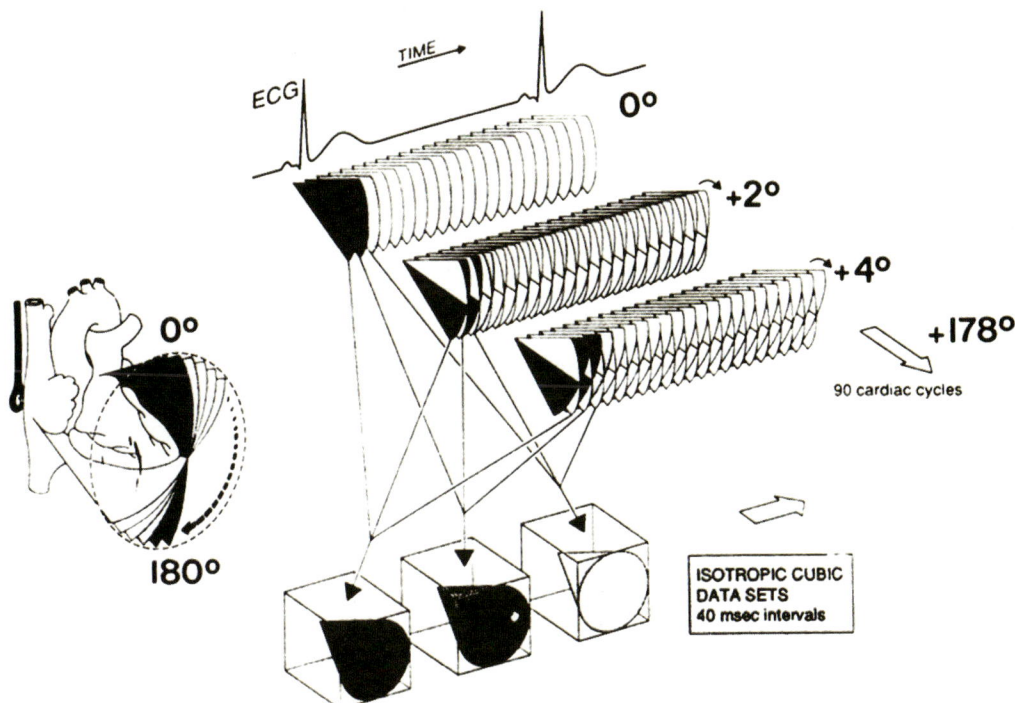

Fig. 5.2: Sequential cardiac images from a fixed point in the esophagus with multiplane transducer at 2-degree steps. Each incremental step is controlled by a steering algorithm. At each scanning plane starting from the longitudinal cross section (0°), images of a complete heart cycle at 40-ms intervals are sampled (25 frames/s). The images are digitized and stored in the computer memory. After recording 90 cardiac cycles to cover (180° at 2° intervals), the cross sections are organized according to their ECG phase and stored in a series of isotropic conical data sets at 40-ms intervals, which are used for dynamic three-dimensional reconstruction

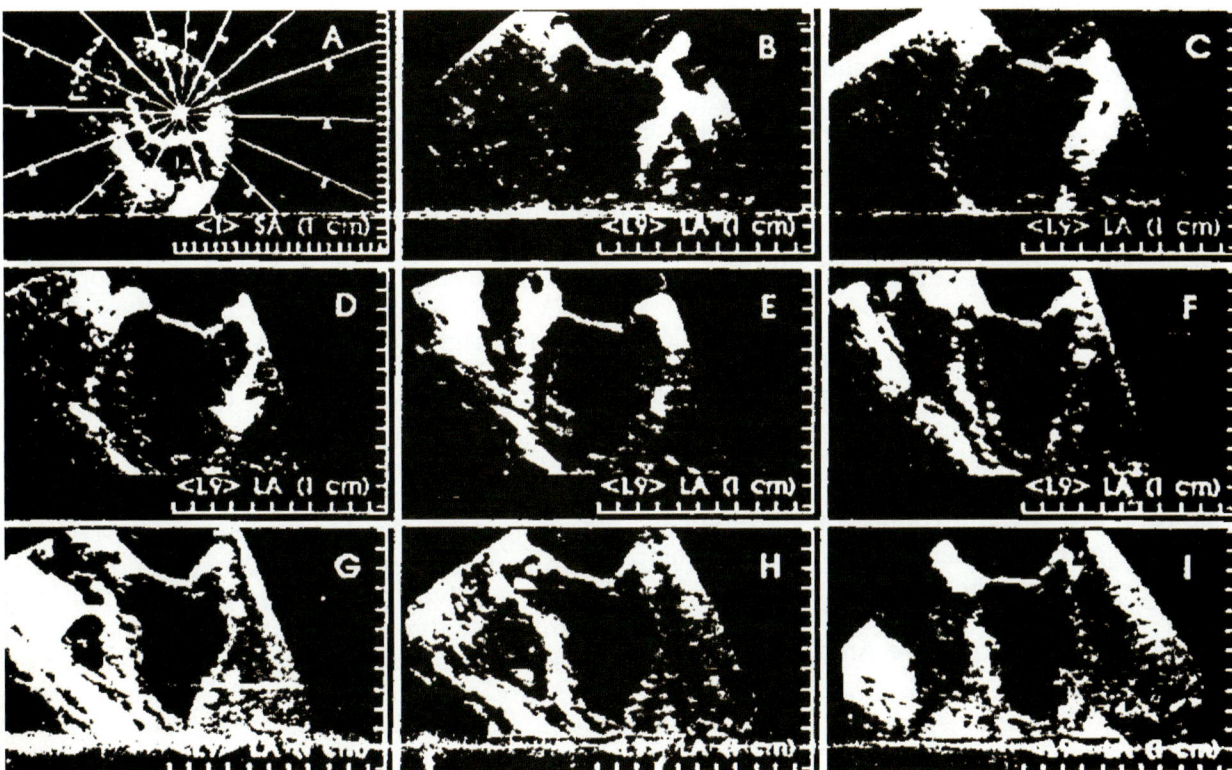

Fig. 5.3: 3-D Dynamic echocardiography showing LV reconstruction by the application of multiplane transesopageal probe (from scans A-I)

recording combined with the volume rendered tissue reconstruction and its dynamic three dimensional display will provide a quantitative assessment of the regurgitant flows or shunts in the future, and greatly enhance the comprehensive assessment of valvular lesions.

Data Acquisition and Analysis

Three-dimensional images are obtained from standard parasternal, apical and sub-costal windows using a Sonos 7500 Live 3-D Echo. Method of data acquisition is based on recommendations of Adhoc 3-D Echo Protocol Working Group endorsed by the International Society of Cardiovascular Ultrasound. Data analysis is acquired using integrated tools for advanced image processing to obtain views with details of endocardial and valvular surfaces and their relationship with adjoining structures. Quantitative assessment was performed on a dedicated personal computer using dedicated software capable of measuring three-dimensional data sets.

Qualitative Analysis (Figs 5.1 and 5.2)

Three-dimensional images are analyzed using integrated software system by cropping in three different colour-coded cutting planes perpendicular to each other. Besides these cutting planes, an additional oblique plane capable of cropping the image in any desired angulation is also employed. This particular plane is advantageous in assessing the intra-cardiac structures placed at an angle other than the perpendicular one. One single 3-D data set acquired in any possible view is sufficient to get all the conventional 2-D. The echocardiographic images are sectioned to obtain the desired cut planes. Brightness, contrast and colour mapping are adjusted to obtain the optimal image quality. These acquired real-time and full volume cine images can be rotated in space to visualise complete anatomy of the structure under study.

Quantitative Analysis

The acquired 3DE data sets are stored on CD-ROM in DICOM format and transferred to a separate work-station for off-line data analysis. Quantitative analysis is done using dedicated software analysis systems (QLAB Advanced Quantification software, version 3.0, Philips Ultrasound, USA, and Tomtec 4-D Cardio-view, version 1.2, Tomtec, Gmbh, Germany) for measurement of distance, area, volumes and angles.

Quantitative Assessment of Valve Area

In order to obtain planimetry assessment of valve area, conventional 2DTTE short-axis view and 3DTTE images are acquired from any available window. Measurements are done using off-line analysis software (QLAB Advanced Quantification software, version 3.0) which

provides a 3-D cine image along with corresponding 2-D images in three modifiable cutting planes. These planes are aligned to the axis of valve opening plane to get short axis image in the plane of shortest valve area enface (Figs 5.3 and 5.4).

Quantitative Assessment of Atrial Septal Defect (ASD) (Figs 5.7 and 5.12)

Patients suffering from ASD are studied with 2DTTE and are registered in the protocol of transcatheter device closure. ASD shape, number and dimensions (major diameter D_1, minor diameter D_2 and area) were determined by 2DTTE, 2DTEE and 3DTTE. During transcatheter closure, balloon occlusive diameter (BOD) which is considered as the gold standard for selection of the size of any device, was measured using standard technique and is correlated with echoderived measurements by different techniques.

Quantitative Assessment of Ventricular Volumes: Analysis of left ventricular volume is carried out by using a semi-automated border detection software (Tomtec 4-D LV Analysis v.1.2, Tomtec, Gmbh, Germany). The original 3DTTE pyramidal volume, acquired encompassing the complete left ventricle (LV), is used to calculate global as well as segmental volumes, actual stroke volume and ejection fraction (EF). EF is calculated off-line from time volume curve of entire reconstructed cast. This cast can be subdivided into conventional 17 segment model of LV with estimation of individual segmental motion and volumes in time-volume curve. Wall motion abnormalities and LV dyssynchrony can also be detected and analyzed by the segmental time-volume curve.

Right ventricular volume and EF analysis is performed on optimal 3-D images encompassing the complete right ventricle (RV) volume using Tomtec Cardio-view software. The images are cropped in three orthogonal cutting planes to obtain best possible image of RV in long axis. Endocardial borders are manually traced in eight contiguous volumetric slices of tagged end-systolic and end-diastolic frames with formation of volume-rendered holographic cast. End-systolic volume, end-diastolic volume and EF are calculated from these images.

3-D Echocardiography and Valvular Heart Disease: There is no doubt that conventional 2-D echocardiography is the most commonly used modality for assessing valvular heart disease. The routine planimetry of mitral valve orifice by 2-D echocardiography, pressure half time, continuity equation and proximal iso-velocity surface area (PISA) are the acceptable methods for assessment of mitral valve area (MVA), however they have their own drawbacks and so are the Doppler-based methods as they are heavily dependent on hemodynamic variables and coexisting valvular

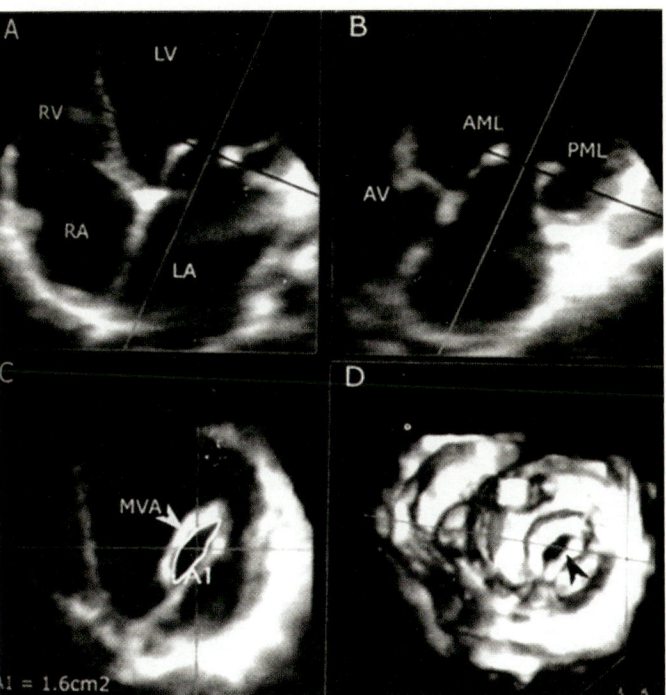

Fig. 5.4: Apical 4C window has been employed in obtaining full volume 3-D data set with three orthogonal cutting planes (D) along with conventional two dimensional images in respective planes A. B and C. The C cutting plane was aligned to the opening plane of the mitral valve in A and B images to visualize the shortest mitral valve opening area (arrow head) in image C for measurement

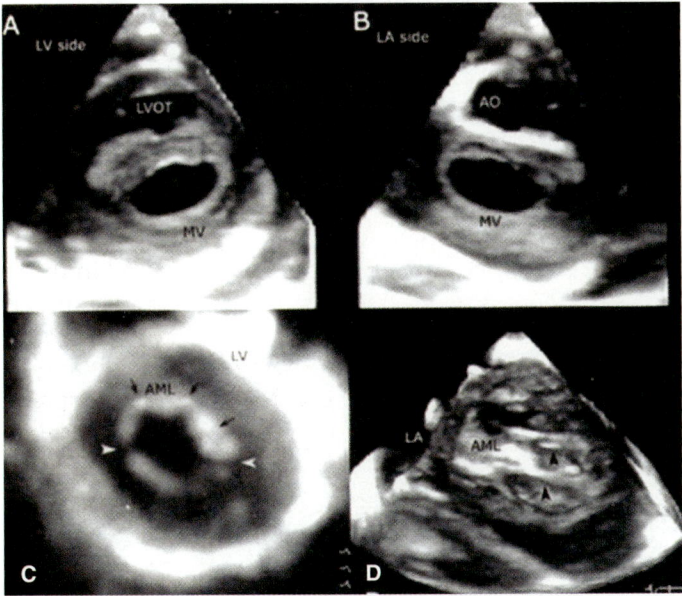

Fig. 5.5A to D: Zoomed view of mitral valve has acquired from LV side by employing real time 3-D TTE data set from parasternal window. **(A)** and LA (side **B**) depicting the surface of the thickened mitral valve with unfused commissures (arrow heads) and three scallops of anterior mitral leaflet A1, A2 and A3 (black arrows). **(C)** Full volume 3-D data set is aquired from parasternal window .Anterolateral left ventricular wall was cropped to visualize mitral apparatus with subvalvular structures. Thickened chordae have also been seen **(D)**

lesions. Various workers have claimed the success rate of planimetry as low as 75%. However, others have reported an overestimation of MVA in the range of 63% for a small deviation of 6° from the optimal plane. This error further increases with a small change of transducer position, angulations and rotation. Difficulty in defining the correct imaging plane that displays the true mitral valve orifice is a major limitation. On the contrary, 3-D echocardiographic estimation has overcome most of the limitations as it measures actual anatomical valve area in an ideal short axis plane and is independent of hemodynamic variables. By using the oblique plane on the 3-D acquired data set, one can correctly ascertain the plane of the opening of the valve and by cropping the image in that particular plane at a level, one can get the smallest opening area of the leaflets and the actual mitral valve orifice area. Applebaum *et al.*, have also demonstrated the value of visualising the mitral valve commissural splitting and leaflet tears in reconstructed 3-DTEE which are not visualised on conventional 2-D images in patients who underwent balloon mitral valvotomy (BMV) for mitral stenosis. Now with real time imaging, the correlation is found to be even better with high reproducibility. The other practical use of this new technique has been in the cases of mitral valve prolapse, which is frequently under or over-estimated using M-mode and 2-D techniques because of its non-planar leaflet-annular relations. Enface visualisation of mitral valve from ventricular and atrial side along with clear demarcation of scallops of valvular leaflets incorporated in prolapse is possible in volume-rendered images acquired using 3-DTTE. Quantification of severity of mitral regurgitation is also a challenging task while deciding for operative management. Real time 3-D echocardiography has theoretical advantage over conventional methods by incorporating entire regurgitant jet area in spatial orientation. It provides unique information about direction and extent of jet which are useful in eccentric jets. Clinical feasibility of this technique for assessment of valve functions has been validated by previous studies, but for any clinical significance it requires standardisation and further validation. Planimetry measurement of the area of vena contracta and mitral regurgitation area is also possible by this technique and correlates well with conventional Doppler-based methods.

Two-dimensional echocardiography is very well established in diagnosis of mitral and aortic stenosis. Their role in the diagnosis of rheumatic tricuspid stenosis is still being defined as interpretations are based on indirect evidences and not the actual measurement. Recently, 3-DTTE technique, assessment of tricuspid valve had been now possible with clear delineation of all the three leaflets in enface view. By the application of this technology one can actually measure tricuspid

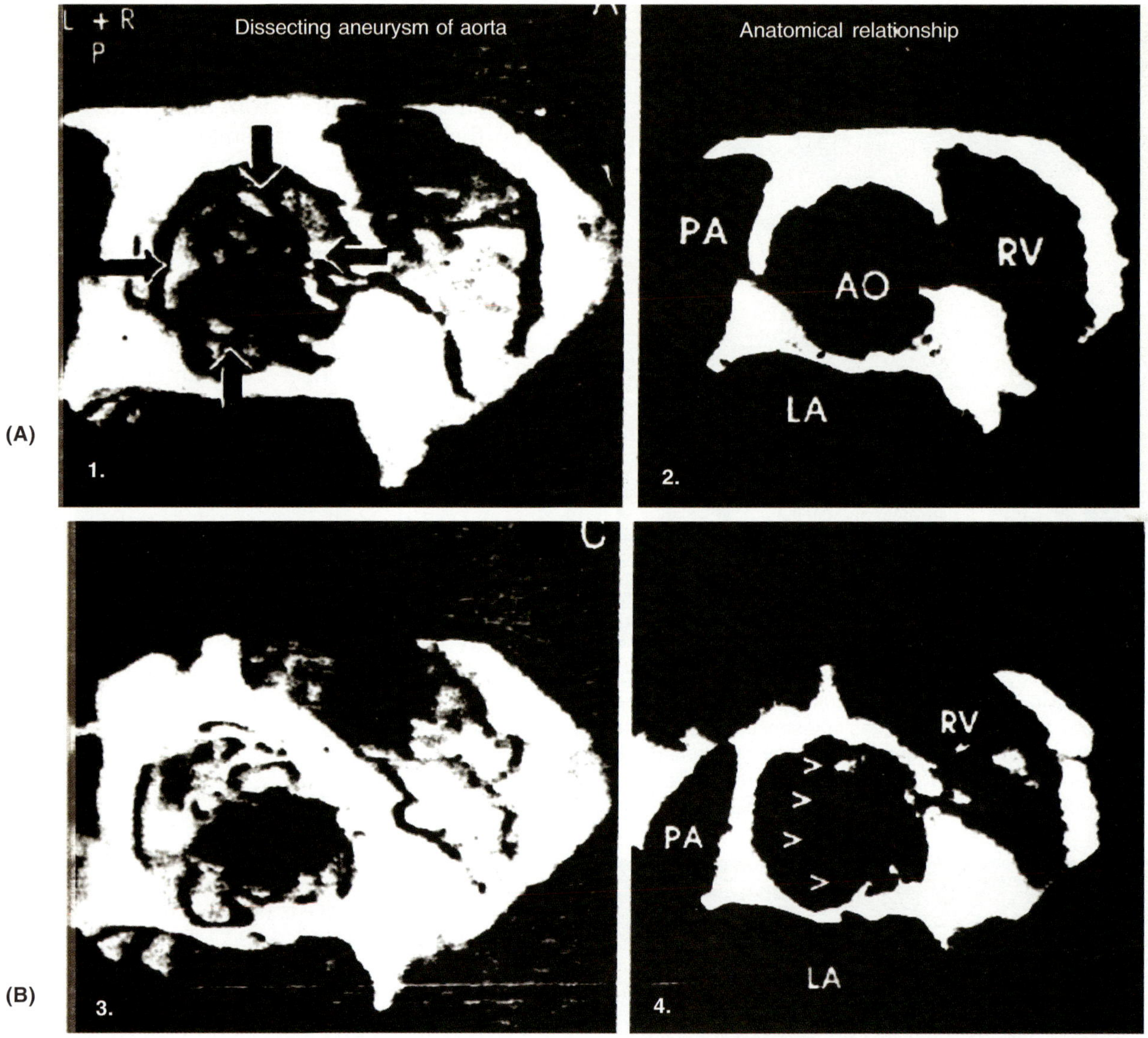

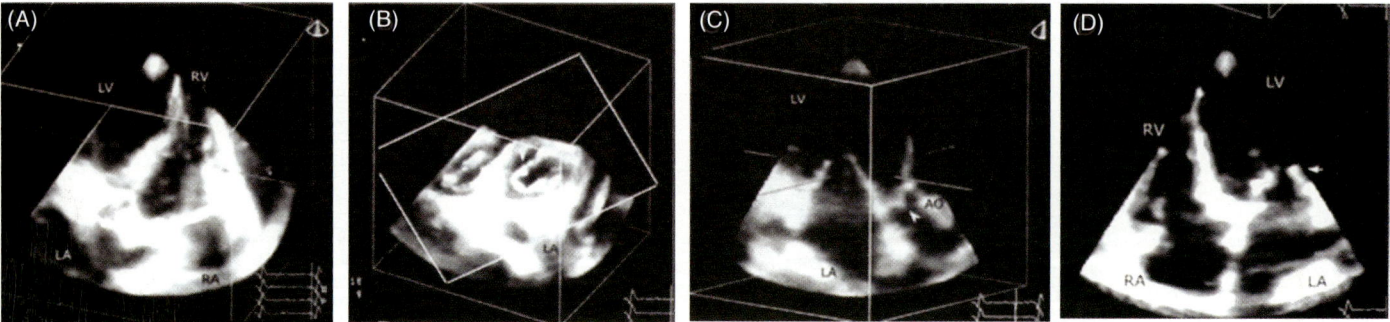

Fig. 5.6A and B: (A1) 3-D showing aneurysm of ascending aorta (arrows) **(A2)** Anatomical relationship between surrounding structures as inscribed on the scan. **(B3 and 4)** Showing circular reflection represented aortic wall. In cavity of aorta some week and thin echoes represented intima of dissecting aorta (arrows) D = Dissection aorta

Fig. 5.7A to D: From apical window full volume 3-DTTE echocardiographic image has been acquired with four ECG triggered sequential data sets. Full volume 3-D data set has been shown with three orthogonal cutting planes shown by lines in the cube **(A)**. The same image has been cropped from apex to base of the heart using oblique cutting plane to obtain the modified short axis view which was not perpendicular to the orthogonal cutting plane **(B)**. The same image has been cropped using three orthogonal cutting planes to obtain the conventional four chamber view with clear visualization of four cardiac chambers and two atrioventricular valves (arrow) **(C)**. Conventional three chamber view with clear visualization of aortic mitral relationship. Closed aortic valve **(D)**

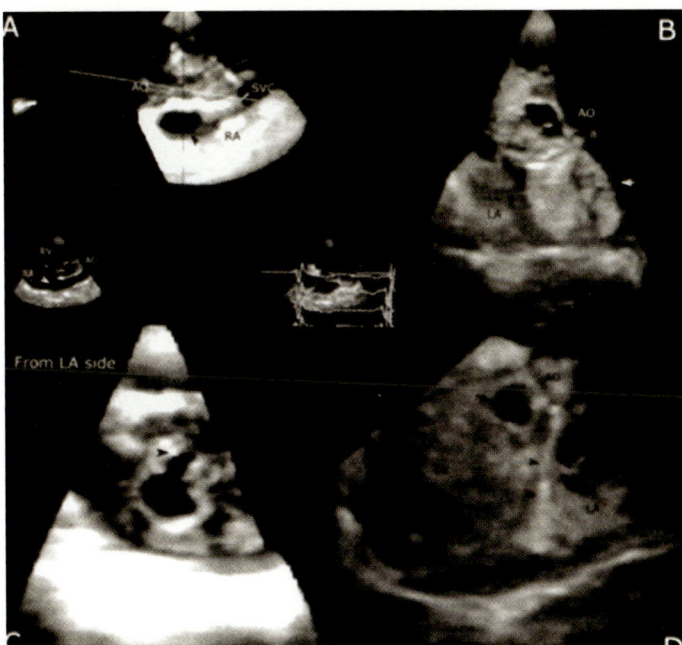

Fig. 5.8: 3-D view of ASD secundum visualizing shape of the defect and its relation with adjacent structures (A), same patient with Amplatzer device in situ (B) Enface view of cleft mitral valve (C) and ventricular septal defect (arrow) and its relation with aortic valve and mitral annulus (D)

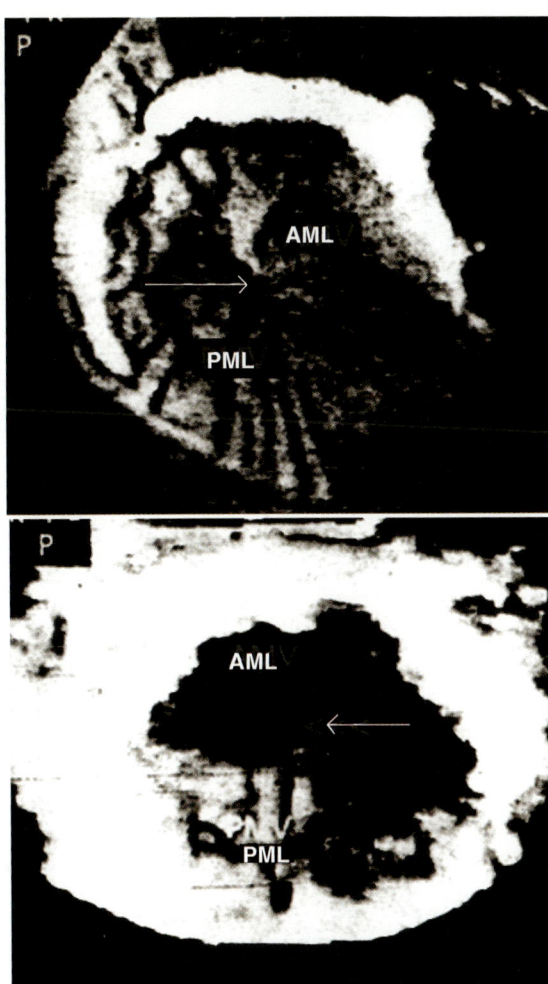

Fig. 5.10: B.3-D1 and 2. Showing anterior mitral leaflet (AML) protruding (arrow) from left ventricle into left atrium in patient with mitral valve prolapse syndrome as seen from bird-eye view from above

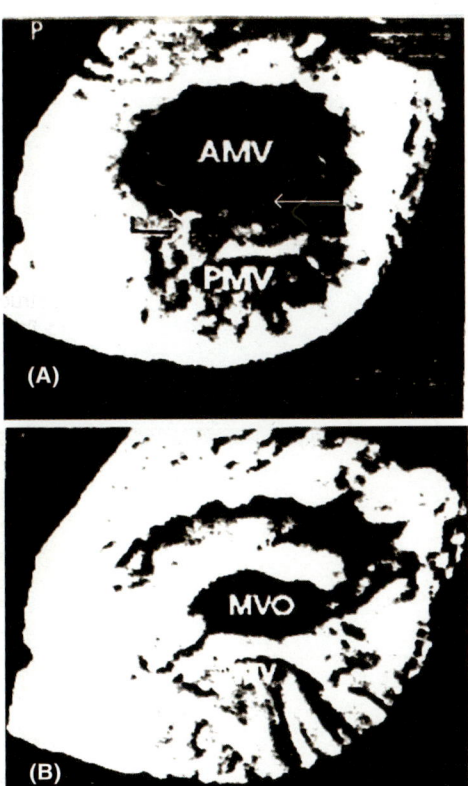

Fig. 5.9A and B: (A) 3-D Reconstruction of LV in short axis view showing anterior mitral leaflet (AML) and posterior mitral leaflet (PML). **(B)** Thickened both AML and PML in mitral stenosis. (MVO = Mitral valve stenosis)

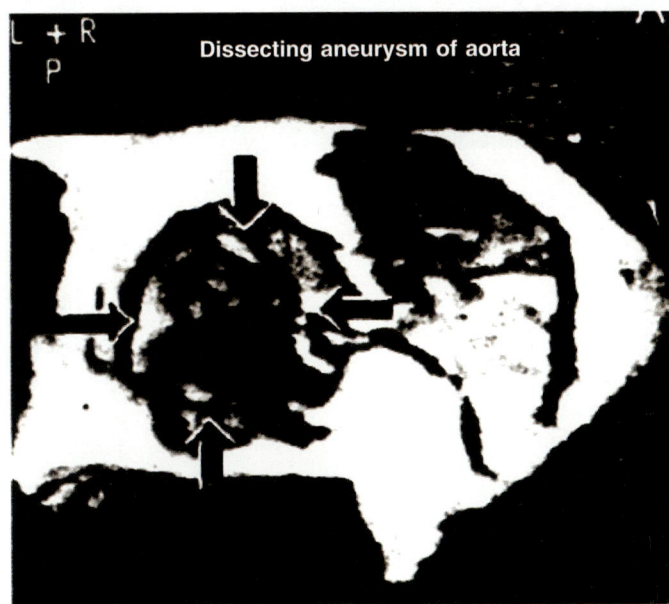

Fig. 5.11: 3-D Showing aneurysm of ascending aorta (arrows)

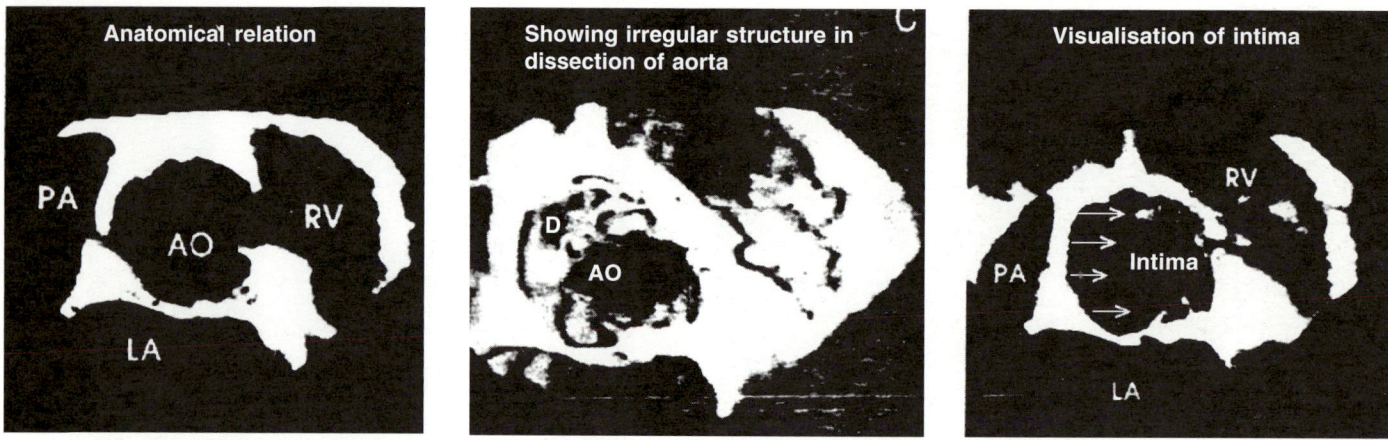

Fig. 5.12A to C: (A) Anatomical relationship between surrounding structures as inscribed on the scan. **(B)** Circular reflection represented aortic wall. **(C)** In cavity of aorta some week and thin echoes represented intima of dissecting aorta (arrows) D = Dissection aorta

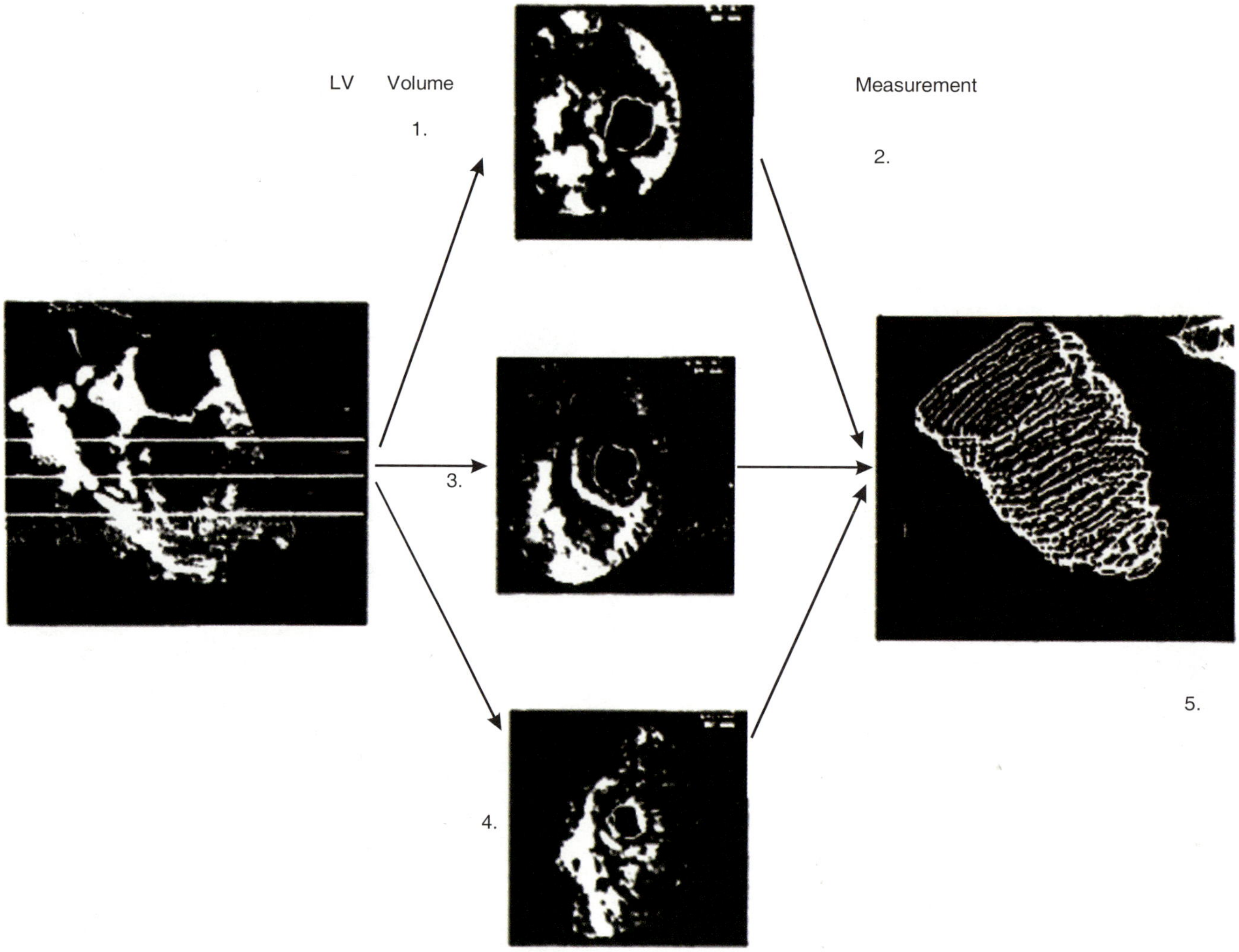

LV   Volume

1.

Measurement

2.

3.

4.

5.

Fig. 5.13: A volume measurement from the 3-D database, long axis cut plane of the heart in selected (left panel 1). Short axis cut planes (perpendicular to the long axis) at predetermined distance are selected and the corresponding images are depited. Three representative short axis images are shown in the middle panel (2, 3, 4). For each short axis image, the endocardial contour is drawn and the calculation of the volume of each slice is automatically done by the computer. Slice by slice the computer does a summation of the corresponding subvolumes (5). Finally LV volume can be determined to its nearest appropriate value

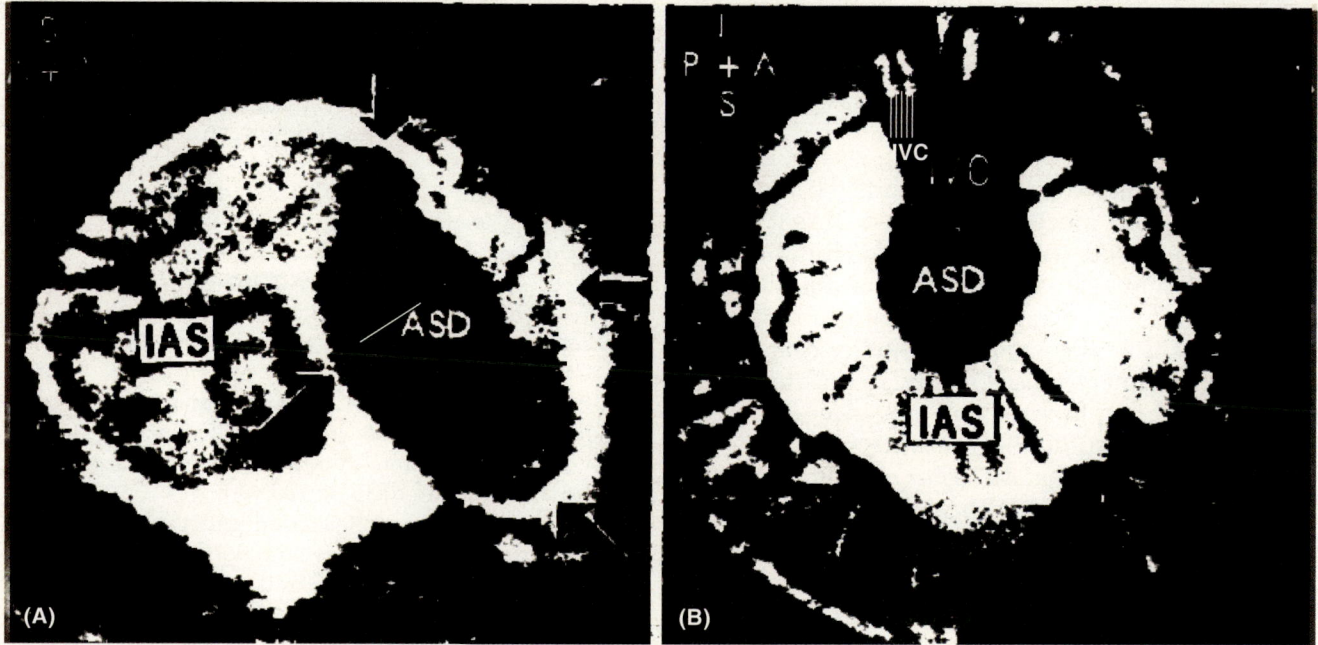

Fig. 5.14: (A) 3-D Dynamic echocardiography showing size, shape and location of the defect in IAS as shown in classical ASD secundum. **(B)** ASD located adjacent to inferior vena cava (IVC). It is like bird eye view from left atrium

valve area by planimetry along with greater details about valvular morphology, and has been accepted as gold standard in absence of any other modality after standardisation with autopsy studies. 3-dimensional echocardiography also provides reproducible images of entire tricuspid regurgitant jet along with actual measurement of regurgitant valve area but requires further confirmation before being used for clinical assessment .

Aortic Valve Disease (Figs 5.6 and 5.7)

3-DE, by overcoming the limitations of conventional echocardiography and correctly ascertaining the actual valve area and effective regurgitant valve area, one can reduce the need for transesophageal echocardiography, but it needs further experience with larger studies.

3-D Echocardiography in Patients with Prosthetic Heart Valves: 3-D echocardiography gives 'enface' view of prosthetic valves along with position of struts and opening and closing motion in a single image, especially in patients with peri-prosthetic leak in which it was very difficult to localize the site and shape of leak by conventional echocardiography.

3-D Echocardiography in Congenital Heart Diseases: In the assessment of congenital heart disease one may require mental conceptualisation of planar 2DE images in 3-D construction of cardiac anatomy by integrating observation from adjacent views, something that is possible only for an experienced echocardiographer. The emerging real time 3-DE has eliminated need for imaginary reconstruction of cardiac structures and their

anatomical relation by different observers. In patients with complex congenital lesions, 3-DTTE had given additional information by providing the spatial orientation of the anatomical structures (Fig. 5.8).

3-D Echocardiography in Assessment of Ventricular Function: LVEF has been accepted as the only important marker for prognostic assessment in patients with LV dysfunction. In the recent past, 2DE has been globally accepted for serial evaluation of EF which is done by eyeballing and is subjective with limited test-retest reliability. But with the introduction of 3-D echocardiography, objective assessment of quantitative measurement of dimensions, areas, volumes and function is now possible more convincingly as compared to conventional 2-D echocardiographic measurements and is highly reproducible. While quantification of ventricular volumes and mass with 2-D imaging requires geometric assumptions, their determination by live 3-D echocardiography is actual and is not assuming anything to calculate the EF. By analysis of regional wall motion, LV contraction patterns, their cyclic changes and temporal differences in regional wall motion pattern, this technique with higher frame rates can be used for assessment of intraventricular dyssynchrony and feasibility of biventricular pacing.

Right Ventricular Volume Measurement using 3-D Echocardiography

Undoubtedly it is very difficult to determine RV volume because of its complex asymmetrical shape. Real-time 3-DE has led to a revolution in this field as it gives complete assessment of RV geometry and RVEF in a holographic 3-D volume data set and provides new insights into its physiology.

Future Prospects

Real time 3-D echocardiography extends the benefits of more complete and precise information in real clinical decision making. However, it has certain limitations like dependence on available echocardiographic window, lower frame rate (20 Hz), and motion artifacts in full volume acquisition. Respiratory and other beat-to-beat variations also damage image quality. Acquisition angle in real time mode requires technical advances to increase the size of insonated volume and frame rate of acquisition. It appears that 3-D echocardiography is the technology of future, and with wider availability and further technological advancement it has potential to replace 2-D echocardiography as a tool for routine clinical assessment of heart diseases.

Bibliography

1. American society of Echocardiography Committee on Standards, Subcommittee or quantitation of two-dimensional echocardiograms. Recommendations for quantitation of the left ventricle by two-dimensional echocardiography. *J. Am. Soc. Echocardiogr* 1989; 2:358–67.

2. Geiser EA, Ariet M, Conetta DA, Lupkiewicz SM, Christie LG, Conti CR. Dynamic three-dimensional echocardiographic reconstruction of the intact human left ventricle: technique; and initial observations in patients. *AM Heart J* 1982; 103:1056–65.

3. Gosh A, Nanda NC, Maurer G. Three-dimensional reconstruction of echocardiographic images using the rotation method. *Ultrasound Med Biol* 1982; 6:655–61.

4. Handschumacher MD, Lethor JP, Siu SL, Mele D, Rivera JM, Picard MH, *et al*. A new integrated system for three-dimensional transesophageal echocardiographic reconstruction: development and validation for ventricular volume with application in human subjects. *J Am Coll Cardiol* 1993; 21:743-53.

5. Levine RA, Handschumaker MD, Sanfilippo AJ, Hagege AA, Harrigan P, Marshall JE, *et al*. Three-dimensional echocardiographic reconstruction of the mitral valve, with implications for the diagnosis of mitral valve prolapse. *Circulation* 1989; 80:589–98.

6. Nanda NC, Pinheiro L, Sanyal R, Rosenthan S, Kirlio JK. Multiplane transesophageal echocardiographic imaging and three-dimensional reconstruction. *Echocardiography* 1992; 9:667–76.

7. Pandian NG, Nanda NC, Schwartz SL, Fan P, Cao Q, Sanyal R, *et al*. Three-dimensional and Four-dimensional transesophageal echocardiographic imaging of the heart and aorta in humans using a computed tomographic imaging prove. *Echocardiography*. 1992; 9:677–87.

8. Pandian NG, Roelandt J, Nanda N, Sugeng L, Cao Q, Azevedo J, *et al*. Dynamic three-dimensional echocardiography: methods and clinical potential. *Echocardiogrphy*. 1994; 11:237–59.

9. Roelandt JRTC, Thomson IR, Vletter WB, Brommersma P, Born N, Linke DT. Multiplane transesophageal echocardiography:latest evolution in an imaging revolution. *J Am. Soc Echocardiogr* 1992; 5:361–7.

10. 4D LV Analysis, v.1.2: Operating Instructions. Tomtec Imaging System Incorporated 1999; Unterschleissheim, Germany.

11. Applebaum RM, Kasliwal RR, Kanojia A, Seth A, Bhandari S, Trehan N, *et al*. Utility of three-dimensional echocardiography during balloon mitral valvuloplasty. *J Am Coll Cardiol* 1998; 32: 1405–1409.

12. Binder TM, Rosenhek R, Porenta G, Maurer G, Baumgartner H. Improved assessment of mitral valve stenosis by volumetric real-time three-dimensional echocardiography. *J Am Coll Cardiol* 2000; 36: 1355–1361.

13. Franke M, Kohl HP. Second-generation real-time 3D echocardiography: a revolutionary new technology. *Medicamundi* 2003; 47/2: 34–40.

14. Fredman CS, Pearson AC, Labovitz AJ, Kern MJ. Comparison of hemodynamic pressure half-time method and Gorlin formula with Doppler and echocardiographic determinations of mitral valve area in patients with combined stenosis and regurgitation. *Am Heart J* 1990; 119: 121–129.

15. Kasliwal R, Trehan N, Mittal S. A new 'gold standard' for the measurement of mitral valve area? Surgical validation of volume rendered three-dimensional echocardiography. *Circulation* 1996; 94 (Suppl): 1355.

16. Kisslo J, Firek B, Ota T, Kang DH, Fleishman CE, Stetten G, et al. Real time volumetric echocardiography: the technology and the possibilities. *Echocardiography* 2000; 17: 773–779.

17. Levine RA, Handschumacher MD, Sanfilippo AJ, Hagege AA, Harrigan P, Marshall JE, *et al*. Three-dimensional echocardiographic reconstruction of the mitral valve, with implications for the diagnosis of mitral valve prolapse. Assessment of regional wall motion abnormalities with real-time 3-dimensional echocardiography. *J Am Soc Echocardiogr* 1999; 12: 7–14.

18. Martin RP, Rakowski H, Kleiman JH, Beaver W, London E, Popp RL. Reliability and reproducibility of two dimensional echocardiographic measurement of stenotic mitral valve orifice area. *Am J Cardiol* 1979; 43: 560–568.

19. Masura J, Gavora P, Formanek A, Hijazi ZM. Transcatheter closure of secundum atrial septal defects using the new self-centering Amplatzer septal occluder: initial human experience. *Cathet Cardiovasc Diagn* 1997; 42: 388–393.

20. Nakatani S, Masuyama T, Kodama K, Kitabatake A, Fujii K, Kamada T. Value and limitations of Doppler echocardiography in quantification of stenotic mitral valve area: comparison of the pressure half-time and continuity equation methods. *Circulation* 1988; 77: 78–85.

21. Nanda NC, Kisslo J, Lang R, Pandian N, Marwik T, Shirali G, *et al*. Examination protocol for three-dimensional echocardiography. *Echocardiography* 2004; 21: 8: 763–768.

22. Pandian NG, Roelandt J, Nanda NC, Sugeng L, Cao QL, Azevedo J, *et al*. Dynamic three-dimensional echocardiography: methods and clinical potential. *Echocardiography* 1994; 11: 237–259.

23. Rao PS, Langhough R. Relationship of echocardiographic, shunt flow and angiographic size to the stretched diameter of the atrial septal defect. *Am Heart J* 1991; 122: 505–508.

24. Sheikh KH, Smith SW, von Ramm O, Kisslo J. Real-time, three-dimensional echocardiography: feasibility and initial use. *Echocardiography* 1991; 8: 119–125.

25. Zamorano J, Cordeiro P, Sugeng L, Perez de Isla L, Weinert L, Macaya C, *et al*. Real-time three-dimensional echocardio-graphy for rheumatic mitral valve stenosis evaluation: an accurate and novel approach. *J Am Coll Cardiol* 2004; 43: 2091–2096.

26. Zhu W, Cao QL, Rhodes J, Hijazi ZM. Measurement of atrial septal defect size: a comparative study between three-dimensional transesophageal echocardiography and the standard balloon sizing methods. *Pediatr Cardiol* 2000; 21: 465–469.

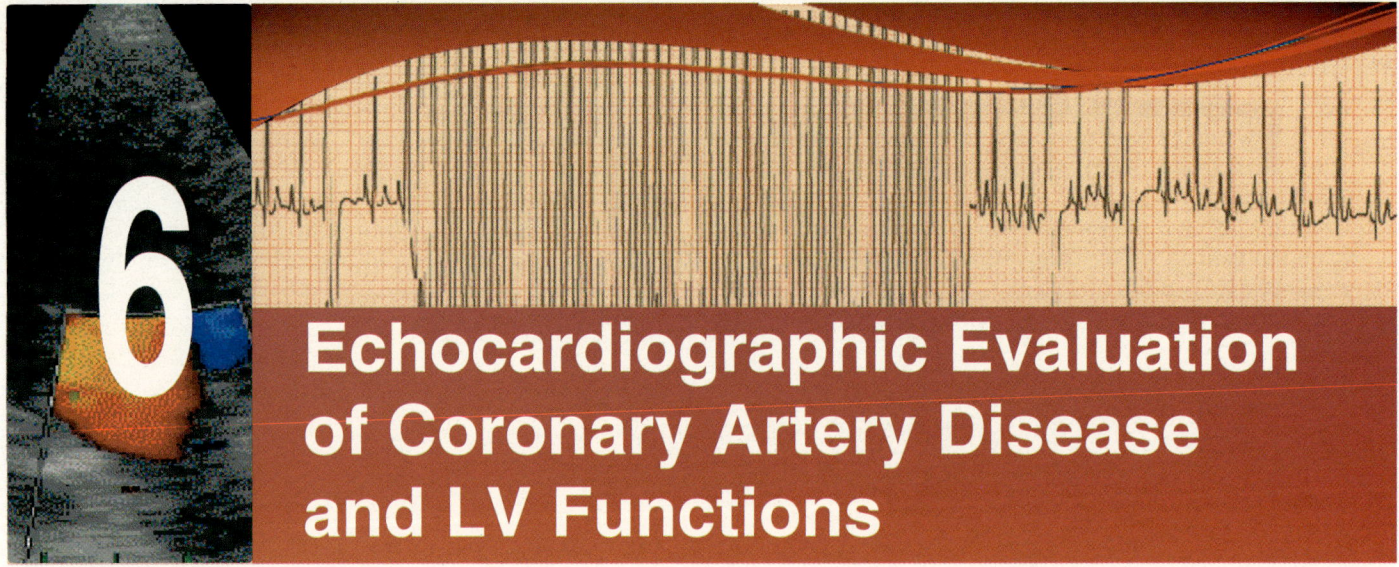
Transthoracic M-mode, 2-dimensional echocardiography and TEE have become indispensable techniques in the evaluation of coronary artery disease and its related complications. It is highly popular among the cardiologists and physicians. It is most accessible repeatable and low risk diagnostic technique that is highly informative in the assessment of typical and atypical chest pain (Table 6.1).

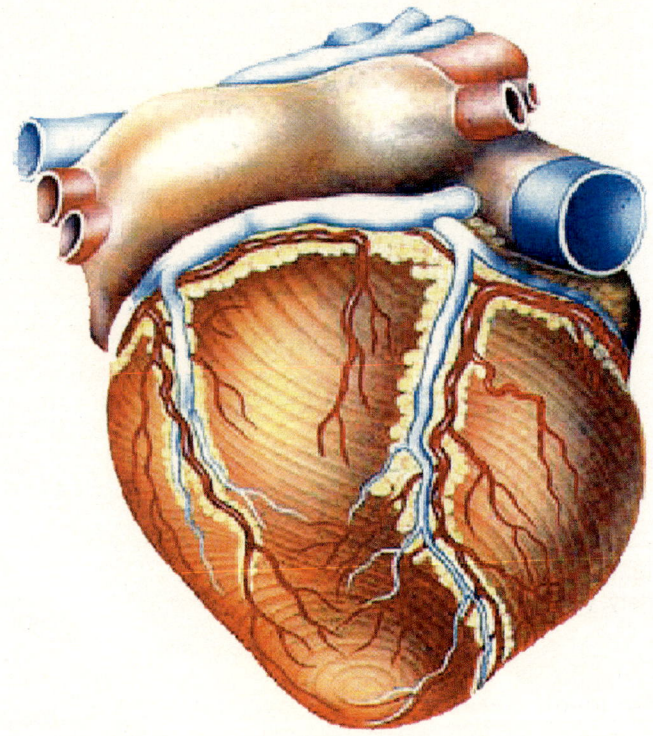

Fig. 6.1B: Cardiaveric diagram back aspect showing circumflex coronary artery along with coronary venus circulation

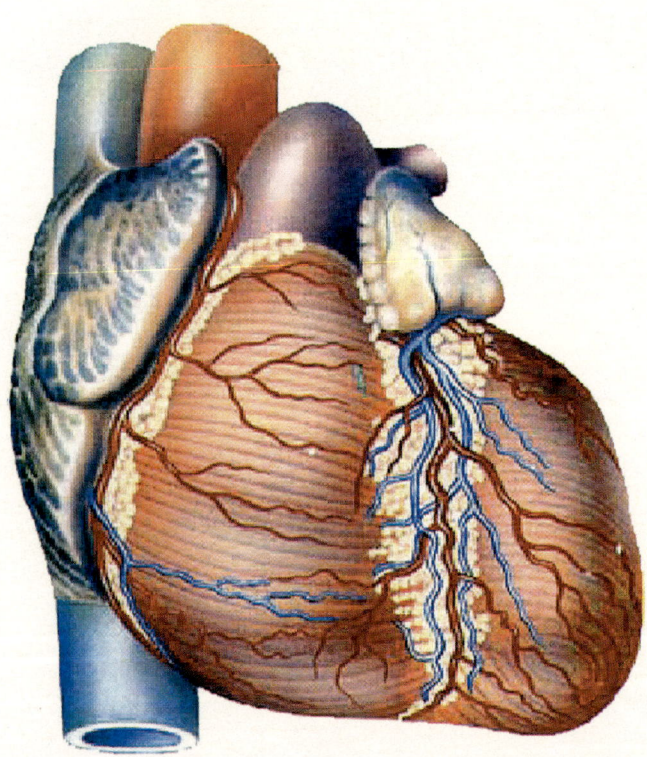

Fig. 6.1A: Cardiaveric diagram showing right coronary and left anterior descending coronary arteries along with their coronary venus circulation

Echocardiography can separate patients with ischemia or infarction from those whose chest pains may be caused by other conditions in the event of a myocardial involvement or the presence of complications may alter the treatment. The extent of left ventricular dysfunction provides a good indication of prognosis after acute myocardial infarction. When combined with stress testing, echocardiography can not only predict the presence of coronary artery disease but

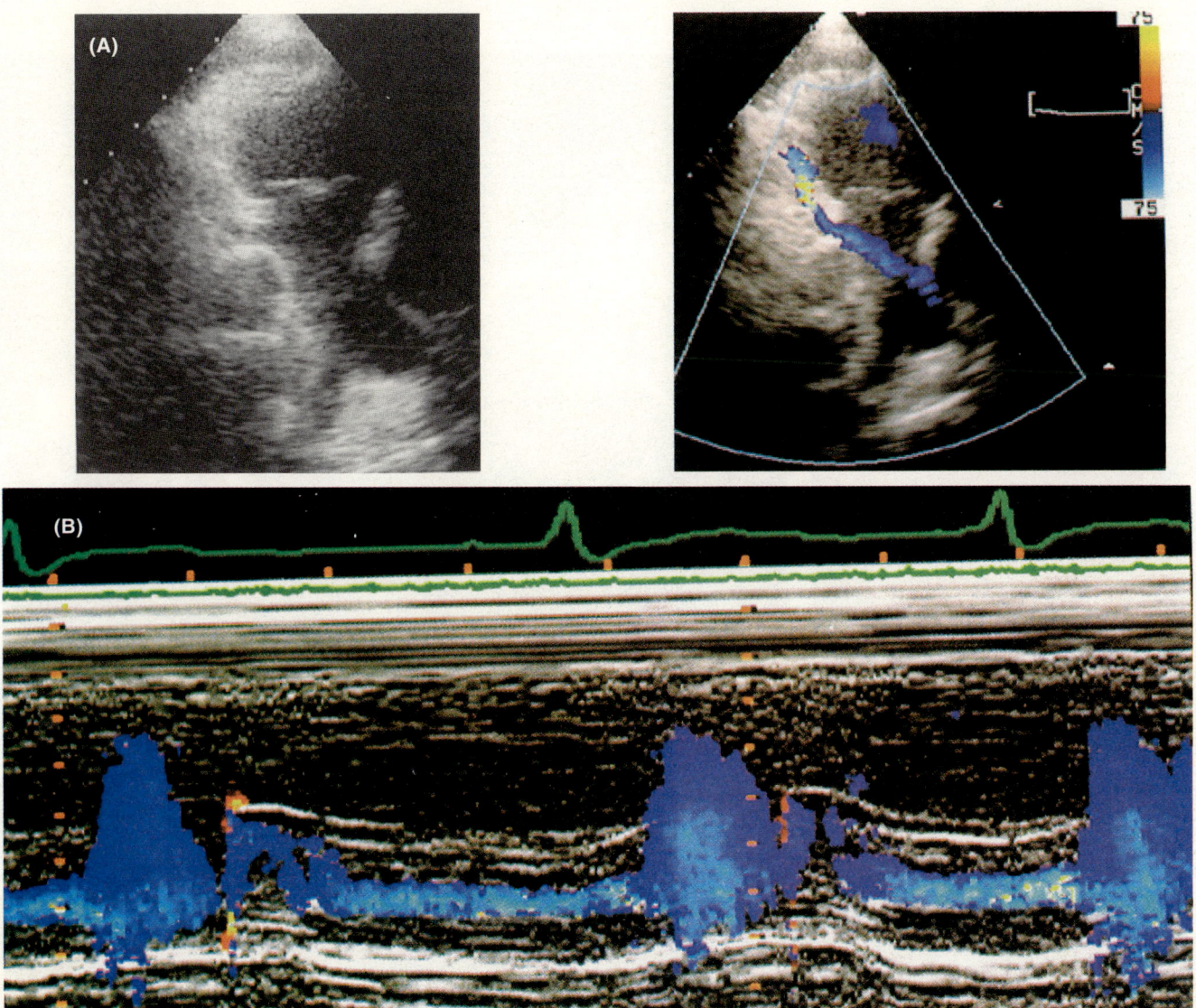

Fig. 6.2A and B: (A) Parasternal short axis view from a patient with anomalous left coronary artery origin, arising from the pulmonary artery. **(B)** Color M-mode scan showing continuous retrograde flow from the coronary artery

also identify areas of myocardium that would besnefit from revascularization. Echocardiography can also provide information on the success of myocardial reperfusion with interventional techniques, such as percutaneous transluminal coronary angioplasty and thrombolytic therapy. Although some limitations do exist, myocardial contrast echocardiography has been shown to be of great value in evaluating myocardial perfusion.

Evaluation of Coronary Artery Disease (Figs 6.1A and B, 6.2, 6.3, 6.4A and B, 6.5, 6.6 and 6.7)

Detection of Ischemic Myocardium

Wall-Motion Abnormalities: Two-dimensional echocardiography is most suited to find out regional wall-motion abnormality by the application of multiple imaging planes. Making division of each echocardiographic view into segments, each segment can be evaluated for the presence and absence of kinetics abnormalities. The results of motion kinetics analysis are classified as normal kinesis, hyperkinesis, hypokinesis, akinesis or dyskinesia. A numeric value can be allotted to each motion category, so each wall segments are totalled and divided by the total number of segments giving rise to a wall motion index which provides us an indication of overall left ventricular functions. In this wall motion index, left ventricle is divided into 22 segments, and numeric values are assigned such as normal kinesis and hyperkinesis = 1, hypokinesis = 2, akinesis = 3, and dyskinesis = 4 (Fig. 6.15A and B).

Although wall motion is sensitive in detecting ischemic muscle, but it carries some drawbacks such as

Anatomical Localization of Normal and Diseased Coronary Arteries by Non-Invasive Method

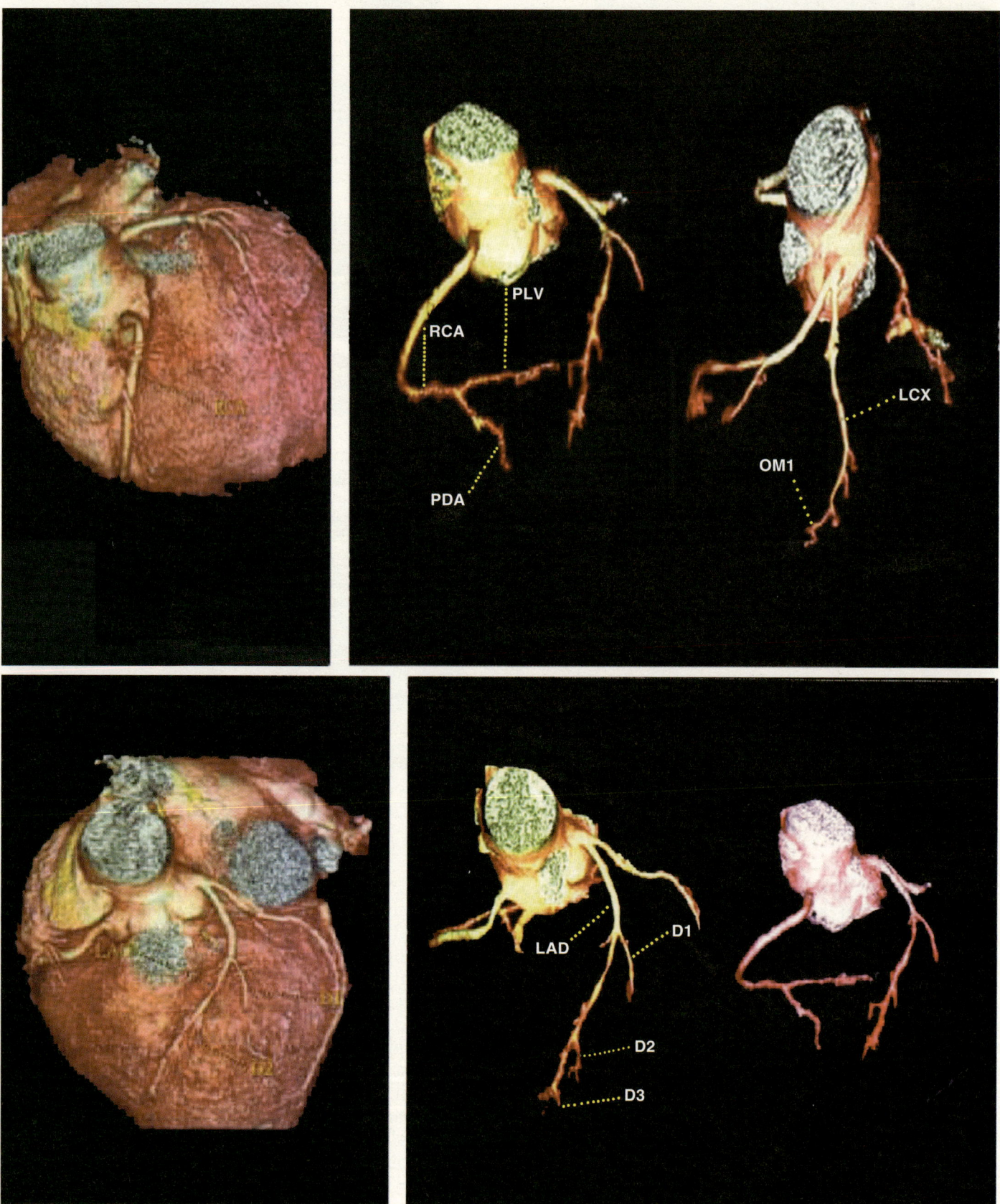

Fig. 6.3: MDCT 32 slices/per sec. scan of the coronary vasculature in elderly patient with chronic heart failure with poor LVEF (<30%)

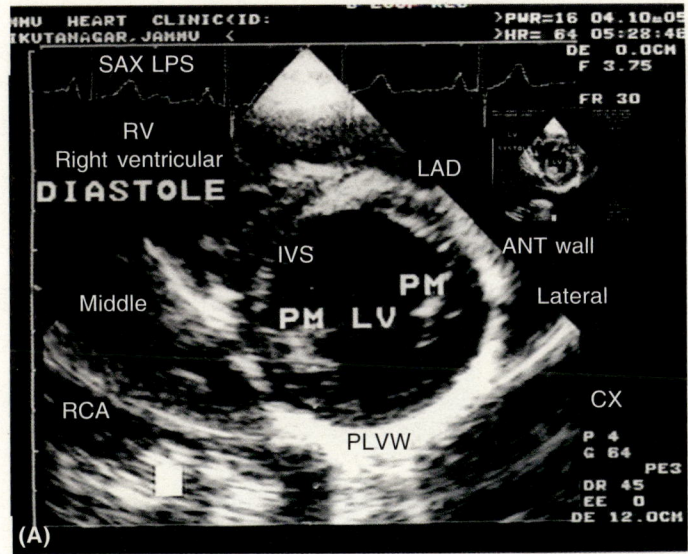

Fig. 6.4A: Short axis view LV showing different segments and their three major arteries

Echocardiographic localisation of different segments of left ventricle in various planes and views

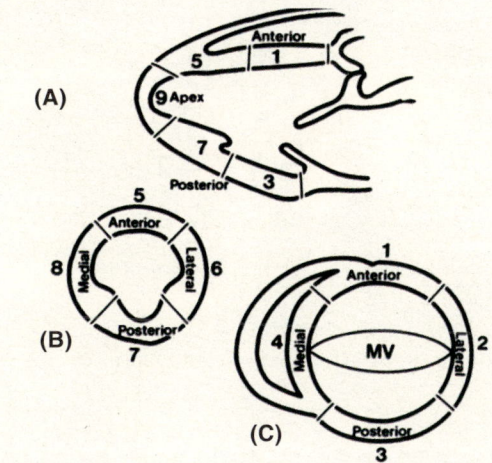

Fig. 6.6A to C: **(A)** L.V. long axis view. **(B)** Short axis LV wall. **(C)** LV short axis at MV

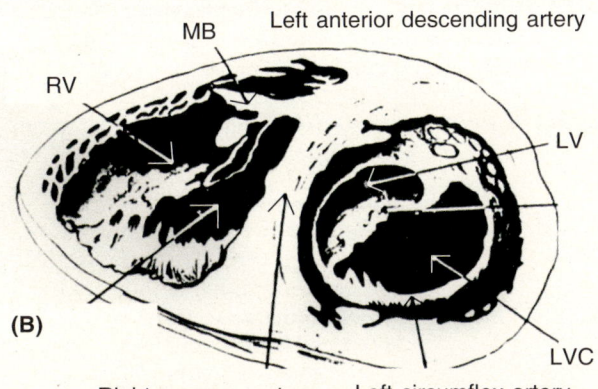

Fig. 6.4B: Short axis view LV showing different segments and their three major arteries (arrows)

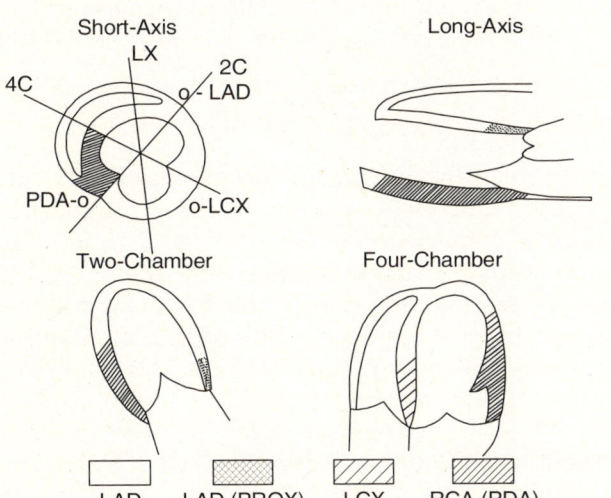

Fig. 6.5: Relationship of two-dimensional views and coronary artery perfusion

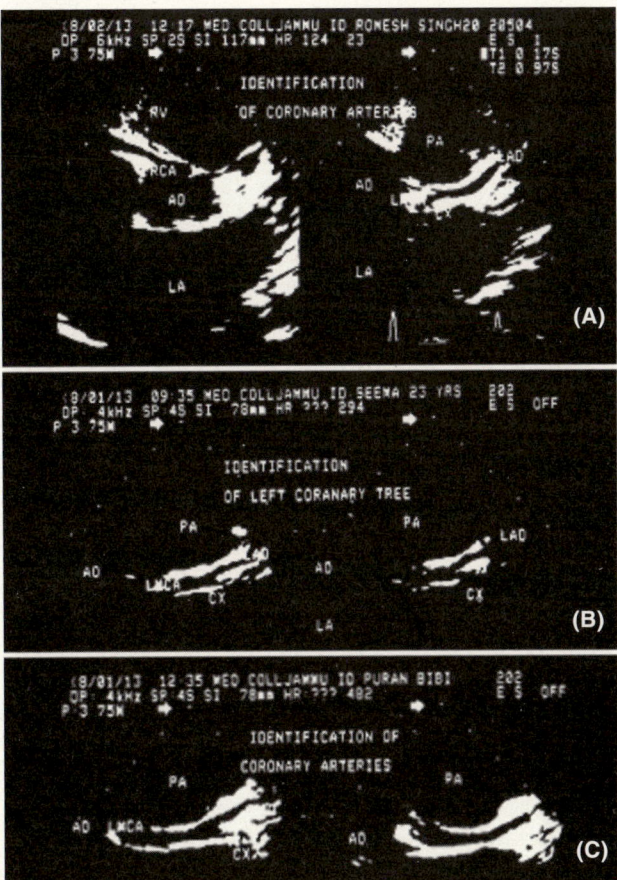

Fig. 6.7A to C: **(A)** Transthoracic short axis view at aorta at subclavicular region showing left main coronary artery and left anterior descending (LAD) and right coronary artery (RCA) in localisation of coronary arteries by the application of TTE. **(B)** Short axis great vessel level view showing LMCA (left) along with well defined left anterior descending artery LAD and circumflex artery (CX). **(C)** It is the repeat of Fig. (B) in identification of left main and its two distinct branches.

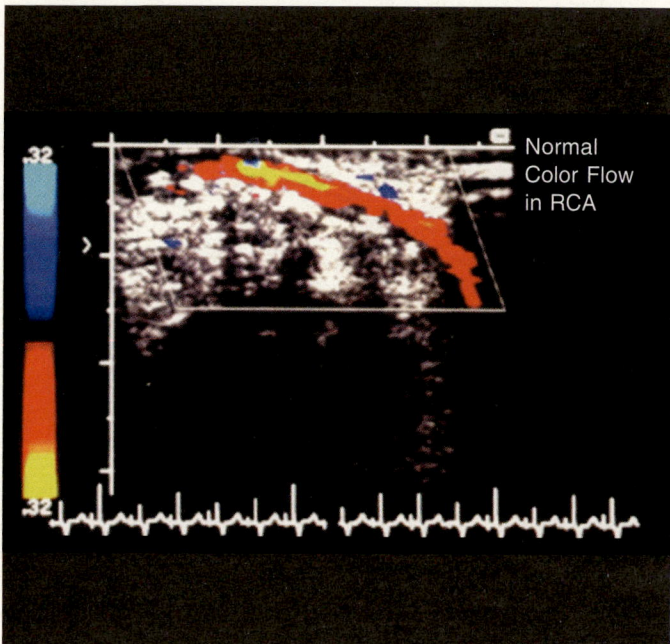

Normal Color Flow in RCA

Fig. 6.8: Color 2-D TEE View showing normal blood flow in right coronary artery in localization of coronary arteries

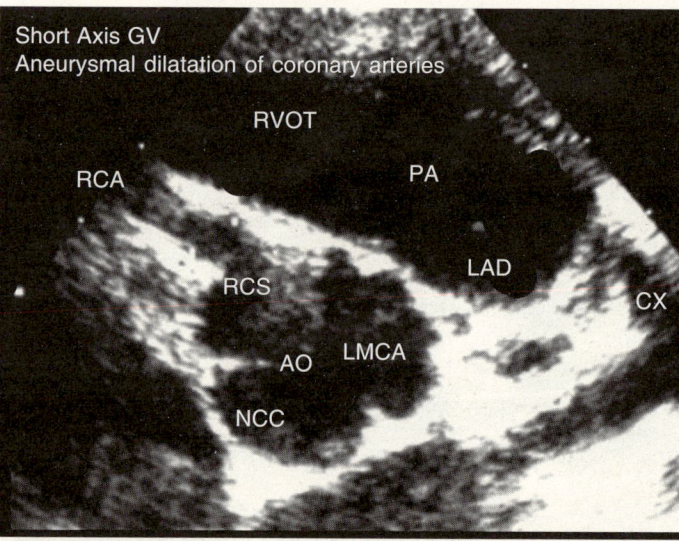

Short Axis GV
Aneurysmal dilatation of coronary arteries

RVOT

RCA   PA

RCS   LAD   CX

AO   LMCA

NCC

Fig. 6.9: 2-D Great vessel view with modified short axis AO showing aneurysmal dilatation of coronary arteries as shown under arrow heads. AO = Aorta, PA = Pulmonary artery, LCS = Left coronary sinus with emerging left main artery. RCS = Right coronary sinus. NCC = Non-coronary cusp, RCA = Right coronary artery, LAD = Left anterior descending artery and CX = Circumflex artery

Table 6.1: *Recommendations for echocardiography in the diagnosis of acute myocardial ischemic syndromes*

Class I	Class II	Class III
1. Diagnosis of suspected acute ischemia or infarction not evident by standard means.	Identification of location/severity of disease in patients with ongoing ischemia	Diagnosis of acute myocardial infarction already evident by standard means 'Transesophageal echocardiography, is indicated when transthoracic echocardiographic studies are not diagnostic.
2. Measurement of baseline left ventricular function.		
3. Evaluation of patients with inferior myocardial infarction and clinical evidence suggesting possible right ventricular infarction.		
4. Assessment of mechanical complications and mural thrombus.		

From Cheitlin MD. *et al.* ACC/AHNASE 2003 Guideline Update for the Clinical Application of Echocardiography: summary article. A report of the American College of Cardiology/American Heart Association Task Force on Practice Guidelines (ACC/AHNASE Committee to Update the 1997 Guidelines for the Clinical Application of Echocardiography). J Am Soc Echocardiogr 2003;16:1091–1110 with permission.
Association Guidelines for Clinical Application of Echocardiography have established areas for which echocardiography is an appropriate diagnostic tool in patients with coronary artery disease.

false negative findings in small subendocardial infarctions, and the tethering effect of dysfunctional areas on the adjacent muscles. It is to be clarified that not all obstructed coronary arteries produce wall-motion abnormalities at rest, as it may be too small to affect adequate perfusion to the region of myocardium. Collateral circulation can sometimes provide adequate blood supply to the region in spite of completely obstructed coronary arteries (Figs 6.8 to 6.12).

Wall-Thickening Abnormalities (Fig. 6.29)

Two-dimensional echocardiography can be employed in the assessment of wall thickness. It is to be known that abnormal myocardial muscle thickness during systolic contraction, is altered in ischemic myocardium. However, some workers have noted systolic thinning of the dyskinetic region in acute ischemia or infarction. It is to be emphasized that combined evaluation of wall motion and thickening by 2-dimensional echocardiography is the best means of detecting ischemic or infarcted myocardium.

Detection of Coronary Artery Disease (CAD)

Stress echocardiography, undoubtedly has become an excellent tool for assessing regional wall-motion abnormalities, as the resting echocardiography has limited

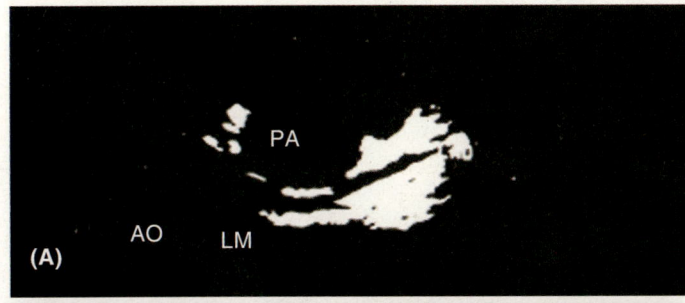

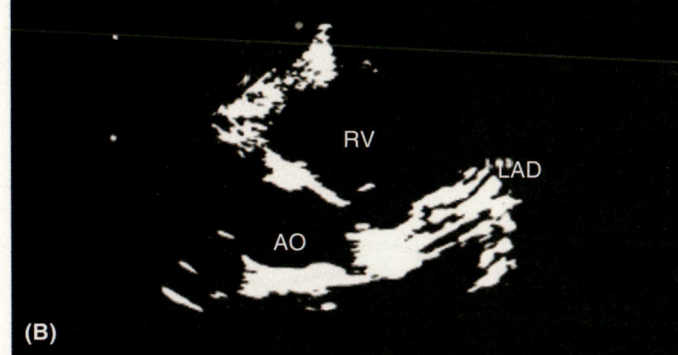

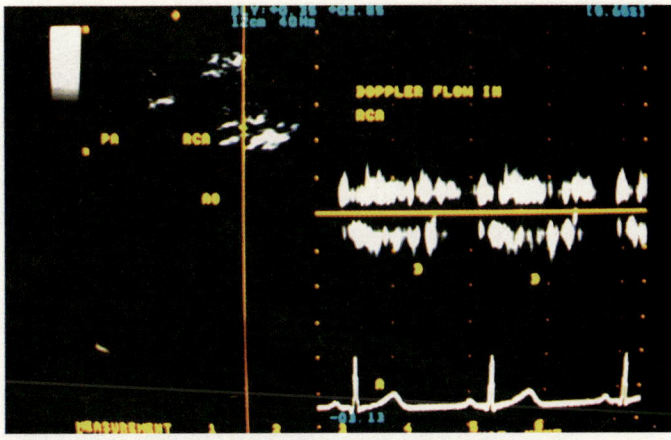

Fig. 6.11B: Doppler flow velocities in right coronary artery (RCA)

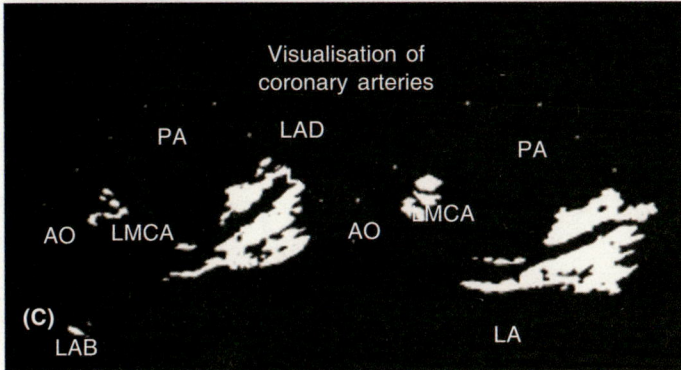

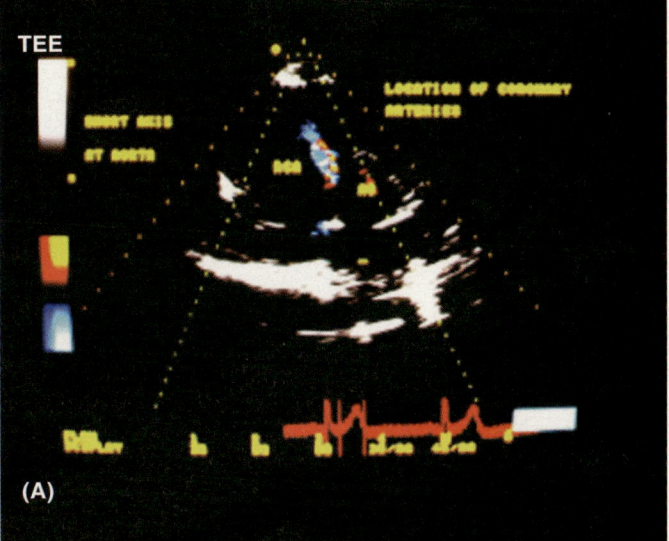

Fig. 6.10A to C: (A) Normal lumen of left main and left anterior descending arteries. **(B)** Normal left main but narrowed LAD and CX arteries. **(C)** Normal LM, LAD but narrowed CX. These observation have been made in a patient with angiographically proved coronary artery disease

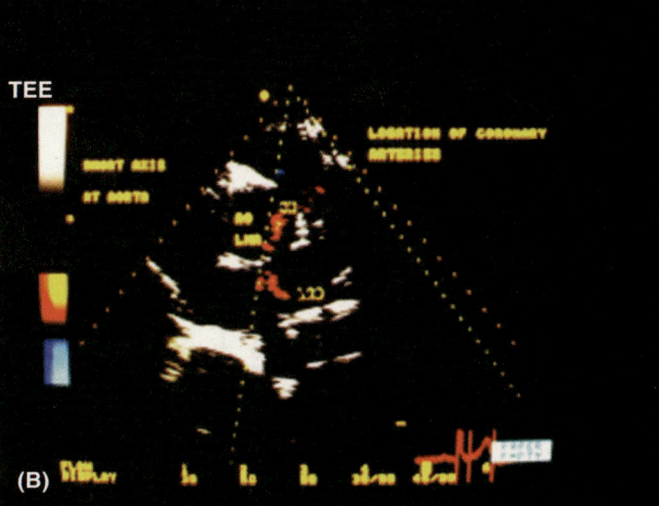

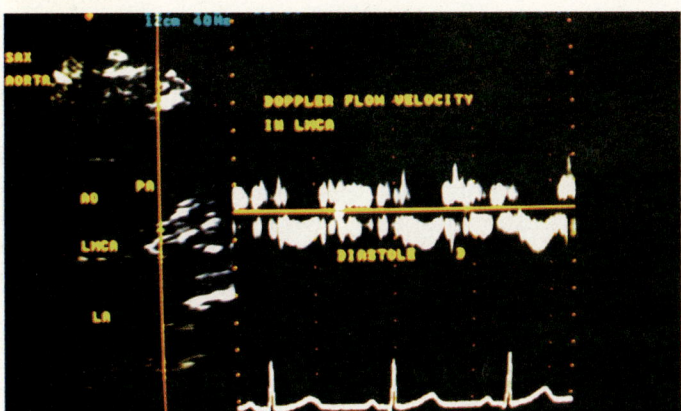

Fig. 6.11A: Doppler flow velocities in left main coronary artery (LMCA)

Fig. 6.12A and B: 2-D Color TEE basal plane at aorta showing identification of right and left coronary arteries as shown on the scans

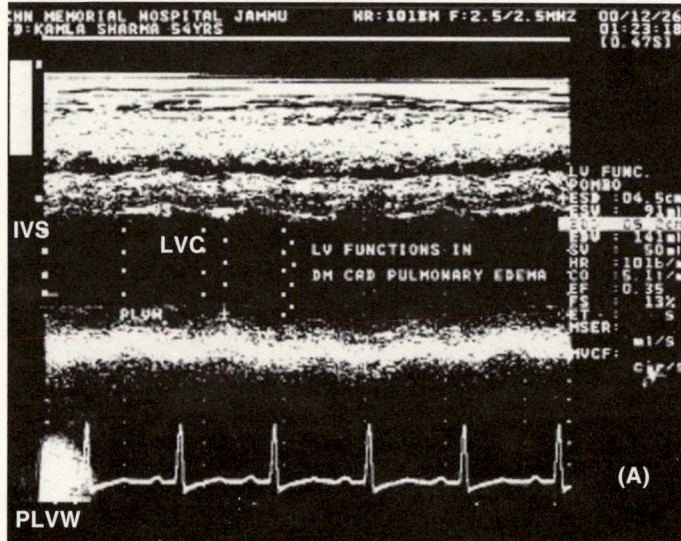

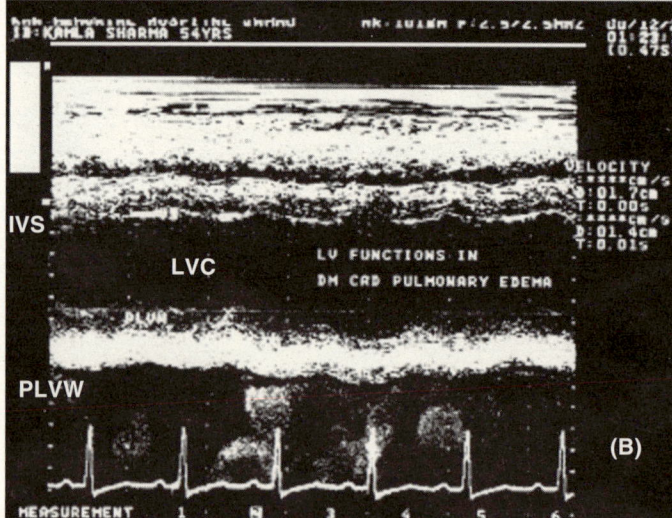

Fig. 6.13 A and B: (A) M-Mode echocardiography showing marked hypokinesia of intraventricular septum (IVS) and posterior left ventricular wall (PLVW) with very poor LV functions as calculated by POMBO method in a patient who had proved CAD, DM and admitted to the hospital with pulmonary edema

REMODELING PHENOMENON IN IHD
Normal Myocardium

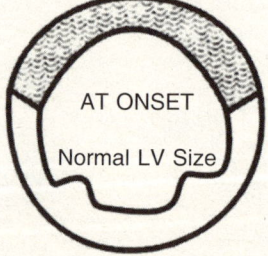

Fig. 6.14A: Diagrammatic representation of antero-septal myocardial infarction with normal thickness and size of myocardium at the onset of myocardial infraction in sequential changes of ventricular wall in remodeling phenomenon

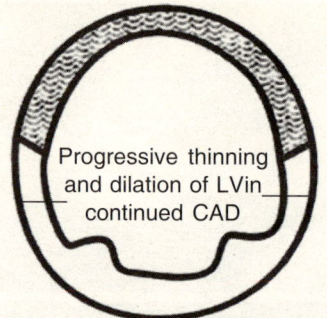

Sub-acute antero-septal wall infarct

Fig. 6.14B: With continued ischemia, there is not only further dilatation and thinning of LV wall but there is involvement of normal myocardial cells resulting into more ischemic burden on the myocardium in sequential changes of ventricular wall in remodeling phenomenon

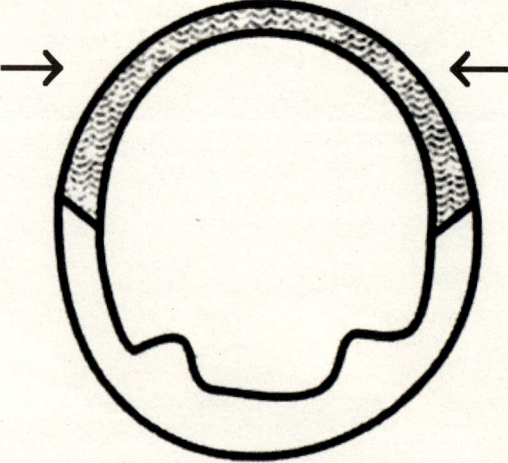

Chronic antero-septal wall infarct

Fig. 6.14C: In continued myocardial ischemia there is further involvement of normal myocardial cells resulting into global thinning and dilatation of LV in remodeling phenomenon. This above described phenomeon may be considered as one of the causes of ischemic cardiomyopathy in progressive deteriorating three vessels coronary heart disease

value in predicting the presence or severity of coronary artery disease. It is to be well understood that ventricular functions may be normal on an echocardiogram taken with patient at rest even in the presence of CAD. Combining echocardiography with stress testing can demonstrate ventricular dysfunction during ischemic conditions. Conventionally two forms of stress testing are primarily used along with two-dimensional echocardiography, i.e. mechanical stress and pharmacologic stress. The treadmill or bicycle is used in mechanical stress echocardiography. The agents most commonly used in pharmacologic stress echocardiography are dobutamine, dipyridamole, and adenosine. The applications and techniques of both these forms have been discussed separately.

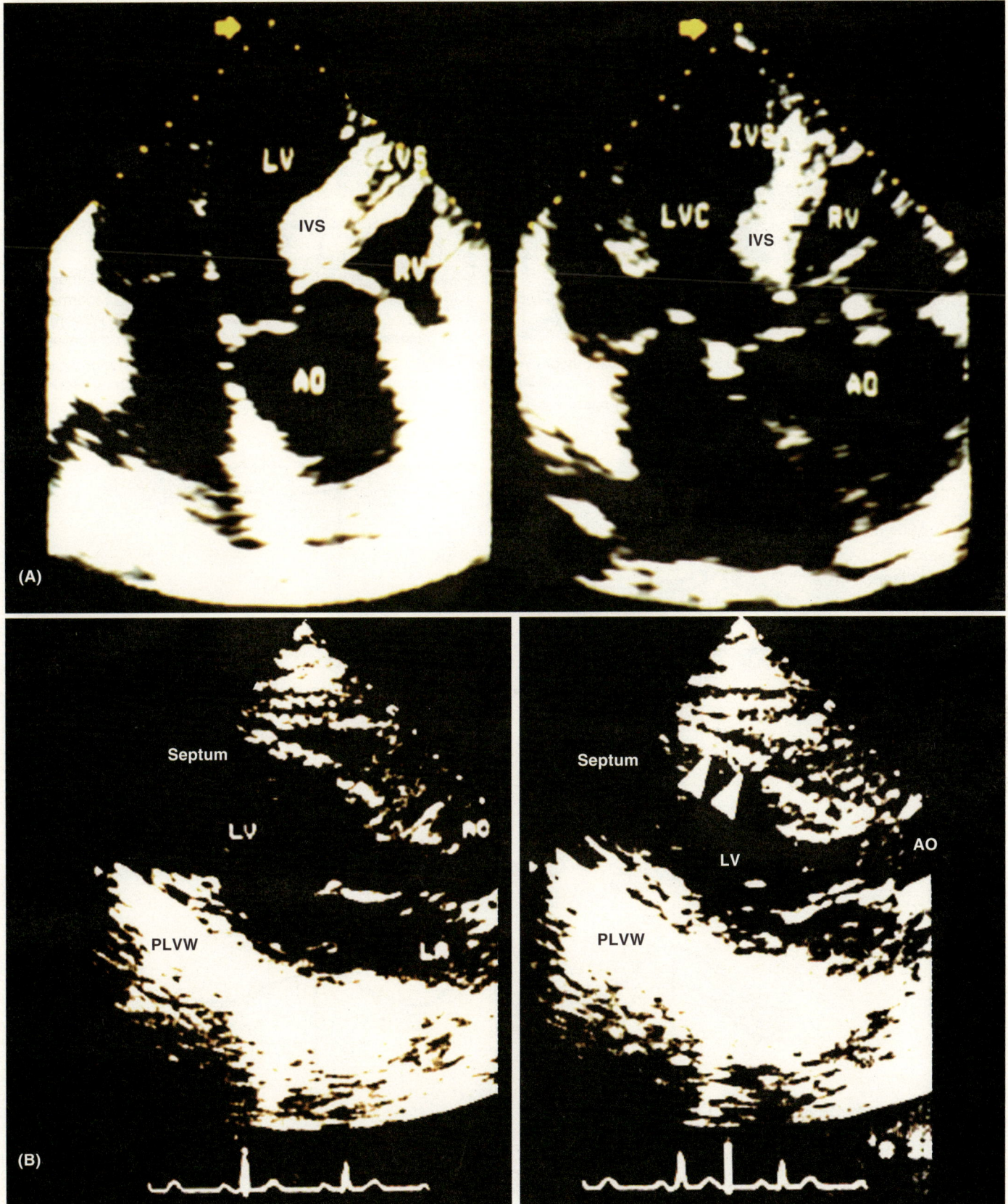

Fig. 6.15A and B: (A) Dual scan 2-D views showing dyskinesia of IVS and dilated ascending aorta in LV aneurysm. **(B)** Long axis left parasternal view showing wall thinning extends from the mid-septum distally as depicted in diastole (left panel). In right panel, it does not either contract or thin down during systole in a patient with coronary heart disease

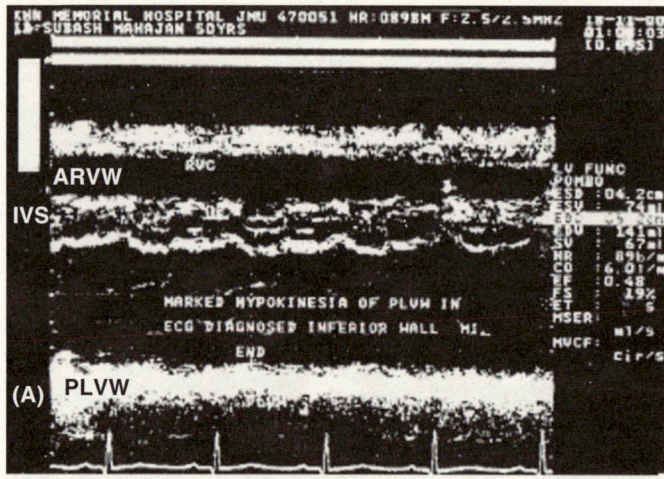 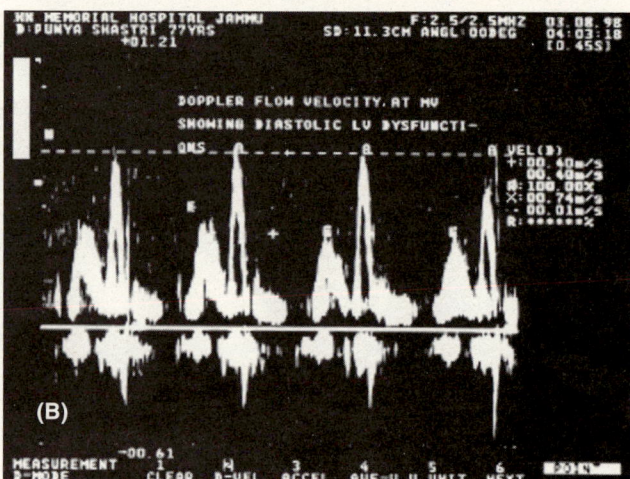

Fig. 6.16A and B: **(A)** M-mode echocardiogram showing hypokinesia of interventricular septum when compared to posterior wall which has retained its thickness on the contrary posterior wall showed marked hypokinesia and thinning in a patient who had inferior wall myocardial infarction. **(B)** Diastolic LV dysfunction in mitral valve (A > E) velocities in patient with coronary heart disease with systemic hypertension

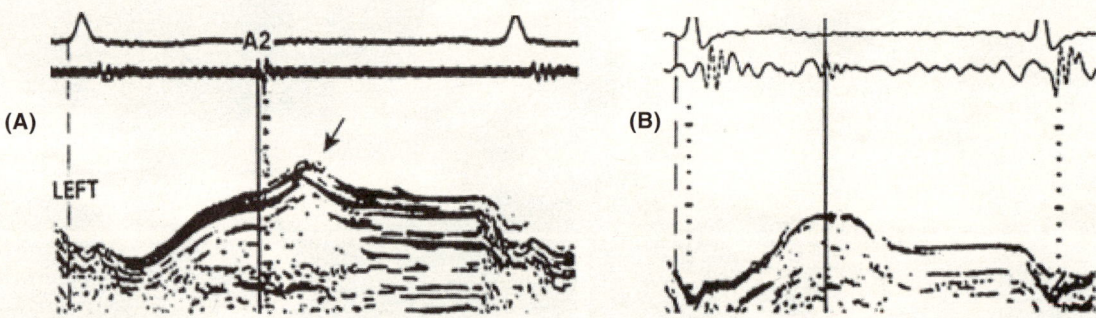

Fig. 6.17A and B: **(A)** Left ventricular free-wall long-axis scan from a patient with coronary artery disease before (A) and after **(B)** coronary angioplasty. Note the remarkable normalisation of the incoordinate pattern (arrow) after procedure

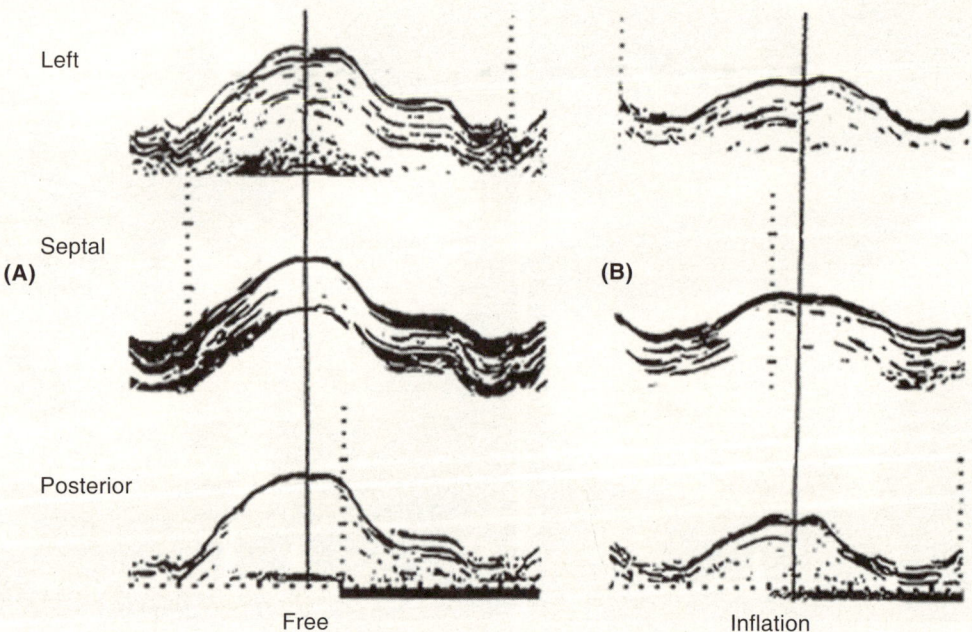

Fig. 6.18A and B: Left ventricular free-wall and septal long-axis scan from a patient during balloon inflation in the proximal left anterior descending artery **(A).** Note the significant fall in long axis amplitude and lengthening velocities **(B)**

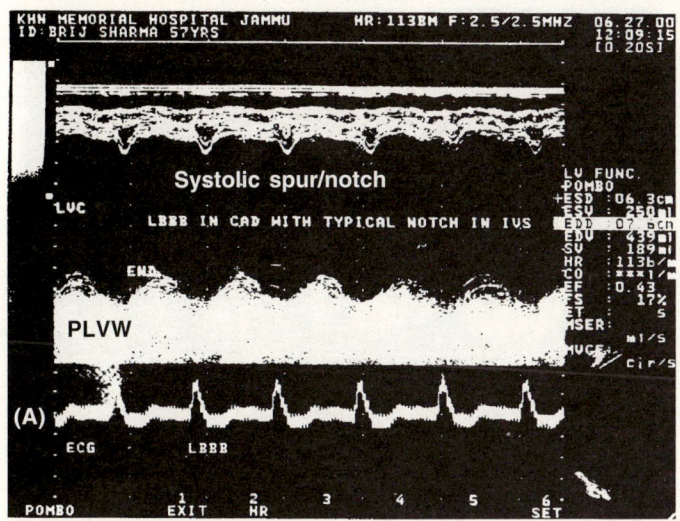 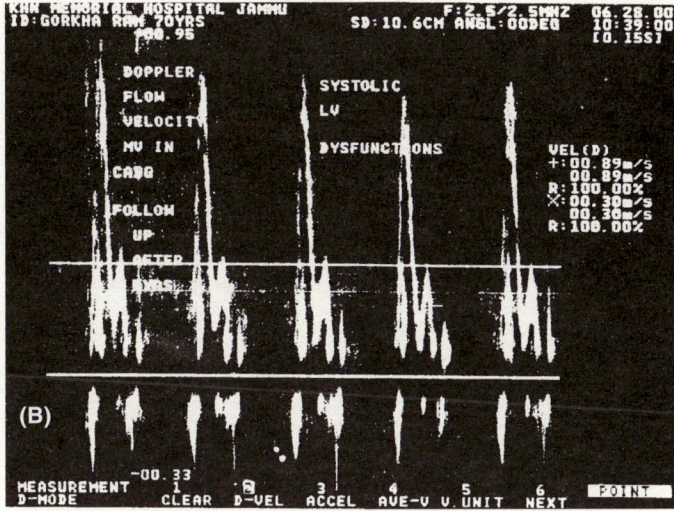

Fig. 6.19A and B: (A) M-mode echocardiogram showing hypokinesia and early systolic beak along interventricular septum in a patient with coronary heart disease with conduction defect (LBBB). **(B)** Systolic LV dysfunctions (E>A) in patient with coronary heart disease

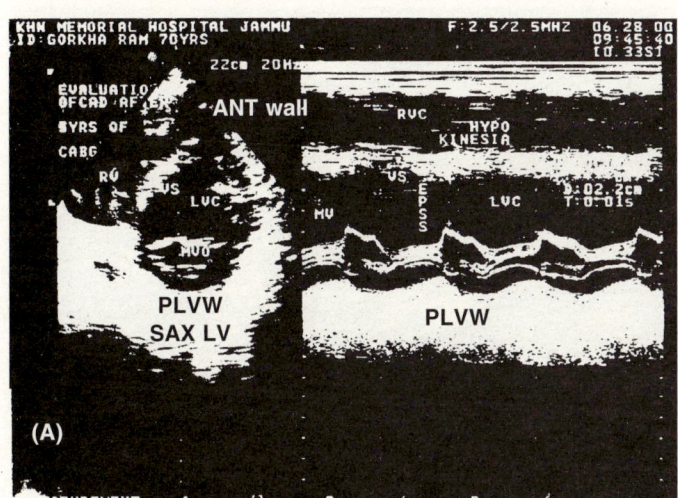 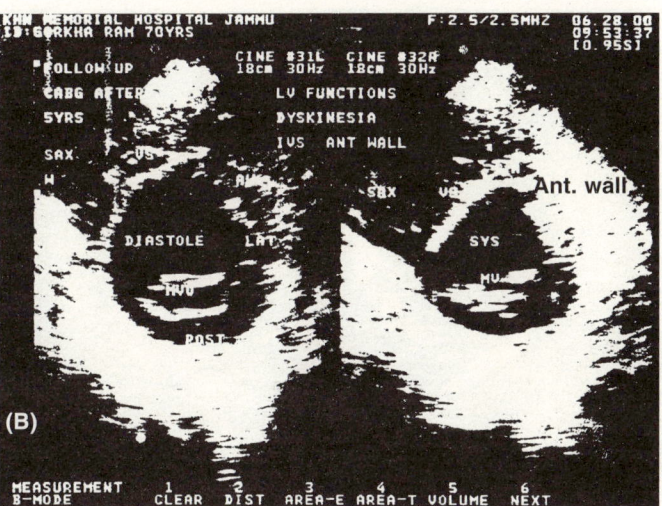

Fig. 6.20A and B: (A) M-mode echocardiogram showing hypokinesia of IVS and PLVW with increased EPSS to 22 mm (distance between E point of mitral valve to the systolic invasination of IVS, Normal = 0–10 mm; increased distance is associated with very low LVEF, as it occurs in ischemic cardiomyopathy). This patient in particular did not improved even after 5 years of 3-vessel coronary bypass grafting. **(B)** 2-D dual scan taken during diastole (left) and systole (right) showed dyskinesia of anterior LV wall as shown in this short axis view in this patient of ischemic cardiomyopathy

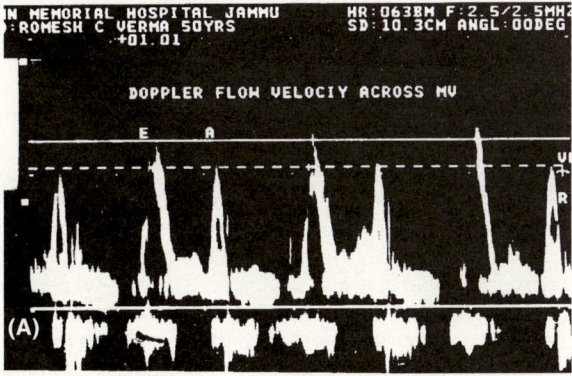 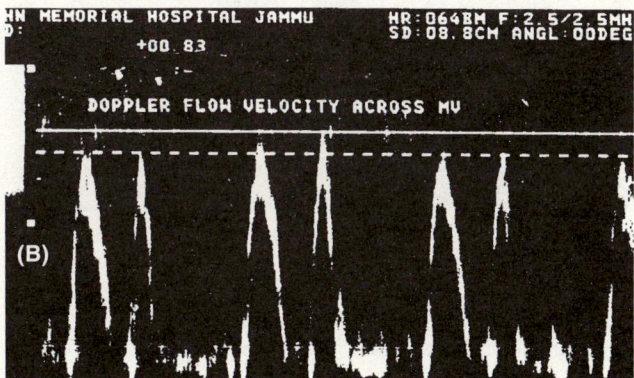

Fig. 6.21 A and B: (A) Normal **(B)** Progressive deterioration of diastolic LV dysfunctions by application of ratio of diastolic E/A velocities

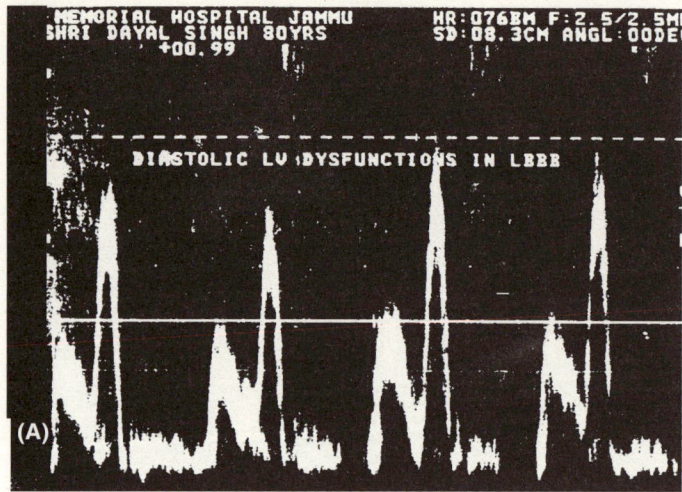
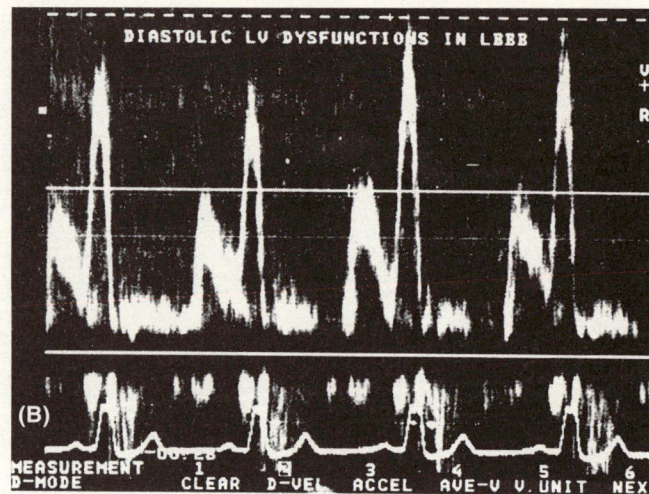

Fig. 6.22B and C: Progressive deterioration of diastolic LV dysfunctions by application of ratio of diastolic E/A velocities. In these patients ratio of A/E is found to be more than unity

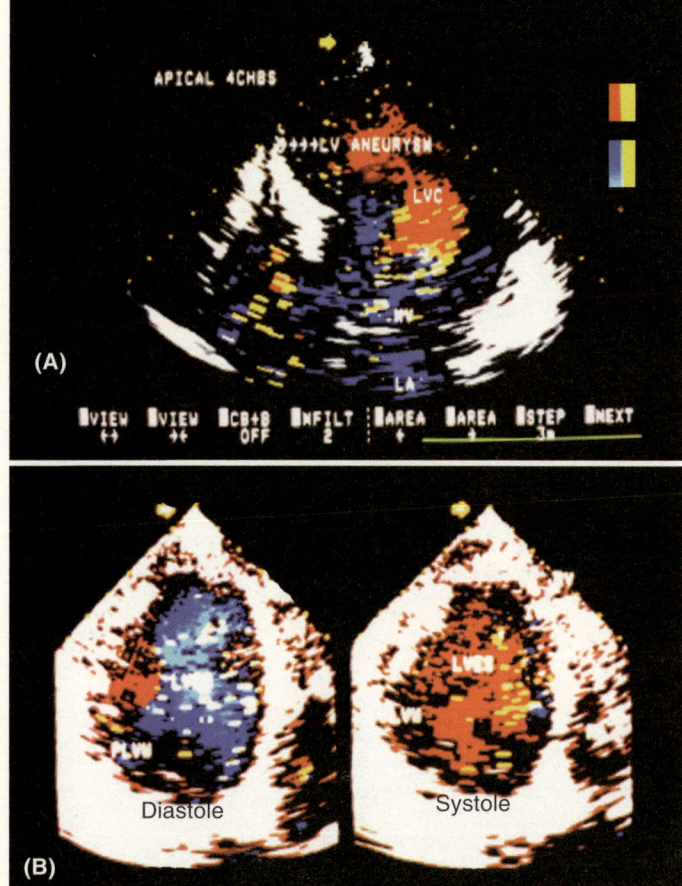

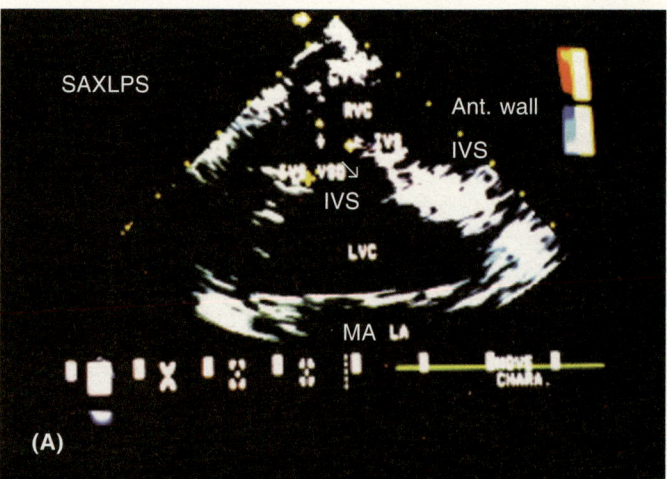
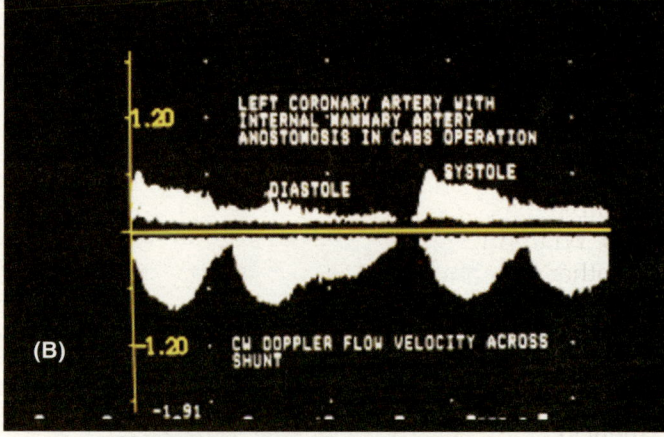

Fig. 6.23A and B: **(A)** 2-D Colour flow apical 4C view showing abnormal colour flow in LV cavity and along the IVS in patient with marked dyskinesia of interventricular septum and aneurysm of LV. **(B)** Short axis view of LV in systole and diastole shows no change in cavity size and abnormal colour flows in a patient with long standing 3-vessels coronary artery disease finally ending with ischemic cardiomyopathy

Fig. 6.24A and B: **(A)** 2-D Short axis view LV showing breakage of interventricular septum near to apex (VSD) (arrow) in patient with acute myocardial infarction with pulmonary edema and pansystolic murmer over 2-3 left parasternal area. **(B)** Doppler flow velocity after anatomosis of left coronary artery with internal mammary artery showing normal shunt flow in both systole and diastole as depicted on the scan

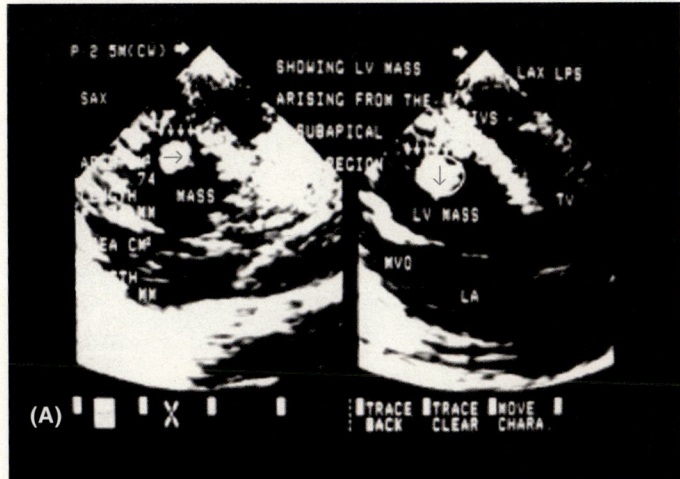

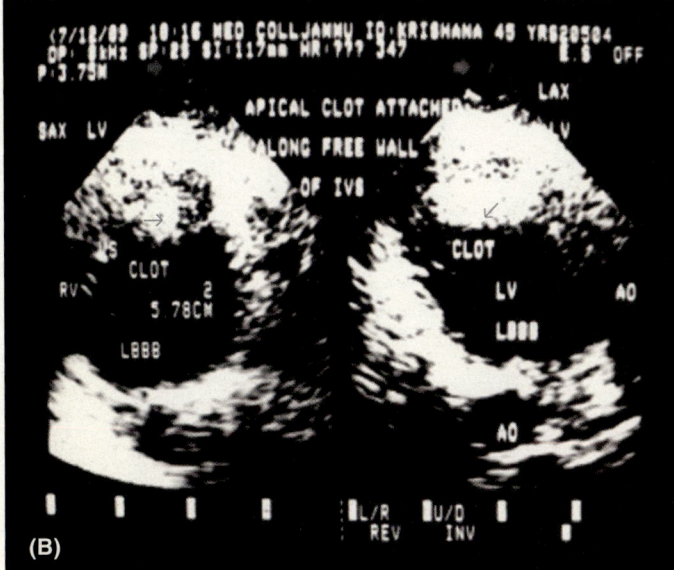

Fig. 6.25A and B: Dual scan 2-D short axis (left) and low long axis (right) views depicting LV clot in apical regions (arrows) with dyskinesia of IVS in patient with coronary artery disease with poor LV ejection function and LBBB

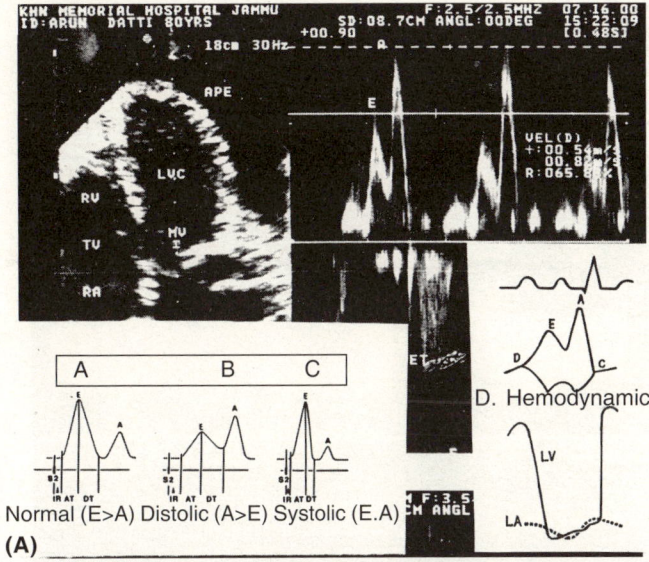

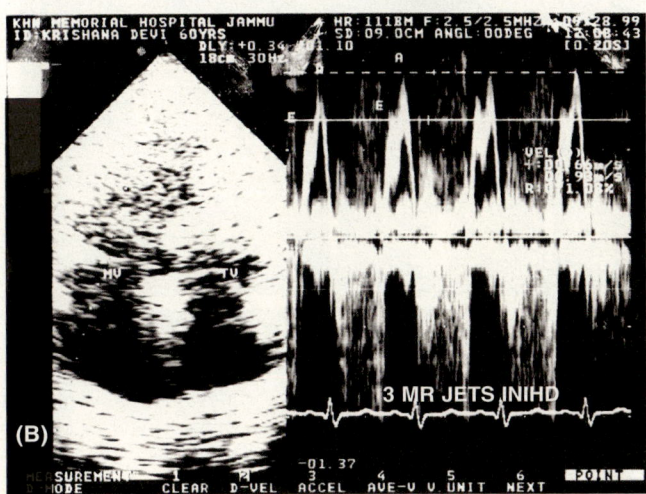

Fig. 6.26A and B: (A) Apical view in Doppler mode showing diastolic defect in relaxation of LV and diagrammatic representation as how progressively LV diastolic function deteriorate (A-C and D shows LV function in comparison with hemodynamic evaluation). **(B)** 2-D Doppler flow in apical 4C view shows diastolic LV dysfunction with gross mitral regurgitation due to papillary muscle dysfunction in patient with hypertension and ischemic heart disease

In the application of two-dimensional echocardiography to detect coronary artery disease, it is imperative to compare images at rest side-by-side with those with stress. When these images are not compared to next to each other, subtle alternations in myocardial contraction induced by ischemia may not be detected. Normal responses to stress testing observed on two-dimensional echocardiography include the decrease in ventricular chamber dimension, increase in wall motion contraction (kinetics), and increase in systolic wall thickening. In patients with abnormal regional response, the location of the arterial obstruction in the corresponding coronary artery or particular branch can be predicted.

In those particular situations, where the myocardium becomes akinetic or dyskinetic with abnormal systolic wall thickening, recognition to these abnormalities is fairly easy and ensured and may predict more significant coronary artery obstructions. When subtle changes are observed, it is not so easy to distinguish the mild abnormalities from the lower limits of normal. In order to detect the subtle changes, long standing experience in wall-motion analysis and correlations to coronary angiograms are needed for their final reporting (Figs 6.13–6.26).

Detection of Reversible Ischemia

In patients suffering from chronic CAD, there is a gradual reduction in blood supply to the heart muscle

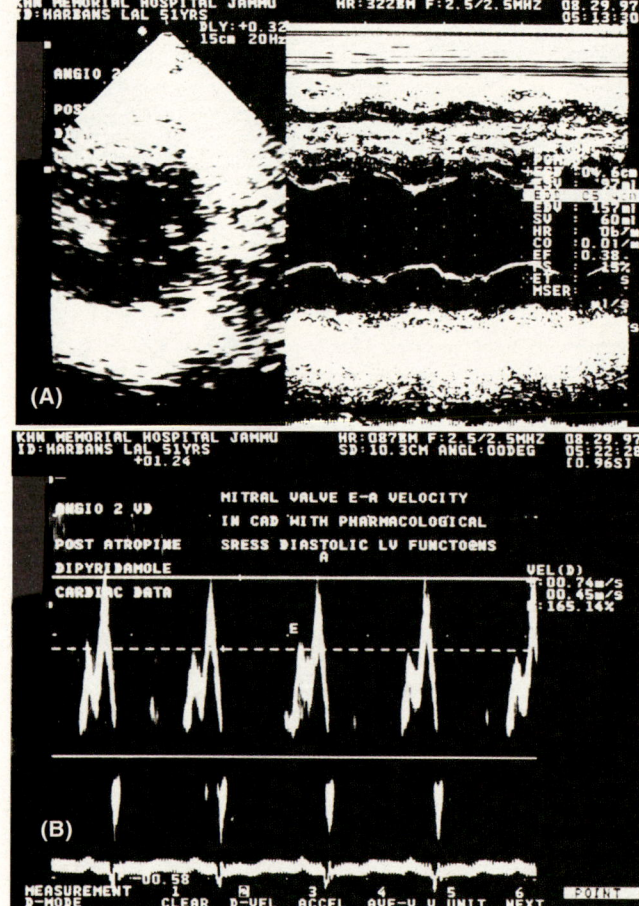

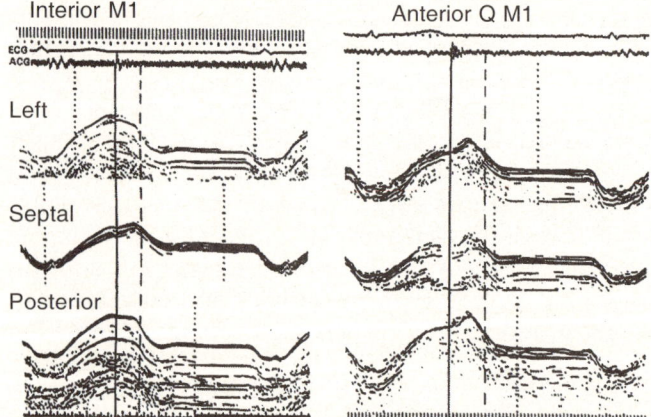

Fig. 6.27A and B: (A) M-Mode echocardiography showing marked hypokinesia of interventricular septum and posterior left ventricular wall in patient with coronary artery disease with very low LV ejection fraction (38%). **(B)** Mitral E and A velocities showing reverse pattern A > E as seen in defect in diastolic relaxation of LV after oral administration of Dipyridamole and injectable atropine in performing pharmacological stress test in the same patient as described in detection of coronary disease and long term prediction of prognosis. His angiogram later revealed two vessel disease

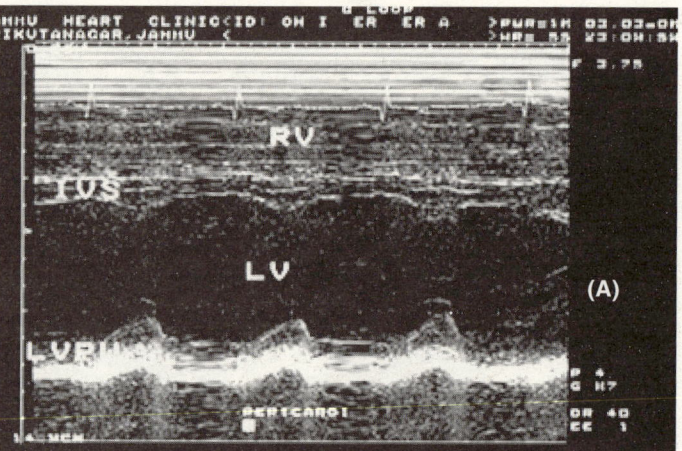

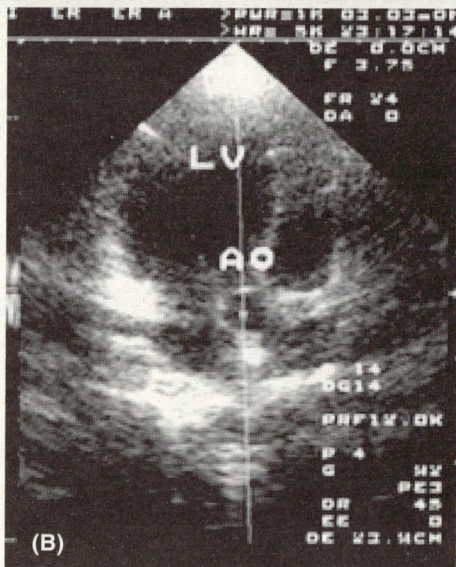

Fig. 6.29A and B: (A) M-Mode echocardiogram showing thinning of IVS and scarred myocardium in patient with obstruction of LAD and RCA. **(B)** Apical 5 chamber view showing scarred myocardium in patient with posterior and basal myocardial infarction with obstruction of RCA and LAD coronary arteries

Fig. 6.28: Left ventricular long-axis recordings of the three segments; left, septal, and posterior demonstrating global incoordination (postejection shortening) in the patient with inferior MI compared with isolated septal incoordination from a patient with anterior M1

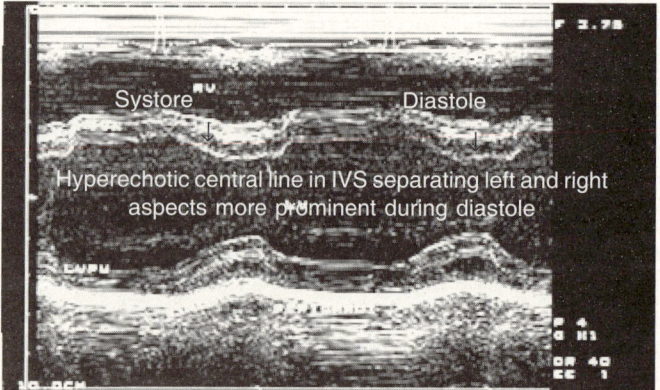

Fig. 6.30: M-Mode echocardiogram showing distinct hyperechotic dense central line separating right and left aspects of interventricular septum (arrow) in a 7 yrs. old child with normal coronary anatomy in left parasternal long axis view

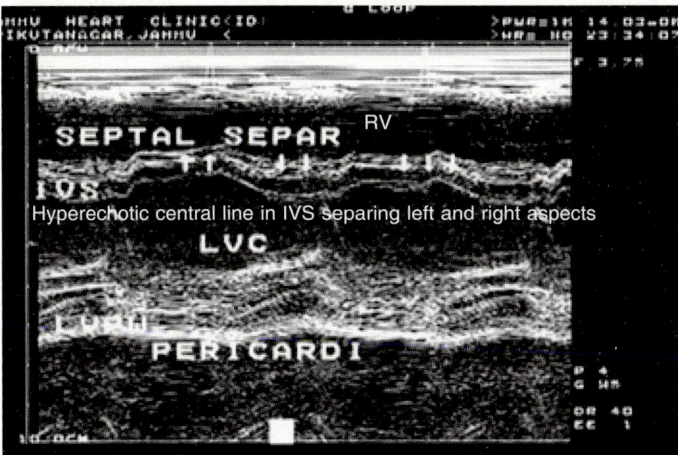

Fig. 6.31A: M-Mode echocardiogram showing distinct hyperechotic dense central line separating right and left aspects of interventricular septum (arrow) in an adult female with normal coronary anatomy in left parasternal long axis view

resulting into hypokinesis, or reduced systolic thickening on resting two-dimensional echocardiography. In such situation the myocardial muscle is still viable and returns to normal activity when blood supply is restored. The term hibernating myocardium has been used to describe these muscles. Such patients suffering from hibernating myocardium are usually benefitted from coronary revascularization. Low dose dobutamine stress echocardiography is very useful test in the identification of hibernating myocardial segments as they show improved myocardial functions with pharmacological stress testing. "Stunned" myocardium occurs when the myocardium has been subjected to a temporary depletion of oxygen supply. Its normal function has been hampered or stunned. With reperfusion, the functions return to normal over a period of time.

Evaluating Reperfusion and Revascularization

In the event of coronary occlusion resulting into infarction, myocardial damage can be reversed or minimized with early interventions, including angioplasty and thrombolytic therapy. Both techniques can produce coronary reperfusion and restore the supply of blood to the infarction prone region. Echocardiography has proved to be a very useful tool in identifying not only a particular arterial occlusion but it can also determine and monitor the results of the intervention. When viable myocardium has been identified, coronary artery bypass surgery or angioplasty may be performed to achieve revascularization. The results of revascularization can then be monitored effectively by serial two-dimensional echocardiography.

Prognosis after Myocardial Infarction

Two-dimensional echocardiography can also be utilised in determining the prognosis after myocardial infarction. Patients who have relatively small, uncomplicated infarction are advised for brief period of hospitalisation. Echocardiography can also identify infarct size, the function of the noninfarcted area and provide information to help identify high risk individuals for their future health planning.

Complications of Myocardial Infarction
Ventricular Aneurysm (Fig. 6.23A)

One of the complications following massive infarction is ventricular aneurysm which can occur in any area, but apical aneurysm is one of the most common among the rest of the complications. Two-dimensional echocardiography is well suited in locating the presence and size of the ventricular aneurysm because of its ability to image from multiple tomographic planes. Apical aneurysm is seen as localized dilation with reduced wall thickness and dyskinesis.

Pseudoaneurysm (False Aneurysm)

The recognition of pseudoaneurysm is of clinical importance as it is often fatal and needs surgical intervention. It results from the rupture of ventricular free wall, leaving blood trapped in the pericardium and forming an aneurysm. Pseudoaneurysm has a fatal consequences as the clotted blood in the aneurysm may predispose to the development of hemopericardium. Both M-mode and 2-dimensional echocardiography can make a clear distinction between the false and true aneurysms by recording the diameter at its entry to the pseudoaneurysm and the size of the cavity in systole. The entrance to the pseudoaneurysm is always small, creating the appearance of a neck. The left ventricular cavity of a true aneurysm contracts in systole, whereas the cavity of a pseudoaneurysm frequently expands.

The major criterion of identification of true and false aneurysm on 2-dimensional echocardiography is that the endocardium and myocardium in pseudoaneurysm have been interrupted or torn but remain intact in true aneurysm provided it is not limited to posterior or basal inferior wall as the interruption at that region is not clearly visualised (Fig. 6.15A).

Rupture of Ventricular Septum (Fig. 6.24A)

Combined approach with 2-dimensional and Doppler flow echocardiography is considered as a very valuable tool in the diagnosis of acquired ventricular septal defect. Acquired VSD of rare occurrence happens when rupture of the myocardium extends to IVS. Its detection in the setting of acute massive myocardial infarction is of clinical importance that it can lead to very high

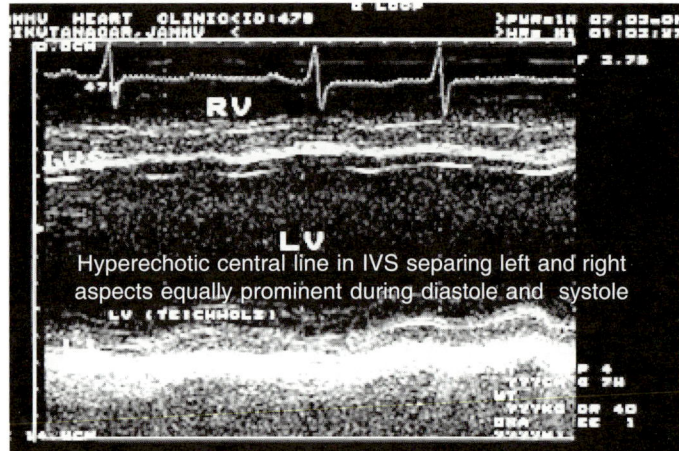

Fig. 6.31B: M-Mode echocardiogram showing distinct hyperechotic dense central line separating right and left aspects of interventricular septum in an adult male with normal cardiac anatomy in left parasternal long axis view

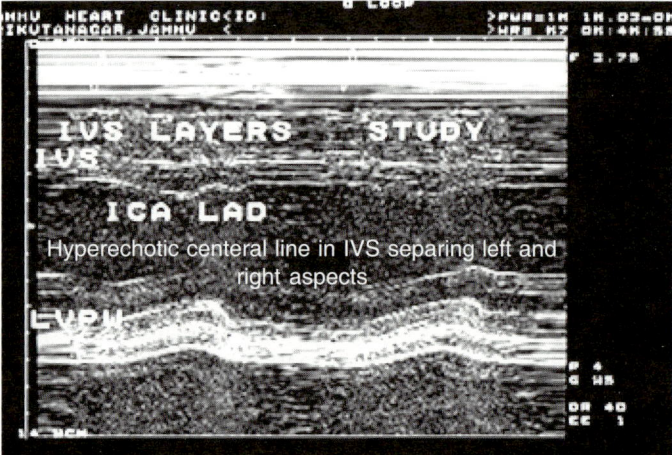

Fig. 6.32: M-Mode echocardiogram showing distinct hyperechotic dense central line separating right and left aspects of interventricular septum with hypolucent area in the left aspect of the septum supplied by the obstructed coronary arteries in an adult male suffering with angiographically proved 2-vessel coronary artery disease (RCA and LAD) with Q-wave inferio-lateral wall myocardial infarction with normal LVEF but mild to moderate mitral regurgitation

mortality (5%) in the follow up course of anterior myocardial infarction. Colour Doppler echo is useful in scanning L-R shunt at IVS level.

Left Ventricular Thrombus (Fig. 6.25A and B)

In the absence of ventricular aneurysm or wall motion abnormalities, it is often difficult to explain its formation visualisation in the presence of LV aneurysm. It may also be very difficult to identify mural thrombi from trabeculation on 2-dimensional echo particularly if images are suboptimal.

Although two-dimensional echocardiography is the technique of choice in identifying thrombi, but it may be difficult to distinguish thrombi from artifacts even with this modality. However, they can be differentiated from each other on echo parameters that thrombi usually occur in areas where the wall motion is abnormal, always attached to the endocardium and move in the same direction as the endocardium and usually have distinct borders with thrombi.

Papillary Muscle Dysfunction (Fig. 6.13 A and B and 6.26)

One of the causes of mitral regurgitation is papillary muscle dysfunction which can occur as a result of acute fibrosis and shortening of the papillary muscle restricting the mitral valve leaflets from closing completely. Occasionally, the papillary muscle or chordae tendineae may rupture in acute myocardial infarction. Ejection fraction can be calculated by the below mentioned formula as:

$$\% \ EF = \frac{LVDV - LVSV}{LVDV} = 100$$

where EF is ejection fraction, LVDV is left ventricular diastolic volume, and LVSV is left ventricular systolic volume. Doppler echocardiography has been used in the assessment of left ventricular diastolic function by determining transmitral diastolic filling characteristics from the mitral flow Doppler velocities. Although the mitral flow velocities reflect the relative change in left atrial and left ventricular pressures, provided sample volume is placed at right side of interrogation. The pulsed wave Doppler sample volume should be placed at or between the tips of the mitral valve leaflets during diastole for maximum velocities. Factors that can alter the filling characteristics include the compliance of the left ventricle, the driving pressure from the left atrium, the loading conditions, and the transmitral pressure gradient, and age of the patient. Some of the parameters using mitral flow Doppler velocities to assess left ventricular diastolic function include peak velocity, flow velocity integral, ratio of early and later filling, deceleration time, and isovolumic relaxation time.

Mitral flow velocity can determine an early diastolic filling E wave and the atrial contraction A wave. The ratio of early filling to atrial contraction can also be calculated for finding out abnormal diastolic filling. The normal value of the E/A ratio is 1.5. Deceleration time (DT) measures the rate of decline in the early mitral velocity (E). It is the time from the early peak filling to an extrapolation of the rate of decline of velocity to baseline. DT increases when myocardial relaxation is delayed or prolonged. Normal value for DT is 199 ± 32 msec for ages 20 to 60. DT is shortened for ages below 20 and lengthened for ages over 60.

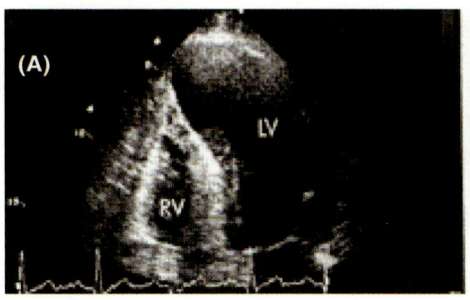 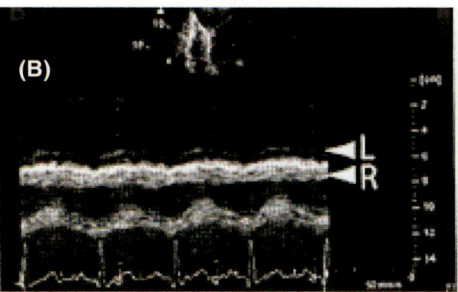 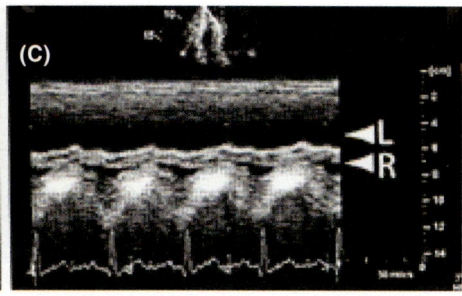

Fig. 6.33A to C: **(A)** Modified four chamber view zoomed in on the septum showing an infarcted apical part of the left-sided septum. **(B)** Anatomical M-mode through the middle part of the septum showing both sides of the septum. **(C)** Anatomical M-mode through the apical part of the septum showing the middle line and the right part of the septum (R) with flattened left part (L)

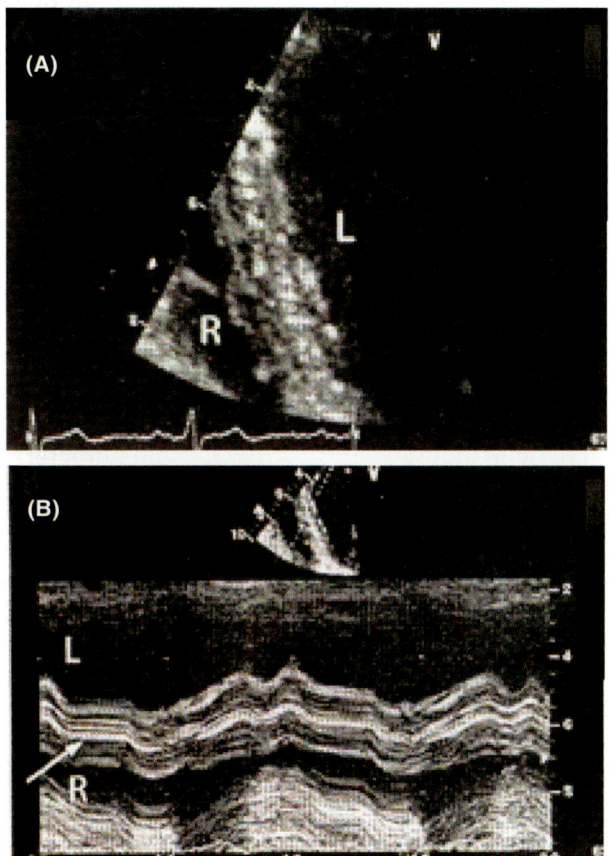

Fig. 6.34A and B: (A) Zoomed B-mode of the interventricular septum in an oblique four chamber view. **(B)** Anatomical M-mode of image A showing the moderately hypertrophied right (R) and normal left (L) part of the septum separated by a bright line of high echodensity (arrow)

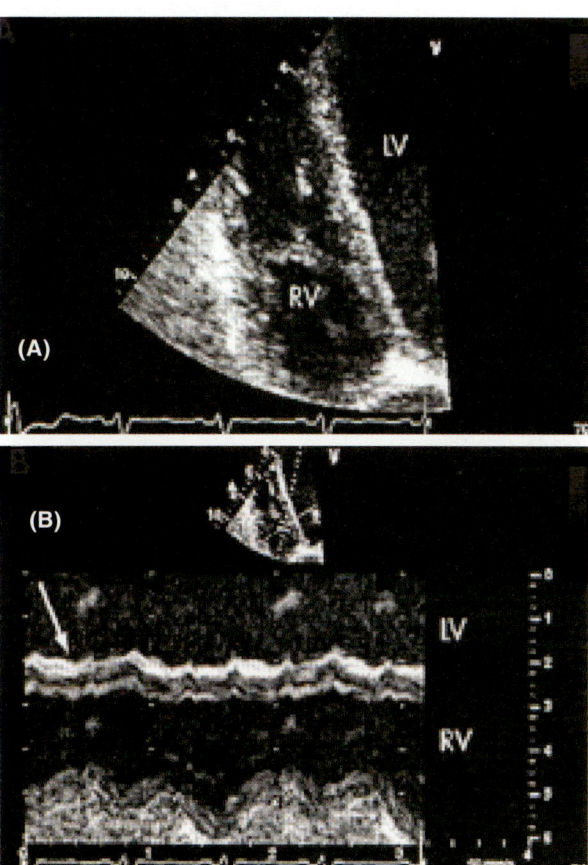

Fig. 6.35A and B: (A) Zoomed B-mode of the interventricular septum in an oblique four chamber view. **(B)** M-Mode of image A showing complete loss of myocardium on the left side of the septum (arrow) in patient with obstructed CAD

Isovolumic relaxation time (IVRT) measures the time from aortic closure to onset of mitral flow. It reflects the rate of myocardial relaxation. IVRT is affected by age. The normal value for less than 40 years of age is 60 ± 12 msec and for over 40 years of age is 76 ± 13 msec. Doppler assessment of left ventricular diastolic function will play an increasingly important role in the evaluation of coronary artery disease and ventricular function (Figs 6.19 and 6.22).

Echocardiographic Evaluation of Newer Aspects of the Ventricular Septum and its Clinical Application (Figs 6.29 to 6.36A and B)

Feigenbaum described a bright line within the interventricular septum (IVS) in a patient with a massively hypertrophied septum. It ran through the middle of the septum and was referred to as an "echo of unknown origin". Although in clinical practice the septum is considered to be one functional unit, with the enhanced

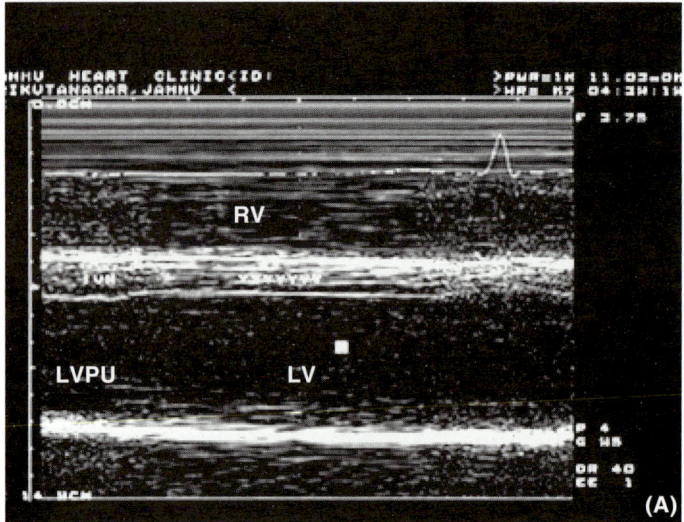

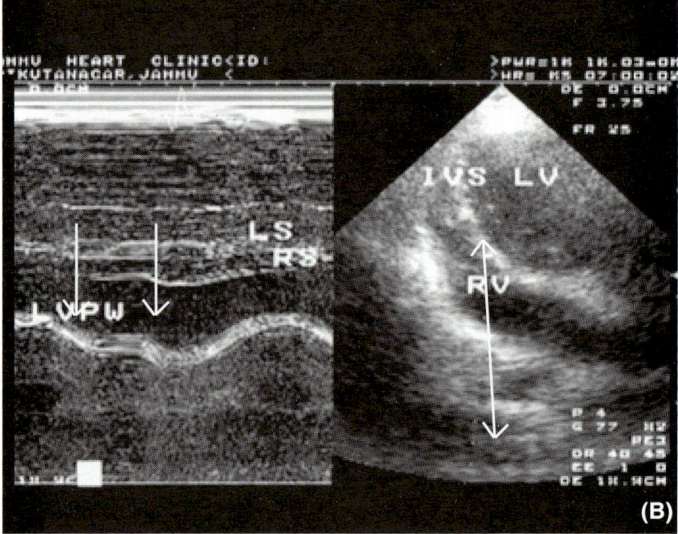

Fig. 6.36A and B: M-mode-echocardiogram (left) taken at higher frame rate in modified 4-C view of LV (right) in the region of apical septum showing less distinct hyperechotic dense central line separating right and left aspects of interventricular septum in an adult patient with old myocardial infarction. Note loss of myocardium in left aspect of the interventricular septum more pronounced during diastole

image quality of the recent generation of echocardiographic equipment and the development of second harmonic imaging, a line with enhanced echogenicity in the IVS can often be seen.

Many investigators have shown that normal right and left ventricles do not act independently of each other and that ventricular interaction occurs. The role of the septum in this interaction is still not fully determined. Some authors have suggested that ventricular interaction is caused by the shared septal wall: whereas others have suggested that the free walls affect the contralateral ventricle independently of the septum. A model developed by Li *et al.*, showed the

impact of septal impairment on ventricular pressure development. Li *et al.* showed that septal dysfunction created by glutaraldehyde injection decreased both left and right ventricular pressures. Transeptal cutting dramatically decreased left ventricular (LV) developed pressure but had no obvious influence on right ventricular pressure. Therefore, the data showed that altering septal function affected both right ventricular and LV function, but not equally. To better understand the interaction of the right sided and left sided part of the septum, Beyar, *et al.* developed a geometrical model. This model evaluated the transmural gradients in stress and strain of the left ventricle and the IVS and showed that the right and left sides of the septum respond differently to various conditions such as a one sided pressure increase by alternate aortic and pulmonary arterial constrictions. In general, there are much greater inhomogeneities in stress between the layers of the septum than between the layers of the LV free wall.

The development of tissue Doppler imaging allowed for evaluation of the differences in regional function within the septum. Fleming *et al.*, assessed total deformation of the septum by narrowest image sector angle possible (usually 30; is used to achieve the maximum colour Doppler frame rate. Three consecutive cycles are recorded during breathholding. For longitudinal deformation, Doppler myocardial imaging data of the septum are obtained in a four chamber view. Careful attention is paid to keep the ultrasound beam aligned perpendicular to the posterior wall and septum when measuring radial deformation and parallel to the septum when measuring longitudinal motion (Fig. 36A and B).

Off-line Analysis

Data are stored in digital format and transferred to a computer workstation for off-line analysis. This allowed the computation of thickening, strain, and strain rate by dedicated software.

Thickness

To quantify the radial thickening of the left and right sides of the septum, M-mode clips of a standard parasternal long axis view are analysed. The borders of both sides of the septum are delineated by the bright line within the septum. Timing information is added by continuous wave or pulsed wave Doppler flow curves of the aorta to define the ejection period (from aortic valve opening to aortic valve closure). Systole is defined from the beginning of QRS to the end of ejection. End of diastole was considered to be at the onset of QRS (ECG tracing). All timing information is aligned through ECG traces. The thickness is obtained at end systole and end diastole. Data are averaged over three consecutive cardiac cycles.

Strain and Strain Rate

From the mean velocity curves, regional strain rate is estimated from the spatial derivative of the myocardial velocity over the computation area. For strain rate, peak values during ejection are calculated. Natural strain profiles are obtained by time integrating the strain rate profile, which was averaged over three consecutive cardiac cycles, with end diastole as the reference point. For radial deformation, parasternal long axis views are used. The sample volumes are manually positioned in both sides of the septum. Motion is tracked throughout the cardiac cycle. To separate the right from the left side of the septum the bright line is used as a boundary. As the averaged end diastolic wall thicknesses of the right and the left sides of the septum are 3.6 mm (right) and 5.5 mm (left), the size of the computation area is fixed to 3 mm for radial analysis. For longitudinal deformation, strain and strain rate data are obtained from a four chamber view. The region of interest is positioned in both sides at the midpart of the septum. Strain and strain rate are calculated as described above. Computation area was fixed to 10 mm for longitudinal analysis. Doppler flow curves of the aortic valve and ECG traces are used for timing as described.

Visualisation of the Septum

Standard two-dimensional and M-mode data sets are obtained for all subjects. The data are uniformly of good quality and allowed subsequent off-line analysis. The bright line within the septum is visualised. This line appeared to divide the septum into a right sided and a left sided layer. The line is best and most consistently visible in the four chamber view and it is more pronounced in diastole than in systole. The line could be followed from the cardiac apex to the aortic root, disappearing at the left aortic cusp (Fig. 6.29A and B).

Conclusion

It shows that the septum can be consistently divided into a left and a right side based on a bright echocardiographic signal. Also, differences in thickening and radial strain between the two sides are observable. These differences are not present in longitudinal motion. Knowledge of fibre architecture with an abrupt change in the middle of the septum, suggests that the septum to be a morphologically and functionally bilayered structure potentially supplied by different coronary arteries. Further studies to evaluate the clinical relevance is advocated.

Bibliography

1. Abraham TP, Belohlavek M, Thamson H, *et al*. Time onset of regional relaxation: feasibility, variability and utility of a navel index of regional myocardial function by strain role imaging. *J Am Coll Cardial* 2002;39:1531–7.

2. Agati L, Voci P, Bilotta F, Luongo R, Autore C, Peno M, *et al*. Influence of residual perfusion within the infarct zone on the natural history of left ventricular dysfunction after acute myocardial infarction: a myocardial contrast echocardiographic study. *J Am Coll Cardiol* 1994; 24: 336–342.

3. Alam M, Thorstrand C, Rosenhamer G. Mitral regurgitation following first-time acute myocardial infarction-early and late findings by Doppler echocardiography. *Clin Cardiol* 1993;16: 30–34.

4. Appleton CP, Hatle LK, Popp RL. Relation of transmitral flow velocity patterns to left ventricular diastolic function: new insights from a combined hemodynamic and Doppler echocardiographic study. *J Am Coll Cardiol* 1988; 12:426–440.

5. Barrett MJ, Charuzi Y, Corday E. Ventricular aneurysm: cross-sectional echocardiographic approach. *Am J Cardiol* 1980;46:1133–1137.

6. Barzilai B, Gessler C, Jr., Perez JE, *et al*. Significance of Doppler-detected mitral regurgitation in acute myocardial infarction. *Am J Cardiol* 1988; 61:220–223.

7. Becker Le, Ferreira R, Thomas M. Mopping of left ventricular blood flow with radioactive microspheres in experimental coronary artery occlusion. *Cardiovosc Res* 1973;7:391–400.

8. Berthe C, Pierard LA, Hiernaux M, *et al*. Predicting the extent and location of coronary artery disease in acute myocardial infarction by echocardiography during dobutamine infusion. *Am J Cardiol* 1986;58(13):1167–1172.

9. Beyar I, Dong SJ, Smith ER, *et al*. Ventricular interaction and septal deformation: a model compared with experimental data. *Am J Physiol* 1993;265: H2044–56.

10. Bhatnagar SK, Moussa MA, AI-Yusuf AR. The role of pre-hospital discharge two-dimensional echocardiography in determining the prognosis of survivors of first myocardial infarction. *Am Heart J* 1985; 109: 472–477.

11. Bishop SP, Whe FC, Bloor CM. Regional myocardial blood flow during acute myocardial infarction in the conscious dog. *Circ Res* 1976; 38:429–38.

12. Bloch A, Morad J, Mayr C, Perrenoud J. Cross-sectional echocardiography in acute myocardial infarction. *Am J Cardiol* 1979;43: 387–395.

13. Block PJ, Popp RL. Detecting and excluding significant left main coronary artery narrowing by echocardiography. *Am J Cardiol* 1985;55:937–940.

14. Bolognese L, Sarasso G, Bongo AS, *et al*. Dipyri- damole echocardiography test. A new tool for detecting jeopardized myocardium after thrombolytic therapy. *Circulation* 1991; 84: 1100–1106.

15. Brecker SJ, Xiao HB, Sparrow J, *et al*. Effects of dual-chamber pacing with short atrioventricular delay in dilated cardiomyopathy. *Lancet* 1992; 340: 1308–1312.

16. Brinker JA, Weiss JL, Lappe DL, *et al*. Leftward septal displacement during right ventricular loading. *Circulation* 1980; 61:626–33.

17. Buda AJ, lotz RJ, Gallagher KP. Characterization of the functional border line around regionally ischemic myocardium using circumferential flow-function maps. *J Am Coli Cardiol* 1986; 8:150–158.

18. Catherwood E, Mintz GS, Kotler MN, *et al.* Two-dimensional echocardiographic recognition of left ventricular pseudoaneurysm. *Circulation* 1980; 62:294–303.

19. Chirillo F, Totis O, Cavarzerani A, *et al.* Transesophageal echocardiographic findings in partial and complete papillary muscle rupture complicating acute myocardial infarction. *Cardiology* 1992; 81: 54–58.

20. Come PC. Doppler detection of acquired ventricular septal defect. *Am J Cardiol* 1985;55:586–588.

21. D'Arcy B, Nanda NC. Two-dimensional echocardiographic features of right ventricular infarction. *Circulation* 1982; 65: 167–173.

22. Douglas PS, Fiolkoski J, Berko B, *et al.* Echocardiographic visualization of coronary artery anatomy in the adult. *J Am Coll Cardiol* 1988; 11:565–571.

23. Drobac M, Gilbert B, Howard R, Baigrie R, Rakowski H. Ventricular septal defect after myocardial infarction: Diagnosis by two dimensional contrast echocardiography. *Circulation* 1983;67:335–341.

24. Drobac M, Gilbert B, Howard R, *et al.* Ventricular septal defect after myocardial infarction: diagnosis by two dimensional contrast echocardiography. *Circulation* 1983;67: 335–341.

25. Duncan AM, Francis DP, Gibson DG, *et al.* Differentiation of ischemic from nonischemic cardiomyopathy during dobutamine stress by left ventricular long-axis function. Additional effect of left bundle-branch block. *Circulation* 2003; 108:1214–1220.

26. Duncan AM, Francis DP, Henein MY, *et al.,* limitation of cardiac output by total isovolumic time during pharmacologic stress in patients with dilated cardiomyopathy: activation mediated effects of left bundle branch block and coronary artery disease. *J Am Coll Cardiol* 2003;41:121–128.

27. Duncan AM, O'Sullivan C, Gibson DG, *et al.* The effect of dobutamine stress on left ventricular long axis and early diastolic filling in patients with coronary artery disease. *J Am Coll Cordiol* 2001; 37:433A.

28. Duncan AM, O'Sullivan CA. Carr-White GS. *et al.* Long axis electromechanics during dobutamine stress in patients with coronary artery disease and left ventricular dysfunction. *Heart* 2001; 86:397–404.

29. Engelsen DJ, Gorgels AP, Cheriex EC, *et al.* Value of the electrocardiogram in localising the occlusion site in the left anterior descending coronary artery in acute anterior myocardial infarction. *J Am Coll Cardiol* 1999;34:389–395.

30. Farrer-Brown G, Rowles PM. Vascular supply of interventricular septum of human heart. *Br Heart J* 1969;31:727–34.

31. Fdva T, Skuistad H, Aolchus S, *et al.* Regional myocardial systolic function during acute myocardial ischemia assessed by strain Doppler echocardiography. *J Am Coll Cardial* 2001; 37:726–30.

32. Feigenbaum H. *Echocardiography,* 3rd ed. Philadelphia: Lea and Febiger, 1981:454.

33. Feneley MP, GaYaghan TP, Baron DW, *et al.* Contribution of left ventricular contraction to the generation of right ventricular systolic pressure in the human heart. *Circulation* 1985;71:473–80.

34. Gibson D. Regional left ventricular wall moon. In:Raelandt JRTC, Sutherland GR, IIiceto S, *et al.* Cardiac ultrasound. Edinburgh: Churchill Livingstone, 1993:241–54.

35. Hashimoto I, Li X, Hejmadi Bhot A, *et al.,* Myocardial strain rate is a superior method for evaluation of left ventricular subendocardial function compared with tissue Doppler imaging. *J Am Coll Cordial* 2003;42:1574–83.

36. Hauser, A, Ghangadharan V, Ramos R, Gordon S, Timmis GC. Sequence of mechanical, electro-cardiographic and clinical effects of repeated coronary occlusion in human beings: echocardiographic observations during coronary balloon angioplasty. *J Am Coll Cardiol* 1985; 5: 193–197.

37. Heger JJ, Weyman AE, Wann LS, Dillion JG, Fiegenbaum H. Cross-sectional echo-cardiography in acute myocardial infarction: detection and localization of regional left ventricular asynergy. *Circulation* 1979;60:531–542.

38. Henein M. Lindqvist P, Francis D, *et al.* Tissue Doppleranalysis of age-dependency in diastolic ventricular behaviour and filling: a cross-sectional study of healthy hearts (the Vmea General Population Heart Study). *Eur Heart* 2002;23: 162–171.

39. Henein MY, Amadi A, O'Sullivan C, *et al.* ACE inhibitors unmask incoordinate diastolic wall motion in restrictive left ventricular disease. *Heart* 1996;76:326–331.

40. Henein MY, Gibson DG. Long axis function in disease. *Heart* 1999;81:229–231.

41. Henein MY, Gibson DG. Normal long axis function. *Heart* 1999;81:111–113.

42. Henein MY, Patel DJ, Fox KM, *et al.* Asynchronous left ventricular wall motion in unstable angina. *Intl Cardiol* 1997;59: 37–45.

43. Henein MY, Priestley K, Davarashvili T, *et al.* Early changes in left ventricular subendocardial function after successful coronary angioplasty. *Br Heart J* 1993;69:501–506.

44. Horowitz RS, Morganroth J, Parrotto C, *et al.* Immediate diagnosis of acute myocardial infareaction by two-dimensional echocardiography. *Circulation* 1982; 65:323–329.

45. Iliceto S, Marangelli V, Memmola C, *et al.* Transesophageal Doppler echocardiography evaluation of coronary blood flow velocity in baseline conditions and during dipyridamole induced coronary vasodilation. *Circulation* 1991;83:61–69.

46. Izumi S, Miyatake K, Beppu S, *et al.* Mechanism of mitral regurgitation in patients with myocardial infarction: a study using real-time two-dimensional Doppler flow imaging and echocardiography. *Circulation* 1987;76:777–785.

47. Jaarsma W, Visser CA, Kupper AJ, *et al.* Usefulness of two dimensional exercise echocardiography shortly after myocardial infarction. *Am J Cardiol* 1986;57:86–90.

48. Jordan RA, Miller RD, Edwards JE, *et al.* Thromboembolism in acute and healed myocardial infarction: Intracardiac mural thrombosis. *Circulation* 1952;6:1–6.

49. Kaul S, Force T. Assessment of myocardial perfusion with contrast two-dimensional echocardiography. In *Principles and Practice of Echocardiography,* 2nd Ed. Editor: Weyman AE. Lea and Febiger, 1993; 687–720.

50. Kaul S, Pandian NG, Gillam LD, *et al.* Contrast echocardiography in acute myocardial ischemia. III. An *in vivo* comparison of the extent of abnormal wall motion with the area at risk for necrosis. *J Am Coll Cardiol* 1986;7:383–392.

51. Kaul S, Stratienko AA, Pollock SG, Marieb MA, Keller MW, Sabia PJ. Value of two-dimensional echocardiography for determining the basis of haemodynamic compromise in critically ill patients: a prospective study. *J. Am Soc Echo* 1994;7:598–606.

52. Kaul S, Tei C, Hopkins JM, Shah PM. Assessment of right ventricular function using two-dimensional echocardiography. *Am Heart J* 1984; 107: 526–531.

53. Kaul S. Doppler echocardiography and Doppler in critically ill cardiac patients. In *Acute Cardiac care. Cardiology Clinics.* Editor: Shah PK. WB Saunders, 1991;711–732.

54. Keller MW, Glasheen W, Smucker ML, *et al.* Myocardial contrast echocardiography in humans. II. Assessment of coronary blood flow reserve. *J Am Coll Cardiol* 1988; 12:925–934.

55. Koenig K, Kasper W, Hofmann T, *et al.* Transesophageal echocardiography for diagnosis of rupture of the ventricular septum or left ventricular papillary muscle during acute myocardial infarction. *Am J Cardiol* 1987;59:362.

56. Koh TW, Carr-White GS, DeSouza AC, *et al.* Effect of coronary occlusion on left ventricular function with and without collateral supply during beating heart coronary artery surgery. *Heart* 1999;81:285–291.

57. Lower I. T radius de corde: ifem de motu and colore sanguinis, el chyli in eumtransitu. Amsterdam: apud Donielem Elzevirium, 1669.

58. Lunkenheimer PP, Redmon K, Florek J, *et al.* The forces generated with the musculature of the left ventricular wall. *Heart* 2004;90:200–7. *Circulation* 1991; 83:1605–1614.

59. Marwick TH, Nemec LL, Pashkow FJ, *et al.* Accuracy and limitations of exercise echocardiography in a routine clinical setting. *J Am Coll Cordiol* 1992;19:74–81.

60. Matsumoto M, Watanabe F, Goto A, *et al.* Left ventricular aneurysm and the prediction of left ventricular enlargement studied by two-dimensional echocardiography: quantitative assessment of aneurysm size in relation to clinical course. *Circulation* 1985;72:280–286.

61. Mclean M, Ross, MA, Prothera J. Three-dimensional reconstruction of the myober pattern in the fetal and neonatal mouse heart. *Anal Rec* 1989; 224:392–406.

62. Meza MF, Ramee S, Collins T, *et al.* Knowledge of perfusion and contractile reserve improves the predictive value of recovery of regional myocardial function post-revascularization: a study using the combination of myocardial contrast echocardiography and dobutamine echocardiography. *Circulation* 1997;96: 3459–3465.

63. Mintz GS, Victor MF, Kotler MN, Party WR, Segal BL. Two dimensional echocardiographic identification of surgically correctable complications of acute myocardial infarction. *Circulation* 1981;64:91–96.

64. Mishra MB, Lythall DA, Chambers JB. A comparison of wall motion analysis and systolic left ventricular long axis function during dobutamine stress echocardiography. *Eur Heart* 2002; 23:579–585.

65. Nissen SE, Gurley JC, Grines CL, *et al.* Intravascular ultrasound assessment of lumen size and wall morphology.

66. O'Sullivan CA, Henein MY, Sutton R, *et al.* Abnormal ventricular activation and repolarisation during dobutamine stress echocardiography in coronary artery disease. *Heart* 1998;79: 468–473.

67. Pasternack RC, Braunwald E, Sobel BE. Acute myocardial infarction. In: Braunwald E, ed. Heart disease. Philadelphia: WB Saunders, 1992:1255–1260.

68. Picano E, Parodi O, Lattanzi F. Comparison of dipyridamole echocardiography test and exercise thallium-201 for diagnosis of coronary artery disease. *Am J Noninvas Cardiol* 1989; 3: 85–92.

69. Picano E. Stress echocardiography. From pathophysiological toy to diagnostic tool. *Circulation* 1992; 85:1604–1612.

70. Pierard LA, De Landsheere CM, Berthe C, *et al.* Identification of viable myocardium by echocardiography during dobutamine infusion in patients with myocardial infarction after thrombolytic therapy: comparison with positron emission tomography. *J Am Coll Cardiol* 1990; 15:1021–1031.

71. Ramonathan KB, Wilson JL, Minis DM. Effects of coronary occlusion on transmural distribution of blood flow in the interventricular septum and left ventricular free wall. *Basic Res Cordiol* 1988; 83:229–37.

72. Rossvoll O, Hatle LK. Pulmonary venous flow velocities recorded by transthoracic Doppler ultrasound: relation to left ventricular diastolic pressures. *J Am Coll Cardiol* 1993;21: 1687–1696.

73. Rueda B, Panidis IP, Gonzales R, *et al.* Left ventricular pseudoaneurysm: detection and postoperative follow-up by color Doppler echocardiography. *Am Heart J* 1990; 120: 990–992.

74. Sabia P, Afrooketh A, Touchstone DA, Keller MW, Esquivel L, Kaul S. Value of regional wall motion abnormality in the emergency room diagnosis of acute myocardial infarction: a prospective study using two-dimensional echocardiography. *Circulation* 1991; 84 [suppl I]:I-85-I-9216.

75. Sakata Y, Kodama K, Adachi T, *et al.* Comparison of myocardial contrast echocardiography and coronary angiography for assessing the acute protective effects of collateral recruitment during occlusion of the left anterior descending coronary artery at the time of elective angioplasty. *Am Cordiol* 1997; 79: 1329–1333.

76. Salustri A, Fioretti PM, Pozzoli MMA, MC Niell AJ, Roelandt JRTC. Dobutamine stress echocardiography: its role in the diagnosis of coronary artery disease. *Eur Heart J* 1992;13: 70–77.

77. Sanchez-Quintona D, diment V, He SY, *et al.* Myoarchitecture and connective tissue in hearts with tricuspid atresia. *Heart* 1999;81: 182–91.

78. Sanlamore WP, Conslantinescu M, Minczak SM, *et al.* Contribution of each ventricular wall to ventricular interdependence. *Basic Res Cardial* 1988;83:424–30.

79. Sanlamore WP, lynch PR, Hackman JL, *et al.* Left ventricular effects on right ventricular developed pressure. *J Appl Physiol* 1976; 41:925–30.

80. Sawada SG, Ryan T, Conley MJ, *et al.* Prognostic value of a normal exercise echocardiogram. *Am Heart J* 1990;120: 49–55.

81. Sawada SG, Segar DS, Ryan T, Brown SE, Dohan AM, Williams R et al. Echo-cardiographic detection of coronary artery disease during dobutamine infusion.

82. Senior R, Labiri A. Role of dobutamine echocardiography in detection of myocardial viability for predicting outcome after revascularization in ischemic cardiomyopathy. *J Am Soc Echocardiogr* 2001; 14: 240–248.

83. Senior R. Role of contrast echocardiography for the assessment of left ventricular function. *Echocardiography* 1999; 16(7. Pt 2): 747–752.

84. Sklenar J, Villanueva FS, Glasheen WP, Ismail S, Goodman NC, Kaul S. Dobutamine echocardiography for determining the extent of myocardial salvage after reperfusion: an experimental evaluation. *Circulation* 1994; 90:1503–1512.

85. Slreeler DD, Spotnitz HM, Patel DP, *et al*. Fiber orientation in the conine left ventricle during diastole and systole. *Circ Res* 1969;24:339–47.

86. Smyllie JH, Sutherland GR, Geuskens R, *et al*. Doppler color flow mapping in the diagnosis of ventricular septal rupture and acute mitral regurgitation after myocardial infarction. *J Am Coll Cardiol* 1990;15:1449–1455.

87. Stoddard MF, Keedy DL, Kupersmith J. Transesophageal echocardiographic diagnosis of papillary muscle rupture complicating acute myocardial infarction. *Am Heart J* 1990;120: 690–692.

88. Torrent-Guasp F, Buckberg GD, Clemenle C, *et al*. The structure and June 60-01 the helical heart and its buttress wrapping: the normal microscopic structure of the heart. *Semin Thoroc Cordiovasc Surg* 200 1; 13:30 1–19.

89. U KS, Sanlamore WP. Contribution of each wall biventricular function. *Cardio Vas JC Res* 1993; 27:792–800.

90. Uematsu M, Miyatake K, Tanaka N, *et al*. Myocardial velocity gradient as a new indicator of regional left ventricular contraction: detection by a two dimensional tissue Doppler imaging technique. *J Am Coll Cardiol* 1995; 26:217–23.

91. Uemotsu M, Nakatoni S, Yamagishi M, *et al*. Usefulness of myocardial velocity gradient derived from two-dimensional tissue Doppler imaging as an indicator of regional myocardial contraction independent of translational motion assessed in atrial septal defect. *Am J Cordial* l997;79:237–41.

92. Urheim S, Edvardsen T, Torp H, *et al*. Myocardial strain by Doppler echocardiography: *valioo* on of a new method to quantify regional myocardial function. *Circulation* 2000;102:115–54.

93. VanDantzig JM, Delemarre BJ, Bot H, Koster RW, Visser CA. Doppler left ventricular flow pattern versus conventional predictors of left ventricular thrombus after acute myocardial infarction. *J Am Coll Cardiol* 1995; 25:1341–1346.

94. Vered Z, Katz M, Rath S, *et al*. Two-dimensional echocardiographic analysis of proximal left main coronary artery in humans. *Am Heart J* 1986; 112:972–976.

95. Visser CA, Kan G, David GK, *et al*. Echocardiographic cine angiographic correlation in detecting left ventricular aneurysm: a prospective study of 422 patients. *Am J Cardiol* 1982;50:337–341.

96. Visser CA, Kan G, Meltzer RS, Koolen JJ, Dunning AJ, Incidence, timing, and prognostic value of left ventricular aneurysm formation after myocardial infarction: A prospective, serial echocardiographic study in 158 patients. *AM J Cardiol* 1986; 57: 729–732.

97. Waller BF, Pinkerton CA, Slack JD. Intra-vascular ultrasound: a histological study of vessels during life. The new "gold standard" for vascular imaging. *Circulation* 1992;85: 2305–2310.

98. Weiss JL, Bulkley BH, Hutchins GM, Mason SJ. Two-dimensional echocardiographic recognition of myocardial injury in man: comparison with post-mortem studies. *Circulation* 1981;63:401–408.

99. Wienreich DJ, Burke JF, Pauletto FJ. Left Ventricular mural thrombi complicating acute myocardial infarction: long term follow-up with serial echocardiography. *Ann Intern Med* 1984; 100: 789–794.

100. Yamagishi M, Miyatake K, Beppu S, *et al*. Assessment of coronary bloodflow by transesophageal two-dimensional pulsed Doppler echocardiography. *Am J Cardiol* 1988;62: 641–644.

101. Yock PG, Fitzgerald PJ, Linker DT, *et al*. Intravascular ultrasound guidance for catheter-based coronary interventions. *J Am Coli Cardiol* 1991; 17 (6 Suppl B):39B–45B.

102. Yoshida K, Yoshikawa J, Hozumi T, *et al*. Detection of left main coronary artery stenosis by transesophageal color Doppler and two-dimensional echocardiography. *Circulation* 1990;81:1271–1276.

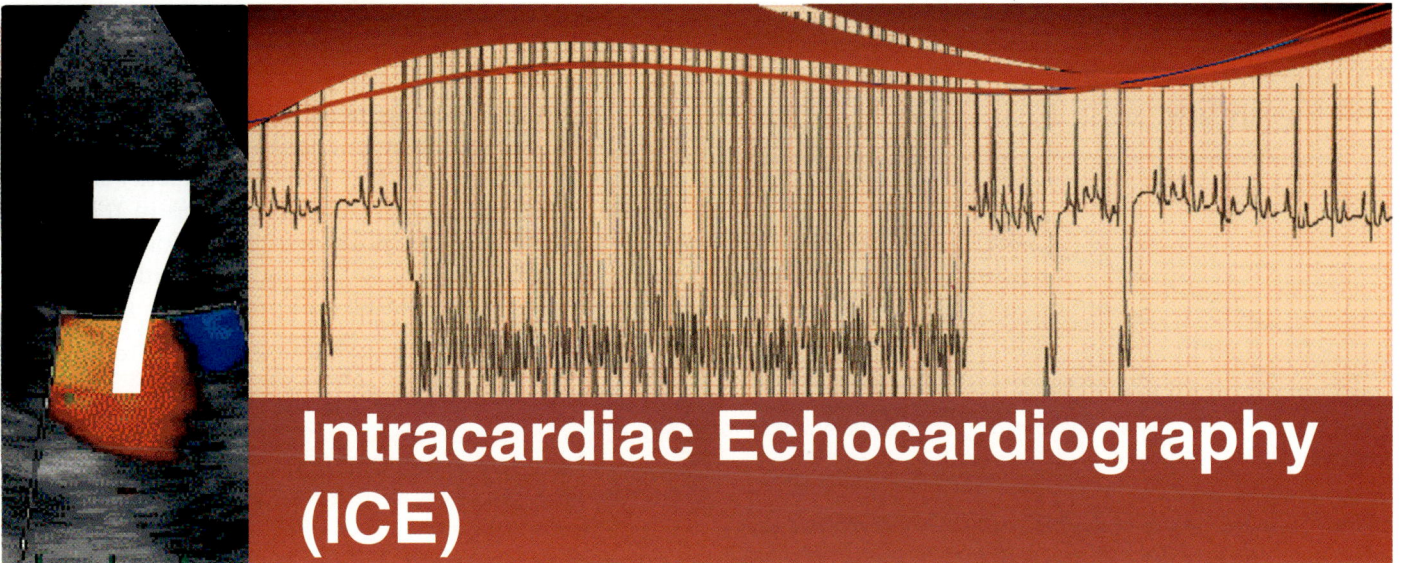

7

Intracardiac Echocardiography (ICE)

Intracardiac echocardiography (ICE) is an imaging technique that is becoming increasingly available as an alternative to transoesophageal echocardiography to guide percutaneous interventional procedures. The probe can be inserted under local anaesthesia and is principally used during closure of atrial septal abnormalities.

Advantages of ICE over Transoesophageal Echocardiography

These include: (Table 7.1)

1. **Elimination of the need for general anaesthesia.**
2. **Clearer imaging.**
3. **Shorter procedure times.**
4. **Reduced radiation dose to the patient.**

Intracardiac echocardiography (ICE) is one of the latest developments in the ever expanding field of cardiac ultrasound and this chapter will try to highlight some of the current applications of ICE and its technique of intracavitary imaging of the heart. Transvenous echocardiography has been described for over 20 years. The initial limitations of poor tissue penetration and difficult manupulation with mechanical intracardiac catheters have been overcome with the development of low frequency transducers and multi-directional steerable devices. The AcuNavTM (Siemens Medical) ICE catheter is a medium calibre (8°F or 10°F), multi-frequency (5–10 MHz), 54-element linear phased array, ultrasound catheter capable of pulsed and colour Doppler imaging. The catheter, provides a 90° sector scan, has tissue penetration of up to 1.0 cm and has four-way head articulation to allow multiple angle imaging. There is a steering lock to maintain angulation of the catheter. The devices are single use only.

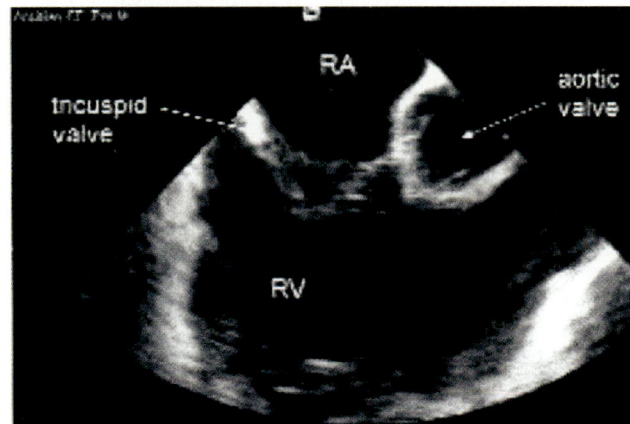

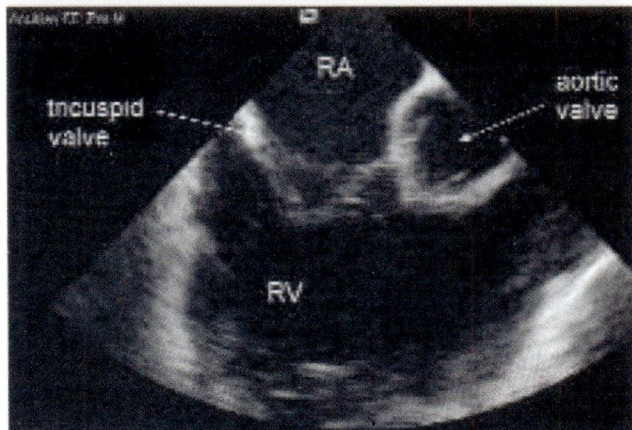

Fig. 7.1: The intracardiac echocardiography (ICE) catheter advanced to the mid right atrium (RA). This provides views of the tricuspid and aortic valves

Visualisation of the Interatrial Septum

ICE is perfectly suited to the visualisation of right heart structures and provides real time imaging of cardiovascular anatomy. The current principal use of the ICE

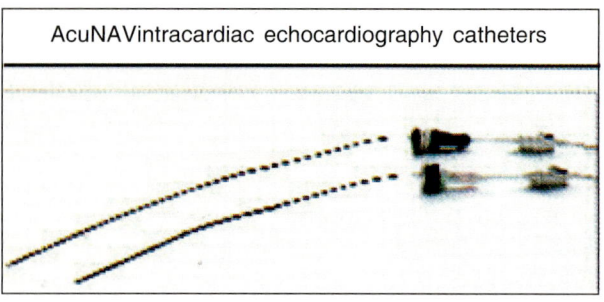

AcuNAVintracardiac echocardiography catheters

Fig. 7.2: AcuNAVintracardiac echocardiography catheters used for obtaining intracardiac views

Table 7.1: *Advantages and disadvantages of intracardiac echocardiography (ICE) compared with transoesophageal echocardiography (TOE) for guiding interventional procedure*

Advantages of ICE	*Disadvantages of ICE*
• Superior imaging safer procedure	• Single-use catheter
• Local anaesthetic no risk from general anaesthetic	• Additional venous puncture
• Less personnel required (no anaesthetist—assistant or echocardiographer) reduced costs	• Initial learning curve
• No risks and discomfort from TOE	
• Less radiation to the patient	
• Shorter procedures	
• Faster turnaround of cases with improved efficiency	
• Quicker patient recovery	
• Day case procedure—cost saving	

catheter is to provide images of the interatrial septum during percutaneous closure of patent foramen ovales (PFOs) and atrial septal defects (ASDs). The catheter is gently advanced to the mid-right atrium from the inferior vena cava and rotated to provide the 'standard view'. In this view the tricuspid valve can be seen directly in front of the transducer. By gently retroflexing the catheter tip and slowly rotating clock-wise, the atrial septum appears directly in front of the catheter tip. Outstanding images of the interatrial septum can then be obtained. This position is then usually extremely stable, so only minute movements of the catheter are required for image optimisation during device development (Figs 7.1 and 7.2).

Closure of Patent Foramen Ovale

A patent foramen ovale (PFO) is an oblique slit-like tunnel formed through lack of fusion of the atrial septum primum and septum secundum and can occur with other abnormalities of the atrial septum including atrial septal aneurysms. Autopsy studies indicate that a PFO is present in approximately one quarter of the population

with significant heterogeneity in the width and size of the defect. There has been considerable interest in the role of a PFO in young patients with stroke or migraine and subsequently an explosion in the use of devices to close PFOs by keen interventional cardiologists. In approximately 40% of patients with ischaemic stroke the cause remains unknown but in younger patients (less than 55 years), the prevalence of PFO is high (50%). Randomised comparisons of medical therapy (with anti-thrombotic therapy) versus percutaneous PFO closure are underway. Similarly, retrospective studies have suggested that percutaneous closure PFOs in migraine sufferers with cryptogenic stroke relieves migraine symptoms in over 50% of patients. A large prospective randomised study has now confirmed that PFO closure may reduce headache burden in some patients with migraine.

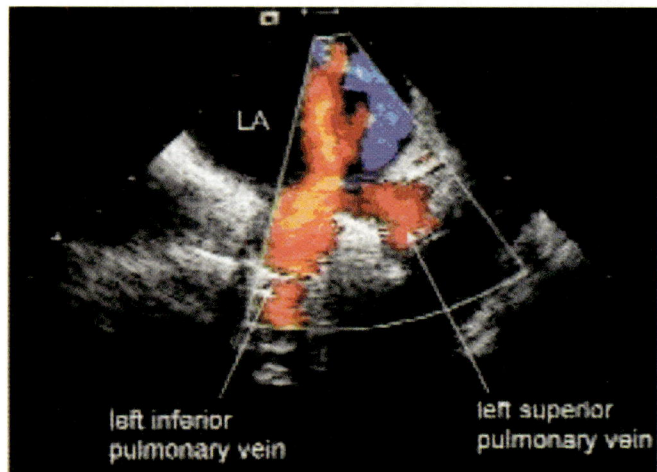

Fig. 7.3: ICE view showing colour-flow echocardiogram of the left-sided pulmonary veins

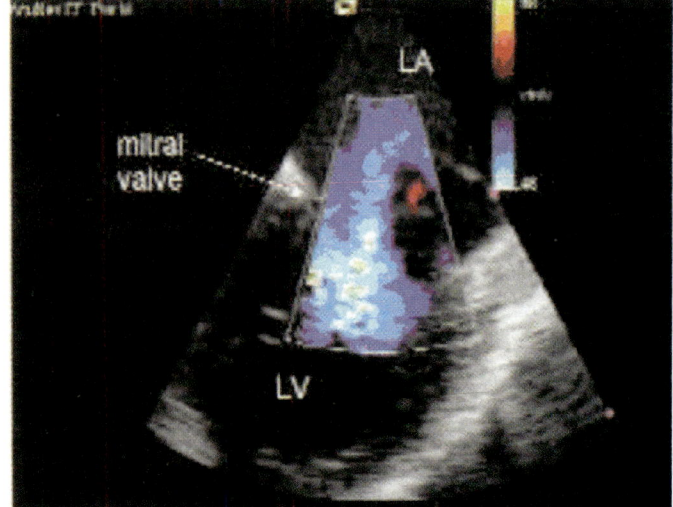

Fig. 7.4: ICE view showing colour-flow echocardiogram of the mitral valve

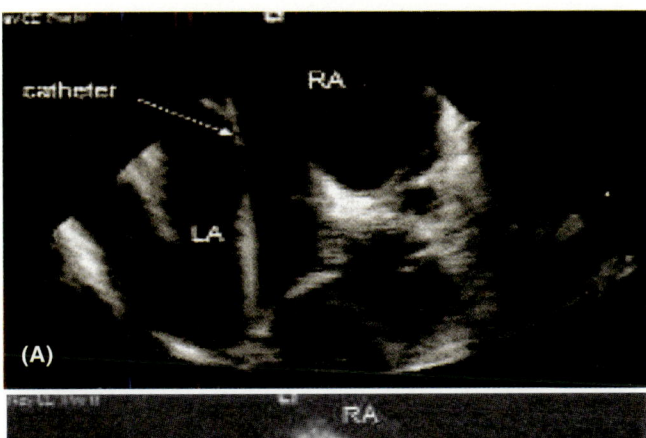

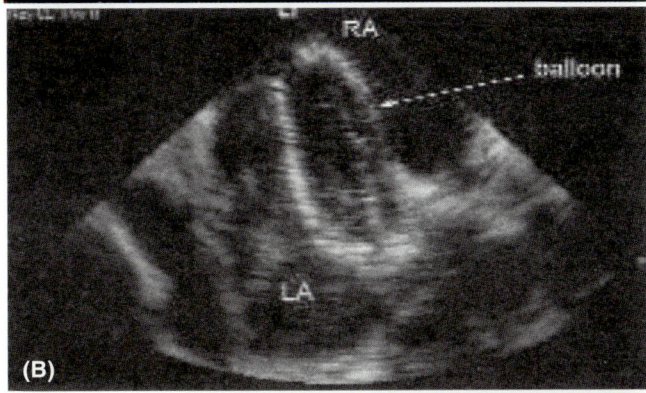

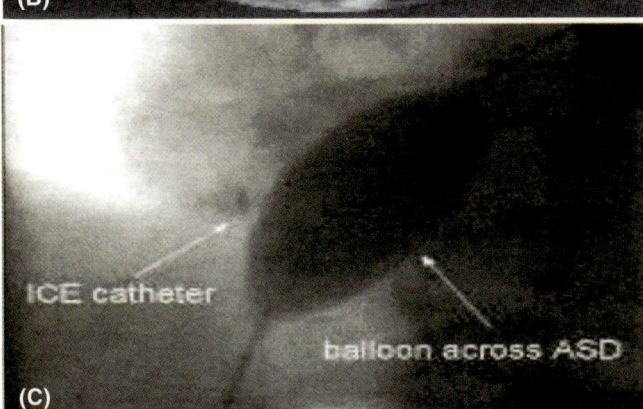

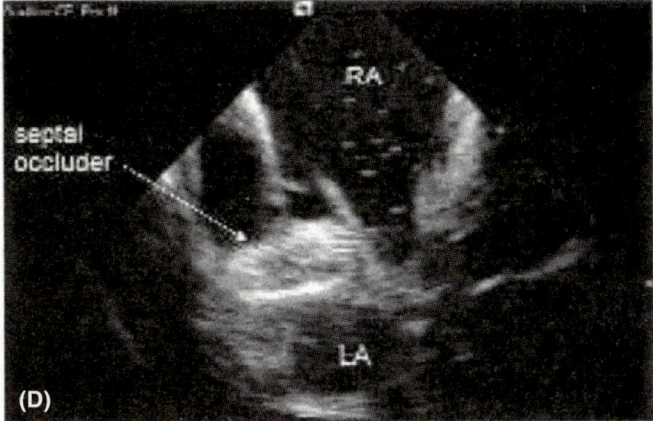

Fig. 7.5: IC Echocardiograms showing **(A)** Catheter through the atrial septal defect (ASD) into the left atrium; LA. **(B)** and **(C)** The view from the right atrium (RA) showing balloon sizing of the ASD. **(D)** Deployment of an atrial septal occluder showing expansion of the LA disc. This was followed by expansion of the RA disc and a good stable position was finally achieved across the ASD

Devices to close PFOs are becoming simpler and quicker to use and the complication rate from these procedures (Fig. 7.5) is falling. The numbers of referrals for closure are already increasing and if the results of studies support PFO closure, then ICE seems perfectly poised for a local anaesthetic approach. Total catheter laboratory procedure and turnaround times are usually less than 30 minutes and the low procedural risk allows PFO closure to be performed as a routine procedure.

Electrophysiological Studies

Internentional electrophysiology has traditionally been performed using fluoroscopic landmarks and electrical mapping catheters. Successful ablation required good delineation of anatomical structures combined with good lesion formation. ICE permits confirmation of stable, complete catheter-tissue contact ensuring more complete electrical isolation and reducing the incidence of catheter clot formation. To prevent tissue overheating (and therefore scar formation, thrombosis or stenosis), operators can deliver ablation until the onset of micro-bubble formation, ensuring maximal safe delivery of therapy. During left atrial ablation for atrial fibrillation, accurate positioning of the catheters is required and ICE is perfectly suited to guide the operator. Additionally, ICE can identify thrombus in the left atrium or left atrial appendage and complications occurring within the pulmonary veins. Use of ICE during ablation of AF to confirm both catheter placement and ablation delivery has been shown to be more successful and with fewer embolic complications than in those cases performed without ICE. One important component of modern ablation techniques is the ability to perform a trans-septal puncture to access the left atrium. Even in the most skilled hands this can be difficult; complications include cardiac tamponade and aortic perforation. ICE provides extremely clear views of the interatrial septum to guide the interventionalist and confirm needle positioning.

Wider Clinical Applications of ICE

There has been work examining the role of ICE to guide closure of perimembraneous ventricular septal defects. Similarly, balloon mitral commisurotomy for mitral stenosis can be performed using ICE guidance as reasonable views can be obtained from the mitral valve. In patients with pacemaker lead endocarditis, vegetations can be difficult to visualise with either transthoracic echocardiography or with TOE. ICE can have an important diagnostic role in suspected lead endocarditis, since identifying the size and location of vegetations may determine if lead extraction is indicated whether by a surgical or percutaneous approach. The small size and versatile nature of the ICE probe has led to its use in a wide variety of interesting imaging roles including guiding left ventricular pacing, atrial septal pacing, imaging the aorta using a transnasal approach, evaluation of cardiac function following cardiac surgery via a modified mediastinal chest drain, fetal TOE guiding septal ablation of hypertrophic cardiomyopathy, diagnosing arrhythmogenic right ventricular cardiomyopathy and guiding the biopsy of cardiac masses.

Traditionally, percutaneous ASD and PFO closures are performed under TOE guidance using general anesthesia. There are clear imaging benefits from visualising the atrial septum from within the heart particularly the visualisation of the inferior rim of the septum. More importantly, as the ICE probe can be inserted percutaneously, only local anaesthetic is required, sparing the patient the risks and costs of general anesthesia. Using a local anaesthetic approach and with the additional imaging quality, atrial septal closure under ICE guidance is performed with lower radiation doses, with shorter procedure times and with faster turnaround than with TOE. There is no reported increase in vascular complications from the additional venous puncture. With smaller 8F catheters being released, this concern should reduced further. Transient atrial arrhythmias have been reported from manipulation of the ICE catheter in the right atrium (Figs 7.3 and 7.4).

Future Concerns

At present the roles of ICE are to provide imaging for PFO and ASD closure and to guide electrophysiological procedures. Benefits compared with TOE include excellent image quality with shorter procedure times reduced radiation exposure and principal uses are to support the percutaneous closure of atrial septal defects/patent foramen ovale and to guide electrophysiological procedures.

Advantages of ICE over transoesophageal echocardiography include the elimination of the need for general anaesthesia, clearer images, shorter procedure times and reduced radiation doses.

The principal disadvantage of ICE is the cost of the catheter. If the PFO trials support device closure, then ICE may prove to be the perfect and cost effective.

Bibliography

1. Alboliras ET, Htiazi ZM. Comparison of costs of intracardiac echocardiography and transesophageal echocardiography in monitoring percutaneous device closure of atrial septal defect in children and adults. *Am J Cardial* 2004; 94:690–2.
2. Bartel T, Konorza T, Neudorf U, *et al.* Intracardiac echocardiography: an ideal guiding tool for device closure of interatrial communications. *Eur J Echocardiogr* 2005; 6:92–96.
3. Boccalandro F, Baptista E, Muench A, Carter C, Smalling RW. Comparison of intracardiac echocardiography versus transesophageal echocardiography guidance for percutaneous transcatheter closure of atrial septal defect. *Am J Cardia* 2004; 93:437–40.
4. Bruce CJ, O'Leary P, Hagler OJ, Seward JB, Cabalka AK. Miniaturized transoesophageal echocardiography in newborn infants. *J Am Echocardiogr* 2002; 15:791–7.
5. Cao OL, Zabal C, Koenig P, Sandhu S, Htiazi ZN. Initial clinical experience with intracardiac echocardiography in guiding transcatheter closure of perimembranous ventricular septal defects: feasibility and comparison with transesophageal echocardiography. *Catheter Cardiovasc Interv* 2005; 66:258–67.
6. Chambers JB, Taylor PR, Reidy JF, Woods C, Carter SJ, Padayachee TS. Transoesophageal ultrasonography: A new approach to imaging the thoracic aorta. *Heart* 2005; 91:245–6.
7. Dalal A, Asirvatham SJ, Chandrasekaran K, Seward JB, Tajik AJ. Intracardiac echocardiography in the detection of pacemaker lead endocarditis. *J Am Sac Echocardiogr* 2002; 15:1027–28.
8. Earning MG, Cabalka AK, Seward JB, Bruce CJ, Reeder GS, Hagler DJ. Intracardiac echocardiographic guidance during transcatheter device closure of atrial septal defect and patent foramen ovale. *Mayo Clin Proc* 2004; 79: 24–34.
9. Glassman E. Kronzon L. Transvenous intracardiac echocardiography. *Am J Cardiol* 1981; 47:1255–9.
10. Hara H. Virmani R, Ladich E, *et al.* Patient foramen ovale; current pathology, pathophysiology, and clinical status. *J Am Coli Cardiol* 2005; 46:1768–76.
11. Homma S, Sacco RL. Patent foramen ovale and stroke. *Circulation* 2005; 112:1063–72.
12. Hynes BJ, Mart C, Artman S, Pu M, Naccarelli GV. Role of intracardiac ultrasound in interventional electrophysiology. *Curr Opin Cardio* 2004; 19:52–57.
13. Jongbloded MR, Bax JJ, de Groot NM, *et al.* Radio-frequency catheter ablation of paroxysmal atrial fibrillation; guidance by intracardiac echocardiography and integration with other imaging techniques. *Eur J Echocardiogr* 2003; 4:54–58.
14. Koenig P, Cao OL. Echocardiographic guidance of transcatheter closure of atrial septal defects Is intracardiac echocardiography better than transesophageal echocardiography? *Pediatr Cardia* 2005; 26; 135–9.
15. Koenig P. Cao OL. Heitschmidt M, Waight DJ, Htiazi ZN. Role of intra-cardiac echocardiographic guidance in transcatheter closure of atrial septal defects and patent foramen ovale using the Amplatzer device. *J Inter Cardio.* 2003; 16:51–62.
16. Marrouche NF, Martin DO, Wazni O, *et al.* Phased-array intracardiac echocardiography monitoring during pulmonary vein isolation in patients with atrial fibrillation: impact on outcome and complications. *Circulation* 2003; 107:2710–16.
17. Mullen MJ, Dias BF, Walker F, Siu SC, Benson LN, McLaughling PR. Intracardiac echocardiography guided device closure of atrial septal defects. *J Am Coli Cardiol* 2003; 41:285–92.

18. Oishi Y, Okamoto M, Sueda T *et al.* Cardiac tumor biopsy under the guidance of intracardiac echocardiography. *Jpn Cric J* 2000; 64:638–40.

19. Pedone C, Vtiayakumar M, Ligthart JM, *et al.* Intracardiac echocardiography guidance during percutaneous transluminal septal muocardial ablation in patients with obstructive hypertrophic cardiomyopathy. *Int J Cardiovasc Intervent* 2005; 7:134–7.

20. Pters S, Brattstrom A, Gotting B, Trummel M. Value of intracardiac ultrasound in the diagnosis of arrhythmogenic right ventricular dysplasia-cardiomyopathy. *Int J Cardiol* 2002; 83:111–17.

21. Salem MI, Makaryus AN, Kort S, *et al.* Intracardiac echocardiography using the ACuNav ultrasound catheter during percutaneous balloon mitral valvuloplasty. *J Am Soc Echocardiogr* 2002; 15:1533–37.

22. Segar OS, Bourdillon PO, Elsner G, Kesler KI, Feigenbaum H. Intracardiac echocardiography–Guided biopsy of intracardiac masses. *J Am Soc Echocardiogr* 1995; 8:927–9.

23. Shalaby AA. Utilization of intracardiac echocardiography to access the coronary sinus for left ventricular lead placement. *Pacing Clin Electrophysio* 2005; 28:493–7.

24. Shalganov TN, Paprika D, Borbas S, Temesvari A, Szili-Torok T. Preventing complicated transseptal puncture with intracardiac echocardiography: case report. *Cardiovasc Ultrasound* 2005; 3:5.

25. Szili, Torok T, Jordaens J, Bruining N, Ligthart J, Roelandt JR. Dynamic three-dimensional echocardiography offers advantages for specific site pacing. *Circulation* 2003; 107:e30.

26. Tsimikas S. Transcatheter closure of patent foramen ovale for migrain eprophylaxis: hope or hype? *J Am Coli Cadio* 2005; 45:496–98.

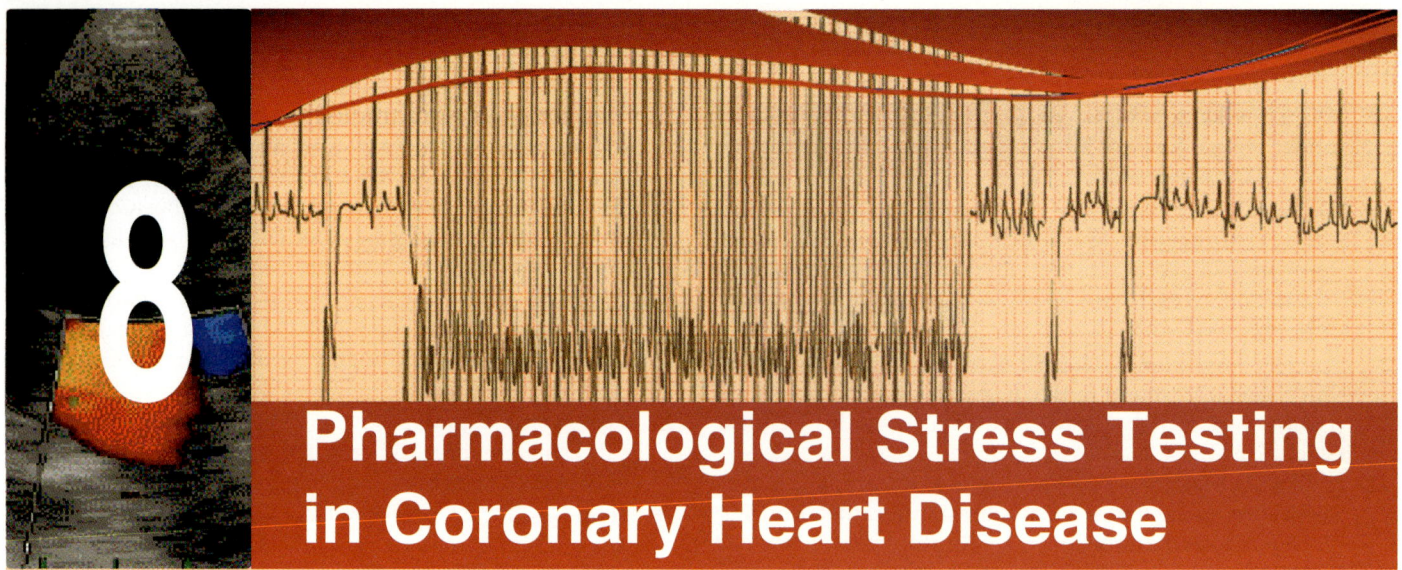

8

Pharmacological Stress Testing in Coronary Heart Disease

Pharmacological stress testing for evaluating suspected or proven coronary artery disease has been widely established particularly in those patients who are unable to perform exercise stress test. Two tests which stand the best among the few screened are dipyridamole-thallium and dobutamine echocardiography stress testing. Each one of them induces a pharmacological cardiac stress which is studied through an imaging technique (Fig. 8.2A and B).

Exercise and pharmacological stress echocardiography have been recently considered important clinical tools in the noninvasive diagnosis of coronary artery disease (CAD). Transient wall motion abnormalities usually indicate an earlier and more sensitive marker of myocardial ischemia than chest pain or ST-segment alterations. Comparing exercise echocardiography, pharmacological stress echocardiography is rated superior as it has the advantage of a better quality of images and can be applied in patients who cannot exercise properly. It has been observed that both dobutamine and dipyridamole echocardiography stress tests have shown a high specificity and sensitivity for the diagnosis of coronary artery disease (Table 8.1).

Physiologic Mechanism of Induction of Ischemia
Dipyridamole

It has been shown that intravenous infusions of dipyridamole inhibits the cellular uptake and block the transmembrane transport of endogenously produced adenosine. It also reduces the deactivation of adenosine by inhibiting the enzyme adenosine deaminase. Collectively, these effects raise serum adenosine levels approximately two fold within 30 minutes of administration. Adenosine is a powerful coronary vasodilator. After dipyridamole administration a drop in coronary

Table 8.1: *The patients in whom echocardiography is done for diagnosis and prognosis of chronic ischemic heart disease*

Indication	Class
1. Diagnosis of myocardial ischemia in symptomatic individuals	I
2. Assessment of global ventricular function at rest	I
3. Assessment of myocardial viability hibernating myocardium for planning revascularization	I
4. Assessment of functional significance of coronary lesions, (if not already known) in planning percutaneous transluminal coronary angioplasty	I
5. Diagnosis of myocardial ischemia in selected patients with an intermediate or high pretest likelihood of coronary artery disease	IIb
6. Assessment of an asymptomatic patient with positive results from a screening treadmill test	IIb
7. Assessment of global ventricular function with exercise	IIb
8. Screening of asymptomatic persons with a low likelihood of coronary artery disease	III
9. Routine periodic reassessment of stable patients for whom no change in therapy is contemplated	III
10. Routine substitution for treadmill exercise testing in patients for whom electrocardiographic analysis is expected to suffice	III

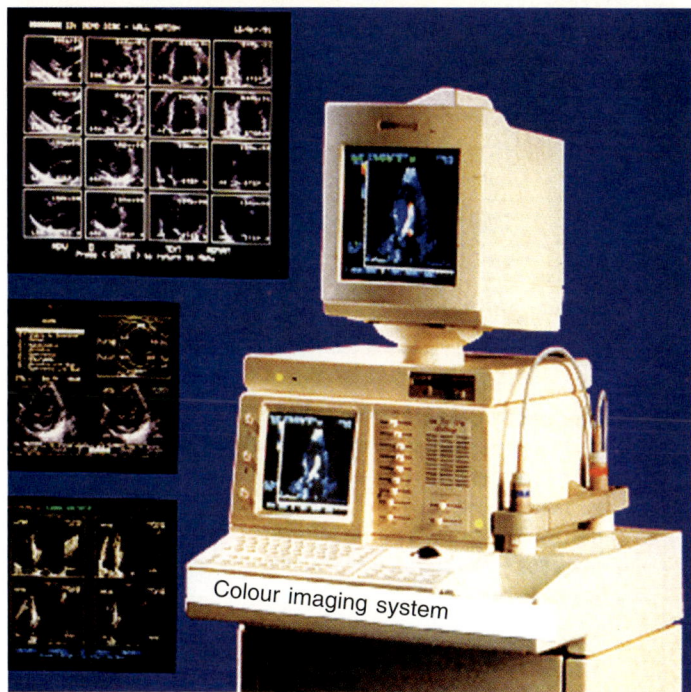

Fig. 8.1: Colour imaging system used for obtaining pharmacological stress test

dipyridamole. Dipyridamole thus creates differences in bloodflow between normal and abnormal coronary artery regions that can be visualised with thallium imaging techniques. Stenosis of 30% to 45% impair only the maximal response to vasodilation, whereas stenosis of 85% impede resting flow as well. Stenosis of 50% result in detectable differences of regional flow by thallium perfusion imaging techniques. If severe coronary artery lesion present, dipyridamole may result in a steal of flow from the subendocardium to the subepicardium and cause ischemia (Fig. 8.4A and B).

Table 8.3: *Wall motion abnormalities score in coronary disease in stress echocardiography*

Change	Standard score	Optional scores
	0	Hyperdynamic
Normal	1	
	1.5	Mildly hypokinetic
Hypokinetic	2	
	2.5	Severely hypokinetic
Akinetic	3	
Dyskinetic	4	
Aneurysm	5	
	6	Akinetic with scar
	7	Dyskinetic with scar

Dobutamine (Table 8.3)

It being a synthetic sympathomimetic amine increases myocardial contractility through stimulation of cardiac B_1 receptors within the myocardium or by indirectly releasing norepinephrine stores. Dobutamine is a synthetic amine based on the structure of isoproterenol and stimulates cardiovascular B_1, B_2 and adrenergic receptors. Dobutamine increases myocardial contractility by directly stimulating cardiac B_1-receptors, resulting in decrease in peripheral vascular resistance. Dobutamine is relatively selective for B_1-receptors; the increase in cardiac contractility that is the primary effect of continuous infusion; causes an increase in stroke volume and cardiac output with a decline in ventricular diastolic pressure and little change in systemic blood pressure at low doses. At doses 20 ug/kg/min., heart rate can increase and peripheral vascular resistance may fall. Dobutamine

Table 8.2: *Wall motion responses during resting period and at stress*

Rest	Stress	Interpretation
Normal	Hypokinetic	Normal
Normal	Hypokinetic/akinetic	Ischemic
Akinetic	Akinetic	Infarction
Hypokinetic	Akinetic/dyskinetic	Ischemic and/or infarction
Hypokinetic/akinetic	Normal	Viable

vascular resistance occurs, resulting in a four fold to five fold increase in coronary artery flow as compared with a potential threefold to fourfold increase during exercise. Dipyridamole undergoes hepatic conversion to a monoglucuronide complex and is excreted in the bile. Its half-life is about 10 hours. Dipyridamole is lipophilic and basic and can be suspended in acidic aqueous solutions. It is generally infused into large arm veins after being diluted several times in normal saline solution or dextrose in water.

Dipyridamole causes equivalent increases in coronary bloodflow in subepicardial and subendocardial regions of normal vessels. Significant coronary artery stenosis blunt this increase in bloodflow. Also, subendocardial vessels beyond severe stenosis may be maximally dilated at rest, precluding a further increase in flow after

Table 8.4: *Emergency drugs required in echo laboratory*

Atropine injection	Tab. Nifedipine
Epinephrine injection	Tab. Verapamil
Dopamine injection	Tab. Captopril
Dobutamine injection	Tab. Nitroglycerine
Adenosine injection	Inj. Lidocaine
Nitroglycerine injection	
Short-acting β-blocker	(e.g. Esmolol)
Inj. Furosemide	
Inj. Theophylline Inj. Sodium bicarbonate	

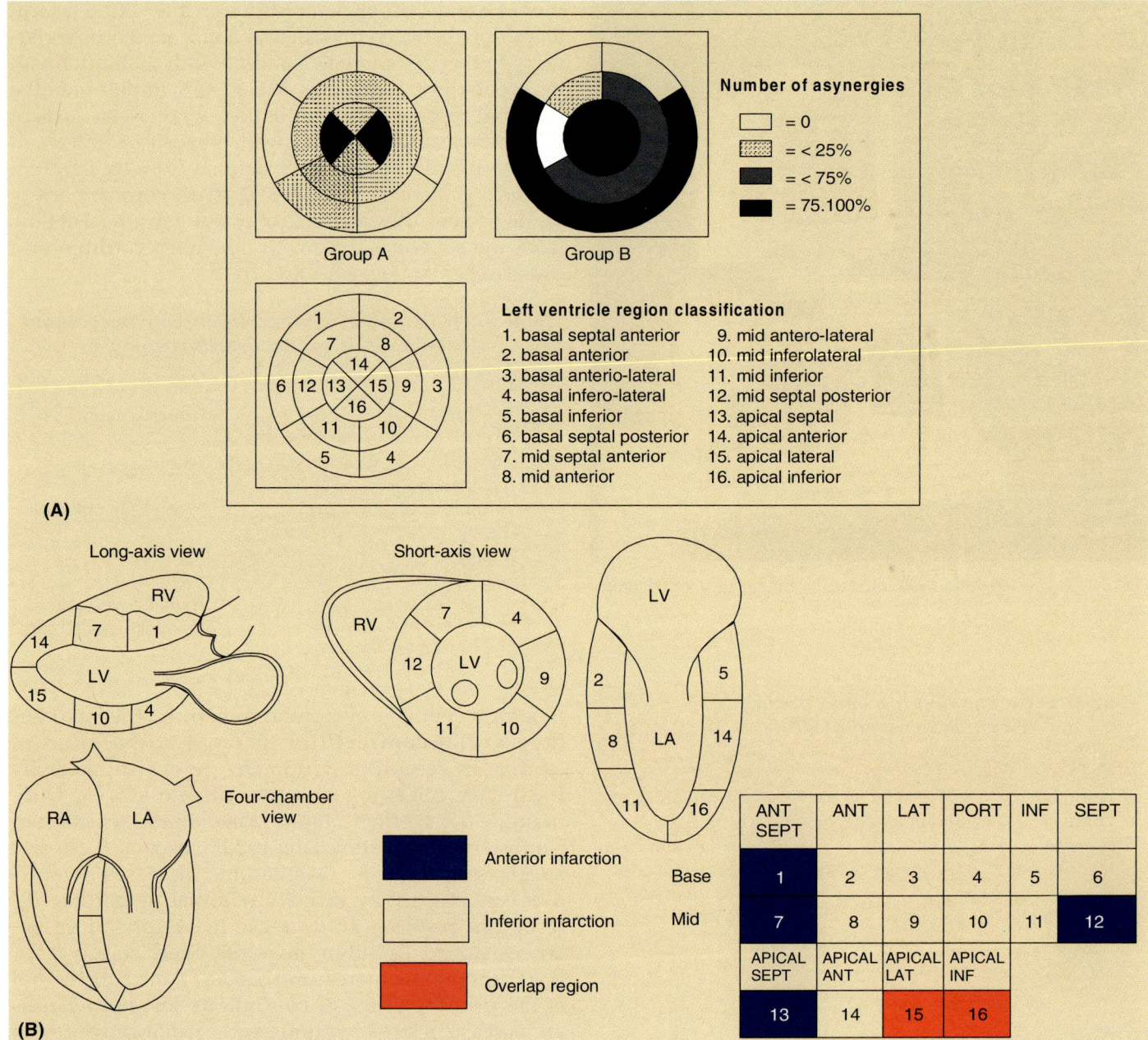

Number of asynergies
- ☐ = 0
- ▦ = < 25%
- ▨ = < 75%
- ■ = 75.100%

Left ventricle region classification

1. basal septal anterior
2. basal anterior
3. basal anterio-lateral
4. basal infero-lateral
5. basal inferior
6. basal septal posterior
7. mid septal anterior
8. mid anterior

9. mid antero-lateral
10. mid inferolateral
11. mid inferior
12. mid septal posterior
13. apical septal
14. apical anterior
15. apical lateral
16. apical inferior

	ANT SEPT	ANT	LAT	PORT	INF	SEPT
Base	1	2	3	4	5	6
Mid	7	8	9	10	11	12
	APICAL SEPT	APICAL ANT	APICAL LAT	APICAL INF		
	13	14	15	16		

■ Anterior infarction
☐ Inferior infarction
■ Overlap region

Fig. 8.2A and B: (A) Diagrammatic representation of sixteen (16) LV regions as compared to recently revised seventeen (17) to be studied in performing wall motion abnormalities on stress test for categoring the severity of coronary heart disease. **(B)** Color coding method in various types of infarctions noted down on different regions of LV taken in different echo windows as shown on colour diagram in the assessment of severity of coronary heart disease

also increases automaticity of the sinus node and augments conduction through the atrioventricular node. At high doses, these may result in acceleration of the ventricular rate during atrial fibrillation or the induction of ventricular arrhythmias. Dobutamine is metabolized in the liver to glucuronide conjugates and 3-0 methylodobutamine and excreted in the urine and faces. Its half-life is only 2 minutes, thus continuous infusions are necessary for sustained effects. Dobutamine has the potential to create ischemia in patients with coronary artery dis-

ease. By increasing contractility (heart rate at higher doses), dobutamine creates a condition of increased oxygen demand. When this conditions occurs in the presence of an impaired oxygen supply, echocardiography can directly visualise myocardial wall motion abnormalities in subjects with fixed coronary stenosis.

Arbutamine Stress Echocardiography

Arbutamine is a recently developed synthetic catecholamine closely related to dobutamine. It has been specifi-

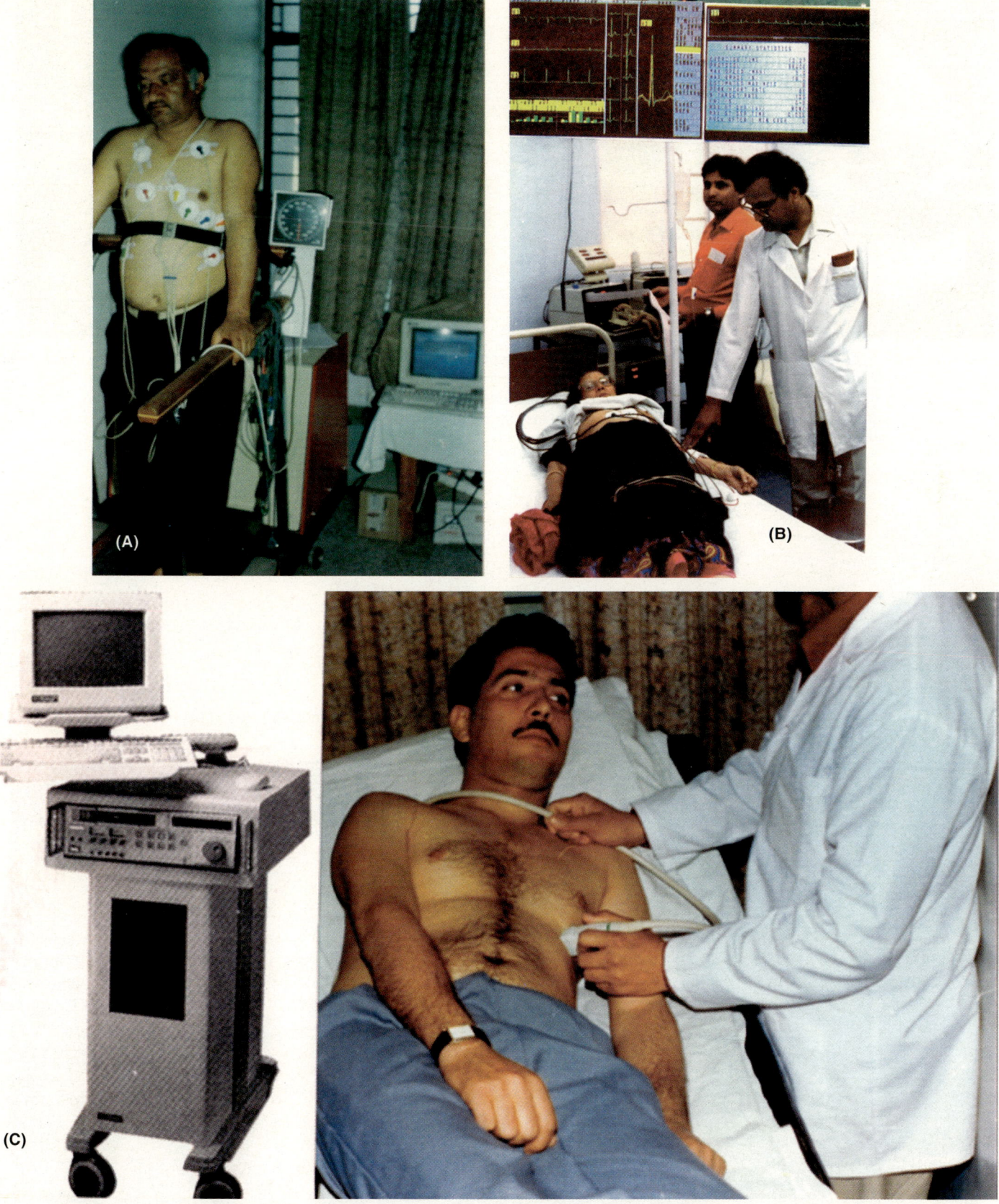

Fig. 8.3A to C: **(A)** Stress test laboratory where patient is being prepared for treadmill test with simultaneous echocardiography. **(B)** Stress test laboratory of Govt. Meidcal College, Jammu where patient under the guidance of author (Dr K C Verma) is being administered I/V Dobutamine. **(C)** Stress Echo. Lab. where volunteer is being examined by a doctor before performing stress echocardiography

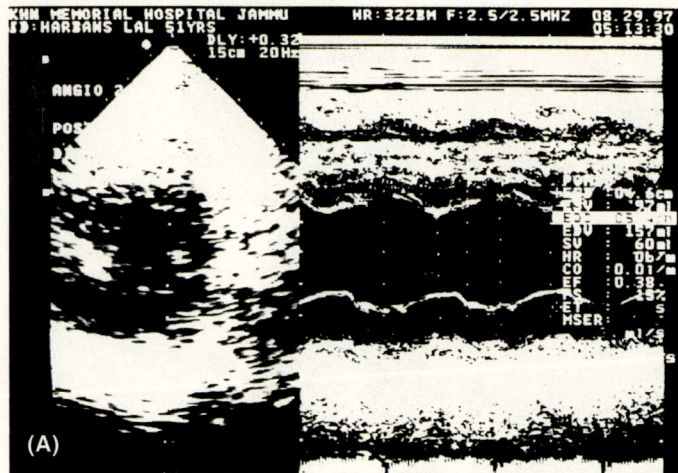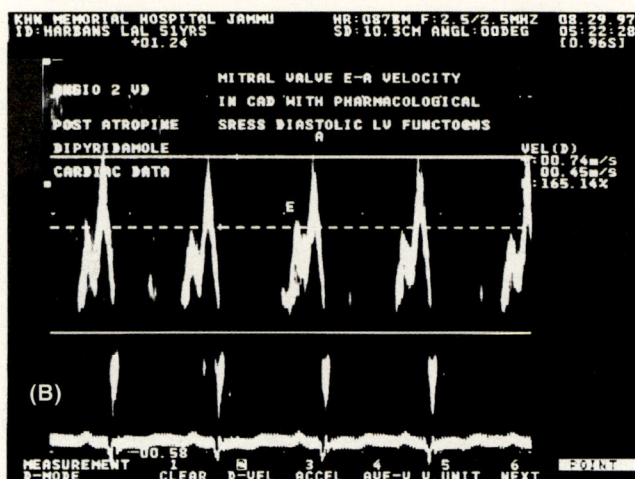

Fig. 8.4A and B: (A) M-Mode echocardiography showing marked hypokinesia of interventricular septum and posterior left ventricular wall in patient with coronary artery disease with very low LV ejection fraction(38%). **(B)** Mitral E and A velocities showing reverse pattern of A >E as seen in defect in diastolic relaxation of LV after oral administration of Dipyridamole and injectable atropine in performing pharamacological stress test in the same patient as described in A for detection of coronary disease and long term prediction of prognosis. His angiogram later revealed two vessel disease

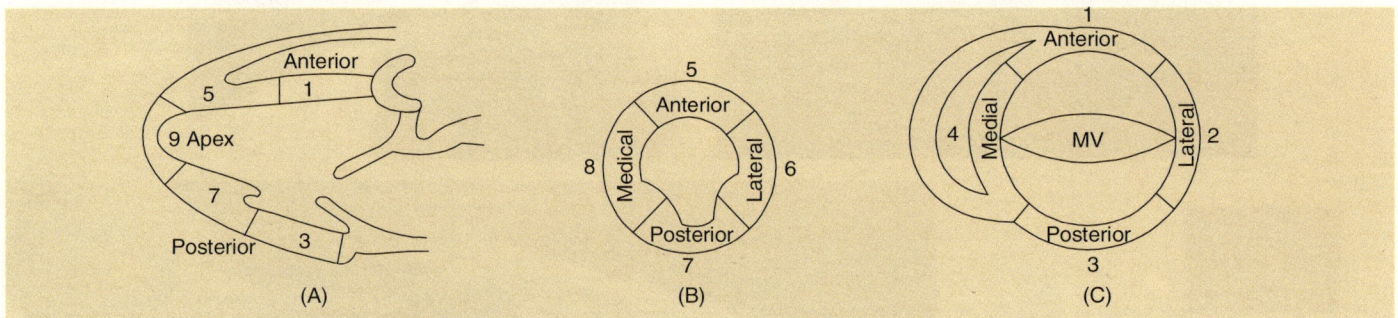

Fig. 8.5A to C: (A) LV long axis view. **(B)** Short axis LV wall. **(C)** LV Short axis at MV

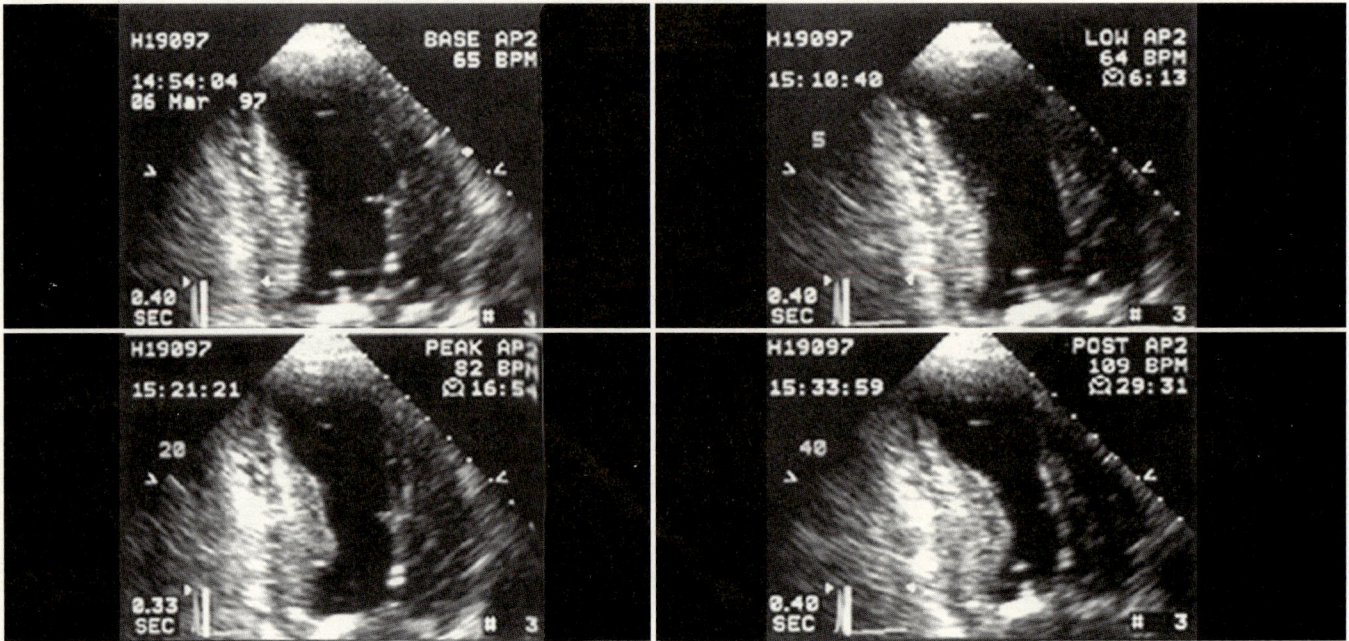

Fig. 8.6: Apical views from a patient with exertional angina at rest (top-left) and peak dobutamine stress (bottom-right). Note the significant development of akinesia of the apex with stress consistent with left anterior descending artery disease

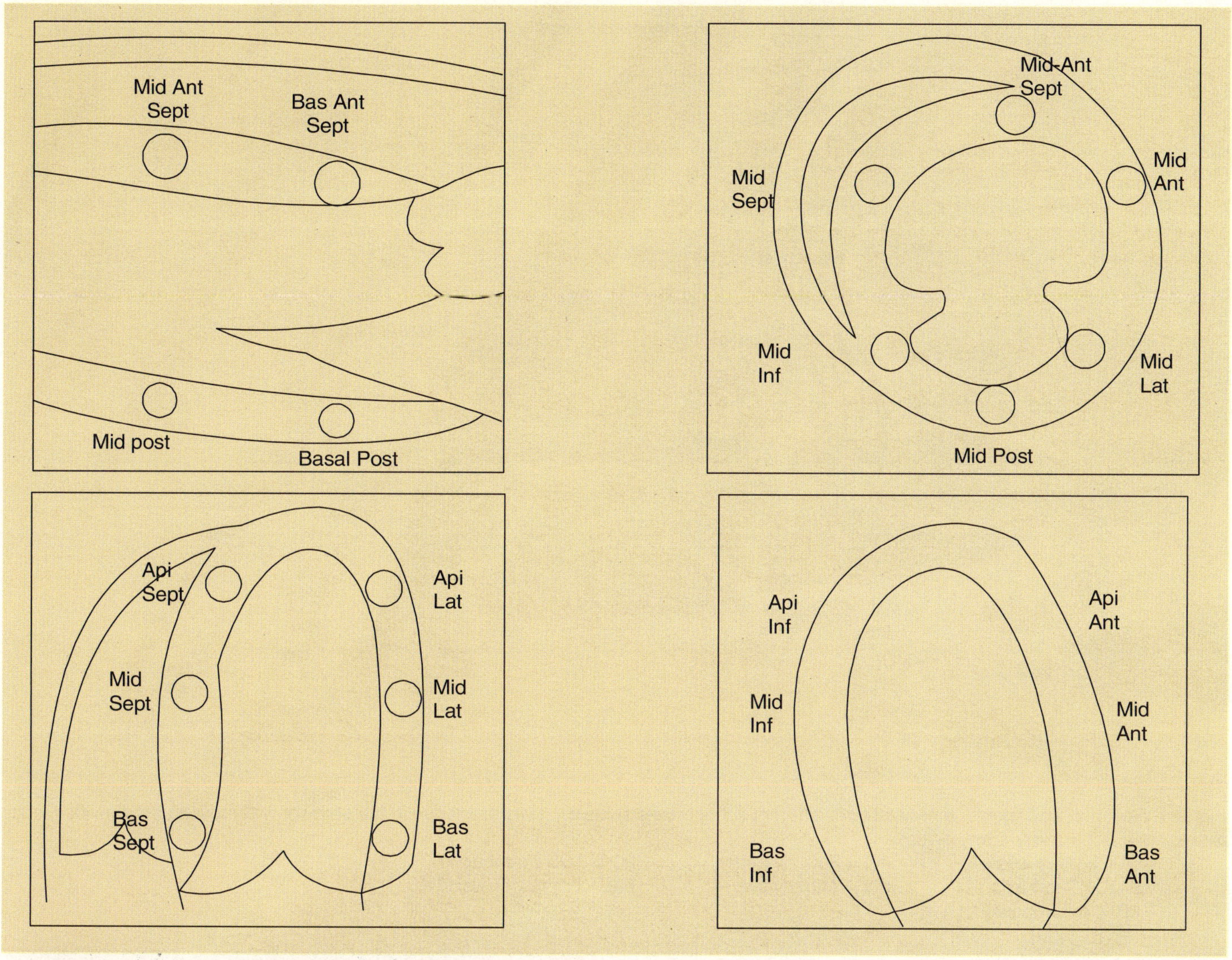

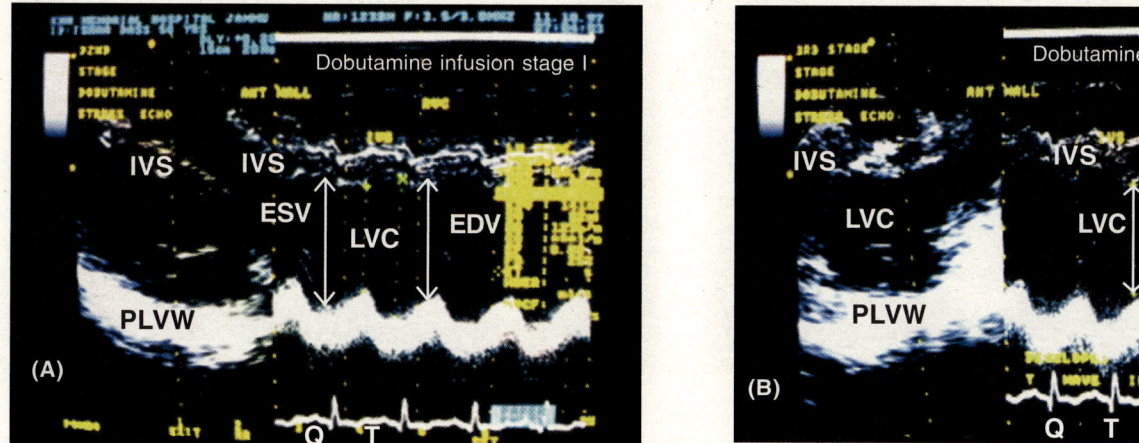

Fig. 8.7: Anatomical localization of different segments of LV wall positioned in various echocardiographic windows for determining wall motion abnormalities and wall motion scoring index in categorizing the severity of coronary heart disease as described on the diagram

Fig. 8.8A and B: **(A)** 2-D and M-Mode echocardiogram showing T-wave inversion (mild) with raised end diastolic volume in dobutamine infusion (stage I × 3 min) in a patient with exertional anginal pain with mild STT changes. **(B)** Stage II of Dobutamine infusion (stage II × 6 min.) showing marked tachycardia, with increased ST segment inversion along with enhancement of Q-wave and increase in end diastolic volume

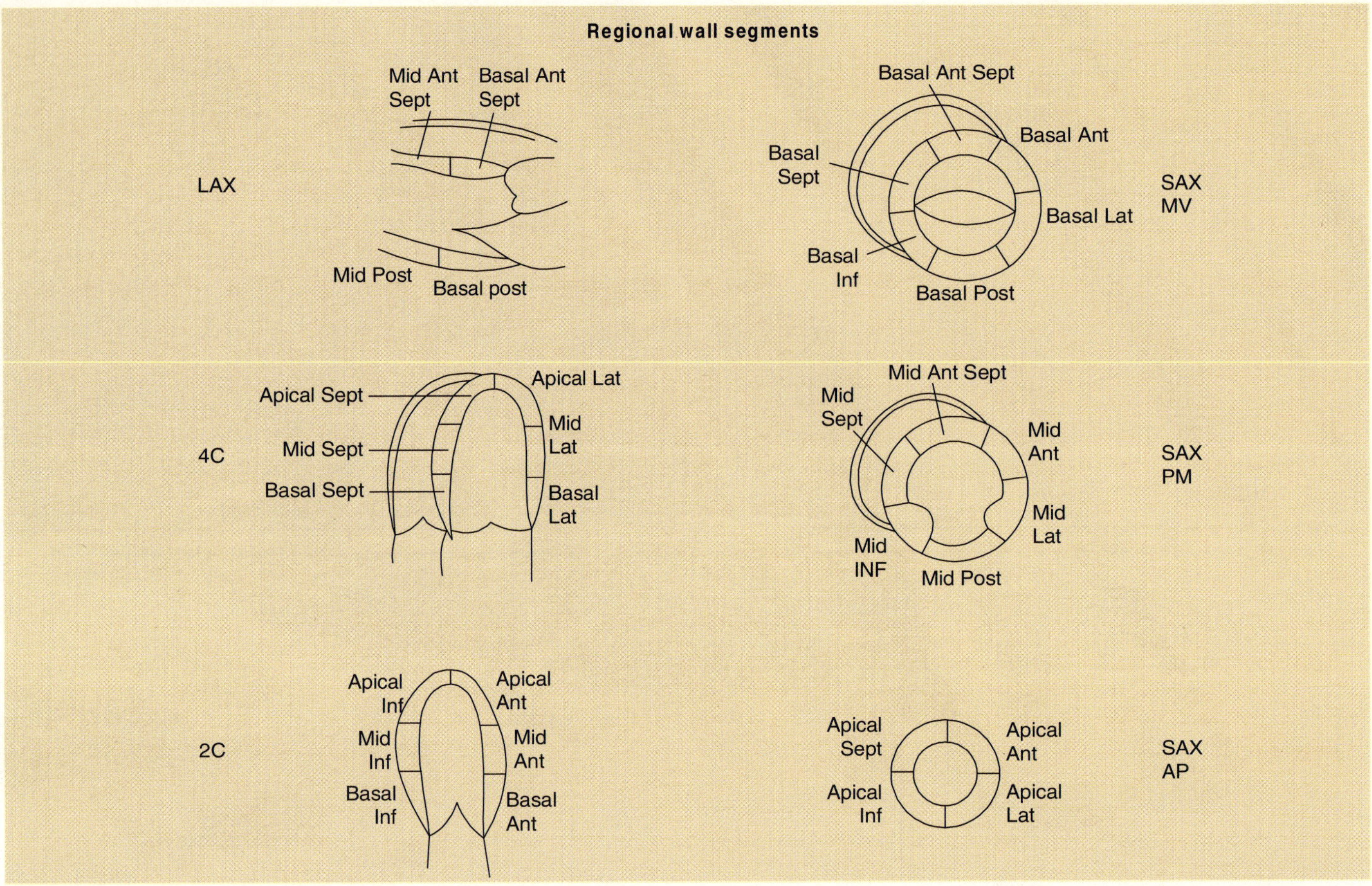

Regional wall segments

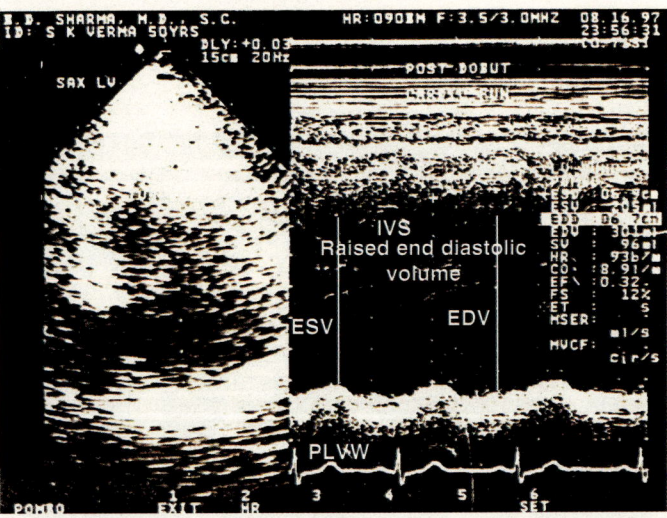

Fig. 8.9: Regional wall segments viewed from different echocardiographic windows employed in the study of wall motion abnormalities in the assessment of coronary artery disease

LAX = Long axis	4C = Four chamber	2C = Two chamber
SAX = Short axis	MV = Mitral valve	PM = Papillary muscle
AP = Anteroposterior		

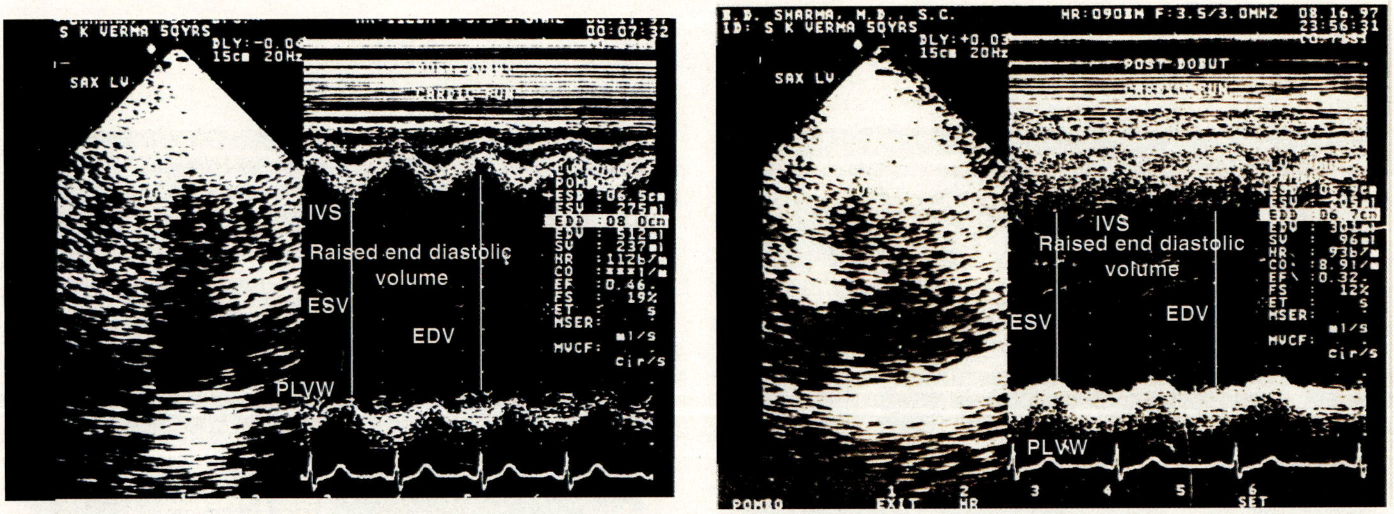

Fig. 8.10: 2-D and M-mode echocardiogram showing thinning and poor contractions of interventricular septum (IVS) and posterior left ventricular wall (PLVW) with raised end diastolic volumes and low left ventricular ejection fraction (LVED). Post-dobutamine study in the same patient showed almost flat movements of IVS and PLVW with dyskinesia and left ventricular ejection fraction reduced from 46 to 32%. His coronary angiogram revealed 2–3 vessel disease. Angioplasty was performed immediately after this test. This procedure worked for nearly 5 years when he suddenly developed full fledged antero-septal infarction with extension to postero-inferior wall. He was later managed with (CABG) internal mammary artery anastomosis. Currently he is doing well (8 years follow up of this patient)

Table 8.5: *Comparison of current (17 segment) and former (16 segment) nomenclature for left ventricular segmentation*

S.no.	New segment no.	New nomenclature	Views of old nomenclature
1.	Basal anterior	PSx, 2C	Same
2.	Basal anterior septal	PSx, PLAX	Same
	Dropped		Basal septal
3.	Basal inferior septal	PSx, 4C	½ basal inferior + ½ basal septal
4.	Basal inferior	PSx, 2C	½ basal inferior + ½ basal post
	Dropped		Basal posterior
5.	Basal inferior lateral	PSx, PLAX	Basal lateral
6.	Basal anterior lateral	PSx, 4C	Basal lateral
7.	Mid anterior	PSx, 2C	Same
8.	Mid anterior septal	PSx,PLAX	Same
9.	Mid inferior septal	PSx, 4C	½ mid septal + ½ mid inferior
	Dropped		Mid posterior
10.	Mid inferior	PSx.2C	½ mid inlerior + ½ mid posterior
11.	Mid inferior lateral	PSx. PLAX	Mid lateral
12.	Mid anterior lateral	PSx. 4C	Mid lateral
13.	Apical anterior	2C	Same
14.	Apical septal	4C	Same
15.	Apical inferior	2C	Same
16.	Apical lateral	4C	Same
17.	True apex	4C/2C	NIA

PLAx, parasternal long axis view; PSx, parasternal short axis view; 4C, four chamber; 2C, two chamber; N/A, not available

Table 8.6: *Echocardiographic detection of regional wall abnormalities in different cardiac dysfunctions*

	Ischemic WMA	LBBB	RV Paced
Maximal location	Distal septum, apex and anterior wall	Proximal/mid anterior septum	Distal septum, often inferior septum
Thickening	Absent or thinning	Partially preserved	Partially preserved
Duration	Usually monophasic	Multiphasic	Multiphasic
Abnormal geometry	Common	Uncommon	Uncommon
Temporal dyssynchrony	No	Yes	Yes

cally developed for use as cardiovascular stress testing agent and is linked to a unique closed-looped delivery system. Genesis of ischemia is similar to that of dobutamine, but it may provide a more balanced chronotropic and inotropic responses. It appears to have equivalent accuracy to exercise echocardiography and dobutamine stress echocardiography. Its accuracy in conjunction with radionuclide imaging also appears equivalent.

Stress Laboratory Protocols

Patients should fast for 4 to 6 hours before stress test, and intravenous access should be obtained through a large arm vein. Heart rate and rhythm are monitored continuously, and blood pressure and 12-lead electrocardiograms are recorded at each stage (or every 1 to 3 minutes) of drug infusion. Monitoring is continued for 5 to 10 minutes after infusion, or until heart rate falls to 100 beats/min. Because stress test may induce myocardial ischemia or arrhythmias, it is important to have equipment and medications for resuscitation readily available (Fig. 8.3A–C).

Dipyridamole-Thallium Testing

Methylaxanthine-containing beverages or medications such as tea, coffee, colas and theophylline should be discontinued for at least 24 hours before testing because methylxanthines prevent vasodilation by dipyridamole. Oral dipyridamole does not affect this procedure; however, antianginal agents may decrease the sensitivity for detecting coronary artery disease. The standard dose of dipyridamole is 0.56 mg/kg infused over 4 minute period; the infusion is prepared by diluting vials containing 10 mg of dipyridamole into 50–60 ml of either 0.9% sterile solution or 5% dextrose in water. The addition of several minutes of low-level exercise after the infusion may reduce side effects caused by systemic vasodilation, increase the frequency of ischemic electrocardiographic (ECG) changes, and improve image quality. Four to six minutes after

Table 8.7: *Echocardiography in risk assessment, prognosis and assessment of therapy in acute myocardial ischemic syndromes*

Class I	Class IIa	Class IIb	Class III
1. Assessment of infarct size and/or extent of jeopardized myocardium	1. In-hospital or early postdischarge assessment of the presence/extent of inducible ischemia in the absence of baseline abnormalities expected to compromise electrocardiographic interpretation.	Assessment of late prognosis (>2years after acute myocardial infarction)	Routine reevaluation in the absence of any change in clinical status
2. In-hospital assessment of ventricular function when the results are used to guide therapy	2. Reevaluation of ventricular function during recovery when results are used to guide therapy.		
3. In-hospital or early postdischarge assessment of the presence/extent of inducible ischemia whenever baseline abnormalities are expected to compromise electrocardiographic interpretation	3. Assessment of ventricular function after revascularization.		
4. Assessment of myocardial viability when required to define potential efficacy of revascularization			

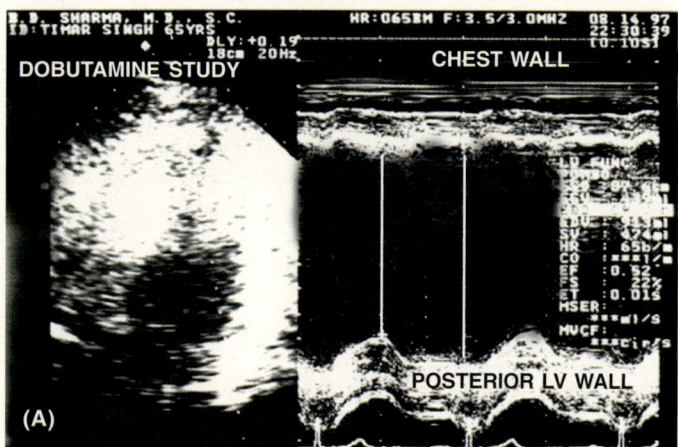 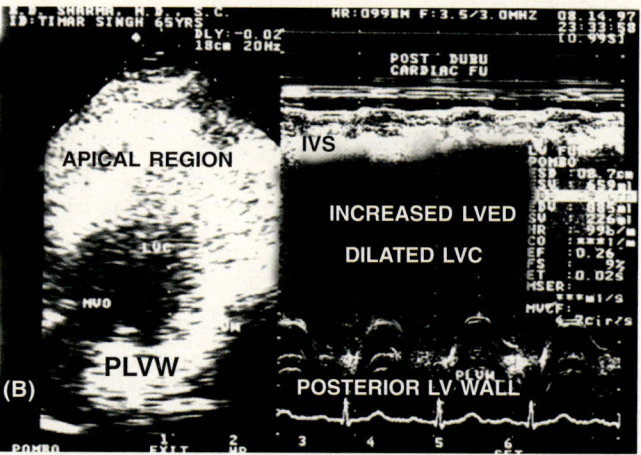

Fig. 8.11: (A) Pre-dobutamine resting 2-D M-mode echocardiogram showing marked hypokinesia of IVS, apical and posterior LV wall hypertrophy in patient with old antero-inferior myocardial ischemia with hypertension. In this scan he had left ventricular ejection fraction of 52%. **(B)** In the same patient Post-dobutamine echocardiogram showing increased hypokinesia of IVS with thinning and dyskinesia of both IVS and posterior LV wall with left ventricular ejection fraction less than 26% (POMBO Method)

completing the dipyridamole infusion 2 to 3 mCi of thallium—201 are injected intravenously, and imaging is begun 3 to 4 minutes later. Aminophylline (75 to 100 mg) can be slowly administered intravenously, to reverse the side effects of dipyridamole which may include anginal pain hypotension, or ECG alterations, such as bradyarrhythmia or tachyarrhythmia.

Some laboratories routinely administered aminophylline 5 mins. after thallium is injected. Additional aminophylline (up to 200 mg) can be administered if adverse effects persist. Sublingual nitroglycerine can also be used to reverse symptoms of ischemia.

Protocol for Dobutamine Stress Echocardiography
(Figs 8.6, 8.8, 8.10 and 8.11)

Patient is prepared for standard stress testing. Intravenous access is obtained. Digital images are acquired at baseline (these loops are displayed and used as reference throughout the infusion. Continuous electrocardiogram and blood pressure monitoring are established. Dobutamine infusion is begun at a dose of 5 or 10) µg/kg/min. The infusion rate is increased every 3 minutes to doses of 10, 20, 30 and 40 µg/kg/min.

The echocardiogram, electrocardiogram, and blood pressure are monitored continuously.

Low-dose images are acquired at either 5 or 10 μg/kg/min (at the first sign of increased contractility).

Atropine in doses of 0.5 to 1.0 mg can be given during the mild and high-dose stages to augment the heart rate response. Mild dose images are acquired at either 20 or 30 μg/kg/min. Peak images are acquired before termination of the infusion. Post-stress images are recorded after return to baseline. The patient is monitored until he or she returns to baseline status.

The various experimental studies have shown that dipyridamole has created more alterations in myocardial bloodflow than dobutamine, but dobutamine induces wall motion abnormalities more frequently than dipyridamole. Thus combining dipyridamole with perfusion based imaging such as thallium and coupling dobutamine with wall-motion-based imaging such as echocardiography should maximize the ability of these tests to detect coronary artery disease.

Dobutamine Echocardiography

Antianginal drugs are usually discontinued 24 to 48 hours before testing to achieve better results. Before dobutamine is administered, patients are placed in the best position for acquiring echocardiographic images, and baseline images of the heart are obtained. Dobutamine is diluted and placed in an infusion pump for delivery at 5 μg/kg/min initially. Continuous echocardiographic imaging allows the early detection of wall motion abnormalities and visualisation of the overall response to inotrophic stimulation. The infusion rate is increased every 3 minutes to 10, 20 and a maximum of 40 μg/kg/min unless end points develop. These end points include the development of new wall motion abnormalities, severe angina pectoris, or other severe side effects, such as ischemia (1 mm of ST-segment depression or elevation) ECG changes, hypertension (systolic 200 mm Hg), symptomatic hypotension, ventricular tachycardia supraventricular tachycardias, or the attainment of 85% of the maximal predicted heart rate (220 minus age in years). Atropine may be administered (0.5 mg doses, upto 2 mg) when heart rate fails to rise in response to dobutamine (such as in subjects treated with B-blockers. In order to revert adverse effects quickly intravenous metoprolol, atenolol, or esmolol can be administered after the dobutamine infusion is stopped (Table 8.7).

Termination of Test

1. Detection of a new or worsening wall motion abnormality;
2. Angina pectoris requiring use of sublingual-nitroglycerine;
3. Systolic blood pressure 220 mm Hg or diastolic pressure 120 mm Hg;
4. Decrease in systolic blood pressure of 20 mm Hg;
5. Major ventricular arrhythmias;
6. Achievement of the target heart rate of 85% of the age-predicted maximal heart rate (220-age in yrs.);
7. ST-segment shift equal or greater than 2 mm;
8. Symptoms unacceptable by the patient.

Echocardiographic Images

The various studies have shown that abnormalities of ventricular contraction detected by echocardiography precede ECG signs or symptoms of ischemia. Thus continuous imaging of the heart to detect new wall motion abnormalities is performed during the infusion of dobutamine. Direct digital and video tape recordings of images are made at rest, mid infusion (10 to 20 μg/kg/min). During each infusion phase, images are obtained from the parasternal long and short-axis planes and from the apical two and four-chamber planes, permitting analysis of motion in 16 myocardial segments. The display of digitized R-wave-gated cine loops facilitates side by side comparisons of wall motion from rest and stress phases. Wall motion is qualitatively graded according to the degree of endocardial motion or dyskinetic response. During stress phases the normal response of the myocardium is hyperkinesis with a marked decrease in end-systolic cavity size (volume): failure of a segment to develop accentuated thickening is also a sensitive marker for coronary artery disease (Tables 8.5 and 8.6).

An additional marker of coronary artery disease includes an increase in ventricular cavity size during stress, which generally indicates three-vessel, proximal left anterior descending, or left main coronary artery obstructions. Electrocardiographic changes may be detected and are specific but insensitive for detecting coronary artery disease. Dobutamine echocardiography takes about 60 minutes to perform and interpret; results are available immediately after the studies are performed, allowing a review of the findings with patients and attending physicians.

Adverse Effects and Limitation of Stress Tests
Dipyridamole-Thallium

The administration of dipyridamole in the standard dose of 0.56 mg/kg is generally well tolerated. It has been observed that patient who received dipyridamole in the dosage range of 0.56 to 0.65 mg/kg major adverse events occurred in only 0.26% and minor adverse reactions are observed in 46.5% of patients. The administration of dipyridamole is relatively contraindicated in patients with a history of bronchospastic diseases of lungs such as asthma and in patients with unstable angina pectoris. However, some patients have tolerated dipyridamole in doses upto 0.84 mg/kg for thallium or echocardiographic imaging. Dipyridamole has been found quite safe among elderly patients. Thallium should be given immediately to patients who develop chest pain suggestive of angina or with significant ST changes followed a few minutes later by intravenous aminophylline. Sublingual nitroglycerin can also be given if symptoms persists despite aminophylline administration.

The limitations of this test is due to its ability to correctly identify coronary artery disease. The inability of patients to lie still may produce motion artifacts or suboptimal image resolution as a result of an increased distance between the heart and the gamma camera. This is mostly related with SPECT studies, because a longer time is required for imaging. Image quality may also be degraded by soft-tissue attenuation, artifacts produced by significant obesity, pendulous breasts, or an elevated hemidiaphragm. The majority of these problems are easily overcome by an experienced worker.

Dobutamine Echocardiography

The administration of dobutamine is frequently associated with mild side effects such as chest tightness, dyspnea, flushing, nausea, headache, paresthesias, chills, anxiety, or palpitations. Symptoms of any degree are seen in approximately 33% of patients, and chest pain suggestive of angina occurs in about 18% of patients. Hypertension is uncommon (0.8%); however, hypotension is more frequent (4% in pooled data, upto 20%) and has several potential mechanisms with unstable angina pectoris, recently active ventricular arrhythmias, and uncontrolled atrial fibrillation where significant increases of ventricular rate may occur.

Limitations of echocardiography should be considered when selecting patients for stress studies. Chest wall deformities, emphysema, and severe obesity limit visualisation of the heart with transthoracic probes, and patients with these characteristics (about 5% to 10% of all patients) may not be suitable for transthoracic echocardiographic imaging. Many patients with these features may be successfully imaged during dobutamine stress, however only 0.9% of the studies are found unsatisfactory for analysis.

Bibliography

1. Afridi I, Kleiman NS, Raizner AE, Zoghbi WA. Dobutamine echocardiography in myocardial hibernation. *Circulation* 1995;91:663–670.
2. Berth C, Pierard LA, Hiernaux M, Trottenur G, Lempereur P, Carlier J, *et al.* Predicting the extent and location of coronary artery disease in acute myocardial infarction by echo-cardiography during dobutamine infusion. *Am J Cardiol* 1986;58:1167–1172.
3. Boccaneli A. Diagnostic value and safety of dobutamine echocardiography in diagnosis of coronary artery disease. *Cardiol* 1993;19–28.
4. Bourdellon PDV, Broderick TM, Sawada SG, Armstrong WF, Ryan T, Dillion JC, *et al.* Regional wall motion index for infarct and non-infarct regions after reperfusion in acute myocardial infarction. Comparison with global wall motion index. *J Am Soc Echocardiogr* 1989;2:398.
5. Coma-Canella, Abascal P, Sensitivity and specificity of dobutamine echocardiography test to detect multivessel coronary artery disease after acute myocardial infarction. *Eur Heart J* 1990; 11:249–57.
6. Crouse LJ, Harbrecht, JJ, Vacek JL, Rasmond TL, Kramer PH. Exercise echocardiography as a screening test for coronary artery disease and correlation with coronary angiography. *AM J Cardiol* 1991; 67:1213.
7. Distane A, Moscavelli E, Moralis MA, Latranze F, Reisenhoffer B, for the assessment of coronary artery disease. *Echocardiography* 1991; 8: 99.
8. Johnson LL, Seldin DW, Keller Ana, Wall RM, Bhatia K, Bingham C, *et al.* Dual isotope thallium and indicum antimyosine SPECT imaging to identify acute infarct patients of further ischaemic risk. *Circulation* 1990; 81:37–45.
9. Krivokapich J, Child JS, Walter DO, *et al.* Prognostic value of dobutamine stress echocardiography in predicting cardiac events in patients with known or suspected coronary artery disease. *J Am Coll Cardiol* 1999; 33:708–716.
10. Kuntz KM, Fleischmann KE, Hunink MG. *et al.* Cost-effectiveness of diagnostic strategies for patients with chest pain. *Ann Intern Med* 1999;130:709–718.
11. La Canna G, Alfieri O. Glubbini R, *et al.* Echocardiography during infusion of dobutamine for identification of reversibly dysfunction in patients with chronic coronary artery disease. *J Am Coll Cardiol* 1994; 23:617–626.
12. Lalka SG, Sawada SG, Dalsing MC. *et al.* Dobutamine stress echocardiography as a predictor of cardiac events associated with aortic surgery. *J Vase Surg* 1992; 15:831–840.
13. Langan EM III, Youkey JR. Franklin DP, *et al.* Dobutamine stress echocardiography for cardiac risk assessment before aortic surgery. *J Vase Surg* 1993; 18:905–911.
14. Ling LH. Pellikka PA. Mahoney DW, *et al.* Atropine augmentation in dobutamine stress echocardiography: role and incremental value in a clinical practice setting. *J Am Coll Cardiol* 1996; 28:551–557.
15. Luotolahti M, Saraste M, Hartiala J. Exercise echocardiography in the diagnosis of coronary artery disease. *Ann Med* 1996;28:73–77.
16. Marcovitz PA, Armstrong WF. Accuracy of dobutamine stress echocardiography in detecting coronary artery disease. *Am J Cardiol* 1992;69:1269–1273.
17. Mamick TH, Anderson I: Williams MI, *et al.* Exercise echocardiography is an accurate and cost-efficient technique for detection of coronary artery disease in women. *J Am Coll Cardiol* 1995;26:335–341.
18. Mannering D, Crepps T, Leech G, Menta N, Valentine H, Gilmour S, *et al.* Dobutamine stress test as an alternative to exercise testing after acute myocardial infarction. *Br. Heart J* 1988;59(55): 521–526.

19. Marangelli V, Fiiceto S. Piccinni G., *et al*. Detection of coronary artery disease by digital stress echocardiography: comparison of exercise, transesophageal atrial pacing and dipyridamole echocardiography. *J Am Coll Cardiol* 1994; 24:117–124.

20. Marcovitz PA, Armstrong WF, *et al*. Accuracy of dobutamine stress echocardiography in detecting coronary artery disease. *Am J Cardiol* 1992;69:1269.

21. Martin TW, Seaworth JF, Johns JP, Pupa LE, Condos WR, Comparison of adenosine, Dipyridamole and dobutamine in stress echocardiography. *Ann Int Med* 1992;116:190

22. Martin TW. Seaworth JF, Johns JP, *et al*. Comparison of adenosine. dipyridamole and dobutamine in stress echocardiography. *Ann Intern Med* 1992;116:190 196.

23. Marwic TH, Nemac JJ, Pashkow FJ, Stewart WJ, Salcedo EE. Accuracy and limitation of exercise echocardiography in routine clinical setting. *J Am Coll Cardiol* 1992;19:74.

24. Marwick T, Willemart B, AM D' Hondt AM, *et al*. Selection of the optimal nonexercise stress for the evaluation of Ischemic regional myocardial dysfunction and malperfusion. Comparison of dobutamine and adenosine using echocardiography and 99mTc. MIBI single photon emission computed tomography. *Circulation* 1993;87:345–354.

25. Marwick T. D'Hondt AM. Baudhuin T, *et al*. Optimal use of dobutamine stress for the detection and evaluation of coronary artery disease: combination with echocardiography or scintigraphy or both? *J Am Coll Cardiol* 1993;22:159–167.

26. Marwick TH, Torelli J, Hatjal K, *et at*. Influence of left ventricular hypertrophy on detection of coronary artery disease using exercise echocardiography. *J Am Coll Cardiol* 1995;26:1180–1186.

27. Marwick TH. D' Hondt AM, Mairesse GH. *et al*. Comparative ability of dobutamine and exercise stress in inducing myocardial ischaemia in active patients. *Br Heart J* 1994;72:31–38.

28. Marwick TH. Mehta R. Arheart K, *et al*. Use of exercise echocardiography for prognostic evaluation of patients with known or suspected coronary artery disease. *J Am Coll Cardiol* 1997;30:83–90.

29. Mason SJ, Weiss JL, Weisfeldt ML *et al*. Exercise echocardiography: detection of wall motion abnormalities during ischemia. *Circulation* 1979;59:50–59.

30. Mazeika PK, Nadazdins A, Oakley CM, *et al*. Dobutamine stress echocardiography for detection and assessment of coronary artery disease. *J Am Coll Cardiol* 1992;19:1203.

31. Marcovitz PA, Shayna V, Horn RA *et al*. Value of dobutamine stress echocardiography in determining the prognosis of patients with known or suspected coronary artery disease. *Am J Cardiol* 1996;78:404–408.

32. McCully RB, Roger VL. Mahoney DW, *et al*. Outcome after abnormal exercise echocardiography Cor patients with good exercise capacity: Prognostic importance of the extent and severity of exercise-related left ventricular dysfunction. *J Am Coll Cardiol* 2002:39:1345–1352.

33. McCully RB. Roger VI. Mahoney DW, *et al*. Outcome after normal exercise echocardiography and predictors of subsequent cardiac events: follow-up of 1325 patients. *J Am Coll Cardiol* 1998;31:144–149.

34. Mertes H, Sawada SG, Ryan L, *et al*. Symptoms, adverse effects, and complications associated with dobutamine stress

35. Mertes H, Sawanda SG, Ryon T, Segar DS, Kovacs R, Leigenbawn H, *et al*. Symptoms, side effects and complications during dobutamine stress echocardiography. (Abstract) *Circulation* 1992;86:1–126.

36. Mertes H. Erbe1 R. Nixdorff U., *et al*. Exercise echocardiography for the evaluation of patients after nonsurgical coronary artery revascularization. *J Am Coll Cardiol* 1993; 21: 1087–1093.

37. Nihoyannopoulos P, Marsonis A. Joshi J, *et al*. Magnitude of myocardial dysfunction is greater in painful than in painless myocardial ischemia: an exercise echocardiographic study. *J Am Coll Cardiol* 1995;25:1507–1512.

38. Olmos U. Dakik H. Gordon R., *et al*. Long-term prognostic value of exercise echocardiography compared with exercise 201TI. ECG. and clinical variables. In patients evaluated for coronary artcl)" disease. *Circulation* 1998; 98:2679–2686.

39. Ostojic M, Picano E, Beleslin B. *et al*. Dipyridamolc-dobutamine echocardiography: A novel test for the detection of milder forms of coronary artery disease. *J Am Coll Cardiol* l994;23:1115–11 22.

40. Pellikka PA. Roger VL. Oh JK, *et al*. Safety of performing dobutamine stress echocardiography in patients with abdominal aortic aneurysm diameter. *Am J Cardiol* 1996; 77:413–416.

41. Picano E, Lattanzi F. Masini M. *et al*. High dose dipyridamole echocardiography test in effort angina pectoris. *J Am Coll Cardiol* 1986;8: 848–854.

42. Picano E. Sicari R. Landi P. *et al*. Prognostic value of myocardial viability in medically treated patients with global left ventricular dysfunction early after an acute uncomplicated myocardial infarction: a dobutamine stress echocardiographic study. *Circulation* 1998;98: 1078–1084.

43. Pierard LA, De Landsheere CM, Berthe C. *et al*. Identification of viable myocardium by echocardiography during dobutamine infusion in patients with myocardial infarction after thrombolytic therapy: comparison with positron emission tomography. *J Am Coll Cardial* 1990;15: 1 021–1031.

44. Pingitore A. Picano E, Colo MQ, *et al*. The atropine factor in pharmacologic stress echocardiography. Echo Persantlne (EPIC) and Echo Dobutamine International Cooperative (EDIC) Study Groups. *J Am Coll Cardiol* 1996;27:1164–1170.

45. Plotkin JS, Benitez RM. Kuo PC, *et al*. Dobutamine stress echocardiography for preoperative cardiac risk stratification in patients undergoing orthotopic liver transplantation. *Liver Trampl Surg* 1998;4:253–257.

46. Poldermans D, Arnese M, Fioretti PM., *et al*. Improved cardiac risk stratification in major vascular surgery with dobutamine-atropine stress echocardiography. *J Am Coll Cardiol* 1995;26:648–653.

47. Poldermans D, Fioretti PM, Boersma E. *et al*. Long–term prognostic value of dobutamine-atropine stress echocardiography in 1737 patients with known or suspected coronary artery disease: a single center experience. *Circulation* 1999;99:757–762.

48. Poldermans D, Fioretti PM. Forster T., *et al*. Dobutamine stress echocardiography for assessment of perioperative

cardiac risk in patients undergoing major vascular surgery. *Circulation* 1993;87: 1506–1512.

49. Poldermans D. Arnese M. Fioretti PM, *et al*. Sustained prognostic value of dobutamine stress echocardiography for late cardiac events after major noncardiac vascular surgery. *Circulation* 1997;95:53–58.

50. Porter TR, Xie F, Silver M, *et al*. Real-time perfusion imaging with low mechanical index pulse inversion Doppler imaging. *J Am Coll Cardiol* 2001;37:748–753.

51. Quinones MA,. Verani MS. Haichin RM, *et al*. Exercise echocardiography versus 20111 single-photon emission computed tomography in evaluation of coronary artery disease. Analysis of 292 patients. *Circulation* 1992;85:1026–1031.

52. Rallidis L, Cokkinos P, Tousoulis D, *et al*. Comparison of dobutamine and treadmill exercise echocardiography in inducing ischemia in patients with coronary artery disease. *J Am Coll Cardiol* 1997; 30:1660–1668.

53. Ruffalo RR. Review. The pharmacology of dobutamine. *Am J Med Sci* 1987; 294:244–248.

54. Upton MT, Rerych SK, Newman GE, Port S, Cobe FR, Johns RH. Detecting abnormalities in left ventricular function during exercise before angina and ST segment depression. *Circulation* 1980; 62: 341–349.

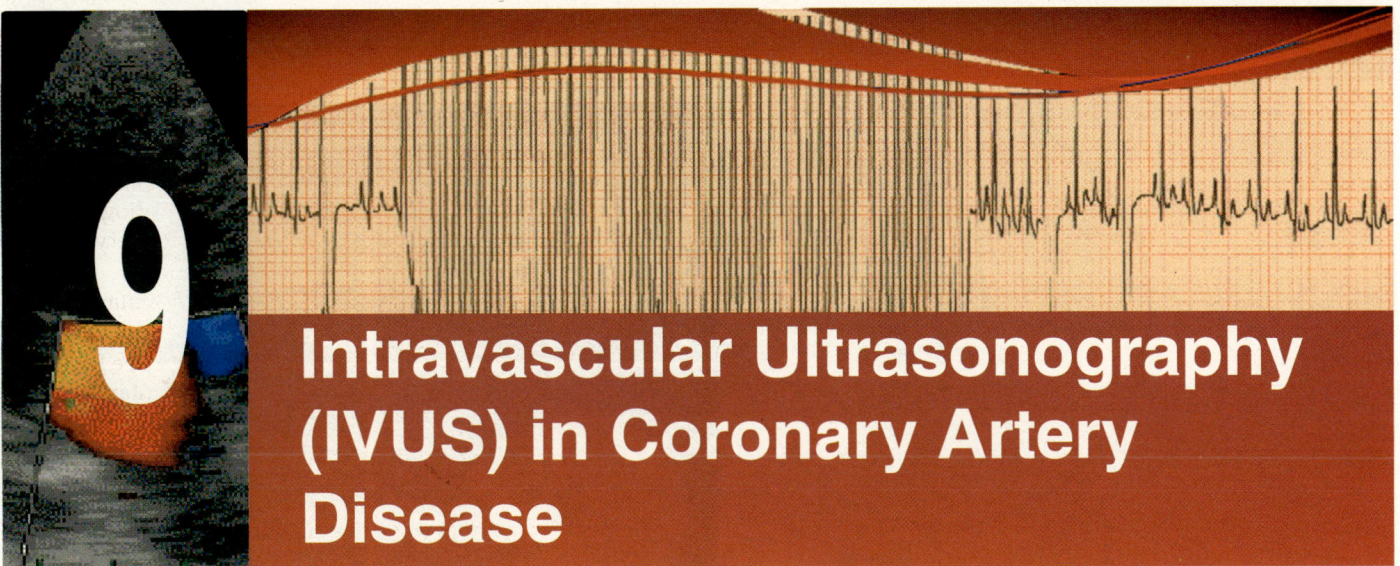

9

Intravascular Ultrasonography (IVUS) in Coronary Artery Disease

Intravascular coronary artery ultrasonography is a unique versatile technique which has already established its place in the diagnosis of coronary atherosclerosis with greater sensitivity. Striking atherosclerotic abnormalities are occasionally evident in patients with totally normal coronary arteries by an angiography. This, therefore, reveals that a patient should not be absolutely declared atherosclerotic free based exclusively on angiographic report. It being relatively a new imaging modality, intravascular ultrasound (IVUS) yields elaborate high resolution pictures of the vessel wall, enabling visualisation of atheromas regardless of whether they narrow the lumen. This incremental diagnostic information is proving revolutionary in understanding the pathophysiology of coronary disease, the effects of pharmacological therapy and the effects of interventional devices. Intravascular ultrasound has also been applied to evaluation of angiographically normal coronary arteries following cardiac transplantation, often revealing occult initimal thickening.

Historical Background

The year 1913 was the beginning of angioscopy when two research workers, i.e. Rhea and Walker used a rigid illuminated tube in an attempt to visualise the endocardium. Sixty years later, interest in angioscopy was revived by using a flexible device to perform endoscopy to visualise the great vessels. The first report of coronary angioscopy was published in 1985 by Spears *et al.*, and Sherman *et al.*, who, in 1986, demonstrated the superior sensitivity of intraoperative angioscopy over preoperative angiography for detecting the presence of complex atherosclerotic plaques and intracoronary thrombi in patients with unstable angina undergoing coronary bypass surgery.

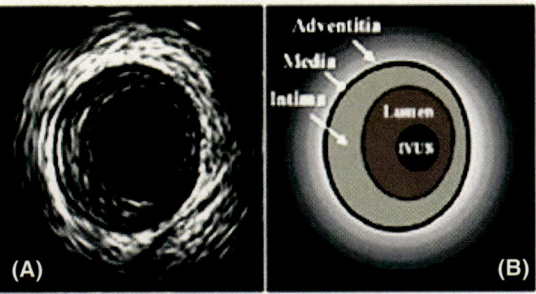

Fig. 9.1A and B: (A) Ultrasonographic features of coronary artery. **(B)** Lumen, catheter inside the lumen and three layers of artery. From inner to outside as intima, media and adventia respectively

Technique of IVUS in CAD

Angioscope: The angioscope (imagecath), is a kind of catheter which houses another catheter inside the outer one. The delivery catheter externally resembles a conventional angioplasty balloon catheter. The inner catheter contains the imaging fibres and is guided within the coronary artery over a 0.014 inch angioscopy guidewire. The outer catheter measures 4.5 French in diameter and has a lumen for inflating and deflating the occlusion balloon at its distal tip. The occlusion balloon is a compliant balloon that achieves a variable final diameter depending on the volume of liquid introduced by hand injection upto a maximum diameter of 5.0 mm. The image bundle may be withdrawn independently of the outer catheter, a distance of 6 cm, so that longer segments of the vessel can be visualised.

Angioscopy was developed with subsequent advances made in coronary balloon catheters and miniaturization of fiberoptic technology. The percutaneous coronary angioscope consists of two basic components, the imaging system and the delivery catheter. The imaging system is made up of illumination

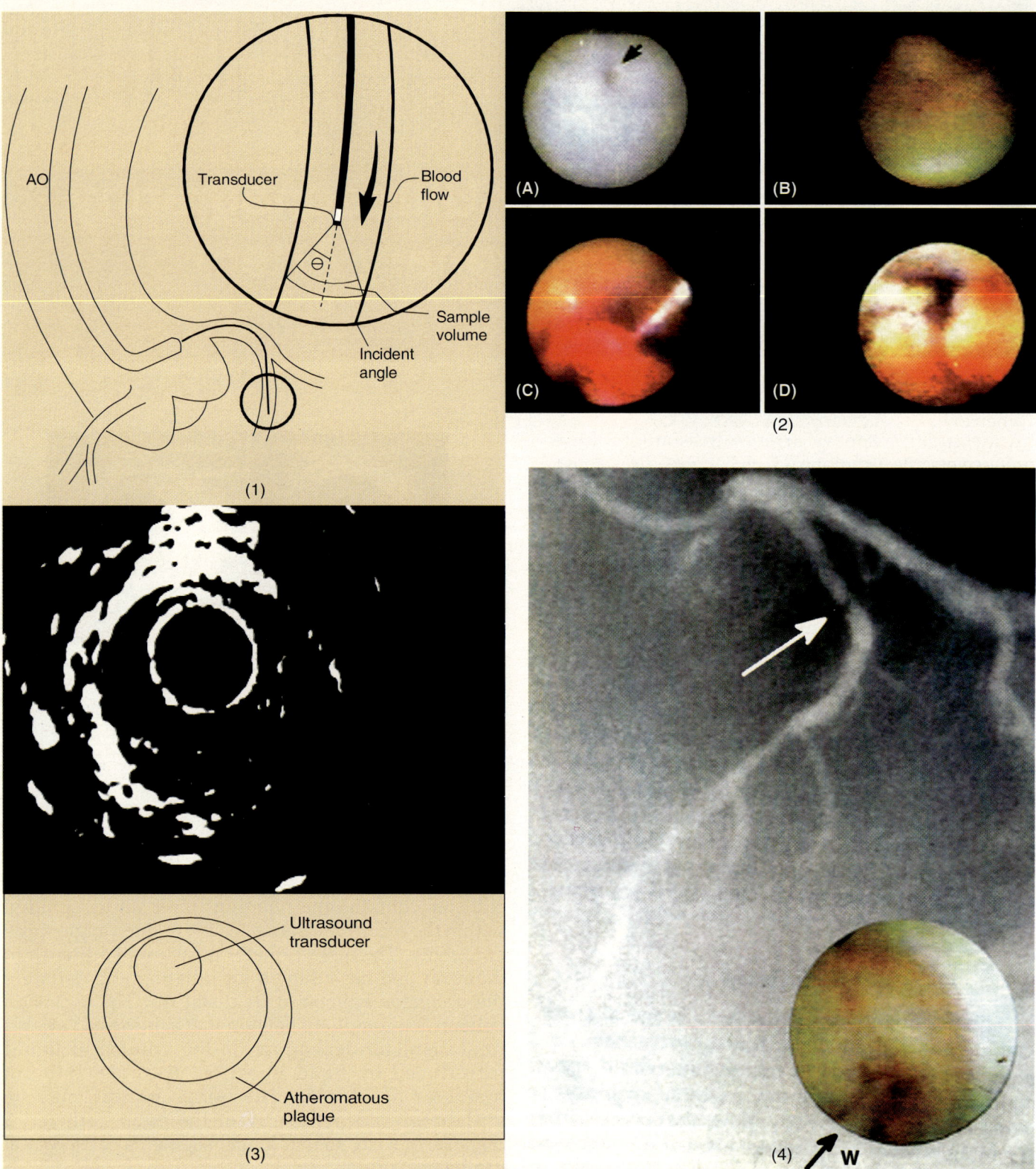

Fig. 9.2: 1. Flowire placed in its proximal left anterior descending coronary artery. Depicted here is the broad sample volume and minimal angle of incidence. **2A.** Angioscopic features of a white plaque in patient with restenosis. **2B.** Yellow plaque. **2C.** Intramural red thrombus along with silverguide wire **2D.** Plaque rupture with small element of mural thrombus present with in a patient with unstable angina **3.** Large crescentic coronary plaque extending from the 1°clock to 7°clock positions resulting into marked reduction in coronary lumen. **4.** Angiographic left anterior oblique view of the left coronary artery showing hazy appearance of lesion in the left anterior descending coronary artery (arrow) indicating the presence of intracoronary thrombus. The insert at the bottom depicts the angioscopic view of the dissection without intracoronary thrombus with guidewire (arrow)

fibres, imaging fibres, a video camera and monitor, and a video recorder. The illumination source provides a high intensity "cold" light to avoid thermal damage to the vessel wall. The imaging bundle, measuring 0.08 inches, consists of at least 2000 optical fibres with a miniature lens attached to its distal end.

In this technique an 9-French conventional angioplasty guiding catheter is advanced to the coronary ostium, and 1,000 units of heparin are administered. After performing angiography to act as a guiding tract for delineating the coronary anatomy and identifying specific areas of interest, a 0.014 inch guide wire is placed into the distal portion of the vessel under examination. The angioscope, which is a "monorail" design, is advanced over a guide wire into the coronary artery proximal to the segment of the vessel visualised. The lumen of the angioscope is connected to a power injector for infusion of warmed lactated Ringer's solution at a rate of 0.5 to 1.0 ml per second after the occlusion balloon is inflated with a 1 ml syringe, filled with a 50:50 mixture of saline and radiographic contrast to create a blood free field. One should always be careful not to over inflate the balloon. The inner catheter, or the imaging bundle, is then advanced over the guide wire to view the intraluminal surface of the vessel.

Ultrasound imaging equipment consists of two major components, a catheter with a miniaturised transducer and a console with the electronics to reconstruct the image. Very high ultrasound frequencies are employed for intravascular imaging, typically 20 to 45 MHz, providing excellent theoretical resolution. At 30 MHz, the wavelength is approximately 50 μm (0.05 mm), which permits axial resolution approaching 100 μm. Two technical approaches to transducer design are currently used: mechanically rotated devices and multielements electronic arrays. Currently available ultrasound catheters for intracoronary applications have an outer diameter between 2.6 and 3.5 F(0.87–1.17 mm).

There is always a choice of a interventional cardiologists to use a 7F or 8F guiding catheter, but some of the smaller catheters can be placed through a large lumen 6F guide. For examination, standard interventional techniques are used; intravenous heparin (5000–10000 units) and intracoronary nitroglycerin (100–300 μg) are routinely administered prior to imaging. After engaging the vessel with the guiding catheter, a steerable 0.014 inch angioplasty guidwire is used to selectively cannulate the vessel.

One can employ two technical approaches to imaging, i.e. motorised and manual pullback. However, it is stressed that a single pullback, even when controlled by a motor, may be insufficient for a complete diagnostic evaluation. Irrespective of the pullback method, imaging should include smooth uninterrupted imaging of at least 100 mm of distal reference vessel, actual lesion site and the proximal reference vessel back upto the aorta.

Bringing a little manipulation of the guide wire causes deflection of the angioscope tip and brings the lumen into view. Each imaging sequence lasts approximately 30 to 45 seconds after which balloon is deflated and the flush discontinued. These steps can be repeated several times until the region under study has been adequately investigated. Guiding catheter pressure, ST-segment changes, cardiac rhythm and patient comfort are monitored continuously and most critically during angioscopy (Fig. 9.2).

In case if angioscopy is to be performed in conjunction with a percutaneous intervention such as balloon angioplasty, the angioscope can be exchanged for a therapeutic balloon over the guide wire without the need for recrossing the lesion. The entire sequence from introducing the angioscope to obtaining images can usually be accomplished in less than 15 minutes.

Image Interpretation in IVUS (Fig. 9.3A and B)

Normal Coronary Morphology: Most of our knowledge regarding the anatomical structure of the vessel has been acquired from intravascular ultrasound comparing images obtained in vitro with histologic cross-sections of the same vessel. However, there are important differences between ultrasound anatomy visualised in vitro and in vivo. Because necropsy specimens are not distended by physiologic pressure, elastic recoil can reduce the lumen to a cross-sectional area <33% of in vivo size. In vitro, shrinkage of vessel wall tissues results in a bunching or corrugations of intramural structures, which alters the acoustic properties of the tissue.

Changes in ultrasound morphology in vessels studied (postmortem) can dramatically affect image interpretation. Distended by physiologic pressures in vivo, the intimal leading edge is frequently of minimal acoustic reflectance, particularly for normal segments, but postmortem, study reveals exaggeration of the acoustic interface artifact yielding a more echogenic appearance. In vitro the media assume a prominent sonolucent appearance and ultrasound exhibits distinct acoustic interfaces between intima, media, and adventitia. In vivo, these antomic landmarks are more indistinct and the sonolucent band is reduced in thickness (Fig. 9.1A and B).

Ultrasonographically a distinctly laminar appearance of the normal vessel wall is reported in many, but not all normal persons, although the genesis of these ultrasound layers remains controversial. In some normal subjects, a discrete linear ultrasonic reflectance is observed at the acoustic interface between the lumen and intima. However, other normal subjects sometimes exhibit an intimal leading edge that poorly reflects ultrasound, a phenomenon that leads to dropout of ultrasound signal. This distinct laminations of the vessel wall are absent at 30–50% of the coronary sites in normal persons.

When an intimal leading edge is observed, the maximal thickness average <0.20 mm and most investigators consider a normal value to be <0.20–0.30 mm. These values are larger than the histologic thickness of the intima and reflect the intrinsic axial resolution of the ultrasound device, not precise anatomic boundaries. A distinct subintimal sonolucent layer is often evident in normal segments (50–70%) of normal subjects, with a maximal thickness averaging <0.20 mm. Some of the workers are of the opinion that the characteristic sonolucent zone represents normal media; however, differences in the ultrasound anatomy of muscular (usually laminar) and elastic arteries (usually non-layered) have been reported. It has also been put forth that the disparate findings in normal subjects may also reflect dissimilarities in instrumentation (electronic *vs.* mechanical probes) or selection of normal subjects (young *vs.* old) (Fig. 9.4).

IVUS in Angiographically Normal Coronary Arteries: In most patients with CAD, intravascular ultrasound demonstrates atherosclerotic abnormalities in coronary wall morphology at sites with no lesion present on angiography. In the presence of any angiographic luminal irregularity, intravascular ultrasound frequently demonstrates CAD at all other examined coronary sites. In one study, intravascular ultrasound abnormalities were detected at >75% of angiographically normal sites in CAD patients. The extent of atherosclerosis in angiographically normal confirms the finding, previously reported from necropsy studies, that coronary disease is frequently more diffuse than reported by angiography. In some cases, it is evident that preservation of angiographic lumen size is a consequence of compensatory remodelling of the vessel wall.

Plaque Morphology by IVUS: Coronary artery afflicted with atherosclerosis exhibit a variety of ultrasound features that reflect the severity, composition and distribution of atheroma (Figs 9.6, 9.11, 9.13 and 9.15).

i. low echogenicity (cellular) lesion (soft plaque) with diffuse lipid infiltration,
ii. dense fibrous lesion, which produces brighter ultrasound reflections (fibrous plaque),
iii. calcified lesion, which produces intensely echogenic reflections with acoustic shadowing (calcified plaque) and
iv. mixed (fibrocalcific) plaque. Additionally descriptors include the single or multiple nature of calcium deposits, the circumferential extent of calcification expressed in degrees of arc and length in millimeters and whether the calcium is superficial or deep.

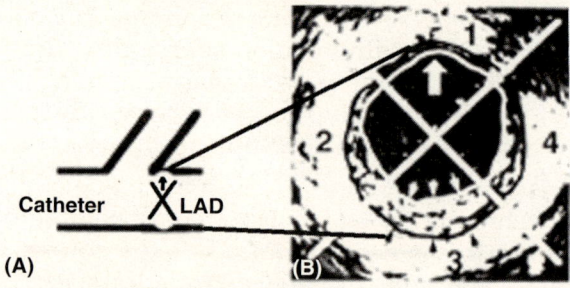

Fig. 9.3A and B: (A) Position in which a cross sectional image is acquired .The image for measurement is obtained at the ostium of the LAD artery. An arrow indicates the direction of the LCx branch. **(B)** Intravascular ultrasound image of the ostium of the LAD coronary artery.The cross section is divided into 4 × 90 degree segments as pointed out by white cross and each quadrant labeled as segment 1 through 4 in a counterclock wise direction.A white arrow indicates the direction of the left circumflex branch (LCx). The planimetry of the inner echogenic ring area and the outer echolucent ring area are enclosed by black and white circles, respectively. Plaque thickness is measured as the distance between the inner echogenic ring and the outer echolucent ring (arrow). Segment 1 = left circumflex artery (LCx) direction; segment 2 = epicardial direction; segment 3 = opposite site of segment 1; segment 4 = myocardial direction

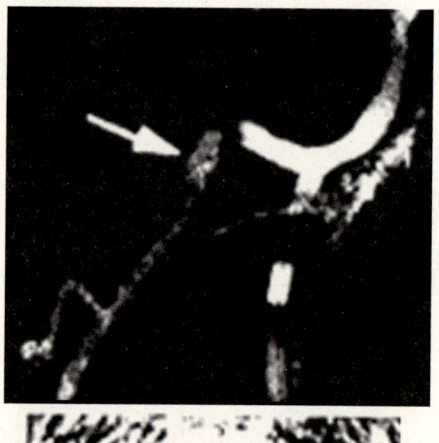

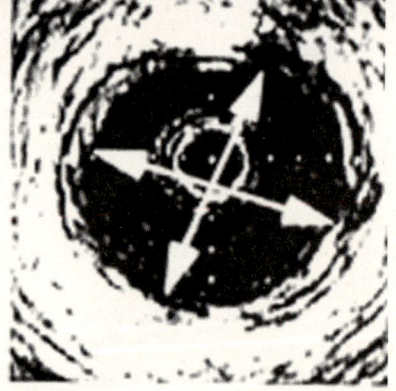

Fig. 9.4: Correlation between IVUS and QCA reference lumen dimensions, and the frequency distribution of the difference between IVUS and QCA refrence lumen. On average, the reference lumen by IVUS is 0.5 mm larger than by QCA; but in a significant number of lesion, the IVUS measurement is larger by 1.0 mm or smaller by 0.5 mm. In this case the guiding catheter was 9F.QCA measured a reference dimension of 3.12 mm. IVUS showed that the reference lumen (double headed white arrow) measured 4.5 × 4.0 mm. A stent was postdilated with a 4.5 mm balloon. The location of the IVUS slice corresponded to the white arrow in the angiogram

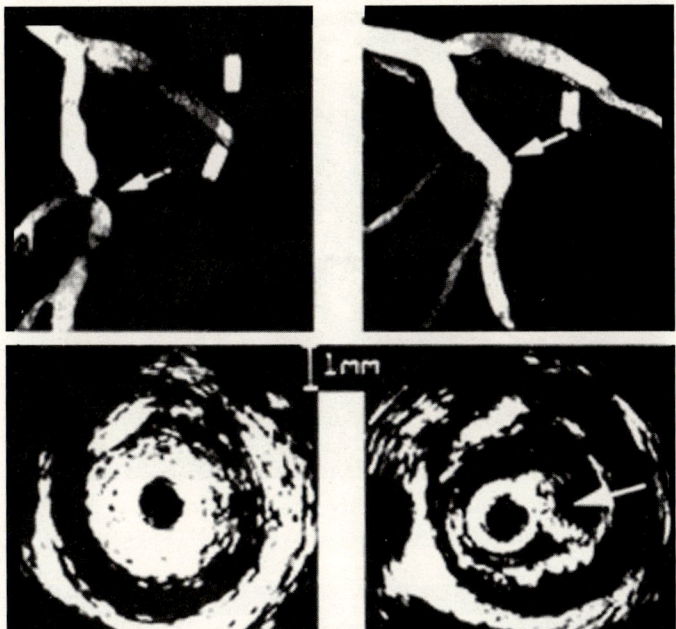

Fig. 9.5: A lesion in the mid-left circumflex which was treated by PTCA. Left pre-intervention; Right, post PTCA. Despite the good angiographic result, IVUS showed multiple dissection planes one of which impinges on the IVUS catheter (white arrow) A stent was positioned in that place

Plaque formations can be eccentric or concentric. Unstable "vulnerable" plaque, can be visualised by IVUS as the thin fibrous cap which is more echogenic with a sonolucent lipid core. Spontaneous plaque rupture is sometimes evident in IVUS examination of culprit lesion in patients with acute coronary syndromes. There are limitations to ultrasound plaque characterisation. IVUS can delineate the thickness and echogenicity of vessel wall structures, but does not provide actual histology. The echogenicity and texture of different histological features may exhibit comparable acoustic properties and therefore appear quite similar by IVUS. A sonolucent plaque may represent intra-coronary thrombus, while a nearly identical appearance may result from an atheroma with high lipid content. Despite these limitations, classification of coronary plaques into soft, fibrous and calcific has significant clinical implications, and the way of response to interventional devices.

Ultrasonic Measurement of Coronary Lumen in CAD:
It is known that atherosclerotic invasion of coronary artery frequently produces far complex and eccenteric lesions. It is therefore, imperative to apply tomographic imaging technique with intravascular ultrasound which might yield measurements that differed significantly from invasive angiography. Quantitative luminal measurement is determined by planimetry of the circumference of the leading edge of the blood-intima acoustic interface. Review of the videotape with the vessel in motion may assist in accurate edge-detection.

The total cross-sectional area (CSA) of the vessel is defined as the area enclosed by the interface between the media and adventitia, the leading edge of the EEM. Minimum lumen diameter (MLD) and maximal lumen diameter are also measured in reference to the central point of lumen.

IVUS Analysis of Area Stenosis

Validation of normal anatomy, plaque composition, and measurements determined using IVUS have been reported. The external elastic membrane (EEM) **cross-sectional area** (CSA) was measured by tracing the leading edge of the adventitia. The lesion site was the **c cross-sectional** slice with the smallest **lumen**; among sections with the same **lumen area,** the one with the most plaque was selected. If the plaque was "packed" around the catheter, the **lumen** was assumed to be the physical (not acoustical) **size of** the catheter. Because IVUS cannot measure media thickness accurately, plaque and media (P and M) were measure of plaque mass. **Cross-sectional** narrowing (CSN) has also been called the plaque burden or percent plaque **area.** The reference segment averaged the most visually normal **cross**-sections (largest **lumen** with least plaque) within 10 mm proximal and distal to the lesion but between major branches; a distal references was used for ostial lesions.

Plaque composition was assessed visually. Calcium was brighter than the reference adventitia, with shadowing of deeper structures; the arc of calcium was measured with a protractor centered on the **lumen**. Hyperechoic, nonclacified plaque was as bright or brighter than the adventitia.

Using computer planimetry (TapeMeasure, Indec Systems), the following lesion and reference measurements were made in diastole: EEMCSA, **lumen** CSA, MLD, P and M (EEM-**lumen** CSA), and CSN (P and M/EEM). The lesion was compared with the reference to calculate **area** stenosis (AS) as shown:

Area stenosis =

$$\frac{\text{Mean reference lumen CSA} - \text{Lesion lumen CSA}}{\text{Mean reference lumen CSA}} \times 100$$

In one of the studies coronary vascular ultrasonography also tries to separate angiographically normal and those patients having atherosterotic pathology. In the normal subjects, the circular shape factor averaged 0.92 ± 0.2, showing the nearly circular lumen shape in patients with normal coronary arteries. In these normal subjects, the correlation between angiographic and ultrasound coronary diameter for normal subjects is very much close, $r = 0.92$. Thus, intravascular ultrasound and angiography yield comparable measurements of lumen size in normal, non-atherosclerotic arteries with a circular lumen profile.

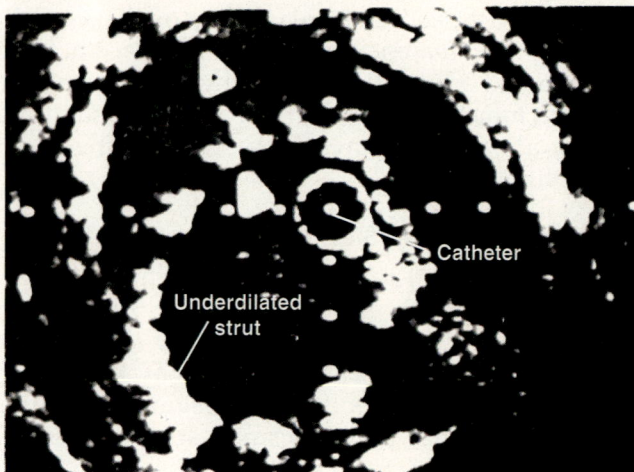

Fig. 9.6: Underdilated/unapposed struts in the coronary artery

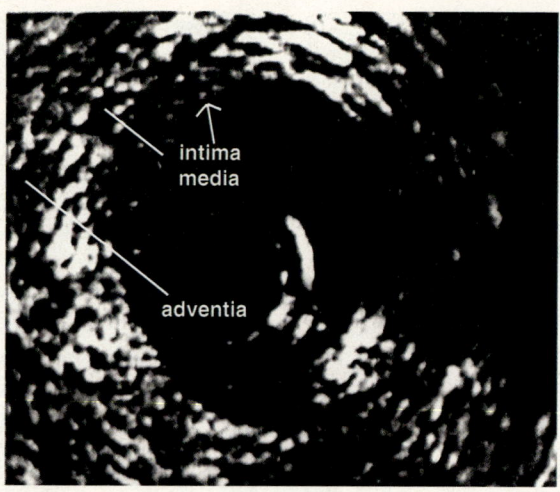

Fig. 9.9: Three layers of coronary artery, i.e from inner to outside are intima,media and adventia as seen in this IVUS image

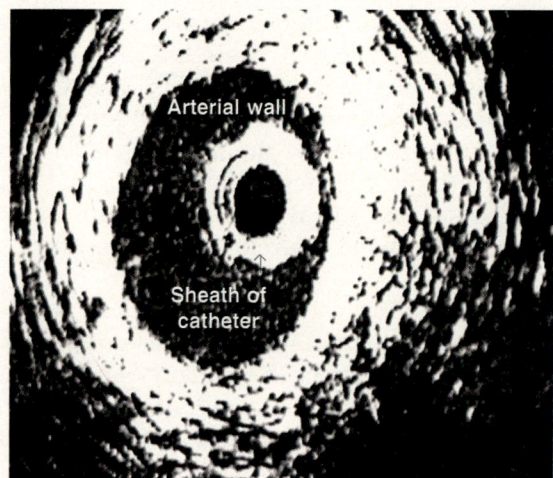

Fig. 9.7: Ultrasound of the normal artery. Inner black circle is the ring artefact due to the catheter sheath (arrow). Outer circle is the interface of the arterial wall

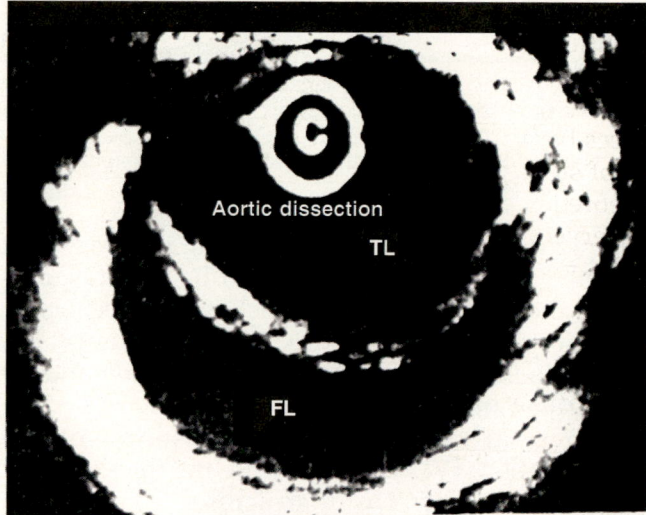

Fig. 9.10: Ultrasound images from aortic dissection C = Catheter, TL = True lumen. FL = False lumen

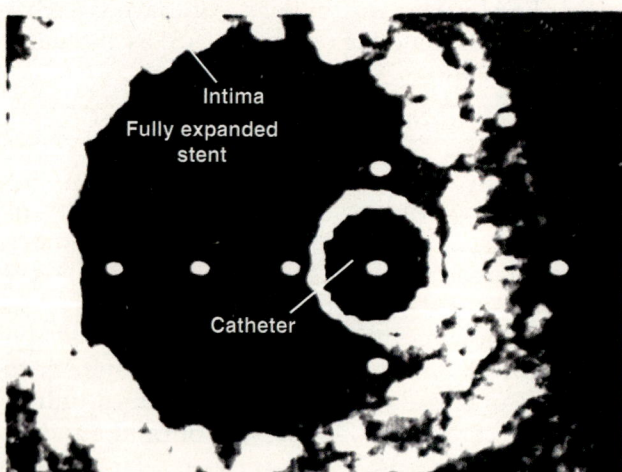

Fig. 9.8: Fully expanded stent in a coronary artery with its struts well apposed in the intima, resulting into large cross sectional area of the lumen

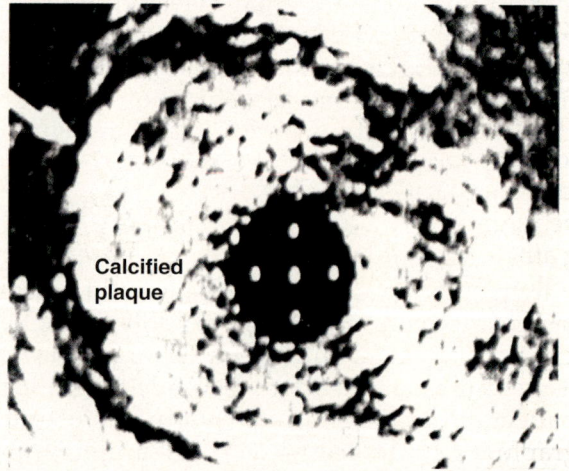

Fig. 9.11: IVUS Showing calcification of an atheromatous plaque in the coronary artery. Arrow marks the echolucent effect caused by absorption of ultrasound waves by calcium

In approximately 67% of CAD segments, the diseased lumen remained concentric in shape (CSF>0.92) and the correlation between ultrasound and angiography is also close, $r = 0.93$. However, the subgroup of CAD patients with an eccentric lumen demonstrated significant disagreement between angiography and ultrasound diameter, $r = 0.78$. This kind of reduced correlation is explained by the irregular, noncircular lumen shape encountered in these atherosclerotic vessels.

Both techniques of angiography and coronary ultrasonography can visualise focal stenosis at 41 sites. Coronary ultrasonography cross-sectional area reduction is estimated from angiography using diameter measurements. At identical sites, stenosis measurements from digitized ultrasound images are performed by planimetry of the lumen. Mean stenosis severity, expressed as percent luminal area reduction, is similar by cineangiography, $48.9 \pm 13.8\%$, and intravascular ultrasound, $52.3 \pm 16.3\%$ ($p = 0.10$). However, the correlation between percent stenosis by cineangiography and ultrasound is only moderate, $r = 0.63$. It therefore, demonstrates that there are important differences between ultrasonic and angiographic assessment of stenosis severity.

Theoretic Perimeter = 9.58 mm
Observed Perimeter = 10.16 mm
CSF = $\frac{9.58}{10.16}$ = 0.88

Clinical Applications of IVU

It can be divided into two categories:

1. Diagnostic Applications (Figs 9.1 and 9.14)

Angiographically Normal Coronary Arteries: In patients with clinical symptoms of CAD and normal angiogram, IVUS commonly detects atherosclerosis in upto half of such patients.

Assessment of Intermediate Stenosis: Coronary angiography underestimates the severity most notably in vessel with 40 to 75 percent luminal narrowing. IVUS can delineate the thickness and echogenicity of vessel wall structures, but not the actual histology.

Coronary Remodelling: This phenomenon was first described by Galgov *et al.*, from necropsy specimens; positive remodelling refers to the increase in EEM area during atheroma development, negative or constrictive remodelling refers to decrease in EEM area, both the processes could be assessed by IVUS.

Assessment of Transplant Vasculopathy: CAD is the major cause of death beyond first year post-transplant. Most patients in this category have silent ischaemia on angiography performed annually, the diffuse nature of the disease impairs the detection by coronary angiography. Accordingly, IVUS has emerged as the optimal method of early detection of intimal thickening in cardiac transplants vasculopathy. Most ultrasound studies define the threshold of transplant vasculopathy as intimal thickness more than 0.5 mm.

Assessment of Ambiguous Lesion: These include (Figs. 9.6–9.11):

1. Left main stem lesion.
2. Ostial lesion.
3. Aneurysmal lesion.
4. Sites with plaque rupture.
5. Filling defect.
6. Hazy lesions.
7. Bifurcation lesions and tortuous vessels. IVUS can provide additional evidence useful in the management plan.
8. Syndrome X, myocardial bridging and coronary artery spasm. A majority of patients with syndrome X have abnormal coronary arteries (atheroma or marked intimal thickening) by IVUS, despite a normal angiogram. Similarly, atherosclerotic plaque frequently detected proximal to bridging segments by IVUS and finally, significant atherosclerotic thickening is shown by IVUS at the site of focal vasospasm (Fig. 9.15A and B).

Assessment Progression Regression of CAD (Fig. 9.14): Angiographic studies in this field have shown minimal changes in luminal dimensions following the antiatherosclerotic treatment. IVUS is ideally suited for atherosclerosis regression-progression studies, because of ability to detect very small changes in atheroma volume. Several large scale IVUS regression/progression studies of atherosclerosis are currently underway, including the Norvasc for Regression of Manifest Atherosclerotic Lesions by Intravascular Sonographic Evaluation of a multicentre trial comparing the effect of atorvastatin and pravastatin on the progression and quantitation of coronary atherosclerotic lesions measured by IVUS.

2. Interventional Applications (Figs 9.12A–D and 9.13A–C)

Target Lesion Assessment: It can be performed pre-intervention, sequentially during the procedure, post-intervention and at follow-up. The small diameter of contemporary ultrasound imaging catheters permits interrogation of most coronary lesions prior to mechanical interventions. This may improve the selection of the length and size of the balloon, especially in a diffuse atherosclerotic involvement. IVUS is a useful adjunct in assessing the result of PTCA. Studies show a poor correlation between ultrasound and angiography in assessing the residual stenosis following angioplasty. Luminal CSA following angioplasty is generally smaller by ultrasound than by angiography.

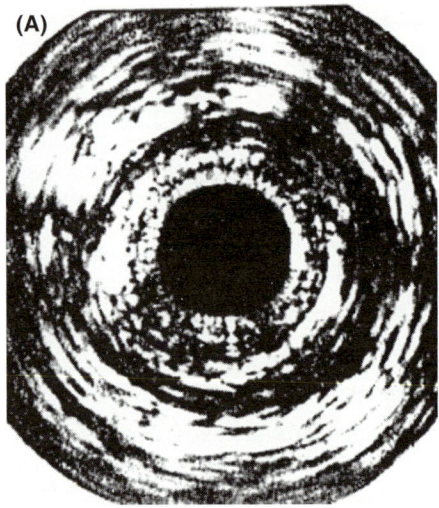

(A)

Before injection of radiographic material

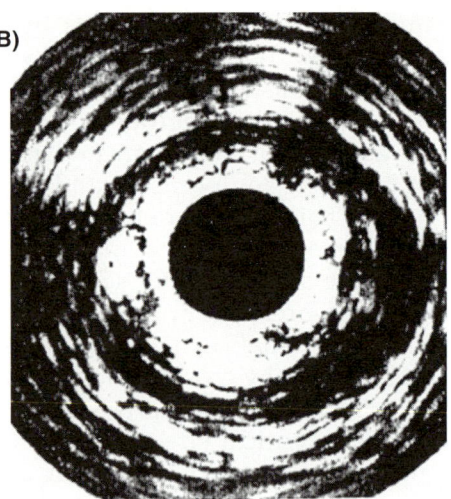

(B)

Enhancement of IVUS image after injection

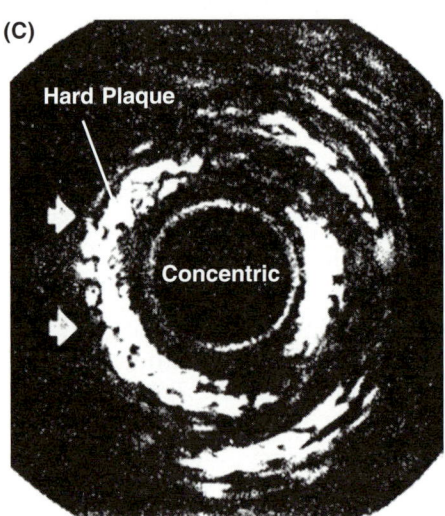

(C)

Hard Plaque

Concentric

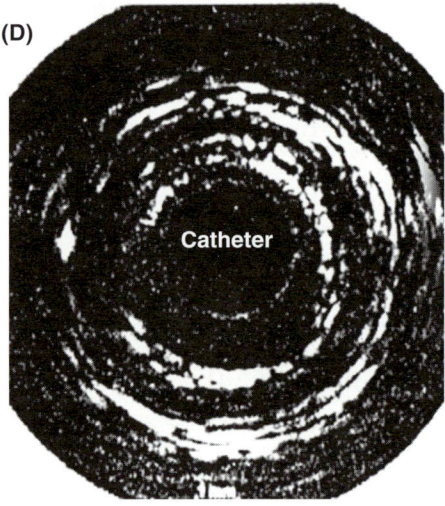

(D)

Catheter

Fig. 9.12 A to D: (A) and **(B)** Intravascular ultrasound before **(A)** and after **(B)** enhancement of luminal opacification by injection of radiographic contrast material. **(C)** IVUS imaging shows dense hard plaque. The arrows indicte a greatly thickened intimal leading edge that obstructs ultrasound transmission, thus shadowing underlying structures. **(D)** IVUS showing diffuse concenteric atherosclerosis. Both the intimal leading edge and sonolucent zone are thickened, resulting in an exaggerated trilaminar appearance to the artery

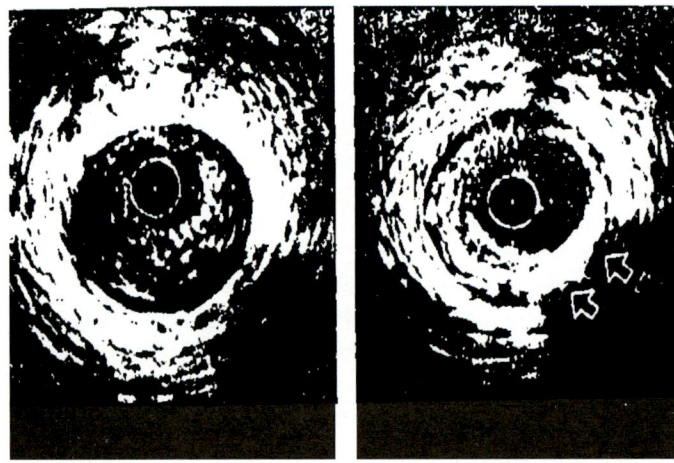

Fig. 9.13A: Right panel shows a mixed fibrocalcific plaque with arrows pointing to the acoustic shadow. Left panel shows a soft plaque

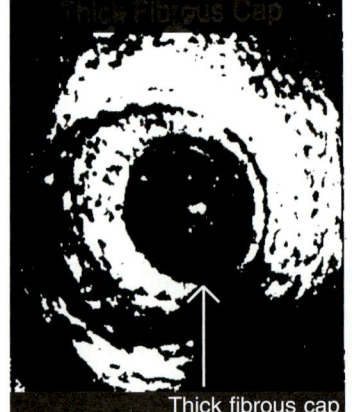
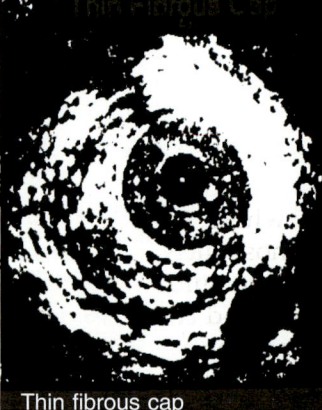

Thick fibrous cap   Thin fibrous cap

Fig. 9.13B: Left panel showing a stable chronic plaque with thick fibrous cap. Right panel shows unstable plaque with the typical thin fibrous cap

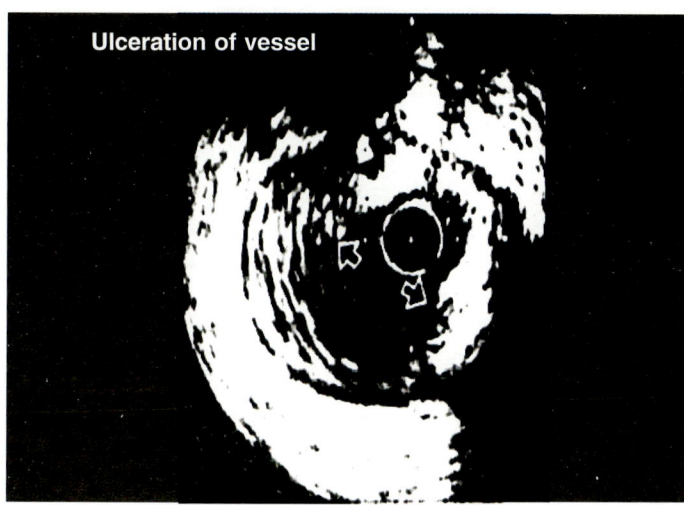

Fig. 9.13C: A ruptured plaque. Arrows pointing to the ulceration edges

Assessment of Lesion Restenosis: To assess the restenotic process, the image slice with the smallest lumen area at follow-up is identified and compared to the same image slice on the post-intervention and pre-intervention studies, using measurements from a fiduciary point or by identifying vascular or perivascular markings. Studies have shown conflicting data regarding the factors predictive of restenosis. Some investigators have suggested that a late reduction in total vessel area (chronic negative remodelling) represents an important mechanism. However, the proportion of lumen loss after intervention produced by vessel shrinkage versus neointimal proliferation remains inadequately defined.

IVUS and In-stent Restenosis: Serial studies both post-intervention and at follow-up can be used to determine whether in-stent restenosis is severe enough to treat and to assess the various mechanisms of in-stent restenosis. These include inadequate stent deployment (under expanded/incompletely opposed), intimal hyperplasia and chronic stent recoil. IVUS has a definite role in detecting complications of intervention. There are many potential complications of percutanous coronary intervention, including, for example, dissection perforation, intramural haematoma, where IVUS represents an ideal imaging tool to diagnose such problems and treat accordingly. It is also useful in guidance of rotational ablation. Rotablator is a diamond coated burr used to debulk plaque within the coronary stenosis. If preinterventional IVUS is available, rotational ablation is commonly employed when the superficial calcium arc exceeds 180 in multiple cross-sections along stenotic segment. Ultrasound can size the vessel and determine the largest burr that can be safely employed (Fig. 9.5).

Ultrasound and Complex Stent Procedures

IVUS is most often used in stenting of small arteries, often corresponding to diffuse disease by ultrasound. Ultrasound guidance is most useful in complex stent procedures such as long stenoses, dissections, or implantation of multiple stents. In these lesions, the additional lumen gain achieved with further ultrasound driven interventions is potentially useful, not only to eliminate subacute thromobosis but also to reduce in-stent restenosis.

IVUS and Brachytherapy: Intravascular ultrasound can be used to study the mechanisms and results of strategies to reduce restenosis, including this new modality. IVUS was used in the Beta Energy Restenosis Trial (BERT) to show the effect of beta radiation in inhibiting the neointima formation. In non-stented lesions, serial (post-radiation versus follow-up) analysis of lesion site and reference segment EEM, lumen and plaque plus media volume is the most accurate approach. In stented lesions, measurements should include serial (post-radiation versus follow-up) volumetric analysis of the stent, lumen, intimal hyperplasia volumes and wherever possible, measurement of serial analysis of EEM volumes as well.

Ultrasound and Complex Stent Procedures: The technology and role for intravascular ultrasound examination of the coronary arteries are still rapidly evolving. Important technical advances include further reductions in the size of imaging catheters and development of improved devices combining a small imaging transducer (l.16 mm) and low profile angioplasty balloon (0.028–0.033 inch) are undergoing large-scale trials. Other investigational approaches include transducers mounted on atherectomy devices and laser delivery systems. If such devices provide practical assistance to revascularization procedures, combination imaging and therapy devices have the potential of becoming the future standard for angioplasty techniques.

Researchers are also busy in manufacturing imaging catheters that incorporate a tip mounted Doppler flow probe to allow simultaneous cross-sectional area and flow velocity measurements. Secondly forward looking probes with ability to examine downstream sites to permit imaging of coronaries with diameters smaller than existing transducers are also under consideration. Other research is examining the utility of 3-dimensional reconstruction of a series of tomographic coronary images. Although visually appealing, 3-dimensional reconstruction are largely artificial because the image are generated during a pull-back through a coronary segment. During the pull-back procedure, the transducer invariable shifts position or angulation in the lumen, a confounding variable not accounted for by current reconstruction techniques unless alternative or its modification is invented in near future.

Limitations of Intravascular Ultrasound

Inspite of considerable technical progress in catheter design, one may find important limitations to intravascular ultrasound imaging of small coronaries or tight stenosis and precludes examination of most lesions prior to balloon angioplasty. The smallest size of currently available coronary imaging devices is slightly more than 1.0 cm. Its further reduction in size may also be limited as it reduces available acoustic power and thus compromises signal to noise ratio.

Currently available vascular ultrasound catheter design is unable to visualise the calcific lesions or plaque as heavily fibrotic or calcified intimal atherosclerosis impedes transmission of the low energy, high frequency ultrasound signals utilised for intravascular imaging. Presence of shadowing plaques may preclude measurement of atheroma area because the full thickness of the vessel wall is obscured.

The mechanical transducers, with their rotational speed may increase or decrease because of mechanical drag, particularly when the drive shaft is bent by a tortuous coronary, resulting into nonuniform rotational velocity which may produce a distinctive and troublesome distortion of the image. Improvements in the mechanical precision of these devices have reduced, but not eliminated, nonuniform rotational distortion.

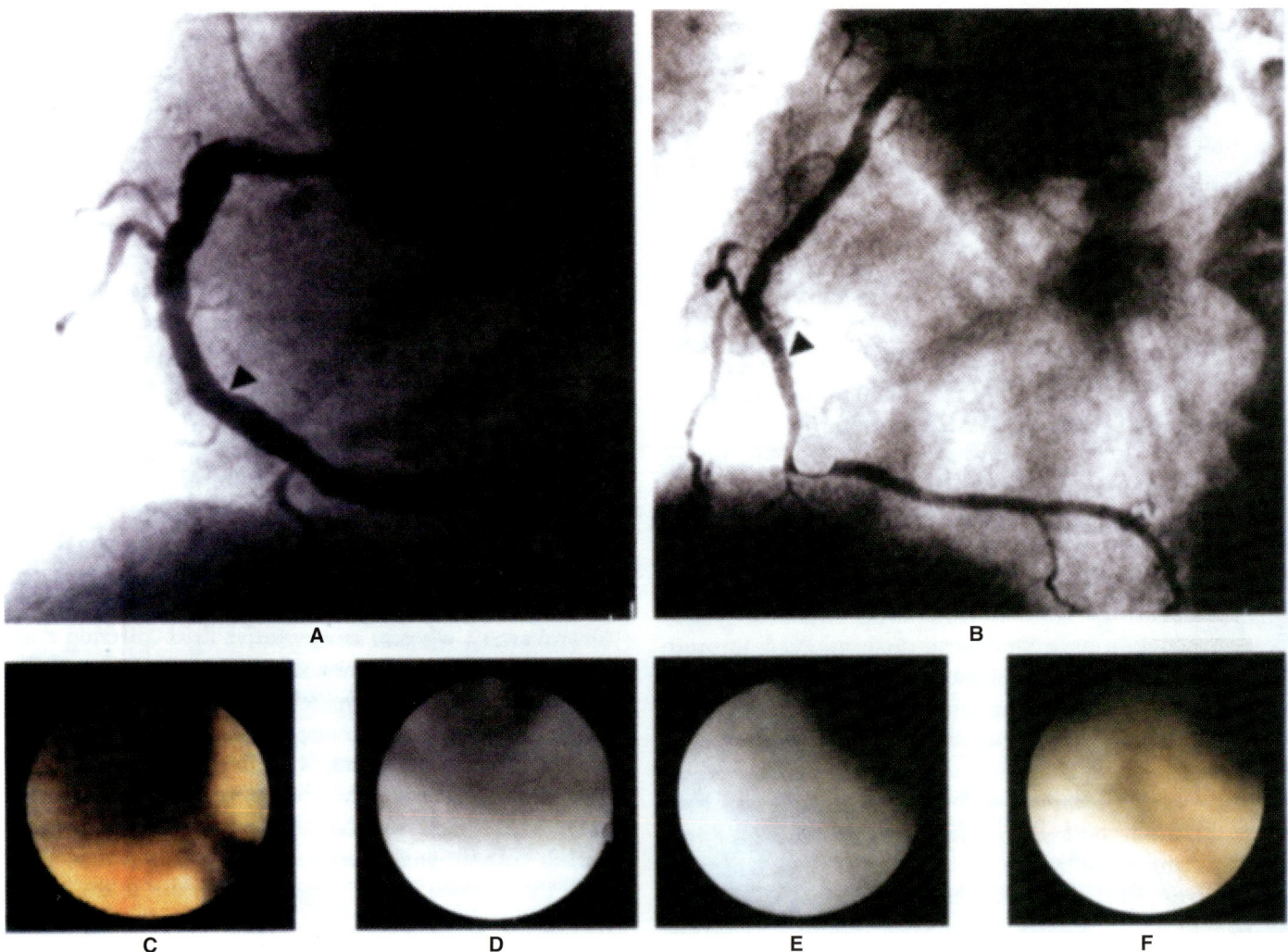

Fig. 9.14A to F: (A) Right coronary angiogram of a patient in atorvastatin study. **(B)** A right coronary angiogram of a patient in the comparison group. **(C)** Yellow plaque in a patient in the atorvastatin group at baseline. Yellow plaque was observed in the mid portion of the right coronary artery at baseline (arrow). The surface of this plaque was smooth, and a thrombus was not found. **(D)** White plaque in a patient in the atorvastatin group at follow up. After treatment with atorvastatin, the yellow plaque changed into a completely white plaque. Both the yellow score and disrupted score were zero. **(E)** Yellow plaque in a patient in the comparison group at baseline. Yellow plaque was observed in the mid portion of of the right coronary artery at baseline (arrow in B) The surface of this plaque was smooth and a thrombus was not noted. **(F)** Yellow plaque in a patient in the comparison group at follow up. After 12 months of follow up neither plaque nor thrombus could be detected. It therefore shows that therapy with atorvastatin in a patient with atheromatous plaque not only can change its morphology but it can sufficiently reduce its size and thrombus may disappear after longterm treatment with atorvastatin in appropriate doses

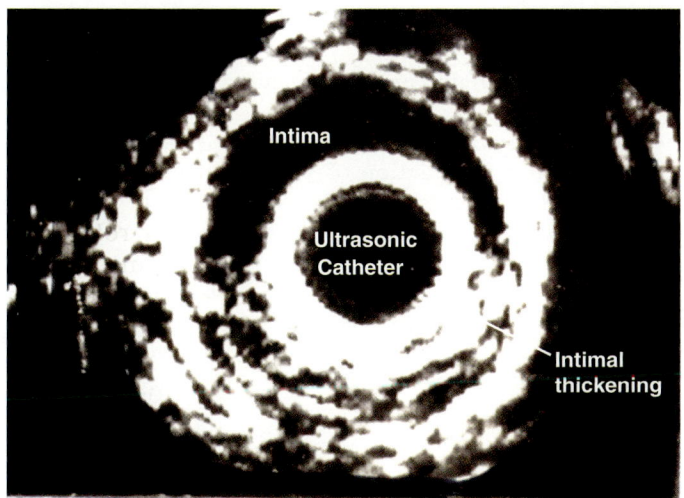

Fig. 9.15A: IVUS of coronary artery showing atherosclerotic thickening of intima and media at 3–9 o' clock position

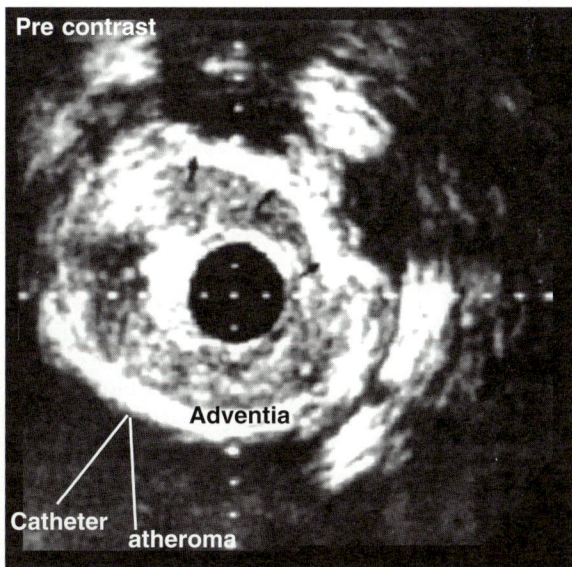

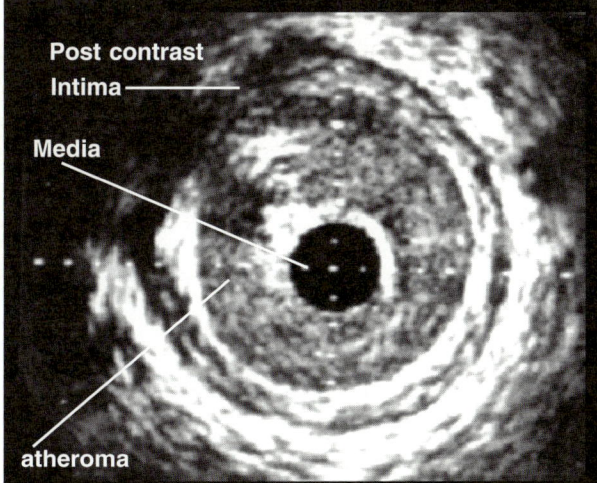

Fig. 9.15B: IVUS comparing pre and post contrast scans. All the three layers of coronary artery are affected by the atherosclerosis which is visualized much better in post contrast scan

All tomographic imaging techniques, including intravascular ultrasound, are vulnerable to distortion produced by oblique imaging planes. Thus, a vessel with circular cross-sectional profile will appear elliptical whenever the transducer is not orthogonal to the long axis of the vessel. This phenomenon can represent a confounding variable in quantitative measurements. However, nonorthogonal orientation is more prevalent in the larger vessels encountered during peripheral vascular imaging; for the small size of the coronaries limits the extent of angulation.

Emerging Applications for Coronary Ultrasound

Published studies support several emerging applications for intravascular ultrasound. Precision measurements of coronary luminal diameter and cross-sectional area may have incremental value in assessment of eccentrically diseased vessels. The tomographic perspective of intravascular ultrasound is likely superior to planar methods such as angiography for cross-sectional area measurement. The advantages of tomographic imaging are particularly evident in the assessment of results of these catheter-based revascularization procedures because it is difficult for angiography to characterise the complex alterations in the vessel wall produced by balloon, laser or atherectomy procedures.

Unlike angiography which depicts only the effects of atheroselerosis on the lumen, intravascular ultrasound permits evaluation of the actual pathologic site of the disease. The ability image atheroselerotic wall abnormalities in vivo has considerable research potential. Coronary ultrasound is currently contributing to scientific understanding of the anatomy and pathophysiology of CAD, including the plaque features associated with conversion from stable to unstable angina. Measurements of the size and morphologic characteristics of plaques will enable more precise quantitation of disease progression, including the effects of pharmacologic or dietary interventions.

Intravascular ultrasound has demonstrated greater sensitivity than angiography in the detection of CAD and commonly detects atherosclerosis in angiographically normal segments. Striking atherosclerotic abnormalities are occasionally evident in patients with totally normal coronaries by an angiography. Based on this finding, it can be argued that a patient should not be dismissed as processing normal coronaries based exclusively on an angiographic images. Intravascular ultrasound has also been applied to evaluation of angiographically normal coronary arteries following cardiac transplantation, often revealing occult intimal thickening.

The indications for intravascular ultrasound during coronary angioplasty continue to evolve. Ultrasound imaging provides precise measurements of the cross-sectional area of the residual lumen and atheroma. The morphology of the vessel wall following revascular-ization may hold important clues to phenomena such as restenosis and abrupt occlusion. However, the ultimate value of ultrasound anatomy in predicting the short and long-term complications of angioplasty is not yet defined. The development of combined imaging and therapy devices will likely expand the utility of ultrasound imaging following PTCA.

The unique tomographic perspective of coronary intravascular ultrasound and the ability to image atherosclerotic plaques directly ensure a prominent role for this technology in the cardiac catheterization laboratory of the future.

Bibliography

1. Bech A, Milic S, Spagnoli AM, Mudinger A, Blum U. The clinical value of percutaneous transluminal angioscopy. Angioscopic findings in primary vascular diagnosis and in interventional radiology. *Clin Radiology* 1989; 131:93–105.

2. Beyer-Enke SA, Zeitler E. Angioplasty and angioscopy . *Curr Opin Radiol* 1989; 1: 183–185.

3. Escobar A, White CJ, Ramee SR, Collins TJ. Coronary angioscopy in ischemic heart disease: insights into pathophysiology (abstr.) *Circulation* 1993; 88: 1–550.

4. Etsuda H, Mizuno K, Arakawa K, Satomura K, Shibuya T, Isojima K. Angioscopy in variant angina: coronary artery spasm and intimal injury. *Lancet* 1993; 342:1322–1324.

5. Giacomino PP, Abela GS, Barbeau GR, Seeger JM, Tomaru T, Akins W, Hawkins IF, Fried ISE. Angioscopy: current techniques. *Dynamic cardiovascular imaging* 1989; 2:178–187.

6. Goldberg SL, Colombo A, Nakamura S, Alamgor Y, *et al.* Benefit of Intracoronary ultrasound in the deployment of Palmaz Schatz stents. *J. Am Coll Cardiol* 1994; 24:996–1003.

7. Gruntzig AR, Senning A, Seegenthaler WE. Nonoperative dilatation of coronary artery stenosis. Percutaneous transluminal coronary angioplasty. *N. Engl J Med* 1979; 301:61–68.

8. Hoskins D. Angioscopy management. *Br. J. Theatre Nurs* 1994; 3:8–9.

9. Itoh A, Miyazaki S, Nonogi H, Daikoku S, Haze K. Angioscopic prediction of successful dilation and of restenosis in percutaneous transluminal coronary angioplasty. Significance of yellow plaque. *Circulation* 1995; 91:1389–1396.

10. Mizuno K, Arai T, SatomuraK, Shibuya T, Arakawa K, Okamoto Y, Miyamoto A, Kurita A, Kikuchi M, Nakamura H. New percutaneous transluminal coronary angioscope. *J Am Coll* Cardiol 1989; 13:363–368.

11. Mizuno K, Arakawa K, Isojima K, Shibuya T, Satomura K, Kurita A, Nakamura H, Arai T, Kikuchi M. Angioscopy coronary thrombi and acute coronary syndromes. *Biomed Pharmacother* 1993; 47: 187–191.

12. Mizuno K. Angioscopic examination of the coronary arteries: what have we learned? *Heart Dis Stroke* 1992; 1: 320–324.

13. Nissen SE, Gurley JC, Grines CL, Booth DC, MC Clure R, Berk M, Fischer C, DeMaria AN. Intravascular ultrasound assessment of lumen size and wall morphology in normal subjects and patients with coronary artery disease. *Circulation* 1991; 84:1087–99.

14. Ramee SR, White CJ, Collins TJ. Percutaneous angioscopy during coronary angioplasty using a steerable micro-angioscope. *J Am Coll Cardiol* 1991; 17: 100–105.

15. Resar JR and Brinker J. Early coronary artery stent restenosis Cathet Cardiovasc Diagn 1992;27:276–279.

16. Rickenbacher PR, Pinto FJ, Lewis NP. Prognostic importance of intracoronary ultrasound after cardiac transplantation. *Circulation* 1994; 90:641.

17. Sumida S, Masuda M, Furuyama M. Visualization and recording of intravascular details by fiberoptic angioscopy: the Sumida cardioangioscope. *J Cardiovasc Surg* 1988; 29:177–180.

18. Uchida Y. Percutaneous coronary angioscopy by means of a fiberscope with a steerable guide wire. *Am Heart* J 1989; 117: 1153–1155.

19. White CJ, Ramee SR, Percutaneous angioscopy during coronary angioscopy before and after angioplasty in acute myocardial infarction: Preliminary results (abtr). *Circulation* 1987.

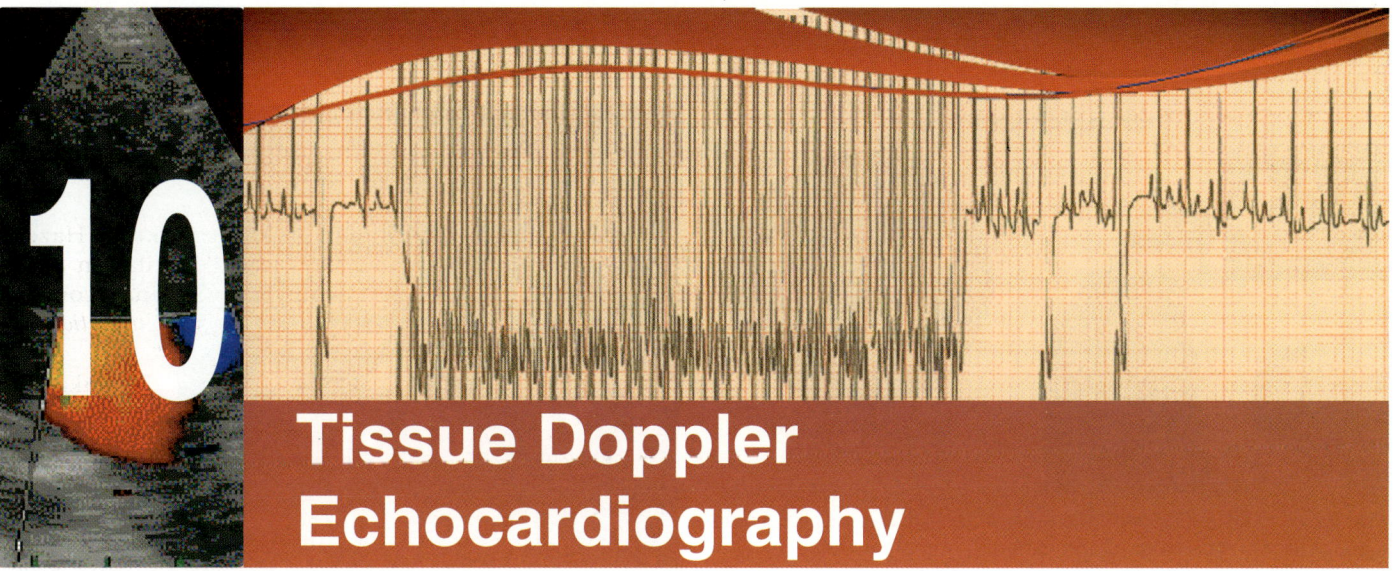

10

Tissue Doppler Echocardiography

Echocardiography is considered as reliable technology for the noninvasive evaluation of regional and global myocardial function. However the existing two-dimensional (2-D) techniques have two noticeable drawbacks:

(a) 2-Dimensional echocardiographic imaging using a grey scale does not always provide effective visualization of the endocardial border for a proper evaluation of regional wall motion in a significant subset of patients.

(b) Analysis of regional wall motion has a considerable learning curve and being semi-qualitative in nature, has substantial inter- and intraobserver variability. Workers have been engaged for many years in searching one of the superior techniques to quantify regional and global myocardial function till they focused their efforts towards a newly described noninvasive technique of tissue Doppler echocardiography. It is a new ultrasound technique that uses shifts in Doppler frequencies for quantifying myocardial motion and it does not depend on the amplitude of the reflected wave. It is possible to get information regarding myocardial wall motion from an area that may not have satisfactory grey-scale information on 2-D echocardiography. In its earlier application, tissue velocity imaging (TVI) was only limited to real-time visualisation of only a single myocardial segment but subsequent technical advancements in colour-coded TVI and other technical improvements had enable us to use superior temporal and spatial resolution for simultaneous quantification of velocity data from multiple segments of the myocardium. Till recently TVI has emerged not only as a nobel technique for quan-

tifying the nature and the extent of myocardial dysfunction in investigation of heart ailments, but it also becomes an important pivot for strain rate imaging.

Technique (Fig. 10.1A, B and C)

In its practical application, Doppler shifts obtained from myocardial tissue motion are of high amplitudes, about 40 dB higher, and move about 10 times slower than the red blood cells with a velocity ranging from 0.06 to 0.24 m/s. It is, therefore, possible to display regional myocardial velocities by using thresholding and filtering algorithms that reject the echoes originating from the blood pool. The velocity information can be displayed as either colour-coded data in real-time or pulse tissue Doppler. Similar to the routine colour flow instrumentation. Colour-coded TVI also uses autocorrelator technique to calculate and display multigated points of colour-coded velocities along a series of ultrasound scan lines within a 2-D sector. The velocity data are then superimposed on the grey-scale images in real-time. Doppler shifts resulting from wall motion are also filtered out to obtain low-velocity tissue motion. When using colour TVI, the 2-D gain settings should be reduced for optimal colour display of myocardial velocities. The displayed colour maps represent mean myocardial velocities rather than peak velocities. The information is stored in an interfoiled format with grey scale during one or several cardiac cycles at high temporal resolution, giving signals that can tolerate mathematical processing such as derivation, integration and Fourier analysis of velocity profiles without distortion. The colour information can also be presented in cine-loops, phase imaging, time-delay imaging, amplitude imaging, acceleration imaging and instantaneous phase imaging. The over-

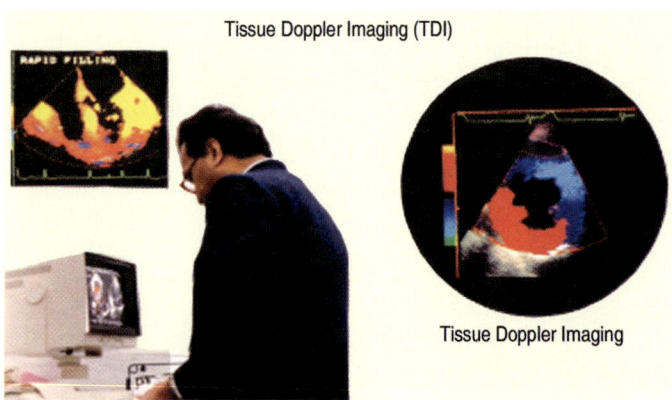

Fig. 10.1A: Tissue Doppler laboratory of the private hospital where most of the records were analysed by the author himself

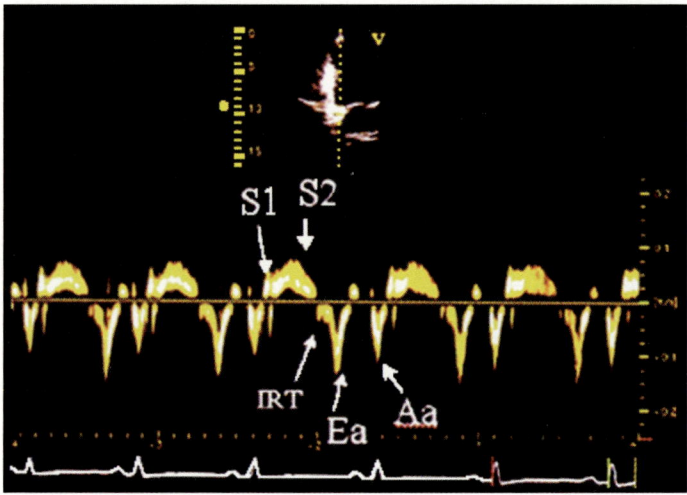

Fig. 10.2A: High frame rate pulsed Doppler myocardial imaging in a normal healthy individual showing longitudinal tissue velocites from the septal corner of the mitral annulus. (S1 Tissue velocity wave in the isometeric contraction period. S2; Velocity wave in ejection period; IRT; Velocity wave in isovolumic relaxation period. Ea; and Aa velocity waves in early and late diastolic relaxation respectively)

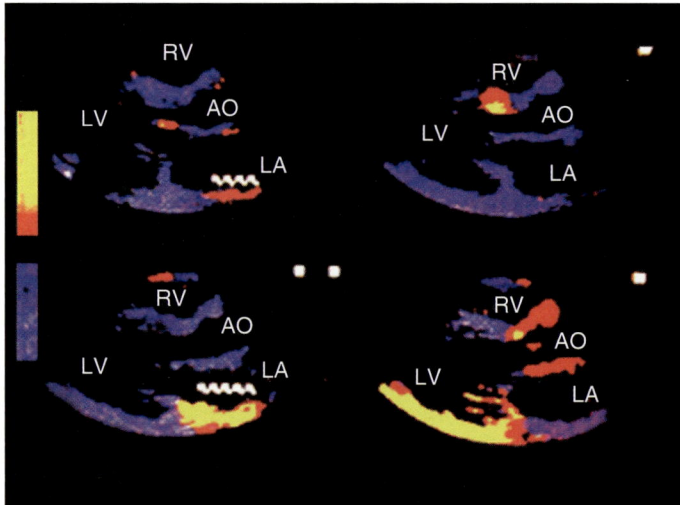

Fig. 10.1B: Quad scan of tissue Doppler imaging showing normal sequence of activation, early diastole, mid diastole, atrial contraction and early systole

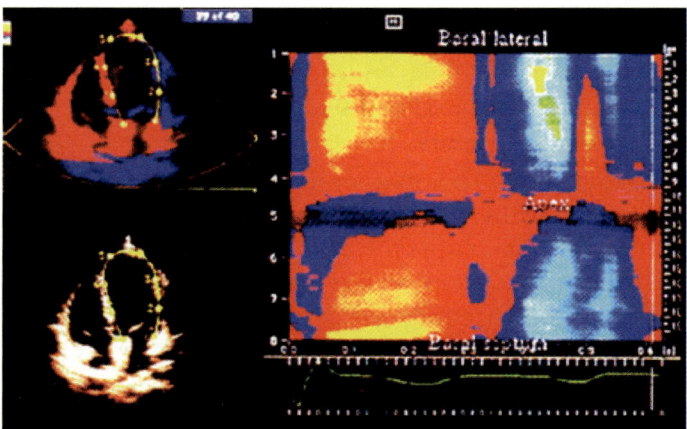

Fig. 10.2B: Offline color Doppler myocardial imaging for obtaining tissue velocity by employing curved M-mode echogram in function of time

all imaging can be optimized by altering one or more of the following parameters—velocity range and nyquist limits, colour gain, pulse-repeating frequency. Several post-processing algorithms are available. Velocity data from a region of interest can be arranged to obtain spectral displays of tissue velocities. These spectral displays resemble pulse tissue Doppler in their waveform but are smaller in peak values, as they are computed waveforms from mean velocity data. Colour data can also be displayed in standard M-mode or curved M-mode for better spatial resolution and correlation. Colour TVI is visually appealing and discloses differential velocities in all layers of the heart. This can be used for calculating myocardial velocity

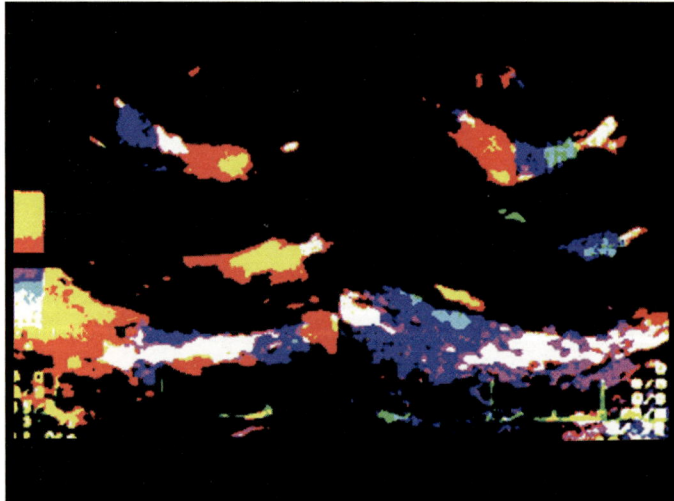

Fig. 10.1C: TDI Scan showing normal characteristics of various intracardiac structure in systole and diastole through left parasternal long axis view

gradients among different layers of the heart. The main disadvantage of colour TVI is the requirement for an off-line analysis for quantifying myocardial velocities, which can be time-consuming.

Pulse wave tissue Doppler provides a spectral display of the peak tissue velocities with tissue velocities in the y-axis and time in the x-axis. A sample gate of about 1 cm is used and directed to assess the region of interest. Appropriate scale, sweep speed and low-gain settings are used for optimizing the spectral display. An advantage of pulsed TVI is an improved temporal resolution and the ability to quantify peak rather than mean myocardial velocities. It does not require off-line analysis and provides instantaneous display of the spectral Doppler information. Its limitation, however, is its inability to obtain data from more than one site at a given time. Also, specific sample placements into the epicardium and subendocardial layers cannot be done simultaneously.

Normal Myocardial Tissue Velocities

Proper recording of tissue Doppler waveforms which are known to vary in their peak velocity and character and inturn are very much dependant upon the angle of the Doppler beam in relation to the axis of the myocardial motion. Velocity is highest if the incident beam is parallel to the axis of cardiac motion. However, myocardial motion is complex and includes longitudinal shortening, radial contraction, rotation, translation and respiratory movements. The origin of tissue velocities can be traced to the specific orientation and arrangement of muscle fibers in the myocardium. It has been shown that the fibers situated in the endocardium and epicardium are longitudinally oriented and result in longitudinal shortening of myocardium. Circumferential fibers are present in the midwall of the myocardium. Tension develops first in the longitudinal fibers during the initial ventricular activation. Shortening occurs first in the longitudinal axis followed by circumferential shortening. However, unlike longitudinal shortening, circumferential fibers also produce rotation of the left ventricle (LV) in its long axis. The waveforms registered in short axis imaging, therefore, represent a summated motion of circumferential shortening and rotatory motion. Since there is hardly any technique which can simultaneously assess all the components of myocardial motion. However, there is a uniform agreement regarding the role of longitudinal shortening which is an integral part of the global contractile function and has a good correlation with the overall ejection performance of the ventricle. Longitudinal movements can be recorded from the apical views and one popular approach is to record the tissue velocities of the mitral annular region as it moves towards the transducer during systole and away during diastole. Mitral annular velocities have been shown to provide an accurate assessment of global left systolic and diastolic function. Two positive waves of myocardial shortening can be recorded in systole. The first positive wave (S_1) occurs as a result of the longitudinal shortening of the myocardial tissue during the phase of isometric contraction. The second wave (S_2) occurs due to left ventricular shortening during LV ejection. The S_1 along the long axis is greater than the S_1 along the short axis. The S_2 along the short axis is greater than that along the long axis. Thus, in healthy subjects the shortening of the longitudinal fibers predominates over that of the circumferential fibers during early systole, whereas the shortening of the circumferential fibers predominate over that of longitudinal fibers in the ejection phase.

During diastole, the first wave that appears is that of isovolumic ventricular relaxation (IVR). The diastolic expansion wave during the early rapid filling phase (Em) is normally of a higher velocity than the atrial contraction wave (Am). A recoil wave can usually be seen after high velocity movements during isovolumic contraction, relaxation or after early diastolic filling and occurs in a direction opposite to initial movement. The Em is greater along the short axis than the long axis whereas the atrial systolic wave along the long axis is greater than that along the short axis. Thus during diastole, the circumferential fibers predominate in the LV expansion at early diastole, whereas the longitudinal fibers predominate at atrial systole.

For acquiring myocardial velocities from the posterior wall and the interventricular septum, short axis view has to be constructed. Posterior wall waves resemble the waveforms of the longitudinal plane with two systolic (Sm1 and Sm2) and three diastolic waves (IVR, Em and Am). The motion of the interventricular septum is more complex as it is shared between the two ventricles. Moreover, there is a hinge point in the septum, proximal to which it moves away from the LV cavity in systole and towards the LV cavity in diastole. The part of the septum distal to it moves in the opposite direction. The tissue velocities in the later part of the septum shows two inward movements in systole, the first (Sm1) being due to isometric contraction and the second (Sm2) due to ventricular ejection. The diastolic waves show a biphasic wave in early diastole (Em' and Em) and a wave of atrial contraction (Am). The systolic and diastolic waves occur earlier in the septum as compared to the posterior wall and are consistent with the pattern of electrical activation of the septum. The reason for the biphasic motion of the septum in early diastole is not known. It may be because of translational and/or right ventricular influences.

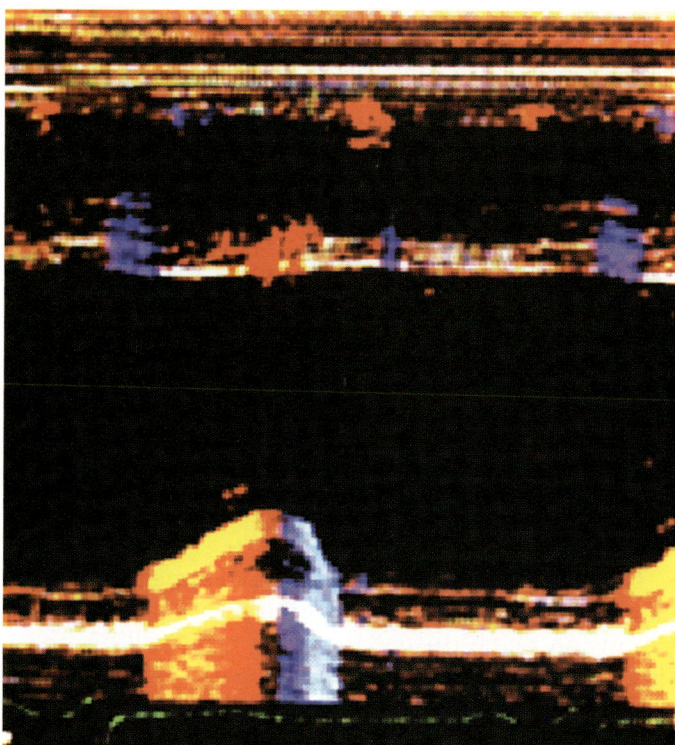

Fig. 10.3A: TDI M-mode scan showing abscence of color coding of IVS and posterior left ventricular wall in antero-septal wall

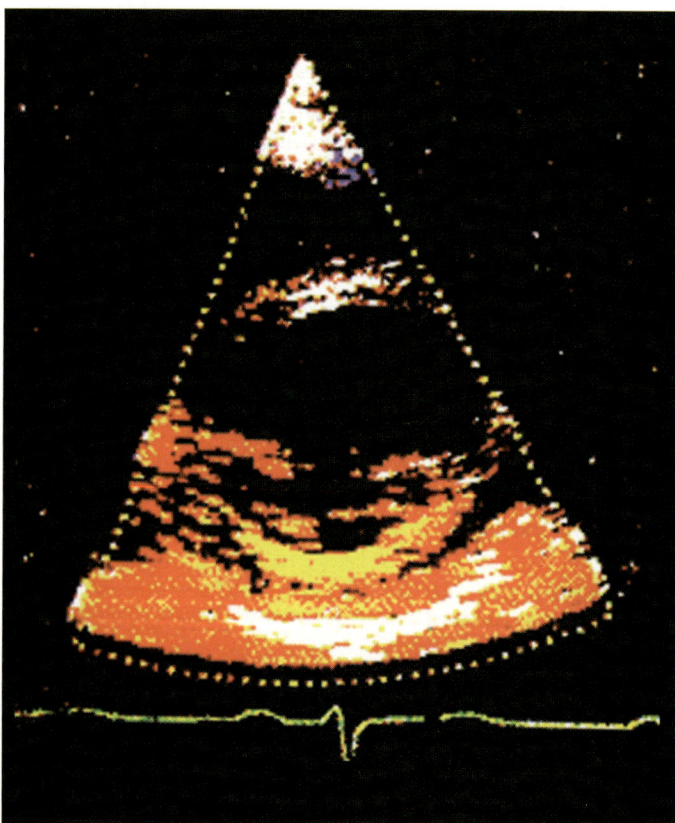

Fig. 10.3B: TDI Short axis LV showing abscence of color coding of antero-septal wall in antero-septal myocardial infarction

Lengthening and shortening velocities vary throughout the entire myocardium. As we move away from the mitral annulus to the apex, the peak systolic and diastolic myocardial velocities gradually decrease, although the Em–Am ratio remains the same. Similarily, in any myocardial segment, a dynamic myocardial gradient exists between the endocardium and the epicardium and can be determined from the velocity profile along a radial line from the centre of contraction. Normally the endocardium has a higher velocity than the epicardium and is altered in the presence of myocardial disease. The myocardial velocity gradient provides a quantitative assessment that is independent of the angle of the Doppler beam and is not affected by myocardial motion. Significant correlation of tissue velocity waves has been seen with age and heart rate. The peak Em velocity decreases proportionally with age and correlates with age-related diastolic dysfunction in the normal population. The peak S_2 wave along the long axis also varies inversely with age such that shortening of the longitudinal fibers in early systole is impaired with increasing age in healthy individuals. This impairment results in an age-related diastolic dysfunction, although global LV systolic function and myocardial contractility are maintained. Systolic myocardial velocity and Em have also been shown to be strongly dependent on both the number of myocytes and the myocardial beta-adrenergic receptor density. However, Am has no significant relation with the beta-adrenergic receptor density and this probably indicates that the late diastolic ventricular motion may be passive in nature and dependent on the atrial function alone.

Assessment of Systolic Function (Figs 10.1A, B, C and 10.2A and B)

One of the significant contributions of any type of non invasive technique would be its determination of left ventricular systolic function but are often limited by technical difficulties, inaccuracy and poor reproducibility. Currently, it is the tissue Doppler technique that has the capability to obtain information that is not completely dependant on the visibility of the endocardial border. The axial and lateral resolution of TVI is 3 × 3 mm, which provides it a resolution sufficient enough to assess the function of most myocardial segments. Although the resolution does not approach that obtained from 2-D data, it has to be realized that TVI depends entirely on Doppler data obtained from frequency shift information rather than from the reflected signal amplitude required for a grey-scale image. Thus TVI can obtain data from subjects with suboptimal echocardiographic windows and has more quantitative and reproducible information, since it decreases the wide inter-and intraobserver variability

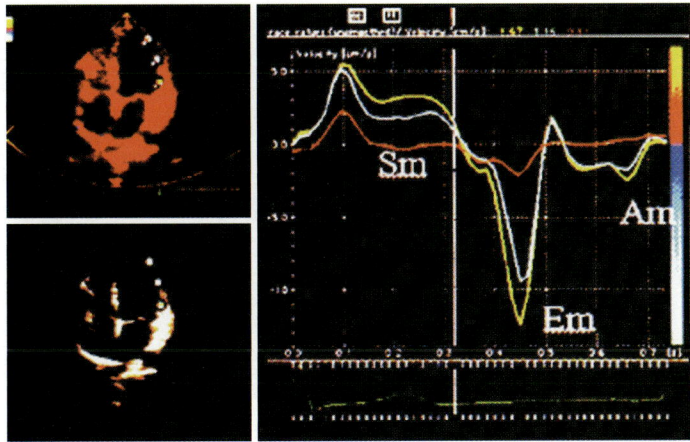

Fig. 10.4A: Color Doppler myocardial imaging data for obtaining spectral representations of mean systolic (Sm) and diastole (Em and Am) myocardial velocities from LV segments in lateral wall. It also points out normal velocity gradients as seen in normal person

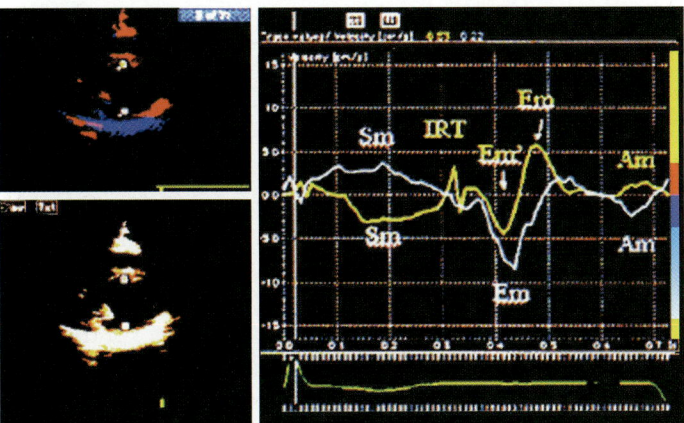

Fig. 10.4B: Short axis mean velocity taken from the IVS and posterior wall of LV showing the opposite polarity of waves from the two walls. Systolic wave in septum (Sm) is followed by a wave in isovolumic relaxation period (IRT), a biphasic wave in early diastolic relaxation period with a initial motion towards the cavity (Em^1) and a second movement away from the cavity (Em) and in late diastolic relaxation (Am)

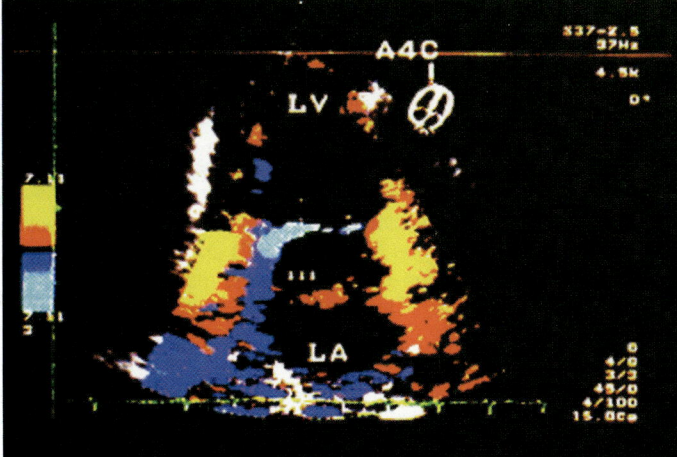

Fig. 10.5A: TDI Apical 2-C view of LV in diastole showing left atrial strand (arrows)

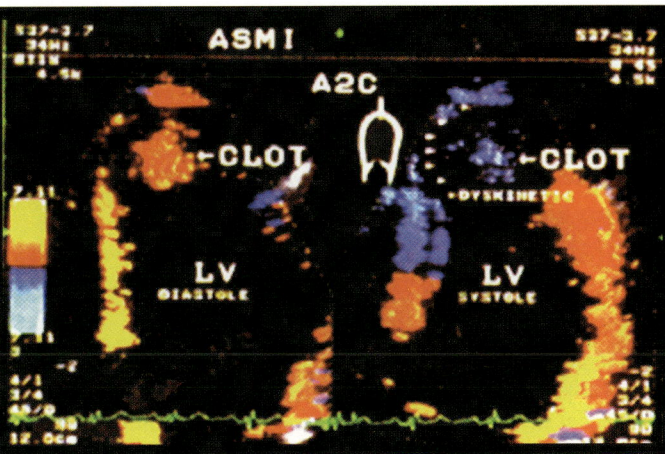

Fig. 10.5B: Color-coded TDI in apical 2-C view of LV in systole and diastole showing LV apical clot as inscribed on scan, and dyskinetic lower half of septal wall of LV

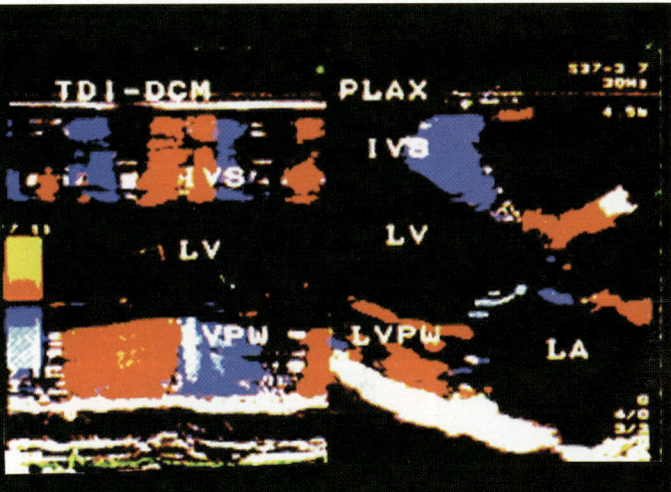

Fig. 10.6A: TDI M-mode and parasternal long axis view showing thin hypokinetic septal and posterior LV wall in dilated cardiomyopathy

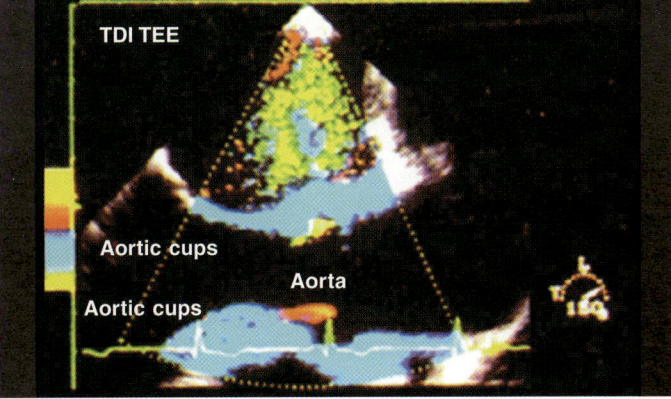

Fig. 10.6B: TEE in combination with TDI showing colors of the aortic cusps in the long axis as they start to close. The green color in LA depicts a very low blood velocity

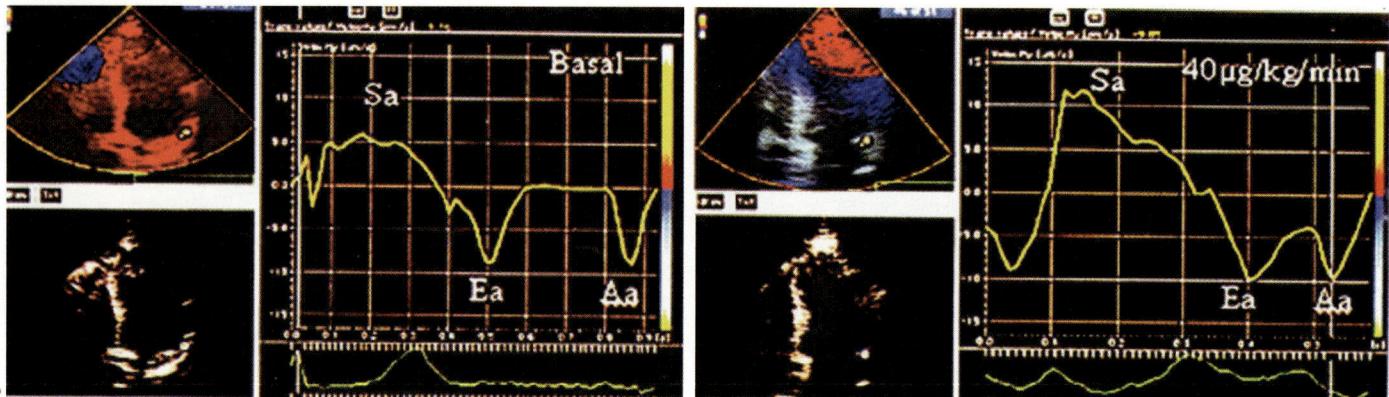

Fig. 10.7A: Myocardial velocities in normal person during dobutamine stress echocardiography taken from the lateral corner of the mitral annulus

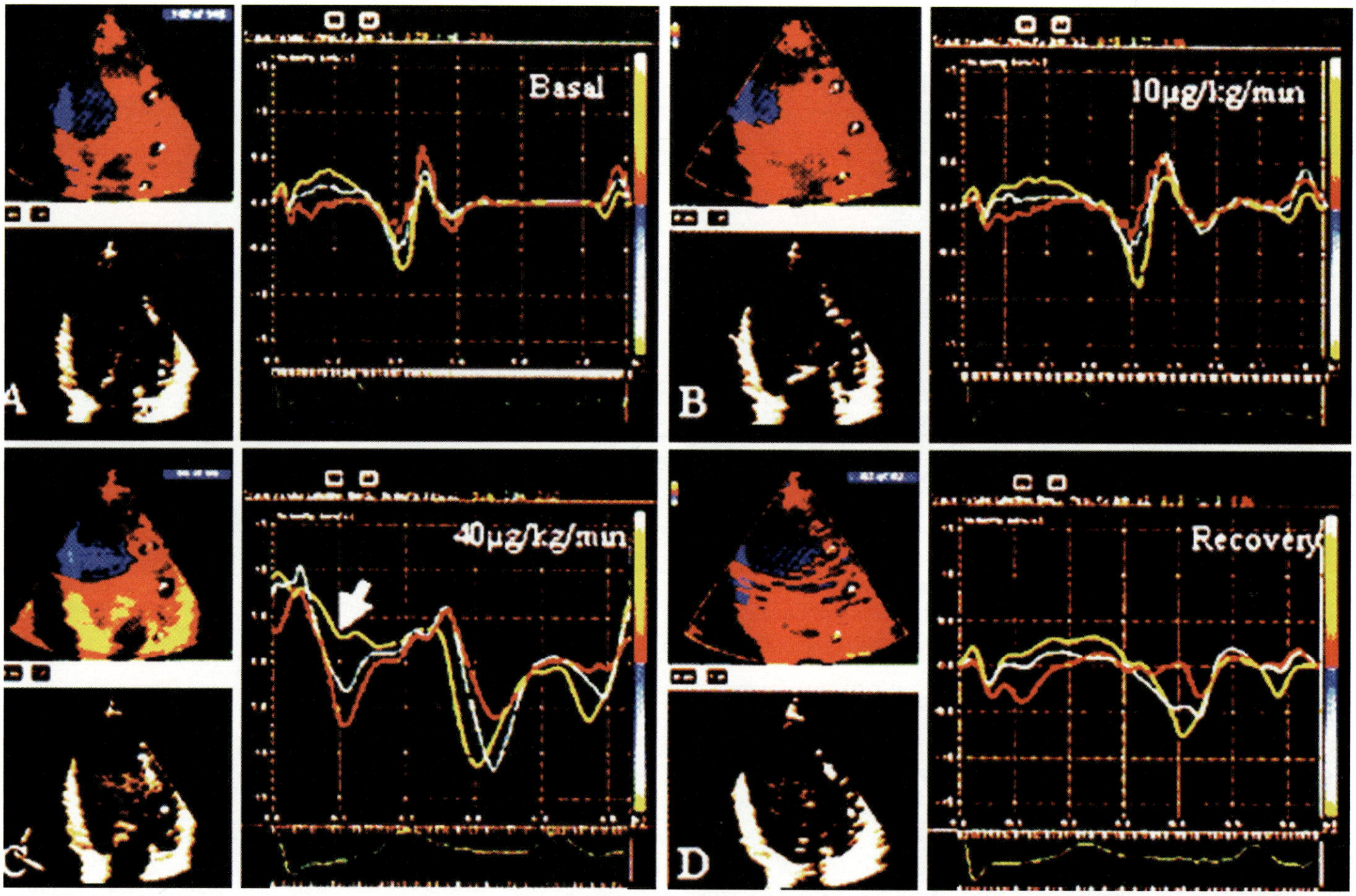

Fig. 10.7B: TDI during stress echocardiography in a patient with coronary artery disease showing systolic myocardial velocities in the ejection period (S2) are recorded normal during resting period. **(A)** but attenuated response observed during peak stress **(C)** and normalised during recovery period. **(D).** He showed 90% ostial lesion of left circumflex artery and 95% proximal lesion in the first obtuse marginal artery

of B-mode imaging. One approach is to quantify the global left ventricular function by measuring the mitral annular displacement velocity. Measurements are made at several sites, for example, the lateral, septal, anterior and inferior corners of the mitral annuli to derive an average figure.

Estimation of Diastolic Dysfunction

In heart failure there is always an alteration of diastolic LV functions and is very well correlated with mitral diastolic flow and hence various studies in the past focused their attention towards mitral diastolic flow and pulmonary venous flow patterns for estimating the left ventricular filling pressures. However, Doppler flow variables are highly influenced by certain physiologic variables like the preload, afterload and intravascular volume. In patients with a mitral Doppler inflow pattern of delayed relaxation, the volume infusion resulted in a change towards normalization with a shortening of the E-wave deceleration time and an increase in the E/A ratio, whereas patients with a normal or pseudonormal filling at baseline demonstrated a significant reduction in mitral inflow E velocity and E/A ratio after nitroglycerine infusion. In contrast there are no changes in Ea velocity, confirming that early diastolic tissue velocity was less load-sensitive than mitral inflow variables. Mitral annular E velocities have been proposed to be preload-independent variables of diastolic function. However, subsequent work by other investigators have debated the load independence of Ea. In day-to-day practice it is often necessary to obtain a noninvasive judgement regarding the left ventricular filling pressures for guiding the management of patients with cardiac diseases. Some workers have proposed a ratio of E/Ea as an important tool for noninvasive assessment of the left ventricular filling pressure. They categorized patients into asymptomatic persons with left ventricular E/A > 1 (normal), E/A < 1 (impaired relaxation) and E/A > 1 but with symptoms of heart failure (pseudonormal). Ea was reduced in patients with impaired relaxation and pseudonormal pattern. The best correlation for pulmonary artery wedge pressure was with E/Ea ratio ($r = 0.87$). Others showed that the ratio of E/Ea could be used to estimate pulmonary artery wedge pressure accurately even in the presence of sinus tachycardia (Fig. 10.4A and B).

Assessment of Coronary Artery Disease

Coronary artery disease leads to myocardial ischemia with changes in regional contraction and relaxation. Patients who suffer with acute heart attacks show not only loss of contractility but also tensile strength and stiffness. These alterations can be quantified by tissue velocity imaging. Diastolic abnormalities also occurred simultaneously and are characterised by a decrease in Em wave and increase in Am wave. The velocity of isometric relaxation and contraction increased and peaked at 1 min. There is a good correlation between decrease of systolic velocity and regional myocardial flow. However, positive isovolumic contraction velocities are able to distinguish segments with different degrees of necrosis. Preserved isovolumic contraction waves in hypokinetic or akinetic segments are associated with smaller infarcts. It is therefore important to note that ischemia and perfusion-induced contractile dysfunction resemble each other and thus cannot be differentiated. Assessment of myocardial perfusion through myocardial velocities, therefore, is only valid

in the situation of ongoing ischemia and not following reperfusion (Fig. 10.7A and B).

In chronic stable angina with normal ejection fraction, minor abnormalities of LV isovolumic relaxation and contraction and longitudinal shortening can be detected on tissue Doppler imaging (TDI). This technique has also been used during stress echocardiography for quantifying regional wall motion abnormalities. Dobutamine stress echocardiography using TDI is also an accurate tool for assessing myocardial viability. Dobutamine TDI, either used alone or in combination with conventional stress echocardiography, had a higher sensitivity and equivalent specificity for the prediction of recovery of dysfunctional segments. Tissue Doppler imaging is thus a useful technique during stress echocardiography for counterbalancing the poor agreement of standard echocardiography for evaluating wall motion. The tissue velocity profile is particularly important in interpreting regional wall motion in the basal segments.

Assessment in Pericardial and Myocardial Diseases
(Figs 10.9 and 10.10)

It has been always difficult to differentiate between restrictive cardiomyopathy and constrictive pericarditis. However, differentiation of these syndromes is important since constrictive pericarditis can be cured with pericardiectomy and an inappropriate surgical exploration of a patient with restrictive cardiomyopathy is undesirable. Doppler echocardiography has been used to demonstrate exaggerated interventricular interdependence in constrictive pericarditis by showing marked respiratory variations in mitral and pulmonary flow Doppler. However, these are not seen in all patients with constrictive pericarditis, hence the search for more accurate noninvasive variables has continued. Tissue Doppler assessment of mitral annular Ea velocity has been proposed to differentiate constrictive pericarditis from restrictive cardiomyopathy. An absolute value of 8 cm/s was shown to differentiate both the groups with no overlap. Some of the workers have compared the tissue velocity waves in short axis with constrictive pericarditis, who were diagnosed by cardiac catheterization, with normal subjects. In the patient group, the motion velocity of the ventricular septum along the short axis showed a "backward" motion with a sharp and marked peak velocity immediately before Em, or a biphasic early diastolic wave; a clear "downward" motion immediately after Em was observed in the motion velocities of the anterior right ventricular (RV) wall, ventricular septum and LV posterior wall along the long axis. These distinctive backward and downward motions were not observed in any of the ventricular walls of the normal subjects. Thus, TVI appears promising for differentiating myocardial from pericardial disease. However, it needs further support with more studies.

Myocardial Hypertrophy (Fig. 10.8)

In order to differentiate between physiological and pathological myocardial hypertrophy myocardial tissue velocities are considered more reliable than any other parameters assessed. Patients with systemic hypertension and HCM had significantly lower long axis systolic and diastolic velocities than athletes. A mean systolic annular velocity of < 9 cm/s had an 87% sensitivity and 97% specificity for differentiating pathologic from physiologic hypertrophy. Regional myocardial velocities have been shown to be altered in HCM septal tissue velocities showed lower peak velocities, E/A ratios, lengthened regional deceleration and isovolumic relaxation times. The tissue velocity in the lateral wall showed a prolonged deceleration and isovolumic relaxation time. Pulsed TDI also differentiates circumferential and longitudinal in fiber dynamics in HCM. It has also been shown to identify subjects who are positive for mutations for HCM but without myocardial hypertrophy (Fig. 10.8).

Heart Failure and Cardiac Transplant

Tissue velocity is one of the finest techniques for quantifying the degree of regional and global dysfunction in patients with critical CHF, monitoring their disease severity on follow-up and studying the outcome of different therapies in improving ventricular function. Preliminary studies have shown that TVI may provide important patho-physiologic information on the degree of LV resynchronization and may thus help in selecting and monitoring patients who may benefit with the use of biventricular pacing. TVI is also being employed in monitoring patients following cardiac transplantation. Many noninvasive techniques for detecting transplant rejection have been investigated but none has been found to be reliable enough to replace endomyocardial biopsies. Some workers have studied TVI as diagnostic tool to detect acute transplant rejection and transplant CAD in patients who underwent endomyocardial biopsies and catheterizations during their follow-up period after cardiac transplant. In all patients with acute rejection, a significant reduction in Em velocity and extension of the S_2–Em interval was obtained from the basal LV posterior wall in the short axis. Absence of such a change can thus be used for practically excluding acute transplant rejection. In the absence of rejection, an Sm value of <10 cm/s had a 97.7% likelihood of CAD, whereas an Sm value of >11 cm/s excluded angiographic CAD with 90% probability. In 91.7% of cases, the pulsed Doppler findings reverted completely during antirejection therapy within 65 hours. Thus, TVI has a potential to be used as an effective screening test for optimal timing of endomyo-cardial biopsies for detecting transplant rejection and transplant CAD, and can thus avoid the need of routine invasive monitoring in these patients.

Strain Rate Imaging

Tissue velocity imaging does not differentiate between active contraction and passive movement of a myocardial segment. Thus rotation and translation movements of the whole heart, as well as active contraction of segments adjacent to the analyzed segment, may affect the determined velocity. The point velocity thus measured does not necessarily reflect the active function of the interrogated segment. The velocity obtained from the apical view represents a cumulative velocity of all segments apical to the analyzed segment. Computing the tissue velocity data for obtaining the local strain and strain rate has circumvented these limitations of TVI.

Strain rate corresponds to the rate of deformation of an object. Local myocardial strain can be calculated from the spatial gradient in velocities recorded from two neighboring points in the same tissue. It is given by the following formula

$$SR = V_b - V_a/l$$

where "a" and "b" are two points and "l" reflects the distance between the two points. Integration of this parameter with time gives myocardial strain. In theory, to characterize regional myocardial function accurately, it is necessary to measure local deformation in three directions longitudinal, radial and circumferential. Current echocardiography transducers acquire only one-dimensional datasets—a parasternal view for radial strain and apical position for longitudinal strain. During radial deformation, a segment thickens in systole and is given a positive value. When it thins, it is given a negative value. In longitudinal direction, as the segment shortens in systole, it is given a negative value. In diastole, it lengthens and is given a positive value. Longitudinal strain and strain rate are homogeneous throughout the septum and all LV walls, which is in contrast to the base–apex gradient found on TVI. Systolic deformation starts virtually simultaneously except at the apex. Lengthening during isovolumic relaxation is generally seen first in the midwall and, at the same time, reciprocal shortening is seen in the neighbouring segments, whereas stretching starts later in the apex. Diastolic deformation of the ventricle occurs during the early and late filling phases and progresses as a wave from the mitral annulus to the apex. For the RV free wall, strain rate is not uniform and is highest at the apex and reduces towards the base, a reversed pattern as compared to the tissue velocity data. Preliminary data have demonstrated that strain rate imaging might be more accurate than planar wall thickening analysis for discriminating regional myocardial function in CAD.

TDI in Combination with MVG. ECG and PCG

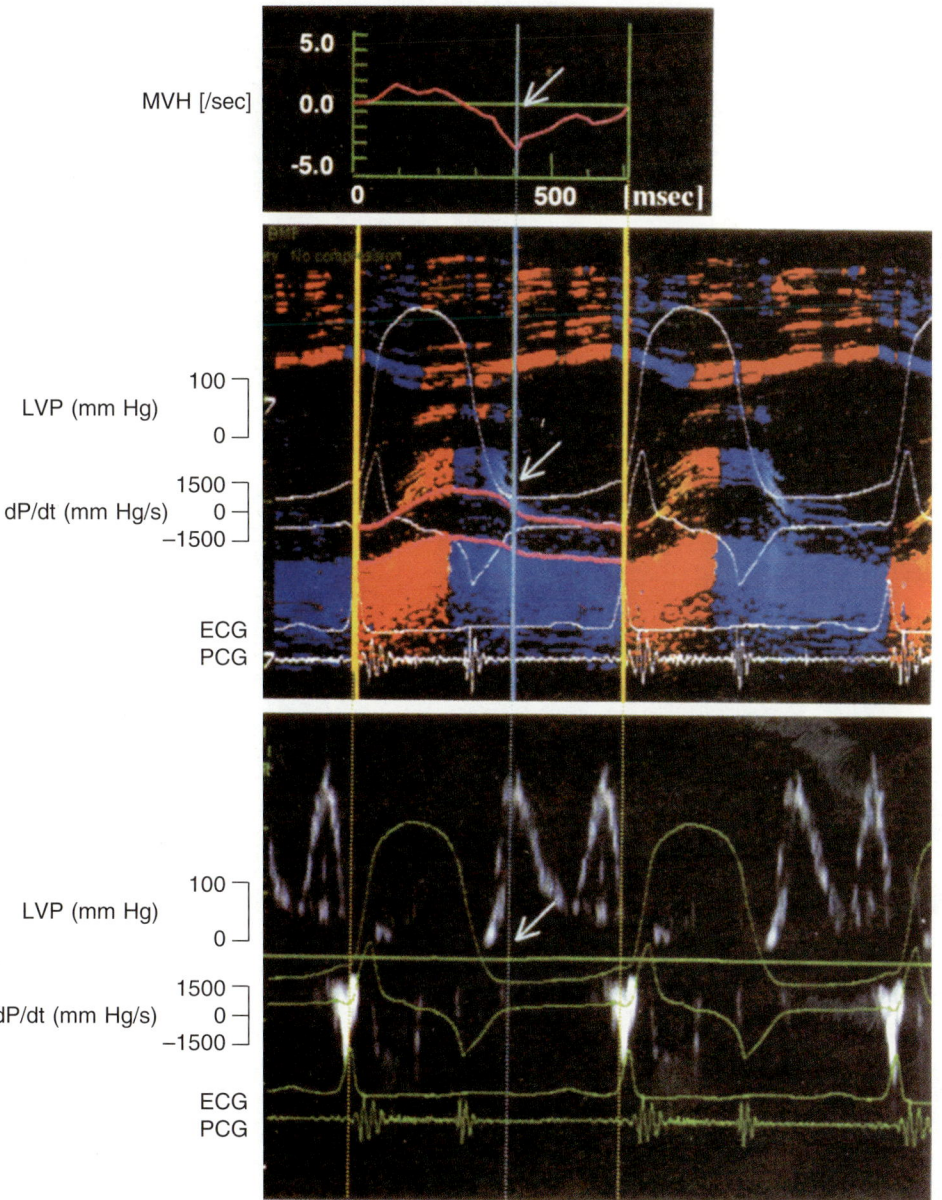

Fig. 10.8: Posterior wall myocardial velocity gradient (MVG) (top), tissue Doppler imaging TDI M-mode images (middle) (bottom) and corresponding transmitral flow velocity patterns with electrocardiogram (ECG) phonocardiogram, (PCG) tracing of left ventricular pressure (LVP) and first derivative of left ventricular pressure for a patient with hypertrophic cardiomyopathy

Changes in strain rate have also been shown to have potential in assessing myocardial viability. It has also been used to assess the degree of segmental asynchrony and asynergy in patients with cardiomyopathies and advanced LV dysfunction. In order to employ it as the most reliable technique for getting incremental value in quantifying regional and global myocardial function, further studies are necessary.

Summary

Tissue velocity imaging has emerged as one of the most finest techniques in the field of cardiac ultrasound that provides quantitative information for analysis of myocardial motion independent of the quality of grey-scale 2-D echocardiography data. It holds promise to reduce inter- and intraobserver variability in regional wall motion interpretation and is likely to improve the accuracy and reproducibility of stress echocardiography and myocardial viability assessment. It also enables regional diastolic function assessment independent of the loading conditions and offers a practical clinical tool to differentiate pathologic from physiologic myocardial hypertrophy, restrictive cardiomyopathy from constrictive pericarditis and for monitoring and selecting

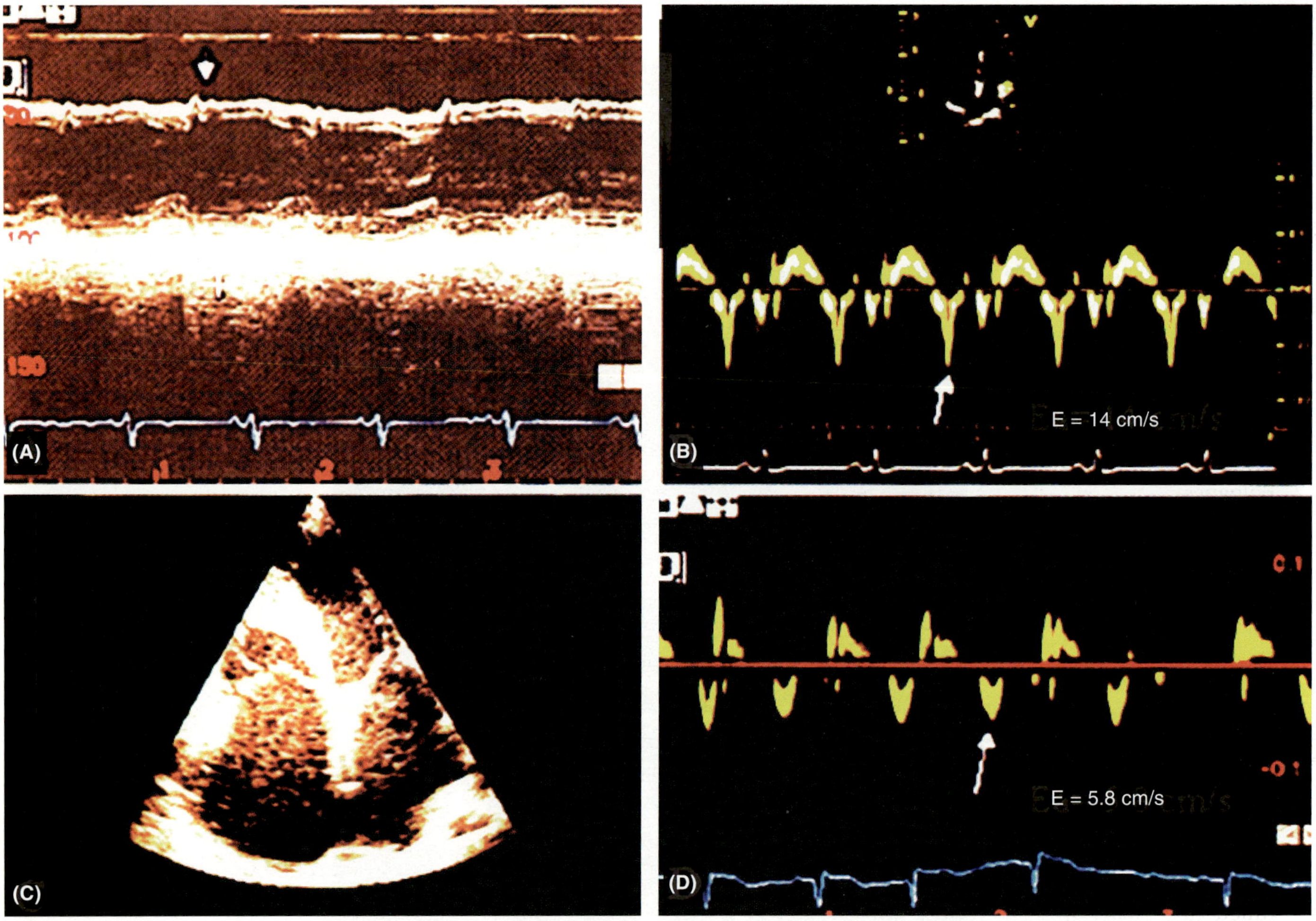

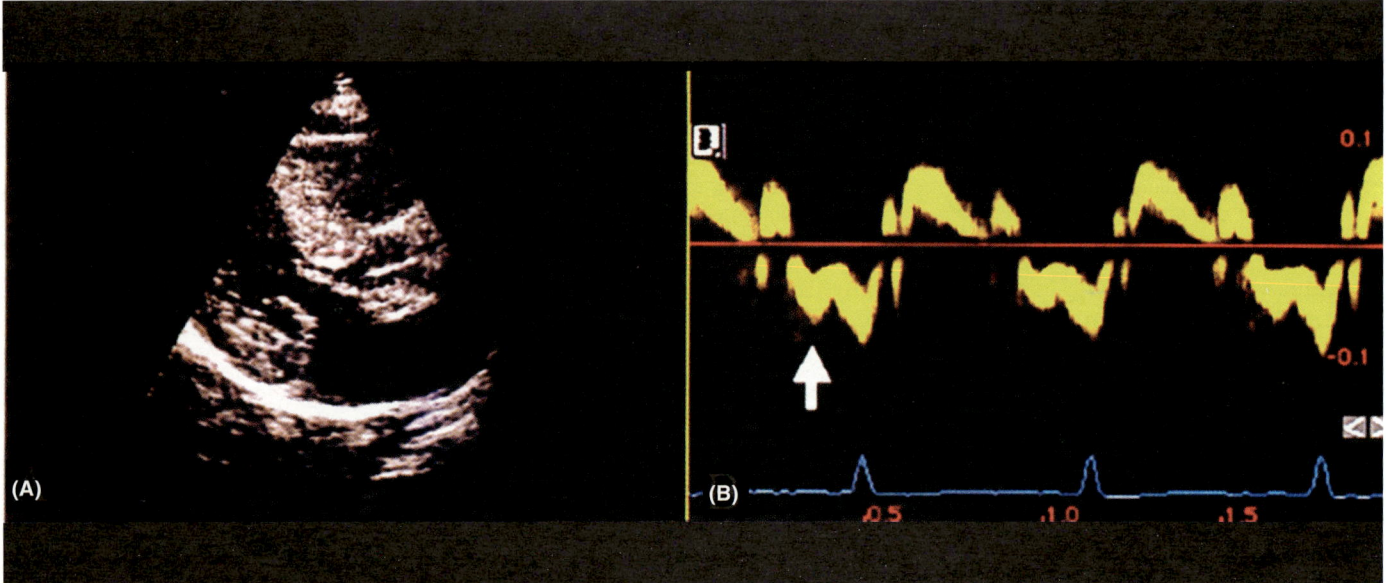

Fig. 10.9: TDI scans showing typical septal bounce (arrow) and pericardial thickening (arrow) in patient with constrictive pericarditis **(A)** Early diastolic longitudinal annular velocity (Ea) recorded by the pulsed Doppler are found normal **(B)** and helps differentiating this condition from that of restrictive cardiomyopaty **(C)** where it is markedly diminished **(D)**

Fig. 10.10: TDI velocity recorded from the interventricular septum showing marked reduction in early diastolic myocardial velocity in quantification of diastolic dysfunction in asymmeterical septal wall hypertrophy

therapies in patients with advanced heart failure. The use of tissue velocity data for myocardial strain and strain rate imaging is likely to circumvent the limitations of tissue velocity in differentiating active and passive motion of a myocardial segment. However, its incremental utility and exact role in improving the diagnostic yield and clinical outcome needs to be addressed in future studies.

Bibliography

1. Arnold MF, Voigt JU, Kukulski T, Wranne B, Sutherland GR, Hatle L. Does atrioventricular ring motion always distinguish constriction from restriction? A Doppler myocardial imaging study. *J Am Soc Echocardiogr* 2001; 14: 391–395.

2. Bolognesi R, Tsialtas D, Barilli AL, Manca C, Zeppellini R, Javernaro A, et al. Detection of early abnormalities of left ventricular function by hemodynamic, echo-tissue Doppler imaging, and mitral Doppler flow techniques in patients with coronary artery disease and normal ejection fraction. *J Am Soc Echocardiogr* 2001; 14: 764–772.

3. Dagdelen S, Eren N, Karabulut H, Akdemir I, Ergelen M, Saglam M, et al. Estimation of left ventricular end-diastolic pressure by colour M-mode Doppler echocardiography and tissue Doppler imaging. *J Am Soc Echocardiogr* 2001; 14: 951–958.

4. Dandel M, Hummel M, Muller J, Wellnhofer E, Meyer R, Solowjowa N, et al. Reliability of tissue Doppler wall motion monitoring after heart transplantation for replacement of invasive routine screenings by optimally timed cardiac biopsies and catheterizations. *Circulation* 2001; 104: 1184–1191.

5. Derumeaux G, Ovize M, Loufoua J, Andre-Fouet X, Minaire Y, Cribier A, et al. Doppler tissue imaging quantitates regional wall motion during myocardial ischemia and reperfusion. *Circulation* 1998; 97: 1970–1977.

6. Fathi R, Cain P, Nakatani S, Yu HC, Marwick TH. Effect of tissue Doppler on the accuracy of novice and expert interpreters of dobutamine echocardiography. *Am J Cardiol* 2001; 88: 400–405.

7. Galiuto L, Ignone G, De Maria AN. Contraction and relaxation velocities of the normal left ventricle using pulsed wave tissue Doppler echocardiography. *Am J Cardiol* 1991; 67: 222–224.

8. Garcia MJ, Rodriguez L, Ares M, Griffin BP, Klein AL, Stewart WJ, et al. Myocardial wall velocity assessment by pulsed Doppler tissue imaging: characteristic findings in normal subjects. *Am Heart J* 1996; 132: 648–656.

9. Garcia MJ, Rodriguez L, Ares M, Griffin BP, Thomas JD, Klein AL. Differentiation of constrictive pericarditis from restrictive cardiomyopathy: assessment of left ventricular diastolic velocities in longitudinal axis by Doppler tissue imaging. *J Am Coll Cardiol* 1996; 27: 108–114.

10. Garcia-Fernandez MA, Azevedo J, Moreno M, Bermejo J, Perez-Castellano N, Puerta P, et al. Regional diastolic function in ischaemic heart disease using pulsed wave Doppler tissue imaging. *Eur Heart J* 1999; 20: 496–505.

11. Garot J, Diebold B, Derumeaux GA, Monin JL, Bosio P, Duval-Moulin AM, et al. Comparison of regional myocardial velocities assessed by quantitative 2-dimensional and M-mode colour Doppler tissue imaging: influence of the signal-to-noise ratio of colour Doppler myocardial images on velocity estimators of the Doppler tissue imaging system. *J Am Soc Echocardiogr* 1998; 11: 1093–1105.

12. Gorcsan J 3rd, Gulati VK, Mandarino WA, Katz WE. Colour-coded measures of myocardial velocity throughout the cardiac cycle by tissue Doppler imaging to quantify regional left ventricular function. *Am Heart J* 1996; 131: 1203–1213.

13. Grant RP. Notes on the muscular architecture of the left ventricle. *Circulation* 1965; 32: 301–308.

14. Greenbaum RA, Ho SY, Gibson DG, Becker AE, Anderson RH. Left ventricular fibre architecture in man. *Br Heart J* 1981; 45: 248–263.

15. Greenberg NL, Firstenberg MS, Castro PL, Main M, Travaglin in patients with hypertrophic cardiomyopathy and provides a novel means for an early diagnosis before and independently of hypertrophy. *Circulation* 2001; 104: 128–130.

16. Gulati VK, Katz WE, Follansbee WP, Gorcsan J 3rd. Mitral annular descent velocity by tissue Doppler echocardiography as an index of global left ventricular function. *Am J Cardiol* 1996; 77: 979–984.

17. Hoffmann R, Hanrath P. Stress echocardiography: the scourge of subjective interpretation. *Eur Heart J* 1995; 16: 1458–1459.

18. Hoffmann R, Marwick TH, Poldermans D, Lethen H, Ciani R, van der Meer P, et al. Refinements in stress echocardiographic techniques improve inter-institutional agreement in interpretation of dobutamine stress echocardiograms. *Eur Heart J* 2002; 23: 821–829.

19. Isaaz K, Thompson A, Ethevenot G, Cloez JL, Brembilla B, Pernot C. Doppler echocardiographic measurement of low velocity motion of the left ventricular posterior wall. *Am J Cardiol* 1989; 64: 66–75.

20. Jones CJ, Raposo L, Gibson DG. Functional importance of the long axis dynamics of the human left ventricle. *Br Heart J* 1990; 63: 215–220.

21. Katz WE, Gulati VK, Mahler CM, Gorcsan J 3rd, Quantitative evaluation of the segmental left ventricular response to dobutamine stress by tissue Doppler echocardiography. *Am J Cardiol* 1997; 79: 1036–1042.

22. Lange A, Palka P, Caso P, Fenn LN, Olszewski R, Ramo MP, et al. Doppler myocardial imaging vs. B-mode grey-scale imaging: a comparative in vitro and in vivo study into their relative efficacy in endocardial boundary detection. *Ultrasound Med Biol* 1997; 23:69–75.

23. Larrazet F, Pellerin D, Daou D, Witchitz S, Fournier C, Prigent A, et al. Concordance between dobutamine Doppler tissue imaging echocardiography and rest reinjection thallium-201 tomography in dysfunctional hypoperfused myocardium. *Heart* 1999; 82: 432–437.

24. Mishiro Y, Oki T, Yamada H, Wakatsuki T, Ito S. Evaluation of left ventricular contraction abnormalities in patients with dilated cardiomyopathy with the use of pulsed tissue Doppler imaging. *J Am Soc Echocardiogr* 1999; 12: 913–920.

25. Miyatake K, Yamagishi M, Tanaka N, Uematsu M, Yamazaki N, Mine Y, et al. New method of evaluating left ventricular

wall motion by colour-coded tissue Doppler imaging: in vitro and in vivo studies. *J Am Coll Cardiol* 1995; 25: 717–724.

26. Nagueh SF, Bachinski LL, Meyer D, Hill R, Zoghbi WA, Tam JW, *et al.* Tissue Doppler imaging consistently detects myocardial abnormalities A, Odabashian JA, *et al.* Doppler-derived myocardial systolic strain rate is a strong index of left ventricular contractility. *Circulation* 2002; 105: 99–105.

27. Nagueh SF, Middleton KJ, Kopelen HA, Zoghbi WA, Quinones MA. Doppler tissue imaging: a noninvasive technique for evaluation of left ventricular relaxation and estimation of filling pressures. *J Am Coll Cardiol* 1997; 30: 1527–1533.

28. Nagueh SF, Mikati I, Kopelen HA, Middleton KJ, Quinones MA, Zoghbi WA. Doppler estimation of left ventricular filling pressure in sinus tachycardia. A new application of tissue doppler imaging. *Circulation* 1998; 98: 1644–1650.

29. Nishino M, Tanouchi J, Tanaka K, Ito T, Kato J, Iwai K, *et al.* Dobutamine stress echocardiography at 7.5 mg/kg/min using colour tissue Doppler imaging M-mode safely predicts reversible dysfunction early after reperfusion in patients with acute myocardial infarction. *Am J Cardiol* 1999; 83: 340–344.

30. Oki T, Tabata T, Mishiro Y, Yamada H, Abe M, Onose Y, *et al.* Pulsed tissue Doppler imaging of left ventricular systolic and diastolic wall motion velocities to evaluate differences between long and short axes healthy subjects. *J Am Soc Echocardiogr* 1999; 12: 308–313.

31. Oki T, Tabata T, Yamada H, Abe M, Onose Y, Wakatsuki T, *et al.* Right and left ventricular wall motion velocities as diagnostic indicators of constrictive pericarditis. *Am J Cardiol* 1998; 81: 465–470.

32. Onose Y, Oki T, Mishiro Y, Yamada H, Abe M, Manabe K, *et al.* Influence of aging on systolic left ventricular wall motion velocities along the long and short axes in clinically normal patients determined by pulsed tissue doppler imaging. *J Am Soc Echocardiogr* 1999; 12: 921–926.

33. Pai RG, Bodenheimer MM, Pai SM, Koss JH, Adamick RD. Usefulness of systolic excursion of the mitral annulus as an index of left ventricular systolic function. *Am J Cardiol* 1991; 67: 222–224.

34. Pai RG, Gill KS. Amplitudes, durations, and timings of apically directed left ventricular myocardial velocities: I. Their normal pattern and coupling to ventricular filling and ejection. *J Am Soc Echocardiogr* 1998; 11: 105–111.

35. Picano E, Lattanzi F, Orlandini A, Marini C, L'Abbate A. Stress echocardiography and the human factor: the importance of being an expert. *J Am Coll Cardiol* 1990; 17: 666–667.

36. Pislaru C, Bruce CJ, Belohlavek M, Seward JB, Greenleaf JF. Intracardiac measurement of pre-ejection myocardial velocities estimates the transmural extent of viable myocardium early after reperfusion in acute myocardial infarction. *J Am Coll Cardiol* 2001; 38: 1748–1756.

37. Rushmer RF, Crystal DK, Wagner C. The functional anatomy of ventricular contraction. *Cir Res* 1953; 1: 162–170.

38. Sahn DJ. Instrumentation and physical factors related to visualization of stenotic and regurgitant jets by Doppler colour flow mapping. *J Am Coll Cardiol* 1988; 12: 1354–1365.

39. Severino S, Caso P, Galderisi M, De Simone L, Petrocelli A, de Divitiis O, *et al.* Use of pulsed Doppler tissue imaging to assess regional left ventricular diastolic dysfunction in hypertrophic cardiomyopathy. *Am J Cardiol* 1998; 82: 1394–1398.

40. Shan K, Bick RJ, Poindexter BJ, Shimoni S, Letsou GV, Reardon MJ, *et al.* Relation of tissue Doppler derived myocardial velocities to myocardial structure and beta-adrenergic receptor density in humans. *J Am Coll Cardiol* 2000; 36: 891–896.

41. Simonson JS, Schiller NB. Descent of the base of the left ventricle: an echocardiographic index of left ventricular function. *J Am Soc Echocardiogr* 1989; 2: 25–35.

42. Sogaard P, Kim WY, Jensen HK, Mortensen P, Pedersen AK, Kristensen BO, *et al.* Impact of acute biventricular pacing on left ventricular performance and volumes in patients with severe heart failure. A tissue Doppler and three-dimensional echocardiographic study. *Cardiology* 2001; 95: 173–182.

43. Sohn DW, Chai IH, Lee DJ, Kim HC, Kim HS, Oh BH, *et al.* Assessment of mitral annulus velocity by Doppler tissue imaging in the evaluation of left ventricular diastolic function. *J Am Coll Cardiol* 1997; 30: 474–480.

44. Sutherland GR, Stewart MJ, Groundstroem KW, Moran CM, Fleming A, Guell-Peris FJ, *et al.* Colour Doppler myocardial imaging: a new technique for assessment of myocardial function. *J Am Soc Echocardiogr* 1994; 7: 441–458.

45. Tabata T, Oki T, Yamada H, Abe M, Onose Y, Thomas JD. Subendocardial motion in hypertrophic cardiomyopathy: assessment from long- and short-axis views by pulsed tissue Doppler imaging. *J Am Soc Echocardiogr* 2000; 13: 108–115.

46. Uematsu M, Miyatake K, Tanaka N, Matsuda H, Sano A, Yamazaki N, *et al.* Myocardial velocity gradient as a new indicator of regional left ventricular contraction: detection by a two-dimensional tissue Doppler imaging technique. *J Am Coll Cardiol* 1995; 26: 217–223.

47. Vinereanu D, Florescu N, Sculthorpe N, Tweddel AC, Stephens MR, Fraser AG. Differentiation between pathologic and physiologic left ventricular hypertrophy by tissue Doppler assessment of long-axis function in patients with hypertrophic cardiomyopathy or systemic hypertension and in athletes. *Am J Cardiol* 2001; 88: 53–58.

48. Weidemann F, Eyskens B, Sutherland GR. New ultrasound methods to quantify regional myocardial function in children with heart disease. *Pediatr Cardiol* 2002; 23: 292–306.

49. Yamada H, Oki T, Mishiro Y, Tabata T, Abe M, Onose Y, *et al.* Effect of aging on diastolic left ventricular myocardial velocities measured by pulsed tissue Doppler imaging in healthy subjects. *J Am Soc Echocardiogr* 1999; 12: 574–581.

50. Yamada H, Oki T, Tabata T, Iuchi A, Ito S. Assessment of left ventricular systolic wall motion velocity with pulsed tissue Doppler imaging: comparison with peak dP/dt of the left ventricular pressure curve. *J Am Soc Echocardiogr* 1998; 11: 442–449.

51. Yamazaki N, Mine Y, Sano A, Hirama M, Miyatake K, Yamagishi M, *et al.* Analysis of ventricular wall motion using colour-coded tissue Doppler imaging system. *Jpn J Appl Physc* 1994; 33: 3141–3146.

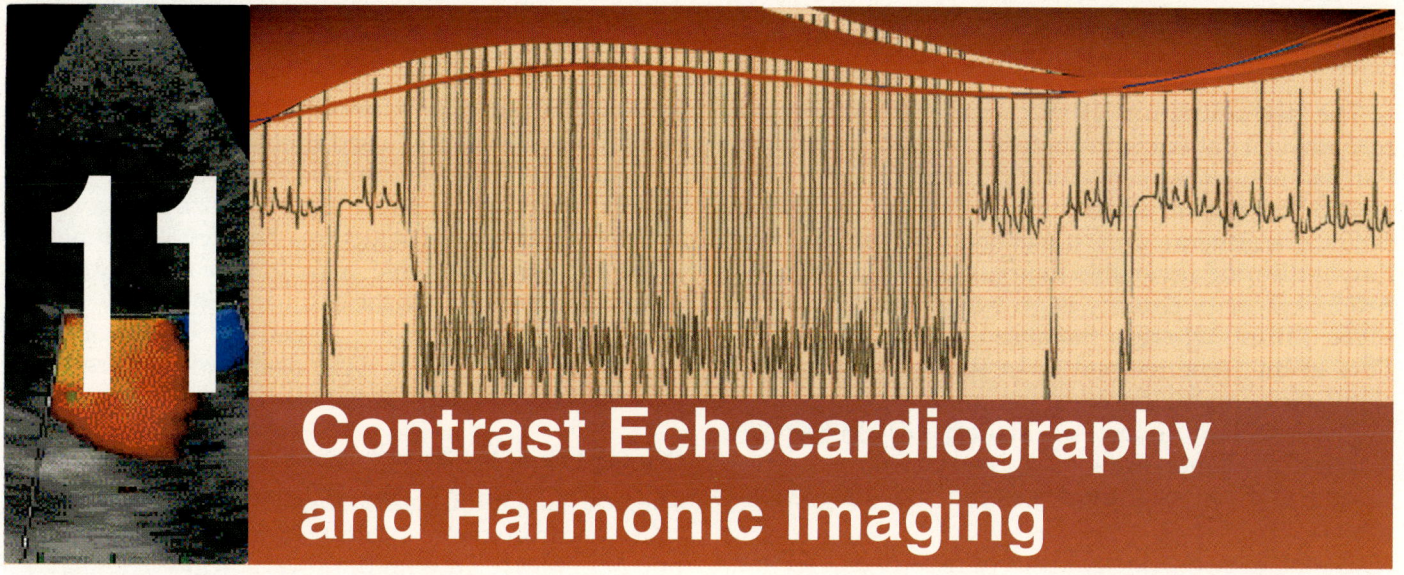

11

Contrast Echocardiography and Harmonic Imaging

The use of an ultrasonic contrast agent in conjunction with echocardiography was reported in the late 1960s. It was used to identify and verify cardiac structures. When injected into the vascular system, an ultrasonic contrast agent produces clouds of echoes visible on the echocardiogram. Soon after the initial application, contrast echocardiogram was used to diagnose intracardiac shunts and valvular regurgitations and to calculate cardiac outputs.

Contrast agents are usually made up of bubbles microbubbles, or encapsulated gas suspended in the liquid being injected. A good contrast agent must be stable enough to reach the target organ. It must also be nontoxic and easily removed by the body. The presence of the bubbles acting as backscatter targets increases the echogenicity of the substance injected intravenously. Thus it is possible to visualise the path of the blood-flow with opacification of the chambers. Substances that have been used for contrast agents include saline, indocyanine green dye, carbon dioxide gas, hydrogen peroxide, dextrose with water, the patient's own blood, sonicated human albumin, a saccharide based microbubble preparation, and emulsions of various chemical compounds. In spite of new contrast agents, agitated saline remains an accepted, economical, and effective means to detect intracardiac shunts (Fig. 11.1).

Agitated saline is admitted accomplished by connecting two 10 to 12 ml syringes to a three way stop cock. One of these syringes is filled with saline and the other one is empty. By rapidly and repeatedly transferring the saline to the other empty syringe, the bubbles are formed. When injected intravenously, the agitated saline opacifies the right atrium and the right ventricle, if there is a right to left shunt at the atrial level, contrast also appears in the left atrium almost instantaneously as the right atrium is opacified.

A frame by frame analysis may help to determine the timing of the contrast appearance. However, if there is a known right to left shunt, care must be taken to exclude any visible large bubbles before injecting the agitated saline. This is to prevent any catastrophies that may occur from the large bubbles blocking the supply of blood into any vessel. To detect a left to right to shunt using contrast from intravenous injections, one relies on the negative contrast effect when flow from a left chamber enters a well opacified right chamber through the shunt.

Drawback of this technique include the inflow from venous return, which may be mistaken for a shunt, and a less than optimally opacified chamber that will not demonstrate a clear negative contrast. With improvements in two dimensional echocardiography and colour-Doppler resolution, most left to right shunts can be detected without using contrast echocardiography.

Although contrast echocardiography has been to detect tricuspid and pulmonic regurgitations, the advance of Doppler techniques has virtually eliminated the need to use intravenous injections of contrast agents to make these diagnoses.

The clinical application of contrast echocardiography with peripheral venous injection is currently limited to the right heart. This is mainly because of the inability of the bubbles to pass through the lungs. Many investigators have been working on developing a contrast agent capable of passing through the capillaries to opacify the left heart. Two of these transpulmonary contrast agents are Albunex, a sonicated human albumin, and Levovist, a monosaccharide based microbubble preparation. It is hoped that these agents will soon be available. The potential application for a transpulmonary contrast agent is the opacification of the myocardium using peripheral venous injection.

The determination of risk area is probably most relevant in a patient with acute MI who present beyond the time-windows for thrombolytic therapy. Myocardial contrast can help to determine the adequacy of collateral flow to the ischemic area. If there is significant collateral flow indicating reversible injury, then interventions to restore coronary patency is probably useful to salvage myocardium, whereas the absence of any significant flow in the ischemic bed or in the border zone may signify irreversible necrosis.

The detection of coronary stenosis by contrast echo is based on demonstration of abnormal coronary flow reserve in the myocardium, subtended by the stenosed artery.

There are two principal uses of myocardial contrast echocardiography in the operating room during coronary artery bypass surgery. Firstly, to guide delivery of adequate cardioplegia especially with retrograde cardioplegia, and secondly to assess the imaging in the clinical setting remains to be tested, but the advent of imaging resolution and the breakthrough development agent with consistent passage through the lungs, holds much promise.

Opacification of the myocardium has been demonstrated using intracoronary or intraaortic injections of contrast agents. The applications of myocardial contrast echocardiography include identifying regional perfusion defects assessing risk area size in acute myocardial salvage after myocardial infarction, assessing myocardial salvage after reperfusion, and, assessing coronary bloodflow reserves in critical coronary stenosis. Although intracoronary injection of contrast in humans has been found to be safe, application of the technique has been limited. Contrast echocardiography becomes available in the noninvasive laboratory routinely and reproducibly using peripheral intravenous injection. The potential clinical applications for this technique include detecting and assessing coronary artery disease, risk stratification for patient management, and assessing cardiac output with videodensitometry. Major advantage of echocardiography is its inherent ability to image solid cardiac structures from blood filled cavities without the need for exogenous contrast materials. Gramiak and Shahi in 1968 used saline contrast opacification of heart chambers to study echocardiographic anatomy using intracardiac injections through catheters positioned in various cardiac chambers. Later workers used this technique to study intracardiac shunts, anomalous communications and valvular regurgitation. It was shown that hand agitated saline was an excellent contrast agent but the contrast bubbles do not cross the pulmonary circulation and hence do not opacify the left heart chambers. Tei *et al.* used direct intracoronary injections of hand agitated saline to study regional

myocardial perfusion abnormalities in experimental animals and Kaul, *et al.* used the same technique in the cardiac catheterization lab. The introduction of contrast agents which cross the pulmonary circulation and opacify the left heart structures have evoked renewed interest in noninvasive echo imaging of not only the left heart chambers but also the coronary blood flow. Newer techniques of visualising selectivity of the contrast opacified blood vessels were designed and are being perfected (Fig. 11.11A, B and C).

Contrast agents (Fig.11.3–11.5)

The first generation contrast agents were hand Agitated saline or cardiogreen. Recently newer agents containing microbubbles filled with fluorocarbon gas (Albunex, FS 069), or dodecafluoropentane, a fluorocarbon which is a liquid at room temperature (EchoGen), or galactose like substances which release air to form microbubbles in the blood (Echovist, Levovist), are being approved for human use. These agents generate microbubbles of less than 10 microns in size, which will cross the pulmonary capillaries and opacify the left ventricle and the coronary circulation. Some of these agents have stable contrast bubbles staying in the circulation for a long time for continued viewing of structures. Contrast echocardiography has an established role for enhancement of the right heart Doppler signals, the detection of intra-cardiac shunts, and most recently for left ventricular cavity opacification (LVO). The use of intravenously administered microbubbles to traverse the myocardial microcirculation in order to outline myocardial viability and perfusion has been the source of research studies for a number of years. Despite the enthusiasm of investigators, myocardial contrast echocardiography (MCE) has not attained routine clinical use and LV opacification during stress has been less widely adopted than the data would support. The purpose of this review is to facilitate an understanding of the involved imaging technologies that have made this technique more feasible for clinical practice, and to guide its introduction into the practice of the non-expert user.

Imaging Technique

Microbubbles (Fig. 11.2): Two aspects of microbubbles are important— their gas content and the nature of their shell. Recently approved microbubbles almost universally involve encapsulation of a high molecular weight gas, which improves the persistence of the bubble, optimising the number available in the left heart chambers. Air has a greater propensity to dissolve into solution and although currently unattractive because of loss of gas before arrival on the right side of the heart, better encapsulation may allow its resurgence—the benefit would be more rapid disappearance when the

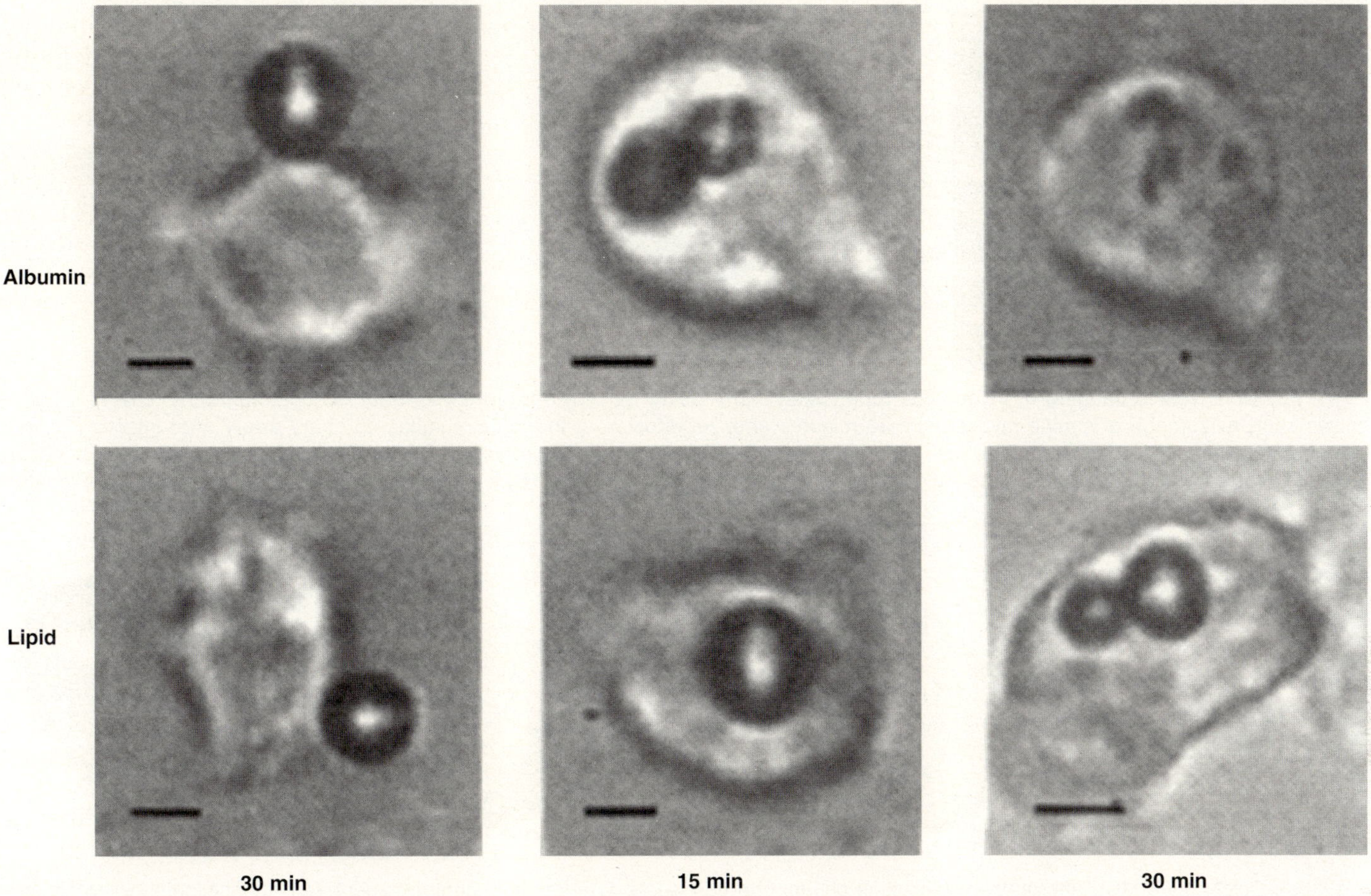

Albumin

Lipid

| 30 min | 15 min | 30 min |

Fig. 11.1: Images as seen through light microscopy of leukocytes at 3 minutes followed by phagocytosis at 15 minutes. Lipid microbubbles remained intact at 30 minutes

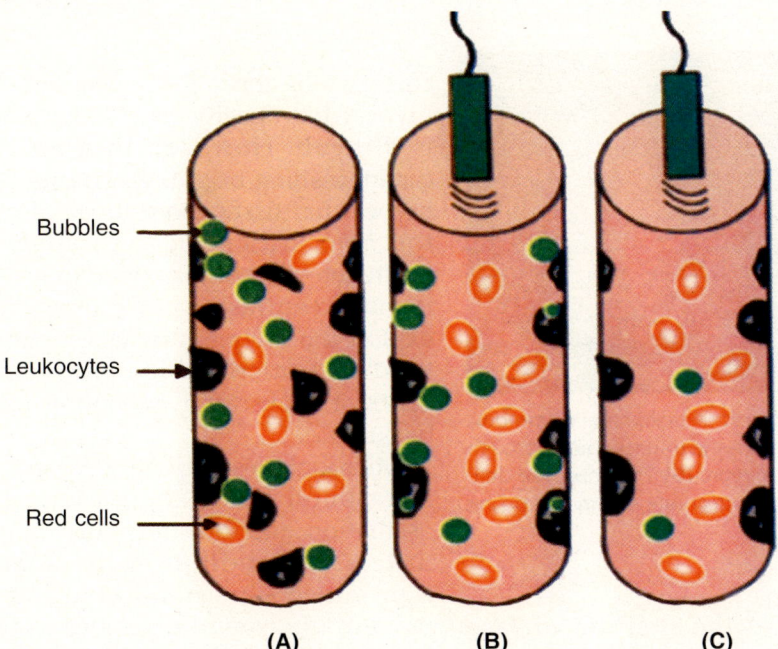

Bubbles

Leukocytes

Red cells

(A)   (B)   (C)

Fig. 11.2: Ultrasound imaging is suspended immediately after injection of bubbles. **(A)** After unbound bubbles have dissipated (minutes), a single frame is obtained. **(B)**. Followed several seconds later by another ultrasound pulse. **(C)** The videointensity differences between B and C is attributable to microbubble adhesion

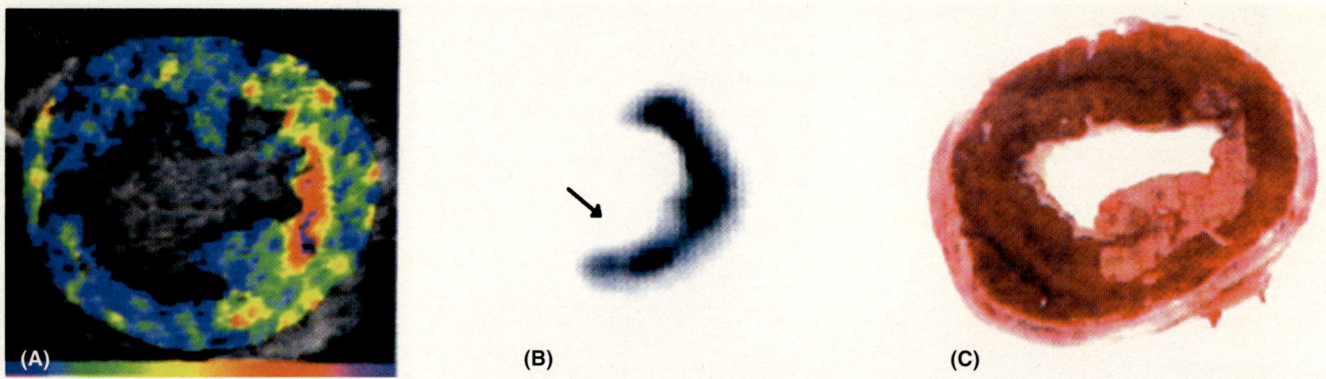

Fig. 11.3: Noninvasive imaging of myocardial reperfusion injury using leukocyte-targeted contrast echocardiography. **(A)** This figure shows short axis image of canine myocardium 60 minutes after reperfusion of the left circumflex coronary artery after injection of lipid microbubbles containing phosphatidylserine to enhance leukocyte binding. **(B)** The region of echo contrast enhancement corresponds in location to the region of leukocyte accumulation as demonstrated with [99M]TcRP517. **(C)** It is greater than the extent of infarction delineated by tetrazolinum chloride staining (C)

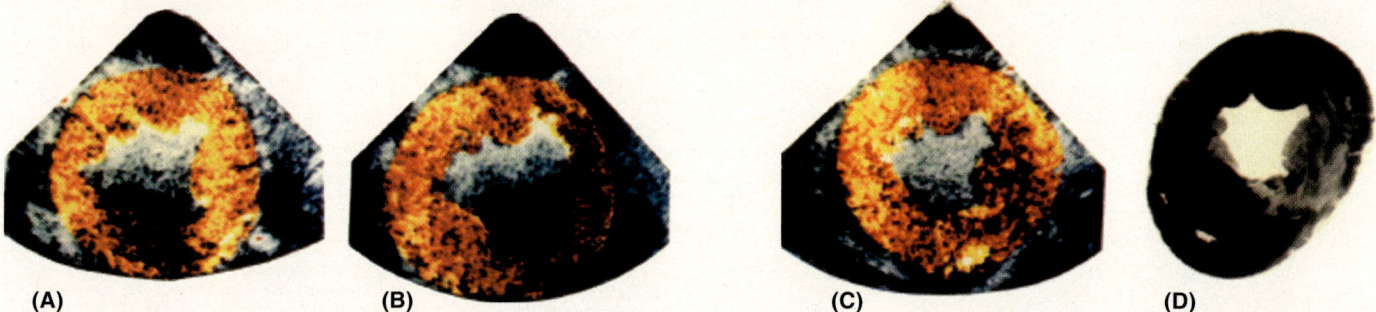

Fig. 11.4: Color-coded MCE after a venous injection of 1 ml of a new second generation contrast agent. **(A)** At baseline showing homogenous contrast effect except for some posterior wall attenuation from the presence of contrast in the left ventricular cavity. **(B)** During coronary occlusion, where the risk area is clearly defined. **(C)** After reflow of where the perfusion defect corresponds in size and topology to the infarction defined on tissue staining **(D)**

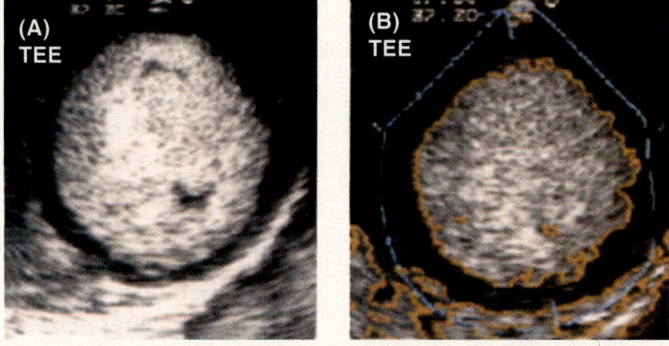

Fig. 11.5A and B: (A) Contrast-enhanced transesophageal harmonic images of the left ventricle obtained from the transgastric approach in a patient who had preserved wall motion. **(B)** The improved definition of the endocardial boundary allows accurate automated online border detection and trackingd

bubble bursts. The nature of the shell or surface modifying agent, which improves stability and prevents dissolution, may become important for new targeted imaging approaches. Even when optimal microbubble delivery to the myocardium is achieved with invasive coronary or aortic root injections. Detection of reliable myocardial opacification using standard 2-D imaging is difficult. However, this partly reflects difficulty distinguishing bright, grey scale echo signals from the myocardial tissue from those of micro-bubbles within the myocardial micro-circulation, the problem is multifactorial and has been overcome by the development of contrast specific imaging modalities, which exploit the unique interaction between the ultrasound field and microbubbles to maximise the received contrast backscatter and minimise myocardial tissue backscatter.

Microbubbles oscillate (expand and contract) in the ultrasound field. The pattern and nature of their oscillation, and thus the nature of the backscatter signal differs, depending on the acoustic power of the transmitted ultrasound field, which is expressed on modern ultrasound machines as the mechanical index (MI). In general, the amplitude of returning backscatter depends on the nature of the insonated structure, and is represented by brightness on the formed image. Most backscatter returns at the same frequency as the

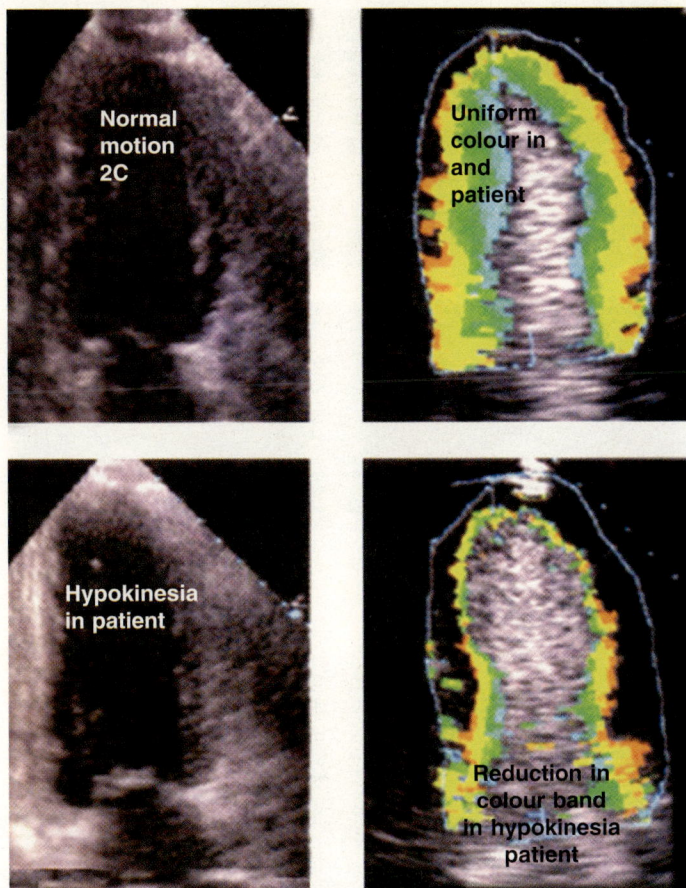

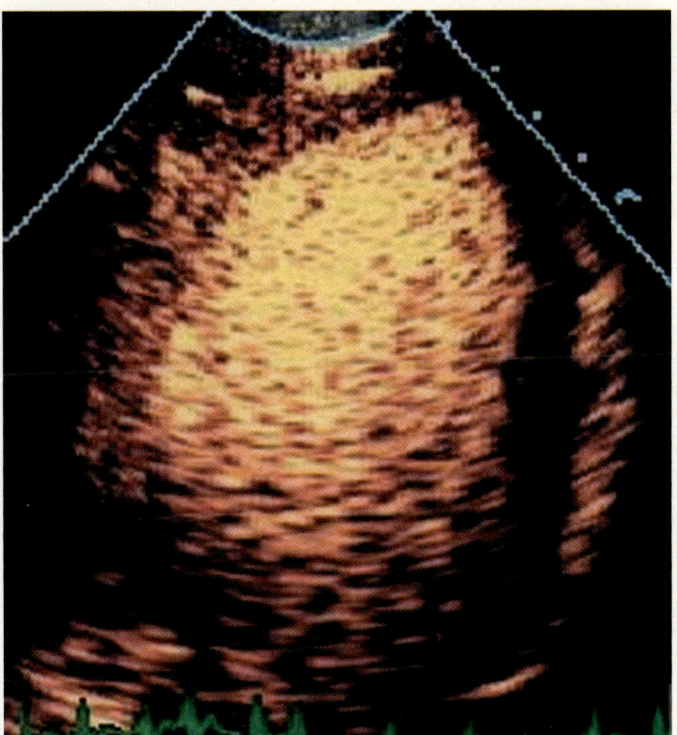

Fig. 11.8: Resting apical 2-chamber view, 10 beats post-flash, demonstrating absent perfusion to the anterior myocardial wall

Fig. 11.6A and B: Apical two chamber images obtained in a patient who had normal wall motion (top) and in a patient who had severe apical hypokinesia (bottom). In the normal patient, the color kinesis overlay in the contrast-enhanced power modulation image (top left) shows a uniform color band reflecting normal wall motion. In contrast in the patient who had hypokinesia, the thickness of the color band is reduced in the apical region (bottom left)

transmitted ultrasound with very low mechanical index imaging (MI <0.1), microbubbles demonstrate linear oscillation, where the contraction and expansion of the microbubbles are equal. All returning micro bubble backscatter remains within the range of the frequency transmitted by the transducer (the fundamental frequency)—as for surrounding structures, low mechanical index imaging (0.1–0.3) generates nonlinear oscillation of the microbubbles whereby expansion is greater than contraction. In addition to the usual backscatter of a particular amplitude within the range of the fundamental frequency, the bubbles also produce backscatter of lesser amplitude as bubbles produce nonlinear echo signals and the summation of returning pulses will not equal zero and a signal will be registered.

Using this technique, processing can theoretically be limited only to signals generated by bubbles. As well as being a grey-scale technique, tissue motion artefacts are a major limitation, as movement of tissue also creates nonlinear signals. Nevertheless the theory behind this technology has led to the development of successful real time imaging.

Ultraharmonic Imaging (Figs 11.6–11.8)

With the development of increased bandwidth transducers, another intermittent high MI technique has been evolved to improve the contrast to tissue ratio of backscatter. While intermittent harmonic imaging demonstrates myocardial perfusion, it is limited by the

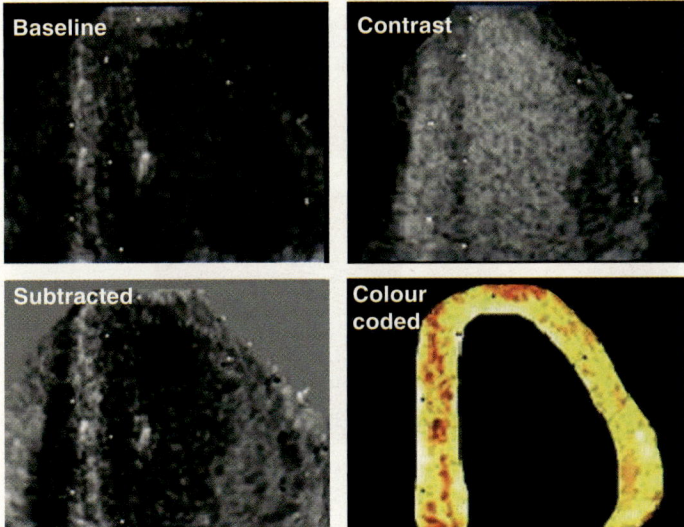

Fig. 11.7: Digital subtraction and colour coding of MCE images acquired using intermittent harmonic imaging

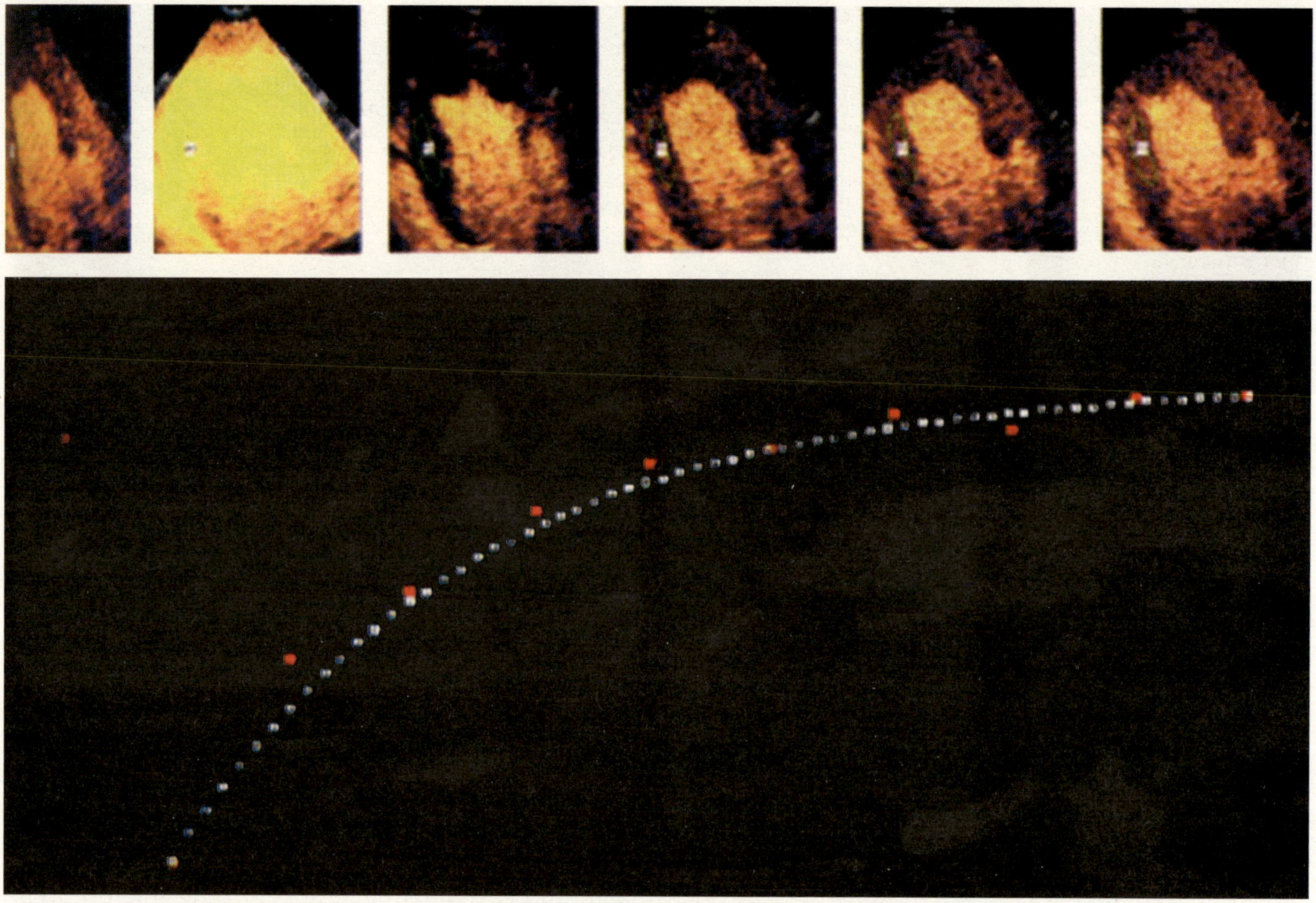

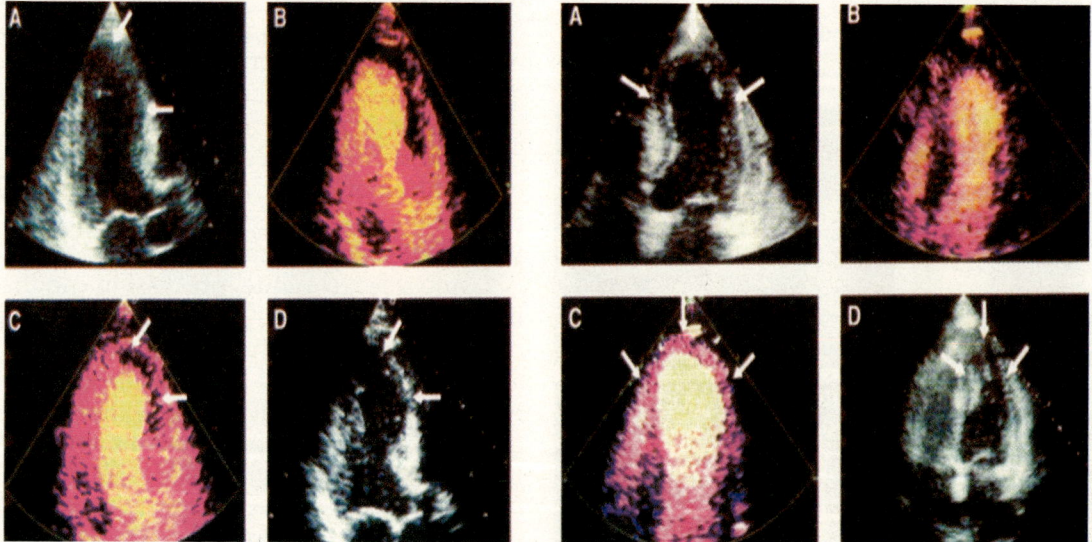

Fig. 11.9: Low MI replenishment curve showing contrast destruction and subsequent refilling

Fig. 11.10: The importance of imaging the abscence of myocardial bubbles in intervals to determine the extent of the perfusion defect in reperfused acute MI (0/2) end-systolic frames of intravenous contrast infusion MCE in the parasternal short axis views, 3 days after primary transluminal coronary angioplasty of the left anterior descending coronary artery LAD with TIMI 3 flow are shown **(A)** the frame immediately before bubble destruction. **(B)** Bubble destruction transient MI of 1/4 **(C)** the frame immediately after bubble destruction. Note the abscence of myocardial bubbles in the LAD region. Subsequently, there is progressive filling of the LAD territory so that the perfusion defect that appears large and nearly transmural at 3-seconds is smaller and non-transmural at 8 seconds

presence of tissue signals at the second harmonic. However, bubble destruction causes backscatter at 3rd, 4th and sub-harmonics. At these higher harmonics the tissue signal is negligible, thus processing only backscatter from these further harmonics enables selective enhancement of the contrast signal. Interestingly, current ultra-harmonic imaging involves processing signals from between the second and third harmonic (Figs 11.9 and 11.10).

The strength of the high MI approaches are their sensitivity for the presence of contrast, because bubble destruction results in the highest amplitude backscatter. The disadvantages are that they lack simultaneous assessment of function, require reliable ECG triggering and image acquisition, and can be both technically challenging and time-consuming (of particular importance for stress imaging). While the difficulty maintaining image position with long triggering intervals has been aided by the use of low MI localisation images, respiratory movement is almost inevitable.

Low Power Techniques

Real Time Imaging: In recent years, these have been developed successfully to exploit the non linear responses of microbubbles, that even low amplitude microbubble backscatter can be isolated from tissue signals for processing. This allows continuous low power imaging to be performed, with limited bubble destruction, enabling simultaneous assessment of wall motion and perfusion in real time (although frame-rate is minimised in order to reduce bubble destruction). Hence, low MI imaging is commonly known as real time imaging.

The use of low MI has two major benefits:
1. The bubbles undergo stable nonlinear oscillation emitting continuous fundamental and harmonic signals.
2. The tissues themselves do not generate harmonic signals at low MI. Like incremental triggered imaging, low MI imaging enables assessment of microbubble replenishment of the myocardium over time after bubble destruction. With low MI imaging, myocardial bubble destruction is achieved by transmission of a series of a high MI pulses (flashes), after which replenishment can be observed in real time. There are 2 major real time techniques.

Power Pulse Inversion Imaging (PPI) (Fig.11.18)

This technique combines the nonlinear detection performance of pulse inversion with the motion discrimination capability of power Doppler. Multiple transmit pulses of alternating polarity are used, and Doppler signal processing techniques are applied to distinguish between bubble backscatter and backscatter from tissue. In a typical configuration, echoes from a train of pulses are combined in such a way that signals from moving tissue are eliminated.

Power Modulation Imaging (Fig. 11.18)

This method utilises the same signal subtraction principles, as PPI, with the transmitted pulses identical in phase but of different in amplitude or power—hence power modulation, one impulse of full power, the other half that power. Echoes reflected from stationary tissue are linear, thus if we subtract two times the lower power from full power, the signals should cancel out whereas a nonlinear oscillation of microbubbles will generate a signal. In power modulation, fundamental imaging is most suited, because the tissue subtraction technique is so effective that the best signal to noise ratio from contrast to tissue is at the fundamental frequency. Both techniques have been validated in animals and utilised for qualitative assessment of perfusion in humans.

Bubble Administration (Figs 11.9 and 11.10)

The decision regarding the use of a bolus or infusion for intravenous administration of microbubbles is dependant on a variety of factors, including the type of microbubble used, equipment and staff available and clinical indication for the test (LVO, qualitative perfusion or quantitative perfusion). For MCE, bubbles should be infused with the aim of LV opacification and adequate myocardial perfusion with minimal/no attenuation of the basal segments. The amount of contrast required for this varies from bubble to bubble, machine to machine and technique used (intermittent or continuous), as well as showing patient to patient variability. Ideally all studies, particularly those assessing perfusion would involve a continuous infusion of micro-bubbles, with a mechanically controlled infusion preferable to a manually controlled one (slow continuous injection). This enables establishment of a true steady state for optimal imaging and in particular quantification.

Left Ventricular Opacification (LVO) (Fig.11.17)

An accurate evaluation of regional and global left ventricular function by echocardiography is dependent on adequate endocardial border resolution. Using fundamental imaging, approximately 20% of resting echoes demonstrate inadequate endocardial definition. While native tissue harmonic imaging enables better endocardial definition than standard fundamental imaging and reduces the number of patients with inadequate studies to 5–10%, contrast induced LVO still confers benefit over harmonic imaging. The most challenging patients have obesity, chronic lung disease or chest wall deformities. Ventilated patients in intensive care also provide significant difficulties because of patient positioning and compliance.

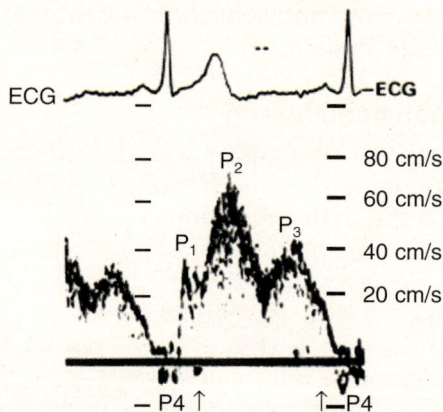

Fig. 11.11A: Pulmonary venus Doppler recording showing two systolic components P1, P2 as well as early diastolic P3 and late systolic reversal P4 waves

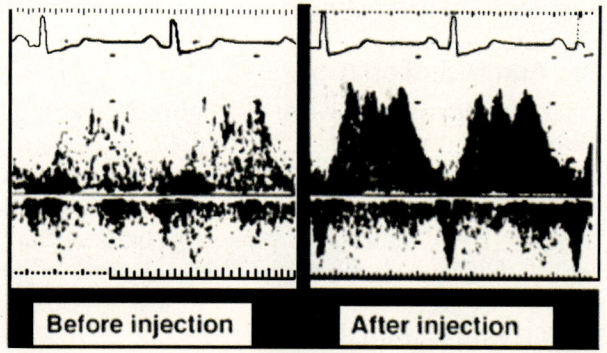

Fig. 11.11B: Pulsed-wave Dopper echocardiogram of the right upper pulmonary vein before and after sonicated albumin injection. Before injection the velocity envelope was not clear enough to determine the peak velocity of systolic, diastolic and atrial reversal flows (left). After injection, the intensity of the Doppler signal was increased and the velocity envelope

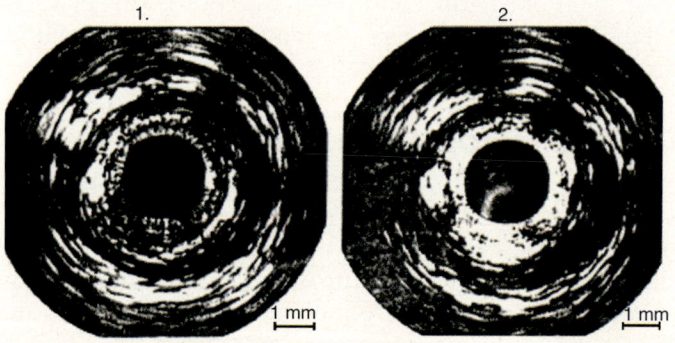

Fig. 11.11C: Intravascular ultrasonography before (1) and after (2) enhancement of luminal opacification by injection of radiogaphic contrast

Techniques that enhance discrimination between myocardial tissue and the blood pool may therefore improve the clinical utility and diagnostic accuracy of echo. Left ventricular opacification (LVO) by contrast

echo enhances this discrimination to better define the endocardial surface.

Contemporary LVO involves administration of perfluorocarbon microbubbles (which show superior duration of opacification and enhancement of endocardial definition compared with air filled bubbles, and intermediate MI harmonic imaging (0.4–0.5) which allows continuous high frame rate imaging, results in reduced bubble destruction, leads to production of microbubble harmonic signals with minimal tissue harmonic production, enabling maximal discrimination between the opacified blood pool and myocardium.

LV Volume Measurement

While there is clear evidence that contrast LVO can improve endocardial border definition, there are theoretical reasons why this may not necessarily translate into more accurate assessment of LV cavity size, volume and function. Attenuation artefacts sometimes obscure the endocardial surface, particularly in the basal segments and myocardial contrast may confuse distinction of the border between the blood pool and the endocardium. Most importantly, the use of any 2-D echo technique to assess left ventricular volumes and ejection fraction (with or without contrast), requires a standard imaging plane. Foreshortened views or views not oriented through the centre of the ventricular cavity will lead to an underestimation of volume no matter how good is the endocardial border definition. Notwithstanding these potential technical limitations, contrast LVO using fundamental imaging improves the correlation between LV volumes obtained with echo and MRI. In addition, accurate classification of systolic function by calculated ejection fraction has been improved from 70 to 94%. A subsequent study confirmed that, even using harmonic imaging, the measurement of LV volumes was optimised with contrast LVO, using electron beam CT as the standard of reference. While the role of LVO for 3-D imaging is currently undefined, it seems likely that this will be an important application of contrast echo.

LVO and Wall Motion Analysis

Enhanced endocardial border definition can improve the accuracy and interobserver agreement for assessment of regional wall motion at rest. Compared with MRI, the number of segments visualised was clearly improved after contrast (86% visualised before contrast, 99% after contrast). In addition, identification of segments with abnormal wall motion improved 82% to 100%; with the clinical utility of the contrast being greatest at the lateral and anterior walls. Importantly, the interobserver agreement for assessment of individual wall segments was significantly improved and

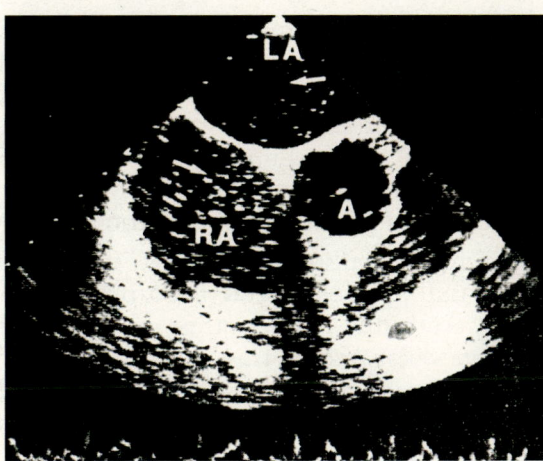

Fig. 11.12: TEE with contrast injection in a patient with patent foramen ovale showing the presence of contrast material in LA (arrow)

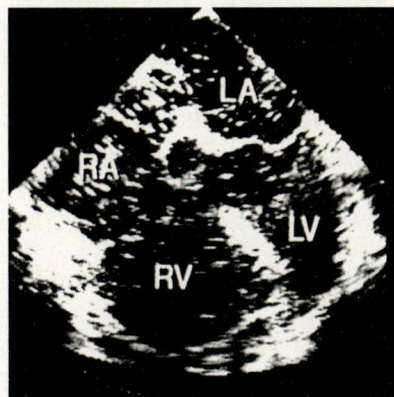

Fig. 11.13: A patient with acute MI in whom injection of agitated saline through a peripheral vein and demonstrates a large right to left shunt. The right sided chambers are enlarged with the bulge of the atrial septum toward the left

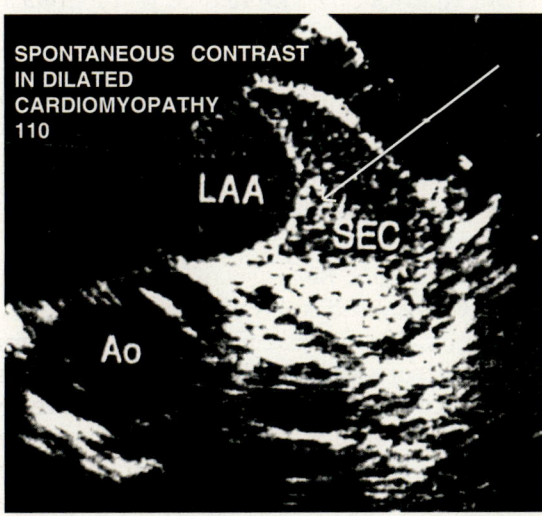

Fig. 11.14: TEE from a patient with dilated cardiomyopathy who had an embolic event. Horizontal plane image at the base of heart showing dense spontaneous echo contrast (SEC) in the left atrial appendage LAA. The aorta (AO) is seen posterior to the left atrium and appendage

contrast also improved intraobserver agreement for determination of normal versus abnormal wall motion and assessment of the severity of wall motion abnormality compared with MRI. The ability of LVO to improve scoring and inter-observer variability of regional wall motion at rest has important implications for stress echocardiography.

Stress Echocardiography is an established clinical tool with a high sensitivity and specificity for the diagnosis of coronary artery disease (CAD). During stress echo, the diagnosis of CAD is based on detection of regional contractile dysfunction, and requires visualisation of all myocardial segments to document or exclude abnormalities definitively. Reduced endocardial border definition is exacerbated during stress because of chest wall movements during hyperventilation and cardiac translational movement during tachycardia. With fundamental imaging, inadequate endocardial definition has been reported in upto 30% of stress echoes. In addition, Hoffman, *et al.* demonstrated that suboptimal studies have worse reproducibility and a poorer interobserver variability, with inter-institutional, institutional observer agreement as low as 43% for studies with poor image quality. Tissue harmonic imaging, digital side-by-side analysis and standardised reporting criteria have alleviated but not overcome this problem (Figs 11.15 and 11.16).

Wall Motion Scoring and reproducibility during stress echo were even improved with air-filled contrast agents and fundamental imaging. Perfluorocarbon filled agents demonstrated almost complete and consistent endocardial border definition, with superiority even to tissue harmonic imaging, and the greatest improvement being seen in patients with poorest image quality. Despite these clear advantages, the critical clinical question of whether LVO actually improves the accuracy of stress echo for diagnosis of CAD remains unanswered. Thus, left ventricular opacification by contrast echo:

1. Improves the visualisation of myocardial endocardial border definition;
2. Improves the accuracy of ventricular volume assessment and estimation of ejection fraction compared with standard fundamental and harmonic imaging;
3. Improves the ability to identify and grade resting wall motion abnormalities;
4. Provides superior endocardial visualisation while imaging at peak dobutamine stress and can enable the accuracy of a dobutamine stress echo in a technically difficult patient to be at least as good as that of a patient with good resting images;
5. Reduces the interobserver variability for all of the above.

From an economic standpoint, the use of contrast agents during stress echo has been calculated to be cost-effective with the cost of the contrast agent itself more than offset by savings incurred by reducing downstream repetitive testing, improved laboratory efficiency and a lower rate of false positive and negatives. However, the calculations are based on a formula incorporating improved accuracy of the technique for the diagnosis of CAD, compared with standard imaging, which remains unproven.

In summary, the use of contrast for LVO is justified for standard or stress imaging of technically difficult patients, and possibly, for calculation of ventricular dimensions in patients whom accurate quantitative serial follow-up is critical, e.g. chemotherapy or valvular heart disease. Other clinical uses of contrast for left ventricular opacification include confirming or excluding the presence of left ventricular thrombus and delineating other left ventricular structures like pseudoaneurysm, apical hypertrophic cardiomyopathy.

Myocardial Contrast Echocardiography

Hypoperfusion precedes wall motion abnormalities, which precede ECG changes and the onset of chest discomfort. Stress echo, which provides an indirect marker of hypo-perfusion by recognition of wall motion abnormalities, is more than 80% sensitive and specific for detection of CAD. The technique has two groups of limitations (Figs 11.17A–D, 11.18–11.20).

1. **Interpretive:** Wall motion analysis is fundamentally subjective leading to the need for specific training and discordance between observers. There are particular problems in the assessment of the inferoposterior wall.

2. Dependence on the induction of ischaemia (increased myocardial oxygen demand) to provide diagnostic information. Many problems spring from this—dependence on performance of adequate stress, influence by beta blockade, limited sensitivity for mild (e.g. single vessel) CAD, poor capacity to identify the extent of CAD (e.g. 50% sensitivity for the detection of multivessel disease. SPECT perfusion imaging is the best-established clinical method to address perfusion directly and theoretically should be more sensitive than stress echo because hypoperfusion occurs earliest the ischaemic cascade. However, the difference between the methods is marginal because of the technical limitations of SPECT scanning, which also relies on subjective interpretation (Fig. 11.17).

If technically feasible, there is clear role for echocardiography to assess myocardial perfusion. Ultra-sound is more widely available, portable, avoids radiation and has a better spatial resolution than SPECT scanning (up to 1 mm, compared with >10 mm). An ideal technique would allow assessment of myocardial perfusion and wall motion simultaneously.

Pathophysiology of Coronary Circulation

Understanding the pathophysiology of normal myocardial perfusion is essential for understanding detection of CAD with MCE. Contrast microbubbles act as pure intravascular tracers, traversing the myocardial vasculature, and contrasting with MRI tracers (which escape into the extravascular space) and radionuclides enter myocytes.

Myocardial Blood Volume: The coronary blood volume (CBV) encompasses the entire coronary system, which includes the epicardial arteries, the arterioles, the capillary network, venules, veins and the coronary sinus. Approximately one-third of the CBV resides within the ventricular myocardium. This myocardial blood volume (MBV) includes "microvessels" of < 300 microns in diameter, with approximately 90% of the total myocardial blood volume lying within the capillaries 6–7 microns in diameter. Assessment of myocardial perfusion with MCE involves processing backscattered signals received from microbubbles within the MBV, so that myocardial opacification almost entirely reflects backscatter from microbubbles flowing through the myocardial capillary compartment.

There are 2 components of this myocardial bloodflow appreciated with MCE:

1. The intensity of the backscatter signal from the microbubbles within the myocardium (brightness of its appearance on echo) related to the myocardial blood volume,

2. The rate of increase in intensity after bubble destruction reflects the red blood cell velocity. Their product represents (myocardial bloodflow). The response of MBF (myocardial bloodflow) and its components to stress is central to the application of perfusion imaging.

Normal Perfusion: Because of the near complete extraction of O_2 from red cells by the myocardium under basal conditions, any increase in myocardial O_2 demand must rapidly translate into increases in coronary bloodflow. In the absence of a coronary stenosis, when myocardial O_2 demand is increased, there is sufficient vasodilator reserve to allow coronary flow to increase by a factor of 4–6 fold above resting levels (Fig. 11.29).

It has shown that the ability to increase coronary flow in response to increased demand is achieved through a process of coronary autoregulation, controlled predominantly by the arterioles. The coronary microcirculation strives to maintain a minimum transcapillary pressure

Rest   Stress

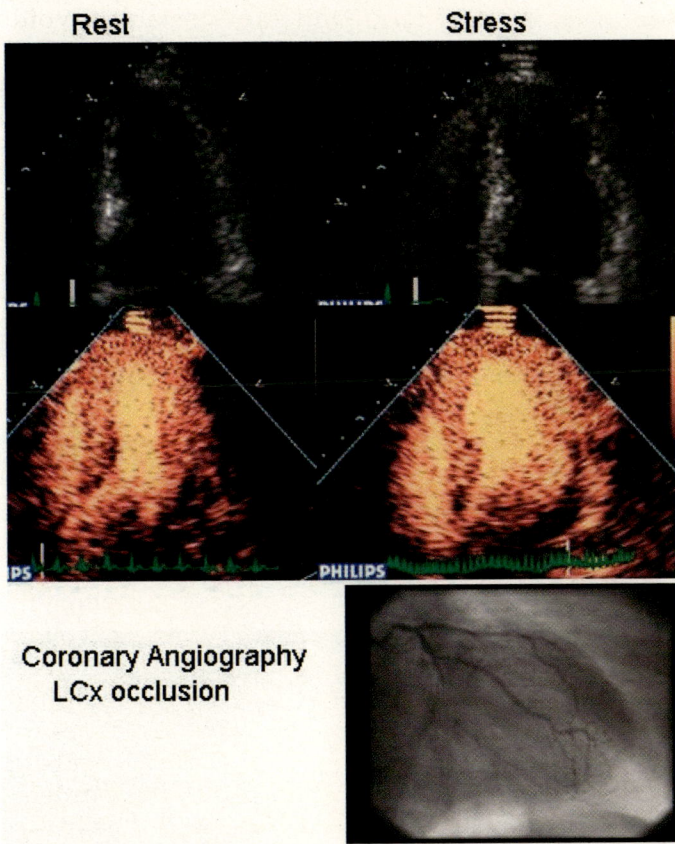

Coronary Angiography
LCx occlusion

Fig. 11.15: End-systolic frames of 4CV at rest (left) and post-stress (right). Note there is no obvious difference in the shape of the cavity on the grey scale images. Importantly, the LVO images demonstrate a clear change in shape with the basal and mid lateral segments lagging, suggestive of LCx stenosis. In addition, the mid lateral segment has a perfusion defect which was not present at rest. Subtotal occlusion of the LCx was demonstrated at angiography

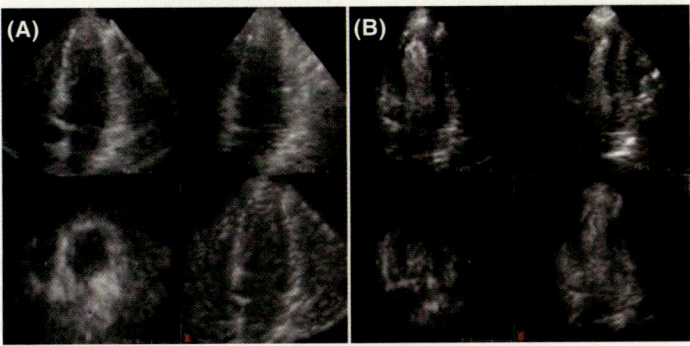

Fig. 11.16: Realtime 3D echocardiography **(A)** and with contrast enhancement **(B)**. There is clear benefit for LV border detection

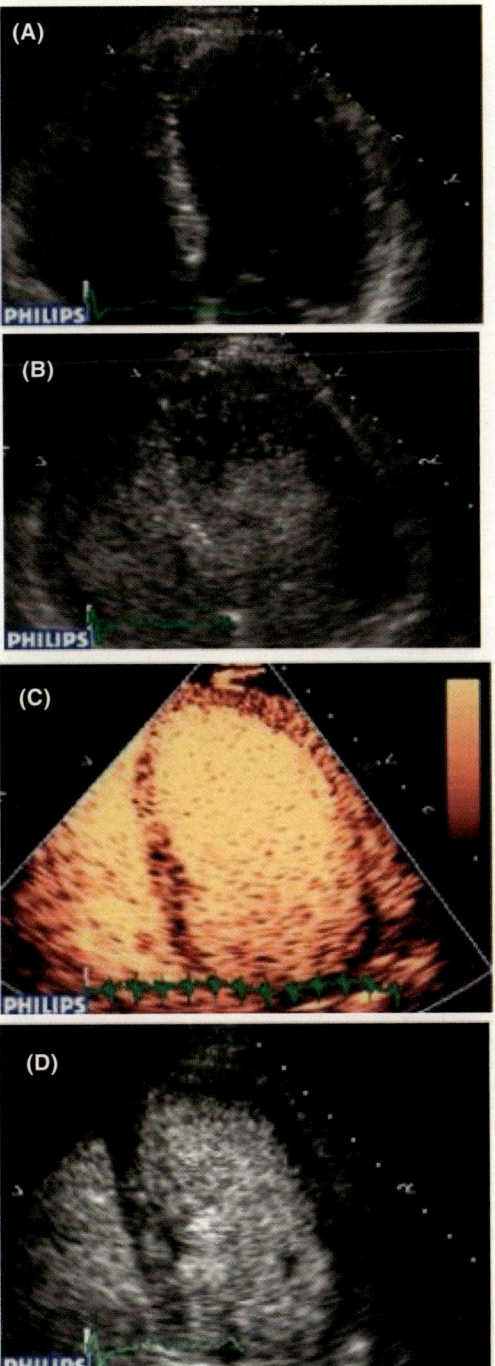

Fig. 11.17A to D: Importance of machine settings for using contrast for LV opacification. **(A)** In this example, endocardial border definition is probably adequate with standard tissue harmonic imaging. **(B)** The use of contrast for LVO with standard diagnostic harmonic imaging machine settings provides worse border definition in the lateral wall, and apical bubble destruction, illustrating the importance of appropriate machine settings. Image. **(C)** shows machine settings for myocardial perfusion imaging – this provides assessment of myocardial perfusion and wall motion, but the frame rate for WMA is 20–25 Hz and thus subtle WMA's could be missed. Therefore, for optimal assessment of WMA image. **(D)** displays specific intermediate MI imaging at high frame rate designed specifically to enhance the endocardial/cavity border. Even in this case there is some apical swirling despite the focal zone set in the mid LV

of approximately 30 mm Hg. In the absence of a coronary stenosis, a resting patient with a mean aortic pressure of 90 mm Hg will have a precapillary pressure of 45 mm Hg. This natural resistance between the aorta and the capillaries is provided by the arterioles which

Harmonic power Doppler 1:1 triggering   Harmonic power Doppler 1:5 triggering

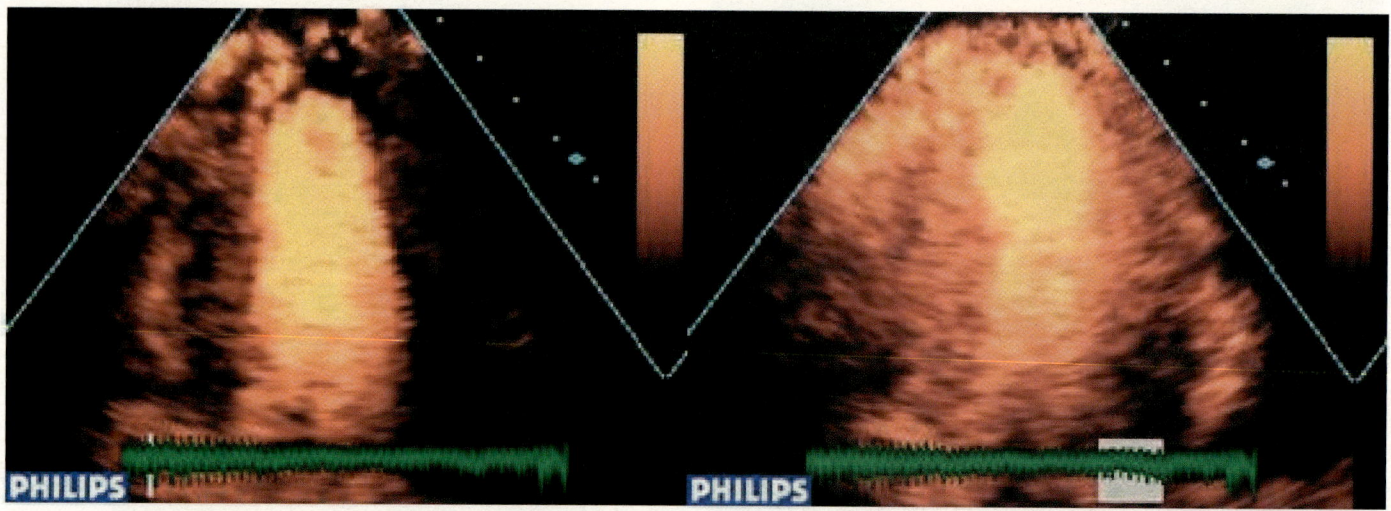

Fig. 11.18: Harmonic power Doppler imaging

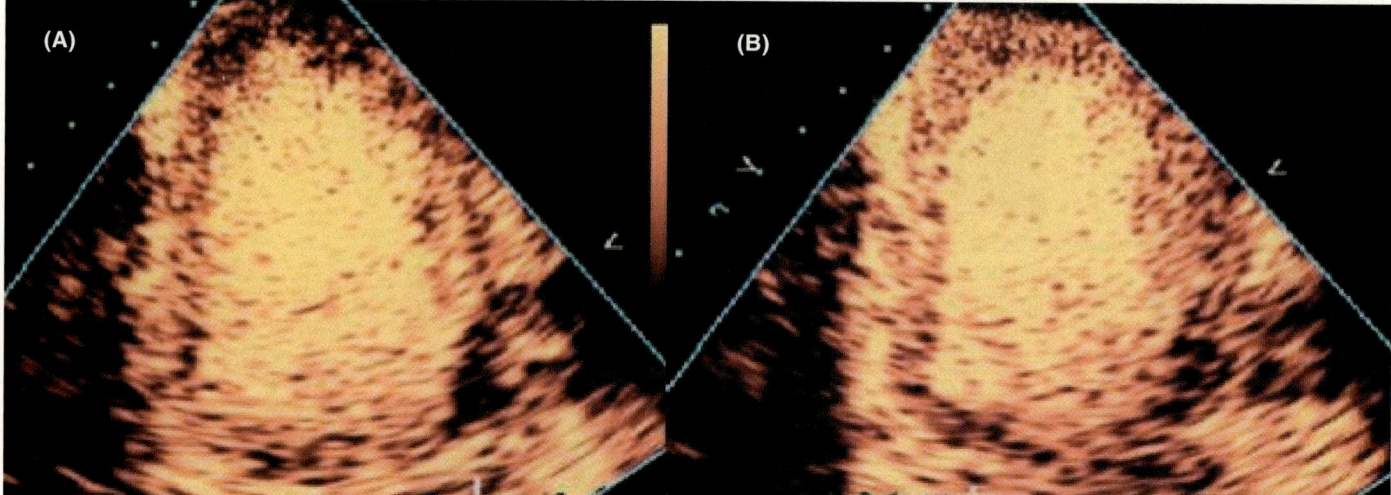

Fig. 11.19: False positive defects with real-time MCE. Pseudo-apical defects are due to apical bubble destruction **(A)**. Relocation of the focus from the base toward the apex **(B)** leads to "resolution" of the apical abnormality, but use of a mid-ventricular focus placement may lead to more problems with definition of the basal segments. This case also exemplifies attenuation of the basal lateral segment by contrast within the LV cavity

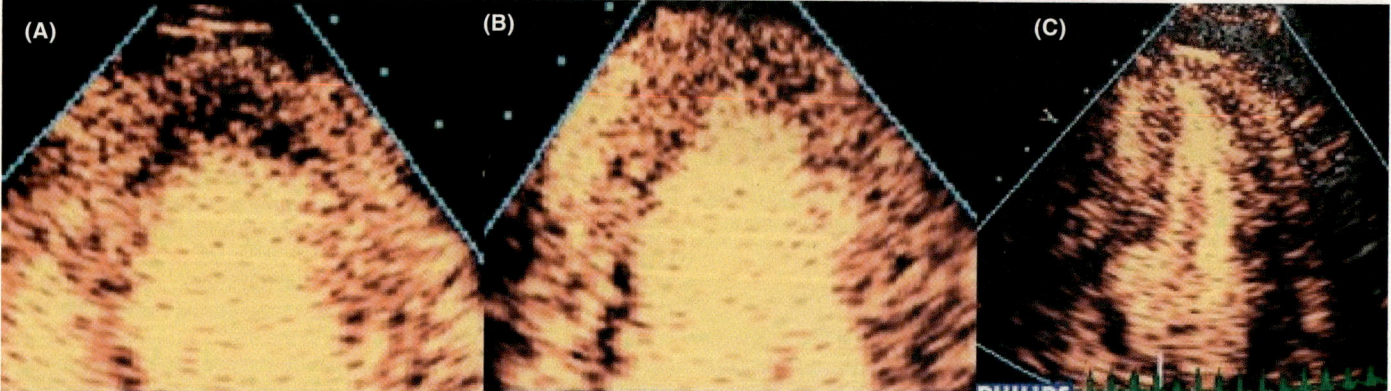

Fig. 11.20: Contribution of regional shape changes to the identification of perfusion defects, including irregular wall contour in the apex **(A)** and mid-inferior segment **(B)**, both associated with subendocardial defects. The C shape of the basal inferior segment complements the diagnosis of a perfusion defect in this segment **(C)**

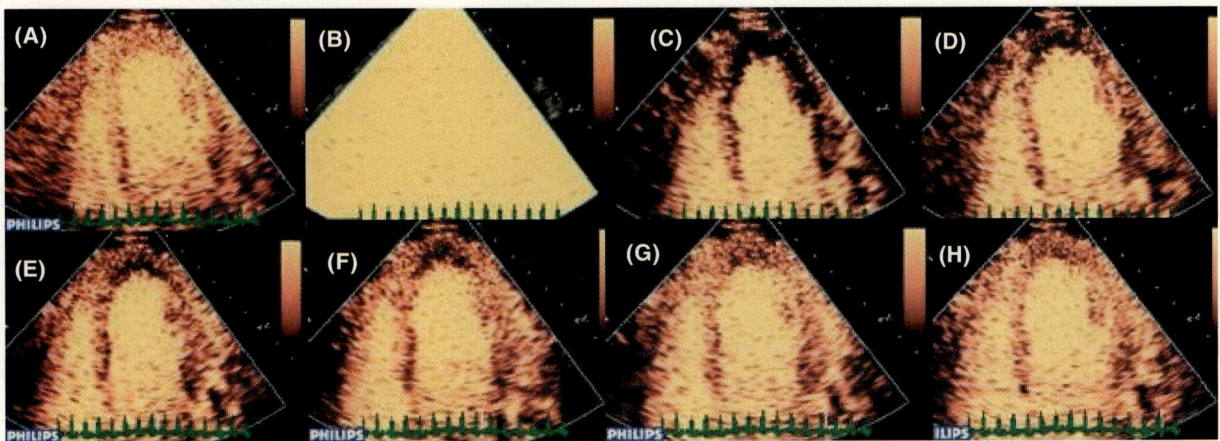

Fig. 11.21: Destruction replenishment imaging with real time MCE

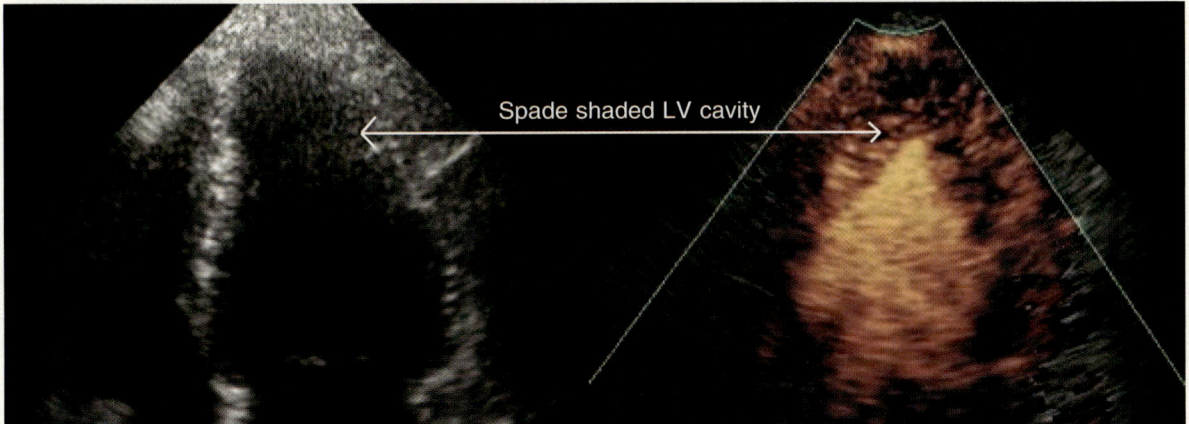

Fig. 11.22: Use of contrast echo to identify a patient with apical hypertrophic cardiomyopathy. Note the 'spade-shaped LV cavity' (arrow) on the contrast image

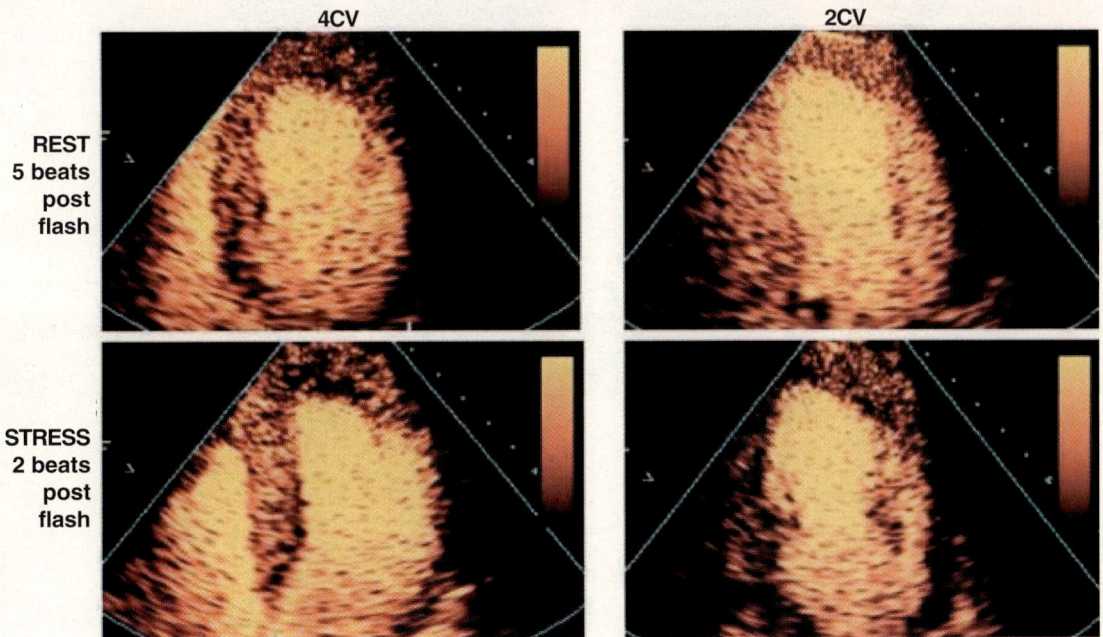

Fig. 11.23: A clear apical defect is evident 2 beats post flash at peak stress (bottom line) which was not evident at rest (top line), consistent with LAD stenosis

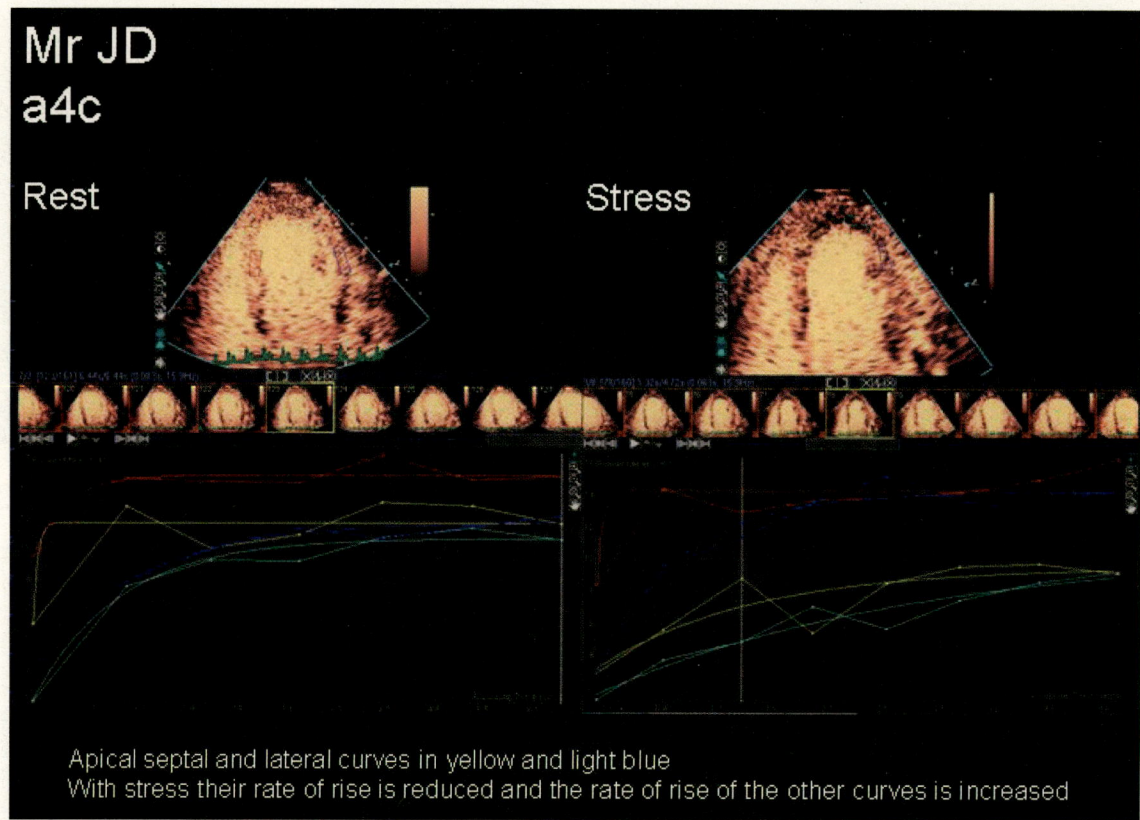

Fig. 11.24: Apical septal and lateral curves in yellow and light blue. With stress their rate of rise is reduced and the rate of rise of the other curves is increased

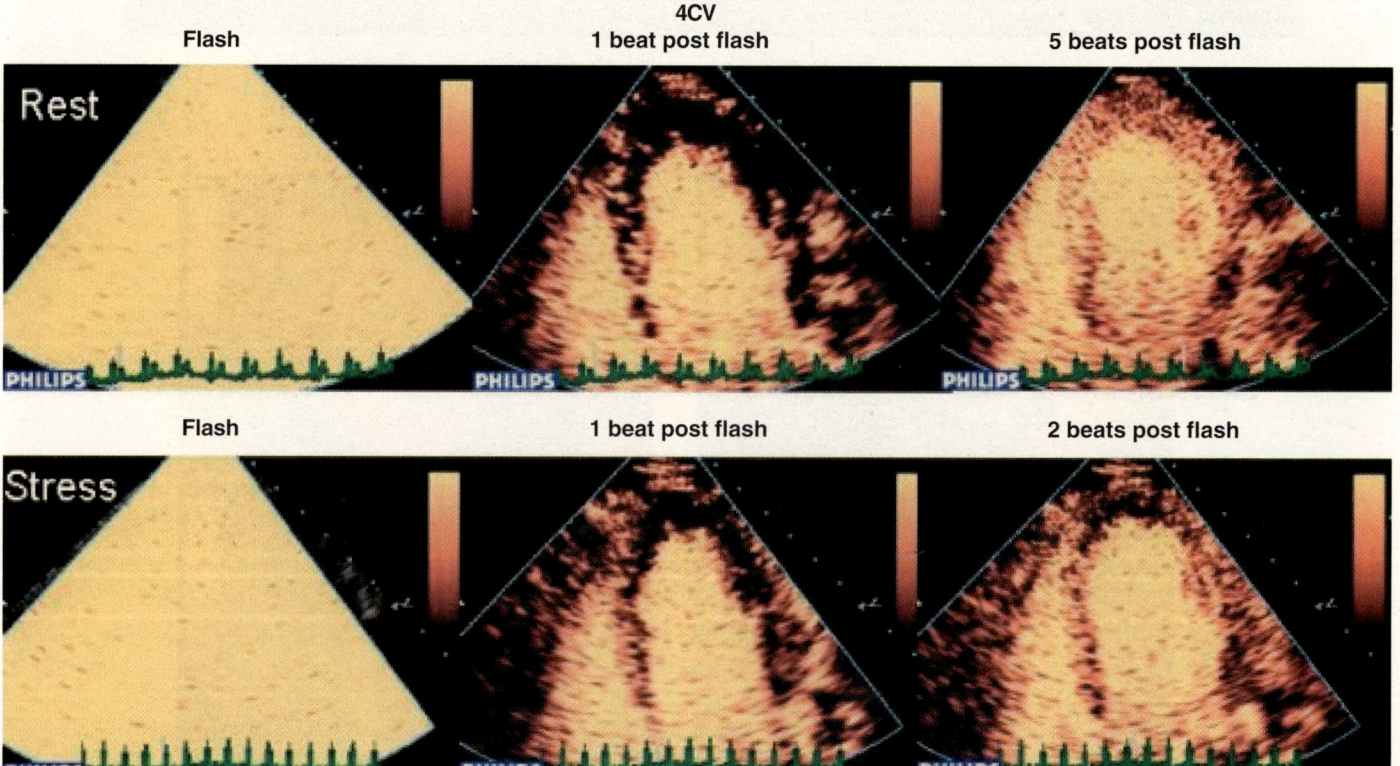

Fig. 11.25: A basal and mid inferior defect is evident 2 beats post flash at peak stress which was not evident at rest, consistent with RCA stenosis

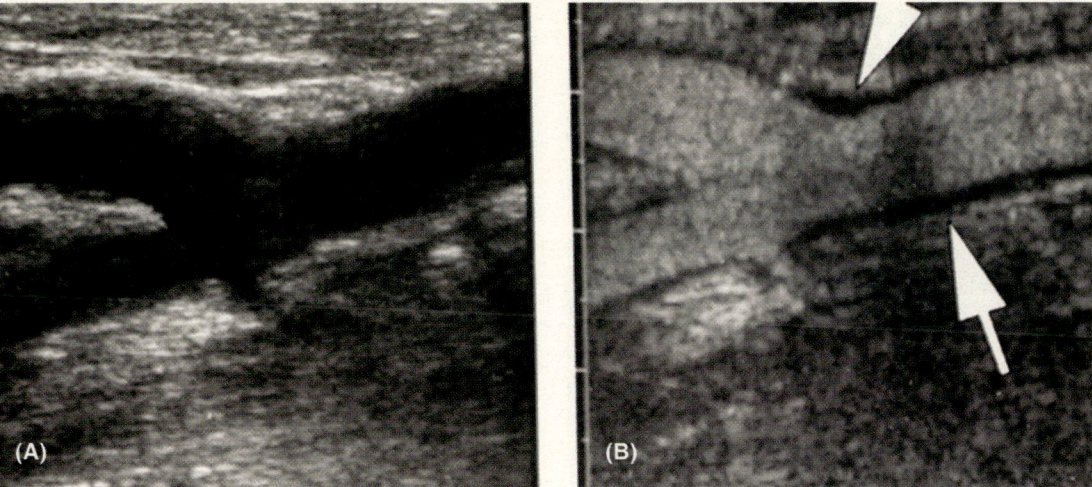

Fig. 11.26A and B: (A) Carotid duplex imaging of a common carotid artery, bulb and bifurcation panel A, shows images without contrast panel. **(B)** Images with contrast agent. Note the dramatic ability to detect intimal and medial thickness arrows accurately which has been underestimated by non-contrast imaging

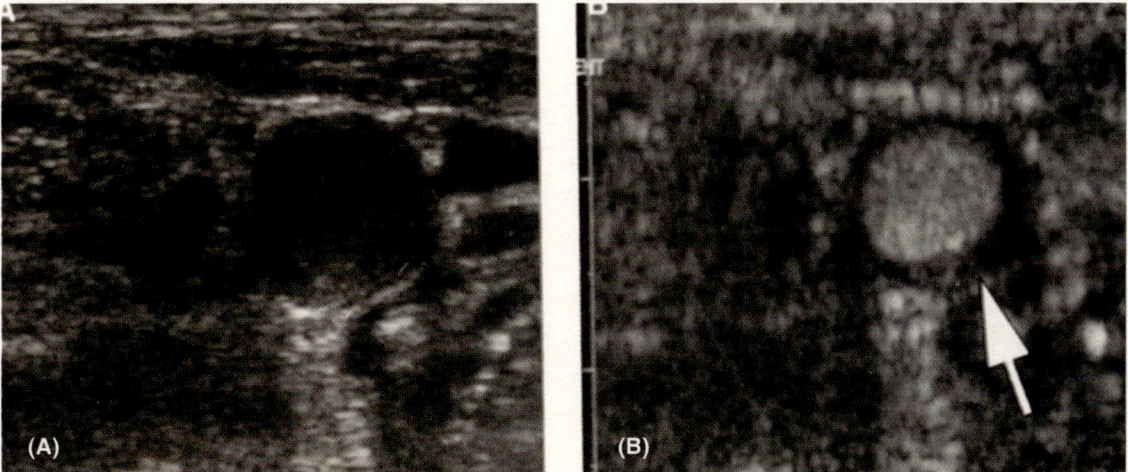

Fig. 11.27: Application of contrast to visualize plaque morphology better (panel A) is a transverse view near the bulb (panel B) is a contrast enhanced transverse image near the bulb, highlighting how the plaque is much better seen by the use of contrast agent (white arrow)

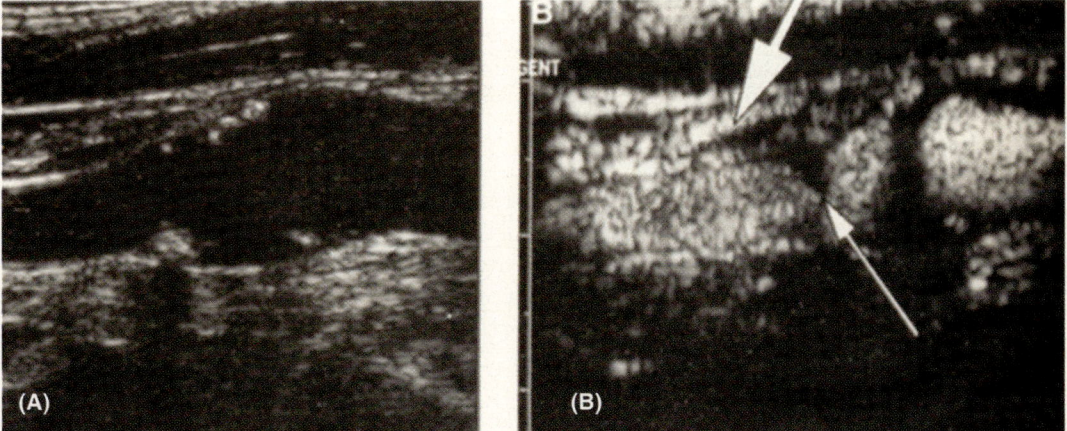

Fig. 11.28: Contrast-enhanced duplex images of a longitudinal scan of the carotid artery (panel A) is a non-contrast enhanced view that suggest of a minimal plaque. (Panel B) is a nonharmonic contrast imaging which depicts a large area of plaque (small white arrow) that was not visualized on non-contrast imaging the large white arrow on (panel B) shows vessel near the advential wall of the carotid, believed to be the vasa vesorum

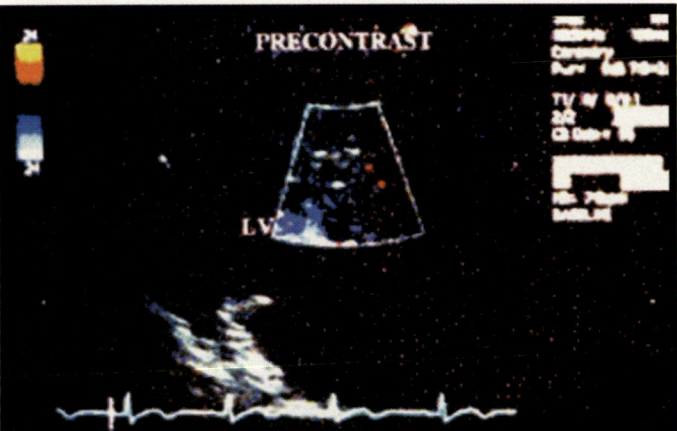

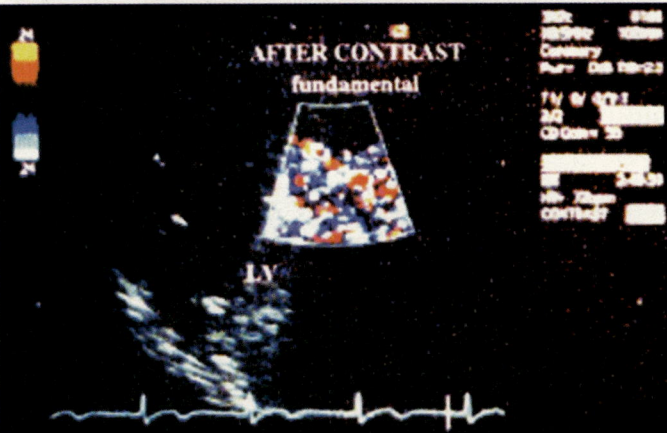

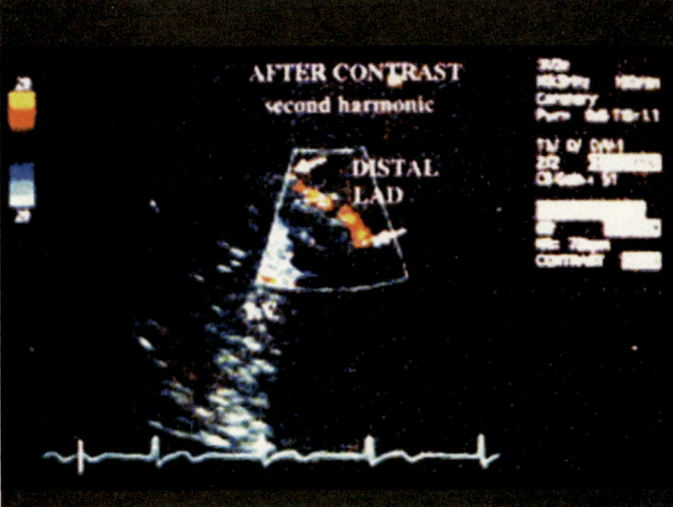

Fig. 11.29: Color Doppler flow mapping in the distal left anterior descending coronary artery (LAD) before (upper panel) and after contrast enhancement using, respectively, fundamental mode (mid plane) and harmonic mode (lower panel). A. modified 2-chamber view has been obtained. Before contrast infusion, (upper panel), faint LAD flow score 2 is detected by color Doppler in fundamental mode in the anterior groove (epicardial side of LV anterior wall). After contrast infusion, blooming and flushing blur color flow Doppler signal from the LAD when fundamental Doppler is used (midplane). Switching to the second harmonic (lower panel) clearly depicts color coded blood flow in the LAD (indicated by arrows). Enhancemet of color Doppler signal in LV cavity is also evident

present up to 60% of the total coronary vascular resistance. In the presence of increased myocardial oxygen demand, there is arteriolar vasodilation, reducing the resistance at the arteriolar level, which enables a higher precapillary pressure, translating into increased red blood cell velocity across the capillary network, and opening dormant capillary networks in order to maintain mean transcapillary pressure, thus increasing the overall myocardial blood volume. Hence overall myocardial bloodflow is increased. Importantly, pure vasodilator stress tends to increase red cell velocity without marked changes in overall myocardial blood volume.

In the presence of a significant, noncritical (60–90%) epicardial artery stenosis at rest, completely normal resting bloodflow is maintained by arteriolar vasodilation. As a result, myocardial perfusion imaging techniques cannot detect defects at rest in patients with noncritical stenosis.

Thus, identification of perfusion defects in the setting of a noncritical coronary stenosis requires stress imaging to induce either ischaemia (increased myocardial oxygen demand) or hyperaemia (pharmacologically induced maximal arteriolar vasodilation). During stress we expect a 4–6 fold increase in flow to areas supplied by non-stenotic arteries, mediated by arteriolar vasodilation, increased red cell velocity and increased myocardial blood volume (opening of dormant capillary networks). Flow in the perfusion bed subtended by a significantly stenosed artery is not augmented, as resting arteriolar vasodilation is present, so limited augmentation of flow can be achieved with hyperaemia. In some cases the precapillary pressure drops significantly due to low distal coronary pressure and steal. With reduced pre capillary pressure the only means of attempting to maintain normal trans-capillary pressure is to shut down capillary networks which were previously open (capillary de-recruitment). The net result is that direct comparison between regions subtended by a significant stenosis and normal territories reveal perfusion mismatch.

In the presence of a critical stenosis, maximal arterial vasodilation maintains perfusion at rest. Any further reduction in distal coronary pressure directly translates into reduced precapillary pressure and reduced myocardial bloodflow. Patients with critical lesions commonly have collateral vessels, making assessment of resting perfusion a complex phenomenon.

Qualitative Assessment of Myocardial Contrast for Diagnosis of CAD

There are three aspects to myocardial contrast opacification—signal intensity (equivalent to myocardial blood volume), pattern of filling and rate of filling (Fig. 11.17).

Signal Intensity: Myocardial blood volume is the easiest parameter to interpret qualitatively, and most studies have addressed differences in MBV between rest and stress in myocardial segments. Perfusion has traditionally been scored using a graded scale; 1 for homogeneous perfusion, 0.5 for reduced perfusion and 0 for absent perfusion. The presence of a stress induced perfusion defect not seen on the resting images indicates ischaemia, but in the absence of destruction-replenishment imaging, may appear normal in mild disease. The presence of a resting perfusion defect signifies infarction or artefact, with an infarction likely if there are associated regional wall motion abnormalities at rest, and if the defect conforms to the distribution of a coronary vascular territory.

False positive defects often reflect technical limitations. Failure to obtain signal from a segment may be due to attenuation by overlying contrast, shadowing by rib or other structure, bubble destruction (especially in the apex) or failure to deliver sufficient contrast to enter the microcirculation.

Perfusion Distribution: While most infarctions are shown as a transmural perfusion defect, stress-induced defects are often restricted to the subendocardium. The detection of this finding allows a greater level of confidence than does a transmural defect, or particularly epicardial defects.

The location of a defect has an important relationship to its likelihood of being a true or a false positive. Generally, defects on the left hand side of the image are most likely to be true positives and those restricted to the right side (anterior, lateral wall) should be considered very critically before they are identified as abnormal, as these are the most common sites of false positives. Fortunately, in our experience the apex is a more sensitive marker of LAD disease than the anterior wall, and is usually well seen. Likewise, a lateral segment should be matched with a posterior wall finding before circumflex disease is reported. The basal segments are also problematic—especially with low MI imaging (Figs 10.15 and 10.16).

The shape of the LV cavity is a clue to true positive findings. A "C-shaped" perfusion defect in the inferior wall is a common distribution with right coronary disease. Irregularities of the walls or apex or apical "beaking" may provide evidence of dyssynchrony, and are often associated with subendocardial perfusion abnormalities (Fig. 11.20).

Rate of Filling: The rate of replenishment after bubble destruction is dependent on coronary flow, and even if this is not quantified, rate of refill is a reliable and sensitive marker of a true positive defect. Using low MI techniques, microbubbles are infused until adequate LVO and myocardial opacification are achieved. Several pulses of high mechanical index are delivered, causing destruction of microbubbles in the beam elevation, such that the previously opacified myocardium is now empty. The replenishment time of microbubbles into the myocardium can be observed qualitatively (Fig. 11.10).

As the mean myocardial microbubble velocity is 1 mm/sec, and the beam elevation is approximately 5 mm, it would take up to 5 seconds (i.e. 5–6 heartbeats at a resting heart rate from 60–80) for homogeneous opacification of the myocardium at rest. With hyperaemia in the absence of stenosis, myocardial bloodflow should increase 4–6 fold. Thus, images taken within 1–2 seconds following bubble destruction (i.e. 2–3 heartbeats at a peak heart rate of 140) should demonstrate complete homogeneous refill within this time frame, and failure to fill in a perfusion defect thus represents reduced myocardial bloodflow. Perfusion defects noted on the post stress images, not evident on the resting images suggest ischaemia for evidence of LAD, RCA and multivessel CAD respectively. Assessment of end-systolic frames is preferable, despite the presence of more coronary flow in diastole, because the myocardium is thicker and there is less risk of contamination by the blood pool, and perhaps also because the capillary network is 'sealed' during systolic contraction with minimal flow in or out of the capillary compartment.

High MI techniques apply the same principles, with infusion until homogenous myocardial opacification. Imaging is then changed to a sequential intermittent mode, beginning with continuous high MI imaging (which results in bubble destruction and empties the myocardium). Images are then recorded intermittently, gated from the ECG (usually end systolic) with an incrementally lengthening triggering interval, i.e. 1:1 an image every cardiac cycle, then 1:2, and image every two cardiac cycles, then 1:3, 1:4 etc. The same principles are used for assessment of perfusion defects.

Validation of Qualitative Contrast Echo for Diagnosis of CAD (Figs 11.23–11.25)

Qualitative assessment of perfusion with MCE was validated in open chest dogs using graded coronary stenosis. The original landmark paper in humans compared MCE (intermittent harmonic MCE with offline digital subtraction and colour coding) with sestamibi SPECT scanning in 30 patients undergoing dipyridamole stress to investigate known or suspected coronary disease. Normal segments showed a 91% concordance, and abnormal segments an 85% concordance, with 90% concordance by vascular territory. There was an overall 86% concordance for the detection of coronary disease. Subsequent studies have validated MCE following vasodilator or dobutamine stress using other imaging modalities, including power Doppler and real time power pulse inversion/power modulation in animals and in humans have produced similar results to SPECT. A recent study using real time imaging was the first to report the use of MCE with exercise stress (which is technically challenging because of cardiorespiratory movement and short duration of hyperaemia) and again demonstrated concordance between MCE and SPECT imaging. There was a 76% agreement between MCE and SPECT and an 88% agreement between the combination of wall motion and MCE with SPECT. This study incorporated the wall motion data from real time imaging, and despite the low frame rate, the results hint at the incremental benefit of combining the approaches.

While numerous studies examining various stress and imaging modalities have demonstrated concordance between MCE and SPECT, there remains a paucity of data using quantitative coronary angiography (QCA) as the gold standard. The presence and extent of CAD by QCA has traditionally been used as the reference standard for the assessment of CAD, but few studies have compared MCE and angiography.

Quantitative Myocardial Contrast Echo for Diagnosis of CAD (Fig. 11.29)

Like stress echo and nuclear perfusion imaging, MCE is also limited by the qualitative nature of the interpretation. Subtle differences in video intensity between vascular beds may not be visually evident, potentially reducing the sensitivity for the detection of stenosis. Quantitative methods may help to alleviate this limitation and possibly reduce intraobserver and interobserver variability in assessment.

The process of quantitative myocardial contrast echo was validated in open chest dogs using intermittent imaging, and the same destruction-replenishment approach is used for contemporary qualitative assessment. At a steady state during continuous intravenous infusion of microbubbles, the number of bubbles entering or leaving any capillary unit is constant and depends on the flow rate of the bubbles. If the microbubbles are destroyed at time zero, the video intensity in a selected myocardial region is close to zero dB (black). With time, bubbles will replenish the beam elevation—the degree of replenishment into the beam elevation increases as the time after destruction is increased until eventually the entire ultrasound beam elevation is replenished and a plateau is reached, whereby no further increase in video-intensity/brightness can occur. Because this relationship was originally described with intermittent imaging, it is usually described in terms of video-intensity *vs.* pulsing intervals.

More recently, the ability of MCE to calculate flow reserves from these measurements in humans using intermittent imaging in 30 selected patients undergoing coronary angiography (11 of whom had no CAD and 19 had noncritical single vessel stenoses) have been studied.

Quantitative MCE and invasive measurement coronary flow (Doppler flow wire) were performed at rest and following vasodilator stress. In the normal subjects, myocardial bloodflow velocity and myocardial bloodflow reserves demonstrated a linear relationship to coronary bloodflow reserve measured invasively. In patients with CAD, there were significant differences in MBF velocity reserves between patients with mild, moderate and severe stenosis, and a MBF velocity reserve of <1.8 indicated a >70% stenosis. Thus MBF reserve appears to be a feasible noninvasive measure of CBF reserve in humans, which may allow noninvasive assessment of CAD and microvascular dysfunction. More recently, Dawson investigated the use of quantitatively derived MBF reserves to diagnose CAD using SPECT as the gold standard. She demonstrated moderate feasibility, with quantitative MBF reserves from both high and low MI imaging able to identify perfusion defects. Low MI imaging had a lower sensitivity (Fig. 11.4).

Contrast Echo and Myocardial Viability in Chronic CAD (Fig. 11.25)

It is now well recognised that regional or global ventricular dysfunction does not necessarily imply irreversible necrosis. Hypokinetic, akinetic or dyskinetic, yet viable myocardium may be stunned or hibernating. Myocardial stunning occurs after a period of acute ischaemia, despite restoration of completely normal bloodflow. The natural history of stunning is of spontaneous improvement in the viable myocardium over time. Hibernating myocardium is the term used to describe the presence of significant ventricular dysfunction in patients with chronic CAD, which recovers after revascularisation. Improvement in function of sufficient numbers of viable but hibernating segments is associated with symptomatic benefit and improved survival. Sadly, many patients with chronic CAD and LV dysfunction have minimal viability, and revascularisation of these patients is associated with significant risk, minimal benefit and possibly worse outcome, hence the need for a reliable test for identification of viability.

Radionuclide Scanning, Dobutamine Echocardiography, MRI and PET Scanning

These are currently available modalities, each with various advantages and disadvantages but similar efficacy for prediction of myocardial functional recovery after revascularization. MCE may also have an important role in this clinical setting. Viable myocardium is associated with preservation of the microvasculature, and as microbubbles act as pure intra-vascular tracers, the presence of myocardial perfusion by any MCE technique at rest implies viability. Using intracoronary injection of bubbles, Nagueh demonstrated that MCE was feasible and had similar accuracy to thallium SPECT and dobutamine echo for identification of functional recovery using intravenous microbubble administration, MCE demonstrated comparable efficacy to SPECT and DSE. Importantly in both of these studies quantitative MCE was superior to qualitative assessment. Unfortunately there remains a paucity of further data in this clinically important area (Figs 11.12, 11.13 and 11.14).

Safety of Contrast Echocardiography

The incidence of reported adverse events in human trials (mainly investigating LV opacification) has been very low. There have been particular theoretical concerns raised about histologic abnormalities and cardiac marker elevation in animals with high MI imaging and whilst serum tropin levels are normal in humans after high MI imaging. Recent work has demonstrated troponin I and myoglobin in coronary sinus samples of humans after high MI imaging.

Conclusion

Advances in microbubble development, combined with the development of contrast specific imaging modalities have enabled not only excellent LVO, but reliable qualitative and quantitative assessment of myocardial perfusion by ultrasound, following intravenous injections of microbubbles. Use of this technology during stress echo increases sensitivity and improves the non-invasive evaluation of cardiac functions.

Bibliography

1. Al Mansour HA, Mulvagh SL, Pumper GM, Klarich KW, Foley DA: Usefulness of harmonic imaging for left ventricular opacification and endocardial border delineation by optison. *Am J Cardiol* 2000, 85:795–9.
2. Allman KC, Shaw LJ, Hachamovitch R, Udelson JE: Myocardial viability testing and impact of revascularization on prognosis in patients with coronary artery disease and left ventricular dysfunction: a meta-analysis. *J Am Coll Cardiol* 2002;39:1151–1158.
3. Becher H, Tiemann K, Schlief R, Luderitz B, Nanda NC: Harmonic Power Doppler Contrast Echocardiography: Preliminary Clinical Results. *Echocardiography* 1997;14:637.
4. Borges AC, Walde T, Reibis RK, *et al.* Does contrast echocardiography with Optison induce myocardial necrosis in humans? *J Am Soc Echocardiogr* 2002; 15:1080–1086.
5. Burns PN: Harmonic imaging with ultrasound contrast agents. *Clin Radiol* 1996; 51 (Suppl 1):50–55.
6. Chen S, Kroll MH, Shohet RV, Frenkel P, Mayer SA, Grayburn PA: Bioeffects of myocardial contrast echocardiography in patients with suspected coronary artery disease: Comparison with quantitative gated Technetium 99m sestamibi single photon emission computed tomography. *J Am Soc Echocardiogr* 2003, 16:1171–1177.
7. Cwajg J, Xie F, O'Leary E, Kricsfeld D, Dittrich H, Porter TR: Detection of angiographically significant coronary artery disease with accelerated intermittent imaging after intravenous administration of ultrasound contrast material. *Am Heart J* 2000;139:675–683.
8. Dawson D, Rinkevich D, Belcik T, *et al.* Measurement of myocardial bloodflow velocity reserve with myocardial contrast echocardiography in patients with suspected coronary artery disease: Comparison with quantitative gated Technetium 99m sestamibi single photon emission computed tomography. *J Am Soc Echocardiogr* 2003; 16:1171–1177.
9. De Jong N, Hoff L: Ultrasound scattering properties of Albunex microspheres. *Ultrasonics* 1993;31:175–181.
10. Dolan MS, Riad K, El Shafei A, *et al.* Effect of intravenous contrast for left ventricular opacification and border definition on sensitivity and specificity of dobutamine stress echocardiography compared with coronary angiography in technically difficult patients. *Am Heart J* 2001; 142:908–915.
11. Firschke C, Wei K, Kaul S: Quantification of the physiological relevance of a coronary stenosis using myocardial contrast echo-cardiography. *Coron Artery Dis* 2000; 11:203–209.
12. Grayburn PA, Weiss JL, Hack TC, *et al.* Phase III multicenter trial comparing the efficacy of 2% dodecafluoropentane emulsion (EchoGen) and sonicated 5% human albumin (Albunex) as ultrasound contrast agents in patients with suboptimal echocardiograms. *J Am Coll Cardiol* 1998;32:230–236.
13. Halmann M, Beyar R, Rinkevich D, *et al.,* Digital subtraction myocardial contrast echocardiography: design and application of a new analysis program for myocardial perfusion imaging. *J Am Soc Echocardiogr* 1994; 7:355–362.
14. Heinle SK, Noblin J, Goree-Best P, *et al.,* Assessment of myocardial perfusion by harmonic power Doppler imaging at rest and during adenosine stress: comparison with (99m) Tc-sestamibi SPECT imaging. *Circulation* 2000, 102:55–60.
15. Hoffmann R, Hanrath P: Stress echocardiography: the scourge of subjective interpretation. *Eur Heart J* 1995; 16:1458–1459.
16. Hoffmann R, Marwick TH, Poldermans D, *et al.* Refinements in stress echocardiographic techniques improve interinstitutional agreement in interpretation of dobutamine stress echocardiograms. *Eur Heart J* 2002; 23:821–829.
17. Hundley WG, Kizilbash AM, Afridi I, Franco F, Peshock RM, Grayburn PA: Administration of an intravenous perfluorocarbon contrast agent improves echocardiographic determination of left ventricular volumes and ejection fraction: comparison with cine magnetic resonance imaging. *J Am Coll Cardiol* 1998;32:1426–1432.
18. Hundley WG, Kizilbash AM, Afridi I, Franco F, Peshock RM, Grayburn PA: Effect of contrast enhancement on transthoracic echocardiographic assessment of left ventricular regional wall motion. *Am J Cardiol* 1999;84:1365–1369.
19. Kaul S, Jayaweera AR: Coronary and myocardial blood volumes: noninvasive tools to assess the coronary microcirculation? *Circulation* 1997;96:719–724.

20. Kaul S, Senior R, Dittrich H, Raval U, Khattar R, Lahiri A: Detection of coronary artery disease with myocardial contrast echocardiography: comparison with 99m Tc-sestamibi single-photon emission computed tomography. *Circulation* 1997, 96:785–792.

21. Leong-Poi H, Le E, Rim SJ, Sakuma T, Kaul S, Wei K: Quantification of myocardial perfusion and determination of coronary stenosis severity during hyperemia using real-time myocardial contrast echocardiography. *J Am Soc Echocardiogr* 2001; 14:1173–1182.

22. Leong-Poi H, Le E, Rim SJ, Sakuma T, Kaul S, Wei K: Quantification of myocardial perfusion and determination of coronary stenosis severity during hyperemia using real-time myocardial contrast echocardiography. *J Am Soc Echocardiogr* 2001; 14:1173–1182.

23. Leong-Poi H, Rim SJ, Le DE, Fisher NG, Wei K, Kaul S: Perfusion versus function: the ischemic cascade in demand ischemia: implications of singlevessel versus multivessel stenosis. *Circulation* 2002, 105:987–992.

24. Lepper W, Nowak B, Franke A, *et al.*, Myocardial contrast echocardiography, single-photon emission computed tomography, and regional function analysis for coronary stenosis description during vasodilator stress. *Am J Cardiol* 2003;91:445–448.

25. Marwick TH, Nemec JJ, Pashkow FJ, Stewart WJ, Salcedo EE: Accuracy and limitations of exercise echocardiography in a routine clinical setting. *J Am Coll Cardiol* 1992;19:74–81.

26. Moir S, Haluska B, Jenkins C, *et al.* Incremental Benefit of Myocardial Contrast to Combined Dipyridamole-Exercise Stress Echocardiography for the Assessment of Coronary Artery Disease. Circulation 2004, in myocardial contrast echocardiography for quantification of coronary stenosis severity and transmural perfusion gradient. *Circulation* 2001;104:1550-1556.

27. Nagueh SF, Vaduganathan P, Ali N, *et al.* Identification of hibernating myocardium: comparative accuracy of myocardial contrast echocardiography, rest-redistribution thallium-201 tomography and dobutamine echocardiography. *J Am Coll Cardiol* 1997; 29:985–993.

28. O'Keefe JH Jr, Barnhart CS, Bateman TM: Comparison of stress echocardiography and stress myocardial perfusion scintigraphy for diagnosing coronary artery disease and assessing its severity. *Am J Cardiol* 1995, 75:25D–34D.

29. Olszowska M, Kostkiewicz M, Tracz W, Przewlocki T: Assessment of myocardial perfusion in patients with coronary artery disease. Comparison of myocardial contrast echocardiography and 99mTc MIBI single photon emission computed tomography. *Int J Cardiol* 2003;90:49–55.

30. PM, Crawford M, *et al.*, Recommendations for quantitation of the left ventricle by two dimensional echocardiography. American Society of Echocardiography Committee on Standards, Subcommittee on Quantitation of Two-Dimensional Echocardiograms. *J Am Soc Echocardiogr* 1989; 2:358–367.

31. Porter TR, Xie F, Kricsfeld A, Chiou A, Dabestani A: Improved endocardial border resolution during dobutamine stress echocardiography with intravenous sonicated dextrose albumin. *J Am Coll Cardiol* 1994; 23:1440–1443.

32. Porter TR, Xie F, Kricsfeld D, Armbruster RW: Improved myocardial contrast with second harmonic transient ultra-sound response imaging in humans using intravenous perfluorocarbon-exposed sonicated dextrose albumin. *J Am Coll Cardiol* 1996;27:1497–1501.

33. Porter TR, Xie F, Silver M, Kricsfeld D, Oleary E: Real-time perfusion imaging with low mechanical index pulse inversion Doppler imaging. *J Am Coll Cardiol* 2001;37:748–753.

34. Rainbird AJ, Mulvagh SL, Oh JK, *et al.* Contrast dobutamine stress echocardiography: clinical practice assessment in 300 consecutive patients. *Am Soc Echocardiogr* 2001;14:378–385.

35. Reisner SA, Ong LS, Lichtenberg GS, *et al.* Myocardial perfusion imaging by contrast echocardiography with use of intracoronary sonicated albumin in humans. *J Am Coll Cardiol* 1989, 14:660–665.

36. Schiller NB, Shah PM, Crawford M, *et al.* Recommendations for quantitation of the left ventricle by two-dimensional echocardiography. American Society of Echocardiography Committee on Standards, Subcommittee on Quantitation of Two-Dimensional Echocardiograms. *J Am Soc Echocardiogr* 1989;2:358–367.

37. Shimoni S, Frangogiannis NG, Aggeli CJ, *et al.* Microvascular structural correlates of myocardial contrast echocardiography in patients with coronary artery disease and left ventricular dysfunction: implications for the assessment of myocardial hibernation. *Circulation* 2002, 106:950-956. Microbubble destruction by echocardiography. *Echocardiography* 2002, 19:495–500.

38. Shimoni S, Zoghbi WA, Xie F, *et al.* Real-time assessment of myocardial perfusion and wall motion during bicycle and treadmill exercise echocardiography: comparison with single photon emission computed tomography. *J Am Coll Cardiol* 2001; 37:741–747.

39. Spencer KT, Grayburn PA, Mor-Avi V, *et al.* Myocardial contrast echocardiography with power Doppler imaging. *Am J Cardiol* 2000, 86:479–481.

40. Stratton JR, Lighty GW Jr, Pearlman AS, Ritchie JL: Detection of left ventricular thrombus by two-dimensional echocardiography: sensitivity, specificity, and causes of uncertainty. *Circulation* 1982; 66:156–166.

41. Thanigaraj S, Nease RF Jr, Schechtman KB, Wade RL, Loslo S, Perez JE: Use of contrast for image enhancement during stress echocardiography is cost-effective and reduces additional diagnostic testing. *Am J Cardiol* 2001; 87:1430–1432.

42. Thomson HL, Basmadjian AJ, Rainbird AJ, *et al.* Contrast echocardiography improves the accuracy and reproducibility of left ventricular remodeling measurements: A prospective, randomly assigned, blinded study. *J Am Coll Cardiol* 2001; 38:867–875.

43. Vandenberg BF, Feinstein SB, Kieso RA, Hunt M, Kerber RE: Myocardial risk area and peak gray level measurement by contrast echocardiography: effect of microbubble size and concentration, injection rate, and coronary vasodilation. *Am Heart J* 1988;115:733–739.

44. Wei K, Crouse L, Weiss J, *et al.* Comparison of usefulness of dipyridamole stress myocardial contrast echocardiography to technetium-99m sestamibi single-photon emission computed tomography for detection of coronary artery disease (PB127 Multicenter Phase 2 Trial results). *Am J Cardiol* 2003; 91:1293–1298.

45. Wei K, Jayaweera AR, Firoozan S, Linka A, Skyba DM, Kaul S: Quantification of myocardial bloodflow with ultrasound-induced destruction of microbubbles administered as a constant venous infusion. *Circulation* 1998;97:473–483.

46. Wei K, Ragosta M, Thorpe J, Coggins M, Moos S, Kaul S: Noninvasive quantification of coronary bloodflow reserve in humans using myocardial contrast echocardiography. *Circulation* 2001; 103:2560–2565.

47. Wei K, Skyba DM, Firschke C, Jayaweera AR, Lindner JR, Kaul S: Interactions between microbubbles and ultrasound: *in vitro* and in vivo observations. *J Am Coll Cardiol* 1997; 29:1081–1088.

48. Zhu H, Muro T, Hozumi T, *et al.* Usefulness of left ventricular opacification with intravenous contrast echocardiography in patients with asymptomatic negative T waves on electrocardiography. *J Cardiol* 2002;40:259–265.

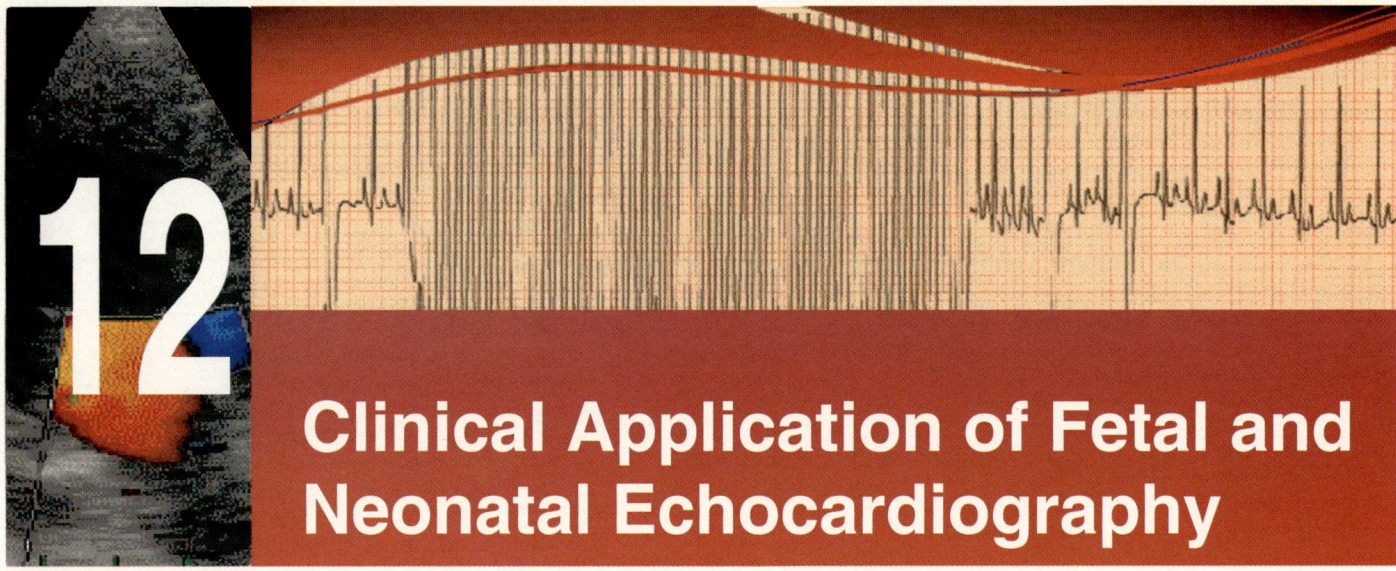

Clinical Application of Fetal and Neonatal Echocardiography

Fetal Echocardiography in Pregnant Women with Congenital Heart Disease

Women with important cyanotic or acyanotic, operated or unoperated congenital heart disease (CHD) have been shown to carry an inherent risk during pregnancy for themselves and for their fetuses. Obstetrical and fetal echocardiography has recently been upgraded by new technical developments in ultrasound machines. These improvements have increased the detection rate of congenital malformations and cardiac anomalies. Obesity or an unfavourable position of the fetus may, however, obscure the imaging quality and cause limitations to visualise the fetal heart from different angles and thus prevent the detection of anomalies. In addition, several cardiac anomalies develop throughout pregnancy and may not yet be present at an early date of screening. While the risk for a congenital cardiac malformation (CCM) in a normal population is 0.8–1%, the recurrence rate for CCM increases to 2–3% when a previous child has been affected but will become significantly higher when genetically determined anomalies have affected a family member or when the pregnant woman (5.8%) has CHD. The aim of fetal screening in women with CCM is to ascertain normal intrauterine growth, to exclude fetal CHD and/or to ascertain a malformation or arrhythmia which has been suspected during an obstetrical screening. The acquired detailed echocardiographic knowledge of the malformation or arrhythmia allows the explanation of a CCM to the future parents, to present therapeutic options during pregnancy or afterbirth and to plan delivery in a tertiary centre that provides early cardiovascular and/or catheter interventions and disposes of intensive care facilities for affected newborns. Under certain conditions, termination can be dis-cussed in early pregnancy. Therapeutic measures in the fetus have been attempted with very limited success so far successful life saving treatment does, however, exist for fetal arrhythmias. Fetal echocardiography has become an important analytical tool in high-risk pregnancies, especially when parents are affected by a CCM. The examination is safe and can be performed with a high predictive and sensitivity rate (Fig. 12.1).

What is Fetal Echocardiography? (Figs 12.1 and 12.2)

Fetal echocardiography is an ultrasound test performed during pregnancy to evaluate the heart of the unborn baby. Echocardiography assesses the heart's structures and function. A small probe called a transducer (similar to a microphone) is placed on the mother's abdomen and sends out ultrasonic sound waves at a frequency too high to be heard. When the transducer is placed in certain locations and at certain angles, the ultrasonic sound waves move through the mother's and baby's skin and other body tissues to the baby's heart tissues, where the waves bounce (or "echo") off of the heart structures. The transducer picks up the reflected waves and sends them to a computer. The computer interprets the echoes into an image of the heart walls and valves. Fetal echocardiography can help detect fetal heart abnormalities before birth, allowing for faster medical or surgical intervention once the baby is born. This improves the chance of survival after delivery for babies with serious heart defects.

When is a Fetal Echocardiogram Necessary?

It is not necessary for all pregnancies to receive an echocardiogram. The prenatal ultrasound tests that are done prior to birth can give information about whether

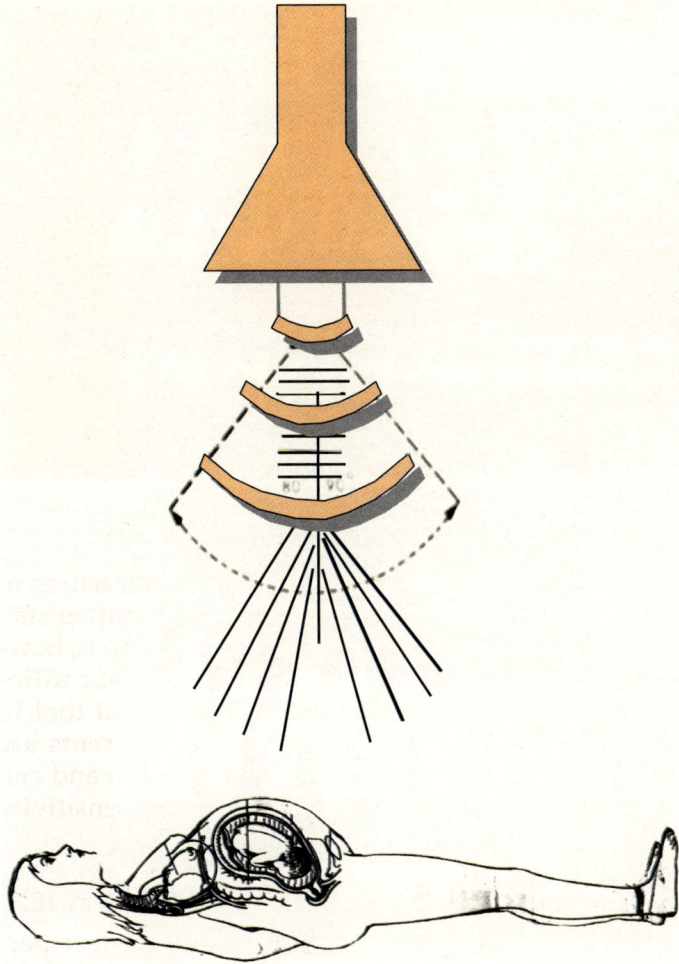

Fig. 12.1: Foetus in the womb of the pregnant women (lower panel) and ultrasound beam is being directed to create the image

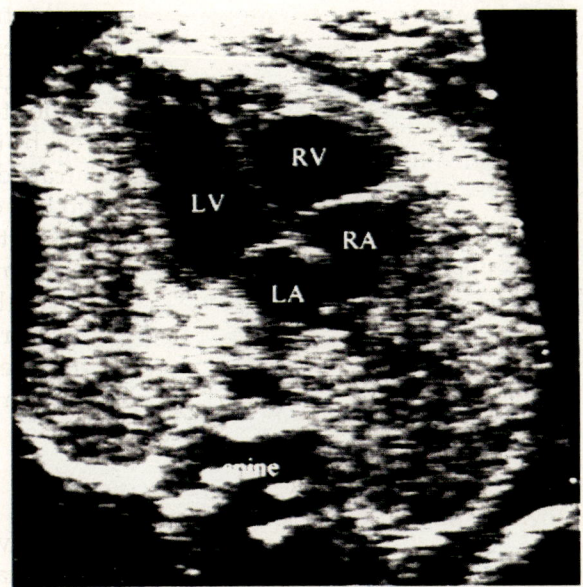

Fig. 12.2: Four chambers view with persistent foramen ovale. RV = Right ventricle, RA = Right atrium, LV = Left ventricle, LA = Left atrium

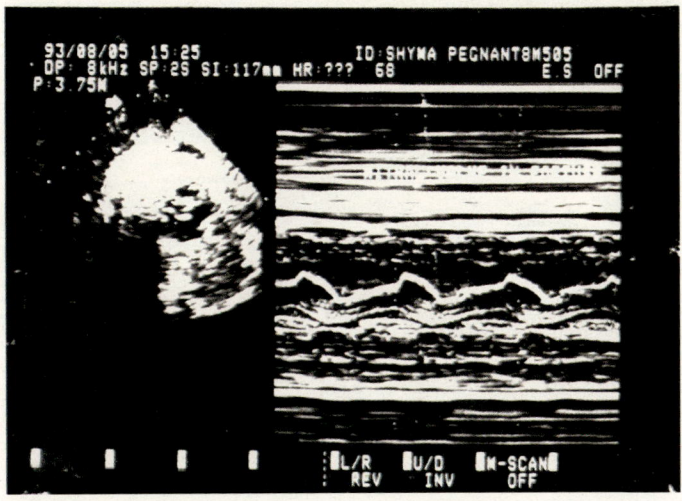

Fig. 12.3: M-Mode echocardiogram showing normal foetal mitral valve

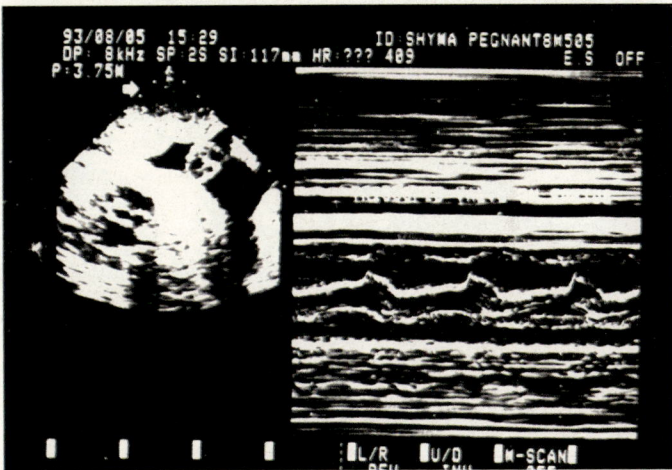

Fig. 12.4: M-Mode echocardiogram showing normal foetal tricuspid valve

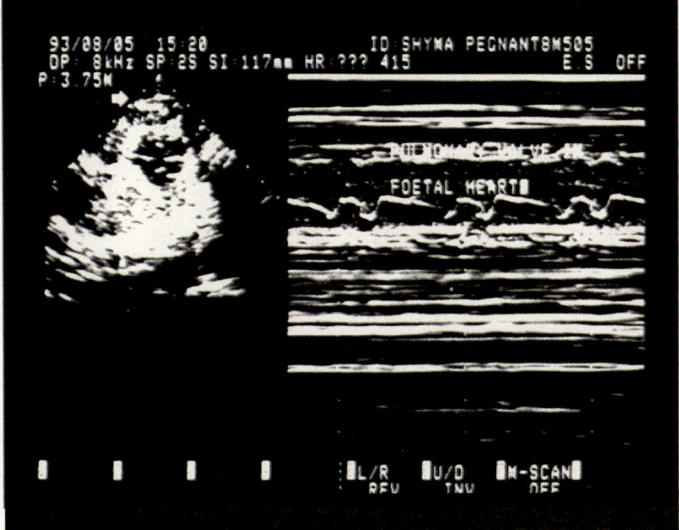

Fig. 12.5: M-Mode echocardiogram showing normal pulmonary valve

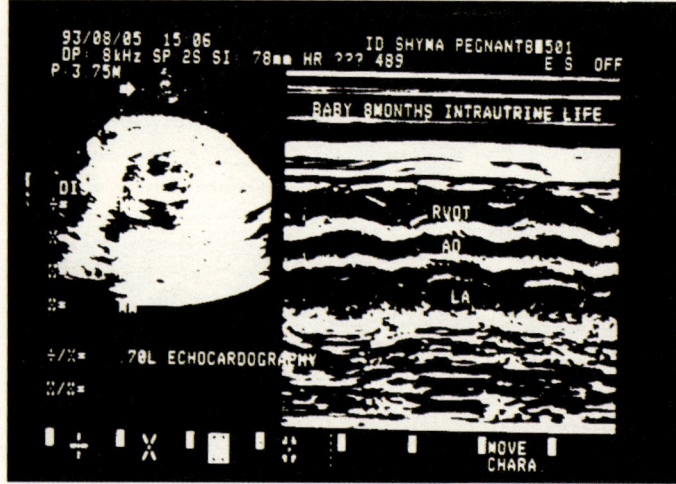

Fig. 12.6: M-Mode echocardiogram showing normal foetal aortic valve

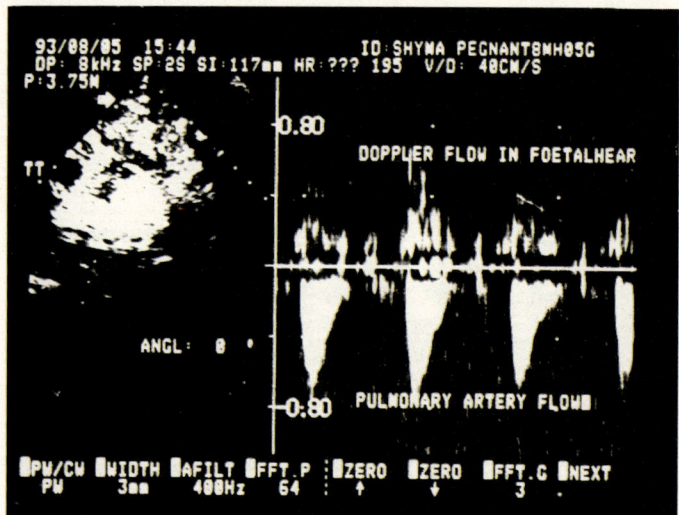

Fig. 12.7: Doppler flow velocity across normal foetal pulmonary valve

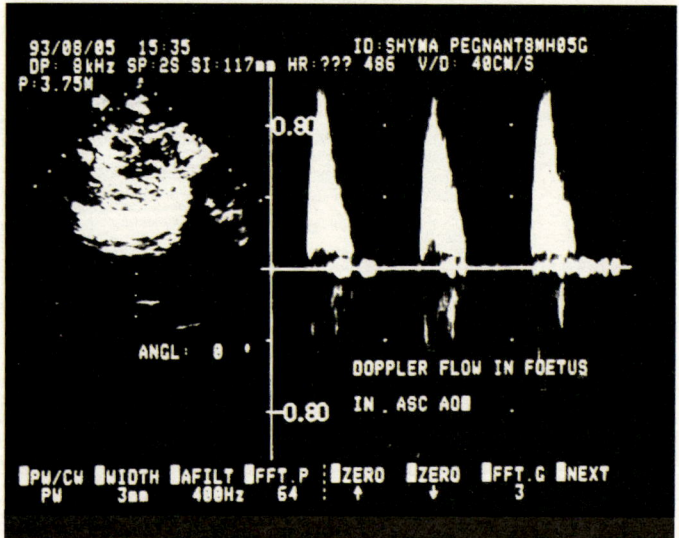

Fig. 12.8: Doppler flow velocity across normal foetal ascending aorta

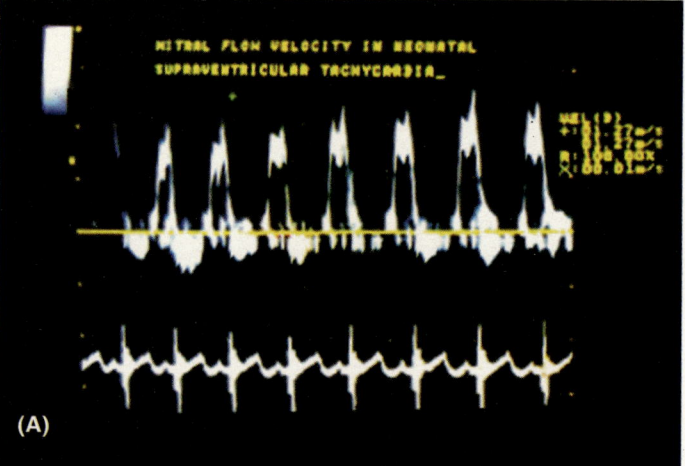

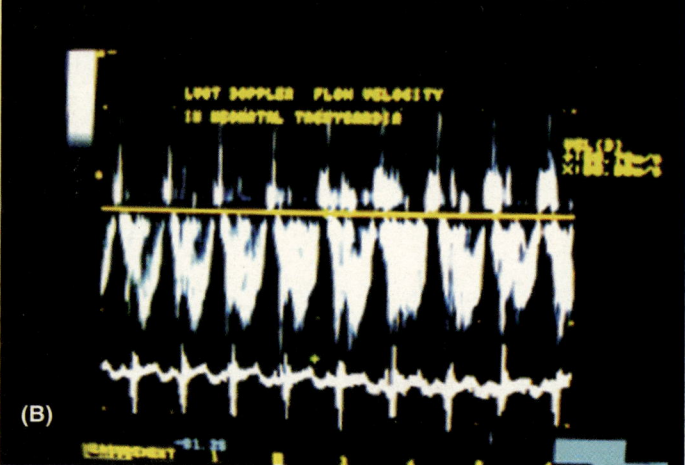

Fig. 12.9A and B: Doppler flow velocity across MV in newborn with supraventricular tachycardia with ventricular rate more than 150 beats/min with A-V conduction of 1;1 (A) Doppler flow velocity across left ventricular outflow tract (LVOT) in newborn with supraventricular tachycardia with ventricular rate more than 150 beats/min with A-V conduction of 1;1 (B)

the fetal heart has developed with all four chambers. Most unborn babies do not require any further testing. Situations in which a fetal echocardiogram may be necessary include, but are not limited to, the following:

1. If a sibling was born with a congenital (present at birth) heart defect

2. A family history of congenital heart disease (such as parents, aunts or uncles, or grandparents)

3. A chromosomal or genetic abnormality discovered in the fetus

4. If a mother has taken certain medications that may cause congenital heart defects, such as anti-seizure medications or prescription acne medications

5. If the mother has abused alcohol or drugs during pregnancy

6. If a mother has diabetes, phenylketonuria, or a connective tissue disease such as lupus
7. If the mother has had rubella during pregnancy, a routine prenatal ultrasound has discovered possible heart abnormalities.

Fetal echocardiograms are usually performed in the second trimester of pregnancy at about 18 weeks. The test is sometimes done earlier in pregnancy using transvaginal ultrasound (the ultrasound probe is inserted in the mother's vagina), but will be repeated later to confirm any findings.

How is a Fetal Echocardiogram Performed?

A fetal echocardiogram is performed by a pediatric cardiologist or a fetal specialist (also called a perinatologist) who is specially trained. The test may be done using an abdominal or transvaginal ultrasound.

Abdominal Ultrasound

In an abdominal ultrasound, gel is applied to the abdomen and the ultrasound transducer glides over the gel on the abdomen to create the image.

Transvaginal Ultrasound

In a transvaginal ultrasound, a smaller ultrasound transducer is inserted into the vagina and rests against the back of the vagina to create an image. A transvaginal ultrasound produces a sharper image than abdominal ultrasound and is often used in early pregnancy.

During the test the transducer probe will be moved around to obtain images of different locations and structures of the fetal heart. Techniques sometimes used to obtain detailed information about the fetal heart include the following:

2-D Echocardiography

This technique is used to "see" the actual structures and motion of the heart structures. A 2-D echo view appears cone-shaped on the monitor, and the real-time motion of the heart's structures can be observed. This enables the physician to see the various heart structures at work and evaluate them (Figs 12.1–12.8).

Doppler Echocardiography

This Doppler technique is used to measure and assess the flow of blood through the heart's chambers and valves. The amount of blood pumped out with each beat is an indication of the heart's functioning. Also, Doppler can detect abnormal bloodflow, which can indicate such problems as an opening between chambers of the heart, a problem with one or more of the heart's four valves, or a problem with the heart's walls.

Colour Doppler

Colour Doppler is an enhanced form of Doppler echocardiography. With colour Doppler, different colours are used to designate the direction of bloodflow. This simplifies the interpretation of the Doppler images.

Fetal echocardiography can help detect fetal heart abnormalities before birth, allowing for faster medical or surgical intervention once the baby is born. This improves the chance of survival after delivery for babies with serious heart defect. Since the time, effective foetal therapy and surgical interventional techniques have been invented for the management of various fetal disorders, foetal physicians have been showing keen interest in fetal echocardiography and have found it being as an effective and sensitive tool for the prenatal diagnosis of cardiac malformations during the mid trimester stage of the pregnancy. Like many other modern techniques; the utility of foetal echocardiography has not been critically assessed and there are conflicting reports in literature about its precise role. However foetal echocardiography has provided useful information of the development of cardiac lesions and foetal physiology. Prenatal screening for congenital heart defects is now possible even in the previable foetus. Most major heart defects can be reliably diagnosed by 18 to 20 weeks of gestation. The indications for prenatal echocardiography include as follows:

1. A previous child with a heart defect.
2. A parent with a heart defect.
3. Maternal diabetes mellitus.
4. A known chromosomal anomaly.
5. Multiple noncardiac anomalies.

If this technique is applied, much the same way as it is in the newborn infant provided the segmental approach is employed; even the complex defects can be diagnosed accurately. Defects that remain difficult or impossible to detect in utero include atrial septal defect patent ductus arteriosus, ventricular septal defect, coarctation of aorta, and some valvular abnormalities. Usually, it is impossible to distinguish between normal patency of foramen ovale and atrial septal defect. Patency of the ductus arteriosus is, of course, normal prior to birth. Even moderate sized VSD may be below the resolution of the imaging equipment. An examination later in gestation (35 weeks) may improve the detection rate of VSD (Figs. 12.30, 12.32 G and H).

Coarctation of aorta may not be apparent until after closure of the ductus arteriosus or may not be detected in utero because of limited resolution. However, a disparity in ventricular size (right ventricle larger than left ventricle) is a sensitive; although not specific marker for coarctation of aorta. The ability to detect heart defects

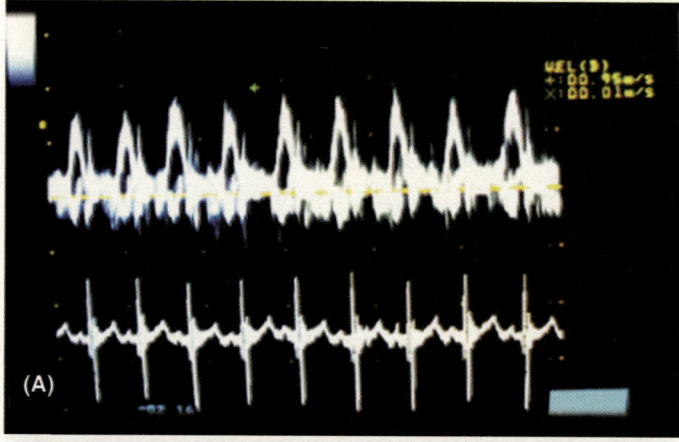

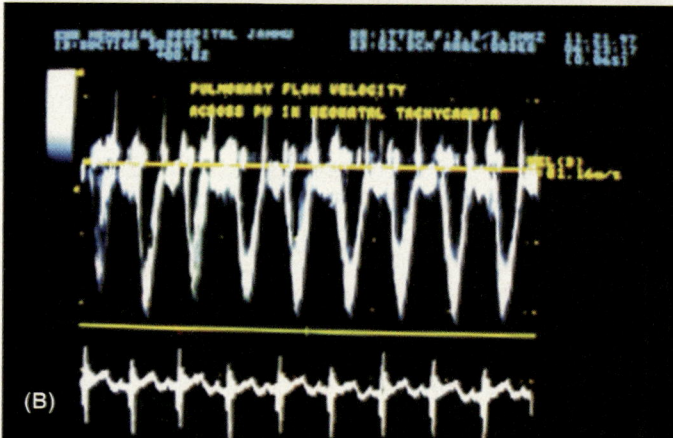

Fig. 12.10A and B: Doppler flow velocity across TV (A) and pulmonary valve (B) in newborn with supraventricular tachycardia with ventricular rate more than 150 beats/min with A-V conduction of 1;1

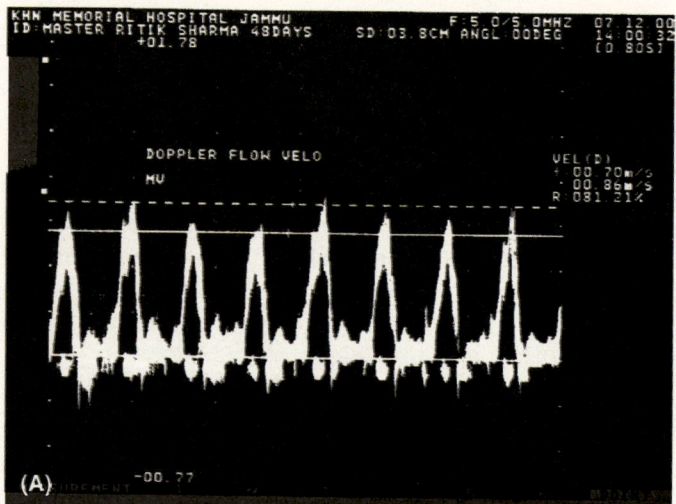

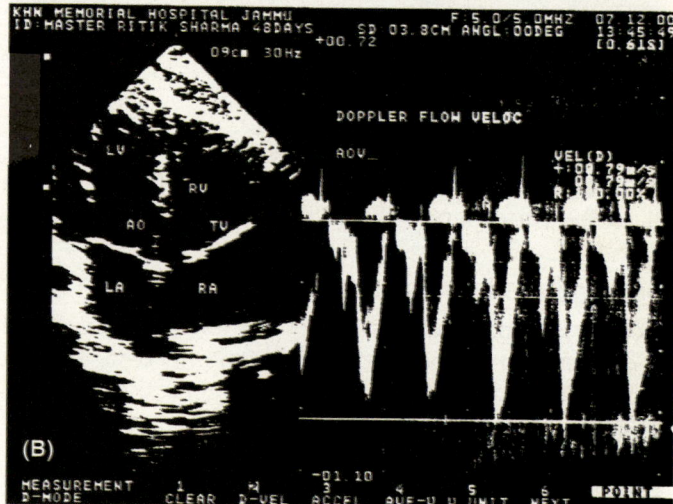

Fig. 12.11A and B: **(A)** Doppler flow velocity across normal mitral valve (MV). **(B)** 2-D Apical 5C (left)for localization of ascending aorta and Doppler flow velocity across normal aortic valve (right) in a 48 days old newborn

in the previable foetus gives the parents an opportunity to terminate the pregnancy. On the other hand, plans can be made to expedite the neonatal management of the foetus known to have a heart defect. Most commonly anxious parents can be assured that the foetus has no detectable heart defect. The other major use of foetal echocardiography is for the management of arrhythmias in the foetus. Atrial premature either conducted or blocked are the most common rhythm disturbance detected in utero. These are almost always benign and only if frequent or associated with short burst of tachycardia do they require specific follow up. Supraventricular tachycardia and atrial flutter are the two most common serious arrhythmias encountered in the foetus. Either may cause congestive heart failure manifested by hydrops fetalis. Both require close follow-up and often pharmacological therapy via the placenta. The diagnosis is made using two dimensionally directed M-mode echocardiography or Doppler examination to demonstrate a rapid regular atrial rate with corresponding ventricular activity at the same rate or with some of atria-ventricular block. Atrial tachycardia should be suspected in any hydrop foetus for which no other cause

is found. Even intermittent tachycardia which can be missed on brief ultrasound examination can cause hydrops. In such cases arrangements should be made for frequent monitoring of the foetal heart rate over a period of several hours; or until tachycardia is detected. Ventricular tachyarrhythmias are rare in the foetus (Fig. 12.22).

Isolated ventricular beats may be distinguished from premature beats of atrial origin by noting the sequence of activation of atria and ventricles on the M-mode strip. Complete heart block is the most common prolonged bradyarrhythmia detected in utero. Diagnosis is made using 2-D or M-mode echocardiography to demonstrate independent contraction of the atria and ventricles. Complete heart block usually occurs in the setting of maternal lupus erythematosus or with some structural heart defects, such as complete common atrioventricular canal or corrected transposition of great vessels. It is

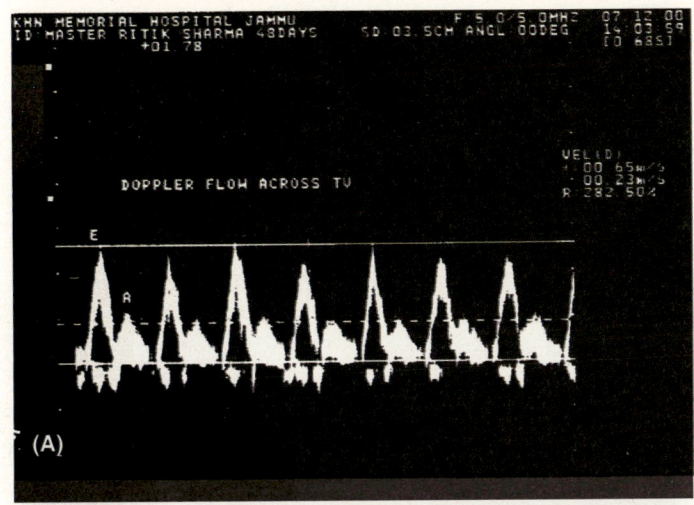

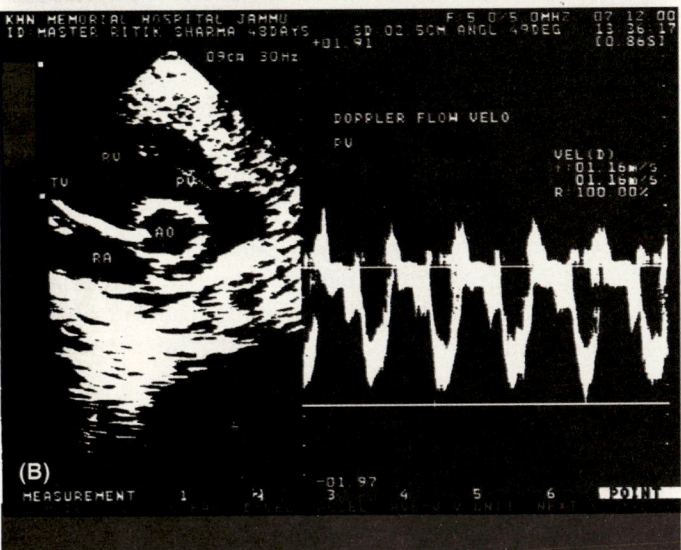

Fig. 12.12A and B: (A) Doppler flow velocity across normal tricuspid valve (TV). **(B)** Short axis view at aorta (AO) for localization of pulmonary valve and Doppler flow velocity across normal pulmonary valve

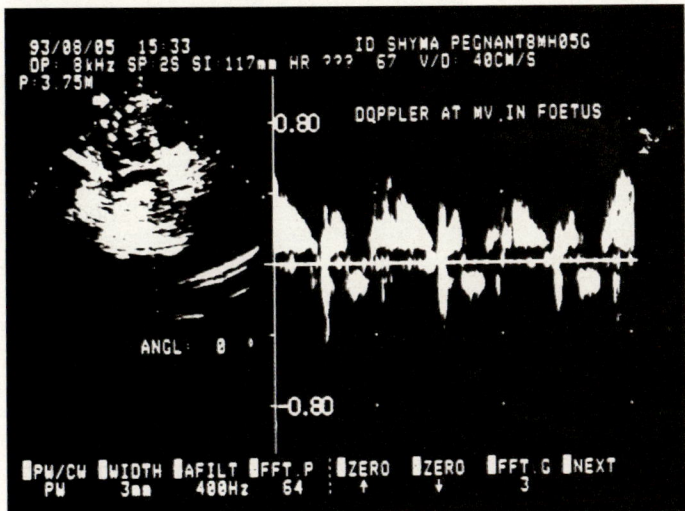

Fig. 12.13: Doppler flow velocity across normal foetal mitral valve

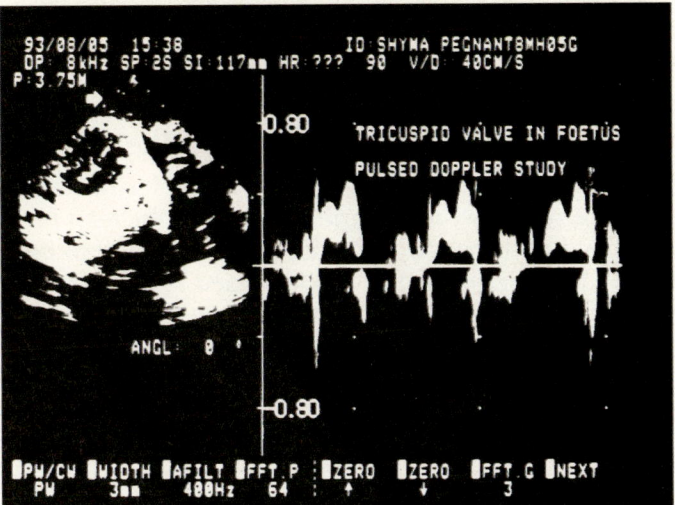

Fig. 12.14: Doppler flow velocity across normal foetal tricuspid valve

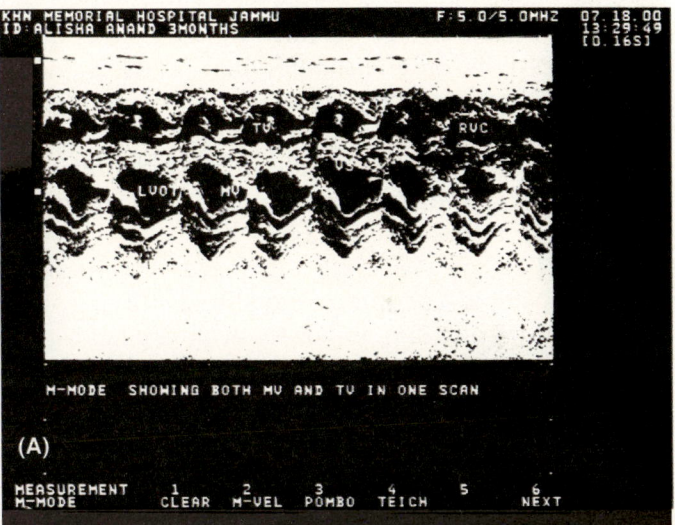

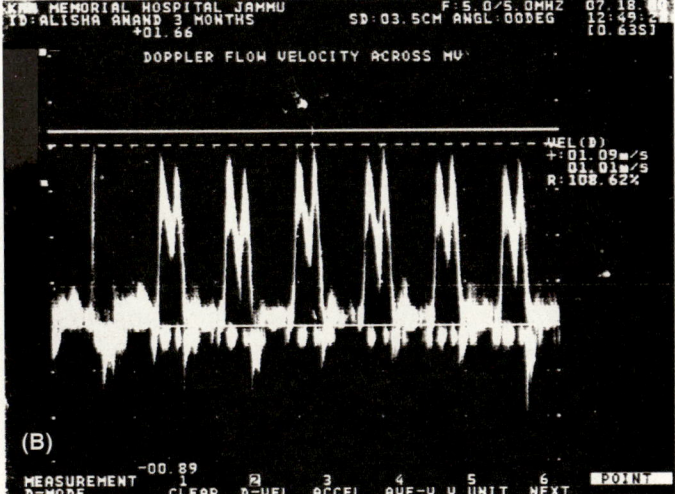

Fig. 12.15A and B: (A) M-Mode echocardiogram showing simultaneous recording of normal mitral and tricuspid valves in single scan. **(B)** Doppler flow velocity across normal mitral valve in a three months old infant

important to distinguish complete heart block from the bradycardia accompanying foetal distress, in order to avoid unnecessary cesarean section.

Technique in Foetal Echocardiography (Figs 12.2–12.8)

It is now possible to apply echocardiographic principles to examine the structure and function of the fetal heart as early as 14 weeks of gestation. Human fetus has been studied with real time M-mode pulsed and continuous wave Doppler; and Doppler colour flow mapping under different planes and views.

Four Chambers View: This view is easiest to obtain in a fetus. Initially the transducer is directed parallel to the spine or the aorta. Once either of these structures is identified, transducer is rotated 90 degree thus imaging the fetal trunk transversely. When the four chambers are viewed, identification of cardiac structural relationships can be divided into two parts (Fig. 12.2):

1. One must find out whether heart lies within left portion of the chest by confirming that the stomach located within the left abdominal cavity is on the same side of the trunk as the fetal heart establishing this orientation, one can reliably exclude situs in versus and displacement of the heart secondary to intrathoracic pathology namely diaphragmatic hernia or intrathoracic mass lesion.

2. It consists of assessing intracardiac structural relationships. A simple method for identifying atrial and ventricular anatomy is to locate the fetal spine and draw an imaginary line to the opposite anterior chest wall. The ventricle lying beneath the intersection of this line and the anterior chest wall is the right ventricle. The ventricle lies on the same side of the fetal trunk as the stomach is inferior and to the left of the right ventricle. However placement of interventricular septum, interatrial septum, mitral and tricuspid valves is almost similar to the examination outside the uterus.

Five Chambers View: The five chambers view can be imaged by directing the ultrasound beam parallel or tangential to the interventricular septum (IVS) cephalad to the four chamber view. This view is very useful for demonstrating continuity of the left ventricular outflow tract (Fig. 12.11B).

Left Parasternal View: When the transducer is rotated 30° from the plane of four-chambers view, the left ventricular inflow and outflow tracts be imaged; once they are recognized, the transducer can be rotated to 90° to image the pulmonary outflow tract (Fig. 12.26).

Short Axis Outflow Tract View: It is imaged by directing the ultrasound beam parallel to the long axis of the trunk. When beam is shifted laterally from the spine, the short axis of the outflow tracts comes into view. In the normal fetus the diameters of the aortic and pulmonary outflow tracts at the level of the semilunar valves are similar in size. After it has been visualised, right ventricular outflow tract should be examined carefully to confirm the bifurcation of the pulmonary arteries medially and the ductus arteriosus laterally.

Short Axis Ventricular View: Further when transducer is moved in lateral direction, circular left and right ventricular chambers with the pulmonary valve and outflow tract emerging from right ventricle can be visualised (Fig. 12.34A).

Aorta

Directing transducer parallel to the spine and angled parallel to the arch; aorta can be imaged with the fetus in either the spine-up or the spine down position. The ascending aorta can be identified because of its "Candy–cane" appearance with brachiocephalic vessels taking origin from the arch of aorta. It becomes easier to image aorta during 3rd trimester of pregnancy when the spine is up because of lack of interference of visceral and skeletal structures (Fig. 12.26).

Inferior and Superior Venae Cavae: For visualisation of these structures, transducer can be directed parallel and to the right of the spine to image the inferior and superior venae cavae as they enter the right atrial chamber.

Mitral and Tricuspid Inflow Tract Velocities: Mitral and tricuspid inflow velocities have been recorded from the apical four-chamber view in which the Doppler sample is placed distally to the tricuspid and mitral valve leaflets parallel to the bloodflow. Maximum flow velocity (A peak) for the tricuspid valve (51 cm/sec) was greater than the mitral valve (47 cm/sec). The E/A ratio has been shown to increase from 0.85 in the fetus to 1.17 in the newborn over 24 hours of age (Figs. 12.13 and 12.14).

Aortic and Pulmonary Outflow Tract Velocities: These can be recorded by directing the ultrasound beam parallel to bloodflow from the apical five chambers (aortic) and short axis outflow (pulmonary) views and characteristic wave forms can be recorded. The maximum flow velocity is greater for the aorta than for the pulmonary artery (1.3:1) suggesting either increased left ventricular contractility when compared with its counterpart right ventricle or decreased resistance of the aortic outflow tract when compared to the pulmonary outflow tract. However temporal mean velocity is the same for both great vessels (Figs. 12.11B and 12.12B).

Ductus Arteriosus Velocity: It can be studied by placing the sample volume distal to the pulmonary valve. It can vary from 50–141 cm/sec (mean 80 cm/sec). It has also been observed that ductal velocities are the highest in the fetal cardiovascular system (Fig. 12.32C and D).

Thoracic Aorta Velocity: Between 28 weeks till full gestation period velocity can be obtained by using a sector scanner in which the Doppler sample volume can be directed to the thoracic aorta (27.7 cm/sec).

Abdominal Aorta: Between 27 weeks to term; temporal mean velocity remained constant at 32.7 cm/sec during 3rd trimester.

Peripheral Vessel Velocities: When evaluating the velocity and flow of blood through the peripheral vessels ultrasonic beam should be directed towards the thoracic and the abdominal descending aorta as well as the intra-abdominal umbilical vein. It must be kept in mind that the descending aorta represents primarily right ventricular output, while bloodflow within the intra-abdominal umbilical vein represents blood returning to the fetus from the placenta.

Velocity Waveforms: It is obtained by placing pulsed Doppler probe attached to a linear array transducer at an angle varying between 30 and 60 degrees to the direction of bloodflow intra-abdominal umbilical vein velocity. Mean velocity is found to be 18.3 cm/sec; whereas the reported value for temporal velocity from 28 weeks to term fetus is 12.8 cm/sec.

Flow Volume

For the calculation of the flow volume, one may require temporal mean velocity (cm/sec) the cross-sectional area (cm^2) of the orifice through which the blood is flowing heart rate per min. From the above, flow volume can be computed by the following formula:

Volume = [Temporal mean velocity (cm/sec) × [area (cm^2)]

Normalized bloodflow (ml/kg/min)

$$= \frac{[(Volume) \times (Heart\ rate/min)]}{Estimated\ fetal\ weight}$$

Although the temporal mean velocity can be obtained as cited above; but cannot measure the cross-sectional area of the orifice of the structure through which the blood is flowing to its accurate value. 2-Dimensional echocardiography has been tried but it again fails to record accurate value. However, an attempt has been made to utilise M-mode and real time echocardiography for obtaining a diameter of the orifice and then deriving the area to its most accuracy. Converting diameter to area, the latter is divided by two and then square the resultant radius. Secondly for normalizing the bloodflow; the per unit of weight value of the weight is required. Since direct weight cannot be obtained in a fetus, hence indirect value is recorded by the measurement of the biparietal diameter, abdominal circumference and femur length.

Tricuspid and Mitral Flow: Between gestational period of 26 and 30 weeks there is difference in values of tricuspid flow (307 ± 30 ml/kg/min) as compared to mitral bloodflow (232 ± 25 ml/kg/min). The orifice area is calculated by measuring the diameter from the endocardium of the right ventricular wall to the endocardium of the interventricular septum from still frames of real time recording.

Pulmonary and Aortic Flow: In fetuses where diameter of the pulmonary artery ranged from 0.8–1.0; the pulmonary bloodflow ranged from 128–218 ml/kg/min and almost similar figure is found in aortic flow as well.

Peripheral Vessel Bloodflow: The ranges of the reported mean bloodflows for the descending aorta (166–246 ml/kg/min) and the intra-abdominal umbilical vein (103–125 ml/kg/min). The deviations in values are so high in both the vessels and therefore cannot be reliably employed for identification of fetal diseases.

List of Various Congenital Malformations which can be Diagnosed by Foetal Echocardiography

1. Absence of aortic valve
2. Acardia
3. Aortic stenosis
4. Atrial hemangioma
5. Bicuspid aortic valve
6. Coarctation of the aorta (Fig. 12.32G and H)
7. Double-outlet right ventricle
8. Dextrocardia
9. Ebstein anomaly
10. Ectopic cardis
11. Endocardial cushion defect (Fig. 12.27)
12. Endocardial fibroelastosis
13. Hypoplastic left ventricle (Figs 12.19 and 12.20)
14. Hypoplastic right ventricle
15. Mitral atresia
16. Pulmonary atresia
17. Ostium premium defect (Figs 12.40 and 12.41)
18. Pericardial hemangioma
19. Pericardial teratoma
20. Rhabdomyoma
21. Single ventricle
22. Single atrium (Fig. 12.21)
23. Tetralogy of Fallot (Figs 12.33 and 12.34)
24. Thoracopagus (single heart)
25. Tricuspid atresia
26. Transposition of great vessels
27. Truncus arteriosus
28. Ventricular septal defect (Figs 12.43 and 12.49)
29. Cardiac arrythmia (Figs 12.22, 12.28 and 12.29)

Table 12.1: *Echocardiographic identification of right and left ventricles from four chambers view*

	Right ventricle	Left ventricle
Position with Thorax	Beneath anterior chest wall	Left side of thorax, above Spine same side of trunk as stomach
Geometrical shape	Conical	Ellipsoidal
Flap of foramen ovale	—	Present within left atrium
Insertion of atrio-ventricular valve leaflets on intervertricular septum	Tricuspid valve is inserted lower than mitral	Mitral valve is inserted higher than tricuspid valve

Neonatal Echocardiographic Left-Right Shunt Ratios

Pulmonary to systemic flow ratios are useful for indicating shunt flow in terms that are relative. The premise for measuring shunt ratios is based on the following assumption for individuals without shunts or valvular regurgitation.

Tricuspid Flow = Pulmonary Flow = Mitral Flow = Aortic Flow

Methodology for determining the shunt ratio reverts back to the flow methodology for each area. Measurement of shunt ratios in individuals with no shunt indicates that ratios of 0.8 : 1 to 1.2 : 1 can be obtained. The following will indicate the general method for computing left to right shunts.

Ventricular Septal Defect (VSD, $Q_p:Q_s$): In patients with a VSD, tricuspid and aortic flows represent systemic flow, and pulmonary and mitral flows contain both systemic flow and the shunt. VSD ($Q_p:Q_s$) ratio can be computed as follows:

$$(VSD)\ Q_p:Q_s = \frac{\text{Pulmonary or mitral flow}}{\text{Tricuspid or aortic flow}}$$

Atrial Septal Defect (ASD, $Q_p:Q_s$): For patients with ASD, shunted flow plus systemic flow passes through both the tricuspid and pulmonary valves. Flow through mitral and aortic valves is equal to that which leaves the left heart and is, therefore, systemic flow. Accordingly, the $Q_p:Q_s$ ratio can be computed as:

$$ASD\ (Q_p:Q_s) = \frac{\text{Pulmonary or mitral flow}}{\text{Aortic flow or mitral flow}}$$

Patent Ductus ($Q_p:Q_s$): For patient with a patent ductus arteriosus (PDA), systemic flow can be best measured as venous return through the tricuspid valve. Pulmonary artery flow in patient with this lesion is frequently unreliable flow here is frequently turbulent and flow varies in different portions of the pulmonary artery, but pulmonary flow is equal to venous return and can be measured at the mitral or aortic level. Accordingly, PDA—$Q_p:Q_s$ ratio can be computed as (Figs 11.44A and B and 11.50):

$$PDA\ Q_p:Q_s = \frac{\text{Aortic or mitral flow}}{\text{Tricuspid flow}}$$

Clearly, more complex and multiple shunts occur, and principles delineated in these examples can be used to solve for shunt ratios in most cases. It was observed that, up to 90% of CHD occurs in pregnancies where there are no known high risk features. For this reason, in 1985 a group based in Paris put forward the idea of teaching the obstetrician to assess the heart in a simplified form during routine obstetric scanning, which was well established at that time in France. As a result, four chamber view scanning became an integral part of the fetal anatomical survey in many countries by the end of the 1980s. In the early 1990s, some authors suggested extending the cardiac assessment to include great artery scanning in order to detect a higher proportion of cases of major congenital heart disease. If cardiac screening is confined to the four chamber view, about 2/1000 studies will be abnormal and would represent about 60% of the major heart disease seen in infants. If the great arteries are also examined, about 3/1000 cases would be abnormal, and over 90% of major heart disease would be detectable prenatally. Therefore, in ideal circumstances, the vast majority of serious heart malformations could be detected before 20 weeks' gestation. Unfortunately, the reality is far from this for several reasons:

1. Differing policies for obstetric scanning
2. Differing guidelines for scanning
3. Differing skill at scanning.

About 2% of live births have fetal structural malformations, the majority of which can be detected by ultrasound. About 25% of these malformations are cardiac in nature and about half of these are serious or life threatening. Despite these facts, and the opportunity during pregnancy for comprehensive evaluation of the fetal anatomy in fine detail, there is no universal agreement as to either the necessity for or the technique of fetal anatomical scanning. Some countries, such as Norway, France, and Germany, have instituted a government-sponsored policy for routine anatomical screening by ultrasound. In the UK, routine screening is generally well accepted but not uniformly adopted or standardised in all parts of the country. In the USA, routine scanning is not recommended but is allowed only for specific indications, although these are fairly all encompassing. In practice, this leads to later scanning in the US and "targeted" scanning rather than a comprehensive anatomical survey.

Where an anatomical survey is performed, the timing of the scan varies. For example, in France it is usually between 20–22 weeks, in Norway 18 weeks. In general, the later in the mid-trimester that scanning is performed, the more successful will be the detection of abnormalities, partly because scanning become easier and partly because some lesions become more evident as pregnancy advances. However, later detection of malformations will limit the options for interrupting the pregnancy or make it much more difficult both emotionally for the parents and technically for the obstetrician. Thus, the ideal policy would be a universal anatomical scan at a compromise time between 18–20 weeks' gestation.

The skill involved in scanning is extremely variable for several reasons. A sonographer, whether a technician, an obstetrician, or a radiologist, needs to train with a high volume of patients to maintain skills continuously with sufficient numbers of patients to be exposed continually to a critical number of abnormal fetuses to be provided with constant feedback and retraining.

In order to achieve and maintain a high level of expertise in scanning, the practitioner should be doing this as a full-time or nearly full time commitment. Where ultrasound is performed in small numbers, the requisite practice necessary is quite unattainable. Nearly all scanning in the UK is hospital based, with delivery numbers usually over 2000 per year. Therefore, the necessary volume of patients is less of a problem in the UK than in the US, where scanning often takes place in private offices in small numbers.

As a result of the differing policies and standards in obstetric ultrasound, the results of the detection of all malformations in the screening setting varies with the organ involved, but is particularly poor in reference to the heart. During screening, reported detection rates vary between 4.5% and 96% for major CHD, with the most papers giving a rate of 15–20%. The rate of detection of four chamber view anomalies prenatally is better, but averages only about 50%, despite the fact that universally nearly all pregnancies are scanned at least once. Thus, the technology and personnel are in place in obstetric care, but they are not used to their maximum capability.

Referral to Paediatric Cardiologists

A common misconception among paediatric cardiologists is that fetal cardiology is the same as paediatric echocardiography, but a bit smaller. Therefore, nearly all paediatric echocardiographers in the US would not hesitate to offer fetal echocardiography as part of their practice. However, it is clear that quite a different spectrum of disease is seen prenatally, and fetal heart scanning is quite a different skill. Success in accurate diagnosis will be partly dependent on technical skills, which again require training and practice. In the US, there are recommended guidelines for training, and a minimum number of scans in order to maintain skills, but these are not commonly known and certainly are not adhered to. Experience of fetal malformations therefore is so diluted that few practitioners have sufficient numbers to maintain a high standard of expertise. In addition, most paediatric cardiologists know little of fetal medicine and obstetric pathology, which have an important influence on fetal cardiac evaluation.

Although the majority of paediatric cardiology centres in the UK now offer fetal echocardiography, this is usually confined to one or two cardiologists and, theoretically, there should be sufficient numbers in each regional centre to provide adequate experience. However, there is no system of independent review or systematic quality control. Indeed, in the US, pathological correlation after termination of pregnancy is quite rare for various reasons, not least being the difficulty in obtaining remuneration for pathological services, despite their vital role in quality control.

Problems and Limitations

Limitations of fetal echocardiography are related to image quality subtle lesions, such as small ventricular septal defects developing or progressive lesions, lesions which are undetectable before birth. Image quality is dependent on the skill and experience of scanning in addition to local factors such as gestational age, fetal position, and the thickness of the maternal abdomen. Maternal obesity is an increasing problem everywhere but particularly in the US, especially in the poorer states. This is the most important limitation to image quality, which in turn, will limit confidence in excluding malformations in the fetus in any anatomical system. Even though the resolution of ultrasound equipment has improved vastly; since the early 1980s, a great deal more detail is also expected during fetal scanning, and there are a significant proportion of patients where detail is just not possible because of the way scanning is presently organised. As upto 10% of adult Americans are said to be morbidly obese, this group should probably be managed with a different strategy, perhaps with early transvaginal scanning instead of transabdominal scans; to date this problem has not been addressed by the ultrasound community. In a small proportion of fetuses, CHD becomes evident or more evident as pregnancy progresses. Thus, the cardiac evaluation can be normal at 18 weeks, although a significant malformation is found later or at birth. This is true of some cases of aortic or pulmonary stenosis, cardiac tumors, or cardiomyopathies. It is rare for a life

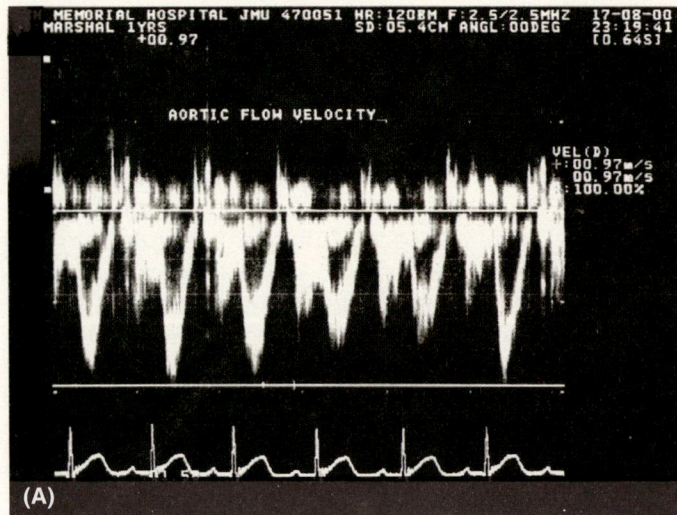

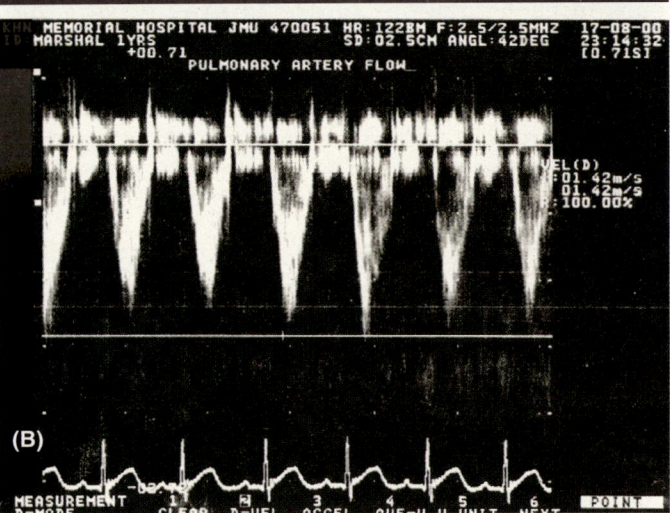

Fig. 12.16A and B: Doppler flow velocities across normal aortic and pulmonary valves in one year old infant

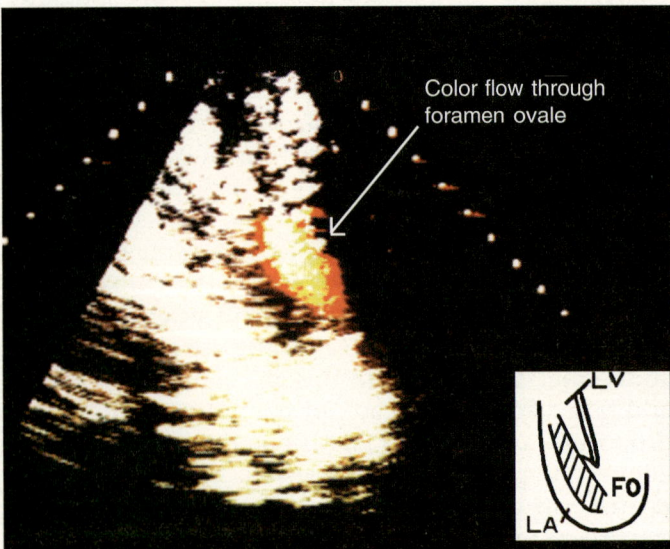

Color flow through foramen ovale

Fig. 12.17: Ultrasonogram showing color flow through patent foramen ovale in normal foetal heart

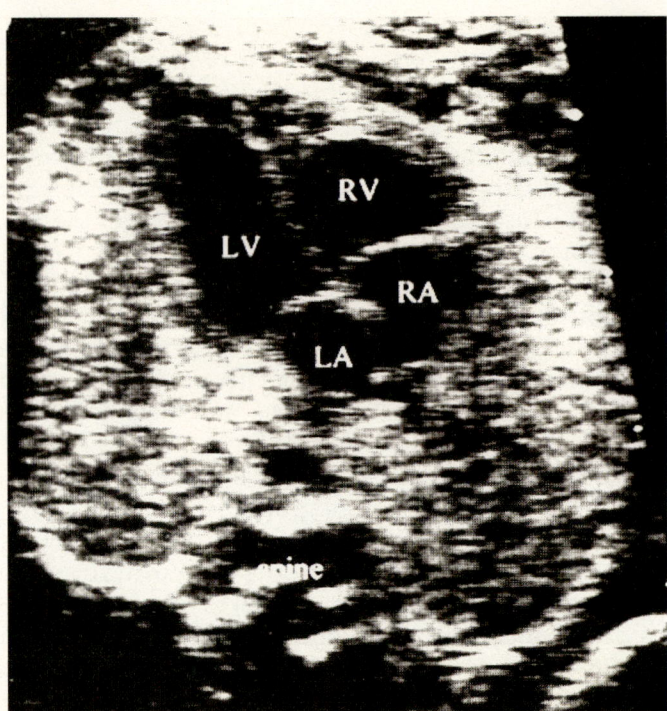

Fig. 12.18: Abdominal ultrasonography showing normal four chamber view showing normal sized heart in its normal position. The size of both atria and two ventricle are normal.There is a cross at the crux of the heart,where the atrial and ventricular septum meet at the insertion of the two atrioventricular valves RV = Right ventricle, RA = Right atrium, LV = left ventricle, LA = Left atrium

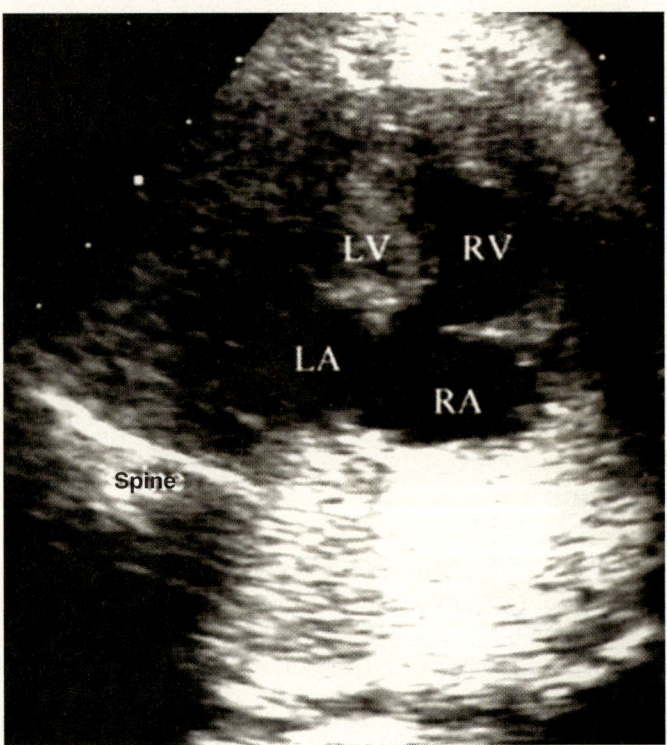

Fig. 12.19: Ultrasonography showing small-sized left atrium, hypoplastic heart forming the apex and atresic mitral valve in an unborn baby with hypoplastic left heart syndrome

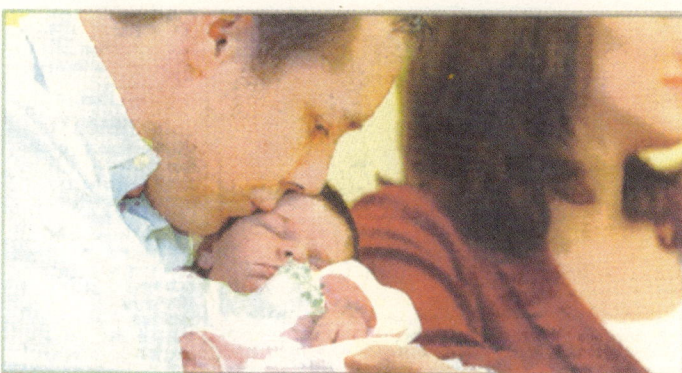

Fig. 12.20: A newborn baby, Grace out of US National couple with mother Angela VanDer-werken of Virginia who became Worlds first baby to receive intra-uterine stent for the treatment of hypoplastic left heart syndrome when this baby was seven months old in the womb of the mother. This surgery was performed by the team of experts under chief surgeon Dr James Lock at children hospital, Boston and Brigham and women hospital, Boston

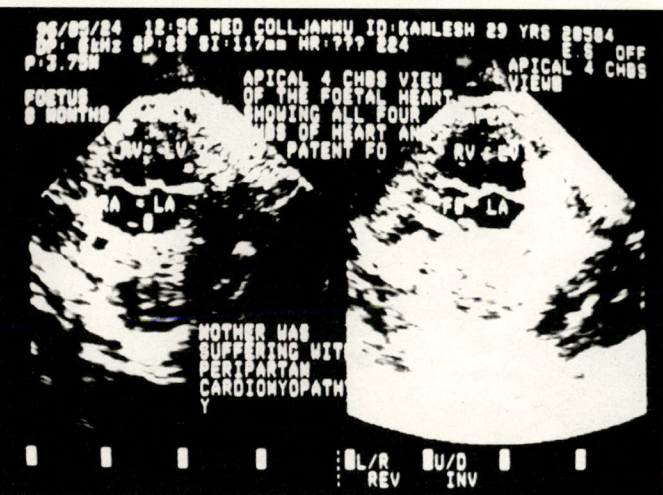

Fig. 12.23: 4C View in foetal heart showing four chambers of the heart with thickening of both mitral and tricuspid valves with persistent foramen ovale in a mother with dilated cardiomyopathy

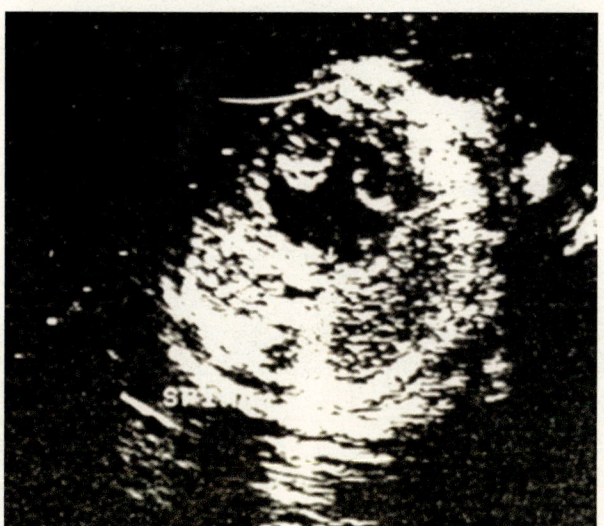

Fig. 12.21: Transverse thoracic echocardiographic section in foetus with right atrial isomerism common atrium, double inlet left ventricle through common atrioventricular valve

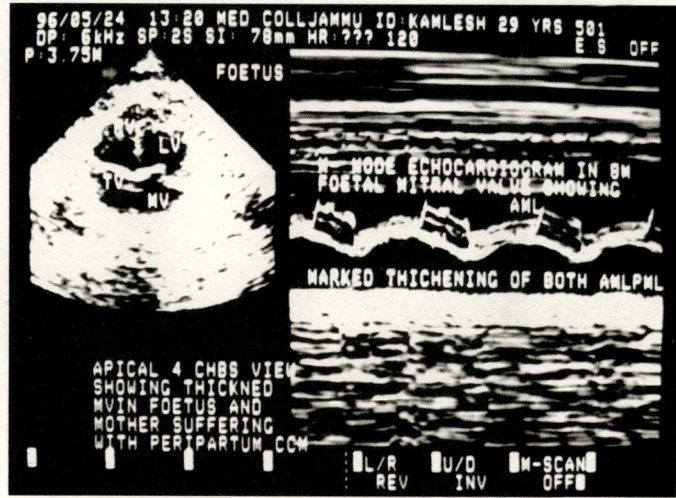

Fig. 12.24: M-Mode echocardiogram in foetal heart showing thickening of mitral valve with mild to moderate mitral stenosis in a mother suffering from dilated cardiomyopathy

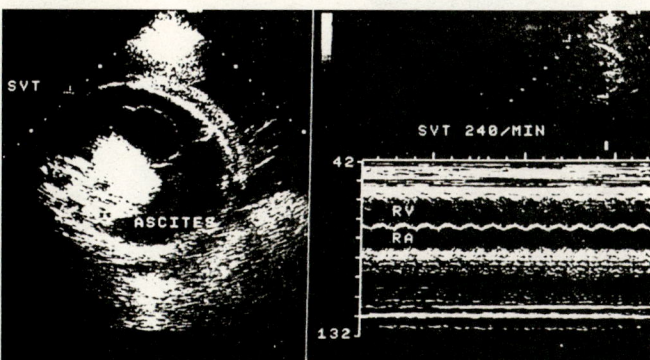

Fig. 12.22: Severe foetal hydrops (left) secondary to heart failure because of sustained atrio-ventricular re-entry tachycardia which is demonstrated by the M-Mode recording of the foetal heart rate (right) There is 1;1 A-V conduction

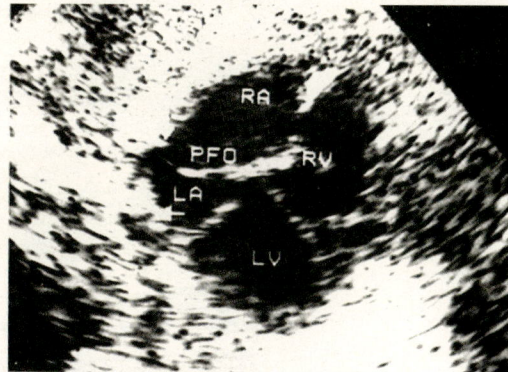

Fig. 12.25: Four-chamber view of a foetal heart showing normal patent foramen ovale (PFO), right ventricle (RV), left ventricle (LV), right atrium (RA) left atrium (LA) Flap of PFO bulges towards the left atrium; this can be used to identify the left atrium

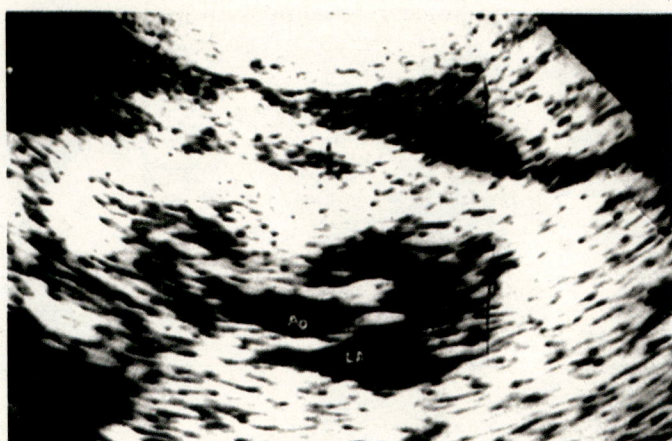

Fig. 12.26: Modified long axis view of foetal heart to outline aortic valve and ascending aorta arising from the left ventricle. AO = aorta, LA = left atrium

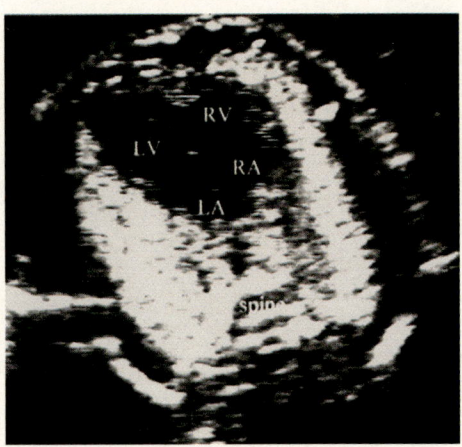

Fig. 12.27: The cross appearance at the crux of the heart is missing due to common atrioventricular junction and a complete atrioventricular septal defect

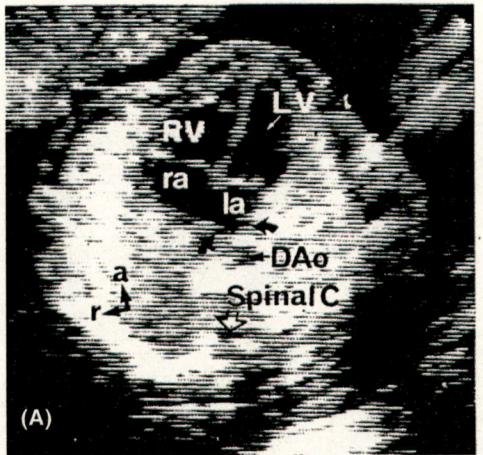

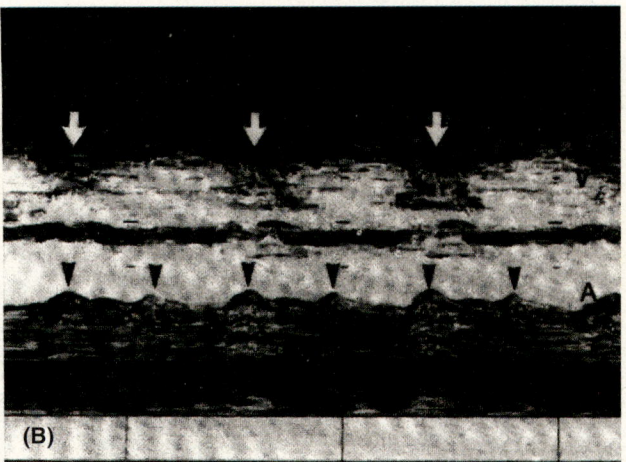

Fig. 12.28 A and B: (A) Foetal four chamber echocardiographic view obtained from a transverse section through the foetal thorax DAo = descending aorta, Spinal C = spinal canal. The curved black arrows indicate pulmonary veins entering left atrium. **(B)** M-Mode tracing of a foetus with complete atrio-ventricular block. The beam passes through the right ventricle (V) and the left atrium (A). The ventricular contractions (white arrows) at a rate of 68 beats/min is independent of atrial contraction (black arrow heads) at a rate of 142 beats/min

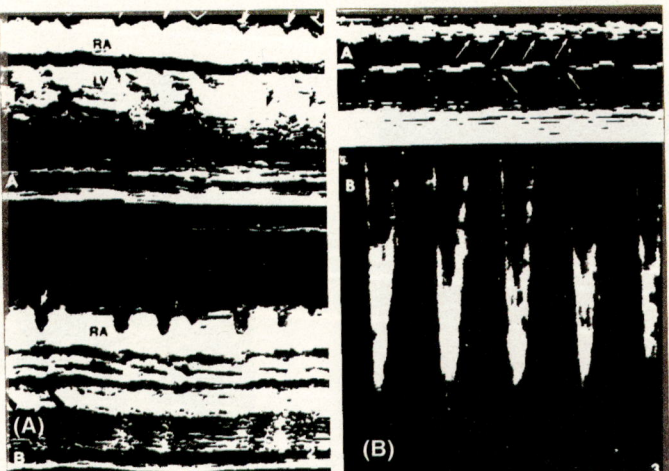

Fig. 12.29A and B: (A) M-Mode cursor passess through the right atrium RA and the left ventricle.After every two regular atrial beats (white arrows) there is PAC (open arrows) which is not conducted as revealed by the absent ventricular contraction (black arrows). The compensatory pause is incomplete. **(B)** Pulsed Doppler of the aortic flow at half of the rate of the atrial contractions

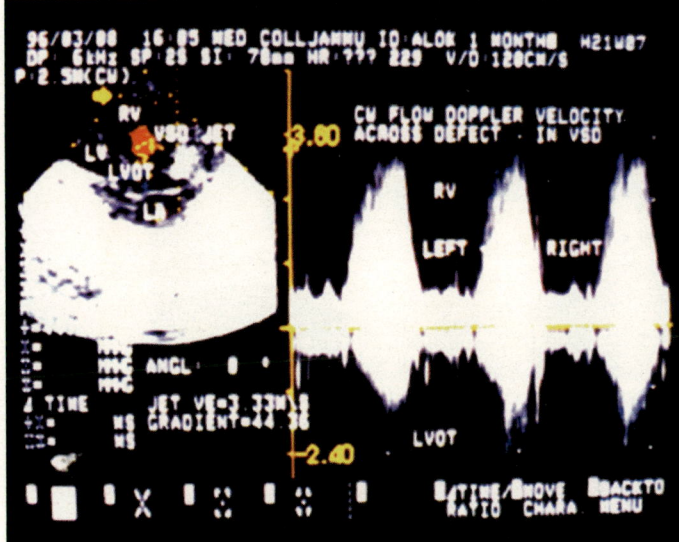

Fig. 12.30: 2-D Doppler echocardiography showing left to right shunt from LVOT to RV in newborn with subaortic ventricular septal defect

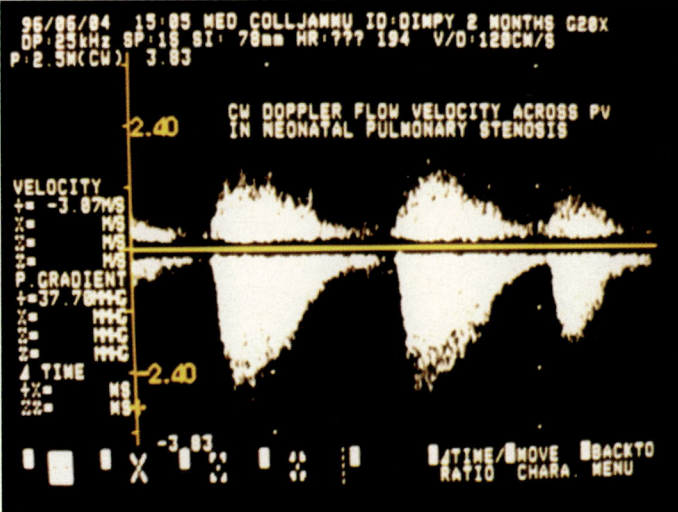

Fig. 12.31: Doppler flow velocity across pulmonary valve in a newborn with native pulmonary valvular stenosis

threatening malformation to arise after 20 weeks' gestation, but it can occur. In addition, minor lesions can be overlooked because of the limits of ultrasound resolution, such as small ventricular septal defects; a persistent arterial duct and an atrial septal defect cannot be predicted prenatally as these communications are always present prenatally. Thus, there are confidence limits with even detailed fetal heart scanning. It is important to realise, however, that confidence limits may be much wider with poor image quality.

Latest Technologies

By 14 weeks' gestation, the cardiac connections can be identified in many patients transabdominally. The connections can be seen in almost all patients at this stage transvaginally, however, and in much finer detail than on the transabdominal scan. Expertise with this technique is essential and the paediatric cardiologist should use the experienced gynaecological technician to display the fetal cardiac images, in a setting where transvaginal scanning is routine. At present, a cardiac scan at 14 weeks is confined to the high risk patient, such as those with a family history of CHD or those whose fetus has been found to have an increased nuchal fold. The data concerning nuchal translucency in early pregnancy (10–12 weeks) are fascinating and intriguing. When the translucent region at the back of the neck is increased in size, there is a high incidence of associated chromosomal anomalies, cardiac malformations, or both, with the incidence of heart disease increasing with increasing nuchal thickness. Conversely, 50% of fetuses subsequently found to have CHD had an abnormal nuchal fold measurement. This may reflect the "insult" which has caused the fetal heart malformation. Extension of the nuchal translucency screening program, which has received little attention in the US so far, is likely to have important implications for the improved detection of both chromosomal and cardiac malformations. In addition, earlier the diagnosis of fetal malformation is made in pregnancy, more likely are parents to choose interruption. If a pregnancy with increased nuchal thickening is continuing, fetal echocardiography is recommended, ideally at 14 weeks, which is the earliest time a cardiac scan can be completely comprehensive.

Impact on Paediatric Cardiology

The impact on paediatric cardiology may include: "reduced prevalence of CHD, especially complex forms improved morbidity after delivery and perioperatively" improved perioperative mortality. Decisions about termination of pregnancy are influenced by many different factors, including gestational age at diagnosis, social circumstances, and socioeconomic group. Generally speaking, however, if complex heart disease is detected in a pregnancy at less than 20 weeks gestation, over half the parents will choose to interrupt the pregnancy. This is true in the UK and the US. Thus, about half of the complex forms of CHD which the paediatric cardiologist would expect to see and treat postnatally may only be seen once in prenatal life. As fetal cardiology preferentially detects the complex forms of heart disease which require long term cardiac care and follow up, this is bound to have an impact on paediatric cardiology in the future. As an example of this, termination of pregnancy has been shown to have lowered the prevalence of pulmonary atresia in England and Wales, compared with Scotland and Ireland where either diagnosis was not made in the fetus or termination

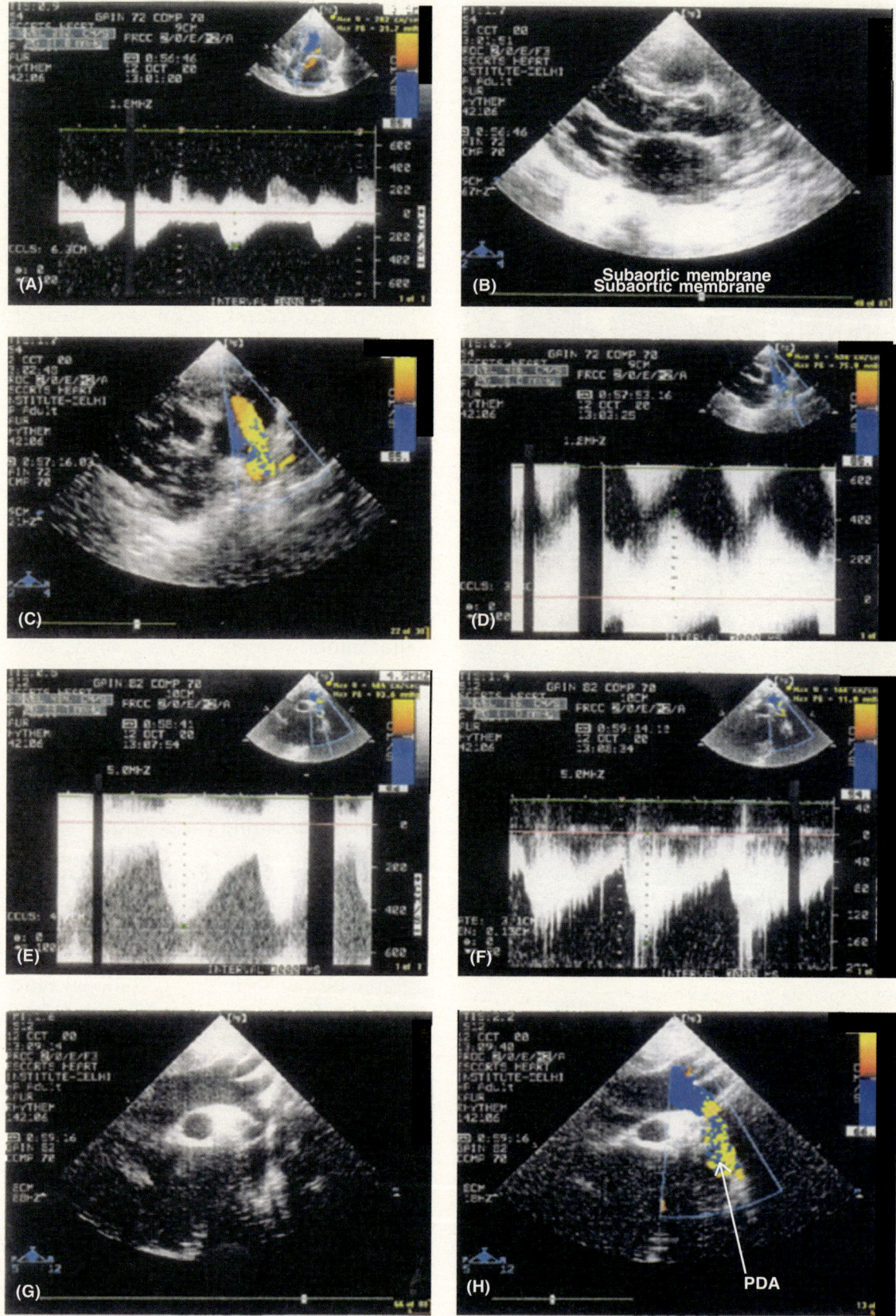

Fig. 12.32A to H: (A) and **(B)** 2D Doppler flow across LVOT showing gradient in subaortic membrane. **(C)** and **(D)** Color Doppler flow velocity across PDA. **(E)** Doppler flow at Coarctation of aorta and **(F)** Doppler flow velocity at preductal area. **(G)** and **(H)** Suprasternal approach at aorta showing coarctation of aorta (G) and color flow across PDA (H) in a newborn baby showing multiple congenital cardiac defects as described above

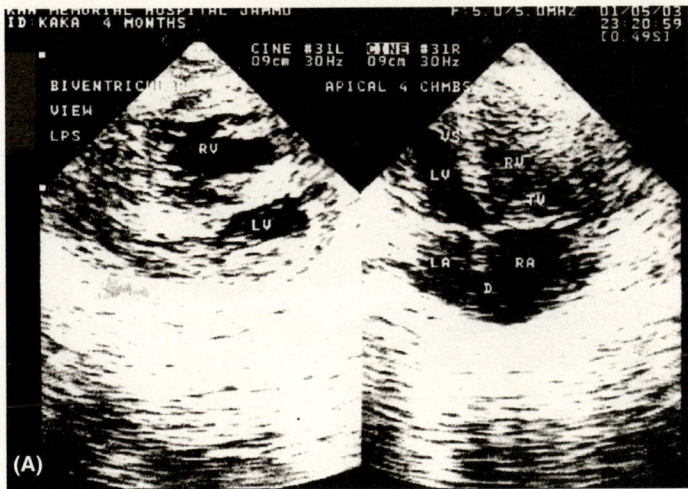
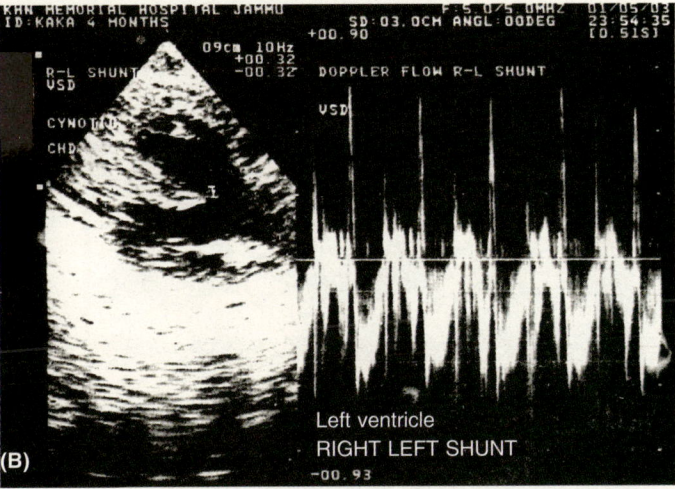

Fig. 12.33A and B: **(A)** Short axis (left) and apical 4C (right) views showing right ventricular hypertrophy, overriding of aorta, and subaortic ventricular septal defect. **(B)** Hypertrophy of RV, Subaortic VSD, Doppler flow velocity across VSD showing right to left shunt in a 4 months baby with cyanotic congenital heart defect (Fallots tetralogy)

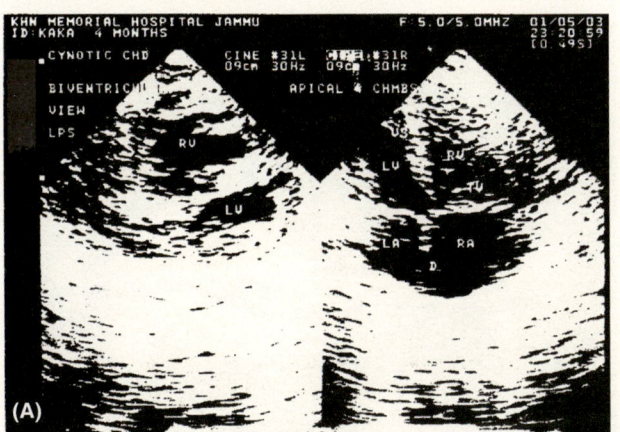
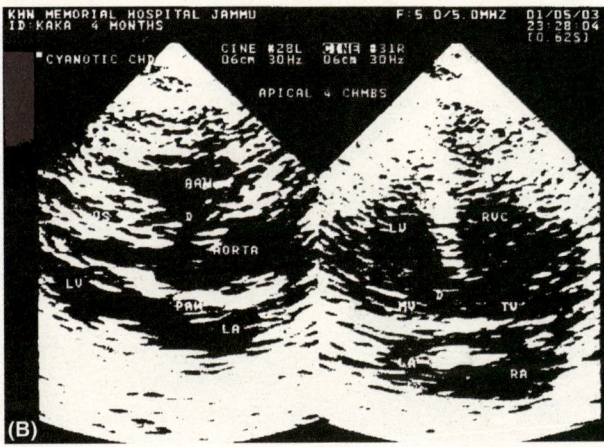

Fig. 12.34A and B: **(A)** Short axis (left) and apical 4C (right) views showing right ventricular hypertrophy, overriding of aorta (AOV), and subaortic ventricular septal defect (D). **(B)** Long axis view (left) depicting subaortic ventricular septal defect (D) overriding of aorta (AOV) and apical 4C view showing a big subaortic ventricular septal defect (VSD). In additon also had pulmonary valvular stenosis in a 4 months old child with Fallots tetralogy

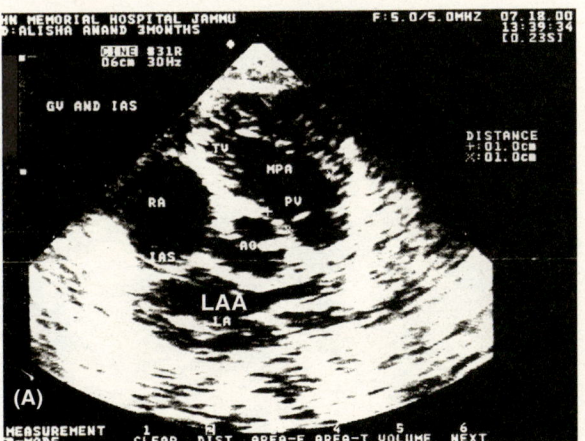
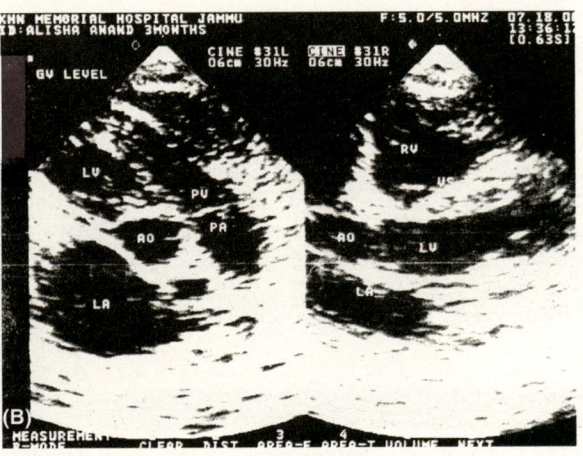

Fig. 12.35A and B: **(A)** 2D echo scan at great vessel level showing anatomical localization of normal aorta (AO) in the centre, pulmonary artery with its valve (MPA) winding around the aorta, interatrial septum (IAS), left atrium (LA) left atrial appendage (LAA), right atrium (RA) **(B)** (left) Great vessel view identifying the same structures as in Fig. A. and (right) biventricular view depicting both right ventricle(RV) LV, AO, LA and interventricular septum (IVS) in a three months old baby

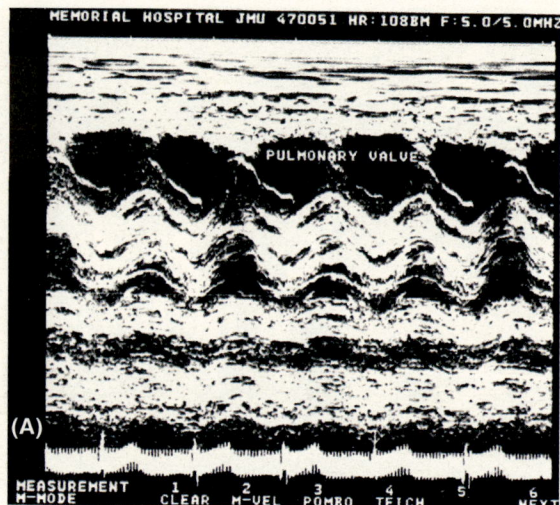
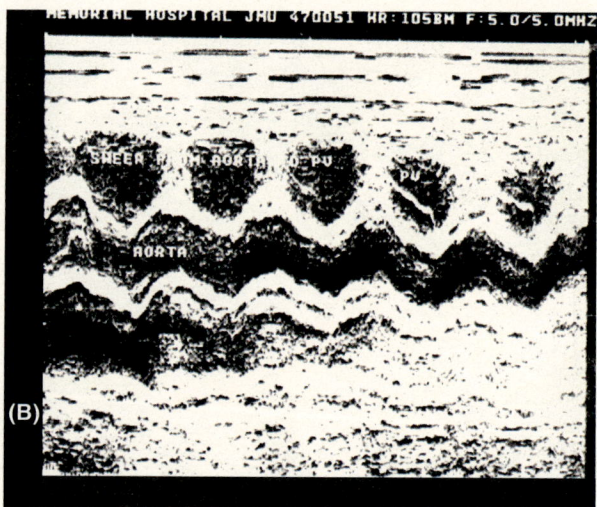

Fig. 12.36A and B: **(A)** M-Mode echocardiogram showing normal pulmonary valve signature in a one month old child. **(B)** M-Mode echocardiogram showing sweep from aorta to pulmonary valve in a one month old normal child

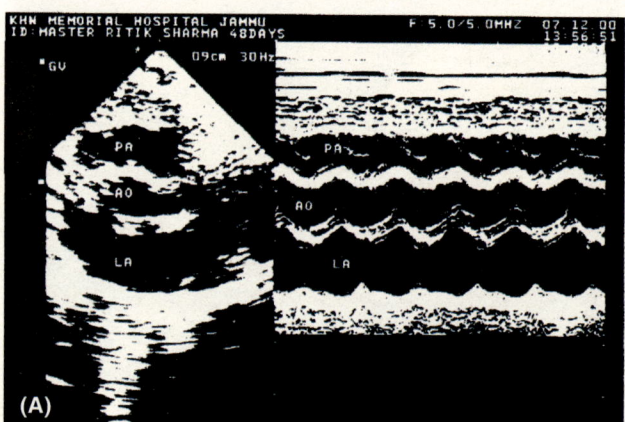
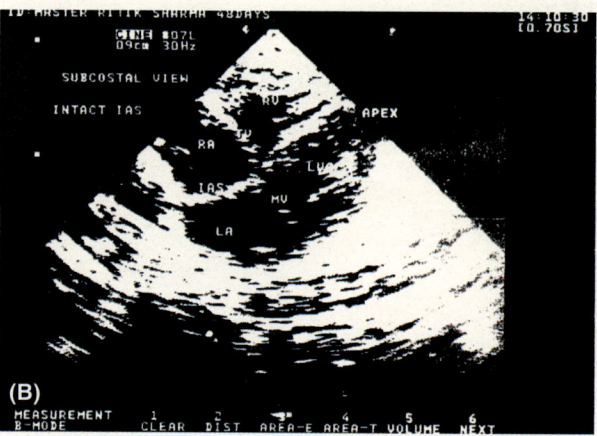

Fig. 12.37A and B: **(A)** Short axis and M-Mode echo scans at great vessel view (L-R) showing anatomical localization of right pulmonary artery(PA), aorta (AO) and left atrium(LA). B.Subcostal view depicting four chambers along with their connecting valves. RA = Right atrium, LA = Left atrium, RV = Right ventricle LV = Left ventricle, TV = Tricuspid valve, MV = Mitral valve and IAS = Interatrial septum in a 48 days old infant

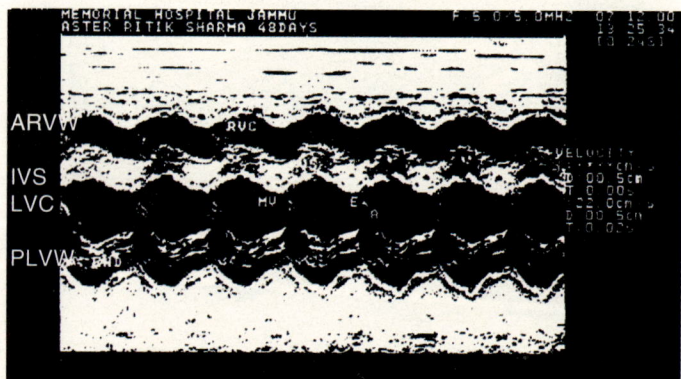
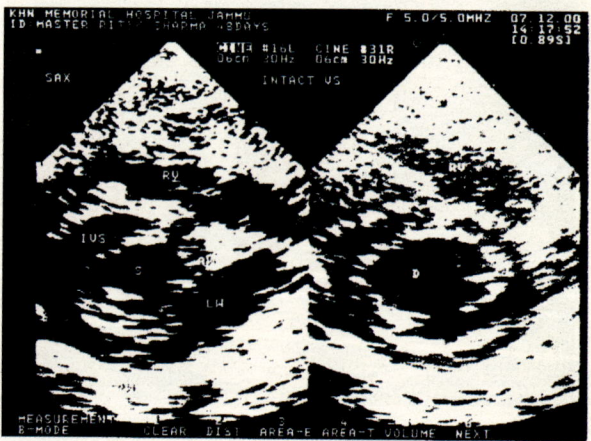

Fig. 12.38A and B: **(A)** M-Mode showing thickened anterior free right ventricular wall (ARVW), right ventricular dominance (RV) and normal interventricular septum (IVS), left ventricular cavity, (LVC) mitral valve and posterior left ventricular wall (PLVW) in a baby with normal heart

Fig. 12.39: Short axis LV views on dual scan during systole (S) and diastole (D) showing anatomical localization of left ventricle (LV) interventricular septum (IVS). AOV = Aortic valve, LA = Left atrium

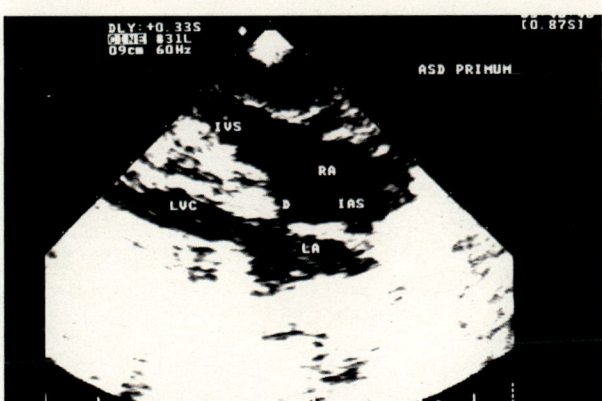

Fig. 12.40: Subcostal biatrial view showing septum primum defect (ASD) In a two months old child. RA = Right atrium, LA = Left atrium, IAS = Interatrial septum, LVC = Left ventricular cavity, IVS = Interventricular septum

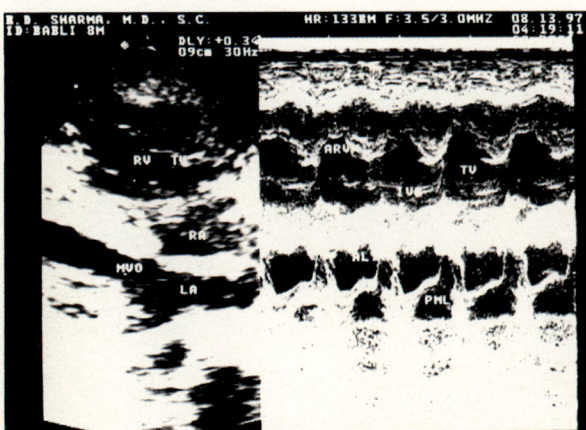

Fig. 12.41: 2D and M-mode echoscans showing simultaneous recording of both mitral and tricuspid valves and traversing of anterior mitral leaflet of mitral valve through interventricular septum in a young baby with septum primum defect. TV = Tricuspid valve, AL = Anterior mitral leaflet, PML = Posterior mitral leaflet

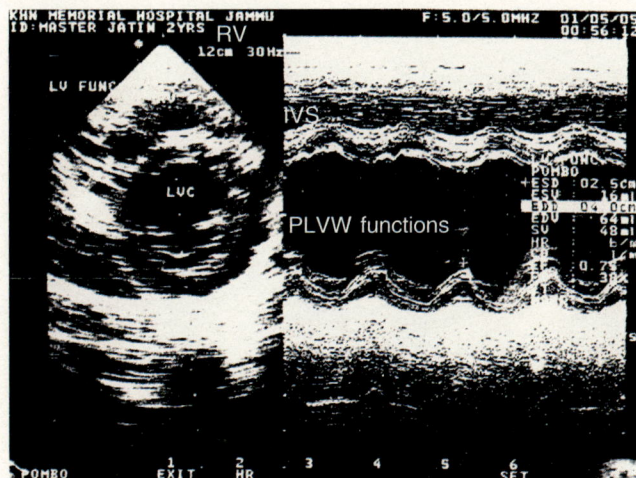

Fig. 12.42: Short axis (left) and M-Mode echocardiogram (right) demonstrating calculation of LV functions by Pombo method in a normal child

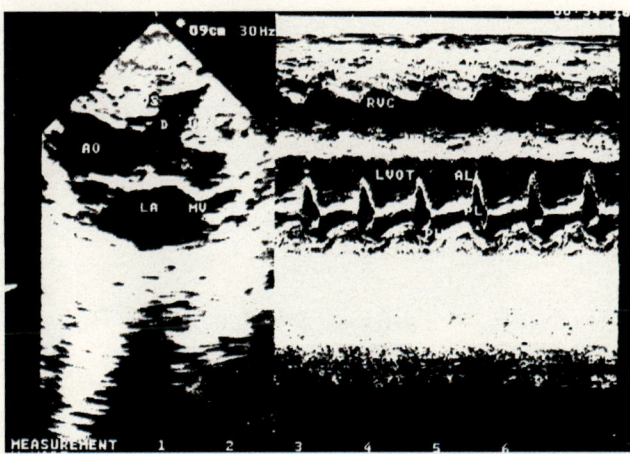

Fig. 12.43: Long axis (left) and M-mode echocardiogram showing a large defect along ventricular septum (D), dilated and hypertrophied right ventricle (RVC) in a 13 days old baby with large ventricular septal defect

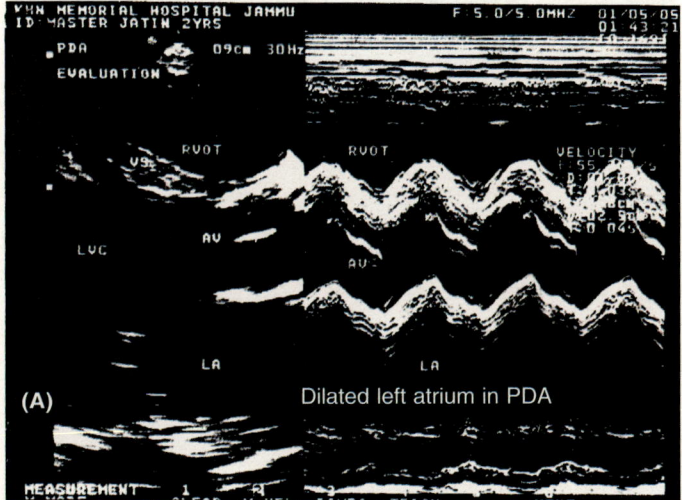

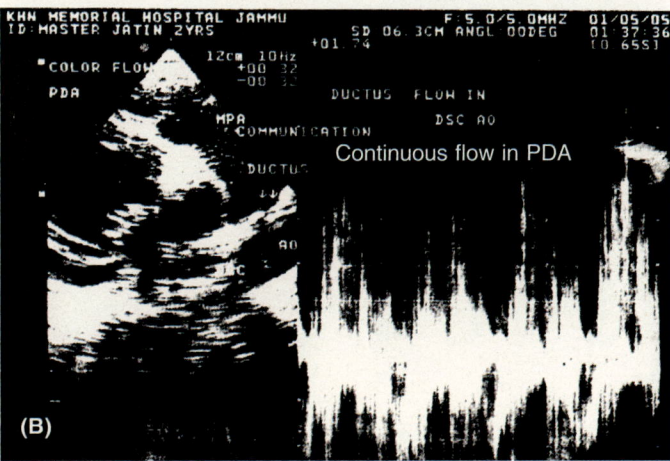

Fig. 12.44A and B: (A) 2 D Short axis aortic and M-Mode aorta views showing normal aortic valve and left atrial and aortic dimension ratio is more than one in a young child with patent ductus arteriosus (PDA). **(B)** 2D and Doppler flow across ductus showing continuous flow during systole and diastole in the same child with PDA

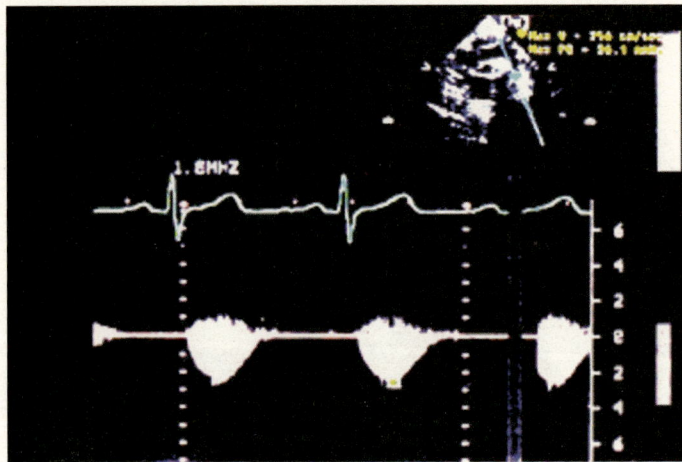

Fig. 12.45: Doppler flow velocity across pulmonary valve showing increased velocity in neonatal pulmonic valvular stenosis

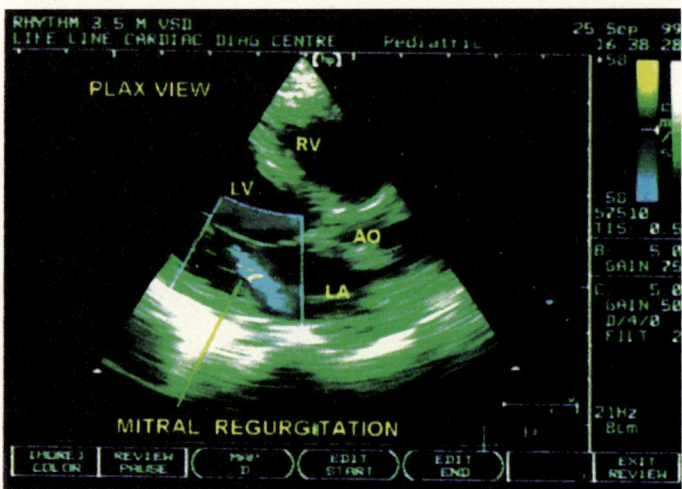

Fig. 12.48: PLAX view showing MR jet into LA in a newborn with VSD and PDA

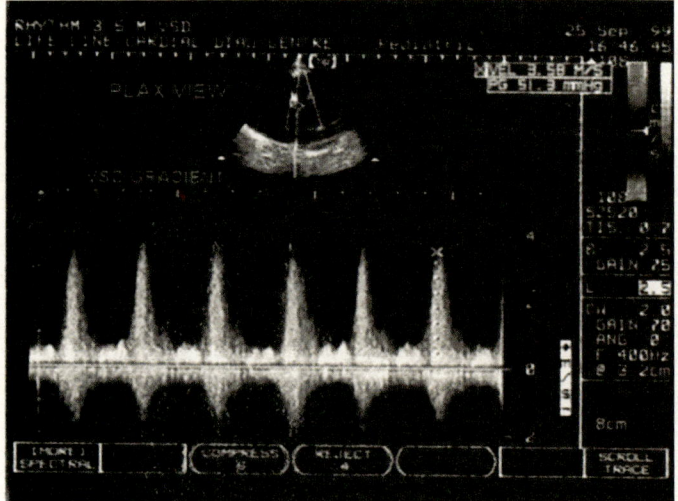

Fig. 12.46: Doppler flow velocity across subaortic defect in an newborn with ventricular septal defect

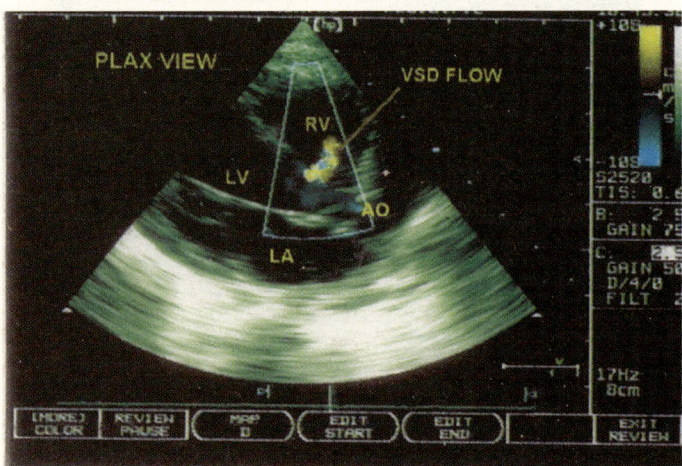

Fig. 12.49: Color Doppler flow across IVS showing color jet entering from LVOT into RV in newborn with ventricular septal defect

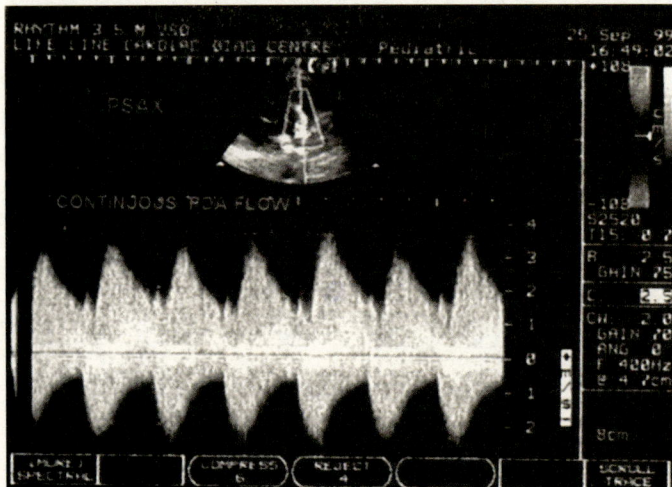

Fig. 12.47: Doppler systo-diastolic flow velocity across ductus arteriosus in an infant with PDA

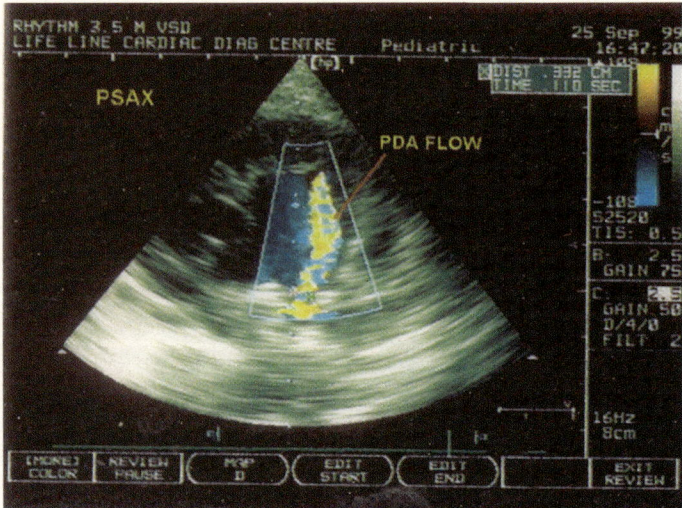

Fig. 12.50: Short axis color flow across ductus connecting pulmonary artery and descending aorta in a neonatal PDA

was not chosen. The frequency of complex one ventricle type cardiac repairs may therefore become less common in the coming years. Some forms of CHD are associated with early decompensation and even death of the infant before the malformation can be recognised and treated. This applies mainly to those where either the pulmonary or systemic circulation is dependent on the patency of the arterial duct, or the lesions which require "mixing" at an adequate atrial septal defect such as transposition of the great arteries or total anomalous pulmonary venous drainage. It appears intuitively obvious that if CHD is recognised prenatally and delivery takes place in or near a paediatric cardiology centre, thus avoiding delay in diagnosis and emergency transfer of a sick neonate, the morbidity for the infant will be minimised. This has been shown in several studies although improvement in mortality has been harder to prove, partly because fetal echo-cardiography preferentially detects more severe forms of CHD which have a higher mortality. However, a recent study of infants with transposition of the great arteries, where there werc adequate numbers to answer this question, showed conclusively that there was a much lower mortality in those cases prenatally diagnosed. Thus, the impact on paediatric cardiology, if fetal heart scanning improved to the ideal level of expertise, would be a decrease in the number of complex malformations, but those patients with CHD who come to surgery would do so in optimum status without prior insult. This would have a potentially significant effect on saving of resources by reducing complex disease and improving both the cardiac and neurological outlook for the survivors.

Bibliography

1. Achiron R, Glaser J, Gelernter I, et al. Extended fetal echocardiographic examination for detecting cardiac malformations in low risk pregnancies. *BMJ* 1992;304:671–674.
2. Alla LD, Maxwell DJ, Carminati M, Tynan MJ. Survival after fetal balloon valvoplasty. *Ultrasound Obstet Gynecol* 1995;5:90–91.
3. Allan LD, Chita SK, Anderson RH, Fagg N, Crawford DC, Tyan M. Coarctation of aorta in prenatal life; An echocardiographic, anatomical and functional study *Br Heart J* 1988; 59;356–360.
4. Allan LD, Crawford DC, Chita SK, Tynan MJ. Prenatal screening for congenital heart disease. *BMJ* 1986; 292:1717–1719.
5. Allan LD, Sharland GK, Miburn A, Lockhart SM, Groves AM, Anderson RH, Cook AC, et al. Prospective diagnosis of 1,006 consecutive cases of congenital heart disease in the fetus. *J Am Coll Cardiol* 1994; 23: 1452–1458.
6. Allan LD, Sharland GK: Hypoplastic left heart syndrome; Effects of fetal echocardiography on birth prevalence. *Lancet* 1991;337:959–961.
7. Allan AD Prenatal screening for congenital heart disease. *Br. Med. J.* 292; 1717–1988.
8. Bonnet D, Coltri A, Butera G, et al. Detection of transposition of the great arteries in fetuses reduces neonatal morbidity and mortality. *Circulation* 1999;99:916–918.
9. Buskens E, Grobbee DE, Frohn-Mulder IM, et al. Efficacy of routine fetal ultrasound screening for congenital heart disease in normal pregnancy. *Circulation* 1996;94:67–72.
10. Chang AC, Huhta JC, Yoon GY, et al. Diagnosis, transport, and outcome in fetuses with left ventricular outflow tract obstruction. *J Thorac Cardiovasc Surg* 1991;102:841–818.
11. Copel JA, Tan AS, Kleinman CS. Does a prenatal diagnosis of congenital heart disease alter short-term outcome? *Ultrasound Obstet Gynecol* 1997;10:237–241.
12. Daubeney PE, Sharland GK, Cook AC, et al. Pulmonary atresia with intact ventricular septum: impact of fetal echocardiography on incidence at birth and postnatal outcome. UK and Eire collaborative study of pulmonary atresia with intact ventricular septum. *Circulation* 1998; 98:562–566.
13. Hyett J, Perdu M, Sharland G, et al. Using fetal nuchal translucency to screen for major congenital cardiac defects at 10–14 weeks of gestation: population based cohort study. *BMJ* 1999;318:81–85.
14. Montana E, Khoury MJ, Cragan JD, et al. Trends and outcomes of prenatal diagnosis of congenital cardiac malformations by fetal echocardiography in a well defined birth population, Atlanta, Georgia, 1990–1994. *J Am Coll Cardiol* 1996;28:1805–1809.
15. Sharland GK, Allan LD. Screening for congenital heart disease prenatally. Results of a 21/2 year study in the south east Thames region. *Br J Obstet Gynaecol* 1992; 99: 220–225.
16. Tegnander E, Eik-Nes SH, Johansen OJ, et al. Prenatal detection of heart defects at the routine fetal examination at 18 weeks in a non-selected population. *Ultrasound Obstet Gynecol* 1995;5:372–380.
17. Todros T, Faggiano F, Chiappa E, et al. Accuracy of routine ultrasonography in screening heart disease prenatally. Gruppo Piemontese for prenatal screening of congenital heart disease. *Prenatal Diagn* 1997;17:901–906.
18. Yagel S, Weissman A, Rotstein Z, et al. Congenital heart defects. Natural course and in utero development. *Circulation* 1997;96:550–555.

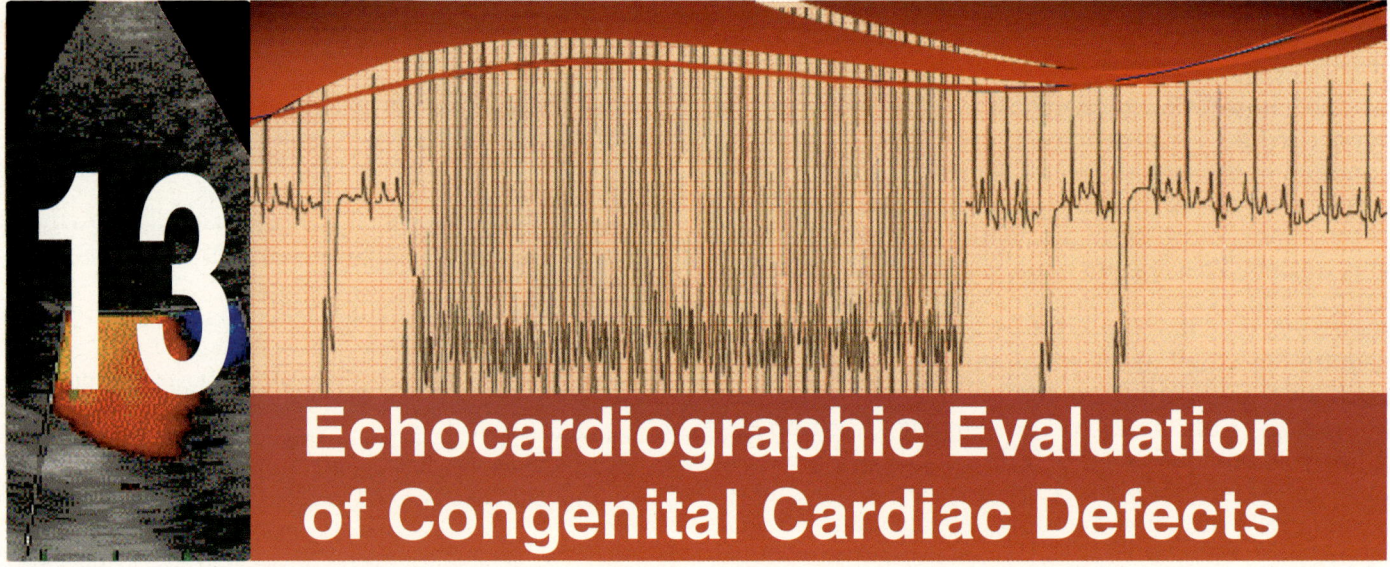

13

Echocardiographic Evaluation of Congenital Cardiac Defects

Examination of a Child Patient

In developing countries of Southeast Asia, the children with congenital cardiac defects are still being examined by a general echocardiographer when compared to technically advanced countries, where examination is performed by a special trained pediatric echocardiographer. The children usually are not accustomed to visit hospital and therefore, very apprehensive and afraid of white coats and multistorey building of a referred medical institution. They are usually made educated either by their parents or social worker about what exactly is likely to happen in a echocardiographic laboratory. They are told that they are going to see the moving coloured pictures of various part of their heart and there would be a great fun in the laboratory besides being served with sweets of their likings. If the child is not consoled, begin the procedure and try to divert his or her attention with toys and different sound producing instruments. Since children seem to be very sensitive to sound, such things as mobiles, music boxes, singing, keys and a variety of rattles and bells may be helpful. For older children, structures can be pointed out on the screen as they appear. These measures would certainly make the task of the cardiac sonographer easier and to ensure that the child remains in a physiologic resting state in order to get accurate measurements of a particular cardiac defect.

Patient Position

It is preferable to keep small infants as warm and comfortable as possible. This can be done with a blanket or a warm air blowing heater. They can be placed entirely on a pillow, which elevates them somewhat and allows positional changes (e.g. left lateral decubitus) with a least of disturbance. Dimming the lights and having a bottle or pacifier hand may often help the infant go to sleep. If the infant has been breast-fed, holding the pacifier under warm water makes it "more like Mom". One can perform echocardiograms on young patients nursing on their moms' laps or in any other position deemed comfortable. The older child usually cooperates and lies quietly on his or her back, or rolls slightly to the left to obtain a good echocardiogram.

Fig. 13.1: The best position for a child under examination is the lap of the mother and tool of examination should be made familiar prior to further examination as shown above

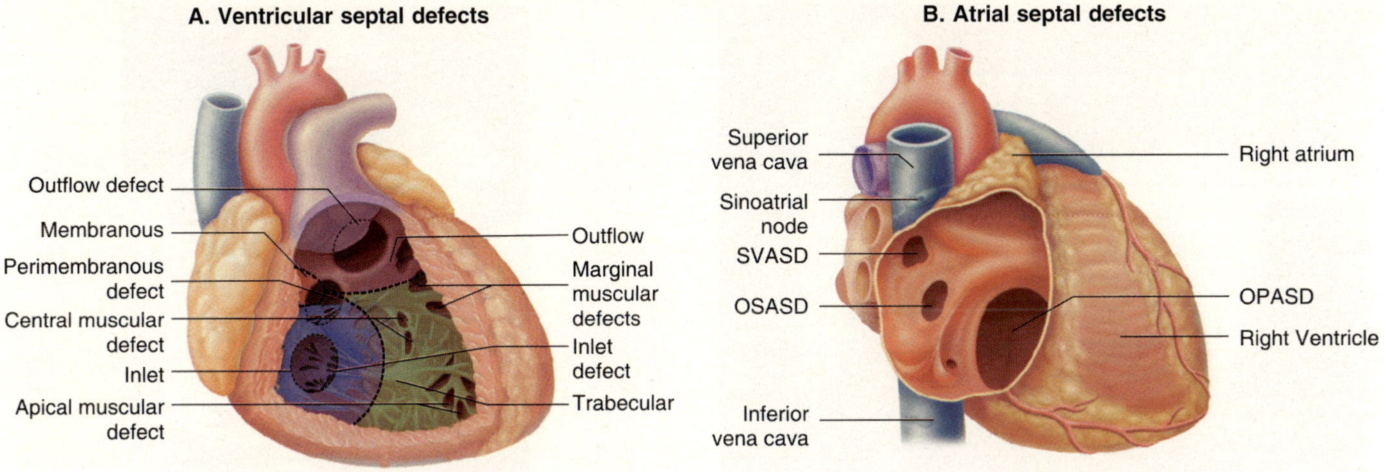

A. Ventricular septal defects

Outflow defect
Membranous
Perimembranous defect
Central muscular defect
Inlet
Apical muscular defect

Outflow
Marginal muscular defects
Inlet defect
Trabecular

B. Atrial septal defects

Superior vena cava
Sinoatrial node
SVASD
OSASD
Inferior vena cava

Right atrium
OPASD
Right Ventricle

Fig. 13.2A and B: Diagrammatic representation of various types of ventricular and atrial septal defects

Segmental approach to congenital heart disease

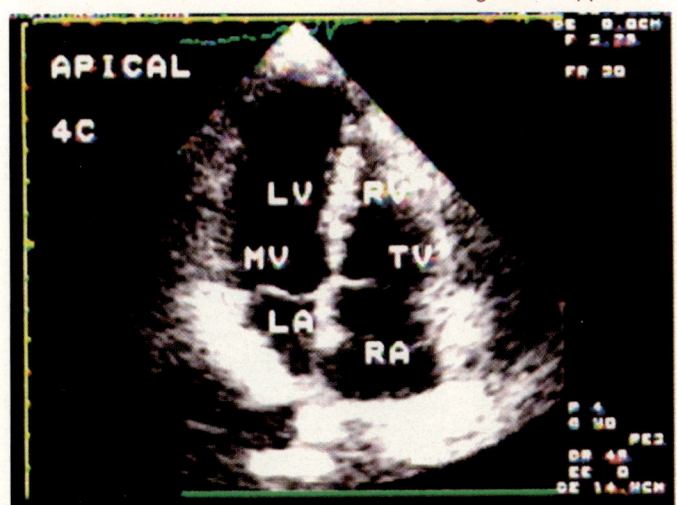

Fig. 13.3: Apical 4C view showing normal anatomical relationship between four chambers of the heart LA = Left atrium, LV = Left ventricle, RV = Right ventricle and RA = Right atrium

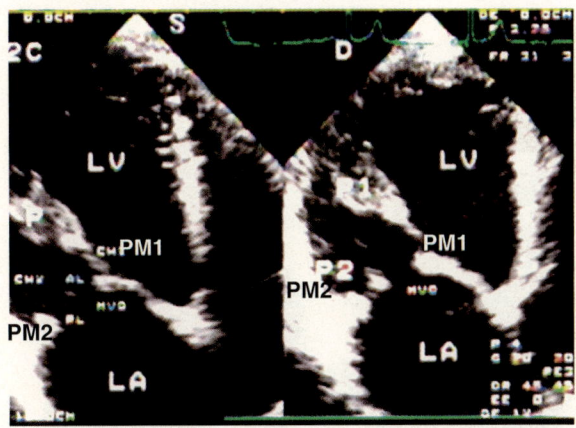

Fig. 13.5: 2C View in dual scan of LV showing normal anatomical relationship of papillary muscles, chordie and their respective attachment in shaping the anatomical structure of mitral valve CH1 and 2 = Chordie1 and 2 and AL = Anterior mitral leaflet, PL = Posterior mitral leaflet, PM1 and 2 = Papillary muscle 1 and 2

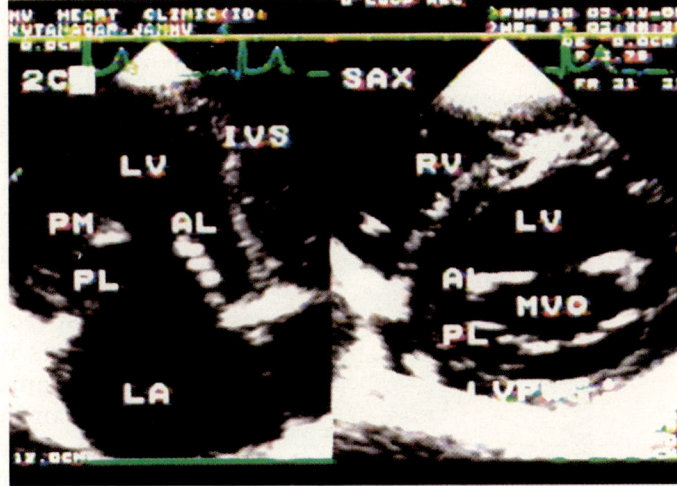

Fig. 13.4: Apical 2C view showing normal anatomical relationship between IVS, LV and LA (left) and short axis view of LV showing morphology of normal mitral valve (right)

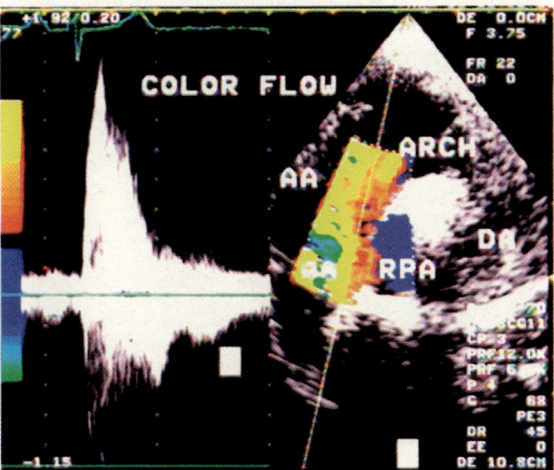

Fig. 13.6: Suprasternal great vessel view showing normal anatomical relationship between ascending aorta, arch, descending aorta and right pulmonary artery

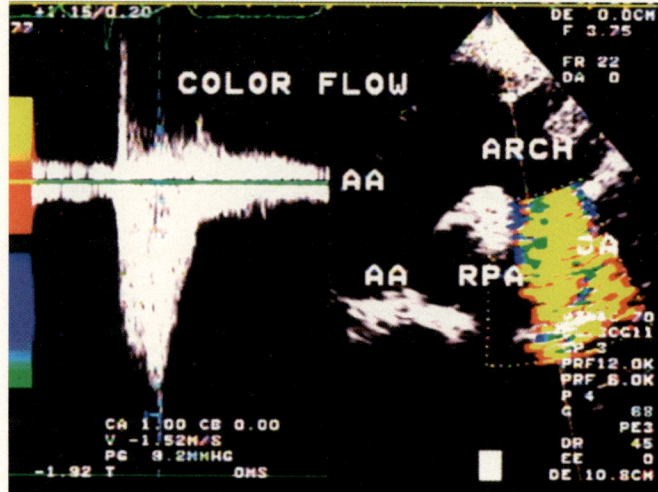

Fig. 13.7: Suprasternal great vessel view showing normal relationship between descending aorta, arch and right pulmonary artery

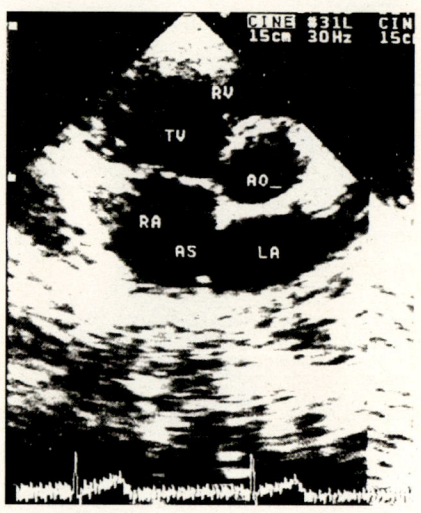

Fig. 13.8: Left parasternal short axis view at aorta showing normal anatomical relationship between aorta, (AO) right ventricle (RV) tricuspid valve, (TV) right atrium (RA), interatrial septum (IAS) and left atrium (LA)

Segmental approach to congenital heart disease

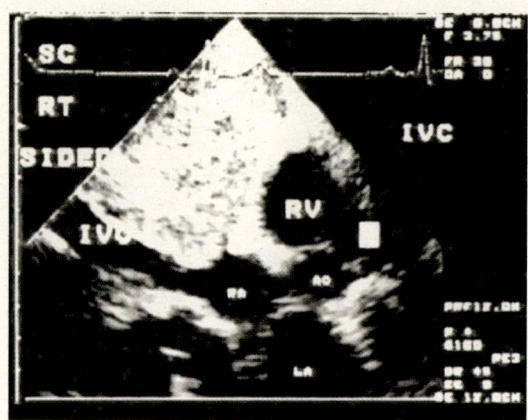

Fig. 13.9: Subcostal view showing right-sided inferior vena cava (IVC) and its normal relationship with right sided liver right ventricle (RV) right atrium (RA) and interatrial septum (IAS) and AO (aorta)

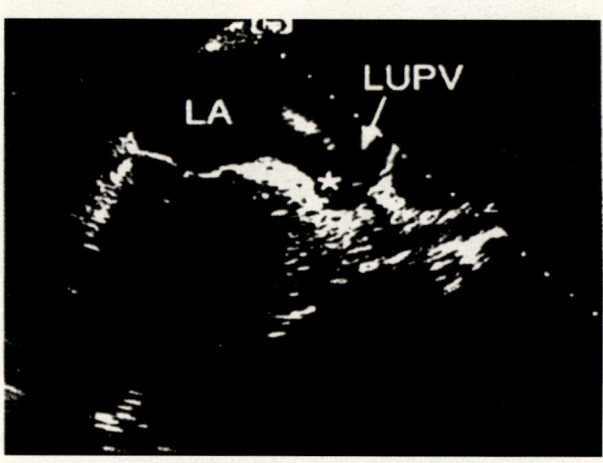

Fig. 13.10: TEE view showing normal relationship between emerging left upper pulmonary vein (LUPV) and left atrium (LA)

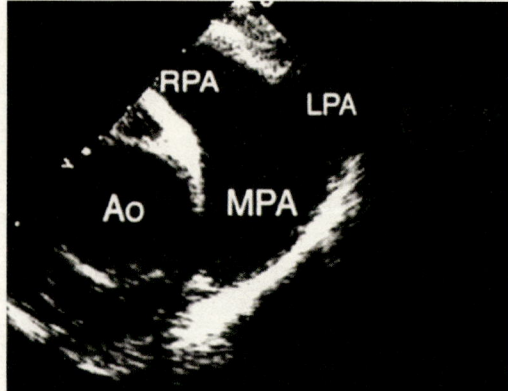

Fig. 13.11: TEE view showing normal relationship between main pulmonary artery (MPA) turning around like a (sausage) and centrally placed aorta (Egg) completely giving a figure of sausage and egg along with its two branches, i.e. right and left pulmonary branches

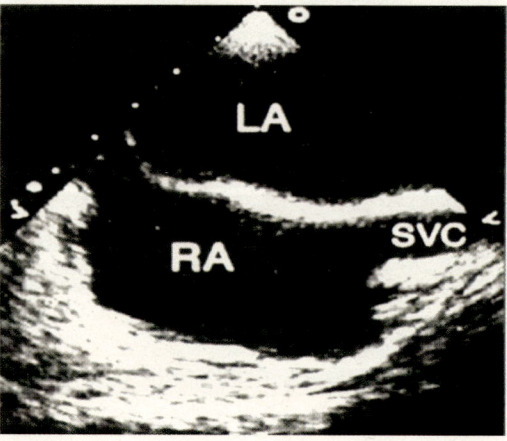

Fig. 13.12: TEE view showing normal relationship between superior vena cava (SVA), left atrium (LA) and right atrium (RA)

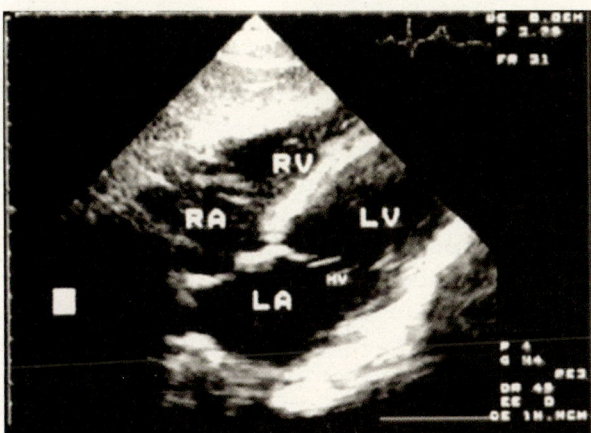

Fig. 13.13: Subcostal oblique 4C showing normal relationship between right atrium (RA), left atrium, (LA) right ventricle (RV) left ventricle (LV) and intervening between right atrium and left atrium is the interatrial septum

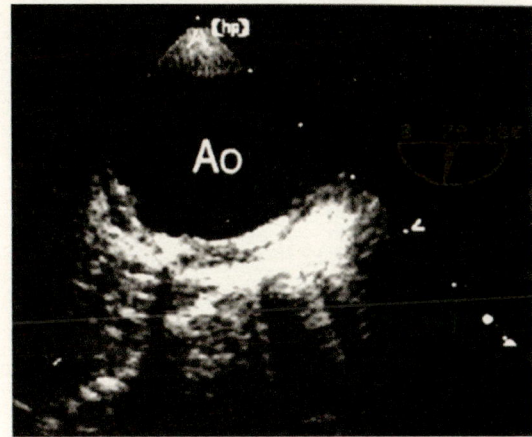

Fig. 13.14: TEE view showing centrally placed round structure aorta (AO) containing all the three normal layers, i.e. intima, media and adventitia

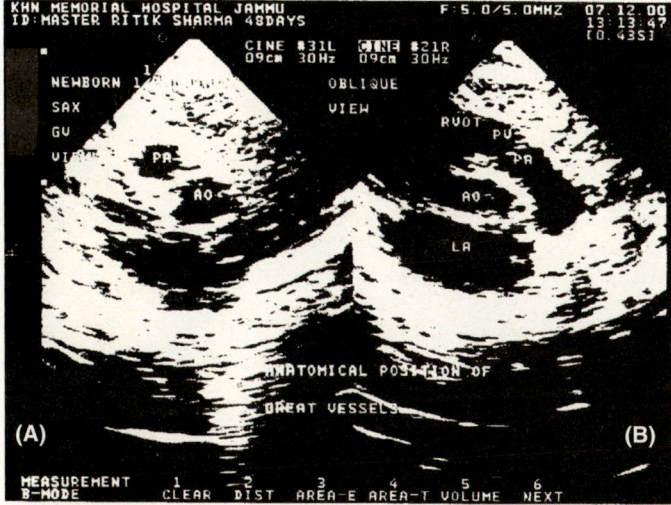

Fig. 13.15A and B: (A) Short axis 2-D view at great vessel level showing normal anteriorly placed main pulmonary atery (PA) and aorta is located posteriorly (AO). **(B)** Short axis and oblique inclination showing relationship between pulmonary artery, aorta left atrium (LA) and right ventricular outflow tract (RVOT)

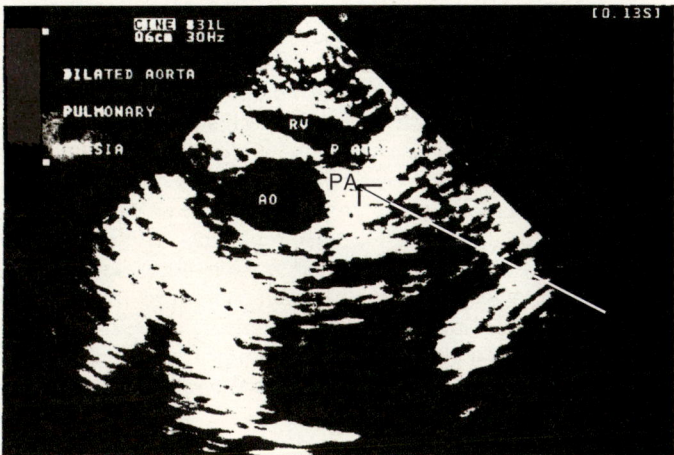

Fig. 13.16: Short axis and slightly oblique view at great vessel level showing dilated aorta (AO) and minimal lumen of the main pulmonary artery as compared to the above described figure (13) in a patient with pulmonary atresia (arrow)

Transducer Selection

On account of small size of the chest of an infant, the structures to be visualized are somewhat superficial, it is important to use a transducer with the best possible resolution. This is achieved by the use of high frequency focused transducers. The transducers usually available are 10 MHz short focus for premature infants, 7.5 MHz medium focus for adolescents and slim adults. One may also occasionally use a 2.25 MHz medium focus for heavier adolescents. To obtain better results, various transducers are often employed to get maximum information during echocardiographic study.

Ventricular Septal Defect (Fig. 13.2A)

Ventricular septal defect is a commonly encountered anomaly of the heart (found in as much as 20% of the congenital heart population. The defect varies in its

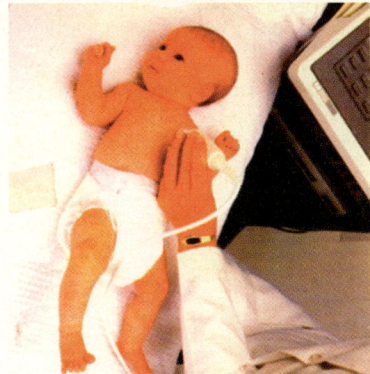

Fig. 13.17: A baby lying on a comfortable examintion table and doctor is performing echocardiography on this infant suffering from heart murmur

Table 13.1: *Segmental approach to cardiac situs and malpositions*

1. *Atrial situs*

   Visceral situs (and visceroatrial concordance)

   Atrial morphology (situs solitus or inversus)

   Venous inflow patterns
2. *Ventricular localization*

   Ventricular morphology (d-loop or l-loop)

   Atrioventricular concordance (atrioventricular valve morphology)

   Base-to-apex axis (levocardia ordextrocardia)
3. *Great artery connections*
4. *Identification of the great arteries*
5. *Ventriculoarterial concordance or transposition*
6. *Spatial relationship between the great arteries and ventricular septum*

anatomic position and may be classified as membranous, muscular, aneurysmal, supracristal, left ventricle to right atrial shunt, or it may involve the endocardial cushion defects.

The most anatomic landmark is the crista supraventricularis, a muscular ridge that separates the main body of the right ventricle, from the outflow (or infundibular) portion. The ventricular septal defect lies either above or below this ridge. The defects that lie above this ridge are called supracristal. These defects are located just beneath the pulmonary orifice so that the valve forms part of the superior margin of the interventricular communication. Defects that lie below the crista are called infracristal and may be found in the membranous or muscular part of the septum, or in the endocardial cushion area.

Table 13.2: *Echocardiography in the adult patient with congenital heart disease*

Indications	Class
1. Patients with clinically suspected congenital heart disease, as evidenced by signs and symptoms such as a murmur, cyanosis, or unexplained arterial desaturation, and an electrocardiogram or radiograph suggesting congenital heart disease	I
2. Patients with known congenital heart disease on follow-up when there is a change in clinical findings	I
3. Patients with known congenital heart disease for whom there is uncertainty as to the original diagnosis or when the precise nature of the structural abnormalities or hemodynamics is unclear	I
4. Periodic echocardiograms in patients with known congenital heart lesions and for whom ventricular function and atrioventricular valve regurgitation must be followed (e.g. patients with a functionally single ventricle after a Fontan procedure, transposition of the great vessels after a Mustard procedure transposition and ventricular inversion, and palliative shunts)	I
5. Patients with known congenital heart disease for whom following pulmonary artery pressure is important (e.g. patients with moderate or large ventricular septal defects, atrial septal defects. single ventricle, or any of the above with an additional risk factor of pulmonary hypertension)	I
6. Periodic echocardiography in patients with surgically repaired (or palliated) congenital heart disease with the following: change in clinical condition or clinical suspicion of residual defects, left or right ventricular function that must be followed, or the possibility of hemodynamic progression or a history of pulmonary hypertension	I
7. To direct interventional catheter valvotomy, radiofrequency ablation valvotomy interventions in the presence of complex cardiac anatomy	I
8. A follow-up Doppler echocardiographic study, annually or once every 2 years, in patients with known hemodynamically significant congenital heart disease without evident change in clinical condition	IIb
9. Multiple repeat Doppler echocardiography in patients with a repaired patent ductus arteriosus, atrial septal defect, ventricular septal defect, coarctation of the aorta, or bicuspid aortic valve without change in clinical condition	III
10. Repeat Doppler echocardiography in patients with known hemodynamically insignificant congenital heart lesions (e.g. small atrial septal defect, small ventricular septal defect) without a change in clinical condition	III

Table 13.3: *Echocardiographic features of right and left ventricles*

Right ventricle	Left ventricle
Trabeculated endocardial surface	Smooth endocardial surface
Three papillary muscles	Two papillary muscles
Chordae insert into ventricular septum, Infundibular muscle band	Ellipsoidal geometry
Moderator band	Mitral atrioventricular valve with two leaflets with
Tricuspid atrioventricular valve with relatively apical insertion	relatively basal insertion

Segmental approach to congenital heart disease

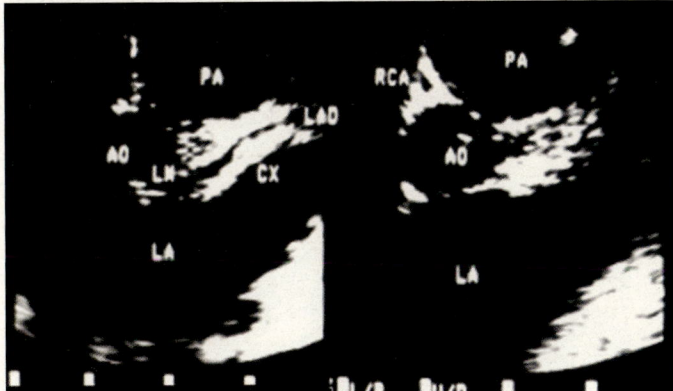

Fig. 13.18: Infraclavicular short axis aorta (AO) and pulmonary artery (PA) for normal anatomical localization of left main coronary artery (LM) along with its circumflex artery (CX) and left anterior descending artery (LAD) as shown on the scan

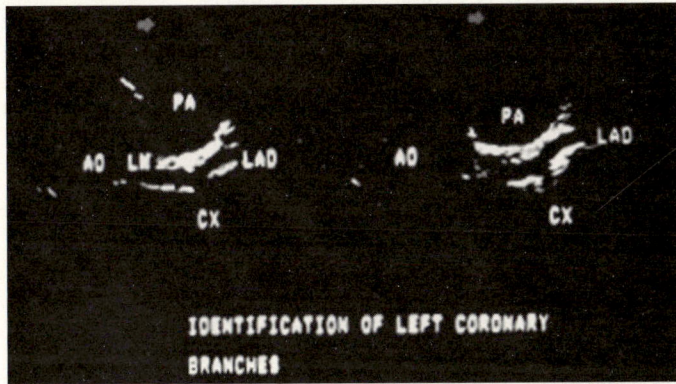

Fig. 13.19: Normal localization of three main coronary arteries with better visualized and normally patent left main (LM), left anterior descending coronary artery (LAD) and circumflex artery (CX) in normal relation to pulmonary artery (PA) and aorta (AO)

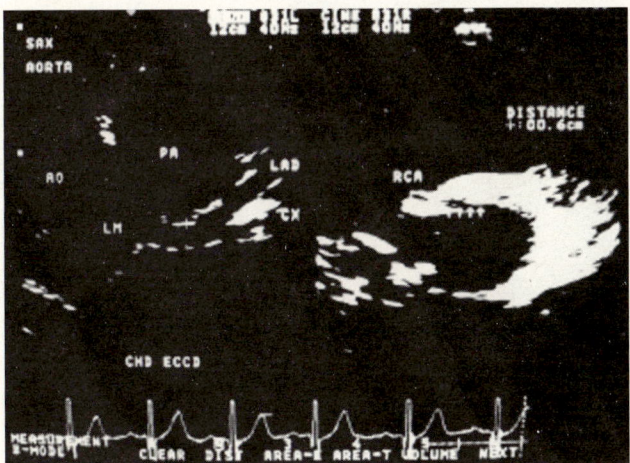

Fig. 13.20: High upper left parasternal in short axis view of great vessels showing normal relationship between left main coronary artery emerging from left coronary sinus of valsalva and branching into LAD and CX arteries, (left) and right coronary artery (RCA) emerging from right coronary sinus of aorta (right panel)

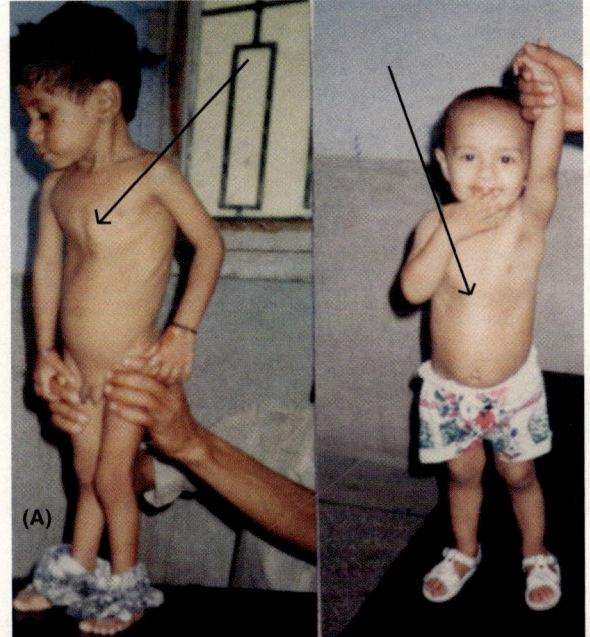

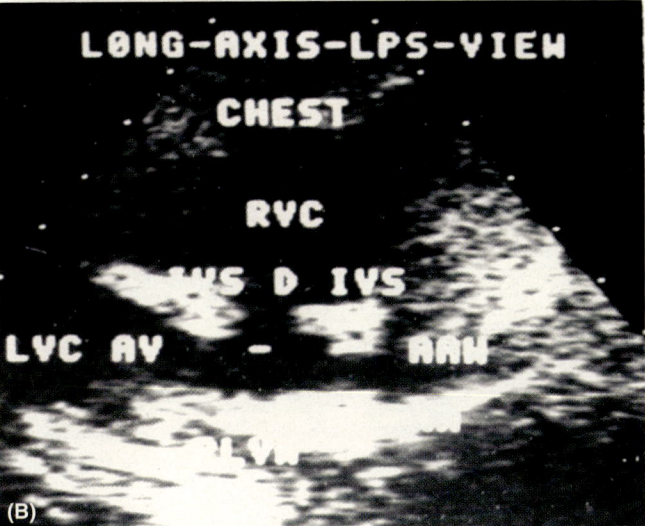

Fig. 13.21A and B: (A) Two children with pigeon shaped-chest deformity (arrows) and stunted growth who were suffering from ventricular septal defect since their birth. **(B)** Long axis LV view focusing at interventricular septum and aorta depicting moderate muscular VSD. RVC = right ventricular cavity, D = Septal defect, LVC = left ventricular cavity

The infracristal defects are the most common type of lesions found, usually in the area of the membranous septum. This defect may be partially hidden by the septal leaflet of the tricuspid valve, and care must be taken with two-dimensional echo to carefully evaluate the area and record Doppler tracings along the septal wall. The membranous defect is found just below the aortic leaflets, and sometimes the aortic leaflet is "sucked" into the defect. A less common infracristal defect is located in the muscular septal wall. These defects may be large or small, or there may be fenestrated defects. These multiple small defects may

Different types and sizes of VSD through different windows of visualization

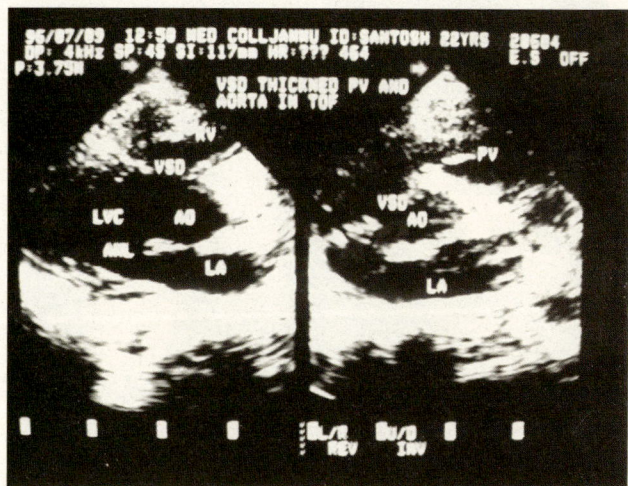

Fig. 13.22: Long axis and oblique view of aorta showing subaortic type of moderate VSD with normal surrounding structures

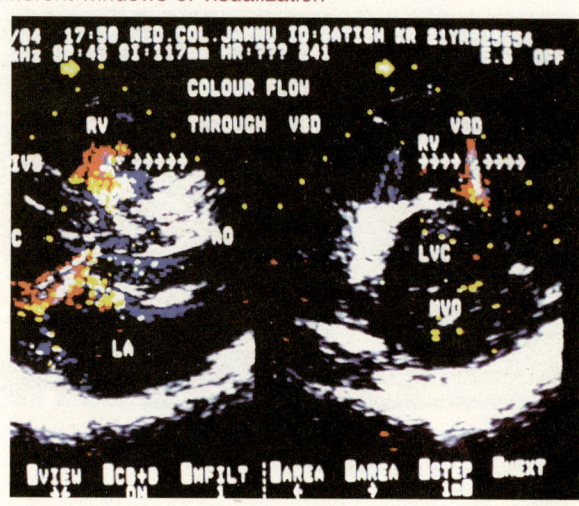

Fig. 13.23: Long axis and short axis views of LV showing small jet of VSD into RV

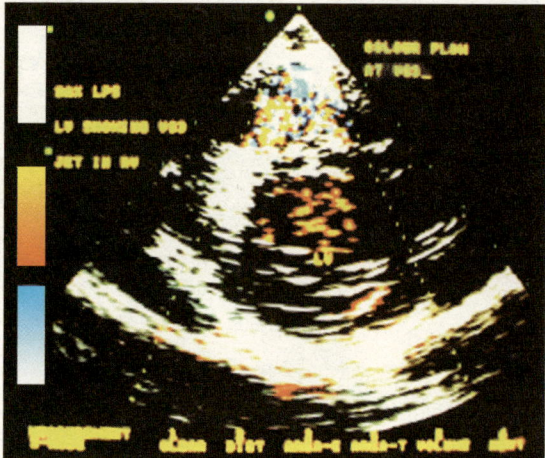

Fig. 13.24: Short axis view LV showing mosaic color jet of VSD into RV

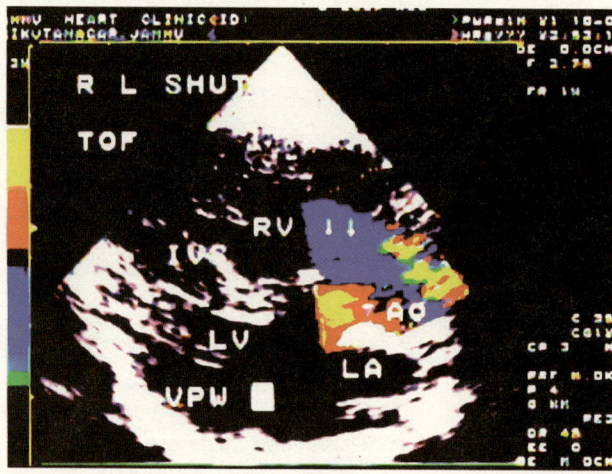

Fig. 13.25: Long axis view of LV showing large VSD with reversal of flow from RV into LVOT in TOF

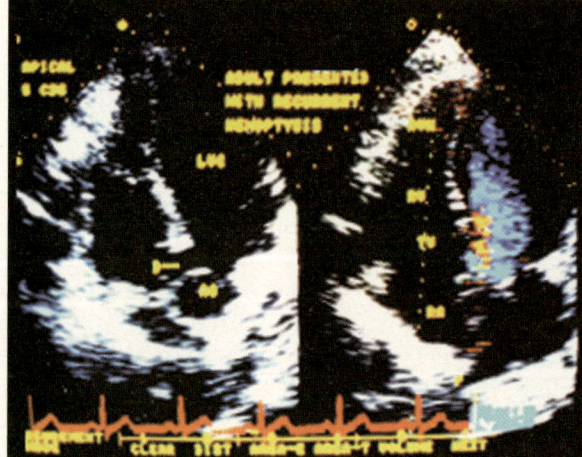

Fig. 13.26: Dual scan frame in apical 5 chamber views showing subaortic VSD with color flow along IVS and blue AR jet into LV as shown in right scan

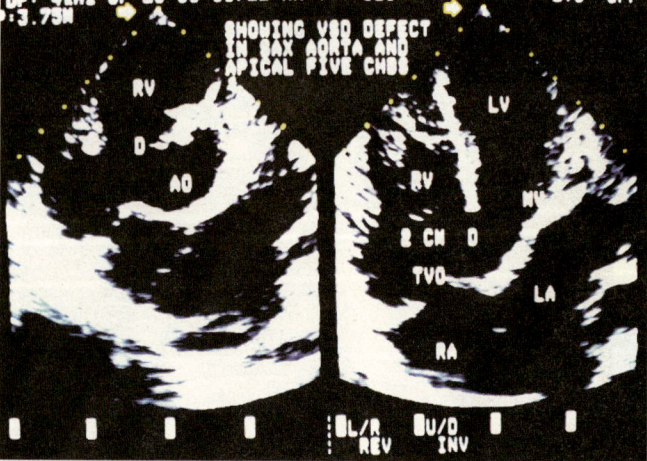

Fig. 13.27: Short axis and apical 4C views showing larger VSD (D) along with septum primum defect in endocardial cushion defect (canal defect)

Different Types and Sizes of VSD Through Different Windows of Visualization

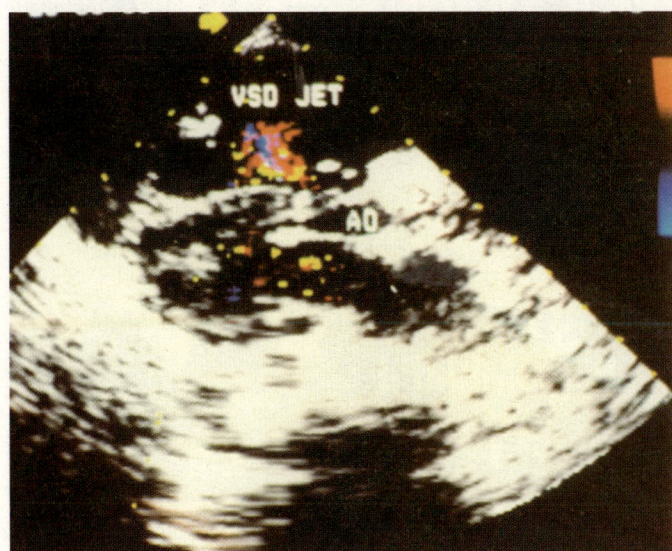

Fig. 13.28: Long axis LV view showing color flow VSD jet from LVOT into RV

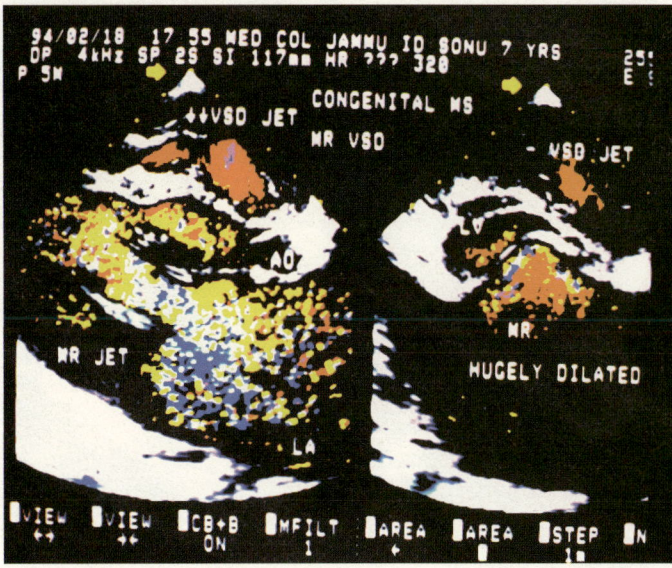

Fig. 13.31: Dual scan frame in long axis LV showing hugely dilated LA, VSD jet into RV with mosaic color flow MR jet into LA

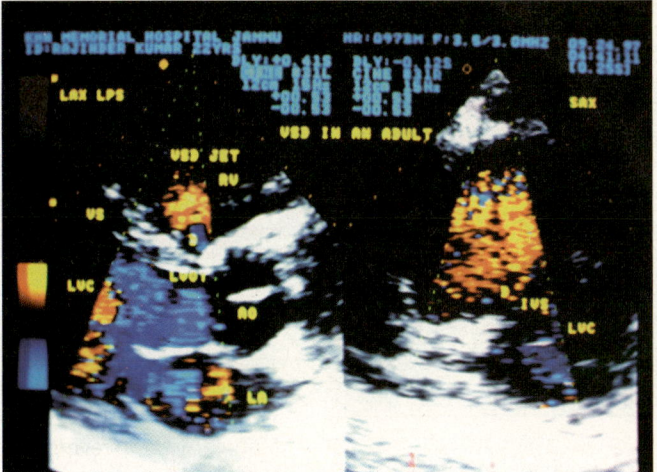

Fig. 13.29: Dual scans in long axis and short axis LV views showing VSD jets along with blue AR and MR.

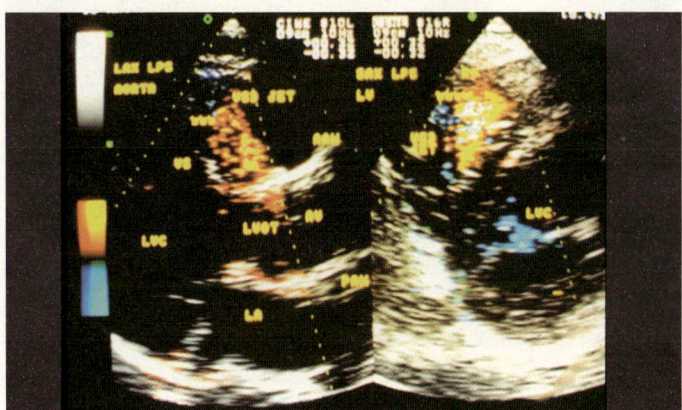

Fig. 13.32: Dual scan frame in long and short axis views of LV showing red and mosaic color VSD jets respectively

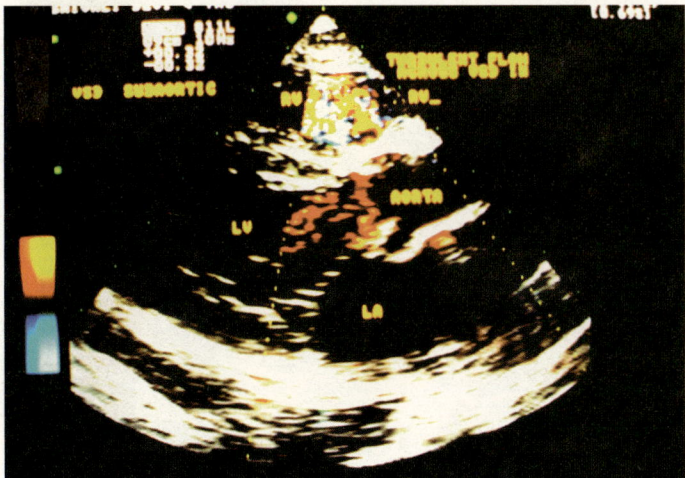

Fig. 13.30: Long axis view LV showing VSD color jet into RV along with dilated LA and LV

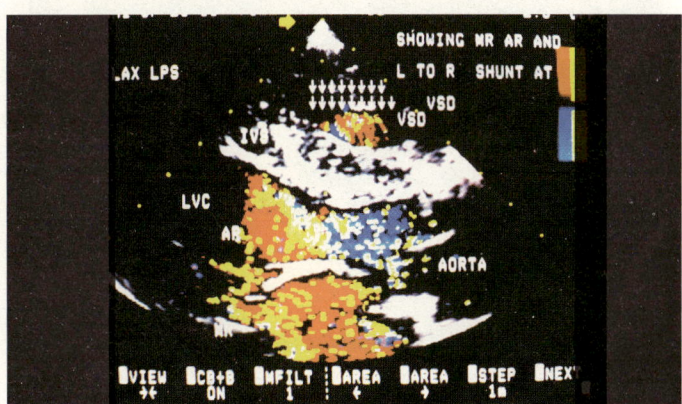

Fig. 13.33: Long axis view LV showing VSD jet into RV and mosaic MR color flow jet into LA

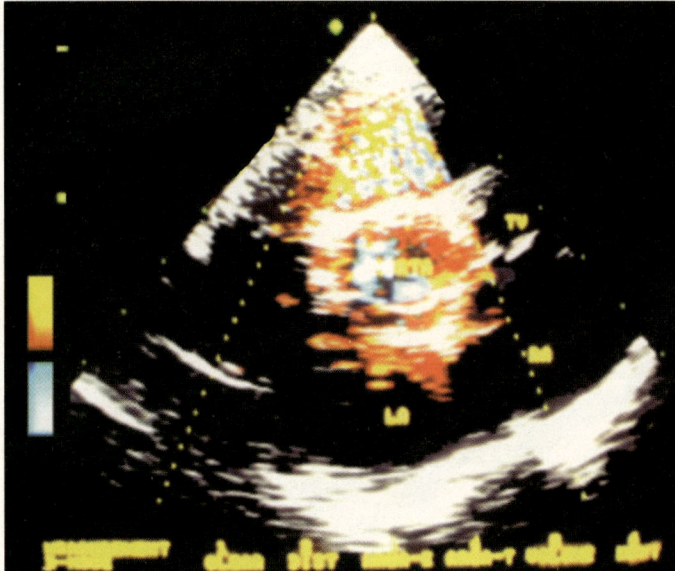

Fig. 13.34: 2-D Short axis view LV showing mosaic color jet from LVOT to RV in moderate sized VSD

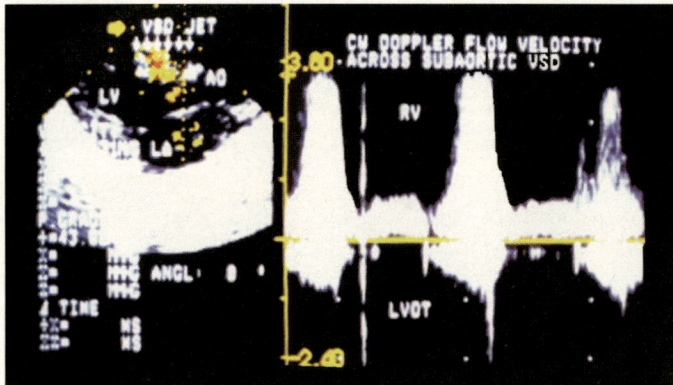

Fig. 13.35: 2-D Color Doppler flow velocity across VSD, left panel shows color jet of VSD from LVOT to RV in long axis view of LV and Doppler flow velocity in subaortic VSD (right panel)

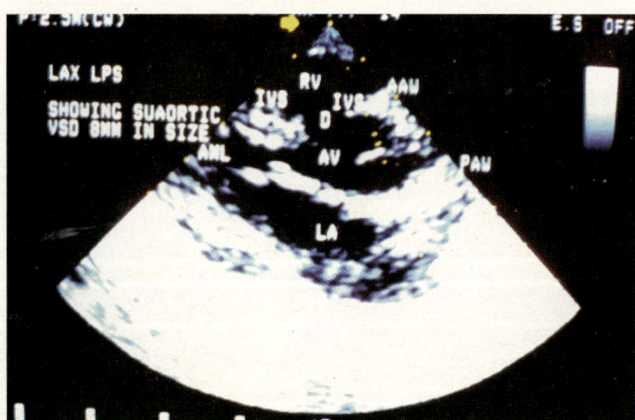

Fig. 13.36: Moderate-sized VSD as shown in 2-D long axis view and also demonstrating the anatomical relationship of nearby structures AV = Aortic valve, LA = Left atrium D = VSD, RV = Right ventricle

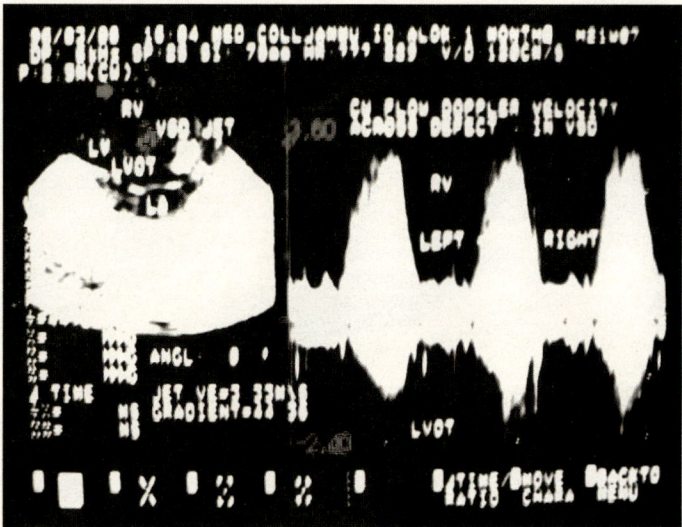

Fig. 13.37: Continuous wave Doppler flow velocity across left to right shunt of VSD (right)

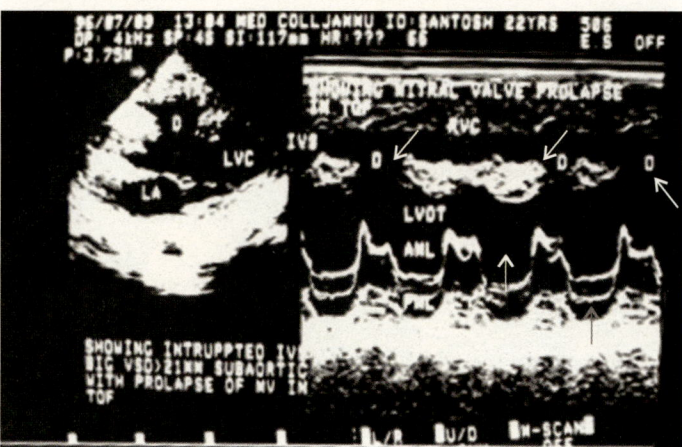

Fig. 13.38: M-Mode echocardiogram showing interrupted echos along the interventricular septum in ventricular septal defect (D) along with mitral valve prolapse as shown in mitral valve echoes during mid systole (arrow)

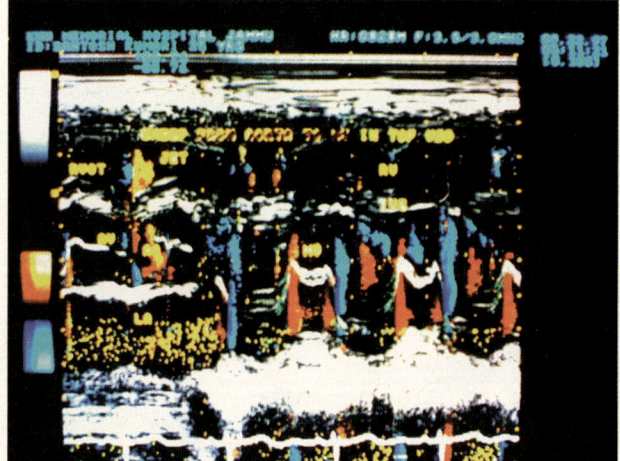

Fig. 13.39: Color M-mode echocardiogram sweep from mitral valve to aorta depicting VSD jet and interrupted echoes along IVS

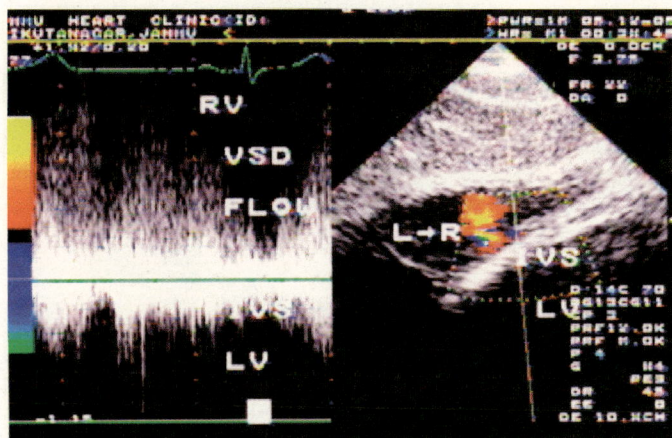

Fig. 13.40: Subcostal long axis LV showing color jet of small muscular VSD in RV (right) along with Doppler waveforms (left) in an adult patient

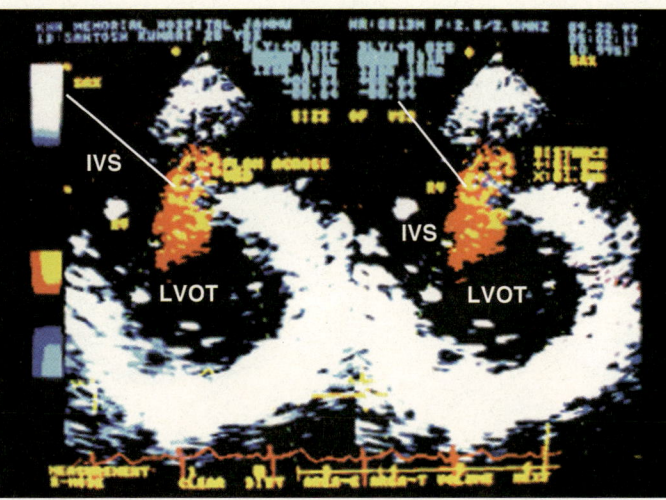

Fig. 13.43: Color 2-D short axis LV dual scan showing a big color jet of VSD emerging from LVOT and going into RV (arrow)

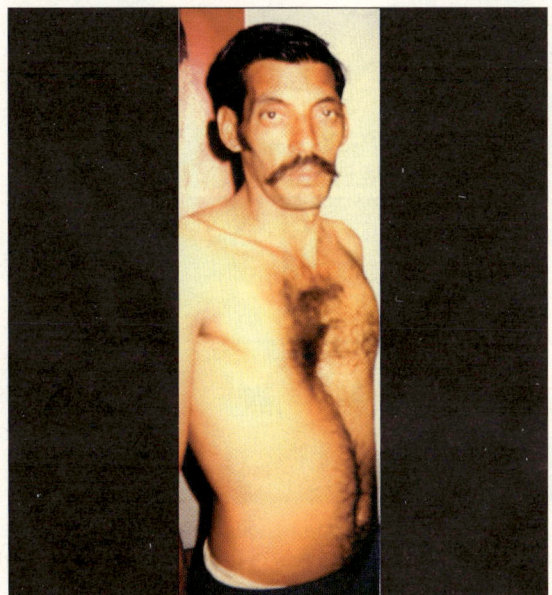

Fig. 13.41: An adult showing chest deformity who had VSD with mitral valve prolapse

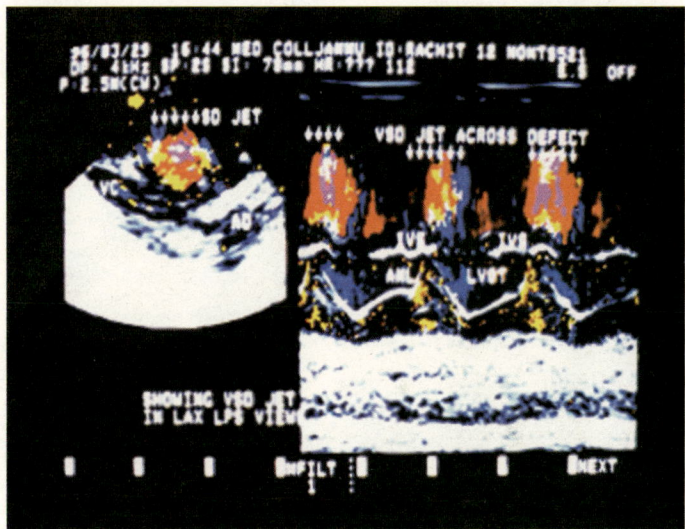

Fig. 13.44: M-Mode showing color jet of VSD traversing from LVOT to RV through IVS

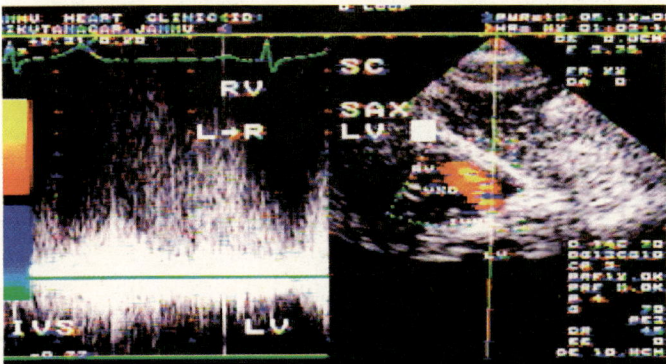

Fig. 13.42: Subcostal short axis LV showing color jet of small muscular VSD in RV (right) along with Doppler waveforms (left) in an adult patient

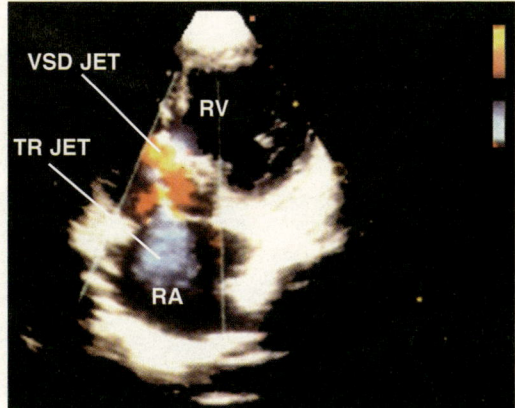

Fig. 13.45: TEE color Doppler echoscan depicting subaortic VSD and moderate blue colored tricuspid regurgitation (TR) jet into right atrium (RA)

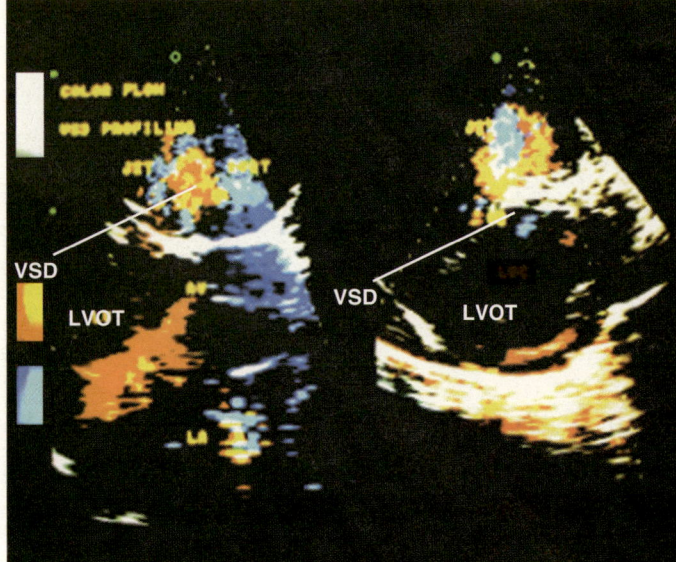

Fig. 13.46: Transthoracic color 2-D long and short axis left parasternal region showing VSD from LVOT into RV in these two planes respectively

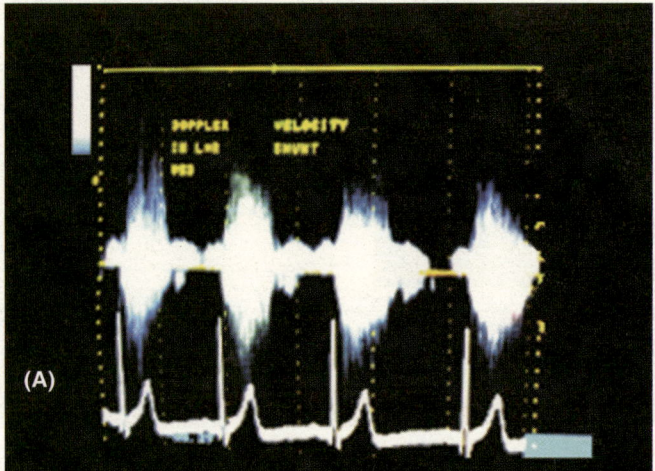

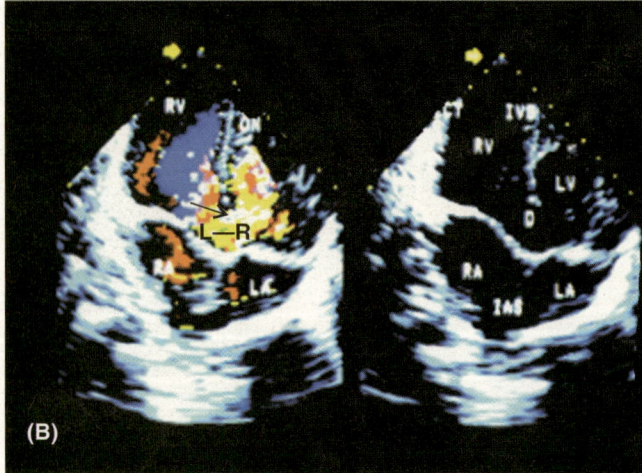

Fig. 13.47A and B: (A) CW Doppler flow velocity across VSD. **(B)** Color flow dual scan view in apical 4C left parasternal region showing color flow from LVOT into RV almost attaining a U configuration (arrow)

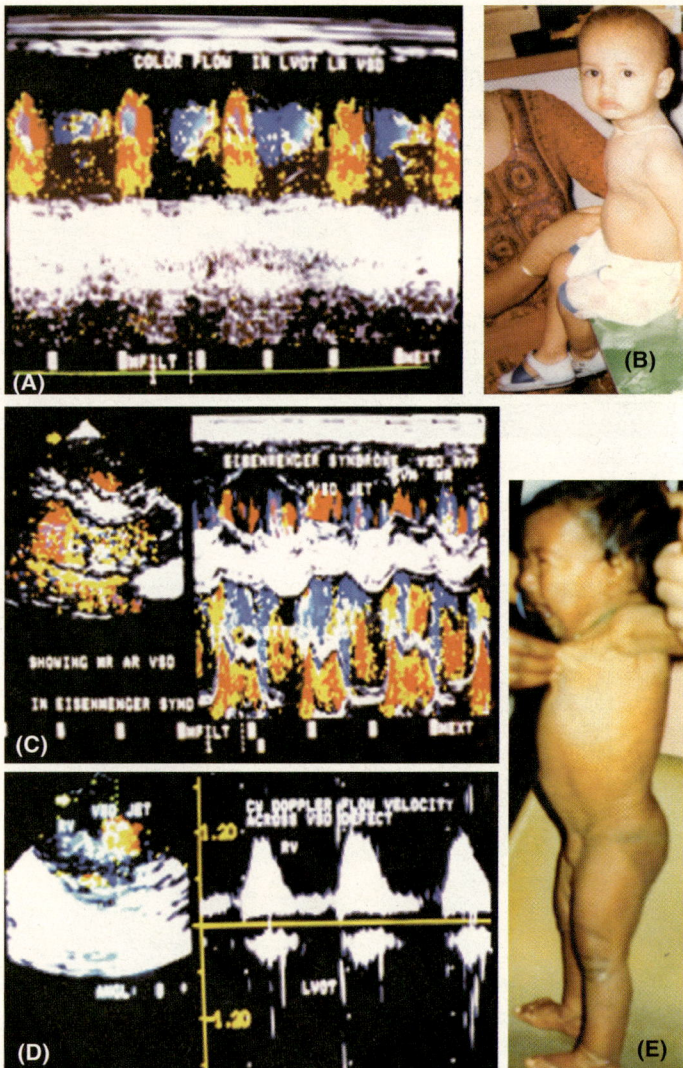

Fig. 13.48A to E: (A) M-Mode echocardiogram showing color jet in VSD traversing from LVOT to RV along with photograph of a child showing stunted physical growth and chest deformity. **(B)** and **(C)** M-Mode color echocardiogram showing VSD jet in RV and severe form of MR and AR jets on AMLof mitral valve. **(D)** Color Doppler echoscan depicts flow velocity across VSD. **(E)** Photograph of a child showing cutis hyperelastica (excessive elastic skin as shown after stretching) with VSD

functionally act as a single large communication. Less commonly an isolated infracristal ventricular septal defect is found in the area of the endocardial cushion and may or may not extend into the ostium primum atrial septum (Figs 13.21–13.53).

While in an attempt to close, VSD may form an aneurysm along the right side of the septal defect. These aneurysms generally bulge into the right heart in one of three directions:

1. Above the tricuspid valve and into the right atrium,
2. Directly into the septal leaflet of the tricuspid valve, or

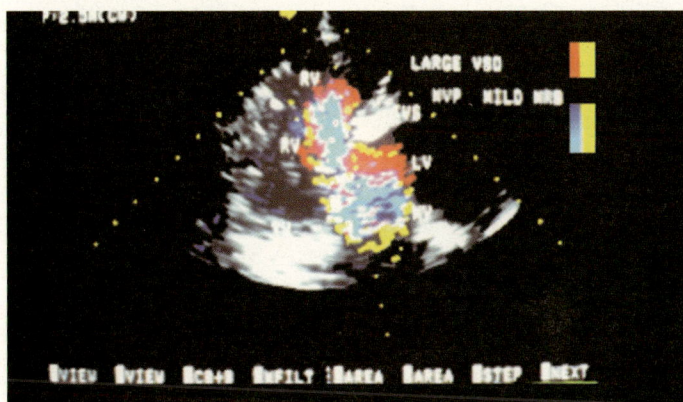

Fig. 13.49: Color flow long axis showing a big VSD with isodirectional shunt between LVOT and RV across IVS through ventricular septal defect in an adult patient with associated patent ductus arteriosus and mitral valve prolapse

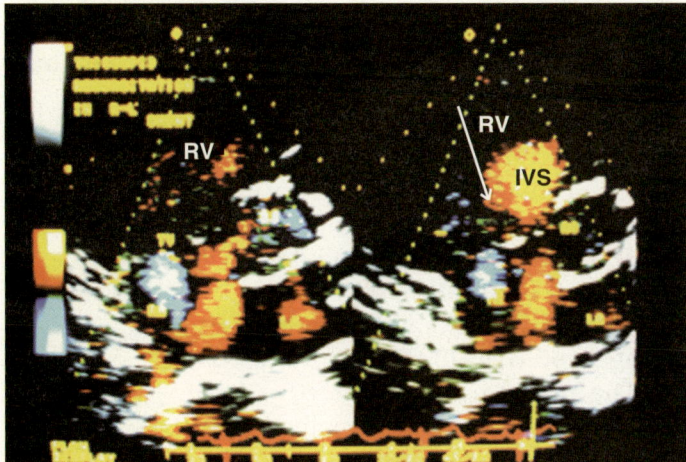

Fig. 13.50: Color 2-D long axis view showing color flow passing from LVOT to RV across the defect like a fountain as indicated (arrow) in a patient with subaortic ventricular septal defect

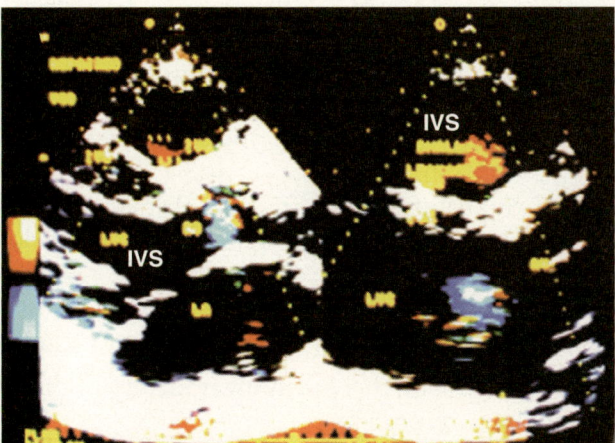

Fig. 13.51: Color 2-D long axis and short axis LV view depicting early entering of blood jet from LVOT into RV (left) and the blood flow is still present in LVOT as seen in scan (right) in patient with almost closed VSD

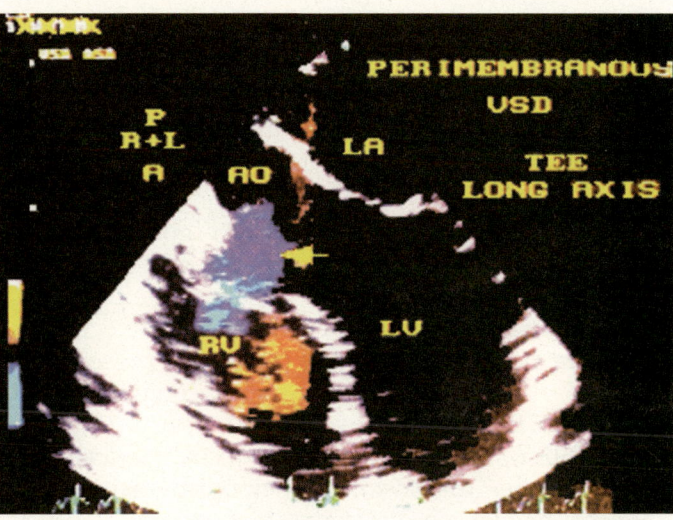

Fig. 13.52: Long axis TEE color flow scan showing perimembranous ventricular septal defect (arrow). AO = Aorta, LV = Left ventricle, RV = Right ventricle

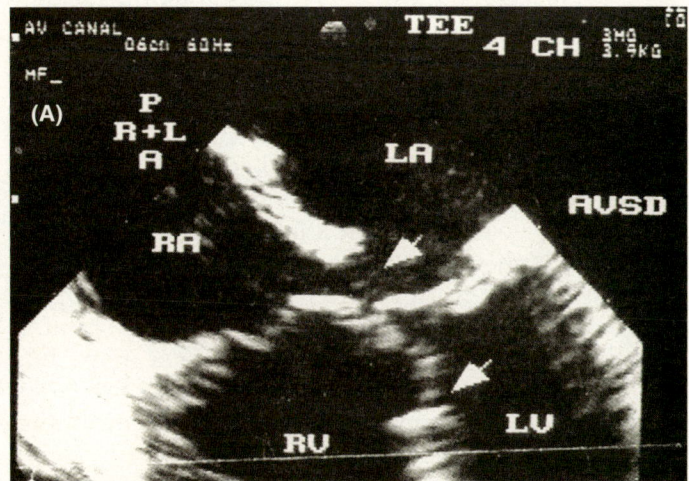

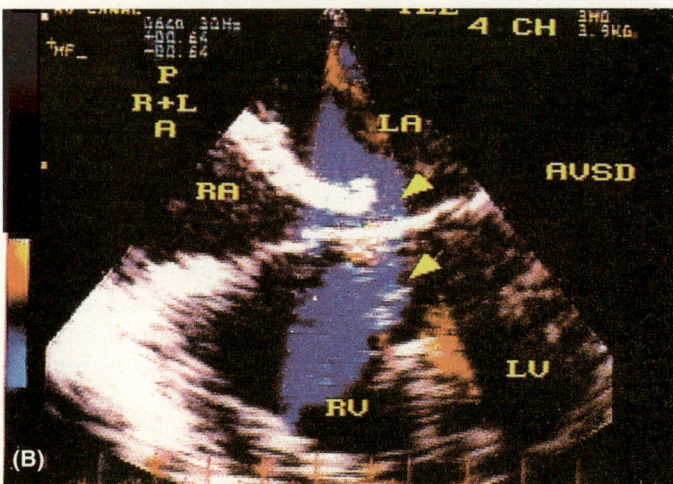

Fig. 13.53A and B: (A) TEE 4C view showing atrio-ventricular (AVSD) as a part of AV canal defect (B) Colour TEE showing atrioventricular defect with blue coloured tricuspid regurgitation as a part of AV canal defect

3.   Below the tricuspid leaflets and into the right ventricular cavity.

They are usually seen as tiny structures, but when they become large they may cause obstruction of the right ventricular outflow tract.

Ventricular septal defects may close with time. Muscular septal defects have a very good chance of closing, if they are quite small. The ventricular septal defects may form aneurysm tissue to help in their closure. A significant number of septal defects close within the first several months of life. The presence of a ventricular septal defect may be seen in conjunction with other cardiac anomalies (i.e. tetralogy of Fallot, transposition of the great vessels, truncus arteriosus, and other complex diseases). Both two-dimensional and transesophageal echocardiography can usually directly visualise the site of the ventricular septal defect. The common views to use are the parasternal long-axis view, the apical four-chamber view, and the subcostal window in 2-D echocardiography. Sometimes the short-axis view is useful to evaluate the extent of a large septal defect.

They are commonly localized in the region of membranous part of the septum, just inferior to the aorta. With careful angulation, the site and size of the defect may be seen on the long-axis view. The Doppler sample volume may be placed along the defects, closer to the right ventricle (with a left to right shunt). An abnormal, high-pitched sound occurs during systole is indicative of left-to-right shunt. Colour flow mapping easily shows the turbulent patterns across the shunt. It also allows one to visualise the presence of more than one defect present in the septum. The septal examination in the apical four-chamber view allows an additional window to image the defect.

Septal aneurysm can be visualised with 2-D echo. An aneurysmal tissue may form in the right ventricle over the area of the defect. Other forms of spontaneous closure may be accomplished by a number of mechanisms, such as direct apposition of the margins of the defect, in growth of fibrous tissue, endocardial proliferation, adherence of the septal tricuspid leaflet to the margins of the defect, or prolapse of an aortic cups through the defect.

The muscular septal defects are sometimes seen with two-dimensional imaging but often are located near the apex of the ventricle and are very small and difficult to image clearly. The Doppler cursor is placed along the septum near the apex of the heart, and the sample volume carefully moved along the septum to record the abnormal flow patterns in systole.

Colour-flow mapping can prove very useful in patients with unusual shunt direction patterns. Instead of the usual left-to-right shunt, one may see the flow to travel from the left ventricle to the right atrium. With Doppler alone, the abnormal flow patterns can be recorded but one may not be able to pin-point exactly where the shunt is flowing. Colour allows one to actually see the turbulent patterns jet into the cavity, and then record the shunt flow.

Proximal isovelocity surface area (PISA) is one of the new modalities for evaluation of VSD shunt. In long axis, left parasternal axis view, VSD is visualised, the indices of maximal flow rate across the defects are developed from both radius and area obtained by planimetry, of the first aliasing based on Doppler colour-flow images. All the indices are correlated for body surface area and compared with shunt flow (Q_p:Q_s) ratio. Proximal isovelocity surface area is a simple and reliable method for quantitative evaluation of shunt across a VSD and correlates well with that obtained at cardiac catheterization

Atrial Septal Defect (Fig. 13.2B)

Echocardiographically, the following are the common types of atrial septal defects which can be easily visualised on both 2-D and 2-D colour-flows: (Figs 13.53–13.66 and 13.72–75).

1. The secundum type, which occurs in the area of the foramen ovale;
2. The sinus venosus type, located in the most superior portion of the atrial septum and usually associated with partial anomalous pulmonary venous drainage; and (Fig. 13.69)
3. The primum type, located just above the atrio-ventricular ring and usually associated with a cleft mitral valve leaflet.

It has been observed by echogram that the area of the foramen ovale is thinner than the surrounding atrial tissue, and hence is prone to signal dropout, particularly in the apical four-chamber view. Therefore any break in atrial septal continuity apparent in the four-chamber view must be confirmed by the subcostal view, in which the septum is more perpendicular to the transducer. Because of beam-width artifacts, the edges of the defect may be slightly blunted and appear brighter than the remaining septum.

Left-to-right shunting at the atrial level manifests itself on M-mode as right ventricular volume overload, which is characterised by the following:

1. Increased excursion of the tricuspid valve,
2. Dilation and hypercontractility of the right ventricle,
3. Enlargement of the pulmonary artery (not from pulmonary hypertension), and
4. Paradoxic to flat septal motion.

Septal motion should be examined at the chordal level, removed from the hinge point near the aorta, since it can appear paradoxic at this site in the normal patients.

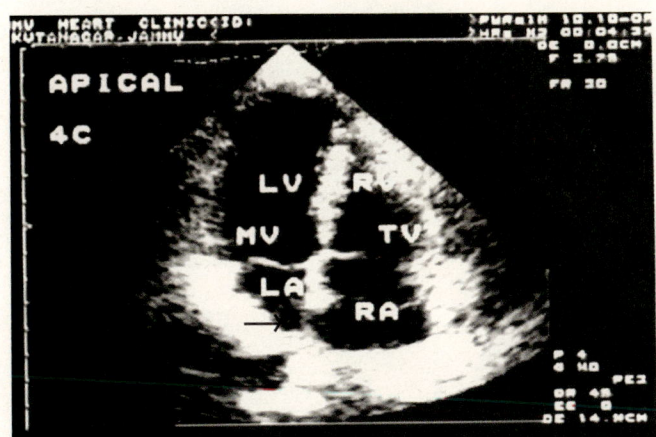

Fig. 13.54: Apical 4C view showing echolucent area along the interatrial septum indicating fosa ovalis type of atrial septal defect (arrow)

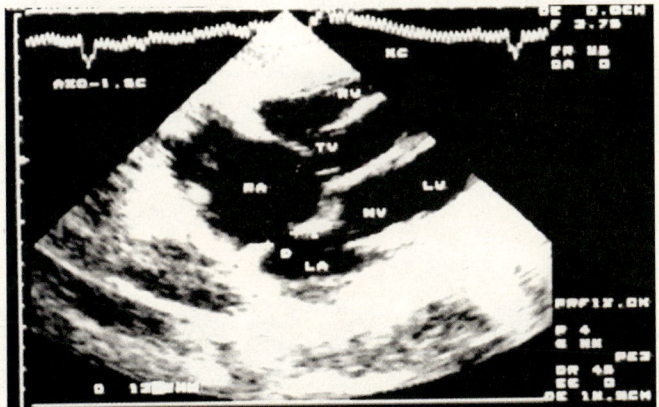

Fig. 13.55: Subcostal 4C view showing all the four chambers of the heart with breakage in interatrial septum in a patient with fossa ovalis type of atrial septal defect (arrow D), subcostal two and four-chamber views is the best out of all other echocardiographic approaches in profiling atrial septal defects

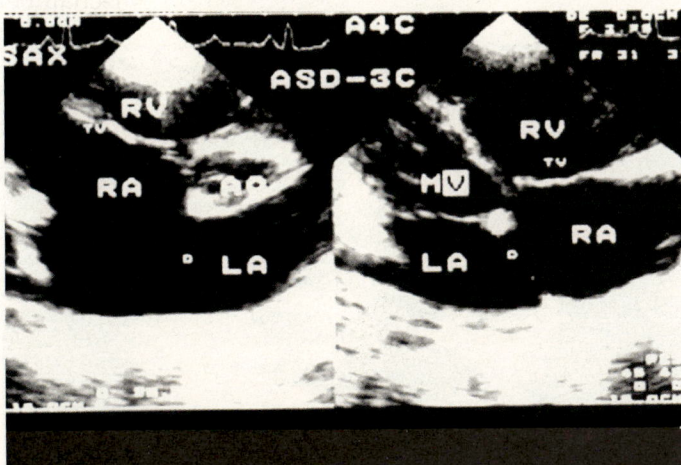

Fig. 13.56: Short axis aortic and oblique 4C views of LV showing echo free space along the location of IAS respectively in echocardiograpic profiling of atrial septal defects (D)

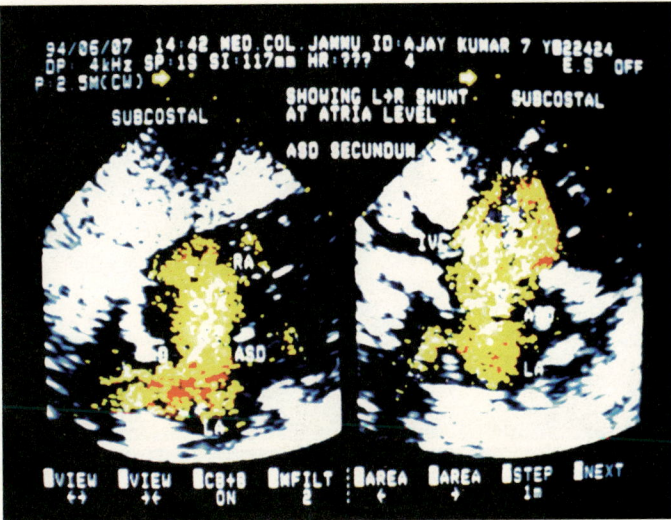

Fig. 13.57: Subcostal four-chamber view showing large ASD secundum (left). Subcostal view showing larger ASD Secundum extending up to inferior vena cava (right)

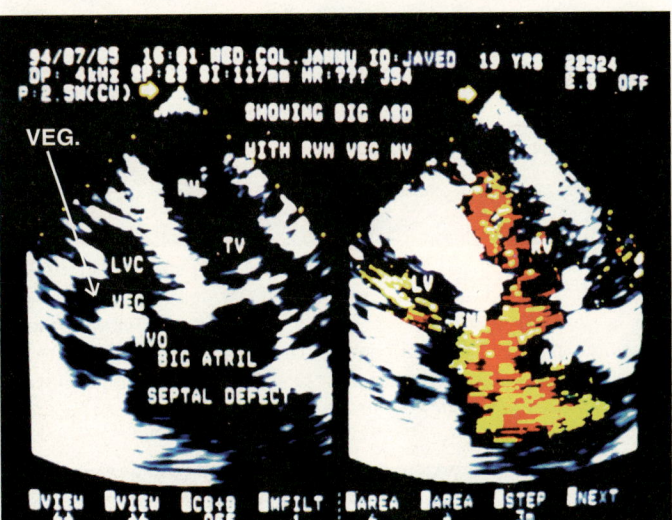

Fig. 13.58: (left) Apical oblique 4C views in a dual scan showing larger ASD secundum with abscence of almost entire interatrial septum (IAS) with dilated RV and vegetation on AML of mitral valve (arrow). Color flow showing filling of entire common atrium and extending right up to tricuspid valve and RV (right)

Contrast echocardiography may be a useful investigation in the diagnosis of an atrial septal defect. If the shunt is right to left, direct visualisation of contrast appearing in the left atrium from a peripheral venous injection is possible. If the shunt is left to right, a jet of nonopacified blood is seen entering the contrast-filled right atrium as the scan is replayed in slow motion and single frame-by-frame action.

Doppler tracings of the atrial septal defect with the sample volume placed at the site of the defect would show a positive flow with a left-to-right shunt and a negative flow with a right-to-left shunt. Colour-flow

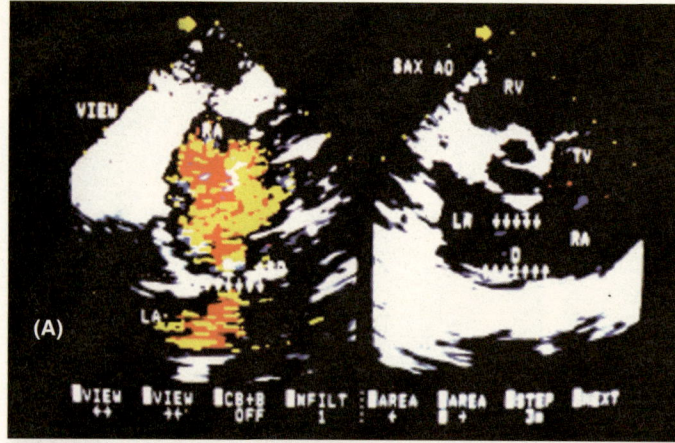

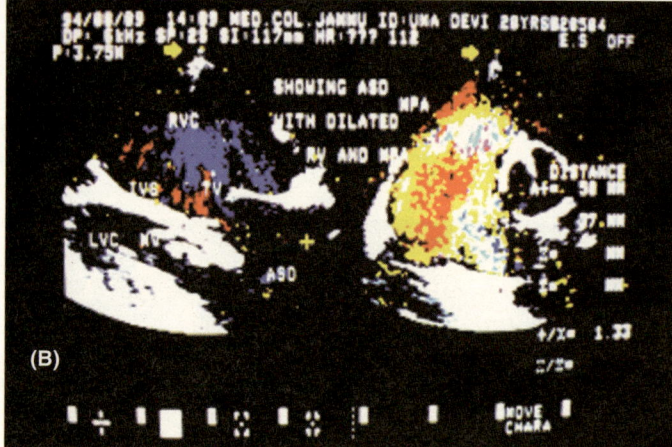

Fig. 13.59A and B: (A) Subcostal 2C view (left) showing color flow from LA to RA and almost filling whole of the right atrium in patient with large ASD secundum. (Right panel) Short axis view at aorta showing a big ASD in a 13 years old boy (arrows). (B) Oblique 4C showing a big ASD (left) and color flow in dilated main pulmonary artery with mosaic color flow in the same patient

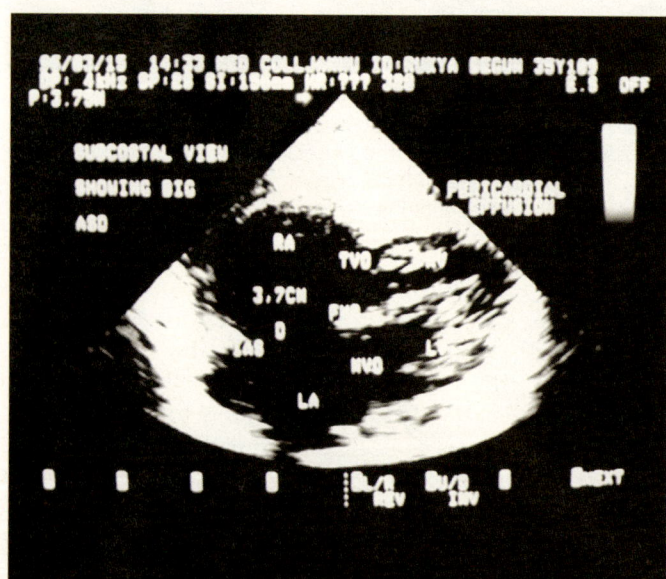

Fig. 13.60: Subcostal 4C view showing a big ASD secundum type of defect

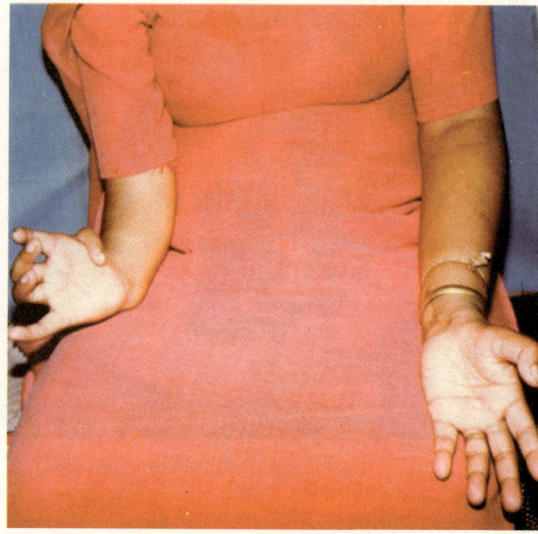

Fig. 13.61: Congenital defect in right forearm with malformation of thumb and fingers in an adult women with ASD of secundum type

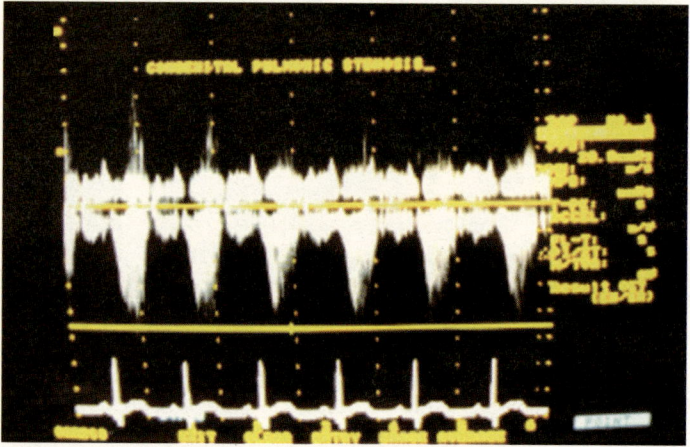

Fig. 13.62: Doppler flow velocity across pulmonary valve showing waveforms of congenital pulmonary valvular stenosis associated with atrial septal defect of secundum type

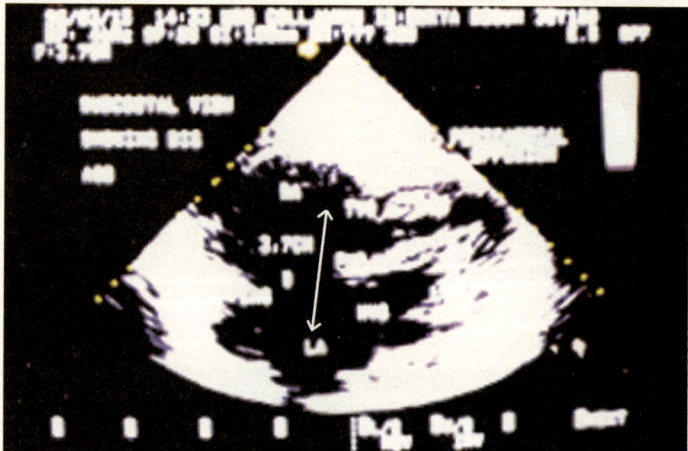

Fig. 13.63: Subcostal 4C view showing large ASD secundum more than 3.0 cm (arrow) there is also dilatation of RA

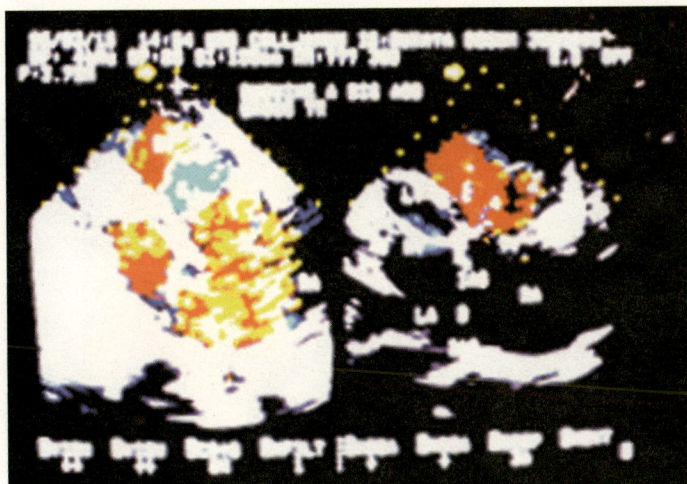

Fig. 13.64: Apical 4C view demonstrating color flow jet across a large-sized ASD secundum almost attaining U-shaped configuration (left panel) and color jet almost filling whole of the right atrium

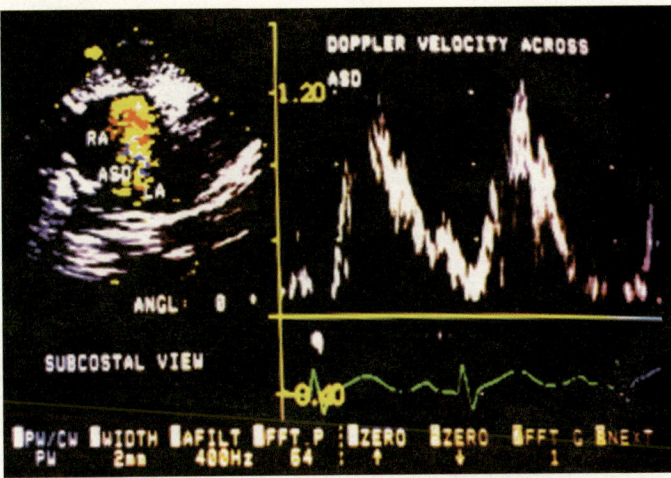

Fig. 13.65: Subcostal color flow 2-C view demonstrating a large left to right shunt (left panel) and pulsed Doppler velocity waveforms across ASD secundum (right panel)

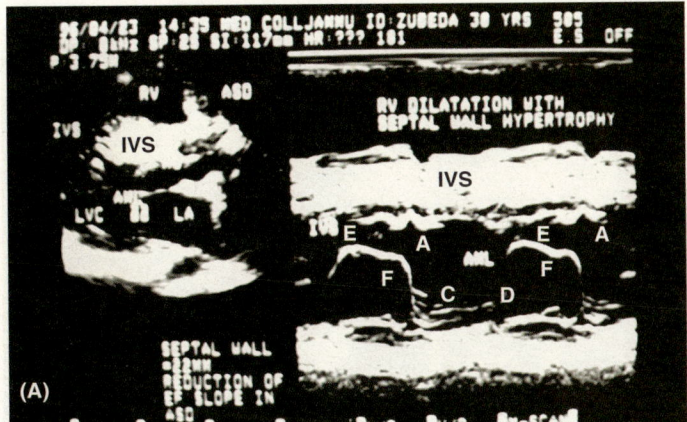

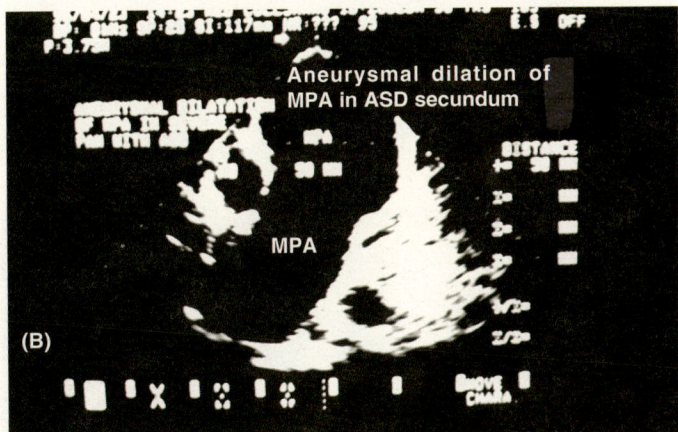

Fig. 13.66A and B: **(A)** M-Mode echocardiogram showing septal wall hypertrophy with reduction of EF slope of mitral valve in a patient with larger ASD with pulmonary arterial hypertension. **(B)** There is aneurysmal dilatation of main pulmonary artery reaching up to 5.0 cm. (Normal size = 11–20 mm) in a patient with larger ASD secundum in an adult patient

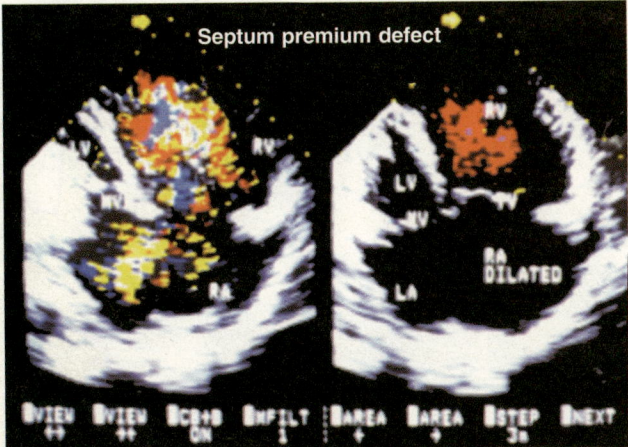

Fig. 13.67: Color flow apical 4C views in dual scan showing large septum primum defect with almost single dilated atrium, dilated LV with gross mitral regurgitation in patient with endocardial cushion defect

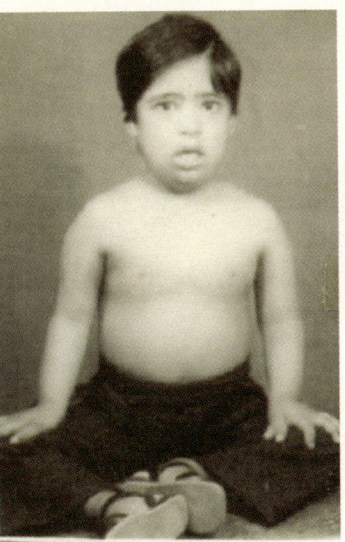

Fig. 13.68: Stunted growth, polydactylism and chest deformity in a child with endocardial cushion defect

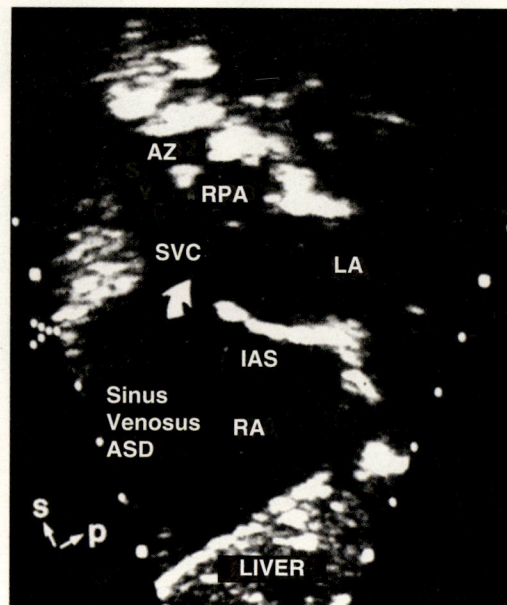

Fig. 13.69: Subcostal parasagittal echoscan depicting a sinus venosus type of atrial septal defect. AZ = azygous vein, RPA = right pulmonary artery, SVC = superior vena cava

CHD, L–R Shunt (ASD²) Profile with Anatomical relationship with surrounding structures

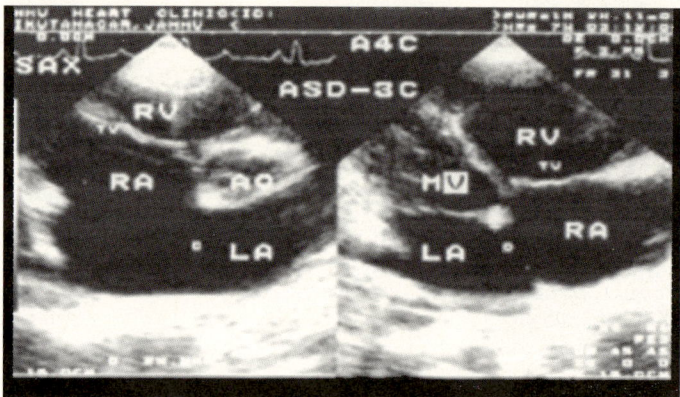

Fig. 13.70: Long axis and oblique 4C views showing thickend tricuspid leaflets diagnosis of ASD associated rheumatic mitral valve valvulitis

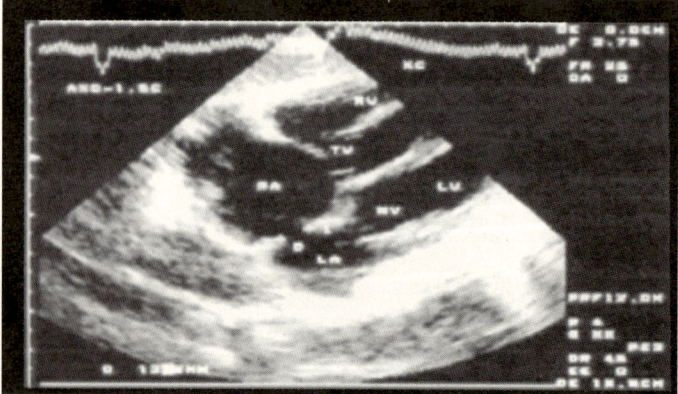

Fig. 13.71: Subcostal view showing ASD in the region of fossa ovalis

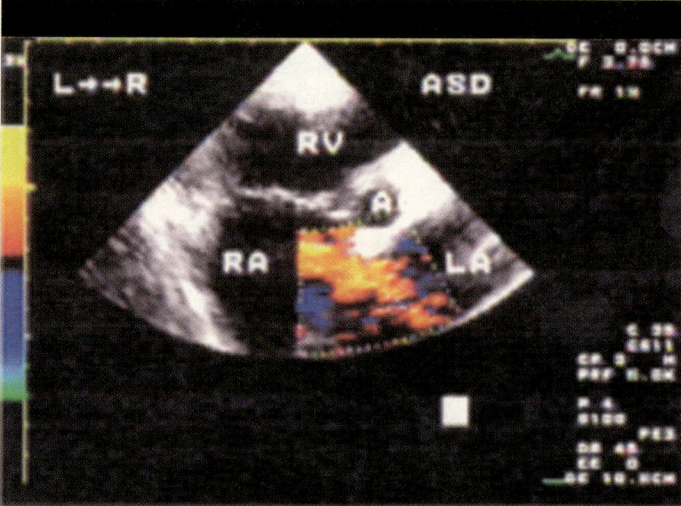

Fig. 13.72: Short axis aorta view showing thickened TV in ASD

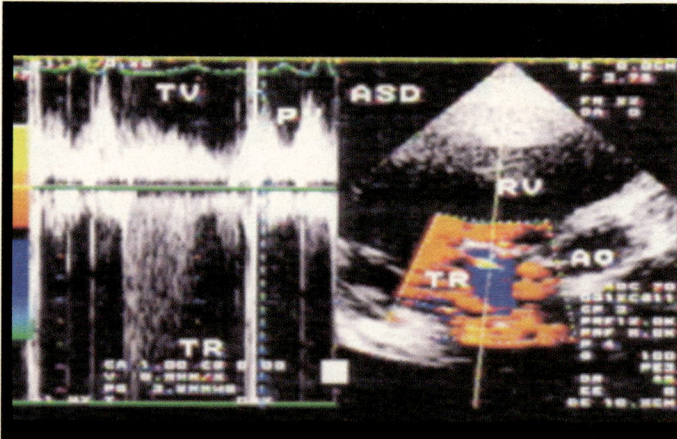

Fig. 13.73: TR in ASD secundum associated with pulmonary arterial hypertension

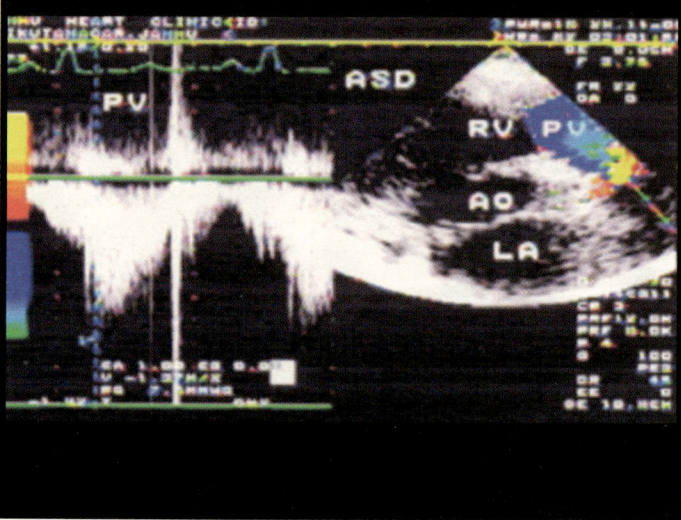

Fig. 13.74: Normal Color Doppler flow velocity across PV

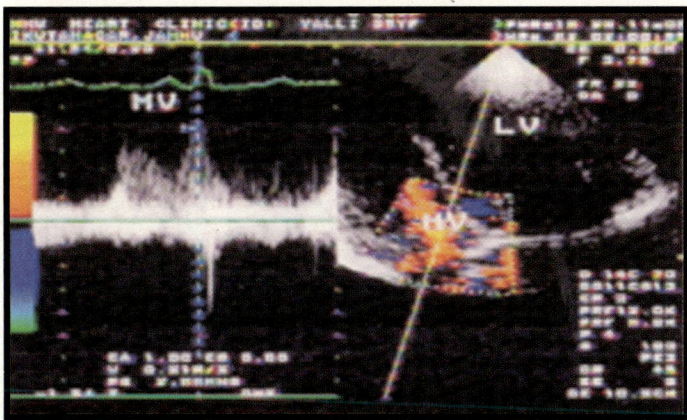

Fig. 13.75: M-Mode echoscan showing thickened mitral valve associated with ASD secundum

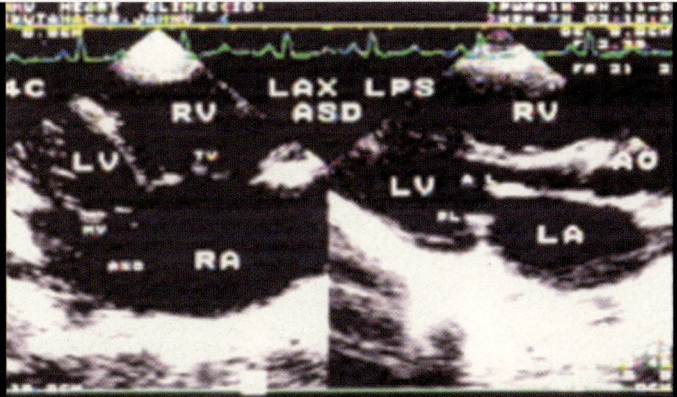

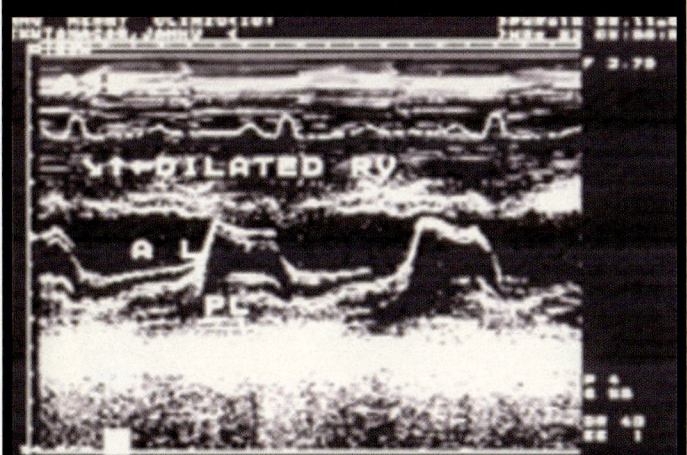

Fig. 13.76A and B: (A) Apical 4C (left) and long axis (right) views showing thickening of MV. **(B)** M-Mode echocardiogram showing reduction in EF slope and thickened MV in patient with ASD secundum (Lutembacher syndrome)

NOTE: It has been observed that atrial septal defect of secundum type is associated with rheumatic valvular pathology resulting into varying grades of mitral valvular stenosis (Lutembacher syndrome). Hence, it is advocated that patient with ASD should be routinely administred prophylactic penicillins for prevention of rheumatic mitral valvular disease.

Doppler is performed in the apical four-chamber and subcostal views and is an excellent techniques to outline the size, number of defects present, and direction of flow as it crosses the atrial septal defect. The flow patterns of the mitral and tricuspid valves would be increased with the shunt flow.

One may encounter difficulty in localizing the sinus venosus atrial septal defect with the help of conventional 2-D echo. This defect lies in the superior portion of the atrial septum, close to the inflow portion of the superior vena cava. This defect is most likely to be visualised with the subxiphoid four-chamber view. If signs of right ventricular volume overload are present, with no atrial septal defect obvious, then care should be taken to study the septum in search for a sinus venosus type of defect. Partial anomalous pulmonary venous drainage of the right pulmonary vein is usually associated with this type of defects; thus it is important to identify the entry site of the pulmonary veins into the left atrial cavity. Colour-flow mapping is useful in this type of problem because it allows the sonographer to actually visualise the venous return to the left atrium and a flow pattern crossing into the right atrial cavity.

Endocardial Cushion Defect (Figs 13.67, 13.68, 13.77 and 13.81)

It is localized in that area where the atrial and ventricular septa join the mitral and tricuspid valves. A complete defect means there is a primum atrial septal defects, a ventricular septal defect, and clefts in the mitral and tricuspid valves. An incomplete defect has an ostium primum atrial septal defect and a cleft mitral valve. Usually, the ventricular septum is intact and the tricuspid valve is normal, although occasionally it may be cleft or underdeveloped valve.

Echocardiograms visualised a long diastolic apposition of the anterior leaflet to the interventricular septum, right ventricular volume overload, and multiple mitral echoes from redundant tissue. The parasternal long-axis views demonstrate the narrowed left ventricular outflow tract that is akin to the gooseneck deformity seen on cardiac characterization (Fig. 13.134).

In its complete form, a ventricular septal defect and abnormal tricuspid valve are seen in conjunction with a primum atrial septal defect and cleft mitral valve. The ventricular septal defect occurs just below the atrioventricular ring and it is continuous with the primum atrial septal defect. Paradoxic septal motion is not seen in a complete canal because of equalized flow and pressure between the ventricles. The Rastelli types A and B are characterized by insertion of the chordae from the cleft mitral valve and tricuspid valve into the crest of the interventricular septum or a right ventricular papillary muscle, respectively. Rastelli type C, the most primitive form, has a single,

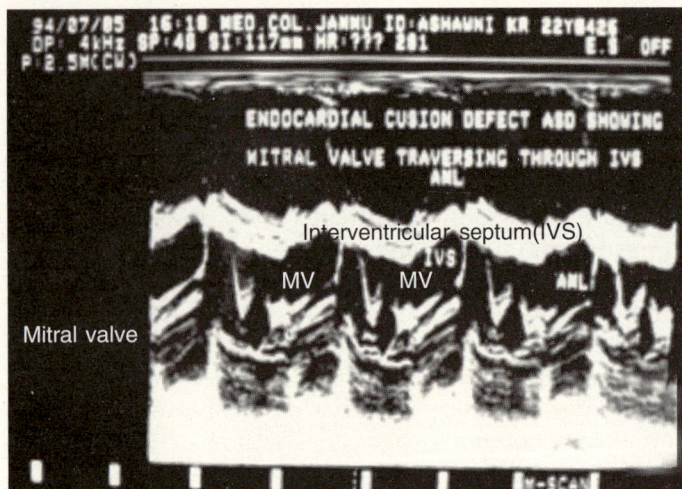

Fig. 13.77: M-Mode echocardiogram depicting mitral valve echo traversing across interventricular septum (IVS) in a patient with septum primum defect

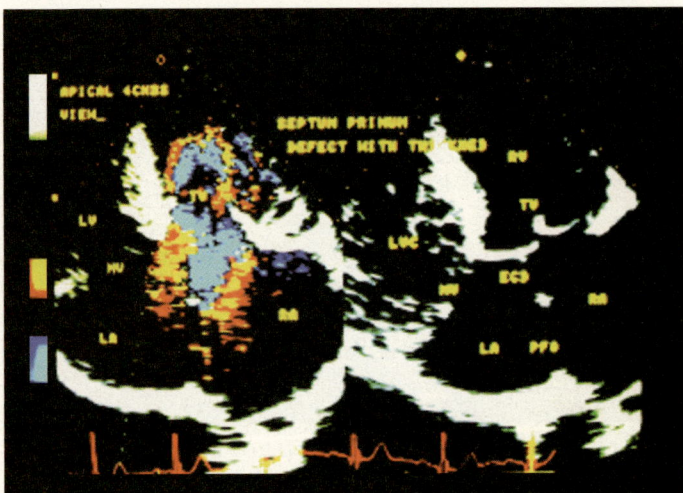

Fig. 13.80: Right and left panels color flow dual scans show a big septum primum defect with large color jet from LA to RA and extending upto TV with tricuspid regurgitation (blue jet) coming from RV to RA in 24 years adult patient

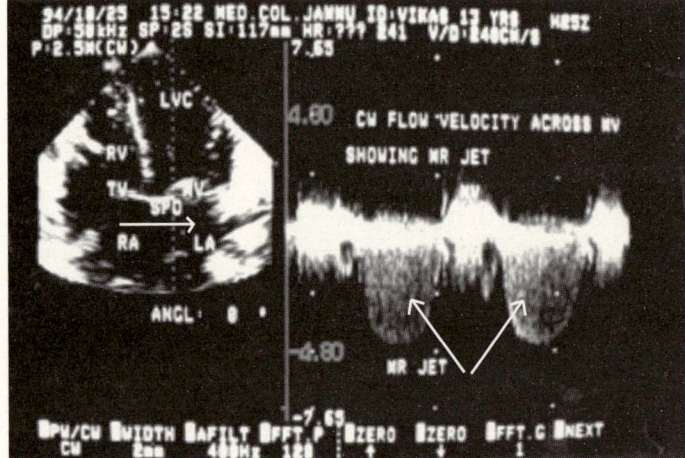

Fig. 13.78: 2-D Apical 4C (left) showing a big septum primum defect and Doppler flow velocity across MV showing very high Doppler regurgitant (MR) flow velocity in severe type of septum primum defect

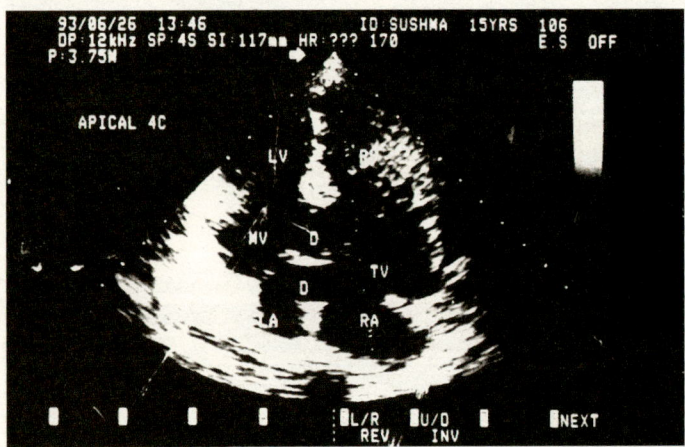

Fig. 13.81: Apical 4C view showing both ASD primum type and subaortic VSD type as a part of endocardial cushion defect

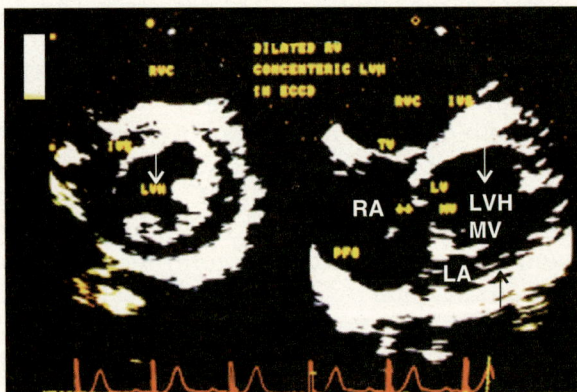

Fig. 13.79: (left) Short axis view of LV showing concentric left ventricular hypertrophy in a patient with endocardial cushion defect. (Right panel) subcostal oblique scan shows dilated RV, RA and hypertrophied LV and septum primum defect (arrow)

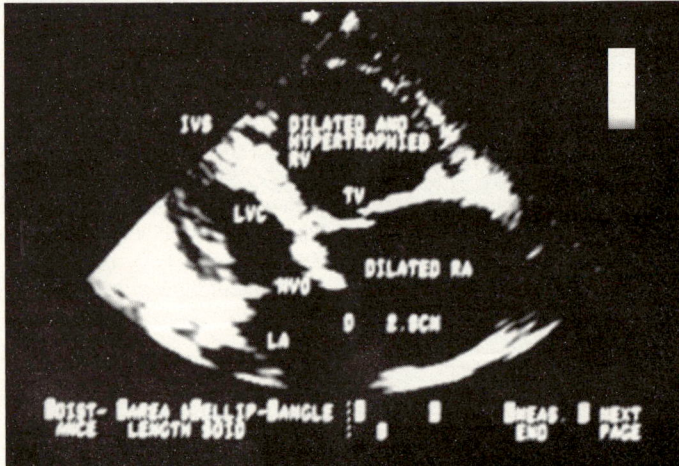

Fig. 13.82: Oblique 4C view showing dilated and hypertrophied RV, dilated RA normal LV, LA and large ASD secundum type of defect

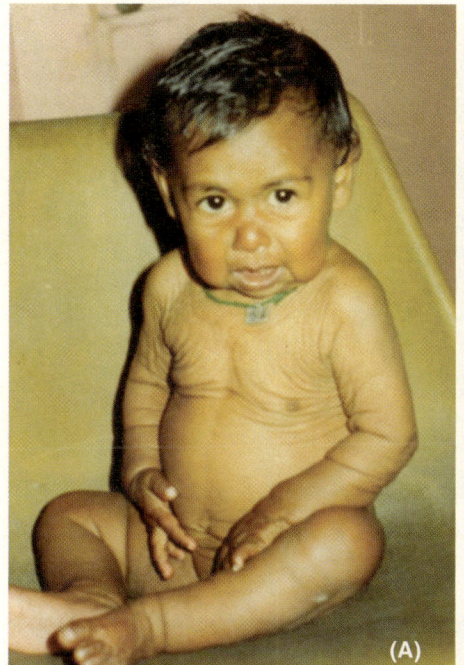
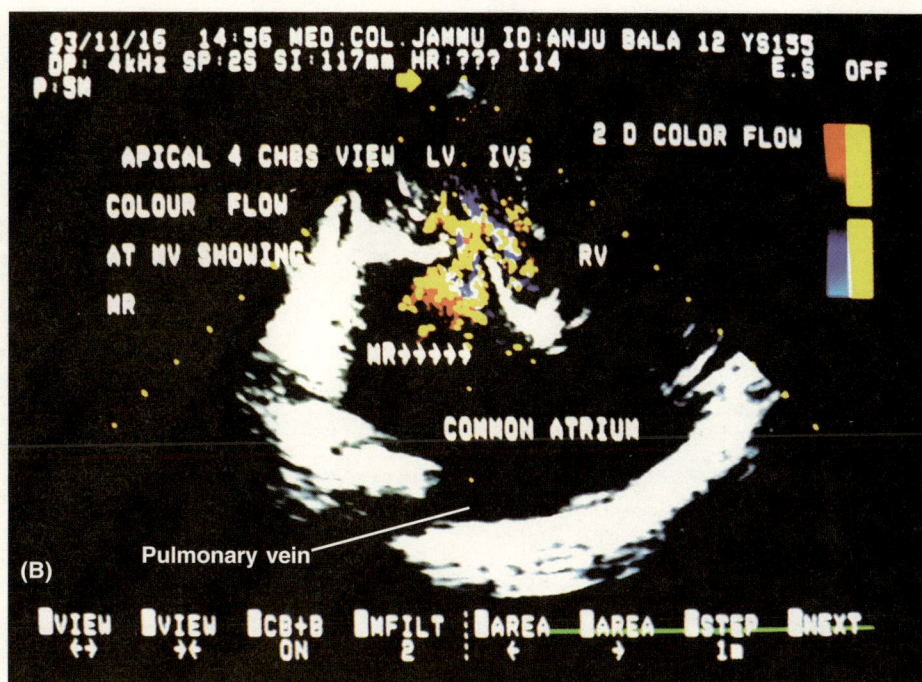

Fig. 13.83A and B: (A) A child suffering from endocardial cushion defect with chronic heart failure and malnutrition. (B) Apical 4C color flow depicting dilated common atrium with mitral regurgitant flow (MR) in canal defect. Pulmonary vein is also seen entering into common atrium

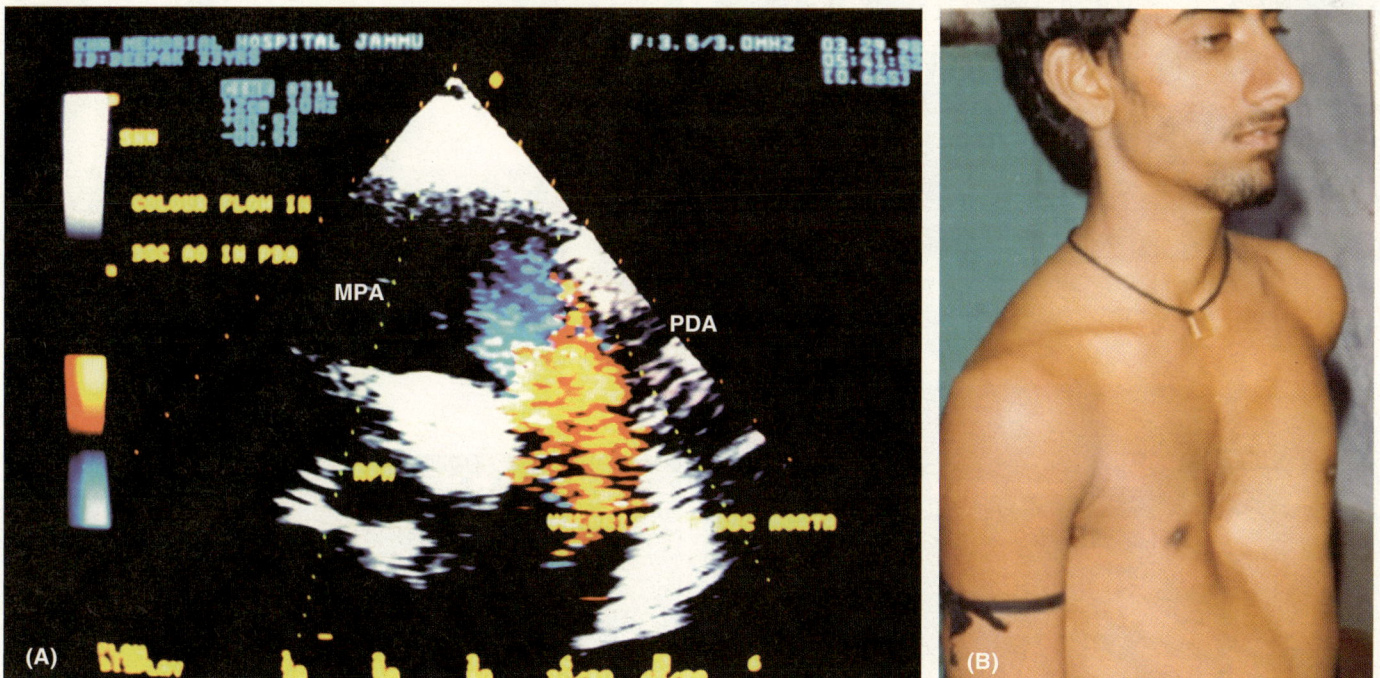

Fig. 13.84A and B: (A) Short axis view at great vessel level showing mosaic color flow pattern in main pulmonary artery in patient with PDA. (B) Chest deformity in an adult patient with PDA

undivided, free-floating leaflet stretching across both ventricles. A sweep from the mitral to aortic valves shows the anterior leaflet of the mitral valve "swinging" through the ventricular septal defect in continuity with the tricuspid valve. The tricuspid valve is said to "cap" the mitral valve. Evaluation of

the pulmonary valve for signs of pulmonary artery hypertension is extremely important in canal patients, since the right ventricular pressure reaches systemic levels very early.

Mitral insufficiency and stenosis associated with repair of the cleft mitral valve are evaluated with

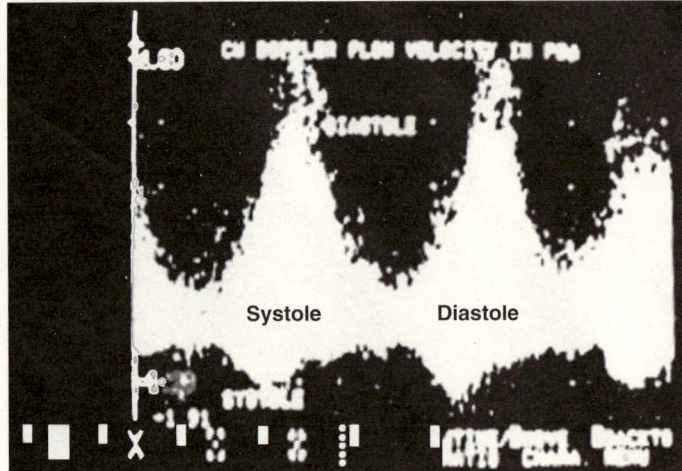

Fig. 13.85A: Continuous wave Doppler flow in both systole and diastole in patient with patent ductus arteriosus

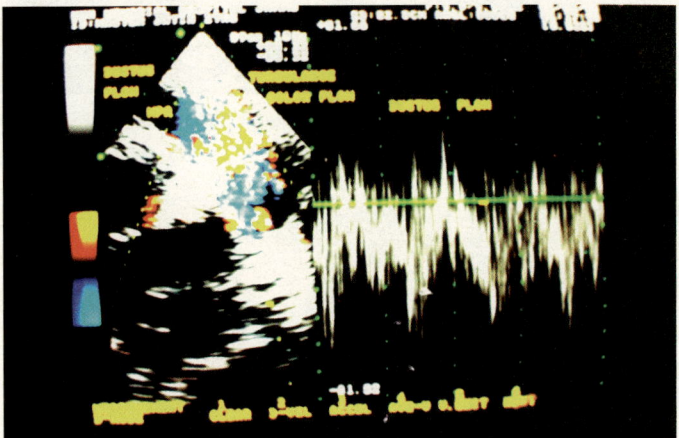

Fig. 13.85B: Continous color Doppler flow during systole and diastole in main pulmonary artery in patient with PDA

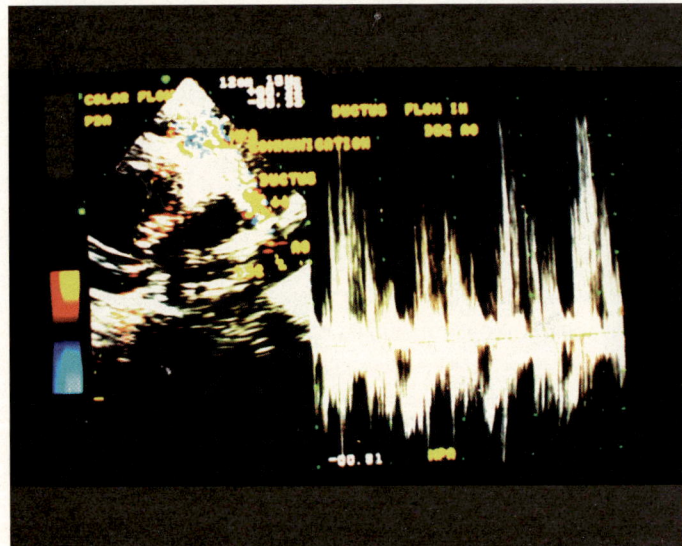

Fig. 13.86: Continous color Doppler flow in ductus as it communicates with descending aorta

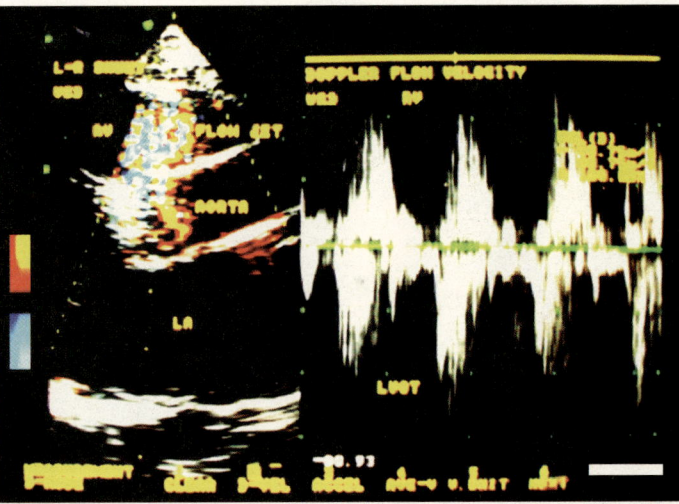

Fig. 13.87: Systolic and diastolic blood flow in PDA associated with VSD

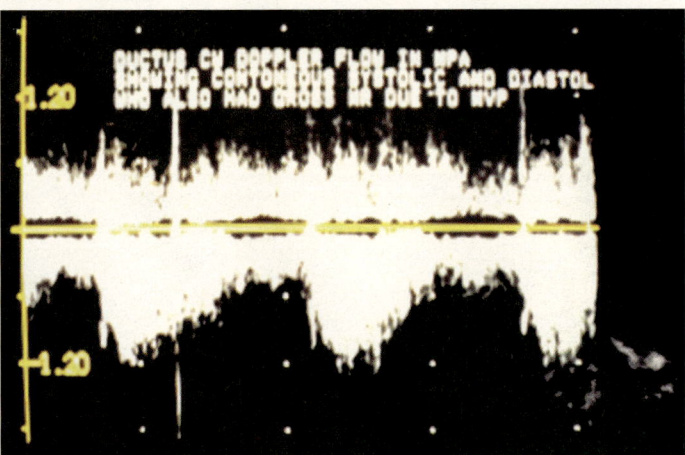

Fig. 13.88: Continuous wave Doppler showing systo-diastolic Doppler flow in patient with ductus arteriosus

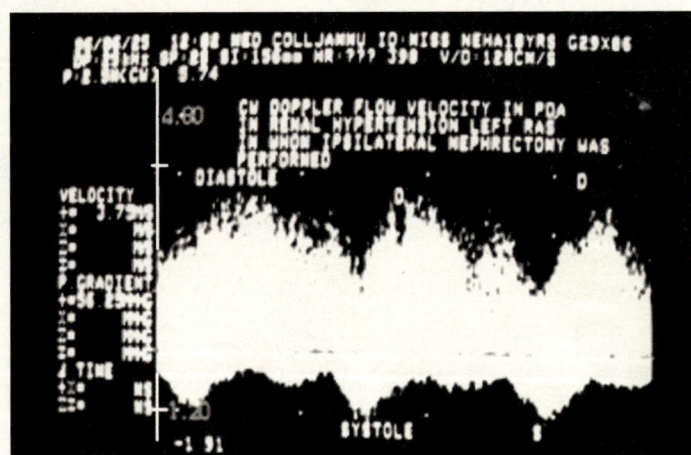

Fig. 13.89: Continuous wave Doppler flow showing continuous systo-diastolic flow in a patient with PDA and renal hypertension (congenital)

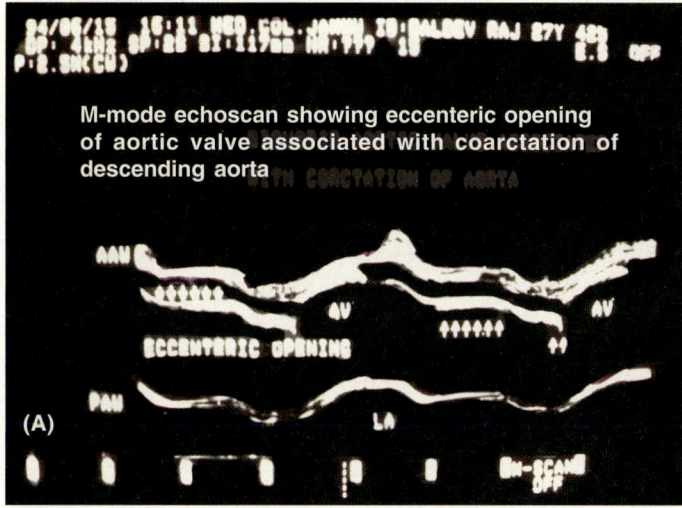

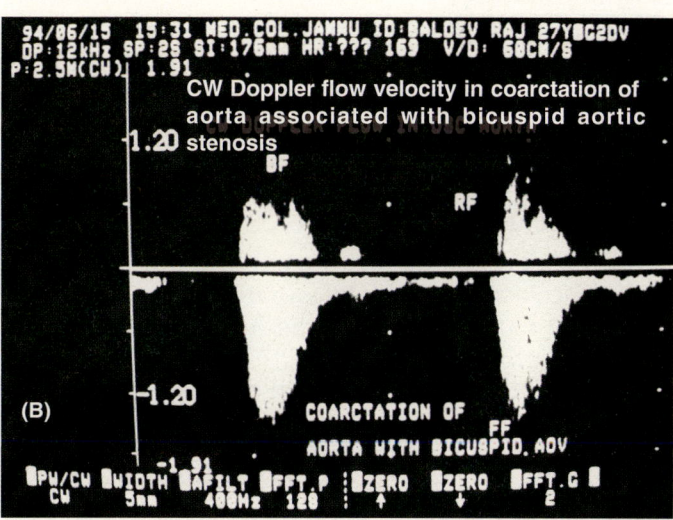

Fig. 13.90A and B: (A) M-Mode echocardiogram showing eccenteric opening of aortic valve in bicuspid aortic valve stenosis. **(B)** Doppler flow velocity showing broad waveform jet in bicuspid aortic valve with coarctation of descending aorta

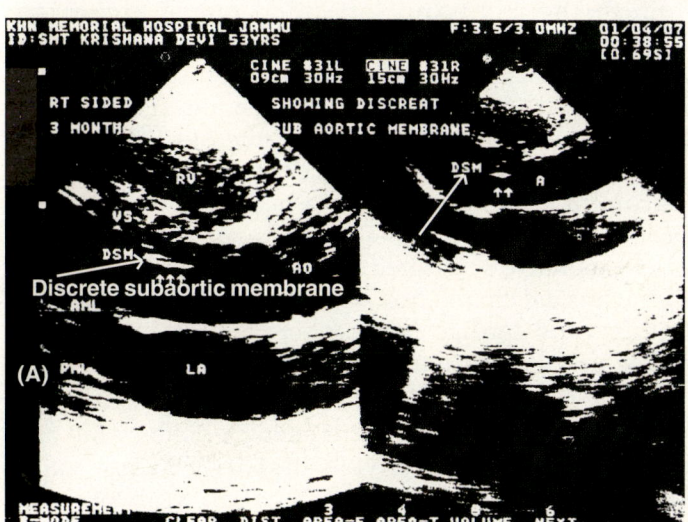

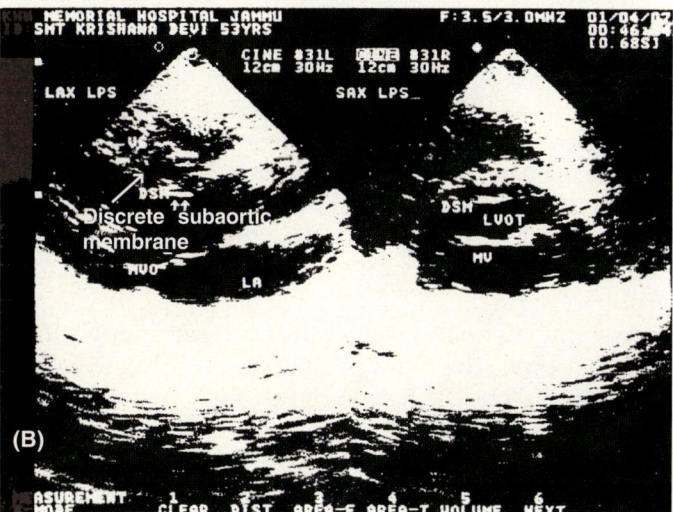

Fig. 13.91A and B: 2-D Long axis and short axis at aorta level respectively showing horizontal long dot-like structure in the LVOT (arrows) as discrete subaortic membrane hemodynamically presenting as subaortic stenosis in 53 yrs old female patient

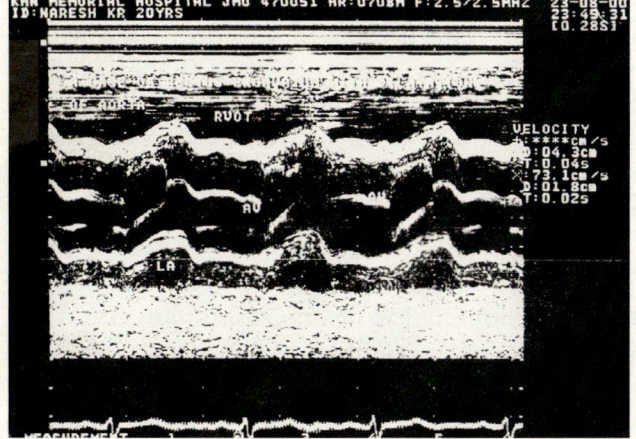

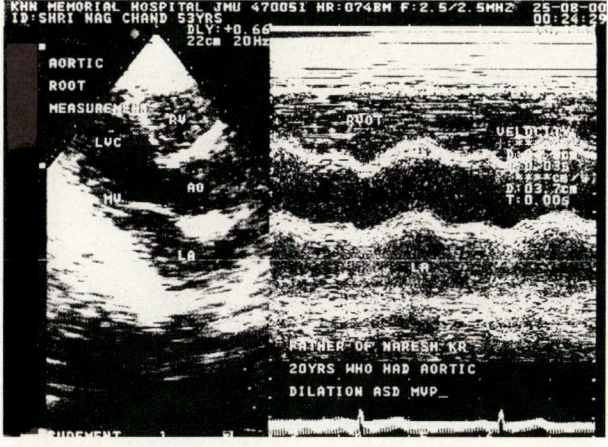

Fig. 13.92: M-Mode echocardiogram showing aortic dilatation in a patient who had ASD secundum MVP and Marfanoid habitus

Fig. 13.93: M-Mode and 2-D echcardiogram showing normal aortic root diameter in his father

echocardiography. Mitral insufficiency remains if the repaired anterior leaflet does not coapt evenly with the posterior leaflet. The Doppler and colour-flow map is useful to evaluate the amount and severity of regurgitation present.

Patent Ductus Arteriosus (Figs 13.84–13.89)

In this type of congenital cardiac defect, there is persistence of a normal fetal vascular channel between the pulmonary artery and the aorta. The ductus is located slightly to the left of the bifurcation of the pulmonary trunk near the origin of the left pulmonary artery.

The parasternal short-axis view is useful to actually image the insertion of the ductus as it flows from the descending aorta to the site near the bifurcation of the main pulmonary artery. With the use of high-frequency transducers, this communication should be adequately visualised in most neonates. Doppler recording carefully angling the beam medial to lateral and superior to inferior to record the maximum flow from the ductus, would be most helpful in the localization of the shunt.

The patent ductus is easily recorded with pulsed-wave Doppler, since the transducer is placed in the high parasternal short-axis view. The sample volume should be placed to the left of the bifurcation of the main pulmonary artery at the mouth of the ductus arteriosus. The left-to-right flow pattern is the most common flow profile observed.

In a given situation where it is larger enough to be bi-directional, the flow is seen in both positive and negative directions. A true right-to-left pattern is seen in neonates with pulmonary hypertension and is best recorded with the sample volume actually in the ductus itself (normally the sample volume is in the lower aspect of the main pulmonary artery).

It can be visualised through yet in another window at suprasternal notch that is sometimes useful in premature infants. The transducer should be able to image the descending aorta to the level of the left subclavian artery (which is the insertion level of the patent ductus). If a ductus is patent, an abnormal flow profile will be seen. The sample volume should be placed at the level of the left subclavian in the descending aorta; a left-to-right shunt would show a positive reflection on the Doppler tracing during diastole.

Coarctation of Aorta (CoA) (Fig. 13.90A and B)

There is a localized deformity in the media of the aortic walls which is shown by curtainlike infolding that eccentrically narrows the aortic lumen. The area of coarctation is usually located just distal to the origin of the left subclavian artery at the site of the ductus. Sometimes, the coarctation occurs as a diffusely narrowed aortic segment that begins distal to the innominate artery and ends in a localized constriction just beyond the left subclavian (termed preductal or infantile coarctation) artery.

Echographically, the site of the coarctation is best visualised from the suprasternal notch window.

While approaching through the suprasternal notch window, the angle of the notch is obtained by propping a pillow or rolled towel under the child's neck so that the head falls back. The transducer is placed in the suprasternal notch and beamed toward the feet to obtain a plane passing between the right nipple and left scapular tip, yielding a long-axis view of the suprasternal notch. By angling the beam posteriorly or anteriorly, a plane should be produced in which lie transverse arch and its brachiocephalic vessels, right pulmonary artery, right main bronchus, and descending aorta are visualised.

Both the right and left-sided aortic arches are differentiated by noticing whether the beam passes through the right or left side of the sternum as the arch is visualised. The arch should be visualised completely beyond the subclavian artery to rule out the presence of a coarctation. Technical officer of the laboratory must be careful not to mistake the echo reflections from the bronchus, right pulmonary artery, or left subclavian artery as narrowed 'shelf' within the arch. The site of the suspected coarctation should be carefully visualised with several cardiac cycles. There is high incidence of aortic valve disease associated with coarctation aorta which should also be looked into critically.

Doppler flow patterns are characteristic in the area of the coarctation. The velocities may be normal to slightly increased in the ascending aorta, with increased velocity occurring as one moves the sample volume closer to the narrowing. At the site of the coarctation the velocity becomes very turbulent with a dropoff in velocity during the latter part of systole and extending into the diastolic segment.

Colour Doppler echocardiography is found to be extremely helpful in visualising the more distal segments of the coarctation. Often it is difficult to see descending aorta with routine two-dimensional imaging, and thus with the colour-flow Doppler, one can follow the turbulent velocity pattern through the site of the narrowing.

Left Ventricular Outflow Tract Obstruction (LVOT)

Left ventricular outflow tract obstruction can occur at three levels (Fig. 13.91A and B):

1. supravalvar,
2. valvar, and
3. subvalvar.

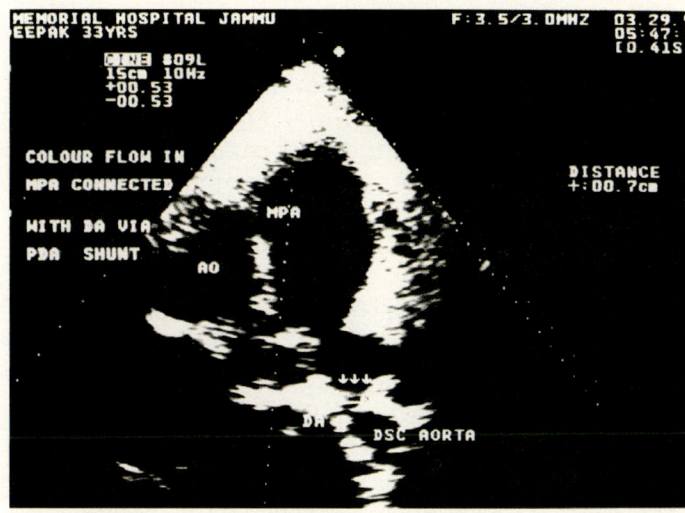

Fig. 13.94: 2-D Echoscan showing ductus communication between main pulmonary artery and descending aorta (arrows)

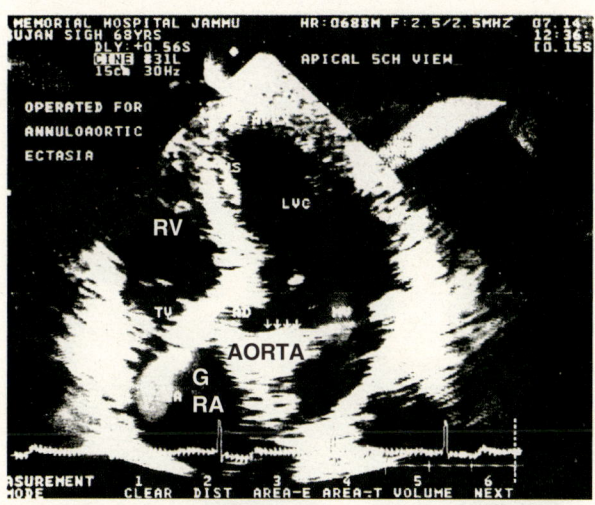

Fig. 13.95: Apical 4C view showing aortic graft (arrows) was applied in a patient with grossly dilated ascending aorta with grade 111 AR and with congenital annulo-aortic ectasia with marfanoid habitus

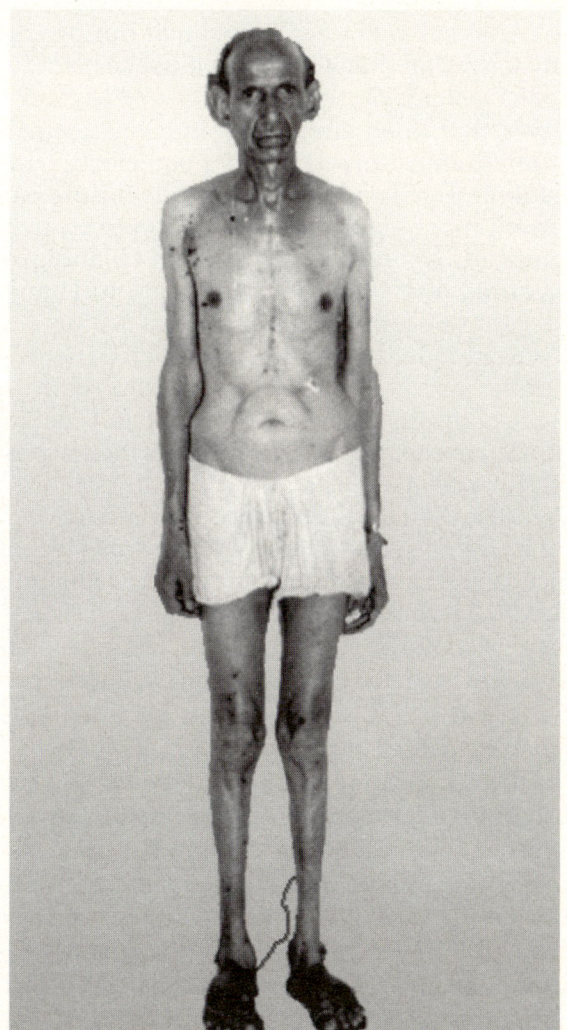

Fig. 13.96: Patient with congenital annulo-aortic ectasia with Marfanoid habitus in whom decran graft was applied to treat aneurysm and gross AR (as shown in Fig. 13.95)

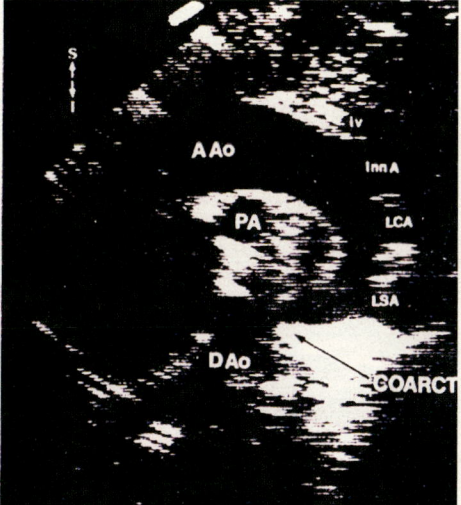

Fig. 13.97: Suprasternal approach showing coarctation of aorta. 1 nnA = innominate artery, IV = innominate vein, LCA = Left carotid artery, LSA = Left subclavian artery, COARCT = Coarctation of aorta

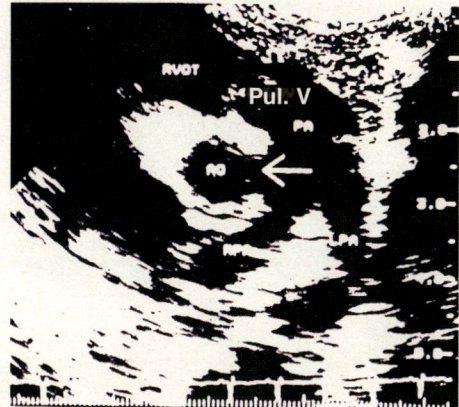

Fig. 13.98: Short axis great vessel view approach showing aorto-pulmonary window (arrow) RVOT = Right ventricular outflow tract, Pul. V = Pulmonary valve, AO = Aorta. PA = Pulmonary artery

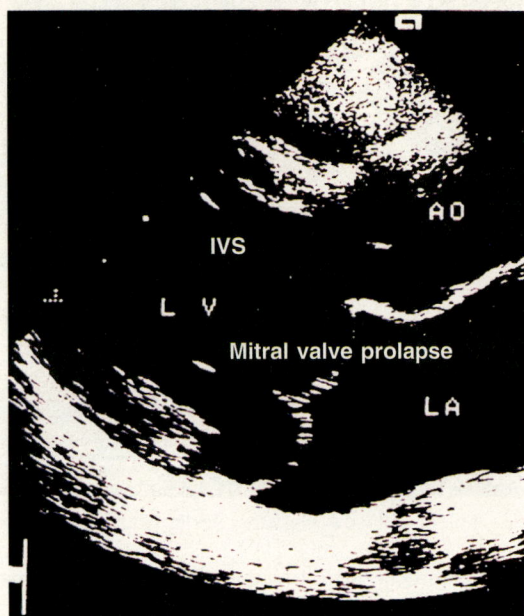

Fig. 13.99: Long axis LV showing mitral valve prolapse and dilatation of the aortic root in Marfan's syndrome

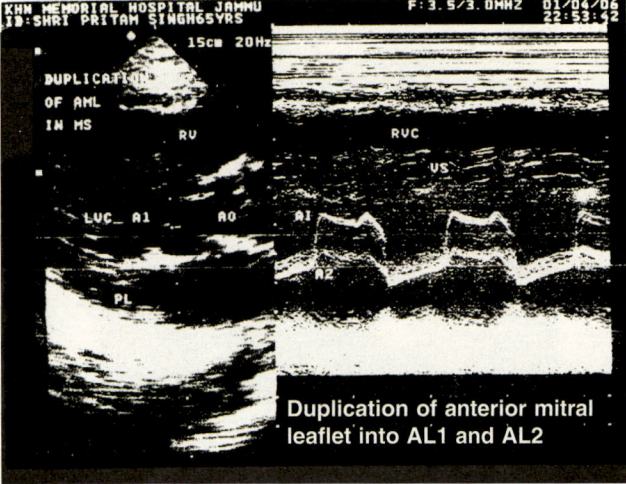

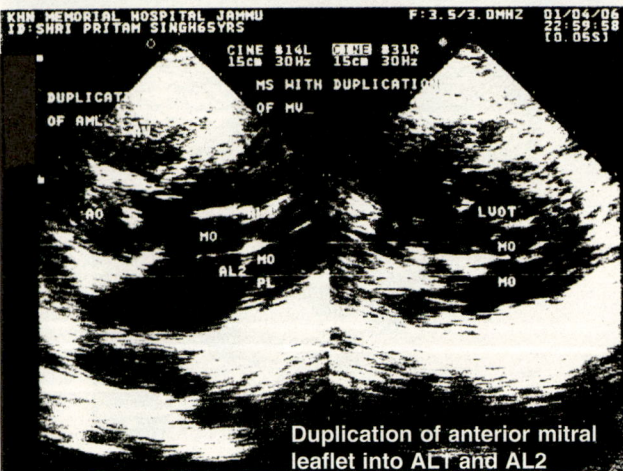

Fig. 13.100A and B: M-Mode and 2-D echoscans respectively showing duplication of anterior mitral leaflet into AL1 and AL2

The stenosis can be either fixed or dynamic in nature. Because auscultation often cannot localize either the site or the severity of a left ventricular outflow tract obstruction, two-dimensional and Doppler echocardiography, with its ability to visualise many planes of the heart, has become very important for qualitative, assessment of this cardiac defect.

a. **Supravalvar aortic obstruction:** It can happen as a narrowing of the aortic root lumen, from anterior and posterior walls, just above the level of the aortic valve. It can be visualised in the parasternal long-axis, apical four-chamber, and subcostal views.

M-mode has proved unreliable in assessing valvar aortic stenosis, because the limited M-mode view may not cut through the tips of the domed aortic valve. Two-dimensional echo, with its ability to visualise the domed aortic leaflets in systole, can be used to quantitate the severity of valvular aortic stenosis in children. The ratio of maximum aortic cusp separation with aortic root diameter against the aortic valve gradients obtained during cardiac catheterization (MaoCS/AoD) must be below 0.5 to predict a significant gradient.

Valves that open superiorly into the aortic root, rather than anteriorly and posteriorly, during systole and show a sagging diastolic closure pattern warrant more vigorous examination to ensure that significant stenosis is not missed. Dilation of the ascending aorta (poststenotic dilation) is another indicator of obstruction.

This technique is not applicable to all patients with stenotic aortic valves. Increased echo return from calcified results in an artificially small maximum aortic cusp separation. The aortic orifice in postoperative patients has been difficult to evaluate reliably. Also a dilated aortic root as found in Marfan's and Turner's syndromes invalidates this technique since it makes the denominator erroneously large (Figs 13.94–13.96).

b. **Congenital aortic stenosis:** Aortic valvular stenosis may give rise to the obstruction in the left ventricular outflow tract. The valve may be unicuspid or bicuspid with restricted mobility.

A bicuspid aortic valve may be the cause of aortic obstruction. The aorta should be carefully evaluated to record the presence of the number of cusps and the opening excursion of such cusps. Depending on how the cusps are divided, the M-mode tracing may show eccentricity in the diastolic segment.

c. **Subvalvar aortic stenosis:** It is considered as a less common type of ventricular outflow tract obstruction. It can occur as a discrete ridge or membrane below the aortic root, a diffuse long tunnel involvement, or a dynamic obstruction resulting

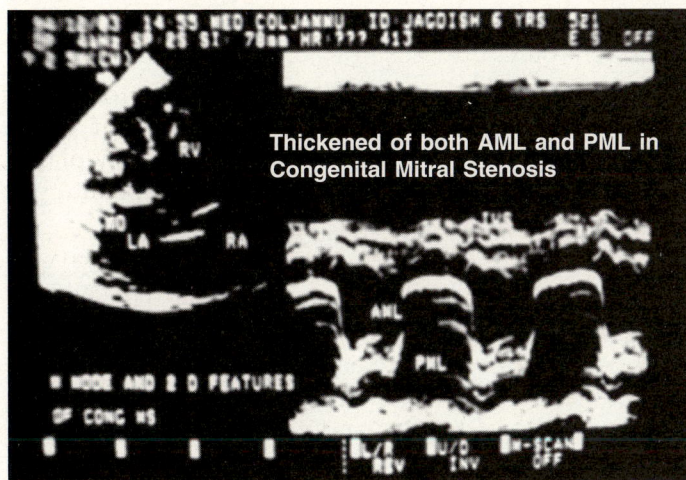

Fig. 13.101: M-mode (right) and 2D (left) echocardiogram showing thickening of AML, reduction of EF slope and paradoxical movement of thickened PML in a young child of 6 yrs old with congenital mitral stenosis

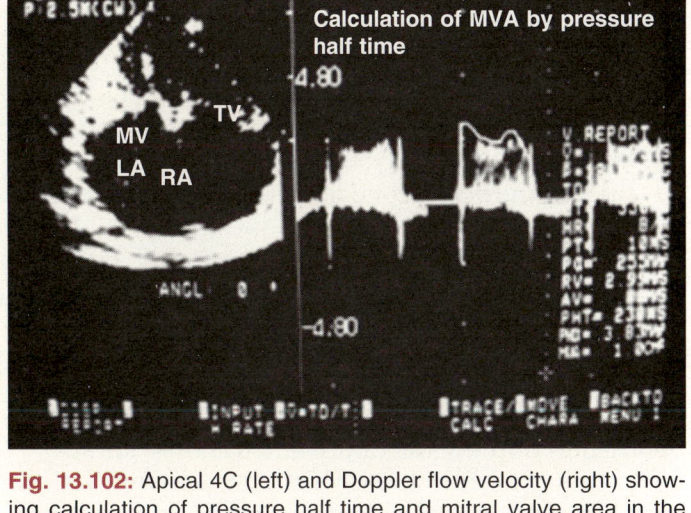

Fig. 13.102: Apical 4C (left) and Doppler flow velocity (right) showing calculation of pressure half time and mitral valve area in the same patient as in Fig. 13.101 in congenital mitral stenosis

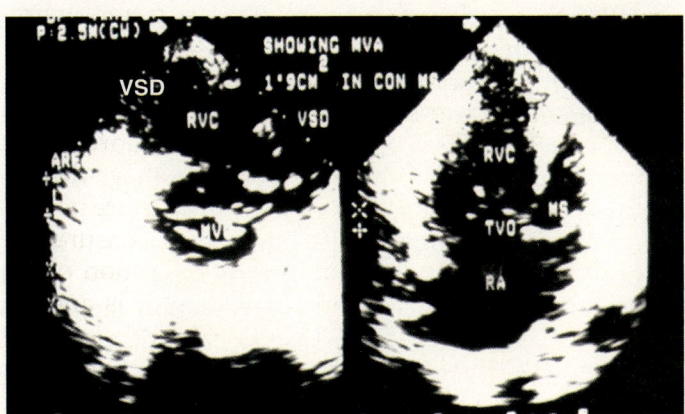

Fig. 13.103: 2-D Short axis (left) and apical 4C (right) showing reduction in mitral valve area (MVA) with ventricular septal defect (VSD) and thickened mitral valve with dilated right atrium (RA) in congenital MS with VSD (arrow)

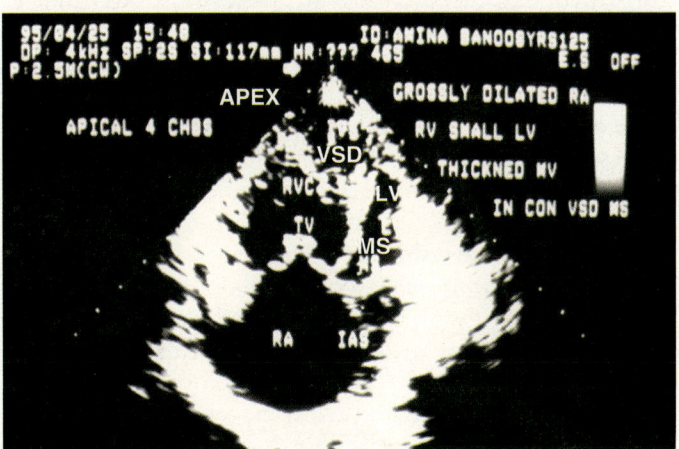

Fig. 13.104: Apical 4C showing markedly thickened MV and mild thickening of TV with apical VSD in patient with congenital mitral stenosis with VSD and dilated right atrium

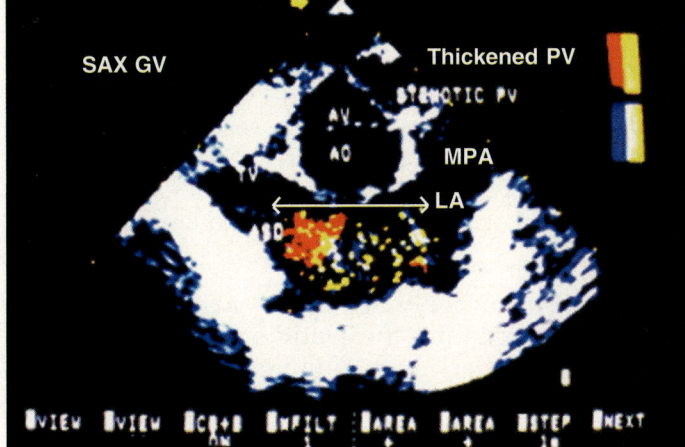

Fig. 13.105: 2-D and color flow short axis view at great vessel level showing thickened pulmonary valve and color flow passing from LA to RA in patient with pulmonary stenosis and ASD secundum

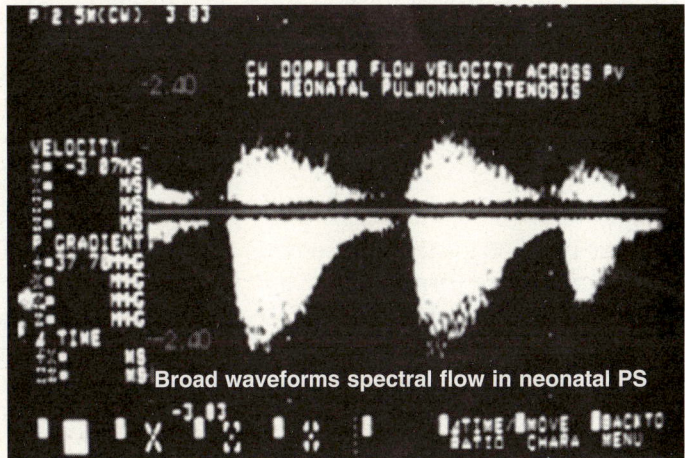

Fig. 13.106: Doppler flow velocity across pulmonary valve in a 2 months old infant showing broad pulmonary waveforms with enhanced velocity in congenital pulmonary stenosis

from systolic motion of the anterior leaflet of the mitral valve. The parasternal long-axis view and the apical four chamber view are probably the best views to visualize this subaortic area. On M-mode studies, early closure of the aortic valve may be seen in systole. There may be concentric hypertrophy of the left ventricle secondary to the pressure overload.

The Doppler study can be extremely useful to evaluate the patient with aortic stenosis. The Bernoulli equation allows one to determine the velocity and thus the gradient across the stenotic area. The best view is generally the apical five-chamber view with the continuous wave sample volume placed at the level of the aortic valve and then carefully moved from the left ventricular outflow tract into the ascending aorta.

The other useful views which can be employed for aortic stenosis include the suprasternal approach and subcostal view. In the supersternal approach the transducer is placed in the suprasternal notch just to the right of the midline. The patient's head should be turned to the left to allow better contact of the transducer and sternal notch. A steep angulation of the transducer is necessary to record the ascending aorta, aortic arch, and descending aorta. If high velocities are recorded, the continuous wave transducer should be used because it is much smaller in diameter and may fit very well into the suprasternal notch. This transducer does not allow the simultaneous two-dimensional visualisation of structures, but with the harsh sound and typical aortic stenosis waveform in the Doppler pattern, the sonographer can determine when the maximum velocity is obtained. The tracing should be smooth and well defined along its maximum border. The audible sound should be turbulent and harsh in its sound when the best window has been found to record the maximum velocity.

In the diagnosis of aortic valvular disease, colour Doppler echocardiography can also be employed as a useful modality. The turbulent pattern is well demonstrated with the colour mapping, provided Doppler is placed in the correct jet stream to record the maximum velocity tracing.

Hypoplastic Left Heart Syndrome

Hypoplastic left heart syndrome is considered among one of the severe forms of left ventricular outflow tract obstruction. This may result from severe tubular hypoplasia of the arch, severe aortic stenosis, or aortic atresia during fetal development. This results into atresia and hypoplasia of left sided structures with poor contractility including atresia of mitral valve. The ascending aorta is usually the smallest part of the aorta while the descending aorta is larger, since systemic cardiac output is maintained via blood ejected from the

right vertricle and circulating right to left through a persistent patent ductus arteriosus.

Congenital Mitral Stenosis (Figs 13.101–13.104)

Congenital mitral stenosis represents with different types of cardiac malformations. One form shows the leaflets to be thickened, nodular, and fibrotic without calcification; the commissures are very small to absent; the chordae tendineae are shortened, thickened, and fused; the papillary muscles are fibrosed. The valve is somewhat tunnel-shaped. Endocardial fibroelastosis may be found in the left ventricle and atrium.

Another form is a "parachute" deformity of the valve, in which normal leaflets and commissures are drawn into close apposition by shortened chordae tendineae that converge and insert into a single large papillary muscle. The interchondral slitlike spaces provide the only access to the left ventricle.

In a rare form of congenital mitral stenosis there is obstruction due to hypertrophy and thickening of the papillary muscles; they cause obstruction while encroaching the subvalvular area.

There is yet another form of stenosis which occurs when the mitral leaflets are normal but the inlet of the left ventricle is encroached on by a circumferential supravalvular ridge of connective tissue that arises at the base of the atrial aspect of the mitral leaflets. This defect may occur alone or with other obstructive lesions (supravalvular ring of the left atrium, parachute mitral valve, subaortic stenosis, and coarctation of the aorta). It can be diagnosed by 2-D echocardiography by visualising the thickened mitral valve to dome on long-axis and four-chamber views. The short-axis view shows the narrow orifice of the anterior and posterior leaflets. The left atrium will be enlarged, mitral regurgitation and enlargement of the left ventricle will also be present. Doppler flow studies should be carefully performed with the sample volume placed at the inlet of the valve and moved slowly into the left ventricle to note the velocity changes with the continuous-wave tracing. The left atrium should be evaluated for the amount and severity of regurgitation present. Colour-flow studies are characteristic of valvular disease. Turbulence in the area of the narrowing demonstrated the stenosis, whereas the jet stream into the left atrium will be easily demonstrated on the four-chamber and long-axis views.

Cor Triatriatum (Fig. 13.111A–D)

When left atrium is divided into two compartments by a partition membrane, the condition is called as cor triatriatum. In this anomaly, pulmonary veins drain into an accessory left atrial chamber that lies proximal to the true left atrium. The accessory chamber is believed to represent the dilated common pulmonary vein of the embryo, therefore, cor triatriatum has also been called stenosis of the common pulmonary vein. The distal

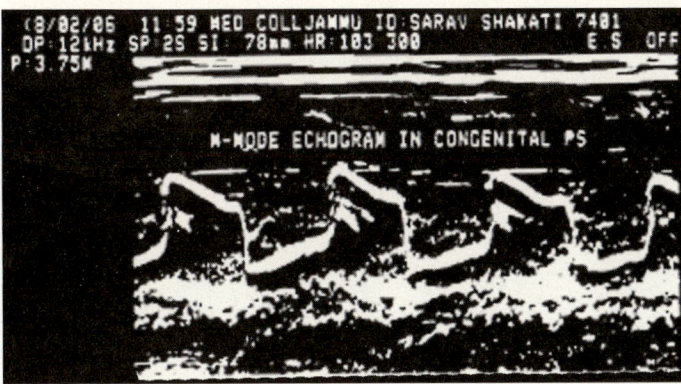

Fig. 13.107: M-Mode echocardiogram showing attenuation of (a) wave of pulmonary waveform at atrio-pulmonary sulcus in patient with congenital pulmonary valvular stenosis

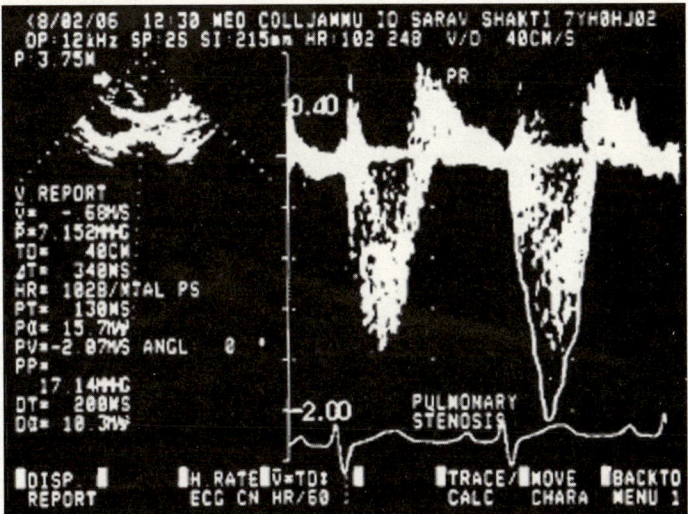

Fig. 13.108: 2-D Doppler echoscan showing enhanced flow velocity across pulmonary valve in congenital pulmonary valvular stenosis

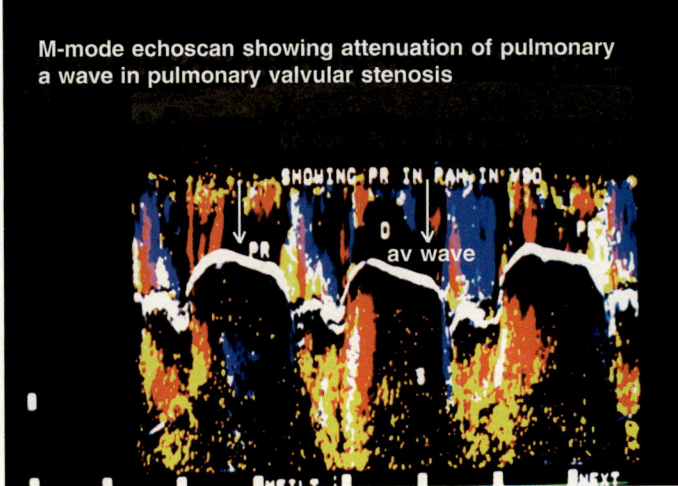

Fig. 13.109: M-Mode color flow at pulmonary valve showing attenuation of a-wave of pulmonary waveform in patient with pulmonic valvular stenosis along with pulmonary regurgitation color jet (PR)

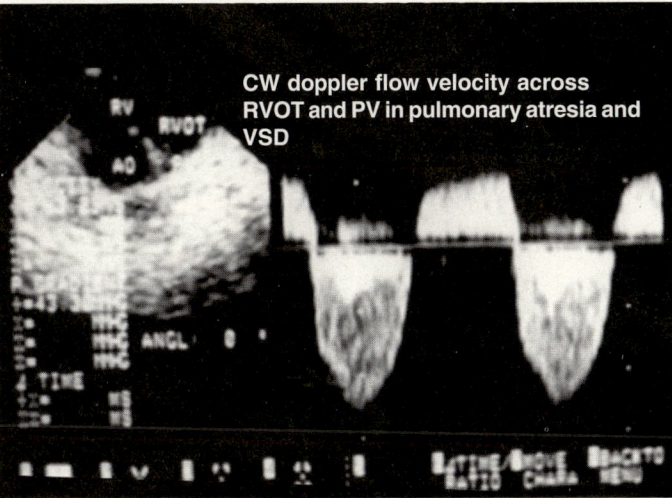

CW doppler flow velocity across RVOT and PV in pulmonary atresia and VSD

Fig. 13.110: Doppler flow velocity showing broad spectral waveform and enhanced systolic flow velocity with regurgitant flow in a patient with severe form of pulmonic stenosis, VSD, R-L shunt in Fallot's tetralogy

compartment communicates with the mitral valve and contains the left atrial appendage and fossa ovalis. The muscular band that partitions the left atrium has one or more openings, and the size of these openings determines the degree of atrial obstruction (Figs 13.110–13.117).

The membranes within the left atrial cavity can be seen on the long-axis or apical four-chamber view as the beam passes through the atrial cavity. Atrial septal defect and pulmonary hypertension and other accompanying congenital cardiac lesions can easily be spotted out with M-mode and 2-D echocardiography. Doppler studies in the area would show an obstructive type of flow through the orifice as the sample volume is placed near the fibromuscular band. Colour-flow Doppler would reveal a turbulent pattern in the left atrial cavity, especially at the site of the diaphragmatic band.

Congenital Pulmonary Stenosis (Figs 13.106–13.110)

Stenosis of the pulmonary valve has been seen as the most common form of right ventricular outflow tract obstruction. In congenital pulmonary stenosis the pulmonary valve cusps are thickened and domed with a restricted orifice. There may be post-stenotic dilation of the pulmonary artery.

The outflow is so restricted that it generates high pressure in right ventricle which can only be decompressed back through the tricuspid valve, resulting in right atrial enlargement and subsequent right-to-left shunting across the foramen ovale. The resultant cyanosis is two-fold in critical pulmonary stenosis and there is diminished pulmonary venous return, which is desaturated and situation still worsens when right to left shunt ensues.

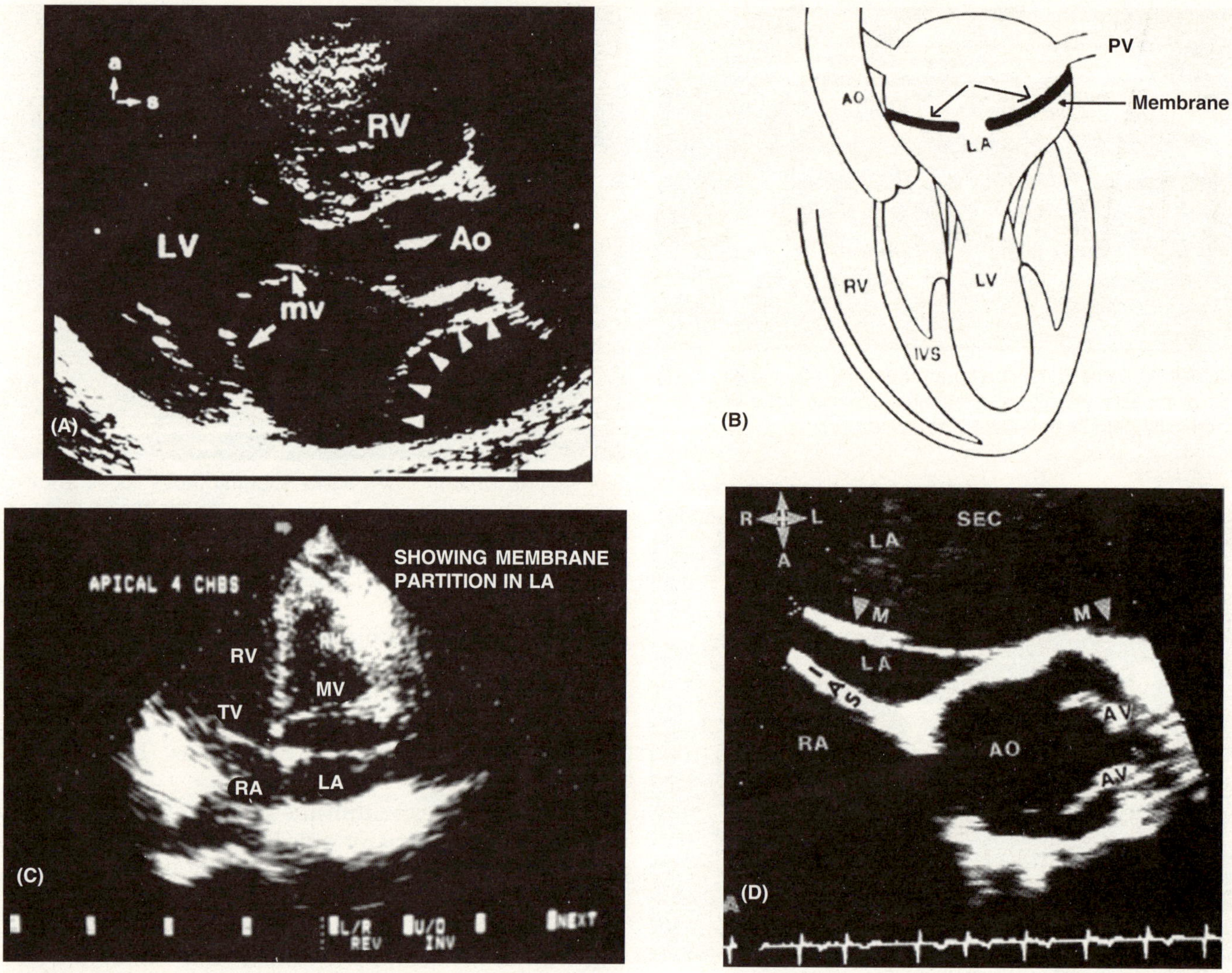

Fig. 13.111A to D: (A) 2-D long axis LV showing membrane in native left atrium dividing the main left atrium into upper and lower divisions in patient suffering from congenital cortriatriatum presenting as LV inflow obstruction. **(B)** Diagram depicting membrane in left atrium (LA). **(C)** Apical 4C view showing membrane in left atrium quite similar to a membrane in LA in a patient with pigeon-shaped chest, MVP and varying grades of cardiac arrhythmia. **(D)** TEE transgastric view showing a membrane (M) in LA in cor triatriatum

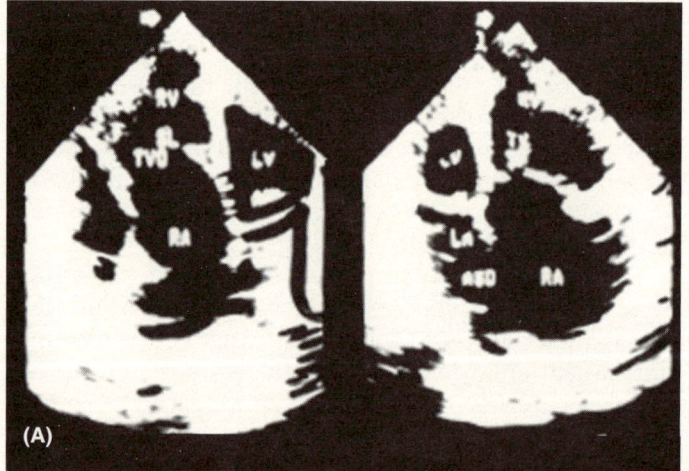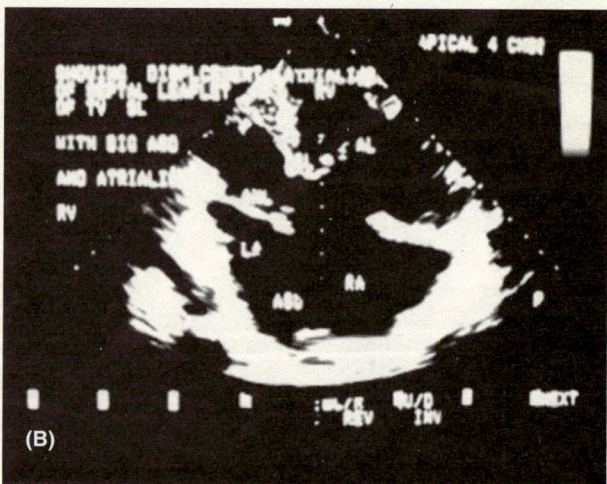

Fig. 13.112A and B: 2-D Oblique 4C view showing large ASD secundum with small LV, atresic MV large TV communicating with large and dilated RA and RV in a cyanosed patient with large ASD secundum with pulmonary arterial hypertension with reversal of shunt

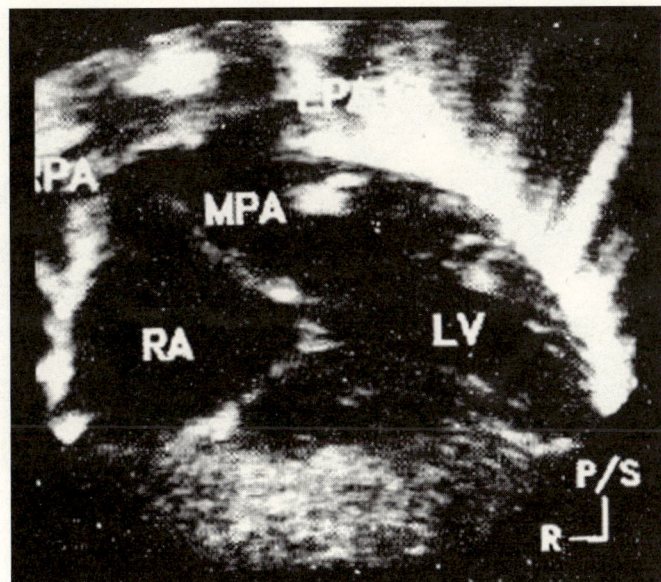

Fig. 13.113: Subxiphoid long axis view showing the bifurcating pulmonary artery aligned with left ventricle in D-type of transposition of great vessels

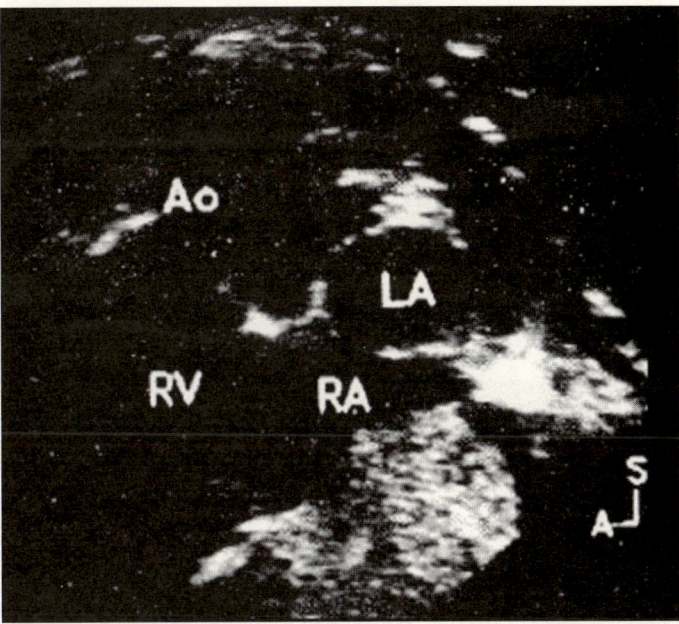

Fig. 13.114: Subxiphoid short axis view depicting the aorta including the arch and the brachiocephalic vessels, aligned with the right ventricle in D-type of transposition of great vessel RPA = Right pulmonary artery, MPA = Main pulmonary artery, RA = Right atrium, LV = Left ventricle, AO = Aorta

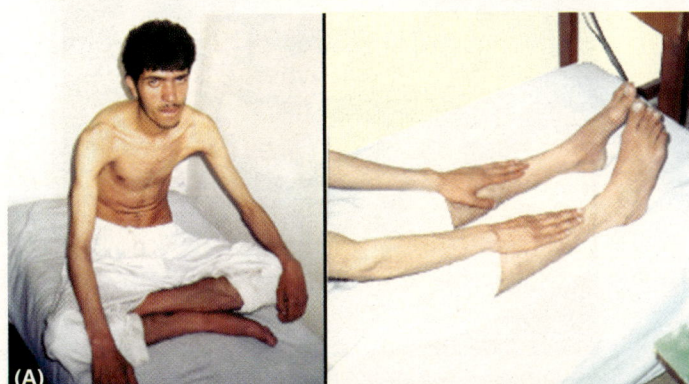

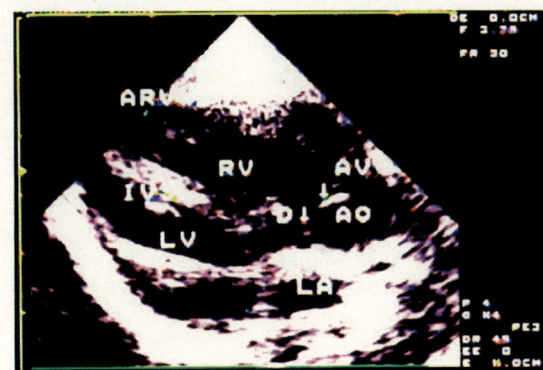

Fig. 13.116: Long axis view showing subaortic ventricular septal defect in Fallot tetralogy

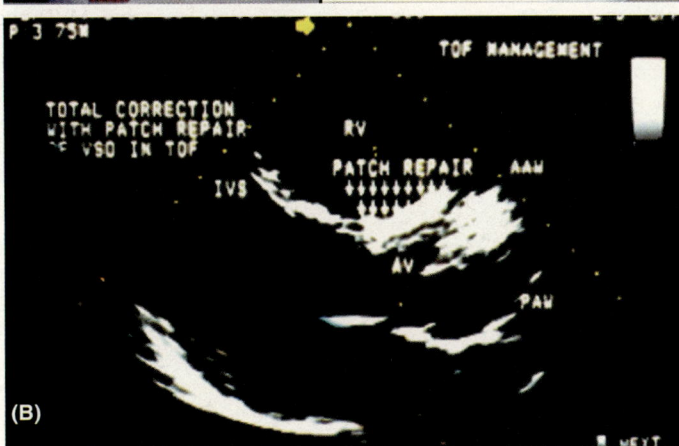

Fig. 13.115A and B: (A) An adult patient with markedly cyanosed extremities in Fallot tetralogy. **(B)** This patient was managed with total correction by patch repair of VSD (arrows) and creation of shunt between subclavian artery and pulmonary artery. This patient is now a govt. employee cyanosis has disappeared fully and is a father of two children. Both graft and shunt is fully patent even after more than 10 years of surgery

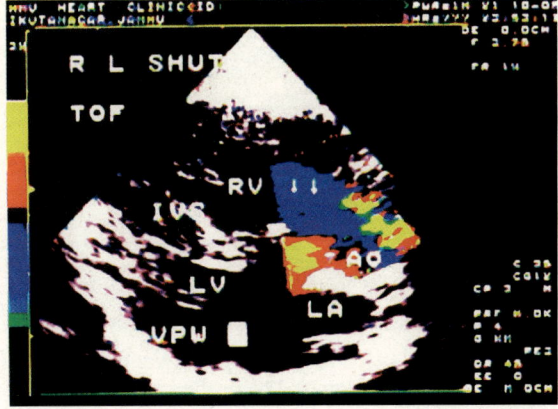

Fig. 13.117: Color flow in long axis view showing R-L shunt with reversal of flow in TOF

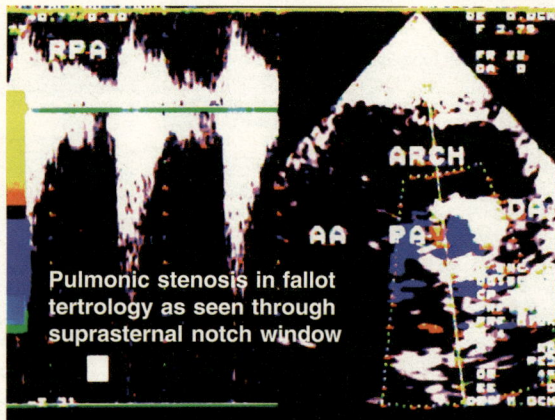

Fig. 13.118: Suprasternal view showing enhanced flow velocity in right pulmonary artery in patient with pulmonary stenosis as a part of Fallot tetrology

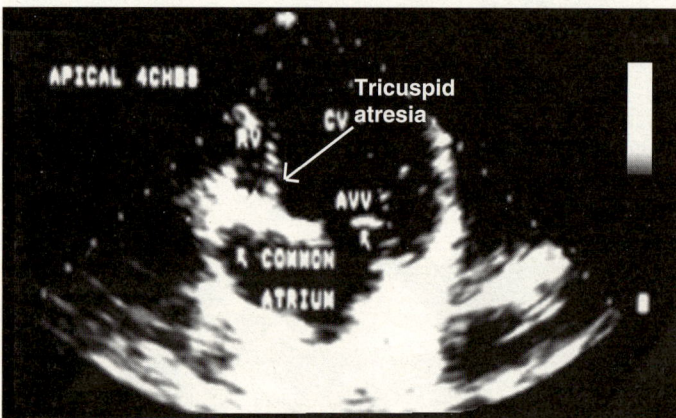

Fig. 13.120: 2-D View in apical 4C plane showing common ventricle (CV) common atrioventricular valve (AVV), common atrium with tricuspid atresia in a child with cyanotic heart disease, single ventricle with tricuspid atresia

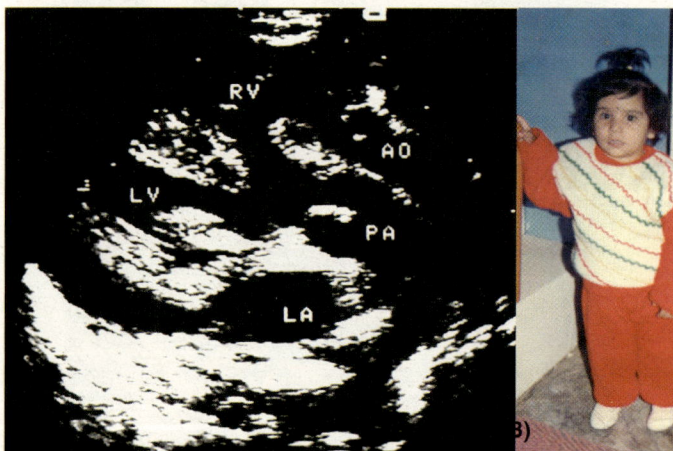

Fig. 13.121A and B: (A) Double outlet right ventricle with sub-pulmonary ventricular septal defect. The pulmonary artery overides the ventricular septum, but slightly more than 50% is committed to right ventricle. **(B)** A young child with stunted growth and cyanosed extremities in DORV

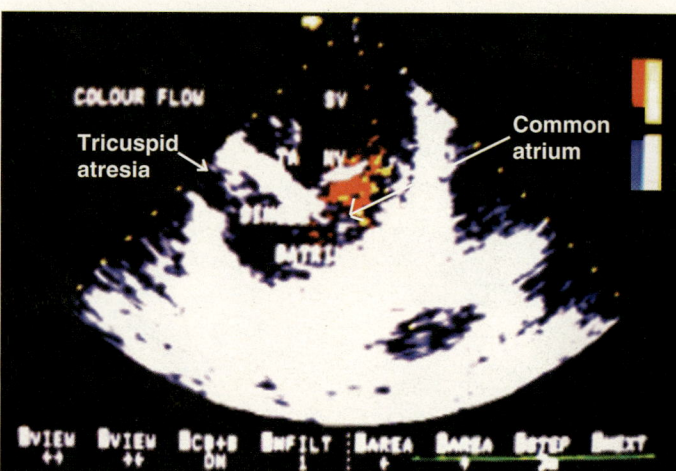

Fig. 13.119: 2-D Apical 4C color flow view showing thickened mitral valve, common atrium, single ventricle and tricuspid atresia with mitral regurgitation and free flow in common atrium, common ventricle and absence of flow through tricuspid valve due to atresia in a child with cyanotic heart disease, single ventricle with tricuspid atresia

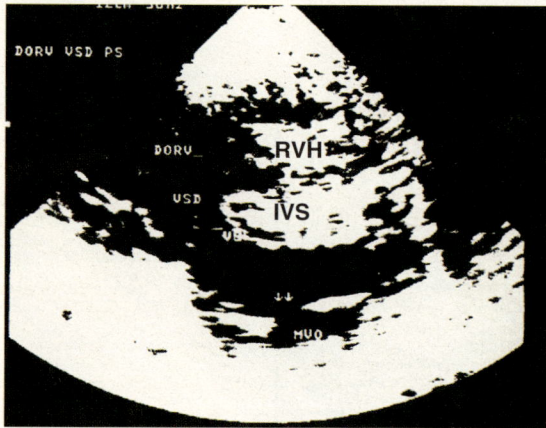

Fig. 13.122: 2-D long axis view. There is subaortic ventricular septal defect (VSD), right ventricular hypertrophy, pulmonic stenosis and absence of mitral-aortic continuity which distinguishes DORV anomaly from that of TOF where it is very well preserved

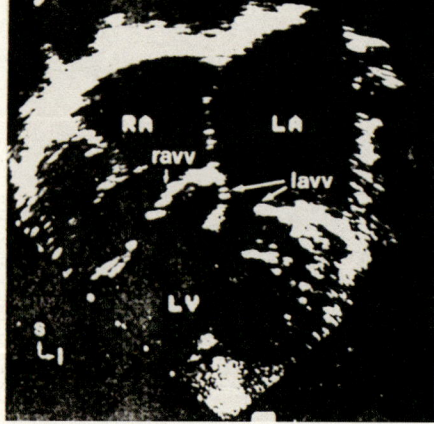

Fig. 13.123: 2-D 4C view showing double outlet left ventricle with two atrio-ventricular valves. ravv = right atrioventricular valve. lavv = left atrioventricular valve, RA = Right atrium, LA = Left atrium, LV = Left ventricle

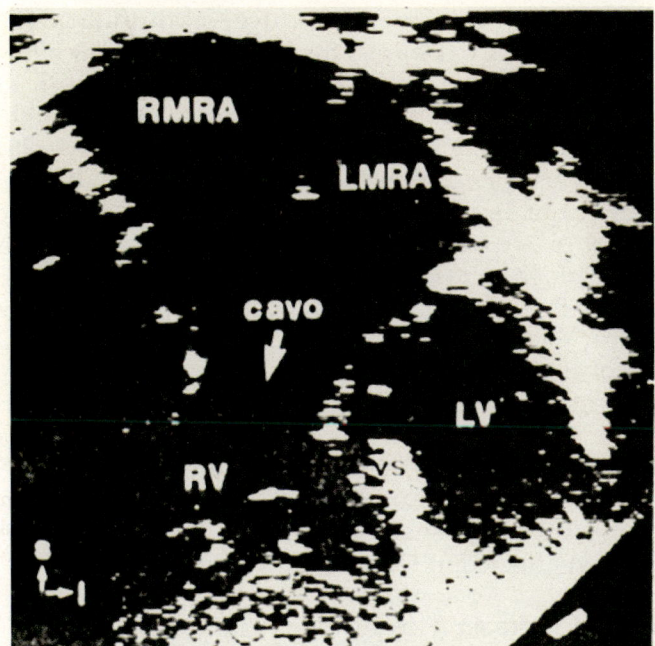

Fig. 13.124: Two 4C view showing double outlet right ventricle with common atrioventriular orifice in a patient with right atrial isomerism, cavo = common atrioventricular orifice. LMRA = Left-sided morphological right atricum. RMRA = right morphological right atrium

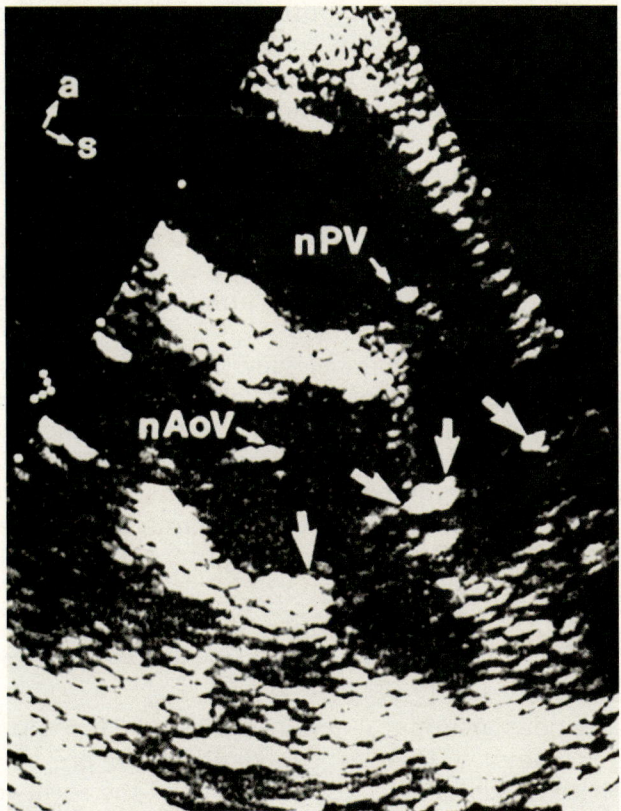

Fig. 13.125: Oblique long axis view in an infant after arterial switch operation for transposition of the great arteries. The large arrows indicate suture lines in the neoaorta and neopulmonary trunk. nAoV = neoaortic valve, nPV = neopulmonary valve

On M-mode echocardiography, the right ventricular pressure overload resulted by the outflow restriction, is characterised by thickening of the right ventricular wall (right ventricular hypertrophy).

Two dimensional echocardiography is the best technique to visualise significant pulmonary stenosis using the parasternal high short-axis and subxiphoid right ventricular outflow tract views. One should look for subpulmonic or suprapulmonic narrowing or hypoplasia. In case of nonvisualisation of pulmonary cusps, there could be a possibility of pulmonary atresia.

Doppler examination of the main pulmonary artery is extremely useful in delineating the degree of stenosis present. Generally a stenotic valve shows a turbulent pattern with the pulsed wave tracing, the continuous-wave transducer must be used to record the maximum velocity.

The Doppler not only determines the gradient across the valve but also determines if any flow is going out, the main pulmonary artery is in critical pulmonary stenosis. One must be careful in the presence of other intracardiac shunts that the velocity is not overestimated because of the increased blood-flow.

Patients with a ventricular septal defect or in tetralogy of Fallot, may cause the pulmonary Doppler flow to be increased.

Pulmonary Atresia with Intact Ventricular Septum

It is visualised with a complete anatomic obstruction to forward bloodflow from the right ventricle into the pulmonary trunk, because the pulmonary valve is imperforate and the ventricular septum is intact.

Pulmonary atresia can be seen in patients with transposition of the great vessels where the pulmonary artery lies more posterior than in the normal great vessel orientation. It may also be associated with a severe form of tetralogy of Fallot or with ventricular septal defect.

The common patterns of pulmonary atresia with intact ventricular septum are observed on echocardiography such as (Fig. 13.16):

1. Sometimes a short distance separates the proximal and right ventricular outflow tract from the main pulmonary artery, with a membranous, bright, immovable echo area between them.
2. In other patients the proximal outflow tract tapers to a dimple, and the pulmonary outflow tract begins some distance distally with a gradual increase in diameter towards the pulmonary artery bifurcation. In the absence of a ventricular septal defect, the right ventricle is usually small, and a right-to-left atrial shunt exists.

Absent Pulmonary Valve Syndrome

In absent pulmonary valve syndrome there is a failure of adequate formation of the cusps, often accompanied by a dilated pulmonary ring with aneurysmal dilation of the main, right, and left pulmonary arteries. Sample volume of the Doppler is placed at the level of the cusps, and a high-pitched blowing sound is heard coming towards the transducer. It is preferable to employ the continuous-wave Doppler to record the maximum velocity of pulmonary insufficiency.

Pulmonary Hypertension and Insufficiency

It has been seen that two most common congenital lesions such as VSD and PDA often predispose to pulmonary artery hypertension. In both pulmonary hypertension and insufficiency the pulmonary artery and ring are dilated. In pulmonary hypertension secondary to lung disease or left-sided heart disease, the typical M-mode tracing shows a dilated pulmonary root and systolic flutter of the posterior cusp (often with early closure or the "flying W" sign). The "dip" which coincides with atrial systole is lost, and the right ventricular pre-ejection period and right ventricular ejection time, ratio, of 0.3 or greater than is often encountered (Fig. 13.112).

With pulmonary insufficiency the pulmonary cusps may be thickened, or there may be dilation of the pulmonary ring. If the amount of insufficiency is significant, there will be right ventricular volume overload with an enlarged right ventricle and paradoxical septal motion.

Tetralogy of Fallot (Figs 13.115–13.118)

Among the category of cyanotic congenital heart defects, tetralogy of Fallot is the most common form of cyanotic heart disease. Its severity varies markedly according to the degree of pulmonary stenosis present. The tetralogy of Fallot has the following four features:

1. A high membranous ventricular septal defect
2. A large anteriorly displaced aorta, which overrides the defect.
3. A smaller pulmonary artery with pulmonary stenosis, (severity determines the degree of cyanosis apparent clinically).
4. Right ventricular hypertrophy develops as a result of the right ventricular outflow tract obstruction.

The pulmonic stenosis can be seen at four different sites: infundibulum, pulmonary valve, pulmonary trunk, and subinfundibular zone.

On echocardiography tetralogy of Fallot can be visualised along the parasternal long-axis view. The aorta is generally quite large when compared with the pulmonary artery and overrides the interventricular septum. A ventricular septal defect is present, the size may vary from small to moderately large. The short-axis view allows one to visualise the small, hypertrophied right ventricle, with a smaller pulmonary artery; and the cusps may be thickened and difficult to

define without some transducer manipulation. A continuous-wave Doppler tracing at this window allows one to assess the degree of velocity shift through the stenotic valve, and thus with the modified Bernoulli's equation, $(4 \times V^2)$ calculate the gradient across the pulmonary valve. (A velocity of 2 m/sec would give a gradient of 16 mm Hg, whereas a velocity of 4 m/sec would give a velocity of 64 mm Hg). The higher the velocity, the more severe the pulmonary stenosis. Colour-flow Doppler would reveal a turbulent pattern within the main pulmonary artery, pointing towards the obstruction of flow across the pulmonary valve. Subcostal short-axis right ventricular outflow tract plane is the preferred view for defining the subvalvular portion of the right ventricular outflow tract and the area of obstruction under the valve which may also allow extensive visualisation of the subpulmonary area so often affected in tetralogy of Fallot.

Tricuspid Atresia (Figs 13.119 and 13.120)

In tricuspid valve atresia tricuspid orifice is always absent, and the only outlet for right atrial blood is by means of an interatrial shunt. Systemic venous blood mixes with pulmonary venous blood in the left atrium. The mitral valve may be large but competent with no regurgitant jet. The left ventricle acts as the primary pumping chamber for both systemic and venous circulations.

Anatomically, the inflow portion of the right ventricle has failed to form, and a membrane or dimple in the floor of the right atrium represents the position where the tricuspid valve should have originated (Figs 13.118–13.119).

Usually a ventricular septal defect is present to help shunt blood into hypertrophied right ventricle. The right ventricular outflow tract and pulmonary artery are reduced to its minimal size.

The apical four-chamber view is best to study the abnormality of tricuspid valve and tricuspid atresia where one may find a dilated left ventricle and the small underdeveloped right ventricular cavity. The tricuspid anulus is seen with no valve movement. On the long-axis and short-axis views, the right ventricle is seen as a slit like cavity just anterior to the interventricular septum.

Complete Transposition of the Great Vessels (TGV) (Figs 13.113, 13.114 and 13.125)

The various anatomical abnormalities which could be seen in complete TGV are: two ventricles are present (a ventricular septal defect may occur) and the aorta and coronary arteries arise from the right ventricle, whereas the pulmonary trunk takes origin from the left ventricle. Both atrioventricular valves are patent and are normally located in right-left heart arrangement. The connections of the systemic, pulmonary and coronary veins are normal. There can also be an interatrial communication, a ventricular septal defect, a patent ductus arteriosus, or large bronchial arteries that join the aorta to the pulmonary bed. Anatomic obstruction to the left ventricular outflow occurs as either valvular or subvalvular pulmonic stenosis. If there is defect in the ventricular septum, pulmonic stenosis is more likely to occur.

One may find different types of TGV depending upon the anatomical placement of ventricles, atrioventricular valves and great vessels connections. There are several varieties of transposition. Those associated with single ventricle, tricuspid atresia, right ventricular aorta with biventricular pulmonary trunk or congenitally corrected, appear as double circles (or two eggs). To visualise pulmonary artery in the anterior great vessel which is located by angling the transducer anterior and towards the patient's left shoulder from a transducer position in transposition.

In dextrotransposition of the great arteries (d-TGA) the truncus septates properly and then spirals in such a manner that the aorta arises from the right ventricle, anterior to the right of the pulmonary artery, which arises from the left ventricle.

Two-dimensional echocardiography allows the direct visualisation of the great vessels and their relationship to one another. On the parasternal long-axis view the aorta normally takes a straight course as it ascends into the arch; however, in transposition the pulmonary artery takes the place of the aorta as the posterior vessel and thus dips downward as it begins to bifurcate into right and left branches.

While visualising through the short-axis view, the right ventricular outflow tract normally "wraps" around the root of the aorta (referred to as the "sausage and eggs" sign). Since the great vessels are parallel in d-TGA rather than wrapping about each other, they surround the anterior great vessel as a complete circle, one moves the transducer more cephalad, the vessel remains as a circle because of its natural superior course. Conversely, the pulmonary artery should bifurcate as it passes posterior to the lungs.

The subcostal view is also very useful in neonates to outline the ventricular outflow tract and great vessel orientation. The pulmonary artery and its bifurcation may be seen to arise from the left ventricle, whereas the aorta, the arch, and its descending branch are seen to arise from the right ventricle. One may consistently find the existence of an interatrial communication and it is important to record how much of a patent foramen or atrial septal defect is present. If necessary, a balloon septostomy may be performed during the cardiac catheterization to open the atrial communication wider so that adequate mixing reveals the aorta (or posterior great vessel). If it is not apparent towards the left shoulder but instead is located by angling towards the right shoulder, a diagnosis of d-TGA should be considered. Alternatively recording of both great vessels from the same transducer position would be of great help in diagnosis of TGV.

The surgical repair of choice in uncomplicated d-TGA is Mustard procedure, which is involved creating a new atria.

The turbulence created by these altered flow paths creates flutter on both atrioventricular valves and can be detected on the M-mode. Because the right ventricle is carrying the systemic pressure, it becomes thick-walled and dilated. The left ventricle may now be relatively smaller and appear pancaked or flattened on the short-axis view.

The baffle can be seen in the apical four-chamber view. The systemic baffle takes a horizontal course across the atrial chambers, whereas the pulmonic baffle takes a "dog-leg" course from the pulmonary venous inflow into the tricuspid orifice. Obstruction may occur at either the caval-systemic venous atrial junction or at the pulmonary vein entry sites, and thus careful Doppler recordings should be taken in these areas. Colour-flow mapping helps in locating the site of turbulence with the baffle so an accurate Doppler tracing can be made. The suprasternal notch window is sometimes helpful to image the superior vena caval-right atrial junction area.

Double-Outlet Right Ventricle (Figs 13.121–13.123)

In this type of malformation of the ventricle, the pulmonary artery arises in its normal position, but the aorta arises entirely from the right ventricle. A ventricular septal defect provides the only outlet for the left ventricle. There may be coexistent pulmonic stenosis. Echocardiographic examination with apical four-chamber view is probably the best window to outline both great vessels as they arise from the right ventricle. The subcostal view may also be useful to delineate the great vessel orientation. The parasternal long-axis view may allow one to outline both great vessels as they assume their parallel course from the right ventricle; in this case a large ventricular septal defect would also be seen just below the transposed pulmonary artery.

Corrected Transposition of the Great Arteries (Corrected TGA)

In this type of cardiac malformation, when the anterior great vessel is to the left of the pulmonary artery, then L-TGA should be suspected. This occurs when the great arteries are transposed, but because of ventricular

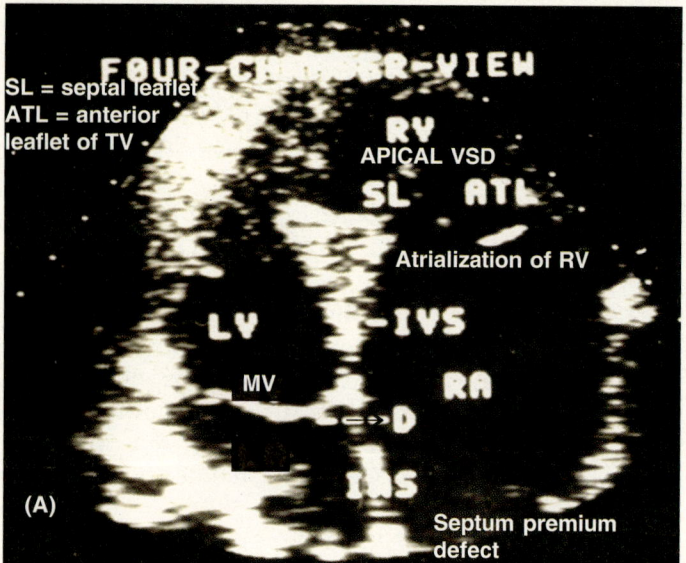
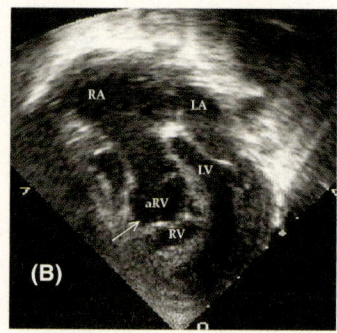
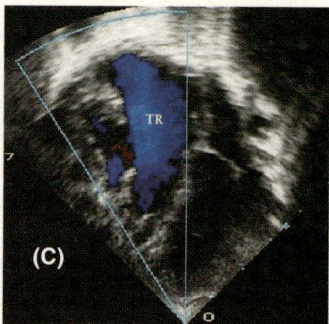

Fig. 13.126A to C: (A) Apical 4C view showing displacement of incompetent tricuspid valve and atrialization of RV with reference to proximally positioned MV. There is also associated septum primum (D) and apical VSD (arrow) in a patient with Ebstein anomaly of TV. **(B)** and **(C)** Atrialization of tricuspid valve (B) and blue jet of tricuspid regurgitation due to incompetent TV (C) in a patient with Ebstein disease of TV aRV = atrialized RV, LA = Left atrium, RA = Right atrium, LV = Left ventricle, TR = Tricuspid regurgitation, ATL = Anterior tricuspid leaflet, SL = Septal leaflet of tricuspid leaflet

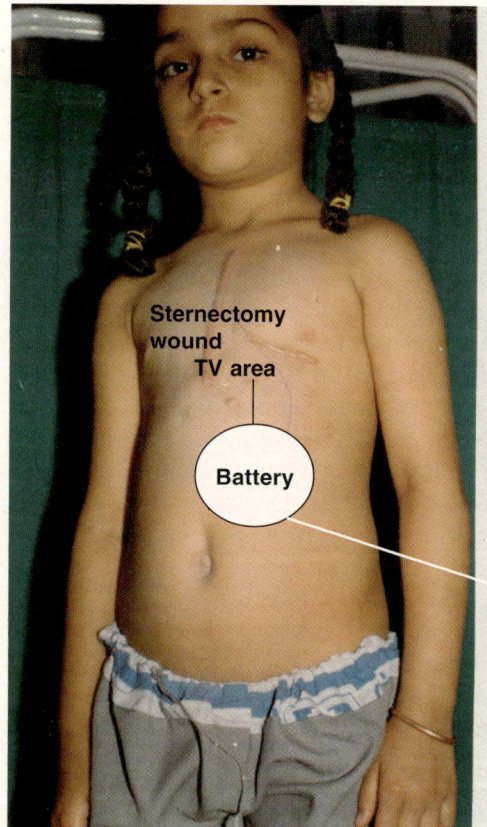
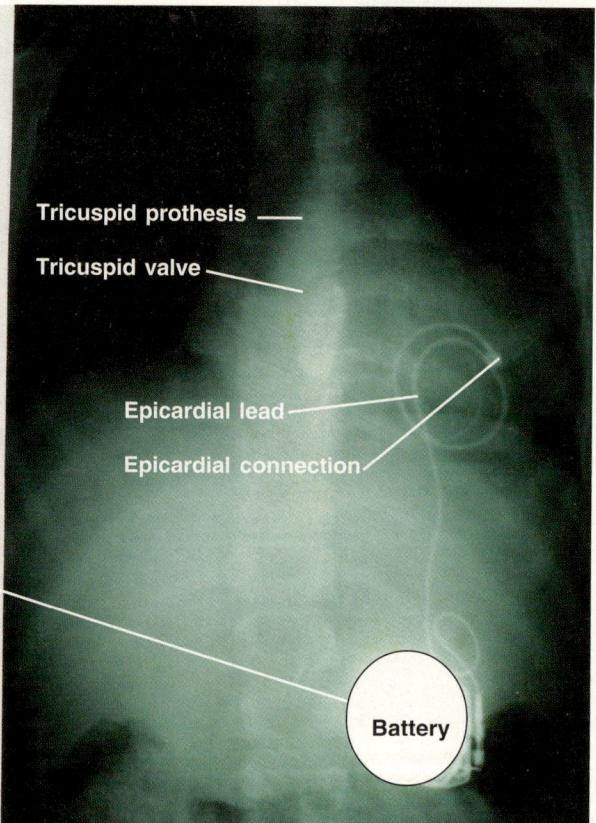

Fig. 13.127A and B: (A) 10 years old girl was suffering from progressive severe form of primary tricuspid regurgitation with CCF with dyspnoea on exertion since her childhood. She was fully investigated and decided to replace tricuspid prosthetic valve, but during operation she developed complete heart block for which epicardial pace-maker was installed. **(B)** X-Ray photograph showing epicardial connection with heart and battery has been placed in the abdominal cavity as indicated with long arrow. She is now 22 years old and is found normal on cardiovascular follow up

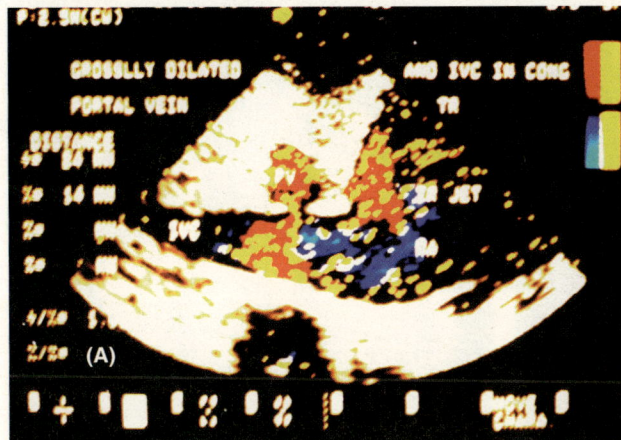

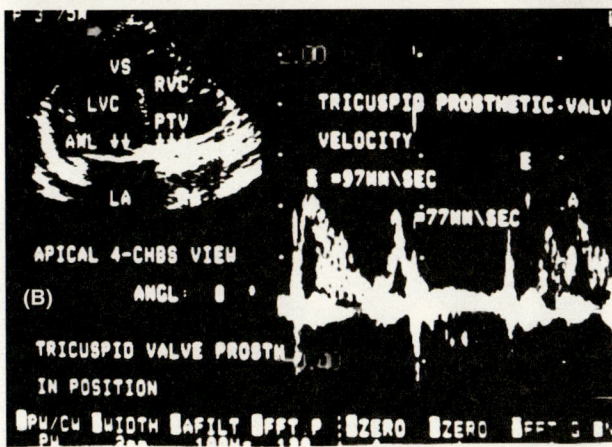

Fig. 13.128A and B: (A) Subcostal transhepatic scan showing dilated IVC and dilated hepatic venous system in above mentioned patient prior to her operative intervention. **(B)** 2-D Doppler echoscan showing normal Doppler flow velocity in tricuspid prosthetic valve which was fitted in this patient

inversion, the circulatory pattern is hemodynamically correct. Each ventricle keeps its respective atrium empty via atrioventricular valve when it inverts. Thus the right atrium empties via the mitral valve into a right-sided morphologic (smooth-walled) left ventricle, which ejects through a posterior pulmonary artery. The left atrium empties via a tricuspid valve into a left-sided morphologic (heavily trabeculated) right ventricle, which ejects through an anterior leftward aorta.

Since the crista supraventricularis separates the aorta from the tricuspid valve, continuity is not seen on the long-axis view between the left-sided atrioventricular valve and the semilunar valve. Visualisation of the septal insertion sites of atrioventricular valves in the four chamber view identifies the inverted ventricles. If the tricuspid valve, which inserts into the septum more inferiorly, is on the left side in the four-chamber view, that left-sided ventricle is identified as a morphologic right ventricle. Ebstein's malformation of left-sided tricuspid valve, ventricular septal defect, and pulmonary stenosis are finding commonly associated with this anomaly.

Ebsteins's Anomaly of the Tricuspid Valve (Figs 13.126 –13.128)

In Ebsteins's anomaly of the tricuspid valve there is displacement of fused, malformed portions of the tricuspid valvular tissue into the right ventricular cavity. The leaflets attach in part to the tricuspid valve and in part below this level. Valvular tissue may be directly adherent to the ventricular endocardium or may be very closely attached to the ventricular wall by multiple, anomalous, short chordae tendineae. The portion of the right ventricle underlying the adherent tricuspid valvular tissue is usually quite thin and functions as receiving chamber analogous to the right atrium. This segment of the right ventricle is referred to as the atrialised chamber because it registers a right atrial pressure pulse on hemodynamic study. The anterior tricuspid leaflet is the largest and least affected of the three leaflets. The septal and posterior leaflets characteristically show the greatest deformity, and the posterior cusp may be rudimentary or entirely absent. The right atrium is usually massively dilated. Often the patients have an incompetent or fenestrated foramen ovale or a secundum atrial septal defect.

The abnormal function of the right heart is related to three factors:

1. The malformed tricuspid valve.
2. The "atrialised" portion of the right ventricle.
3. The reduced capacity of the pumping portion of the right ventricle.

Apical four chamber view is the best to visualise the anatomical malformation seen in Ebstein anomaly. There is apical displacement of septal leaflet of tricuspid valve with resultant tricuspid insufficiency. The atrialised right ventricle is well seen, especially with apical four chamber view. One may find marked displacement of tricuspid annulus towards the apex of the RV.

There is consistent right ventricular dysfunction, which results in an overload pattern of wall motion with paradoxical movement of anterior septum in systole. This right ventricular overload also shows flattening of the septum when viewed in short-axis plane. Doppler tracings are useful to record the amount of tricuspid valvular insufficiency. The sample volume should be placed at the annulus of the tricuspid valve then mapped through the atrialised right ventricle into the right atrial cavity.

Total Anomalous Pulmonary Venous Return (TAPVR) (Figs 13.130–13.132)

In this type of anomaly all the venous blood from both lungs enters the right atrium directly or through one of its tributary veins. The anomalous veins emerge individually from the lungs and either enter directly into

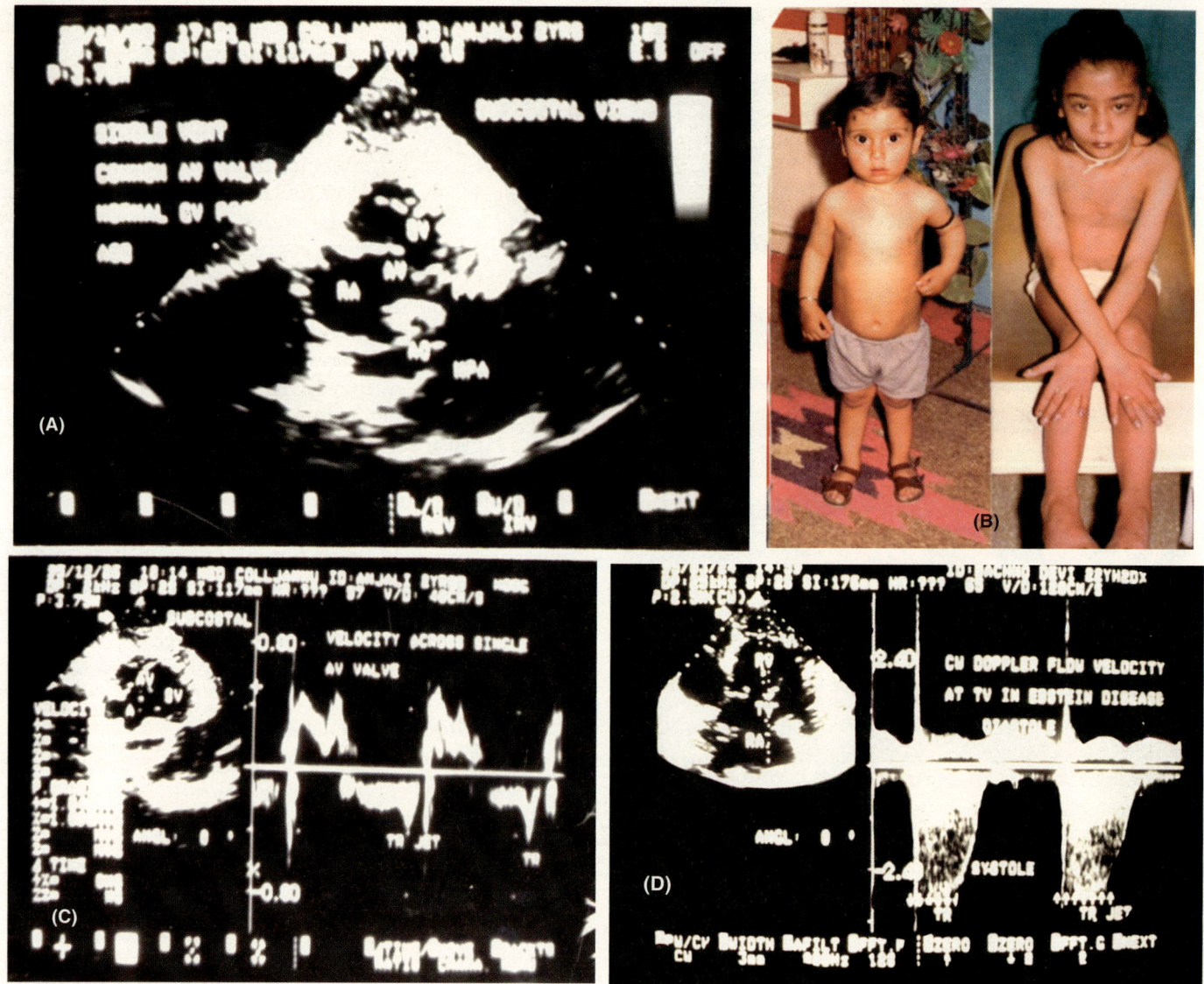

Fig. 13.129A to D: **(A)** Apical 4C view showing single ventricle, pulmonic stenosis with common atrioventricular valve. **(B)** Two children suffering from single ventricle with pulmonic stenosis who died with progressive cardiac decompensation. **(C)** Pulsed Doppler flow velocity in atrioventicular valve showing tricuspid regurgitation (TR). **(D)** 2-D Doppler flow velocity across tricuspid valve showing enhanced velocity >3.0 cm/s in another child with single ventricle with common AV valve

the right atrium or unite in the mediastinum to form a confluence. A separate vascular channel connects this confluence of veins to systemic vein that lies either within the thorax or within the abdomen. Blood from this systemic vein finds its way into the right atrium.

The thoracic or supradiaphragmatic venous channel receives the confluence from one of the following ways:
1. The coronary sinus.
2. The left innominate vein, which communicates with the confluence via an anomalous vertical vein or a left superior vena cava.
3. The right superior vena cava directly or via the azygous vein.
4. Portal venous system.

Less frequently, the pulmonary veins join the systemic venous system below the diaphragm. This vascular channel enters the abdominal cavity through the esophageal hiatus and terminates in the portal vein or its tributaries or in the ductus venosus. Other entry sites have also been described, and occasionally there is more than one entry site.

One may appreciate to note that in TAPVR there exists impedance of flow from the lungs. The most common cause of obstruction is drainage below the diaphragm. In the thorax the obstruction may be compressed when the channel passes between the pulmonary trunk and left bronchus on its way to the left innominate vein.

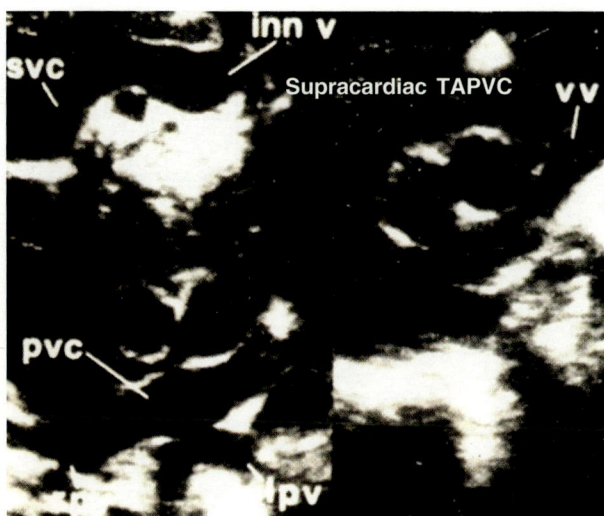

Fig. 13.130: Echoscan taken from suprasternal notch area showing dilated innominate vein and dilated superior vena cava (upper left panel). A pulmonary venous confluence receiving the right and left pulmonary veins (lower left panel). Vertical venous connector draining the venous confluence to the innominate vein (right panel) in a patient with supracardiac total anomalous pulmonary venous drainage pvc = pulmonary venous confluence, rpv = right pulmonary vein, lpv = left pulmonary vein, SVC = superior vena cava, VV = verticle vein

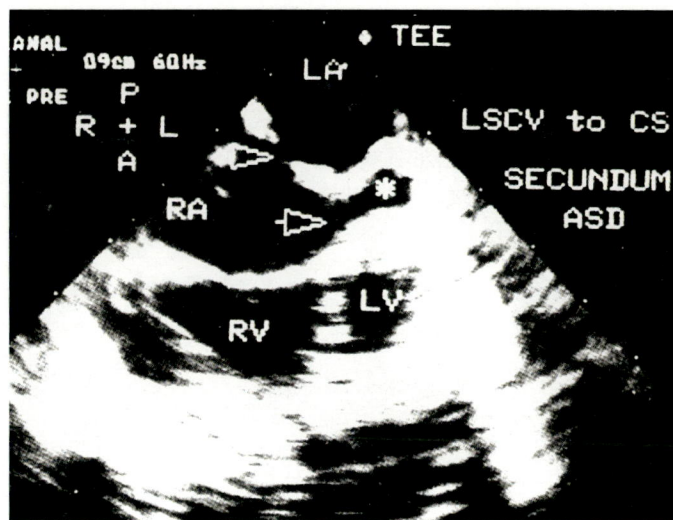

Fig. 13.132: TEE 4C view showing ASD secundum type along with left superior vena cava connected to coronary sinus as a part of partial anomalous venous connection (PAVC). CS = Coronary sinus

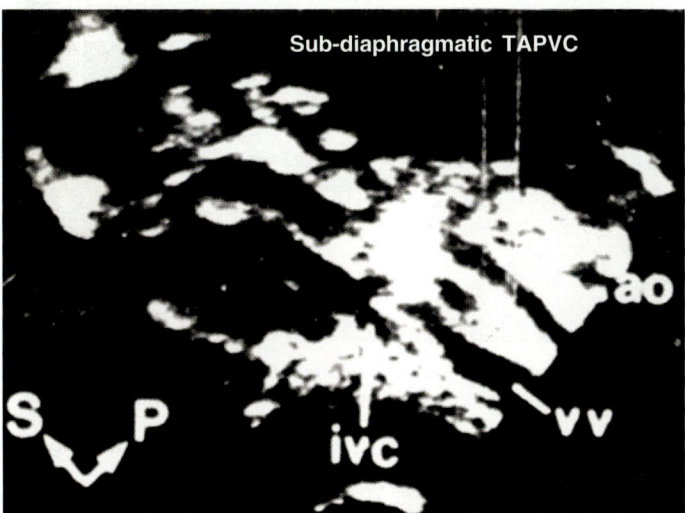

Fig. 13.131: Subxiphoid sagittal plane view showing the verticle venous (VV) connector penetrating the diaphragm between the inferior vena cava (IVC) and the aorta (AO) in a patient with subdiaphragmatic total anomalous pulmonary venous drainage

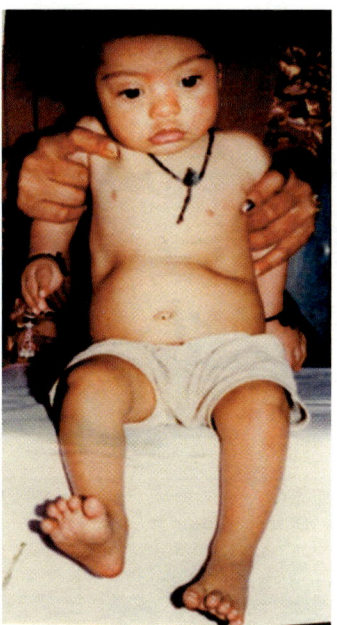

Fig. 13.133: Retardation of both physical and mental milestones with chest deformity in a child suffering with mangolism and endocardial cushion defect

An interatrial communication is critical in total anomalous pulmonary venous return, so blood may reach the left heart. This may be a true atrial septal defect or patent foramen ovale. The wider the defect, the more efficient the interchange between the right and left atrium.

Echocardiographic examination may be some help in the diagnosis of TAPVR in which one may visualise an enlarged right heart, a "common" channel seen posterior to the left atrium, increased flow in the right atrial cavity and interatrial communication. Colour-flow Doppler may help distinguish abnormal venous connections as they drain into the right atrial cavity.

Truncus Arteriosus (Fig. 13.136)

In this type of malformation, a single great vessel leaves the base of the heart through a single semilunar valve associated with a ventricular septal defect. The truncal vessel receives blood from both ventricles. The coronary arteries arise from the truncal vessel. Generally, there are multiple leaflets within the vessel.

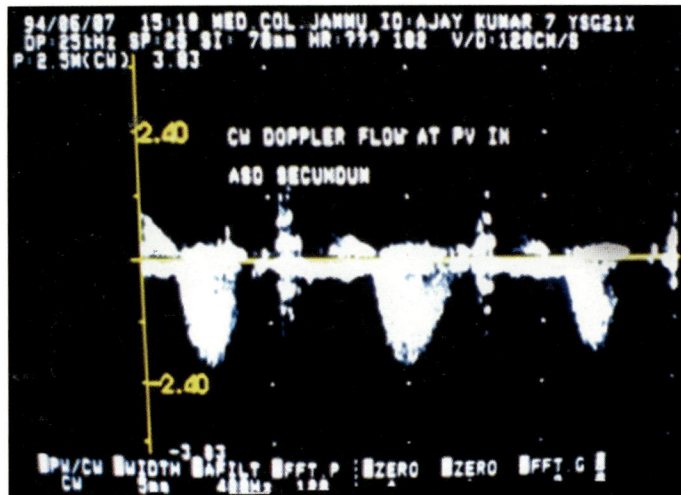

Fig. 13.134: Continuous wave Doppler showing pulmonary wave-forms in a child with congenital pulmonary valvular stenosis associated with ASD secundum

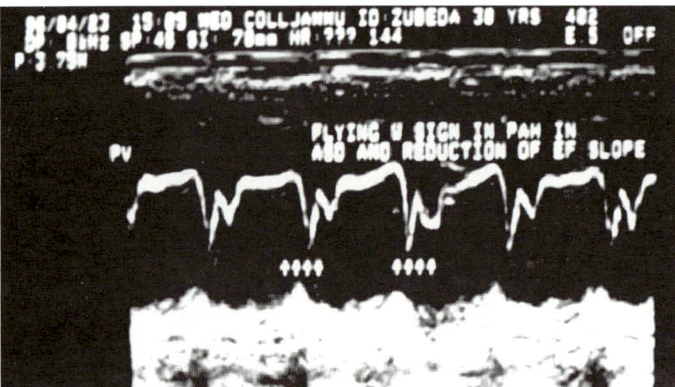

Fig. 13.135: M-Mode echocardiogram showing W type of configuration of pulmonary valve in pulmonary artery hypertension in an adult patient with ASD secundum type of defect

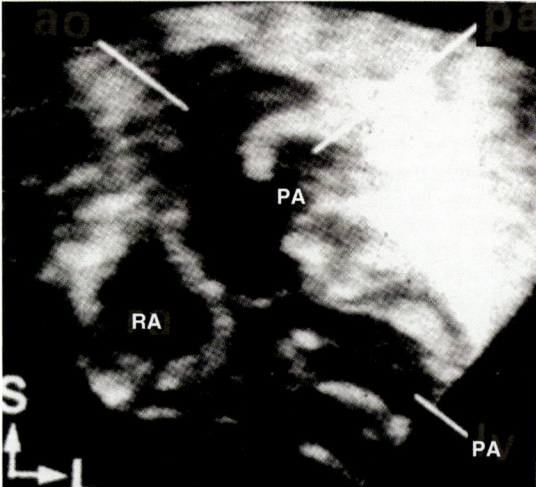

Fig. 13.136: Subxiphoid approach in long axis view showing truncal root branching into ascending aorta in a patient with truncus arteriosus (AO) and the pulmonary artery (PA), LV = Left ventricle, RA = Right atrium

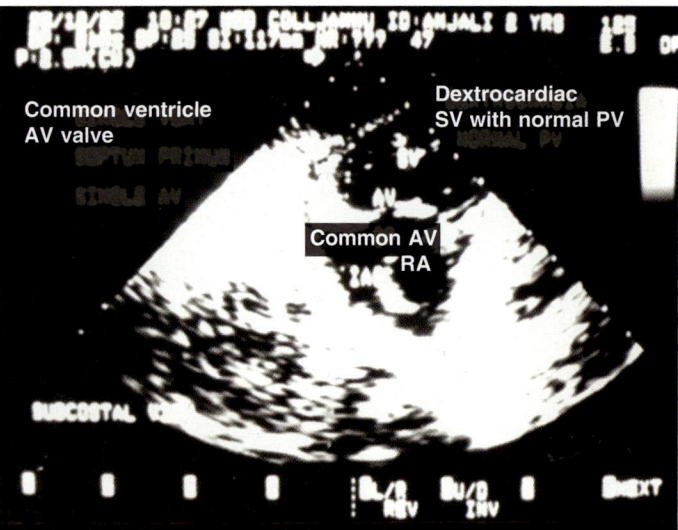

Fig. 13.137: Apical 4C view showing single ventricle, common atrio-ventricular valve, mild form of fossa ovalis ASD defect in a child with cyanotic heart disease with dextrocardia and normal PV

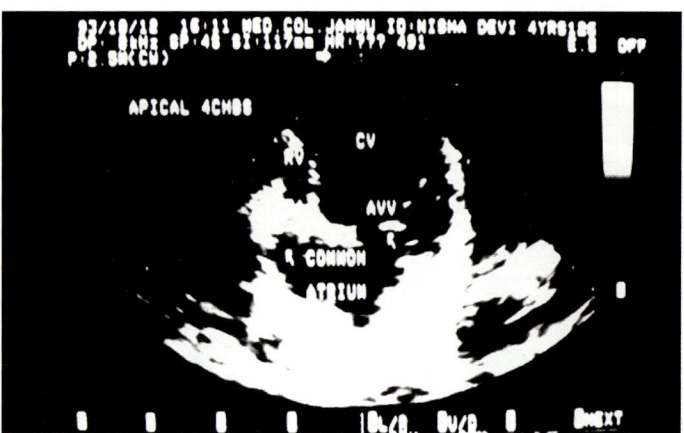

Fig. 13.138: Apical 4C view showing common atrio-ventricular valve (AVV) and common atrium connected with single ventricle

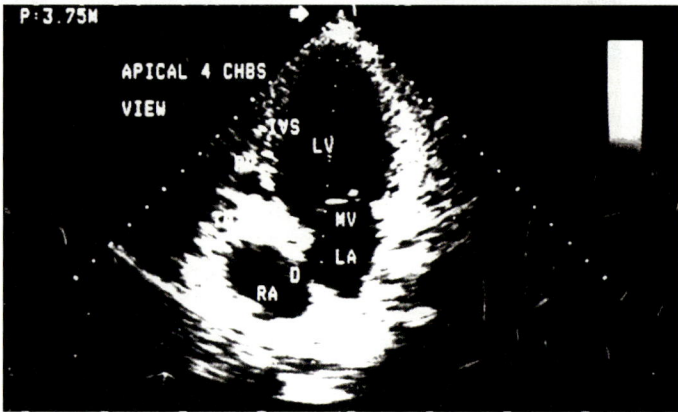

Fig. 13.139: Oblique 4C view showing ASD secundum (D) connected with left atrium (LA) with normal mitral valve (MV) which inturn communicates with dilated LV. Tricuspid valve is atresic with small rudimentary right ventricle (RV)

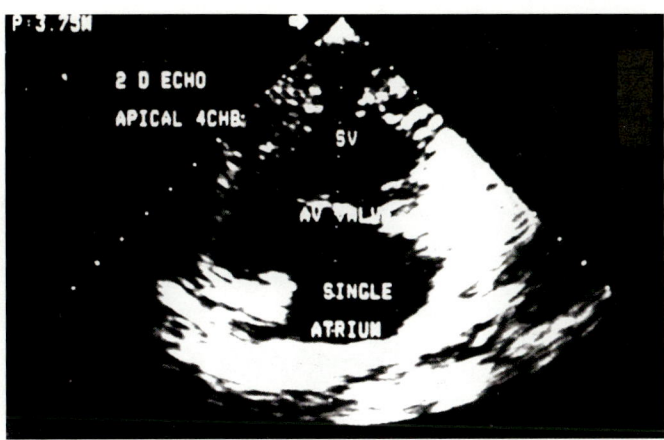

Fig. 13.140: 2-D Apical 4C view showing almost single atrium connected with atrioventricular valve with single ventricle. Tricuspid valve is not developed, and depicts fibro-muscular body as a part of endocardial cushion defect

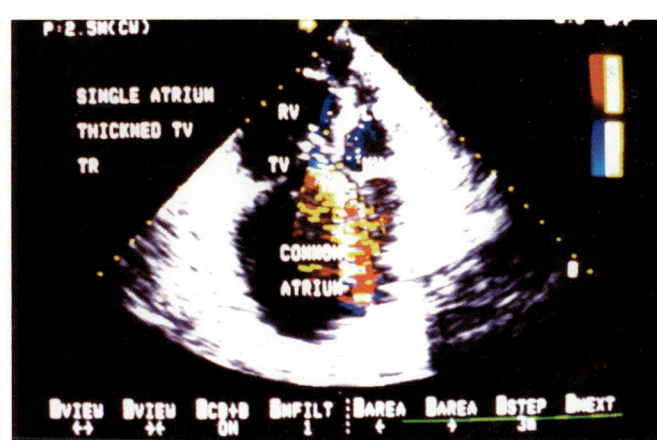

Fig. 13.141: 2-D Color flow scan acquired from apical 4C view depicting common atrium connected to RV and rudimentary left ventricle and color flow demonstrates moderately severe tricuspid valvular regurgitation

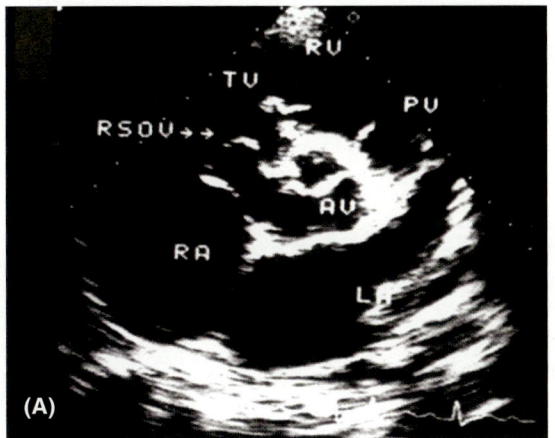

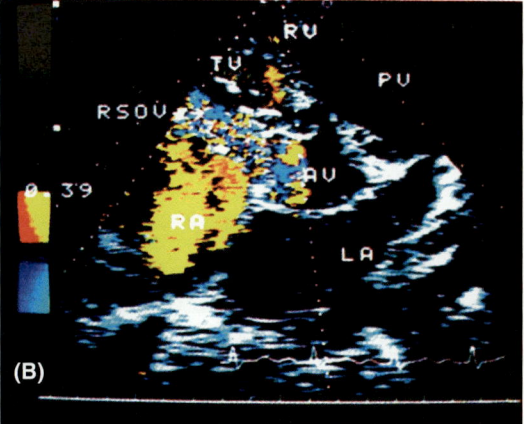

Fig. 13.142A and B: (A) 2-D Short axis view showing breakage in right sinus of valsalva below the tricuspid valve. **(B)** Color flow from aorta to RV through ruptured right sinus of valsalva. RSOV = Right sinus of valsalva, AV = aortic valve, RV = Right ventricle, PV = Pulmonary valve, TV = Tricuspid valve

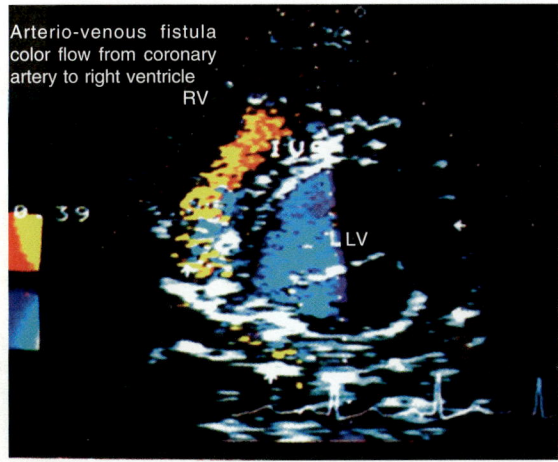

Fig. 13.143: A parasternal short axis view focused at mitral valve shows the color flow from coronary arteriovenous fistula into right ventricle in a patient with coronary arteriovenous fistula. LV = Left ventricle, RV = Right ventricle, IVS = Interventricular septum

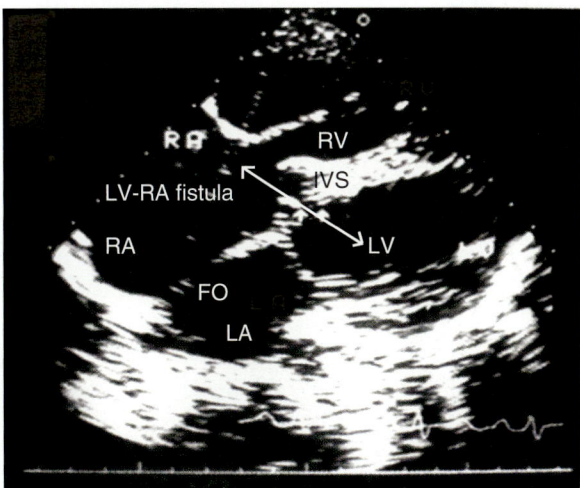

Fig. 13.144: Modified apical 4C view shows the defect in the ventricular septum and septal leaflet of tricuspid valve in a patient with left ventricle to right atrium fistula (arrow)

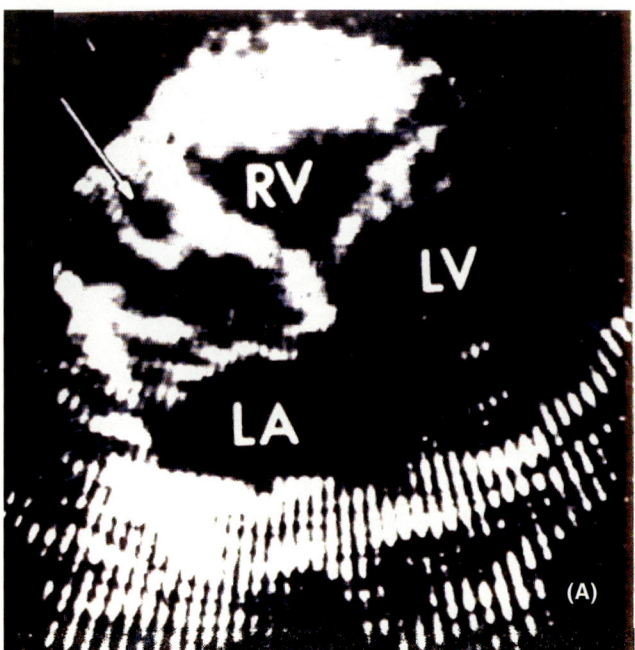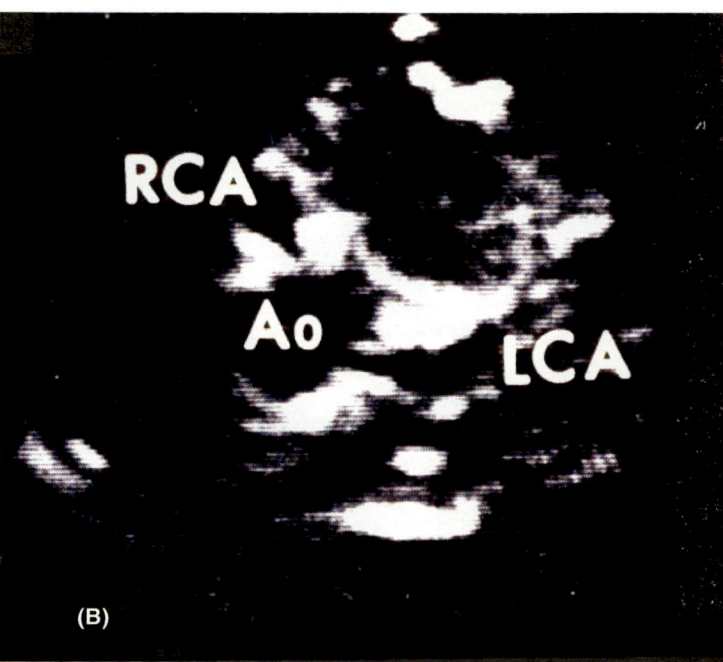

Fig. 13.145A and B: (A) 2-D Frontal echoscan taken at anterior atrio-ventricular valve showing aneurysm of peripheral portion of right coronary artery in a patient with mucocutaneous lymph node syndrome. **(B)** Transverse section of the aortic root in which the most proximal portion of the right coronary artery and left coronary arteries are both clearly visualised in a patient with mucocutaneous lymph node syndrome

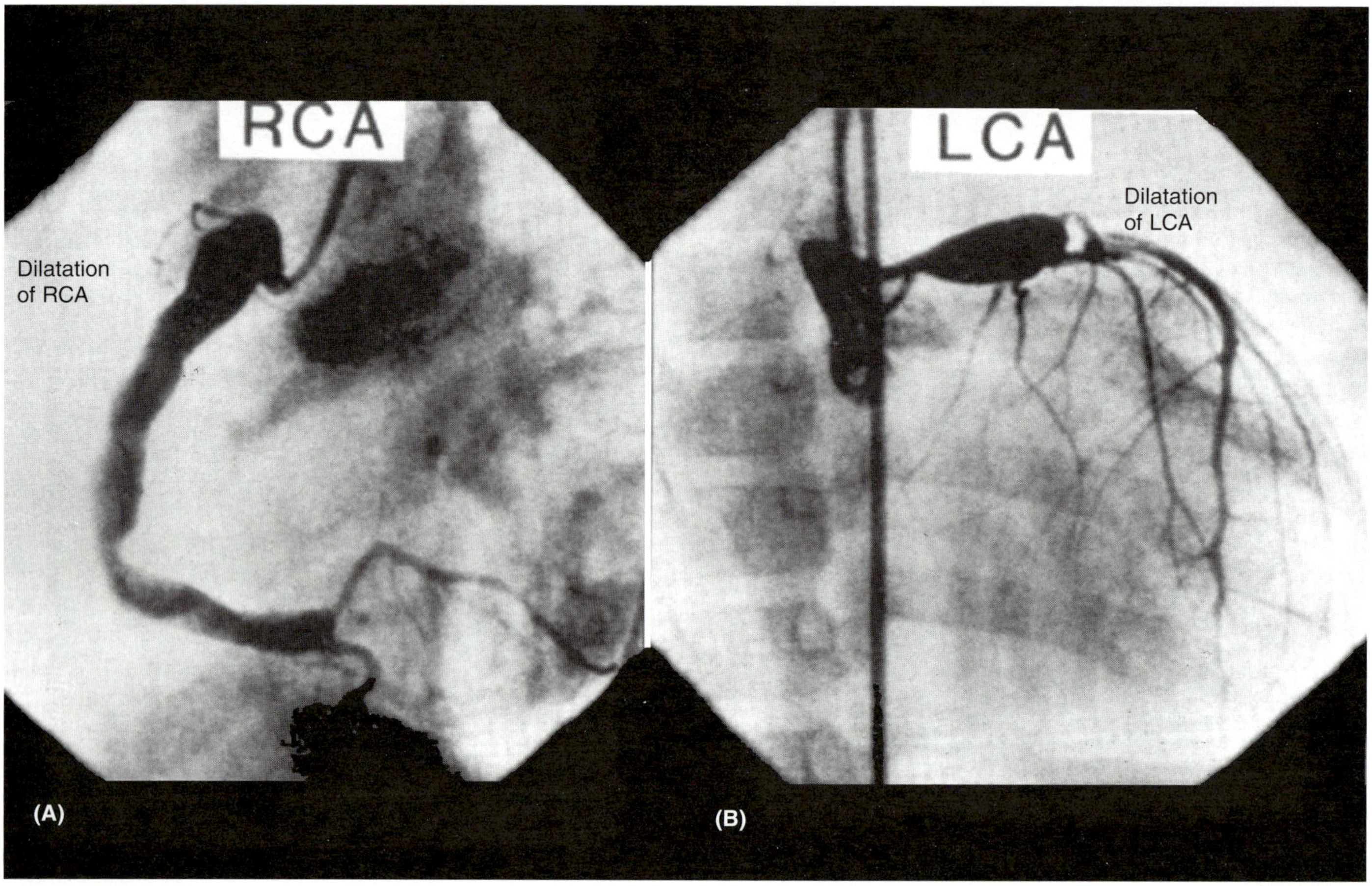

Fig. 13.146A and B: Coronary arterial angiography showing aneurysmal dilatation of left and right coronary arteries in above-studied patient suffering from mucocutaneous lymph node syndrome

Edwards, *et al.* have classified truncal variations into four categories:

Type 1: A short pulmonary trunk emerges from the truncus arteriosus and gives rise to the right midleft pulmonary arteries.

Type 2: The right and left pulmonary arteries arise directly from the posterior wall of the truncus.

Type 3: The right and left pulmonary arteries originate from the lateral walls of the truncus.

Type 4: The pulmonary arteries are absent altogether and the arterial supply to the lungs is through bronchial arteries.

M-mode and 2-D echocardiography is great help in the identification of a very large great vessel with multiple leaflet echoes within. It may be difficult to distinguish the truncal vessel from a tetralogy of Fallot with severe pulmonary stenosis. In order to exclude TOF one should be able to visualise the multiple cusps echoes and identify the truncal origin of the pulmonary artery.

There is increased pulmonary bloodflow in type 1 and 2, in which the pulmonary arteries arise from the truncus. Thus the presence or absence of a pulmonary valve is an important differential point between tetralogy of Fallot and truncus arteriosus.

The subxiphoid right ventricular outflow tract would not be obtainable in truncus arteriosus, but a left ventricular outflow tract scanned superiorly might reveal the pulmonary artery arising from the truncus.

A second differential point is that the left atrium is enlarged in truncus arteriosus because of increased flow through the lungs whereas in tetralogy it is decreased to the lungs stemming from right ventricular outflow tract obstruction.

Single Ventricle (Figs 13.119, 13.129, 13.137 and 13.138)

Single ventricle may be defined as that type of anomaly in which there are two atria but only one ventricular chamber, which receives both the mitral and tricuspid valves. Both atrioventricular valves are patent, and thus mitral and tricuspid valves join to form a common atrioventricular valve.

The most commonly encountered single ventricle consists of a morphologic left ventricle with a small outlet chamber that represents the infundibular portion of the right ventricle (with the body or inflow portion of the ventricle absent).

The right or the left atrioventricular connections may be transposed, along with transposition of great vessels with the aorta arising above the small outlet chamber. If transposition is present, the pulmonary artery lies posterior to the aorta.

The infundibulum lies at the base of the ventricle, communicating with the aorta above and the single ventricle below. If the great vessels are normal, the infundibulum communicates with the pulmonary trunk.

The outlet chambers may be left-sided and anterior or right-sided and anterior, but they commonly lie high on the cardiac silhouette.

Pulmonary stenosis may or may not coexist. If present, the stenosis is usually valvular or subvalvular, the pulmonary trunk is usually slightly smaller than the aortic trunk.

Echocardiographic examination through the apical four-chamber view is probably the most useful window in delineating the cardiac anatomy. One should be careful not to confuse the very prominent papillary muscles with interventricular septum as it can happen with single ventricle where papillary muscles may be quite prominent. With transducers angulation, the chordal structures may be traced for correct delineation. The right ventricle may be just a slitlike cavity as seen on the apical four-chamber view. The position of the great arteries should be assessed, and the aorta and pulmonary arteries should be delineated clearly. There may be regurgitant jets associated with abnormal chordal connections of the atrioventricular valves. Colour Doppler mapping should be used to outline the degree of regurgitation.

Kawasaki's Disease affecting Coronary Arteries (Figs 13.145 and 13.146)

Two-dimensional echocardiographic examination is able to demonstrate the coronary arteries as they arise from the right and left aortic cusp. The right coronary artery may be seen on the parasternal long-axis view as it arises from the aorta and flows along the septal wall.

The left main coronary artery arises from the left coronary cusp at the 4 o'clock position, and with careful angulation, this artery may be followed to its point of bifurcation into the circumflex and left anterior descending branches. A modified short-axis view with extreme angulation towards the pulmonary artery demonstrates a long segment of the pulmonary artery (with cusp) and just below is the left anterior descending artery. The pulmonic cusp marks the distinction between the proximal and distal segments of the vessel. The left posterior descending artery sometimes is seen with a modified apical to subcostal four-chamber view. As the septum is brought into view, the transducer is gradually swept back and forth until the vessel is seen to flow along the posterior surface of the left side of the septum. The coronary arteries should assume a smooth, tubular course as they arise from the aorta. Generally vessels under 3 mm in diameter are considered within normal limits. The presence of an aneurysm may appear to encompass a long segment or short segment of the vessel; they may be single or multiple; and they may occur at any segment of the coronary artery. Thus it is very important to carefully record as much of the proximal and distal segments of each of the coronary artery as possible. If an aneurysm is found, the echocardiography is an excellent method in following the dilation until subsequent resolution of the normal size is obtained. Doppler evaluation of the mitral and aortic valves is also recorded to document evidence of regurgitation. This is best done in the apical four-chamber view at the level of the mitral and aortic valves. M-mode and 2-dimensional echocardiography in the evaluation of the cardiac function and wall motion is also important to asses contractility and the presence of myocarditis, and the presence of pericardial effusion through the parasternal and apical windows.

Bibliography

1. Bc'ilacqua M, Sanders SP, VanPraagh S, *et al.* Double-inlet single left ventricle: Echocardiographic anatomy with emphasis on the morphology of the atrioventricular valves and ventricular septal defect. *J Am Coll Cardiol* 1991;18:559.

2. Berger F, Ewert P, Bjornstad PG, *et al.* Transcatheter closure as standard treatment for most interatrial defects: experience in 200 patients treated with the Amplatzer Septal Occluder. *Cardiol Young* 1999; 9:468.

3. Brandenburg J, Tajik AI, Edwards WD, *et al.* Accuracy of 2-dimensional echocardiographic diagnosis of congenitally bicuspid aortic valve: Echocardiographic-anatomic clation in 115 patients. *Am J Cardiol* 1983; 51:1469.

4. Brickner M, Hillis LD, Lange RA: Congenital heart disease in adults: second of two parts. *N Engl J Med* 2000;342:334.

5. Cantor WJ, Harrison DA, Moussadji JS, *et al.* Determinants of survival and length of survival in adults with Eisenmenger syndrome. *Am J Cardiol* 1999 ;84:677.

6. Carvalho IS, Rigby ML, Shineboume EA, *et al.* Cross sectional echocardiography for recognition of ventricular topology in atrioventricular septal defect. *Br Heart* 11989;61:285.

7. Celermajer DS, Bull C, Till JA, *et al.* Ebstein's anomaly: presentation and outcome from fetus to adult. *J Am Coll Cardiol* 1994;23:170.

8. Cheitlin MD, Alpert IS, Armstrong WF, *et al.* ACCIAHA Guidelines for the Clinical Application of Echocardiography: a report of the American College of Cardiology/American Heart Association Task Force on Practice Guidelines (Committee on Clinical Application of Echocardiography) developed in collaboration with the American Society of Echocardiography. *Circulation* 1997; 95:1686–1744.

9. Chin TK, Perloff IK. Williams RG, *et al.* Isolated noncompaction of left ventricular myocardium: A study of eight cases. *Circulation* 1990;82:507.

10. Cohen M, Fuster V, Steele PM, *et al.* Coarctation of the aorta: long-term follow-up and prediction of outcome after surgical correction. *Circulation* 1989;80:840.

11. Connelly MS, Webb GD, Somerville J, *et al.* Canadian consensus conference on adult congenital heart disease— 1996. *Can J Cardiol* 1998;14:399.

12. Dajani AS, Taubert KA, Wilson W, *et al.* Prevention of bacterial endocarditis: recommendations by the American Heart Association. *J Am Dent Assoc* 128:1142, 1997.

13. Dittman H, lacksch R, Voelker W, *et al.* Accuracy of Doppler echocardiography in quantification of left to right shunts in adult patients with atrial septal defect. *J Am Coll Cardiol* 1988;1l:338.

14. Driscoll D, Allen HD, Atkins DL, *et al.* Guidelines for evaluation and management of common congenital cardiac problems in infants, children, and adolescents: a statement for healthcare professionals from the Committee on Congenital Cardiac Defects of the Council on Cardiovascular Disease in the Young, American Heart Association. *Circulation* 1994;90:2180.

15. Driscoll DJ: Left-to-right shunt lesions. *Pediatr Clin North Am* 1999;46:355.

16. Frommelt PC, Snider AR, Meliones IN, *et al.* Doppler assessment of pulmonary artery flow patterns and ventricular function after the Fontan operation. *Am J Cardiol* l991;68:1211.

17. Gatzoulis MA, Freeman MA, Siu SC, *et al.* Atrial of arrhythmia after surgical closure of atrial septal defects in adults. *N Engl J Med* 1999;340:839.

18. Gentles TL, Calder L, Clarkson PM: Predictors long-term survival with Ebstein's anomaly of the tricuspid valve. *Am J Cardiol* 1992;53:332.

19. Ghai A, Silversides C, Harris L, *et al.* Left ventricular dysfunction is a risk factor for sudden cardiac death in adults late after repair of tetralogy of Fallot. *J Am Coll Cardiol* 2002; 40:1675.

20. Goldmuntz E, Clark BJ, Mitchell , *et al.* Frequency of 22q11 deletion in patients with conotruncal defects. *J Am Coll Cardiol* 1998;32:492.

21. Goyal VS, Fulwani MC, Ramakantan R, *et al.* Follow-up after coll closure of patent ductus arteriosus. *Am J Cardiol* 1999;83:463.

22. Hunter PA, Kreb DL, Mantel SF: Twenty-five years' experience with the arterial switch operation. *J Thorac Cardiovasc Surg* 2002;124:790.

23. Kaulitz R. Stumpel' OFW, Geuskens R. *et al.* Comparative values of precordial and transesophageal approaches in the echocardiographic evaluation of atrial valve function after an atrial conviction procedure. *J Am Coll Cardiol* 1990;16:686.

24. Klcwer SE, Samson RA, Donnerstein RL. *et al.* Comparison of accuracy of diagnosis of congenital heart disease by history and physical examination versus echocardiography. *Am J Cardiol* 2002;89:1329.

25. Kronzon I, Tunick PA, Freedberg RS, *et al.* Transesophageal echocardiography is superior to transthoracic echocardiography in the diagnosis of sinus venosus atrial septal efect. *J Am Coll Cardiol* 1991;17: 537.

26. Lang D, Oberhoffer R, Cook A, *et al.* Pathologic spectrum of malformations of the tricuspid valve in prenatal and neonatal life. *J Am Coll Cardiol* 1991;17:1161.

27. Lipshultz SE, Sanders SP, Mayer IE, *et al.* Are routine preoperative cardiac catheterization and angiography necessary before repair of ostium primum atrial septal defect? *J Am Coll Cardiol* 1988; II :373.

28. Ludomirsl A, Tani L, Murphy DJ. *et al.* Usefulness of colour-flow Doppler in diagnosing and in differentiating supmclistal ventricular septal defect from right ventricular outflow tract obstruction. *Am J Cardiol* 1991;67:194.

29. Lureidini SB, Appleton RS, Nouri S, *et al*. Detection of coronary artery abnormalities in tetralogy of Fallot by two-dimensional echocardiography. *J Am Coll Cardiol* 1998;14:960.

30. Magee AG, Brzezinska-Rajszys G, Qureshi SA, *et al*. Stent implantation for aortic coarctation and recoarctation. *Heart* 1999;82:600.

31. Mail' DD, Hagler DJ, *et al*. Early and late results of the modified Fontan procedure for double-inlet left ventricle: the Mavo Clinic experience. *J Am Coll Cardiol* 1991;18:1727.

32. Martin RP, Qureshi SA, Ettedgui IA, *et al*. An evaluation of right and left ventricular function after anatomical coarctation and intra-atrial repair operations for complete transposition of the great arteries. *Circulation* 1990; 82:808.

33. Marx GR, Allen HD. Accuracy and pitfalls of Doppler evaluation of the pressure gradient in aortic coarctation. *J Am Coll Cardiol* 1986; 7:1379.

34. Mehta RH, Helmcke F, Nanda NC, *et al*. Transesophageal Doppler colour flow mapping assessment of atrial septal defect. *J Am Coll Cardiol* 1990; 16:1010.

35. Meissner MD, Panidis LP, Eshaghpour E, *et al*. Connected transposition of the great arteries: evaluation by two-dimensional and Doppler echocardiography. *Am Heart J* 1986;111:599.

36. Moises VA, Maciel BC, Hornberger LK, *et al*. A new method for noninvasive estimation of ventricular septal defect shunt flow by Doppler colour flow mapping: imaging of the laminar flow convergence region on the left septal surface. *J Am Coll Cardiol* 1991; 18:824.

37. Mullen MJ, Dias BF, Walker F, *et al*. Intracardiac echocardiography guided device closure of atrial septal defects. *J Am Coll Cardiol* 2003;41 :285.

38. Musewe NN, Smallhorn IF, Benson LN, *et al*. Validation of Doppler' derived pulmonary arterial pressure in patients with ductus mletio IUS under different hemodynamic states. *Circulation* 1987:76: 1081.

39. Nihoyannopoulos P, Karas S: Sapsford RN, *et al*. Accuracy of two-dimensional echocardiography in the diagnosis of aortic arch obstruction. *J Am Coll Cardiol* 1987;10:1072.

40. Niwa K, Siu SC, Webb GD, *et al*. Progressive aortic root dilation in adults late after repair of tetralogy of Fallot. *Circulation* 2002;106:1374.

41. Perloff JK, Miner PD: Specialised facilities for the comprehensive care of adults with congenital heart disease. *Congenital Heart Disease in Adults,* 2nd ed. Perloff JK, Child JS, Eds. Philadelphia, WB Saunders Co, 1998.

42. Pieroni DR, Nishimura RA, Bierman Fl, *et al*. Second natural history study of congenital heart defects. Ventricular septal defect: echocardiography. *Circulation* 1993; 87(Suppl1): 1–80.

43. Prendergast B, Newby DE, Wilson LE, *et al*. Early therapeutic experience with the endothelin antagonist BQ-123 in pulmonary hypertension after congenital heart surgery. *Heart* 1999;82:505.

44. Quaegcbeur LM, Sreeram N, Fl'aSer AG, *et al*. Surgery for Ebstein's anomaly: the clinical and echocardiographic evaluation of a new technique. *J Am Coll Cardiol* 1991;17:722.

45. Qureshi SA, Richheimel' R, McKay R, *et al*. Doppler echocardiographic evaluation of pulmonary artery flow after modified Fontan operation: Importance of atrial contraction. *Br Heart J* 1990;64:272.

46. Ramaciotti C, Keren A, Silvlyman NH. Importance of (perimembranous) ventricular septal aneurysm in the natural history of isolated perimembranous ventricular septal defect. *Am J Cardiol* 1986;57: 268.

47. Rosenzweig EB, Kerstein D, Barst RJ: Long-term prostacyclin for pulmonary hypertension with associated congenital heart defects. *Circulation* 1858;1999;99.

48. Sanches-Ugarte T, Keirns C, *et al*. Calcification of patent ductus arteriosus detected by two-dimensional echocardiography. *Am Heart J* 1987; 114:446.

49. Stanger P, Cassidy SC, Girod DA, *et al*. Balloon pulmonary valvuloplasty: results of the Valvuloplasty and Angioplasty of Congenital Anomalies Registry. *Am J Cardiol* 1990;65:775.

50. Suzuki K, Yamaki S, Mimori S, *et al*. Pulmonary vascular disease in Down's syndrome with complete atrioventricular septal defect. *Am J Cardiol* 2000; 86:434.

51. Ueno T, Smith JA, Snell GI, *et al*. Bilateral sequential single lung transplantation for pulmonary hypertension and Eisenmenger's syndrome. *Ann Thorac Surg* 2000;69:381.

52. Wilson NJ, Clarkson PM, Barratt-Boyes BG, *et al*. Long-term outcome after the Mustard repair for simple transposition of the great arteries. *J Am Coll Cardiol* 1998;32:758.

53. Single lung transplantation for pulmonary hypertension and Eisenmenger's syndrome. *Ann Thorac Surg* 2000;69:381.

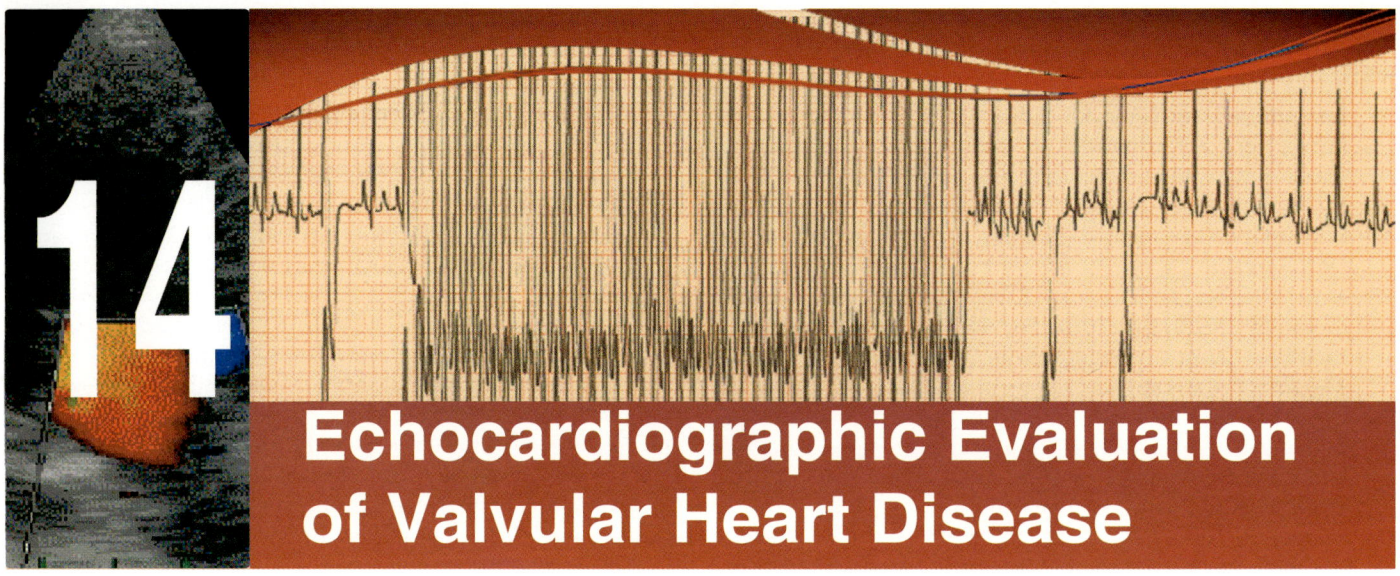

14

Echocardiographic Evaluation of Valvular Heart Disease

Rheumatic fever is a diffuse inflammatory condition usually occuring between the ages of 5 and 15 years, affects the heart, joints, skin and brain. It probably represents autoimmune response to pharyngeal infection with group A hemolytic streptococcus. Mitral valve is the commonest one among the rest of the AV and semilunar valves, affected by this disease.

M-mode and two-dimensional echocardiography represents a significant advance because it has provided the means for comprehensive noninvasive evaluation of both AV and semilunar valvular functions.

Mitral Stenosis (Figs 14.10–14.17)

Mitral valvular area in normal individual is about 5.0 cm^2. When stenosis is present, this orifice measurement is decreased. A valve area of 2.5 cm^2 indicates mild stenosis, whereas an area of 1.0 cm^2 represents moderately severe stenosis, and area less than 1.0 cm^2 is usually considered as severe type of stenosis.

Many workers have found that patients with E-F slopes of less than 10 mm/sec by M-mode criteria would be considered to have severe mitral stenosis. However, when these patients were evaluated by the short-axis real time technique, only two thirds could be expected to have severe mitral stenosis with the criteria of a mitral valve area measuring less than 1.3 cm^2. Some of the workers are of the opinion that where slopes higher than 10 mm/sec are found, the M-mode could not predict the severity of the lesion with good index of sensitivity and specificity.

Evaluation of the mitral orifice (leaflet pliability, thickening, and restriction) should be made in two planes—the short and long axis. The orifice is accessed in the short-axis plane first, and a planimeter measurement is taken at its narrowest point, near the leaflet tips in diastole. The gain settings are then reduced to eliminate reverberations produced by the fibrosis and thickening. Often the mitral orifice has an irregular configuration, hence it should be carefully recorded for the accurate orifice opening (Figs 14.29–14.31 and 14.37).

On M-mode echocardiography, the most consistent finding in mitral stenosis is the reduction of the E-F slope of the anterior leaflet of the valve; in such cases, therefore, the velocity of the E-F slope measures less than 35 mm/sec. Since this slope is an indicator of the rate of left atrial emptying and in mitral stenosis particularly the decreased slope signifies an obstruction caused by the stenotic orifice (Figs 11.41–14.45).

Table 14.1: *Various aetiological factors affecting mitral valve*
Diseases directly affecting the mitral apparatus
Rheumatic heart disease (Figs 14.75 and 14.76)
Congenital mitral stenosis
Congenital cleft mitral valve
Infectious endocarditis (Figs 14.73 and 14.74)
Marantic endocarditis
Libman-Sacks endocarditis
Hypereosinophilic heart disease
Coronary artery disease
Diet drug valvulopathy
Mitral annular calcification (Figs 14.85 and 14.86)
Degenerative
Infiltrative
Carcinoid
Indirect effect on mitral valve function
Dilated cardiomyopathy
Hypertrophic cardiomyopathy
Left atrial myxoma
Myocardial ischemia or infarction

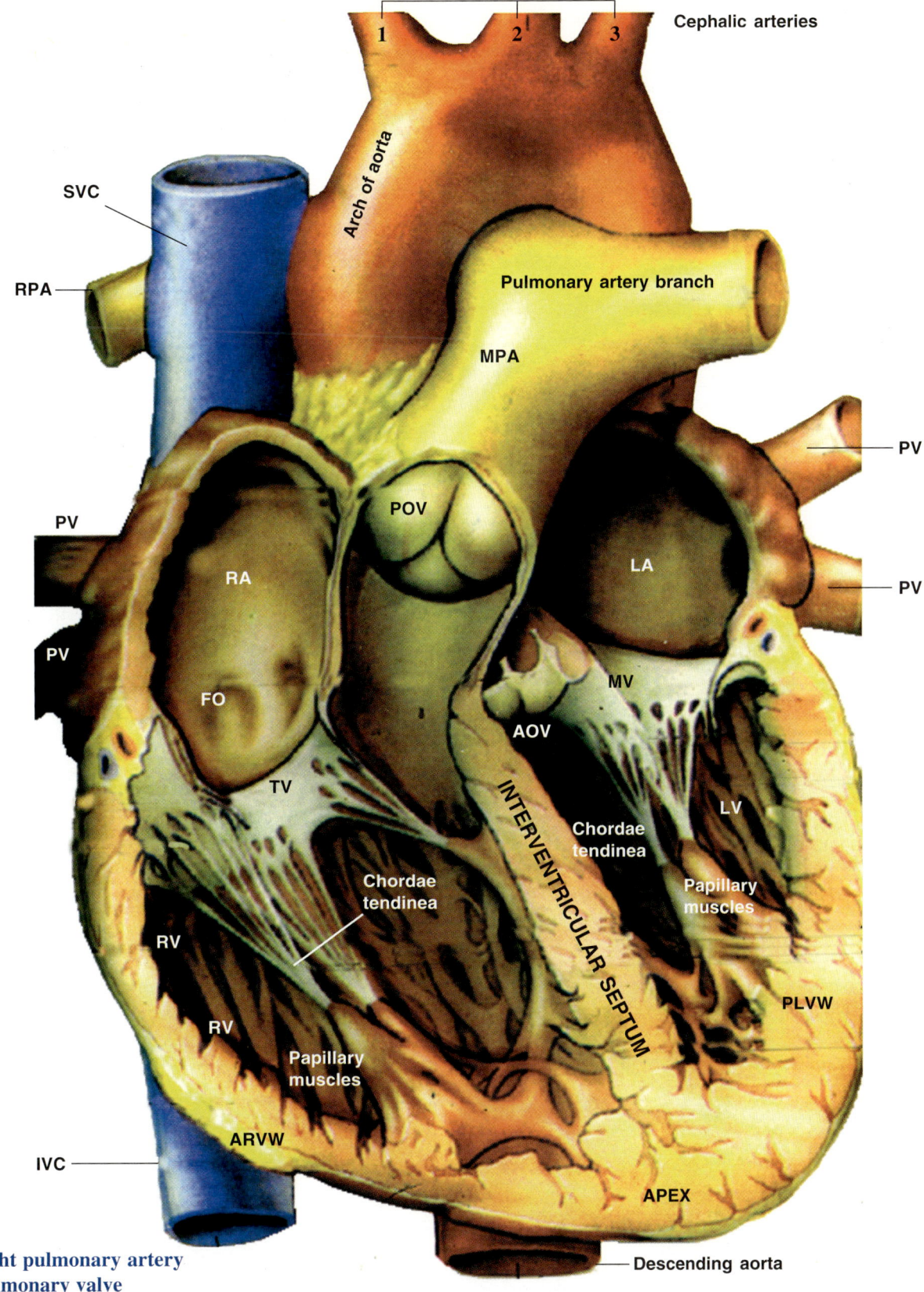

RPA = Right pulmonary artery
POV = Pulmonary valve

Fig. 14.1: Cadaveric diagram showing anatomical location and morphological features of A-V valves, intracardiac structures, myocardium and great vessels of human heart, LV = Left ventricle, RV = Right ventricle, PLVW = Posterior left ventricular wall, MV = Mitral valve, TV = Tricuspid valve, FO = Foramen ovale, AOV = Aortic valve, ARVW = Anterior right ventricular wall, PV = Pulmonary vein, LA = Left atrium and RA = Right atrium. IVC=Inferior vena cava, SVC = Superior vena cava

Visualization of Mitral Valve and its Apparatus by Technique of TTE

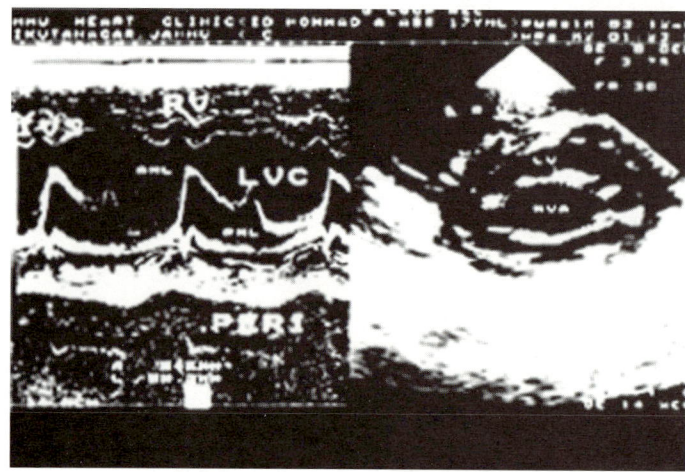

Fig. 14.2: (L-R) M-Mode and 2D scan showing normal morphological features of MV

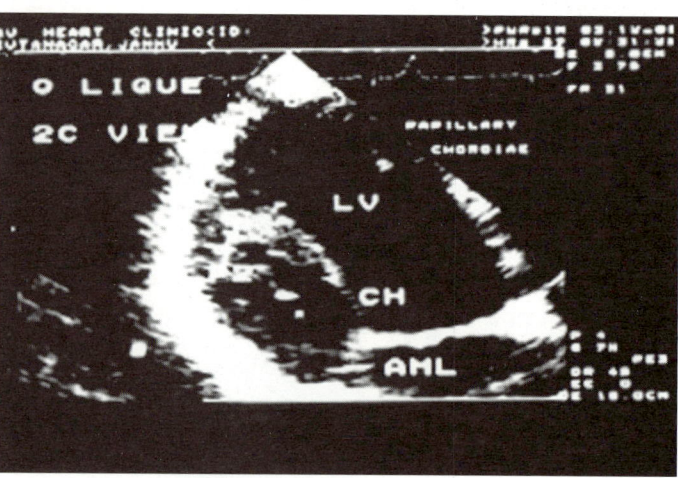

Fig. 14.3: 2-D Oblique in 2C view showing papillary muscle and chordae tendinea (CH) LV = left ventricle

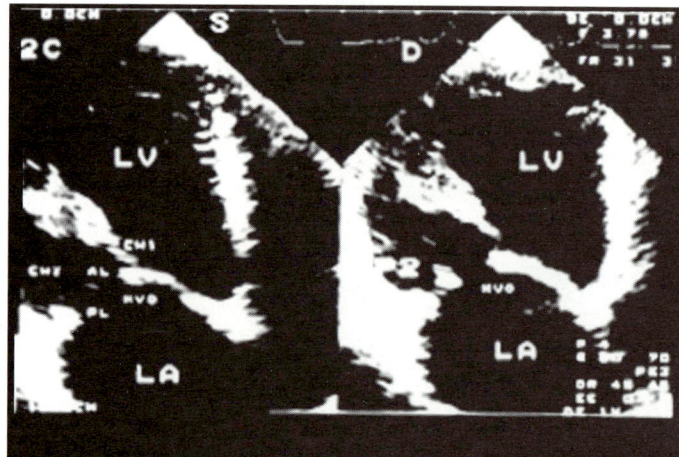

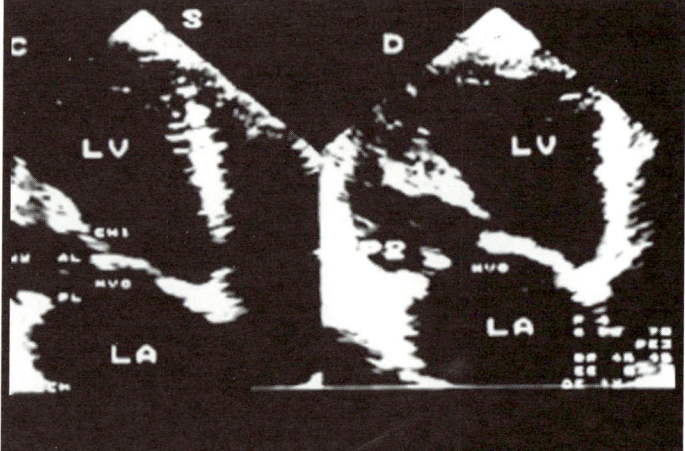

Figs 14.4 and 5: 2D 2C view showing AML, PML and CH1 and CH2 and two major chambers LA and LV PM1= Anterior papillary muscle and PM2 = Posterior papillary muscle. CH1 = Anterior chordie tendinea and CH2 = Posterior tendinea

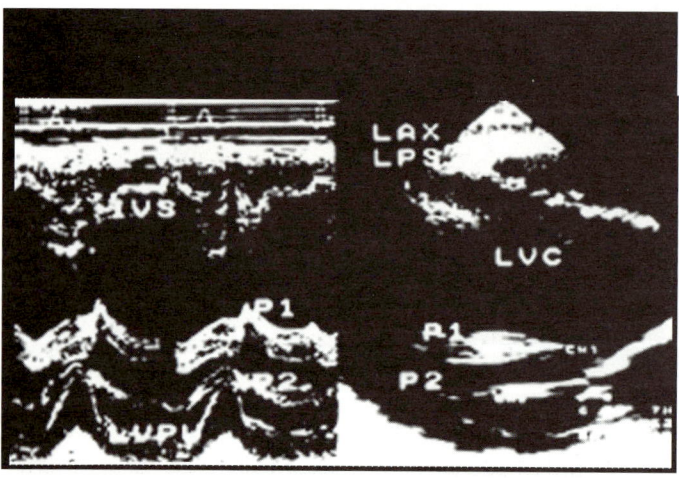

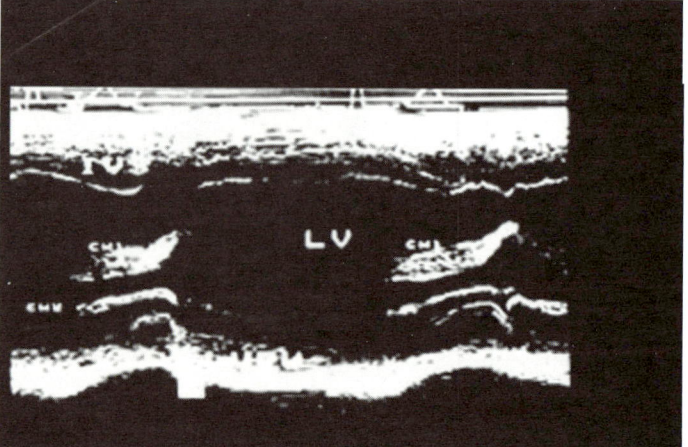

Figs. 14.6 and 7: M-Mode and 2D 2C views (L-R) showing relationship of left ventricular cavity and both anterior and posterior papillary muscles (P1 and P2). Right panel M-Mode echoscan showing attachment of chordea tendinea to posterior papillary muscle (P_2)

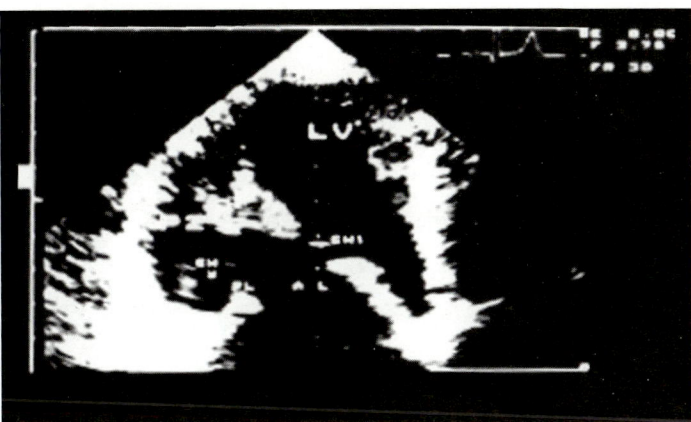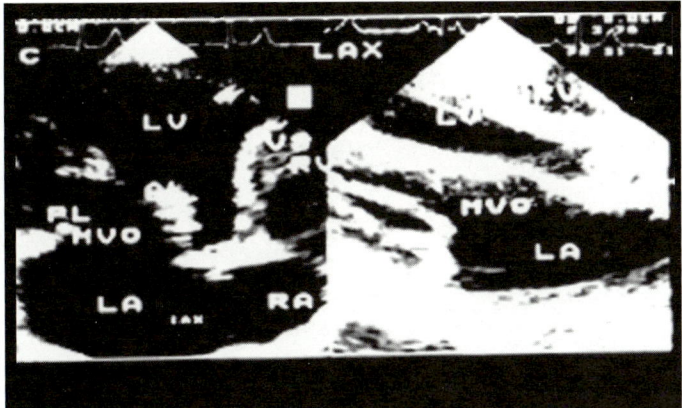

Figs 14.8 and 9: 2-D Oblique view at LV showing normal anatomical relationship between LV, LA chordiae tendiae and papillary muscles MVO = Mitral valve orifice

In addition to the decreased E-F slope, the posterior leaflet moves in the anterior direction just like its fellow partner, anterior leaflet, due to commissural fusion. In very mild cases of mitral stenosis with least thickening or calcification, the posterior leaflet may move in its normal posterior position.

The amplitude, or D-E excursion of the valve measures the degree of mobility or restriction on the leaflet. In a heavily calcified valve, this amplitude is reduced. To assess the maximum mobility of the valve, the examiner must angle the transducer carefully. After the leaflet has been visualised a search is made for its greatest excursion by slight additional angulations of the transducer or by moving the beam up or down through the window already selected (Fig. 14.21).

Increased echoes on the mitral apparatus indicate thickening or the presence of calcification. The gain settings must be carefully adjusted so calcification can be distinguished from reverberation. When the posterior leaflet is well shown, the sensitivity should be gradually reduced to assess the degree of calcification from the remaining echoes (Figs 14.10 and 14.11).

The incidence of atrial fibrillation in mitral stenosis is about 50%. This has serious consequences as it indicates loss of effective coordinated atrial contractions since atrial contraction may contribute 15% to 20% of left ventricular filling. The sudden occurrence of this arrhythmia, with a rapid ventricular rate response, is often accompanied by pulmonary edema. Systemic emboli are common in patients with mitral stenosis because of the relative stasis and diminished flow from the left atrium to the left ventricle and the inflammatory reaction within the left atrial wall (Figs 14.92 and 14.93).

It may also be justifiable to evaluate other cardiac chambers in order to determine the degree of stenosis or rheumatic involvement. In pure mitral stenosis the left ventricle is of normal size. In the presence of mitral regurgitation there exists left ventricle volume load. The left atrium is always enlarged in mitral valve disease; however, with combined mitral stenosis and regurgitation it further increases in dimension, measuring 6 cm or more (Fig. 14.39).

At times it is difficult to assess the posterior movement of the valve in the presence of **a calcified mitral annulus on M-mode echo** alone, hence the leaflet should be accessed with both M-mode and two-dimensional study to separate the posterior leaflet from the calcified annulus (Figs 14.85–14.87).

Decreased Mitral Valve Slope without Mitral Stenosis

1. Decreased contractility of the left ventricle can cause a pseudomitral stenosis, due to a decreased amplitude and reduced E-F, slope of the anterior leaflet of the valve. But the E-F slope usually does not fall below the 35 mm/sec seen in patients with mitral stenosis. The posterior leaflet moves in its normal posterior direction during diastole (Fig. 14.12).

2. Aortic stenosis may also cause a reduced mitral slope and amplitude as a result of the increased pressures within the left ventricle. Calcification of the mitral annulus may make it further difficult to visualise the posterior leaflet, and careful angulation of the transducer should allow the technical officer to separate the posterior leaflet from the calcification of other structures.

3. Hypertrophic cardiomyopathy may cause the anterior leaflet to be decreased amplitude in diastole. In addition, a systolic anterior motion of the mitral apparatus is seen in the obstructive form of hypertrophic cardiomyopathy. The posterior leaflet would be unaffected in these patients. There may be some left atrial enlargement secondary to mitral regurgitation (Figs 14.88 and 14.89).

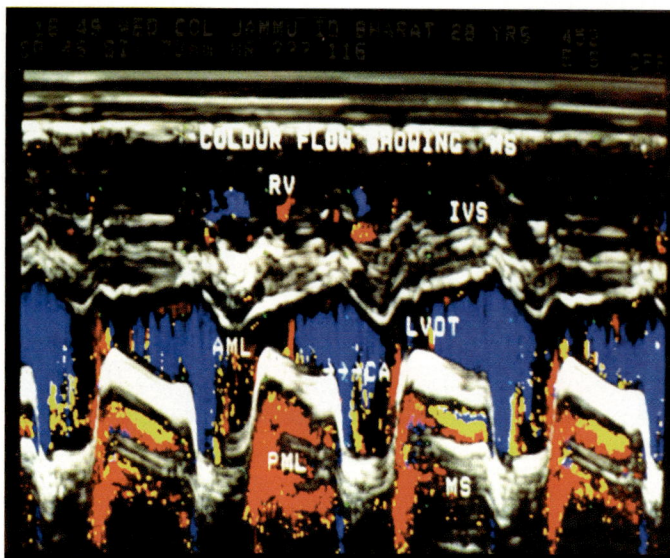

Fig. 14.10: M-Mode echocardiogram in color mode showing mosaic color in stenosed MV during diastole and normal blue color in LVOT in systole in rheumatic mitral valvular stenosis

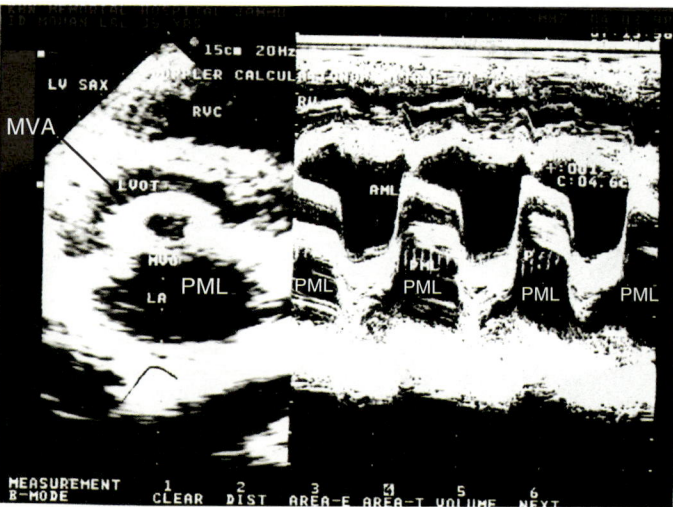

Fig. 14.11: 2D Short axis LV view at mitral valve level (left) and M-Mode echoscan at mitral valve (right) showing reduction of mitral valve area, thickening of both anterior and posterior mitral leaflets with paradoxical movement of posterior leaflet in moderately severe mitral valvular stenosis

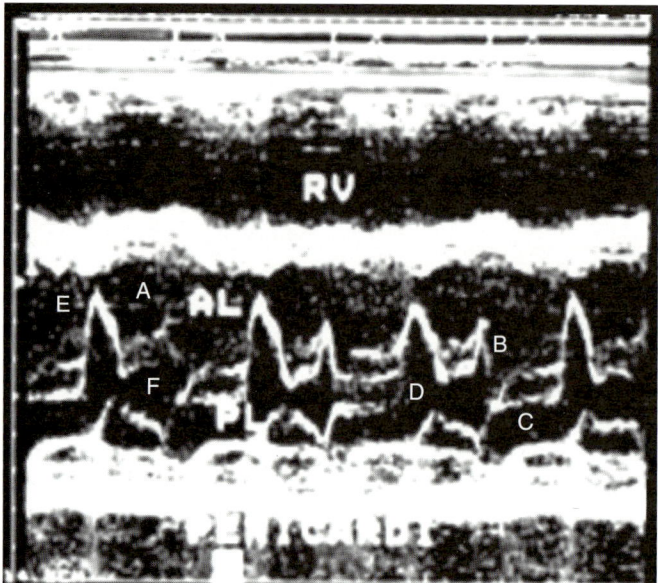

Fig. 14.12: M-Mode echocardiogram showing normal morphological features of mitral valve with A, B, C, D, E and F hemodynamic letters

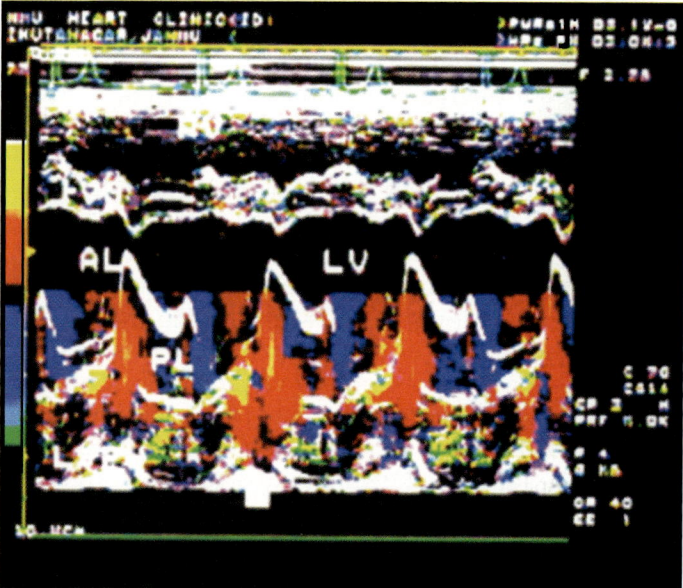

Fig. 14.13: Normal color flow through normal mitral valve. AL = Anterior mitral leaflet and PL = Postrior mitral leaflet, LV = Left ventricle

4. A left atrial myxoma or other such tumor is another form of obstruction to left atrial flow. The tumor may be small or large enough to completely obstruct the left atrial outflow tract. In patients with a myxoma, the tumor is attached to the atrial wall by a pedicle and prolapses into the ventricular chamber shortely after the onset to diastole. It can be distinguished from a severely calcified valve by the early diastolic space occurring after the onset of diastole before the tumor flops posterior to the mitral apparatus. A heavily calcified valve shows increased echoes throughout the diastolic phase.

Doppler Assessment of Mitral Stenosis

Doppler echocardiography can contribute a lot in the evaluation of patients with mitral valve disease. In mitral stenosis, Doppler measurements supplement the two-dimensional echocardiography in the valuation of valvular morphology and its hemodynamic information. After routine two-dimensional and M-mode

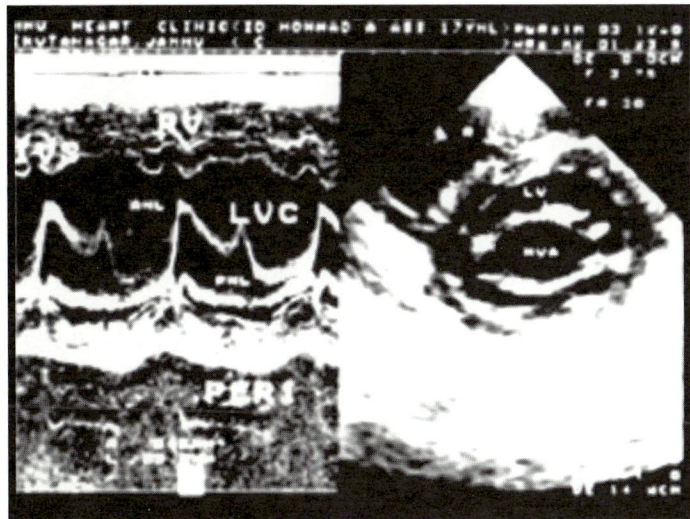

Fig. 14.14: M-Mode and 2D LV views in dual scan frame showing normal features of MV and normal mitral valve area (MVA)

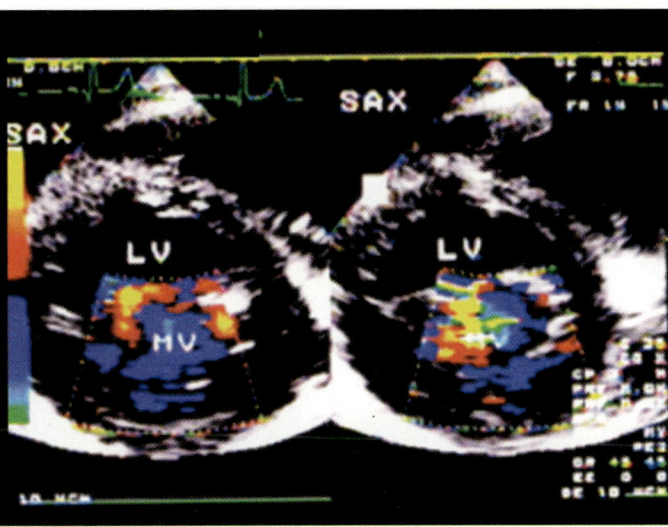

Fig. 14.15: Short axis dual scan in color showing normal color view of mitral valve area. MV = Mitral valve

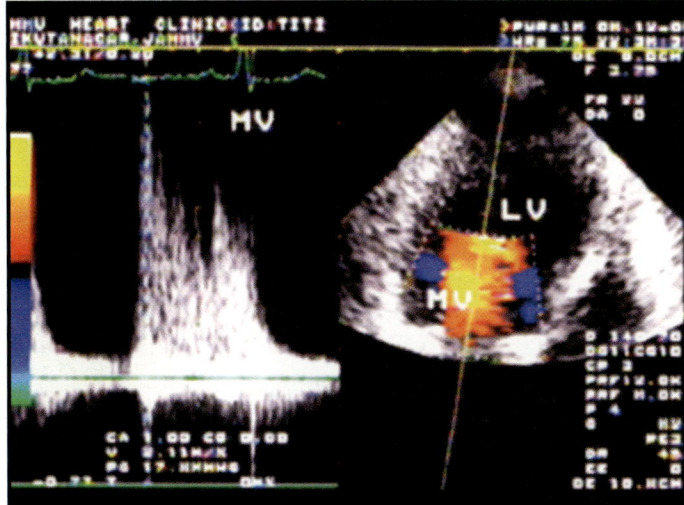

Fig. 14.16: Apical four chamber view in color Doppler mode at MV showing morphological and Doppler velocity features of normal mitral valve

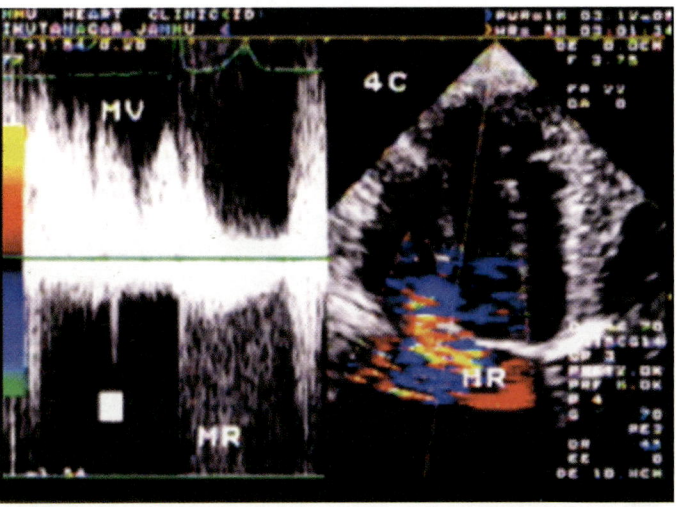

Fig. 14.17: Apical four chamber view in color Doppler mode at MV showing morphological and Doppler velocity features of mitral stenosis (forward flow) and MR (backward flow) with typical MS jet with aliasing

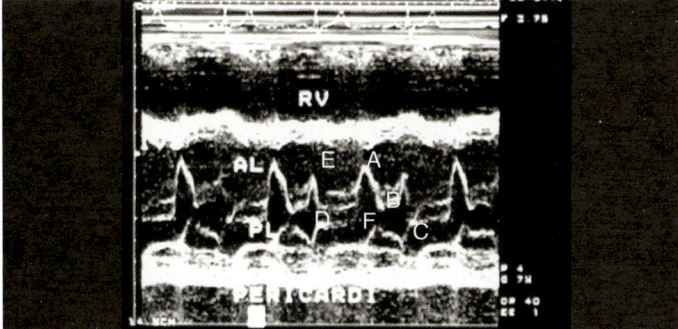

Fig. 14.18: M-Mode echocardiogram showing normal morphological features of mitral valve. RV = Right ventricle. AL = Anterior mitral leaflet and PL = Posterior mitral leaflet and hemodynamic lettering A, B, C, D, E and F

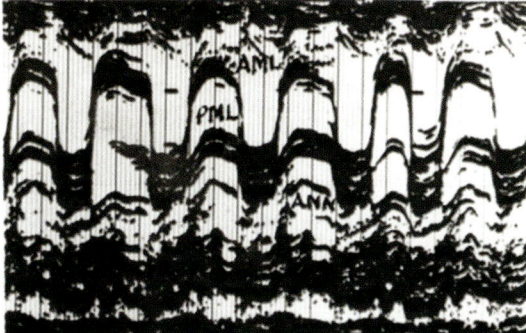

Fig. 14.19: M-Mode echocardiogram showing reduction of EF slope, and thickening of both anterior and posterior mitral leaflets with paradoxical movement of posterior mitral leaflet in mild to moderate mitral valvular stenosis

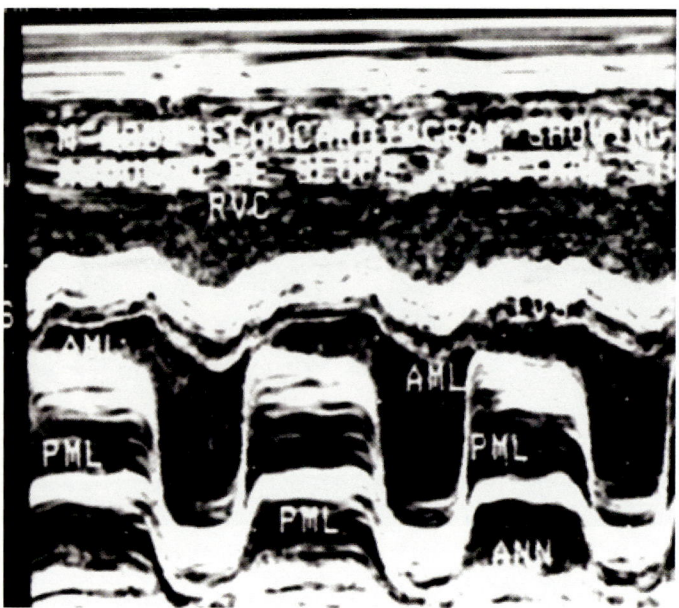

Fig. 14.20: M-Mode echocardiogram showing reduction of EF slope and DE amplitude and thickening of both anterior and posterior mitral leaflets with paradoxical movement of posterior mitral leaflet in moderate mitral valvular stenosis

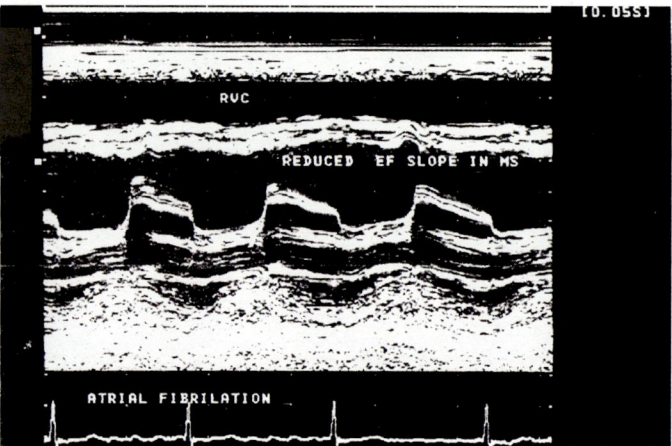

Fig. 14.21: M-Mode echocardiogram showing reduction of EF slope, DE amplitude, calcification of both anterior vand posterior mitral leaflets, with paradoxical movement of posterior mitral leaflet in severe type of mitral valvular stenosis

studies have been performed. Doppler measurements at the inflow, annulus, and outflow tract of the mitral valve should be performed after having visualised the mitral apparatus in apical four chamber views.

The Doppler pattern of a normal mitral valve would demonstrate the maximum velocity to be under 100 cm/sec, or less than 1 m/sec. There is rapid deceleration of the velocity after an early diastolic filling. In patients with mitral stenosis the Doppler maximum velocity would be greater than 1 m/sec, and there would be a slower deceleration of blood velocity after the early diastolic filling phase.

This pressure gradient is proportional to the orifice size and to the flow across the mitral valve. The severity of mitral stenosis can be estimated by calculating the mitral valve orifice by different methods such as 2-D mitral valve area the planimetry, pressure half time, and proximal isovelocity surface area (PISA).

Pressure Half Time Method (PHT) (Figs 14.32–14.36)

The pressure half time indicates the measurement of the time required for the peak early diastolic transmitral gradient to fall to one half of its initial value to estimate the mitral orifice area. This can be calculated from the Doppler tracing as follows:

1. Measure the initial peak velocity from the tracing, and draw a vertical line through it. Do not include the outline of the wave velocity.

2. Estimating the velocity, which represents half the initial pressure gradient, is done using the following rationale: (Figs 14.47–14.50)

   (a) The pressure difference is proportional to the velocity squared:

$$P_1 - P_2 \propto V^2$$

   (b) One half the pressure difference is proportional to the maximum velocity squared divided by two:

$$\frac{P_1 - P_2}{2} \propto \frac{V}{2}$$

   (c) Since it can do the same thing to both parts of a fraction without changing

$$\frac{P_1 - P_2}{2} \propto \frac{V^2}{2} = \frac{V^2}{1.4}$$

   Thus the velocity representing half the initial pressure gradient is established by dividing the peak velocity by 1.4. This point is marked on the tracing, and a horizontal line representing that velocity is drawn.

3. To estimate the pressure halftime, a line is drawn along the slope of the maximum velocities, and a vertical line drawn where the calculated velocity crosses the outline. The distance between the two vertical lines is measured, and the time is then calculated from the timing marks at the edge of the trace.

4. Estimating valve orifice area, pressure halftime remains relatively constant for an orifice over a wide range of flows. For a valve area of 1.0 cm², the pressure halftime ($P_{1/2}$) is 220 milliseconds (msec). The effective orifice can be obtained by dividing the actual $P_{1/2}$ into 220 msec.

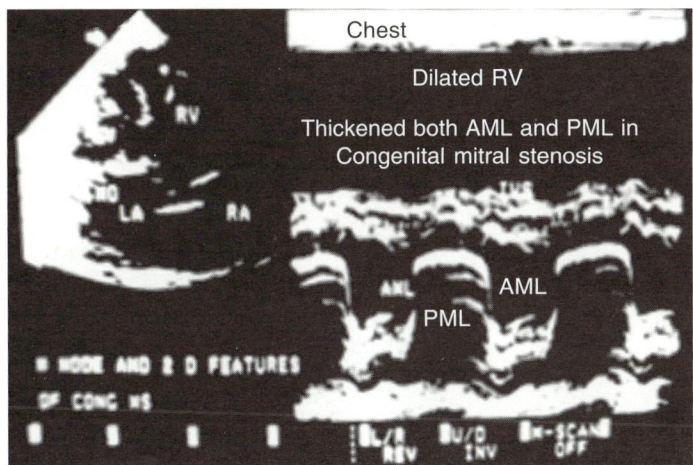

Fig. 14.22: M-Mode (right) and 2D (left) echocardiogram showing thickening of AML, reduction of EF slope and paradoxical movement of thickened PML in a young child of 6 years old with congenital mitral stenosis

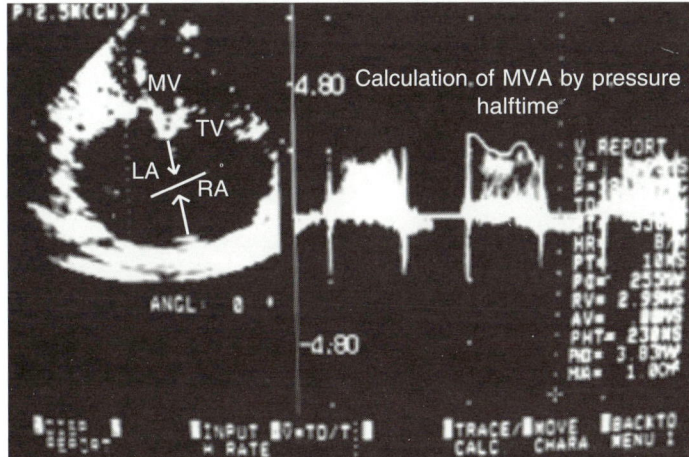

Fig. 14.23: Apical 4C (left) and Doppler flow velocity (right) showing calculation of pressure half time and mitral valve area in the same patient as in Fig. 14.22 in congenital mitral stenosis

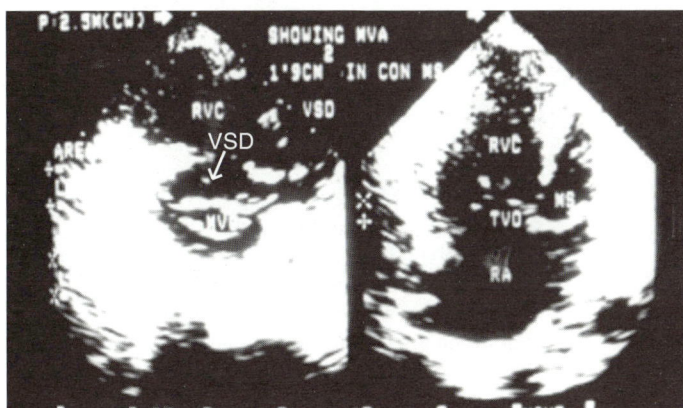

Fig. 14.24: 2-D Short axis (left) and apical 4C (right) showing reduction in mitral valve area (MVA) with ventricular septal defect (VSD) and thickened mitral valve with dilated right atrium (RA) in congenital MS with VSD (arrow)

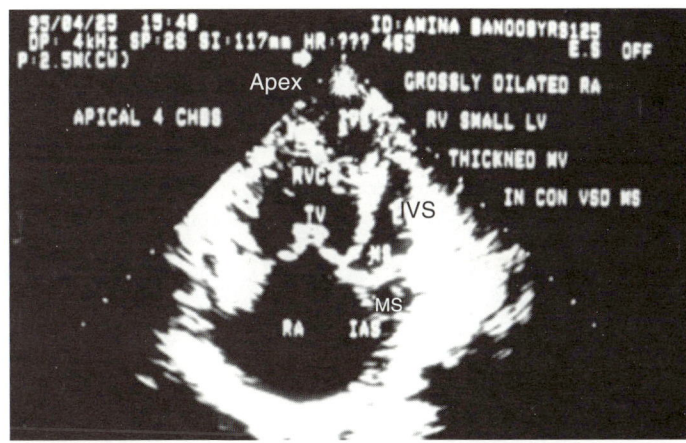

Fig. 14.25: Apical 4C showing markedly thickened MV and mild thickening of TV with apical VSD in patient with congenital mitral stenosis with VSD with dilated right atrium

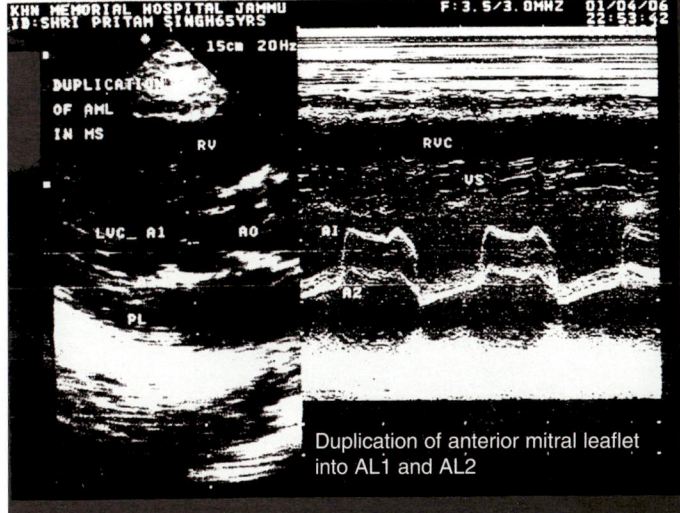

Duplication of anterior mitral leaflet into AL1 and AL2

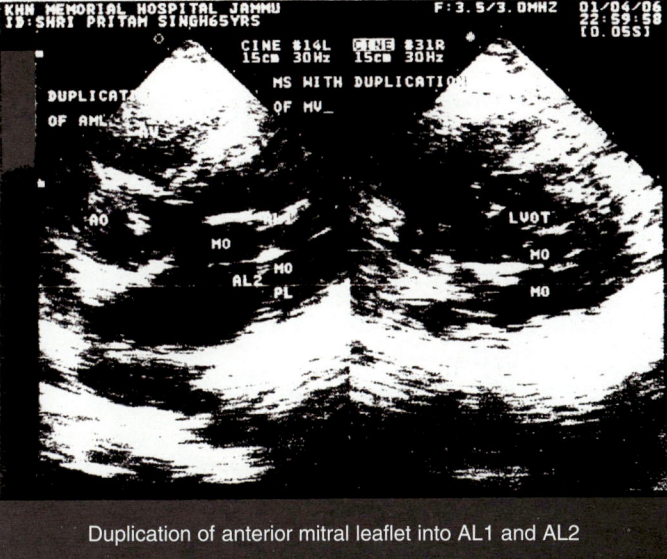

Duplication of anterior mitral leaflet into AL1 and AL2

Fig. 14.26A and B: M-Mode and 2-D echoscans respectively showing duplication of anterior mitral leaflet into AL1 and AL2

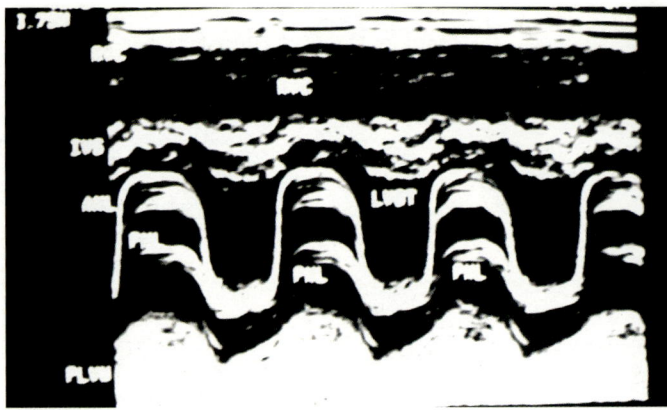

Fig. 14.27: M-Mode echocardiogram showing thickened both anterior and posterior mitral leaflets with paradoxical movement of posterior mitral leaflet in patient with moderate mitral valvular stenosis

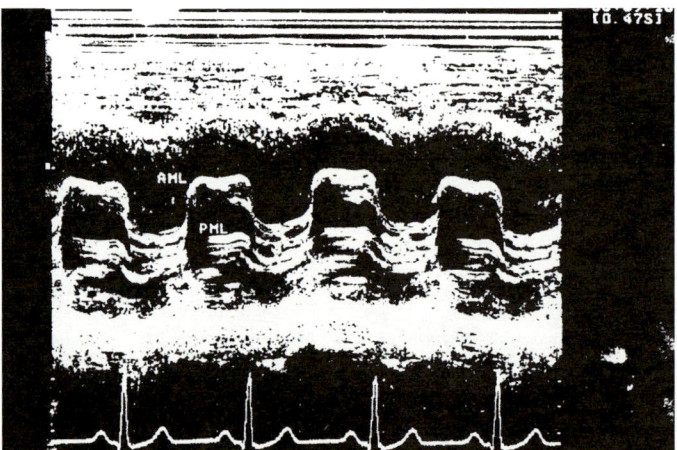

Fig. 14.28: M-Mode echocardiogram showing thickened both anterior and posterior mitral leaflets with paradoxical movement of posterior mitral leaflet thickened subvalvular area, reduction in DE amplitude and EF slope as compared to Fig. 14.27 in patient with severe type of mitral stenosis

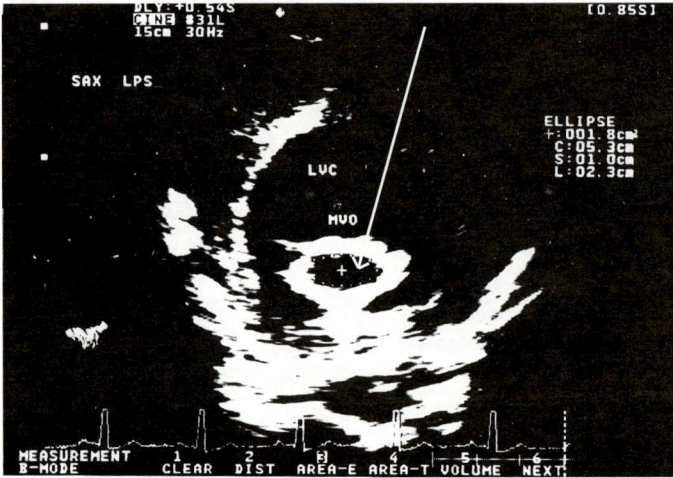

Fig.14.29: Short axis view LV showing calculation of mitral valve area by trace method

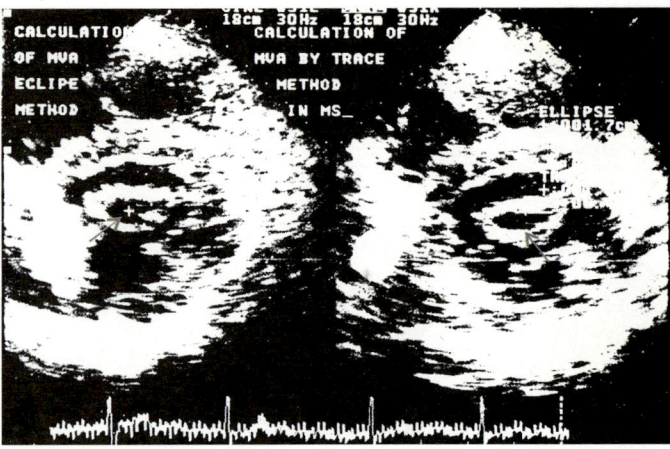

Fig. 14.30: 2-D dual scan in short axis view of LV showing calculation of mitral valve area by trace method (arrow in left panel)

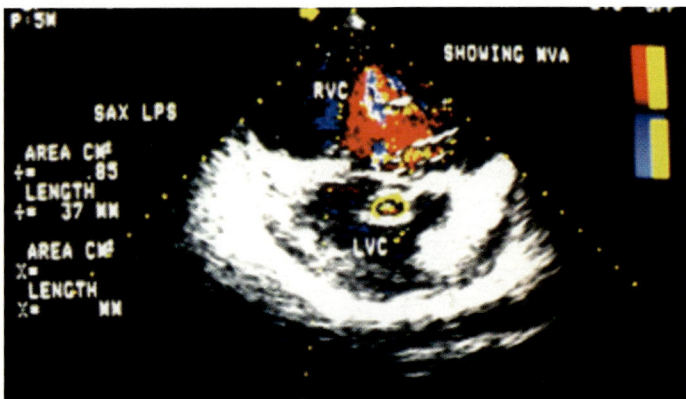

Fig. 14.31: 2-D Short axis view of LV in color mode showing color flow jet of mitral valve stenosis (MVA = 0.85 cm^2)

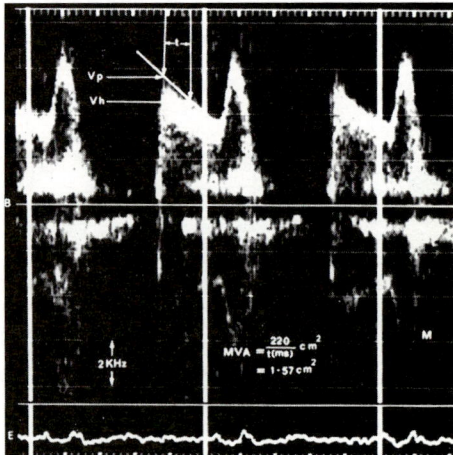

Fig. 14.32: Calculation of mitral valvular area by determining pressure half time as shown on scan. Vp = velocity flow Vh = during half time

t = time taken during fall of velocity in diastole. In this case for example mitral valve area has been calculated as

$$MVA = \frac{220}{t} = 1.57 \text{ cm}^2$$

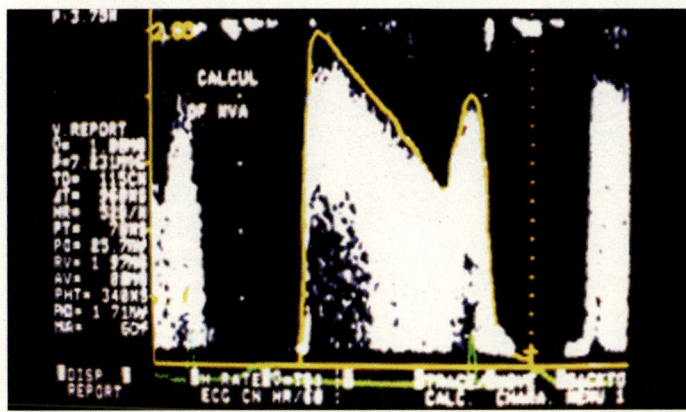

Fig. 14.33: Doppler flow velocity across mitral valve for computer assisted calculation of mitral valve area by just marking the area during diastole with the help of computer provided cursor. The various values are automatically shown on left side of the main graph including peak velocity, pressure gradient pressure half time and finally mitral valve area

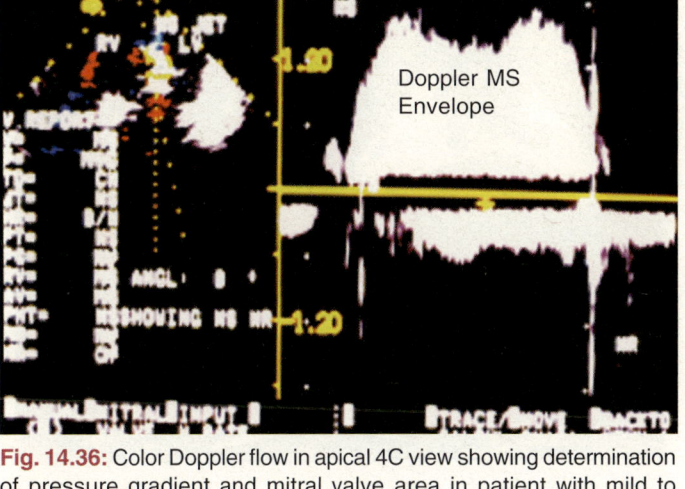

Fig. 14.36: Color Doppler flow in apical 4C view showing determination of pressure gradient and mitral valve area in patient with mild to moderate mitral stenosis

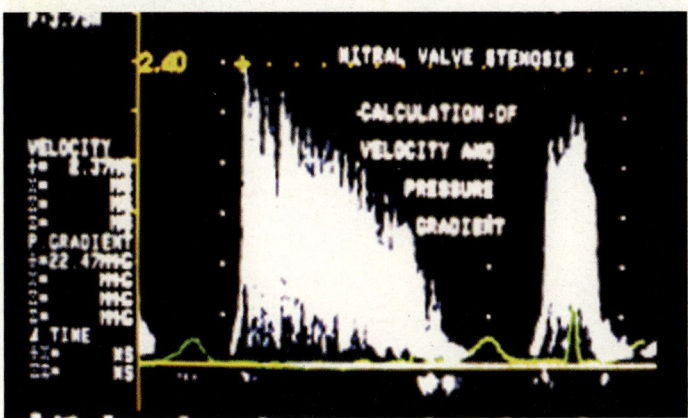

Fig. 14.34: Automatic Computer assisted Doppler method of calculating mitral valve area by determining peak velocity, pressure half time and finally mitral valve area as various values appear on left side of the main graph

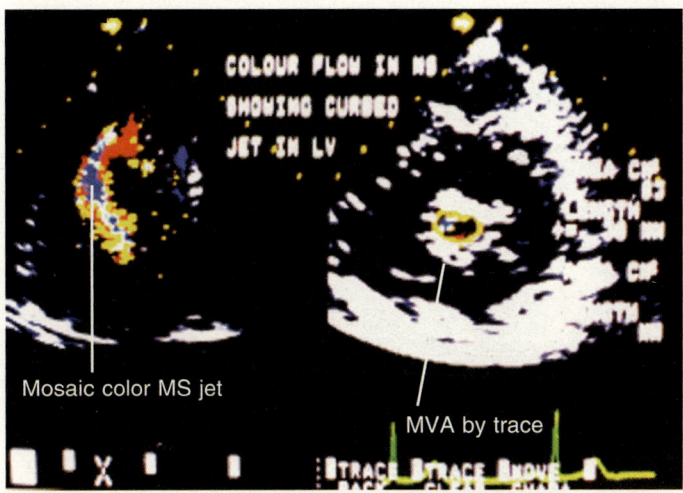

Fig. 14.37: Color flow apical 4C LV view (left) showing C shaped/curved mitral stenotic jet. Right panel shows short axis LV view showing mitral valvular area as a circular trace measurement in patient with severe type of mitral stenosis

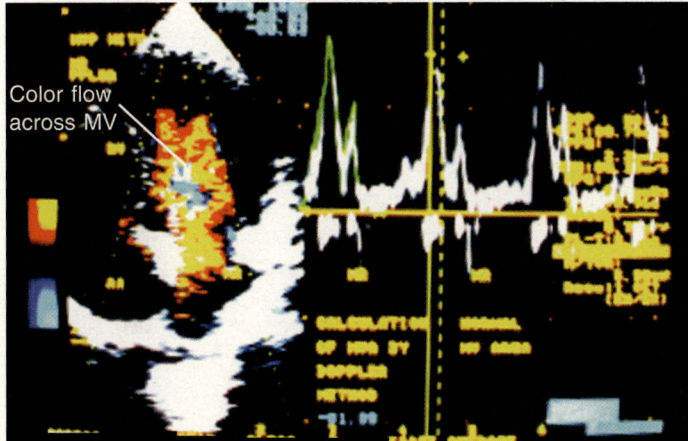

Fig. 14.35: Color Doppler flow in apical 4C view showing determination of pressure gradient and mitral valve area in patient with mild to moderate mitral stenosis

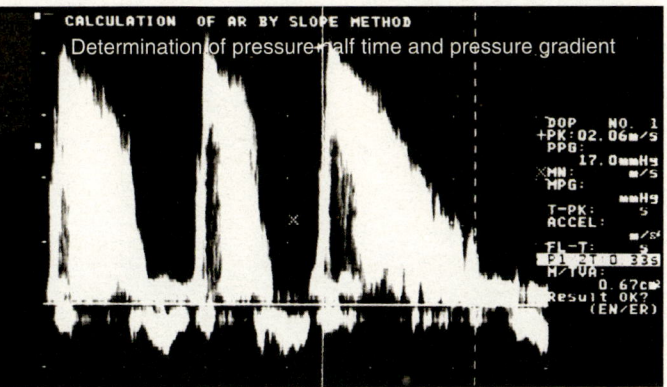

Fig. 14.38: Calculation of pressure gradient and pressure half time in patient with mitral stenosis with atrial fibrillation with fast ventricular response (values of five cardiac cycles should be taken for calculation of data in atrial fibrillation)

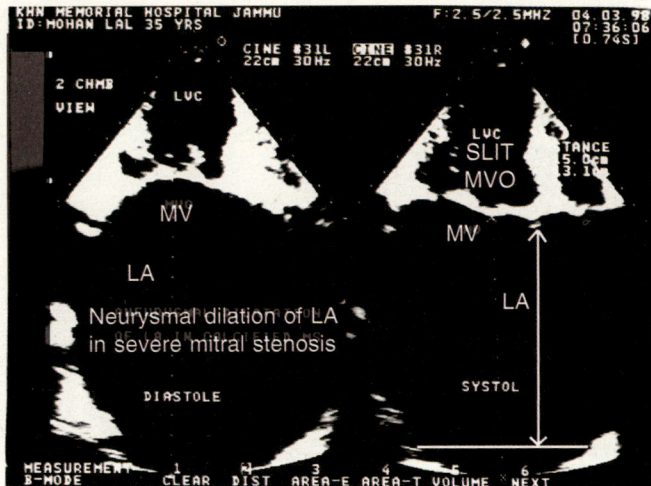

Fig. 14.39: Apical 4 C dual scan view at LV level during systole and diastole showing aneurysmal dilatation of left atrium reduction in LV size, slit type of mitral valve opening in severe form of chronic calcified rheumatic mitral valvular stenosis

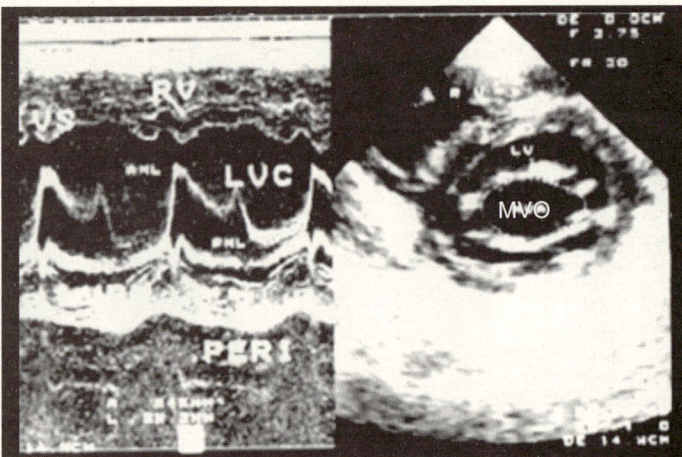

Fig. 14.42: M-Mode and short axis dual scan frame showing normal mitral valve area

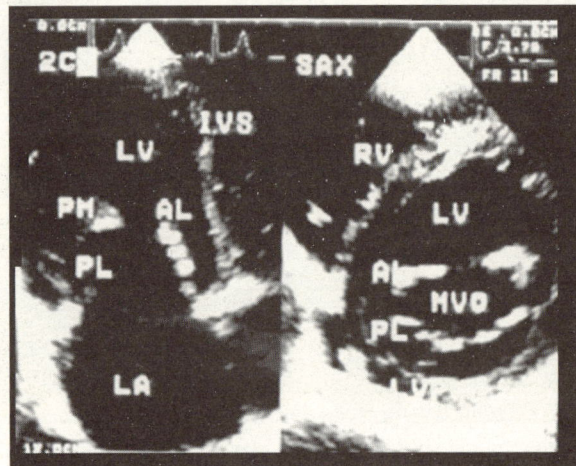

Fig. 14.40: (L-R) 2D 2C and short axis LV show in normal mitral valve orifice (MVO)

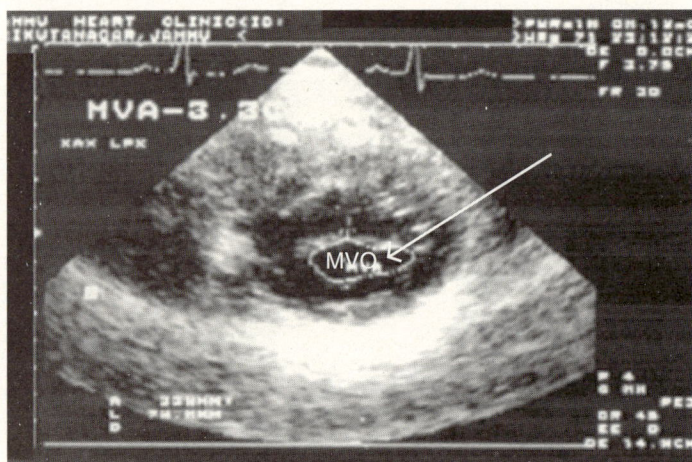

Fig. 14.43: Short axis view taken at left parasternal region showing mild reduction in mitral valve orifice in patient with mitral stenosis (3.3 cm^2)

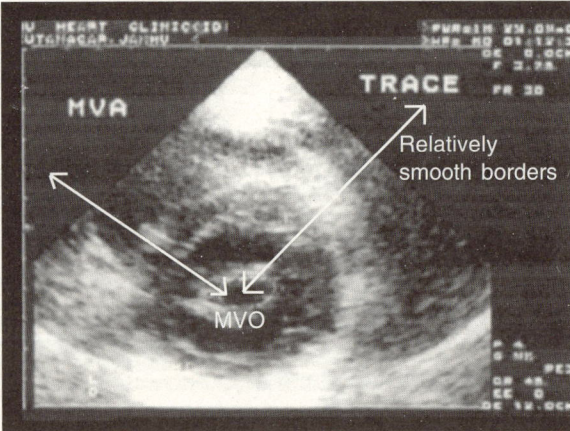

Fig. 14.41: Short axis LV view showing mild reduction in mitral valve orifice in MS (<3.0 cm^2)

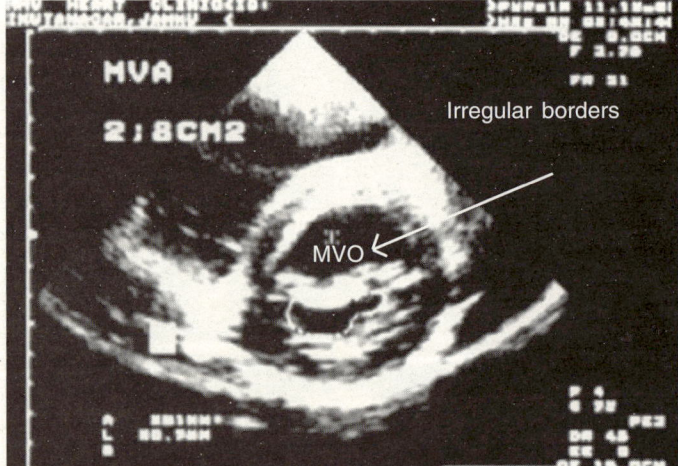

Fig. 14.44: Short axis view LV at left parasternal region showing moderate severe mitral valvular stenosis. MVA = 2.8 cm^2 with irregular and shaggy borders

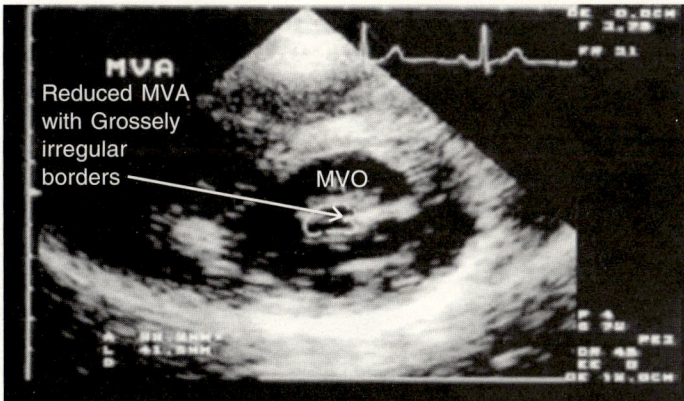

Fig. 14.45: Short axis view LV at left parasternal region showing severe mitral valvular stenosis (MVA = <1.0 cm^2)

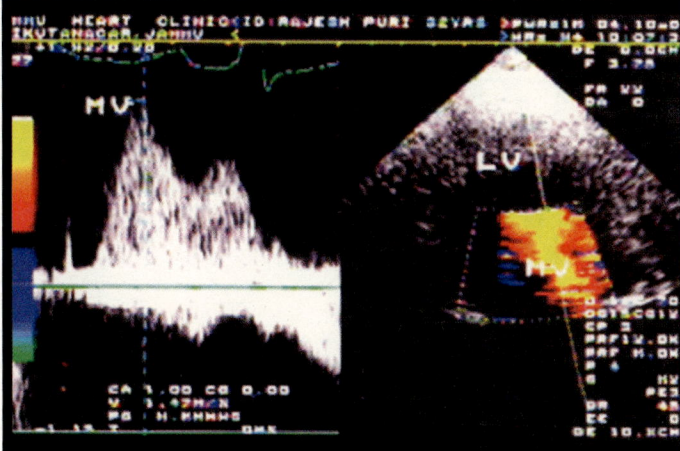

Fig. 14.46: Apical four chamber color Doppler flow velocity across MV showing normal velocity with wide spectral wave form in Doppler mode in a patient with rheumatic mitral valvulitis

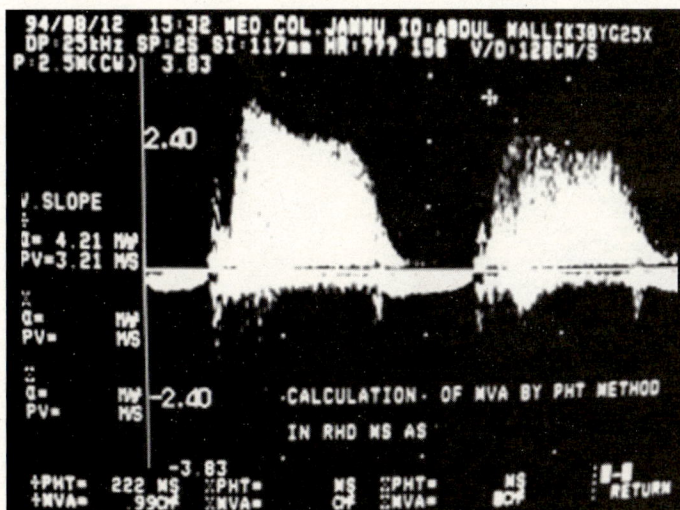

Fig. 14.47: Calculation of pressure gradient across MV by measuring magnitude of Doppler flow velocity by the formula Pressure Gradient = 4 x V^{2i} in patient with moderately severe mitral stenosis

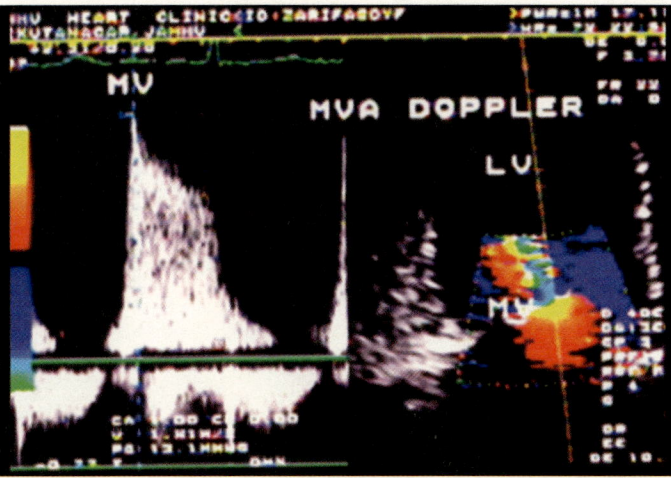

Fig. 14.48: Color Doppler flow velocity across MV showing color jet of MS (right) and velocity flow across MV (left)

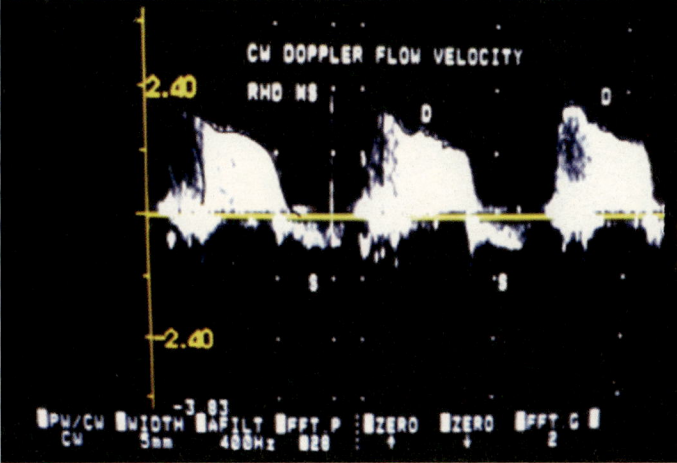

Fig. 14.49: Calculation of pressure gradient across MV by measuring magnitude of Doppler flow velocity by the formula Pressure Gradient = 4 x V^2 in patient with cacified severe mitral stenosis

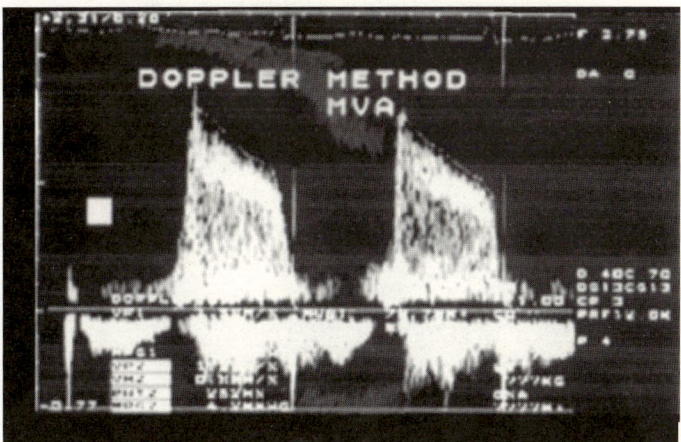

Fig. 14.50: Doppler flow across MV showing calculation of MVA and its severity by pressure half time in patient with moderately severe non-calcified mitral stenosis

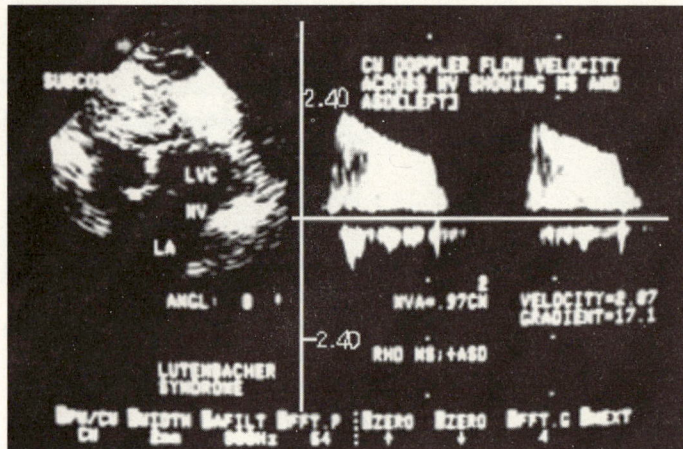

Fig. 14.51: Doppler flow across MV showing further reduction in DE amplitude and enhanced gradient in patient with severe type of calcified mitral stenosis

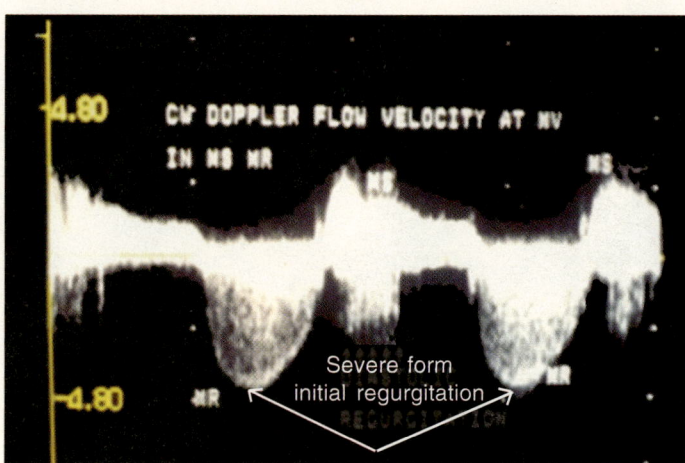

Fig. 14.54: CW Doppler flow velocity across MV in patient with mitral valve stenosis with regurgitation

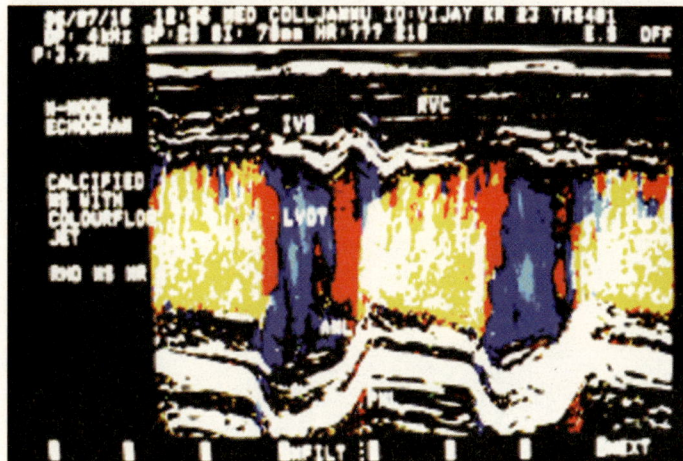

Fig. 14.52: M-Mode echocardiogram in color mode showing pale color jet of thick calcified anterior and posterior mitral leaflets of stenosed mitral valve entering into LV cavity

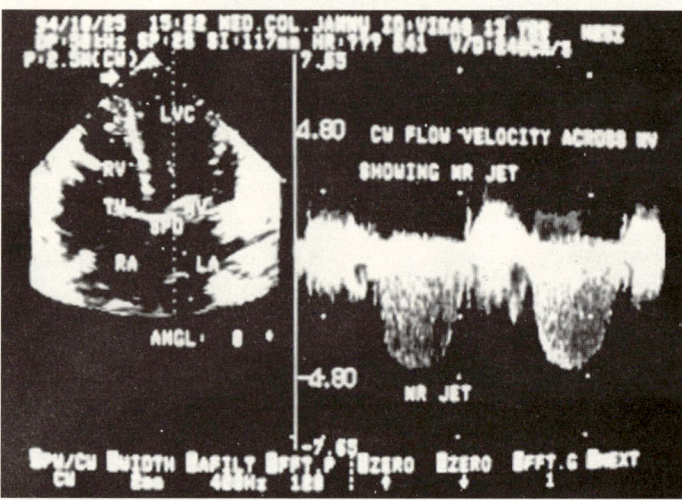

Fig. 14.55: 4C Doppler flow velocity across MV showing mitral stenosis and mitral regurgitation

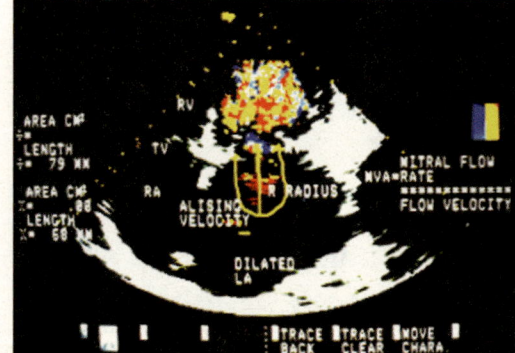

Fig. 14.53: Apical four chamber view in color mode showing derivation of proximal isovelocity surface area and its application for calculation of mitral valve area in a patient with mitral valve stenosis. It also demonstrates the visualization of aliasing velocity(traced cup) and transverse line as radius of velocity. MVA = peak forward Mitral flow rate/ peak mitral flow velocity

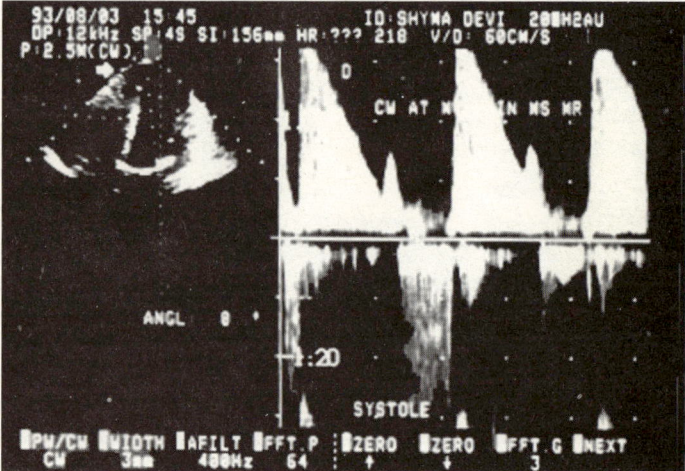

Fig. 14.56: Apical 4C and Doppler flow velocity across MV showing mild form of mitral senosis with mild to moderate mitral regurgitation

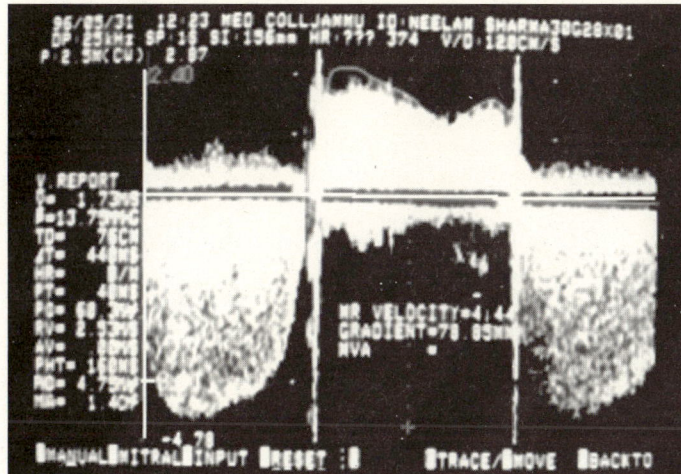

Fig. 14.57: CW Doppler flow velocity across MV showing severe form of mitral regurgitation in patient with moderate mitral stenosis. She had systolic pressure gradient of >75 mm Hg

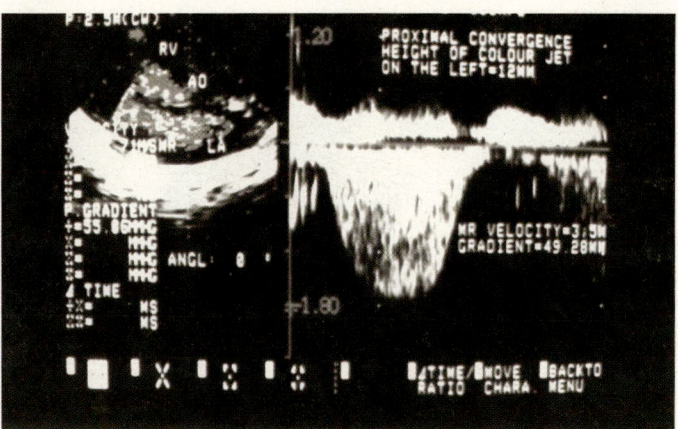

Fig. 14.60: Doppler flow velocity across mitral valve showing gross mitral regurgitation with proximal convergence height of jet on left panel = 12.0 mm and MR velocity = 3.5 m/s with gradient of >49 mm Hg in patient with rheumatic mitral stenosis and regurgitation (for details see text)

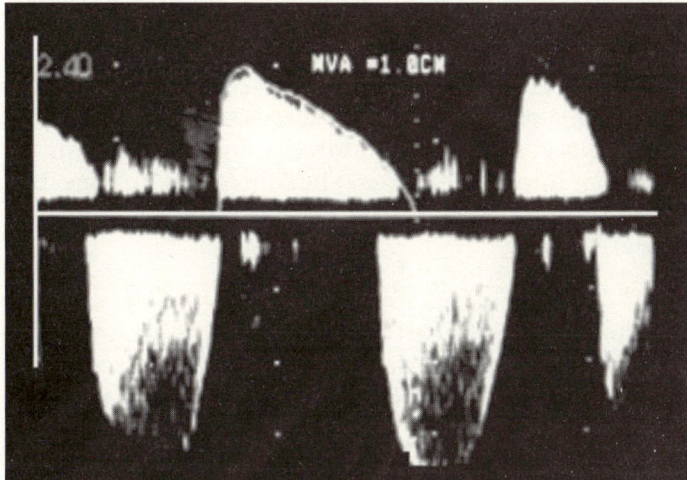

Fig. 14.58: Doppler flow velocity across mitral valve showing moderate mitral regurgitation associated with moderate type of mitral stenosis

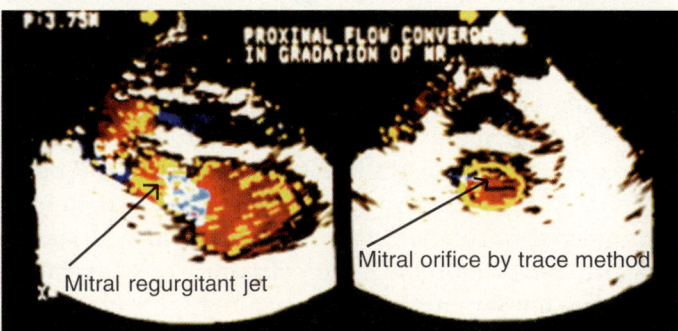

Fig. 14.61: Left parasternal long axis LV view and 2D short axis in Color flow mode showing calculation of severity of mitral regurgitation by proximal flow convergence which can be well correlated with angiographically evaluated mitral valvular regurgitation in this patient the height of mitral jet = 11.0 mm and size of jet =19 mm and mitral valve orifice calculated was 1.85 cm^2

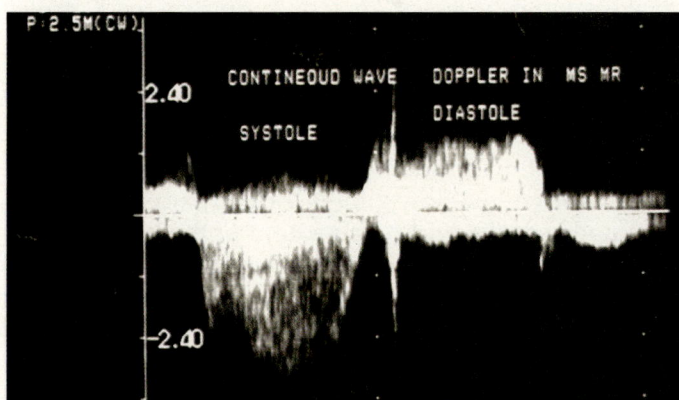

Fig. 13.59: CW Doppler flow velocity across MV showing moderate mitral stenosis with mitral regurgitation with regurgitant velocity of > 3.0 m/s

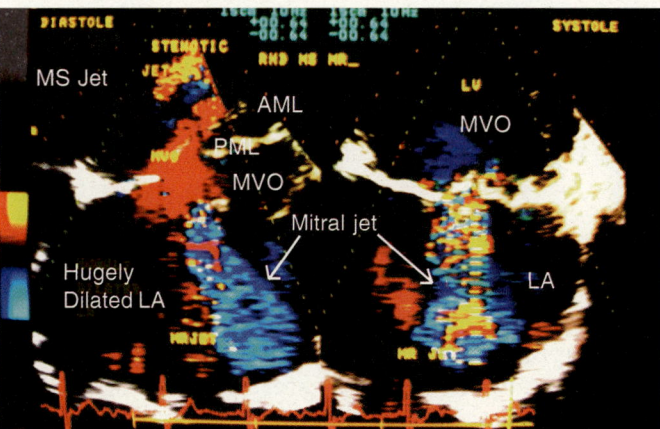

Fig. 14.62: Dual scan left parasternal oblique 2C view showing height and size of regurgitant jet for the application of proximal flow convergence for gradation of mitral regurgitation and regurgitant volume. MR jet is almost reaching upto the roof of the left atrium (grade 3–4)

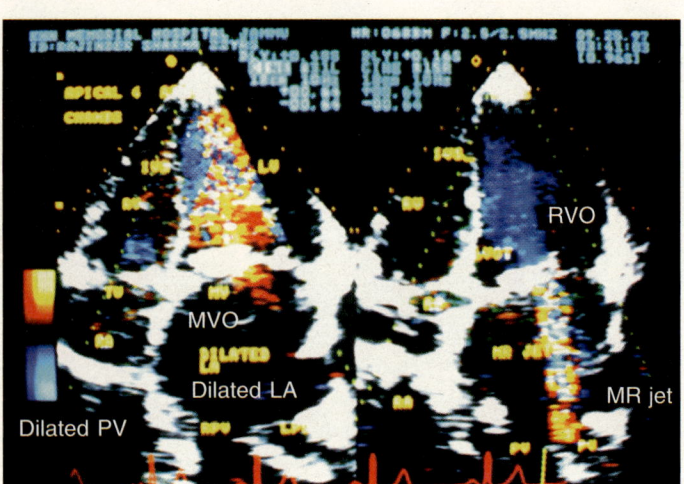

Fig. 14.63: Apical 4C color flow in left parasternal window showing mosaic color jet as bigger to reach up to the roof of the hugely dilated LA. Left panel echoscan showing mosaic color jet of mitral stenosis into LV cavity in patient with moderately severe mitral stenosis with mitral regurgitation

This measurement technique should be performed with high paper speeds (50 to 100 m/sec). If the patient is in sinus rhythm, an average of 3 to 5 beats should be used for measurements. If the patient is in atrial fibrillation, then one should use at least 5 to 10 beats to obtain a more accurate measurement. In the latest models of echocardiographic machines, sonographer only has to guide the software in its technique, the calculated values are usually depicted on the monitor screen.

2-D Mitral Valve Area by Planimetry (Figs 14.29–14.31, 14.37, 14.41, 14.43, and 14.44)

Two dimensional mitral valve area was measured near the tips of the mitral leaflets in the parasternal short axis view with an appropriate setting of gain attenuation. Three measurements were taken for each patient and an average was taken as the final value in patients with sinus rhythm while in patients with atrial fibrillation, an average of 10 measurements was taken.

Proximal Isovelocity Surface Area (PISA) (Figs 14.53 and 14.70)

Mitral inflow region was imaged from the apical window using the apical four chamber view. Colour-flow mapping is done with the colour gain adjusted to eliminate random colour in areas without flow. From the images so obtained, one can measure the angle and radius of flow convergence.

The aliasing velocity is reduced by shifting the colour baseline to maximize the area and this velocity is noted as the first aliasing velocity. The maximal radius of the proximal flow convergence region was measured in early diastole from the first aliasing line to the tips of the mitral valve in a direction parallel to the flow. Using the following formula, the mitral valve area can be calculated effectively.

Forward peak flow rate was calculated by the following formula

$$2\pi r^2 \times \frac{\text{The angle } a}{180} \times \text{first aliasing velocity}$$

Once the flow rate has been obtained, the mitral valve area is derived by dividing the peak flow rate by the peak inflow velocity measured from the continuous wave Doppler tracing.

$$\text{Mitral valve area} = \frac{\text{Peak forward flow rate}}{\text{Peak mitral flow velocity}}$$

Limitations of PISA

Proximal flow convergence may have its own limitation in subjects with limited temporal resolution of colour-flow mapping. Secondly, the angle correction applied may not correct completely the potential variation in the leaflet angle measurements, especially if the valve area is greater than 1.5 cm^2. The area calculation by PISA method is based on the continuity equation presuming a circular mitral valve area. The mitral valve orifice may be elliptical in case of a deformity and the area may be underestimated.

Mean Mitral Valve Pressure Gradient (Figs 14.33–14.36)

These calculations can be performed by dividing the diastolic flow into five to nine equally spaced segments, averaging all the velocities, and then calculating the gradient using the average velocity. This can be done at rest and with exercise.

The Doppler tracings are generally made initially with the pulsed-wave crystal in an effort to record the sharp spectral outline of the stenotic valve and the presence of mitral regurgitation. To combine the higher velocities and the spectral pattern, the continuous-wave crystal should be used. The continuous wave Doppler shows more spectral broadening and is useful in recording the maximum velocities from both the stenotic and regurgitant mitral valve.

The use of colour-flow mapping can be very helpful in detecting the turbulent flow across the stenotic mitral orifice. The colour-flow allows the cardiac echographer to actually see the width and extent of the jet caused by the obstructed valve, and thus a simultaneous Doppler tracing can then be placed at the ideal site to record the maximum velocities across the valve. The pressure and extent of mitral regurgitation is also well demonstrated with the colour-flow technique. Colour-flow is also useful in obtaining the proximal isovelocity surface area as required to calculate mitral valve area in mitral stenosis.

Reconstruction of three dimensional transthoracic images in different Planes of MV in health and disease

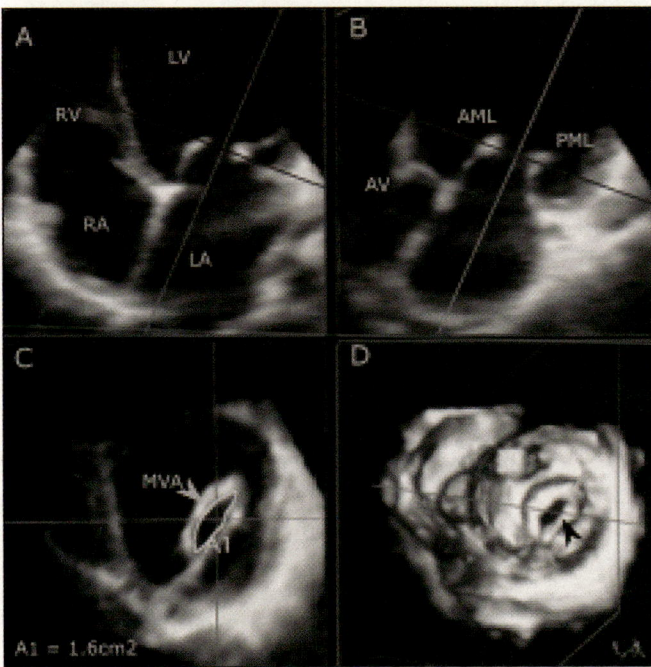

Fig. 14.64: Full volume 3DTT data set has been obtained from apical window shown with three orthogonal cutting planes (D) along with counter part two dimensional images in the respective planes A, B, C. The C cutting plane is aligned to the opening plane of mitral valve in A and B images to visualize the shortest mitral valve opening area in image C for measurement

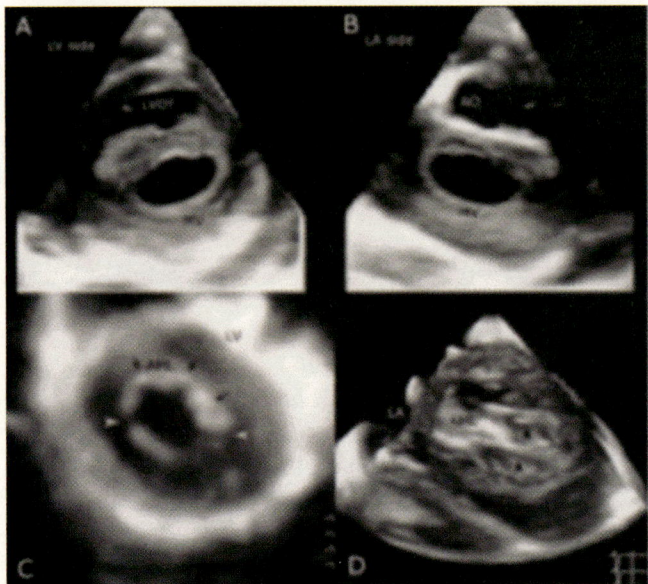

Fig. 14.65: Real time 3DTTE data set taken from parasternal window showing mitral valve viewed from LV side (A) and LA side (B) showing the surface of the thickened anterior and posterior mitral leaflet. (C) Full volume 3D data set acquired from parasternal window. Anterolateral left ventricular wall has been cropped to visualize mitral apparatus with subvalvular structures

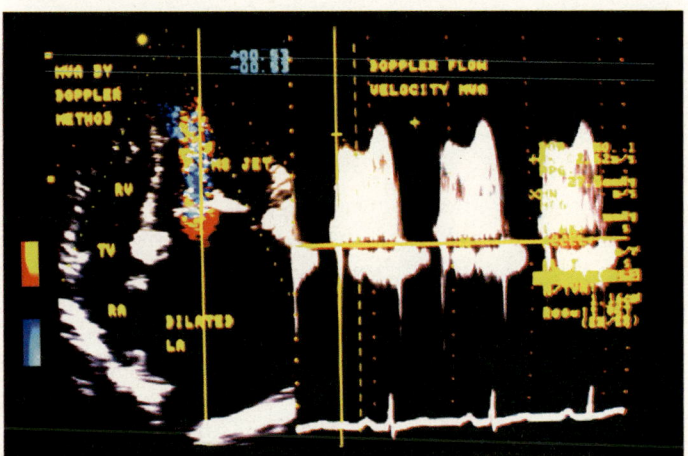

Fig. 14.66: Apical 4C color Doppler flow through left parasternal window shows normal sized LV, dilated LA, mosaic color jet of mitral stenosis (left) and enhanced Doppler flow velocity of mitral stenosis (right)

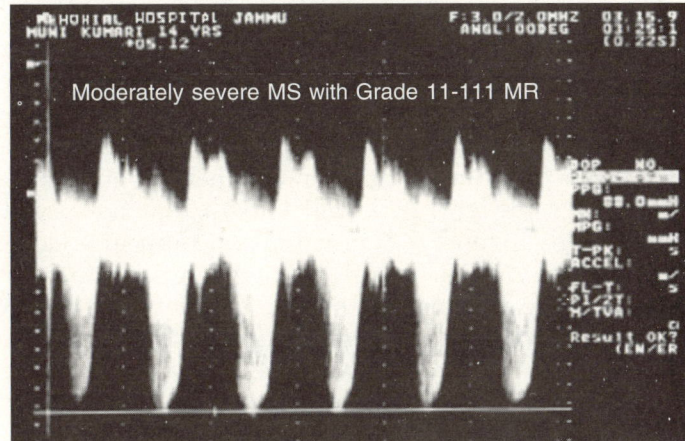

Fig. 14.67: Doppler flow velocity across mitral valve with grade II–III MR in patient who had rheumatic moderately severe mitral valvular stenosis

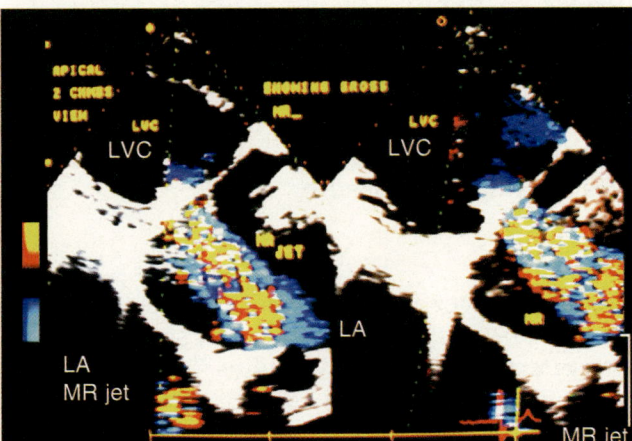

Fig. 14.68: Left parasternal window 2C colour dual scan view showing mosaic color jet of severe mitral regurgitation almost touching the roof of the left atrium

Velocities are performed with the narrowest sector angle (30°) to maximize the colour-flow imaging frame rate (15 to17 Hz). Colour gain is adjusted to eliminate random colour in areas without flow.

Bicuspid Aortic Valvular Stenosis (Fig. 14.143)

Although this anomaly is congenital in origin, with imposition of two leaflets instead of conventional three, it can also be due to rheumatic valvulitis where two leaflets can fuse together resulting into biscuspid morphology as seen in congenital malformation. There are two types of bicuspid valves. In the first the cusps are located to the right and left with the commissures anterior and posterior. If a raphe or false commissures is present, it always is in the right cusp. A coronary artery arises from behind each cusp. In the second type the cusps are located anterior and posterior and the commissures are to the right and left. If a raphe is present, it is always in the anterior cusp and both coronary arteries arise in front of the anterior cusp. Aortic stenosis is the most common complication of this congenital malformation.

The cusps of all aortic valve close concentrically in diastole, whereas those of the bicuspid valve close eccentrically. It is important to record the aortic cusps in various positions to ascertain whether this abnormal conditions present. It is well known that the beam angulation can cause the normal cusps to appear to close eccentrically. It is, therefore, most appropriate to evaluate the patient in a supine and left decubitus position and carefully search for the aortic root area to determine the accurate appearance of the aortic cusps. At times it is difficult to ascertain bicuspid morphology in a calcified valve due to the increased echoes within the aortic root. The possibility that a valve is bicuspid cannot be ruled out completely by echo, but if the eccentricity is shown and only two cusps are demonstrated on the two-dimensional image, the valve is probably bicuspid.

The two-dimensional study provides an additional method of evaluating aortic cusp closure. In the normal patient the short-axis view shows normal trileaflet configuration (simulating an inverted Mercedes Benz insignia), whereas the bicuspid valve clearly demonstrates eccentric cusp closure.

Acquired Aortic Stenosis (Figs 14.16–14.20)

Rheumatic fever is one of the important causes of valvular aortic stenosis and stands second to mitral valve in term of rheumatic valvulitis. The aortic valvular area in an adult measures 2.5 to 3.5 cm^2. As the valve narrows, the left ventricular pressure becomes higher than the aortic pressure to maintain adequate cardiac output. This increased pressure causes left ventricular hypertrophy. The left ventricle is less distensible than

normal, resulting into higher end diastolic pressure, which causes a higher left atrial pressure. It is to be explained that left atrium must maintain an end systolic pressure as high as the left ventricular end-diastolic pressure. The latter leads to hypertrophy of the left atrium.

Calcified Aortic Stenosis

In this type of stenosis the aortic obstruction is caused by calcium deposits that present the cusps from retracting adequately during ventricular systole. 'The wear and tear on the aortic valve probably induces calcification in the aortic wall to extend into the mitral annulus (Figs 14.131 and 14.132).

Echocardiographic Features in Aortic Valvular Disease

Echocardiography is the best means of evaluation of calcification and the thickness of the aortic wall and cusps. As the aortic root is demonstrated on the M-mode sweep, its motion can be observed swinging forward or anteriorly in systole and moving posteriorly in diastole. A lack of motion indicates the presence of atherosclerotic heart disease and calcification. The fine echoes from the anterior and posterior aortic walls should have intensified equal to or less than those from the left atrial wall. As the gain is decreased, the wall echoes disappear. In patients with calcification the echoes are very dense and do not disappear as readily when the gain is reduced. As the transducer beam sweeps from the calcified aortic root to the area of the mitral valve, calcification of the mitral annulus will be demonstrated as thick continuous echo arising from the posterior aortic wall and extending throughout the mitral apparatus. In a normal person, native aortic valve cusps are thin with fluttering echoes within the aortic root. As thickening and fibrosis, ensues echoes, increase their intensity and lose their characteristic flutter. The wide systolic opening of the cusps diminishes with the degree of calcification. If the valve is severely calcified, the systole component of the aortic cusps is difficult to separate from the diastole, on account of many increased echoes within the aortic root.

In many cases, mitral valve is spared in the presence of AS. Pathological changes can be demonstrated on the echo that result from increased pressures in the left ventricle. The amplitude of the mitral valve becomes reduced, and the E-F slope flattens according to the severity of the stenosis. The posterior leaflet of the mitral valve continues its normal posterior motion, and the kick of the anterior leaflet is generally still clearly seen. Concentric hypertrophic changes in the left ventricle have also been visualised in patients with severe aortic stenosis and increased left ventricular pressure. The left ventricle exhibits decreased contractility with decompensation.

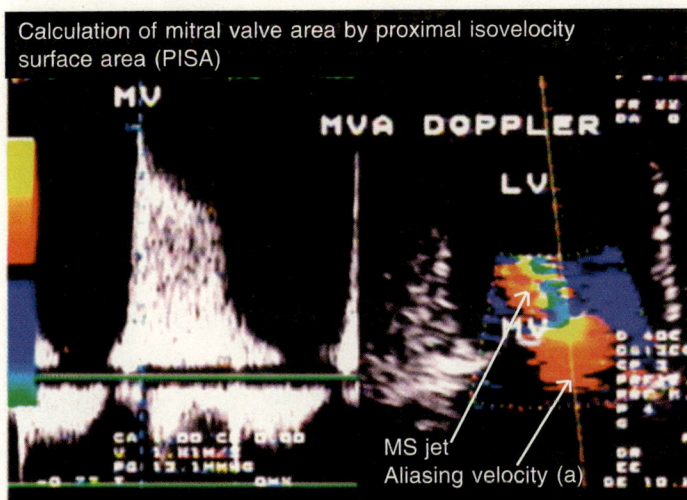

Fig. 14.69: Color Doppler mode at MV in apical 4C left parasternal plane showing enhanced peak velocity of mitral valve with wide spectral waveform (left) and mosaic color jet of LV inflow obstruction directed towards LV cavity due to stenosed mitral valve (right). This scan also reveals aliasing velocity just posterior to the mitral leaflets

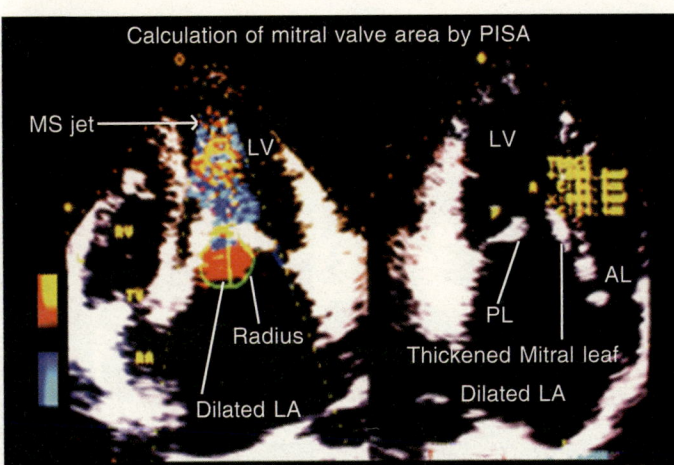

Fig. 14.70: (right panel) Apical 4C Color mode at left parasternal region showing thickened both anterior mitral leaflet (AL) and posterior mitral leaflet (PL) in mitral valvular stenosis left panel shows mosaic color jet of mitral stenosis entering into LV cavity, aliasing velocity (a) and radius of velocity (r) in calculation of mitral valve area by the application of proximal isovelocity surface area (PISA) equation (see text for detail)

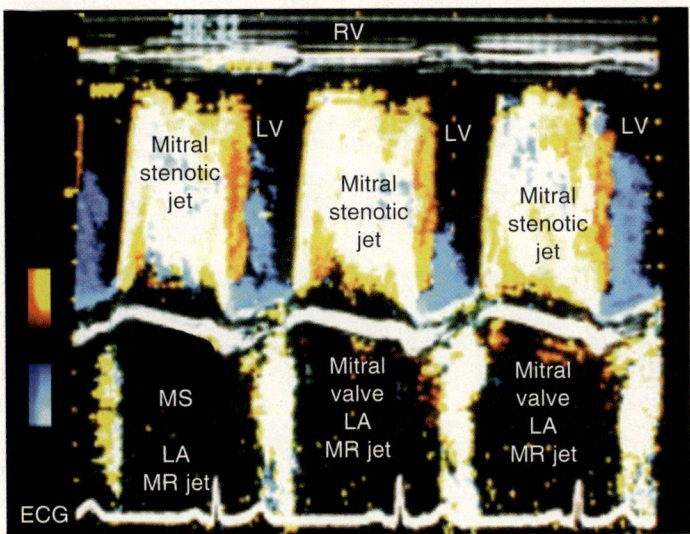

Fig. 14.71: M-Mode echocardiogram in color mode shows yellowish mitral stenotic flow jet traversing through LV cavity and mosaic mitral regurgitant jet into LA across mitral valve orifice

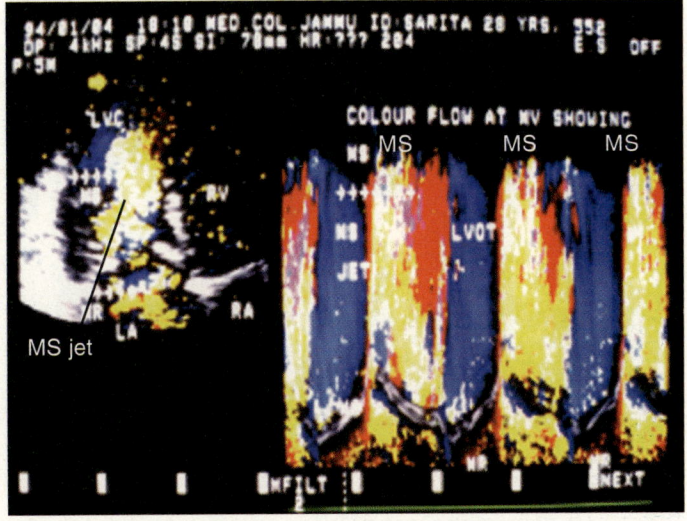

Fig. 14.72: Apical 4C color flow (left) and M-Mode echocardiogram in color mode (right) showing color flow jet of mitral stenosis and alternate blue normal flow jet in LVOT and mosaic jet of mitral stenosis respectively in patient with moderate mitral valvular stenosis

Doppler Flow Assessment of Aortic Stenosis (AS)

Doppler flow echocardiography is an excellent mode in evaluating aortic stenosis; however, the severity of valvular stenosis has been more easily applied in younger patients than in adults because of the secondary effects of decreased left ventricular function as result of the aortic disease. Continuous wave (CW) Doppler is the most useful technique in estimating pressure gradient in aortic stenosis (Figs 14.114, 14.115, 14.123 and 14.132).

One should be very careful while assessing the aortic flow with Doppler mode. The angle of incidence is very important to record the maximum velocity. It may be difficult to find the direction of flow through the stenotic aortic valve, and thus the maximum flow may be underestimated. However, with the advent of colour-flow Doppler, the Doppler beam may be positioned in the exact place to record the maxmium flow velocity so that the actual gradient coincides closer to the cardiac catheterization data than with just the conventional two-dimensional or blind continuous-wave probe. It is also

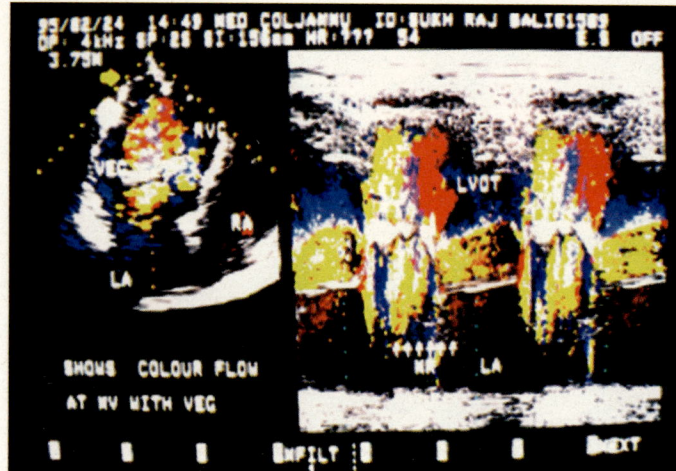

Fig. 14.73: Color 2-D Apical 4C (left) and color M-Mode echo-cardiogram r mode showing vegetation on anterior mitral leaflet resulting into mosaic color jet of mitral regurgitation (arrows) in both views respectively. LVOT = Left ventricular outflow tract, LA = Left atrium Veg = vegetation

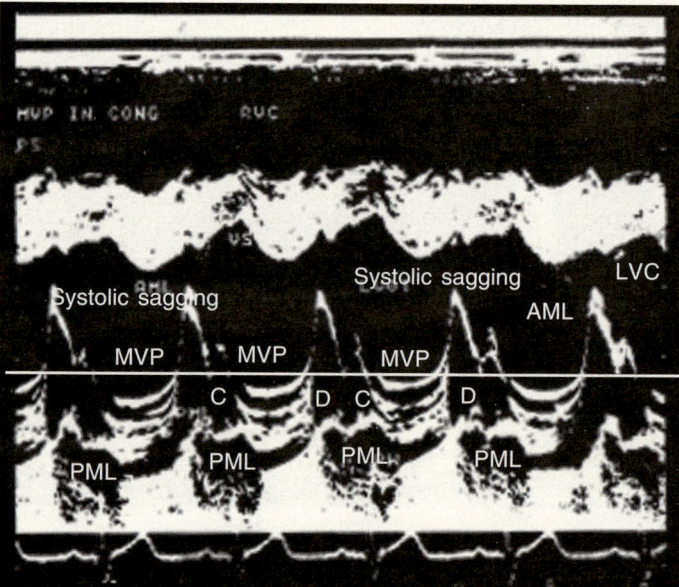

Fig. 14.75: M-Mode echocardiography showing systolic sagging from an imaginary line from C—D points of both anterior and posterior mitral leaflets into LA cavity during mid and late systole due to mitral valvular prolapse syndrome in a young patient with congenital pulmonic stenosis

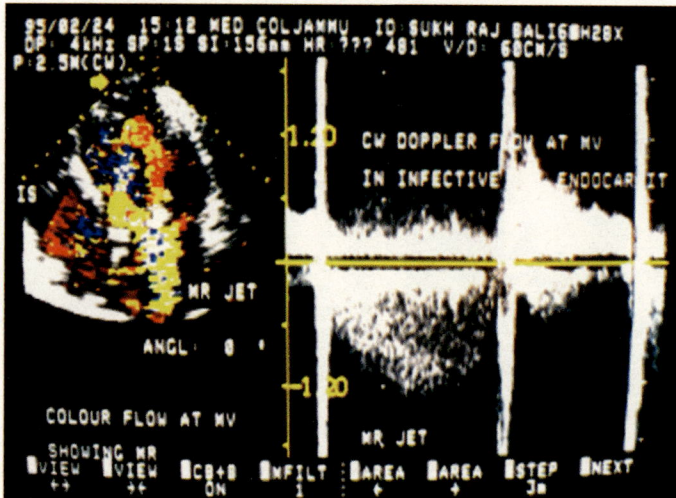

Fig. 14.74: (left panel) Color flow Apical 4C left parasternal view and Doppler flow velocity across mitral valve showing mosaic jet of mitral regurgitation into left atrium (arrow) and regurgitant velocity flow on Doppler study (right panel) in patient with infective endocarditis of mitral valve with clinical mitral regurgitant murmur

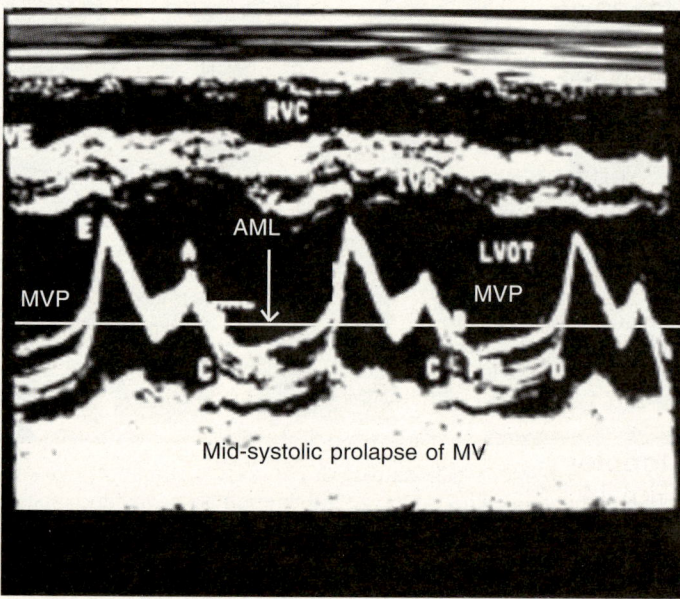

Fig. 14.76: M-Mode echocardiography showing systolic sagging from an imaginary line from C—D of both anterior and posterior mitral leaflets into LA cavity during mid systole due to mitral valvular prolapse syndrome in an adolescent patient with rheumatic mitral valvulitis

a pertinent point to remember that Doppler measures the peak instantaneous gradient, and cardiac catheterization measures the peak pressure gradient (i.e. the peak aortic pressure subtracted from the peak left ventricular pressure). Thereafter a transvalvular gradient of 50 mm Hg represents significant aortic stenosis. The finding of a gradient less than 50 mm Hg does not rule out the diagnosis, since the patient may have severe left ventricular dysfunction, and thus the aortic gradient would be underestimated.

Aortic Regurgitation (AR) (Figs 14.122, 14.125, 14.127 and 14.128)

Aortic regurgitation may be due to number of causes such as rheumatic fever, bacterial endocarditis, syphilis, aneurysm of the ascending aorta, ruptured aortic cusp, myxomatous degeneration of the aortic cusps, and hypertensive dilation of the aortic root. The various factors which come into play in determining the significance of aortic regurgitation, include the size of the diastolic aperture, the compensation and diastolic stretchability of the left ventricle, and the peripheral resistance.

Time to peak velocity measurement in systole:

Time to peak velocity = 160 m sec

Time to left ventricular ejection 280 m sec = 0.50

Time to peak values in mild obstruction = <0.50

Severe obstruction = >0.55

During diastole, if there is aortic valve regurgitation, the left ventricle competes with the peripheral vascular resistance for the blood in the aorta. During systole it must eject whatever extra blood it has received. Critical aortic regurgitation is present when the amount of leak is two to four times the effective cardiac output and the orifice size is 0.3 to 0.7 cm^2.

Aortic cusps may be independently affected by the inflammatory process of rheumatic fever leading to altered morphology of fibrosis and reduction in valvular area. The aortic insufficiency may produce flutter on the anterior leaflet of the mitral valve during diastole. The amplitude and E-F slope of the mitral valve may also be reduced secondarily to the increased pressures in the left ventricle. If the mitral apparatus is calcified, the fine flutter will be difficult to detect by echo and may be seen on the left side of the septum.

Aortic regurgitation may give rise to left ventricular dilation with a hyperdynamic contractile state, dilation of the aortic root (as seen in cystic medial necrosis and Marfan's syndrome) and premature closure of the anterior leaflet of the mitral valve secondary to acute aortic insufficiency. In such patients the PR-ac interval would be foreshortened, indicating the rapid increase in left ventricular pressure from the valve leakage.

Doppler Flow Assessment of Aortic Insufficiency
(Figs 14.122–14.130)

Doppler flow technique is very useful and sensitive technique for detecting aortic regurgitation. Apical five chamber view is an ideal window for this purpose by the application of either pulse wave or continuous wave (CW) modes in cases of moderate to severe insufficiency, the continuous-wave probe records the maximum velocity better than the pulsed-wave probe. Aortic regurgitation is recorded as a diastolic flow reversal in the left ventricular outflow tract or ascending aorta. One may also see increased systolic aortic velocities of 1.5 to 2.5 m/sec with increased velocities beginning in the left ventricular outflow tract.

1. Mild extends just below the aortic leaflets into the left ventricular outflow tract.
2. Moderate extends midway to the septum into the left ventricle.
3. Severe extends to the apex of the left ventricle.

However, with the application of colour-flow Doppler one can precisely record the severity of the flow by mapping out the exact velocity pattern as it extends into the left ventricle. One can also trace the path of the regurgitant jet which, in turn, is influenced by the amount of calcification on the aortic leaflets; thus, although most jets "hug" the septal wall may take bizarre pathways into the left ventricular cavity and may be seen with multiple transducer angulations and various cardiac windows. Parasternal long-axis view is considered as the best option to see a particular regurgitant jet.

Colour-Flow Mapping Studies in AR

Doppler echocardiography is the most common non-invasive method used to quantitate aortic regurgitation. In early studies both pulsed and continuous-wave Doppler were shown to be accurate methods of quantifying aortic insufficiency when compared to results of cardiac catheterization studies. Doppler colour-flow mapping has become the standard for the quantitation of aortic insufficiency because good correlation between colour-flow Doppler parameters and the angiographic grading of aortic insufficiency has been shown. The most commonly used colour-flow parameters have been validated in small series of patients. In most echocardiographic laboratories, both echocardiographic Doppler modalities (i.e. continuous-wave and colour-flow mapping) are used in conjuction to quantitate aortic regurgitation (Figs 14.66–14.68, 14.83 and 14.84).

The height of the regurgitant jet (JH) is defined as the anteroposterior diameter of the jet at its origin in the left ventricular outflow tract, and is measured from the parasternal long axis. The same frame at the same location at which the JH is obtained is used to measure the anteroposterior diameter of ventricular outflow tract (LVOH). The JH/LVOH ratio is calculated in each case. From the parasternal short-axis view, the area of the regurgitant jet (JASA) is planimetered. The same frame at which JASA is obtained is used to measure the area of the left ventricular outflow area (LVOA). The JASA/LVOA ratio is calculated. The apical four-chamber view is used to measure the area of the regurgitant jet (JA). The area of left ventricle (LVA) from the same frame is measured, and the JA/LVA ratio is calculated for each patient. The individual values of the above-mentioned variables corresponding to three cycles are averaged in patients with sinus rhythm. In patients with atrial fibrillation, five cardiac cycles are averaged.

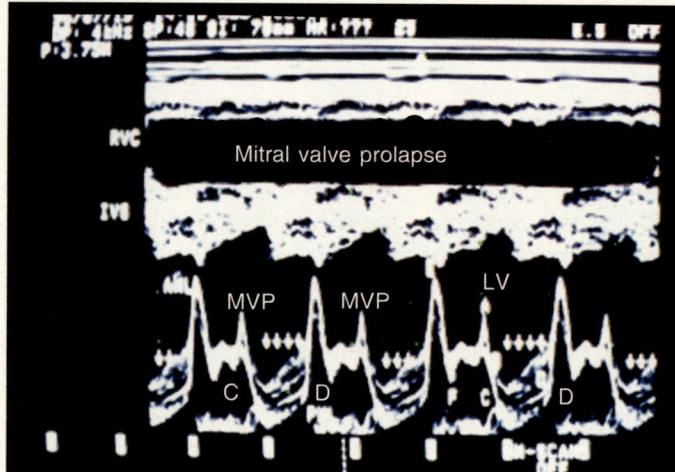

Fig. 14.77: M-Mode echocardiography showing systolic sagging from an imaginary line from C—D points of both anterior and posterior mitral leaflets into LA cavity during an early and mid systole due to mitral valvular prolapse syndrome in a young patient with Marfanoid syndrome

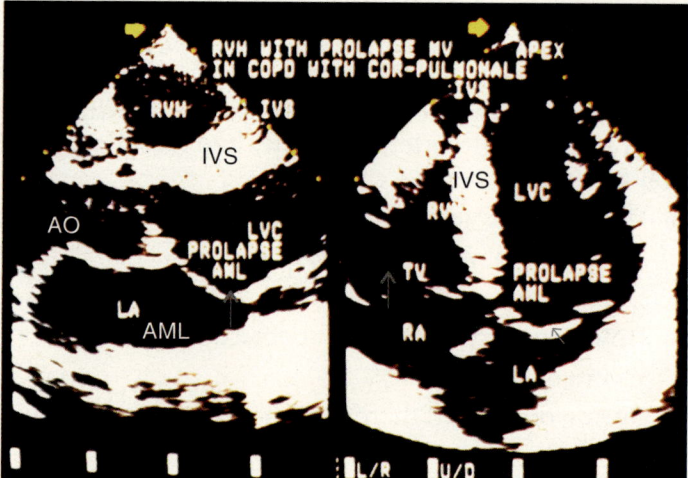

Fig. 14.79: Long axis modified (left) and apical 4C (right) 2-D dual scan views from left parasternal window shows prolapse of anterior mitral leaflet into left atrial cavity along with hypertrophy of right ventricle and dilatation of right atrium in patient with chronic obstructive lung disease. AML = Anterior mitral leaflet, PML = Posterior mitral leaflet AO = Aorta, RVH = Right ventricular hypertrophy

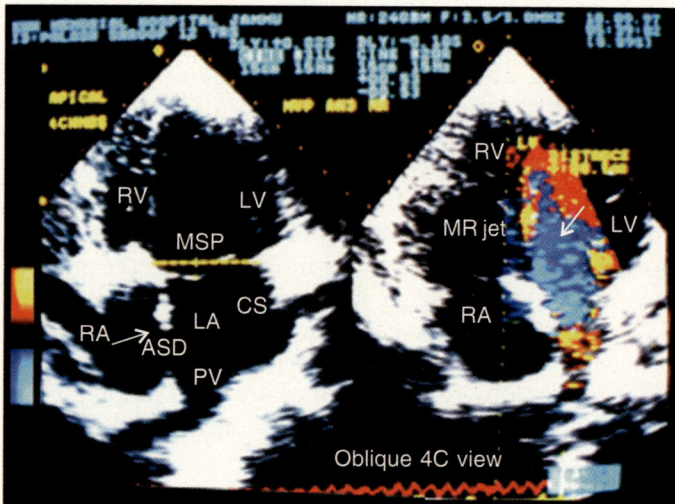

Fig. 14.78: Left panel: Apical 4C view showing systolic sagging from an imaginary line drawn from C—D points of both anterior and posterior mitral leaflets into LA cavity during mid systole due to mitral valvular prolapse syndrome in a young patient with atrial septal defect. Right panel shows blue jet of mitral regurgitation in mitral valve prolapse (arrow) with atrial septal defect of secundum type

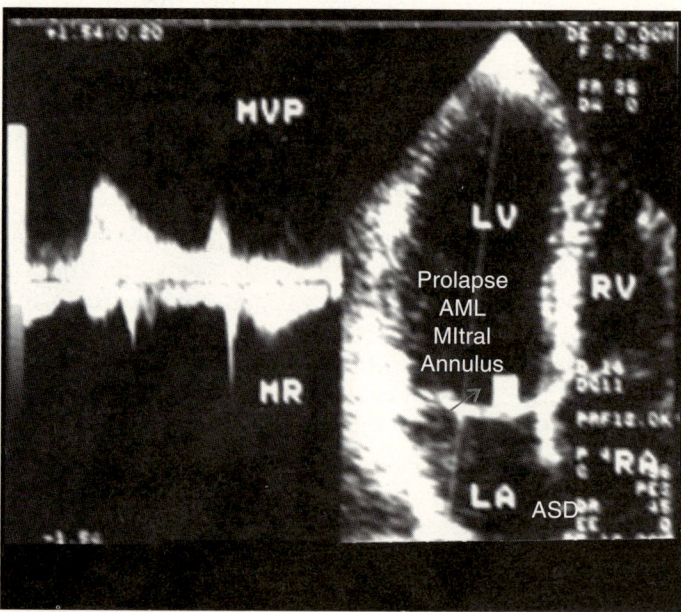

Fig. 14.80: Doppler flow at mitral valve (left) and 4C left parasternal views showing mitral regurgitation (MR) and Doppler flow velocity. Right panel shows dilated LV and LA along with prolapse of anterior mitral leaflet into LA cavity in patient with congenital pectus excavatum with ASD secundum and supraventricular tachyarrhythmia

Continuous-wave Doppler Analysis

Continuous-wave Doppler recordings are obtained from the cardiac apex from either the apical five-chamber or the apical long-axis view. Colour-flow is used to align the Doppler beam parallel to flow. Continuous-wave Doppler signal of early diastolic flow reversal is defined as aortic insufficiency. The slope of diastolic deceleration is determined as the slope of a straight line drawn along the peak velocities throughout diastole. Pressure half-time is defined as the time required for the initial early diastolic transvalvular pressure gradient to be halved. All values for the continuous-wave Doppler parameters are the average of three consecutive beats in patients with sinus rhythm. In patients with atrial fibrillation, five cardiac cycles are averaged.

Colour-Flow Doppler measurements vs. Angiographic Grading

Significant correlations were found between the colour-flow Doppler parameters and the degree of aortic regurgitation assessed by the aortic root angiograms. The best correlation is obtained with the ratio of the maximum JH to the LVOH expressed as a percentage ($r = 0.91$, $p = 0.0001$). By using 25% and 40% as cut-points for the JH/LVOH ratio, a good discrimination among regurgitation groups is obtained. A 40% cut-point for JH/LVOH ratio provided a very good discrimination between angiographic 1 to 2 + and 3 to 4+ groups. However, 25% as another cut-point for the JH/LVOH ratio also permits a very good separation of mild aortic regurgitation from moderate and severe forms.

The simple measurement of absolute JH at the left ventricular outflow tract has a strong correlation with angiographic severity of aortic regurgitation ($r = 0.89$). A cut-point of 0.8 cm for JH provides very good discrimination between the angiographic 1 to 2+ and 3 to 4+ groups. It is highly sensitive (97%), highly specific (98%), and highly accurate (97%) to separate 1 to 2+ from 3 to 4+ aortic regurgitation.

The JASA/LVOA ratio also correlates highly with the angiographic grading ($r = 0.86$, $p = 0.0001$). For this ratio, the best cut-point obtained is 25%, which provides good discrimination between groups 1 to 2 and 3 to 4 aortic regurgitation (although is considerable overlap). The cut-point of 25% for JASA/LVOA also provides a good separation between the angiographic 1 to 2+ and 3 to 4+ groups, with sensitivity 92%, specificity 97%, and accuracy 93%.

Among other colour-flow parameters, the JA/LVA ratio is quite variable in all grades of aortic regurgitation, with a very wide range of values within the groups. However, there is a significant and fairly good correlation with the angiographic grading ($r = 0.75$, $p = 0.0001$). No cut points provides a good discrimination among groups for JA/LVA ratio.

Continuous-Wave Doppler Parameters vs. Angiographic Grading

Deceleration Slope (Figs 14.122 and 14.142)

There is a good correlation ($r = 0.70$, $p = 0.0001$) between the angiographic degree of regurgitation and the deceleration slope. The slopes were significantly lower in patients with mild aortic insufficiency (1.95 ± 0.47 m/sec^2) than in patients with angiography graded 3 to 4+ (3.08 ± 0.7 m/sec^2) aortic insufficiency ($p < 0.01$). With previously established conventional cut-points of 2 m/sec^2 and 3 m/sec^2, the separation of different angiographic groups is not excellent, although an increasing deceleration slope is observed with increasing regurgitation severity. Patients with 4+ aortic regurgitation had

significantly greater slopes than those with moderate and mild aortic regurgitation (3.68 ± 0.50 m/sec^2). However, 3 m/sec^2 as a cut-point for separating severe aortic regurgitation from mild and moderate forms is highly specific (97%) and accurate (86%) (Fig. 13.144B).

Pressure Halftime

There is a fair although significant correlation between the pressure half-time and the severity of aortic regurgitation ($r = -0.62$, $p = 0.0001$). Although this parameter does not allow good separation of different degrees of regurgitation, the patients with mild aortic regurgitation has longer pressure halftimes than patients with moderate or severe regurgitation (353 ± 99 vs 232 ± 58 m sec, $p < 0.001$).

The measurement of the jet as its origin (JH) will provide the most accurate estimation of aortic regurgitation in obtaining either JH/LVOH or JASA/LVOA ratios. In proving this hypothesis, Switzer, *et al.* used an in vitro model to find JH, when measured at its origin, is the best predictor of regurgitant volume.

It has been observed that short axis is the only acoustic window that allows approach of the jet relatively as deflection of two planes; therefore the values from the short-axis view should be superior to the values obtained from the parasternal long-axis view, which is a deflection of only one plane. However, adequate images should be obtained more frequently from the parasternal long-axis than from the parasternal short-axis views.

It is, therefore, concluded that the colour Doppler echocardiography is superior to continuous wave Doppler parameters for the quantification of aortic regurgitation. The ratio of the JH at its origin in left ventricular outflow tract to left ventricular outflow tract diameter obtained from the parasternal long-axis view is found to be the best predictor of aortic regurgitation when compared to angiography. The measurement of the absolute JH at its origin appears to be the simplest and the most practical method not only to detect aortic regurgitation, but also to discriminate accurately between mild and moderate or severe aortic regurgitation. JA/LVOH ratio is very helpful as a predictor of severity of angiographic grading. However, this parameter is limited by technical difficulties. Planimetry is required, which should be considered a disadvantage of the method. The deceleration slope as found with continuous Doppler parameter, has a high predictive accuracy for severe aortic regurgitation, but it has an inferior discriminating power compared to the colour-flow Doppler parameters.

Echocardiographic Evaluation of Valvular Regurgitation

Improvements in outcomes for heart valve surgery, in particular mitral valve repair, have strongly advocated a need for better assessment of valvar regurgitation. Whereas in the past, surgery was delayed until the patient's symptomatic status required intervention, patients today are often sent to the operating room while still asymptomatic or minimally symptomatic. Before committing an asymptomatic patient to open heart surgery, however, it is essential that the severity of valvar regurgitation be quantified to ensure the surgery is actually required. Doppler echocardiography has emerged as a nobel way of assessing valvar regurgitation, as it allows characterisation of valve morphology, severity of regurgitation, and secondary effects, such as left ventricular dysfunction, left atrial enlargement, and pulmonary hypertension. This section will outline current methods available to the echocardiographer in assessing valvar regurgitation, focusing on simple practical ways that true quantitative information can be obtained in a clinical laboratory. Techniques that are generally applicable in all forms of valve regurgitation will be introduced first, followed by specific techniques for mitral and aortic regurgitation.

Colour Jet Area Method (Figs 14.124, 14.125 and 14.128)

The most common way of assessing the severity of valvar regurgitation is to inspect the area of the colour Doppler jet in the down stream chamber. The advantage of this approach is that it is fast, easy, and also provides information on the mechanism of regurgitation, as the jet is generally directed away from the most severely affected leaflet. However, jet area alone is impacted by many factors other than regurgitant flow rate, and an understanding of these will aid in its utilisation.

Determinants of Colour Jet Doppler Area

The physical parameter that is most predictive of the size of a regurgitant jet by colour Doppler is jet momentum, given by the product of regurgitant flow rate multiplied by velocity. Since jet velocity is directly related to the driving pressure across a regurgitant orifice (by the Bernoulli equation), the patient's blood pressure will have an important impact on jet size and so should be recorded at the time of the echo examination. Obviously a jet, which is directed centrally into the left atrium, cannot extend further than the superior wall of the atrium, but chamber constraint is even more important for eccentrically directed jets that hug the chamber wall. In general, such a wall jet will appear much smaller (as much as 60% smaller) than the equivalent centrally directed jet because it is flattened against the wall and cannot recruit stagnant flow into the jet from all sides, the way a centrally directed jet can. The final factor impacting colour jet area size is the

instrumentation set-up of the echocardiograph. Increasing either the transmitted power of the instrument or the receiver gain will result in a larger jet, as weaker echoes on the periphery of the jet are detected. In general, colour gain should be increased until random colour pixels begin to appear in the tissue and then the gain reduce just slightly. The scale of the colour Doppler display (determined by the pulse repetition frequency) can have a profound effect on jet size as low velocity motion at the periphery of the jet will be encoded at low scales.

Table 14.2: Echo-Doppler parameters involved in the genesis of MR

1. Anatomic/Chambers
2. Left ventricular dimensions/size
3. Left atrial dilation
4. Left ventricle volume and stroke volume
5. Valve perforation
6. Doppler Colour flow
7. Jet area
8. Jet area indexed to left atrium
9. Central vs. eccentricities
10. Vena contract a width
11. Proximal isovelocity surface area
12. Size/qualitative

For most purposes, the scale should be set at the highest limit allowed by the combination of imaging depth and interrogation frequency (and usually selected automatically by the instrument). Transducer frequency can have a dual effect on jet size. Because the Doppler shift is more profound at higher interrogating frequencies, jets tend to appear larger with higher frequency imaging. However, higher imaging frequencies are also prone to greater tissue attenuation and so the jets may appear smaller. In general, for transoesophageal imaging the Doppler enhancing effect of the higher imaging frequency dominates while for transthoracic imaging the attenuation factor predominates, causing jets to appear smaller at higher interrogating frequencies. Increasing the wall filter of the instrument will decrease the size of jets, by excluding velocities below a certain cutoff value, while increasing the ensemble length (sometimes referred to as the quality of the Doppler map) will yield a larger jet as lower velocities can be displayed by the finer colour maps. The best rule of thumb is to standardise the instrument set-up within a given laboratory and leave these constant for all examinations. Unfortunately, regardless of the care that is taken in assessing the colour jet area, this method can only yield a semiquantitative assessment of regurgitant severity, with perhaps 4–6 distinct grades of severity detectable. Modern assessment of valvar regurgitation requires a more quantitative approach.

Quantitative Techniques

A variety of techniques have been described for the echo Doppler quantification of valvar regurgitation. Among the key parameters to be determined by these methods are the following:

1. Regurgitant volume, the amount of blood leaking through the valve in each cardiac cycle (given in ml);
2. Regurgitant flow rate, the maximal rate of leakage through the valve (given in ml/s);
3. Regurgitant fraction, the percentage of left ventricular stroke volume that leaks back through the valve; and
4. Regurgitant orifice area, the actual anatomic area of the regurgitant lesion and perhaps the best physical descriptor of valve disruption.

Volumetric Approach to Quantification (Fig. 14.83)

In general the approach to regurgitant quantification can be divided into two broad areas—volumetric assessment and direct assessment. The volumetric assessment relies on measuring stroke volume in two regions of the heart, one of which includes the regurgitant volume, the other of which includes only the systemic stroke volume. The difference between these two stroke volumes is the regurgitant volume through the valve. For example, in the case of mitral regurgitation, measuring stroke volume across the mitral annulus and left ventricular outflow tract and subtracting the latter from the former will yield the mitral regurgitant stroke volume. The stroke volumes can be obtained in a variety of fashions. Flow through the left ventricular outflow tract can be calculated by multiplying the area of the left ventricular outflow tract ($D^2/4$, where D is the diameter of the left ventricular outflow tract measured just below the aortic valve in the parasternal long-axis view) by the time velocity integral of the pulsed Doppler velocity measurement obtained in the same location. A similar approach can be used for measuring flow across the mitral annulus, by measuring the mitral annular area and multiplying this by the time velocity integral of the velocity obtained at that location. Alternatively, stroke volume can be obtained from two dimensional echocardiography by subtracting left ventricular end-systolic volume from end-diastolic volume, calculated by using Simpson's rule or the area-length formula from the left ventricular apex. It is also possible to obtain stroke volume in an automated fashion, by integrating colour Doppler velocities across the left ventricular outflow tract or mitral annulus throughout space and time. Such an approach, unfortunately, is only available on one manufacturer's instrument at the current time. While these volumetric methods are theoretically sound and have been well validated in many carefully performed

trials, they have not achieved widespread use within the clinical echocardiographic community for a variety of reasons. First, they are time-consuming to implement, requiring multiple measurements from a variety of echocardiographic imaging windows and multistage calculations. Furthermore, they are exquisitely sensitive to the error in the primary measurements, and an error in any of these will be propagated throughout all the calculations. This is compounded by the need to subtract two fairly large numbers from each other to obtain a much smaller number at the end of the process. The absolute value of the uncertainty in the measurement rises as the square root of the sum of the squares of the component uncertainties, but the relative uncertainty rises even more.

Proximal Convergence Method (Figs 14.124–14.126)

The proximal convergence method is a more direct approach to the quantification of valvar regurgitation. As blood rushes into a regurgitant orifice, it forms concentric shells of increasing blood velocity and decreasing surface area. Since blood is incompressible, if we could measure flow through any one of the shells, that would yield the instantaneous flow through the regurgitant orifice itself.[8] Fortunately, there is a straightforward way to estimate flow through one of the shells. Fluid dynamics theory demonstrates that for a small orifice in a flat plate, these isovelocity shells are hemispheric in shape, with an area of $2r^2$, where r is the distance of the shell from the regurgitant orifice. Multiplying this area by the velocity v of the isovelocity shell will yield the flow rate. This radius and velocity can most easily be obtained by using the aliasing of the colour Doppler display, as blood rushes into the orifice. Schematically as blood velocity increases, there is an abrupt change from yellow to blue at which point one can know the blood is moving at 42 cm/s and where we can easily measure the radius from the regurgitant orifice. Once flow rate is obtained as $Q = 2r^2v$, then the regurgitant orifice area (ROA) is obtained by dividing this by the maximal velocity through the valve measured with continuous-wave Doppler: $ROA = Q/v_{max}$. This approach has been well validated in a number of experimental and clinical studies.[9] It has advantages over the volumetric approach, in that all measurements are obtained from a single imaging window, typically one of the apical windows, and the flow rate is measured directly, not requiring subtraction of two large quantities from each other as in the volumetric approach. Nevertheless, there are some limitations to the proximal convergence method, also known as the PISA (proximal isovelocity surface area) method, which the reader should be aware of. Additionally, there is an important simplification to this method that will greatly aid in its clinical application.

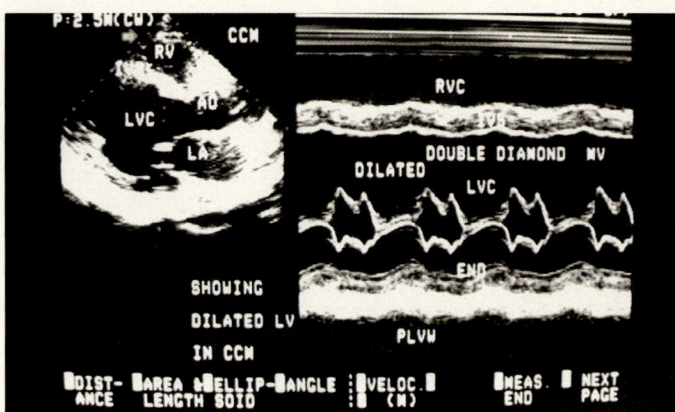

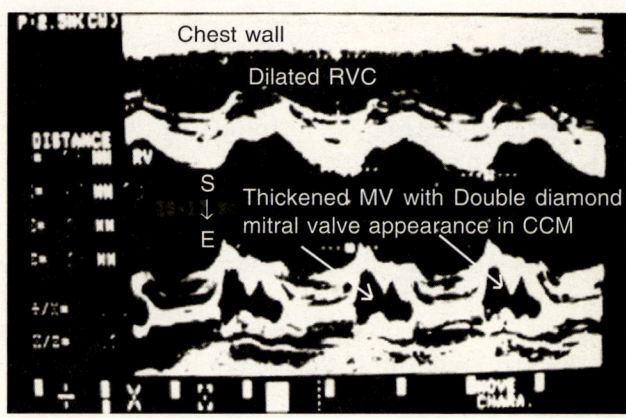

Fig. 14.81: 2D Long axis (left) and M-mode echo scan (right) showing double diamond type of mitral valve configuration in dilated cardiomyopathy

Fig. 14.82: M-Mode echoscan showing dilated right and left ventricles with increased E point septal separation (EPSS = 17MM) and double diamond configuration of thickened mitral valve leaflets in patient with dilated cardiomyopathy

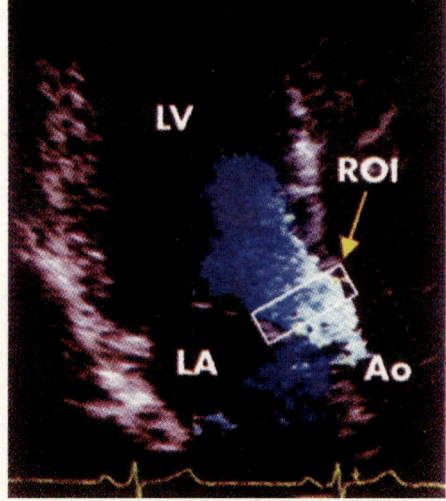

(A) Long axis view

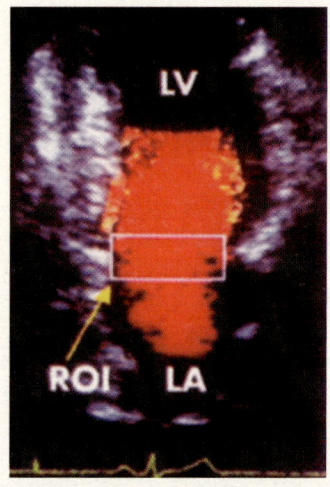

(B) 2-Chamber view

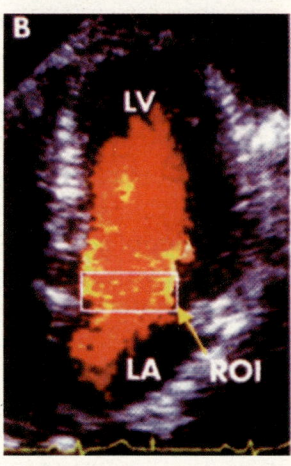

(C) 4-Chamber view

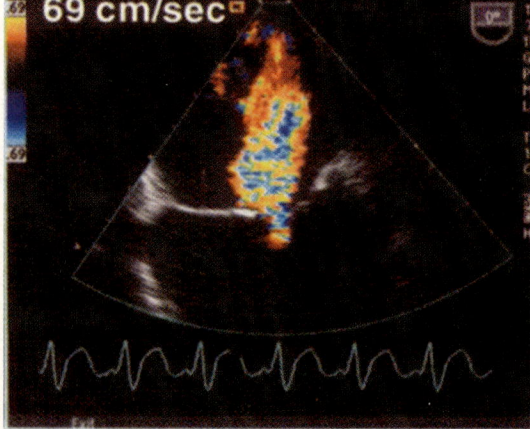

(D) Color Doppler jet size by pulse repetition frequency

Fig. 14.83A to D: (A) An example of measurement of aortic outflow volume in the long axis view by the automatic cardiac flow measurement (ACM) method. Region of interest set of the aortic annulus on the display to obtain the velocity profile. Flow volume rate is obtained by spatial integration of the velocity profile throughout the systolic period. **(B, C** and **D)** An example of measurement of mitral inflow volume in the 2-and 4-chamber view respectively by the ACM method. Flow volume is measured by the temporal integration of the flow volume rate obtained by spatial profile integration of the velocity profile throughout the diastolic period. LA = Left atrium, LV = Left ventricle RA = Right atrium, RV = Right ventricle

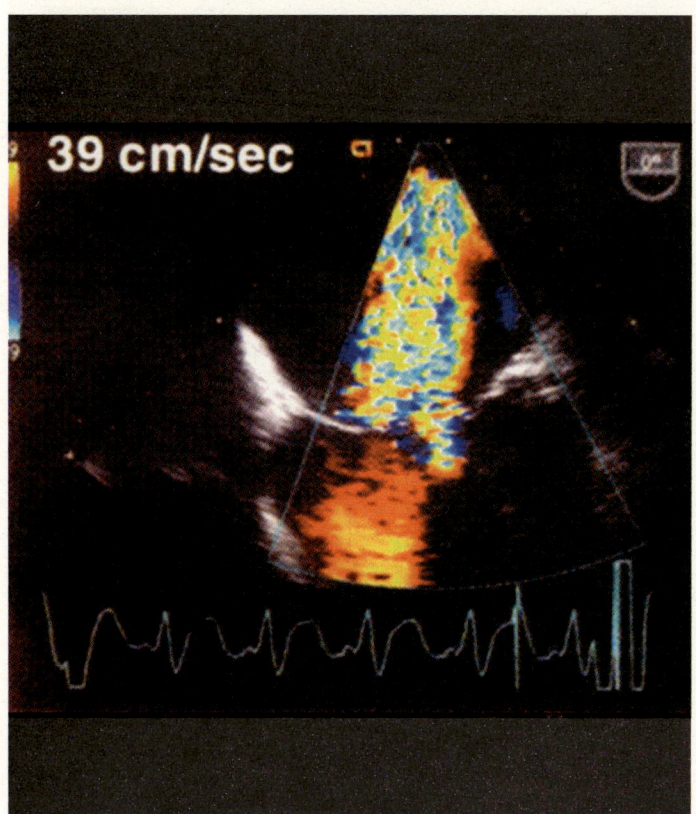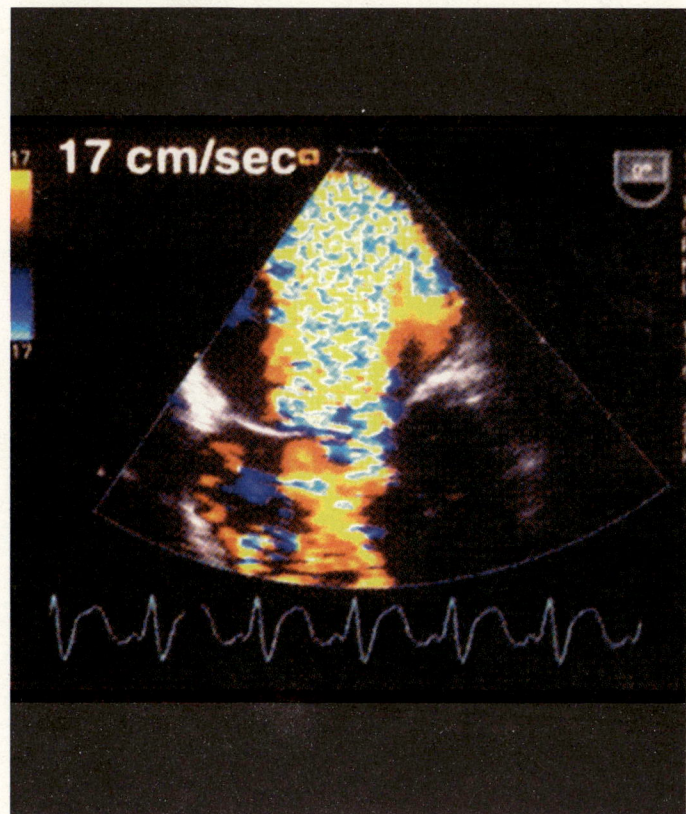

Fig. 14.84: Impact of scale pulse repetition frequency on color jet size. Because the color Doppler processor records approximately 16 levels of red and 16 levels of blue, the lowest velocity encoded is approximately 1/16 of the maximal velocity. Thus the minimal velocities recorded in the above images are approximately 4 cm/s and 1 cm/s as the scale is reduced from 69 to 39 to 17cm/s

Table 14.3: *Doppler criteria in assessing severity of aortic regurgitation*

Modality	Parameter	Criteria for severe	Example of limitations
1. Colour flow	Jet area Jet height PISA	> 60% LVOT area > 60% LVOT height Effective regurgitation Orifice > 0.3 cm²	Instrument (gain) dependent, eccentric jet, temporal Variability Multiple measurements, technically Challenging
2. CW Doppler imaging	Signal density P~I/2t Slope Regurgitant volume	Nonquantitative < 250 ms > 400 cm/s² > 60 mL	Affected by other factors, e.g. blood pressure Pressure, LV Compliance, acuity
3. Pulsed Doppler imaging	Regurgitant fraction Descending aortic Flow reversal LV end-diastolic dimension LV	> 50% Holodiastolic retrograde Flow Flow > 7 cm	Requires multiple measurements, assumes no regurgitation at reference valve limited quantitative information;
4. 2D echocardiography Systolic dimension		> 4.5 cm	affected by sample volume location Non-specific affected by multiple factors

CW = Continuous wave, PISA, Proximal isovelocity surface area; $P_{1/2}t$, Pressure half time LV, Left ventricle

Limitations to the Proximal Convergence Method

There are four important limitations to the proximal convergence method: flattening of the contours near the orifice, constraint of the flow by proximal structures, uncertainty in localising the regurgitant orifice, and variability in the regurgitant orifice throughout cardiac cycle.

Contour Flattening of the Orifice

Since the regurgitant orifice is in fact not infinitely small, the hemispheric shape of the isovelocity contours is not maintained all the way into the orifice; rather, they flatten out on approach to the orifice, and if flow were calculated using the standard formula, flow underestimation would ensue. An in vitro and computational study has shown that this underestimation is closely related to the aliasing velocity used in calculating the flow rate. For example, if an aliasing velocity (v_a) that is 10% of the orifice velocity is used, then approximately 10% of the flow will be missed with the standard formula. This underestimation can be corrected by multiplying the calculated flow rate by the quantity $v_{max}/(v_{max} - v_a)$. Fortunately, for left sided lesions (aortic and mitral regurgitation), this correction factor is rarely needed, since the aliasing velocity usually is less than 10% of the orifice velocity. The correction may be necessary for tricuspid regurgitation, where the aliasing velocity is a larger proportion of the orifice velocity and the underestimation of flow would be more significant.

Flow Constraint by Proximal Structures

A more important limitation is the distortion in the isovelocity contours caused by encroachment of proximal structures on the flow field. It is clear that the proximal convergence zone cannot form full hemispheric contours, and thus is pushed outward from the orifice. Applying the standard formula in this case would lead to significant flow overestimation, but again a simple solution to this exists. By simply excluding from the calculations an amount of flow approximately equal to the geometric reduction in the orifice shape from a hemisphere, most of this overestimation can be eliminated. Ideally, a full three dimensional analysis of the flow-field would allow refinement of the method, but until such methods are widely available, the simple "eyeball" approach works reasonably well. Simply multiplying the calculated flow rate by the ratio/180 will permit estimation of the true flow rate.

While it is generally quite easy to see where the colour Doppler display changes from blue to red, it is often not so easy to see exactly where the centre of the regurgitant orifice is located. This is an important issue, as the radius is defined on the basis of that orifice location; and since the radius is squared in the proximal convergence formula, a 10% error in radius measurement will cause more than 20% error in flow rate and regurgitant orifice area calculations. When the images are being obtained live on the echo machine, it is possible to freeze the image and toggle colour display on and off, improving the anatomical delineation of the regurgitant orifice. Once the images are stored off either digitally or on videotape, however, the colour generally is a fixed overlay on the black and white anatomy and cannot be removed. While some automated methods have been proposed to localise the orifice automatically from the full velocity field, these have not reached clinical use yet. Another alternative is to look not at the first aliasing radius but rather to look at the separation between the first and second aliasing contours. Clinical experience with this interaliasing distance method is limited, but it may prove helpful, particularly for moderate to severe mitral regurgitation where a second aliasing contour is visible.

Variable Regurgitant Orifice

In many patients the degree of regurgitation is not constant throughout systole or diastole in the case of aortic regurgitation, and categorising the regurgitant severity on the basis of the maximal regurgitant orifice area may give a misleading overestimation of the haemodynamic impact of the regurgitation. For example, in cases of classic mitral valve prolapse, the severe regurgitation is often confined to the latter half of systole. Conversely, it has been shown in some cases of functional mitral regurgitation in dilated cardiomyopathy that the most significant regurgitation occurs early in systole and then again during isovolumic relaxation with relatively little flow in mid systole, as ventricular pressure is sufficient to keep the valve closed. One way of addressing this issue is to image the proximal convergence zone with colour Doppler M-mode echocardiography, which shows a temporal display of the velocity through the valve throughout cardiac cycle. While methods have been proposed for using the colour M-mode display in a quantitative fashion, it is often possible to use it in a semiquantitative fashion simply to adjust the clinical judgement of the severity of regurgitation based on the duration of the leakage.

Simplified Proximal Convergence Method

While the proximal convergence method is considerably simpler than the previous volumetric methods, it is still considered by some to be too complex for routine clinical application. In its better understanding some of the workers have devised a simplification to the proximal convergence method that allows the mitral regurgitant

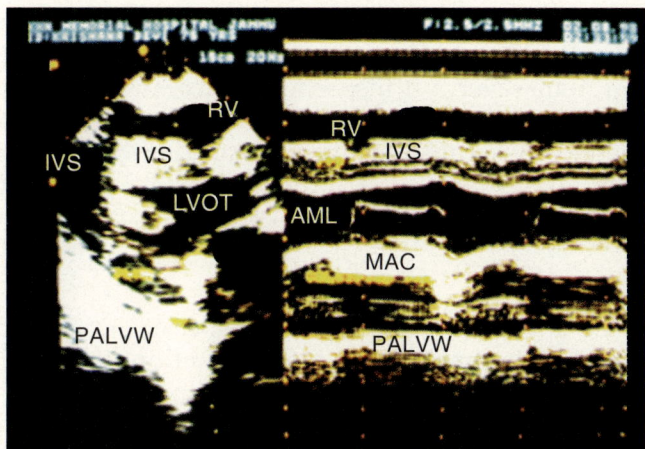

Fig. 14.85: 2D Long axis and M-mode echo scans showing mitral annular calcification (MAC) in patient with insulin dependant diabetes mellitus hypertension and non-obstructive hypertrophic cardiomyopathy (see normal AML = anterior mitral leaflet)

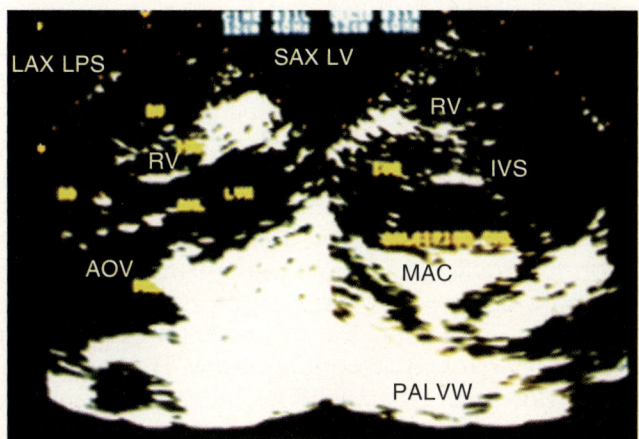

Fig. 14.86: 2D Long axis (left) and Short axis LV (right) echo scans showing mitral annular calcification (MAC) in patient with insulin dependant diabetes mellitus hypertension and non-obstructive hypertrophic cardiomyopathy (see normal AML = anterior mitral leaflet)

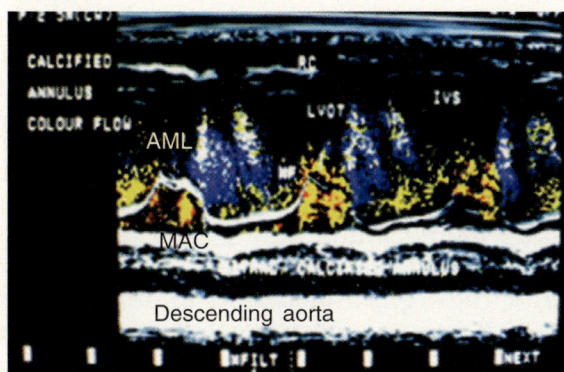

Fig. 14.87: M-Mode in color mode demonstrating mitral annular calcification (MAC). It also shows normal anterior mitral leaflet and normal color flow in left ventricular outflow tract (LVOT) in an elderly patient with hypertension and NIDDM

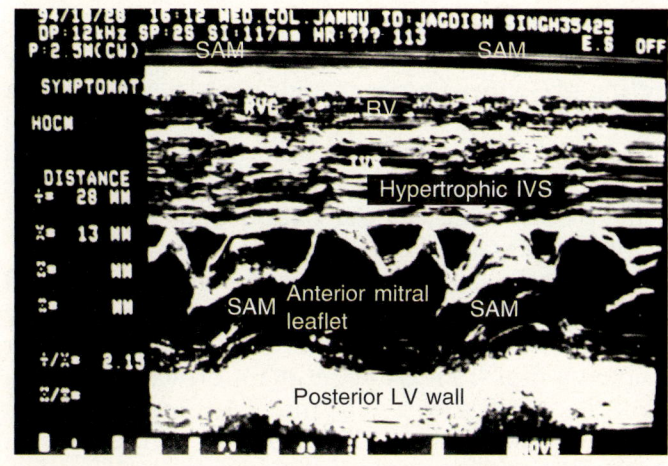

Fig. 14.88: M-Mode echocardiogram showing systolic anterior motion (SAM) of anterior mitral leaflet in patient with hypertrophic obstructive cardiomyopathy (HOCM)

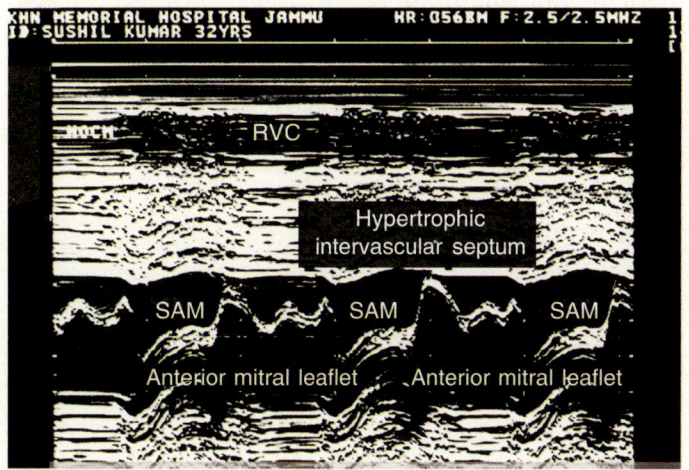

Fig. 14.89: M-Mode echocardiogram showing systolic anterior motion (SAM) of anterior mitral leaflet in another patient with hypertrophic obstructive cardiomyopathy (HOCM)

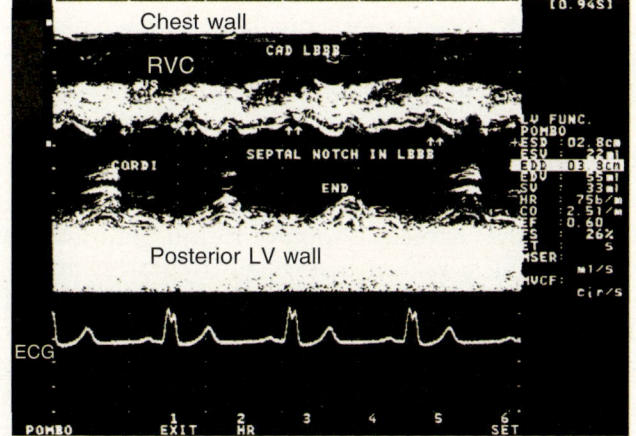

Fig. 14.90: M-Mode echocardiogram showing marked hypokinesia of interventricular septum in patient with three vessel coronary artery disease with wide QRS LBBB

orifice area to be estimated with only one measurement. Underlying this simplification is an assumption that the driving pressure between the left ventricle and the left atrium is 100 mm Hg (which would yield a 5 m/s mitral regurgitant jet). With this assumption, if the aliasing velocity is set to approximately 40 cm/s and the radius of the first aliasing contour obtained, then the regurgitant orifice area is stated quite simply as: ROA = $r^2/2$. After zooming on the proximal convergence zone and baseline shifting to an aliasing velocity of 38 cm/s (close enough to 40 for this application), the aliasing contour is noted 8 mm from the regurgitant orifice, yielding a regurgitant orifice area of 32 mm^2. A recent validation study has shown that this simplified method yields results that are almost the same as the more complete proximal convergence method. Naturally, to the extent that the left ventricle to left atrium pressure difference differs from 100 mm Hg, there will be some intrinsic error in the calculations, but over a pressure range between 64–144 mm Hg, this error should not exceed 20% or 25%. Using the simplified method, it is possible to add quantitation to the assessment of mitral regurgitation with only a minute or two of extra imaging and calculation.

Vena Contracta Method

Another direct approach to quantifying the regurgitant orifice area is by direct visualisation of the vena contracta, the narrowest portion of the regurgitant jet just behind the leaking valve. This has a role in the assessment of aortic regurgitation and has recently been proposed for mitral regurgitation. While this approach is theoretically sound, it is limited by the lateral resolution of colour Doppler echocardiography, which frequently is inadequate to distinguish minor variations in the width of the vena contracta.

Method Specific to Individual Valves

In addition to these general quantitative and colour jet area techniques, there are several parameters that are useful for only the mitral or aortic valve.

Mitral Valve

Assessment of pulmonary venous flow is a useful adjunct in the characterisation of mitral regurgitation. Normally the S wave (during ventricular systole) is larger than the D wave. With progressive degrees of mitral regurgitation, however, the maximal velocity of the S wave is reduced, becoming frankly reversed when mitral regurgitation is severe. Unfortunately, the intermediate pattern, where the S wave is merely blunted (smaller than the D wave but not reversed) is very non-specific. It may be an indicator of moderately severe mitral regurgitation, but it also occurs in situations of left ventricular dysfunction and atrial fibrillation. Another useful adjunct in assessing mitral regurgitant severity is inspection of the transmitral flow pattern. It is almost impossible to have haemodynamically significant mitral regurgitation without having an elevated E wave through the mitral valve (Figs 14.45–62, 14.67, 14.68, 14.73, 14.74, 14.78 and 14.80).

Aortic Valve

For the aortic valve there are two special indices that are useful in characterising regurgitation: the aortic pressure half-time, and flow reversal in the aorta. The aortic pressure half-time is obtained from the continuouswave Doppler recording of reversed flow across the aortic valve in diastole. By measuring the time required for the aorta-to-left ventricle pressure difference to fall by half, one gets an indication of the severity of regurgitation, with values less than 250 ms typically indicating haemodynamically significant regurgitation. However, the pressure halftime depends critically on the chronicity of the regurgitation, with acute aortic regurgitation leading to much shorter values than longstanding leakage, in which case the ventricle has dilated with increased compliance. In addition, the halftime also varies with systemic vascular resistance, such that patients who are treated with vasodilators may shorten their half-time even as the aortic regurgitant fraction improves, in contrast to the usual expectation of this parameter. When aortic regurgitation is haemodynamically significant, flow reversal may be visualised in the aortic arch and descending aorta. The ratio of the reversed flow to the forward flow velocity time integral may be taken as an estimate of the aortic regurgitant fraction. Indeed, if one is to be given only one piece of data upon which to decide whether aortic regurgitation was haemodynamically significant or not, a pulsed Doppler recording in the distal aortic arch would probably be the best one (Figs 14.94 and 14.122–14.130).

Summary

Careful quantification of valvar regurgitation is critical for deciding on the need and success of medical management as well as determining the timing of surgery. The colour Doppler jet area method, despite its many limitations, is still useful for separating regurgitation into several broad degrees of severity. However, any patient with a significant degree of regurgitation should undergo a formal quantification study, which in general can most easily and accurately be done using the proximal convergence method. Combining this with observations of chamber size and function, pulmonary artery pressure, and adjunct parameters such as pulmonary venous flow and aortic flow, will give the

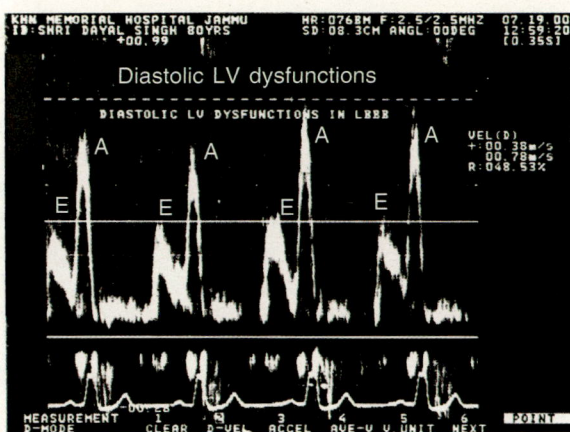

Fig. 14.91: Doppler flow velocity across mitral valve showing enhanced A velocity as compared to E velocity as a Doppler feature of defect in diastolic relaxation of LV in above-described patient with coronary artery disease and wide QRS LBBB

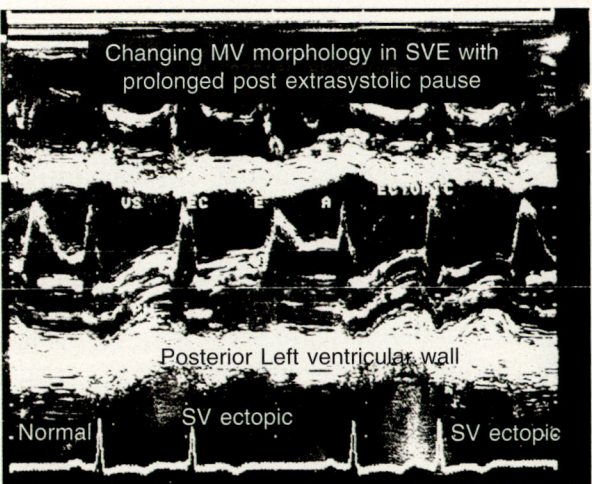

Fig. 14.92: M-Mode echocardiogram showing changing morphology of mitral valve in premature supraventricular ectopics in a patient with sick sinus syndrome

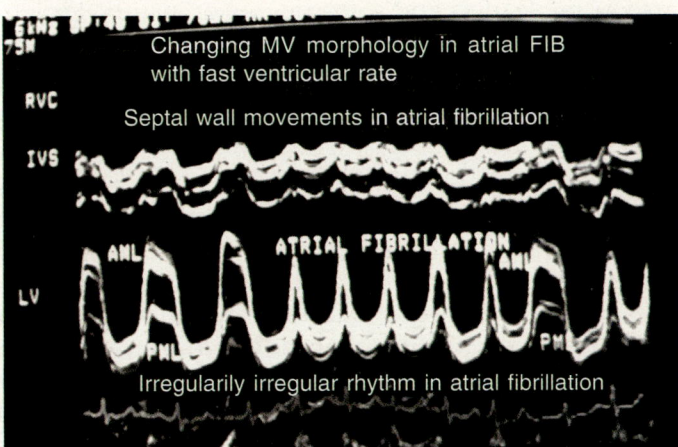

Fig. 14.93: M-Mode echocardiogram showing grossly abnormal configuration of mitral valve in atrial fibrillation with fast ventricular response in a patient with rheumatic mitral stenosis

echocardiographer much improved confidence in the proper assessment about the regurgitation.

Automated Quantification of Aortic Regurgitant Volume and Regurgitant Fraction using the Digital Colour Doppler Velocity Profile Integration Method in Patients with Aortic Regurgitation

In patients with aortic regurgitation, accurate evaluation of the severity of the regurgitation is important in determining whether surgical correction is required. Colour Doppler visualisation of aortic regurgitant jets has been used clinically for this purpose. However, the area and length of the regurgitant jet depends not only on the regurgitant volume and flow rate but also on the flow velocity (pressure difference), chamber compliance, and wall constraint. Because of this, several different methods have been applied to quantify the severity of aortic regurgitation by measuring the regurgitant volume or regurgitant fraction (RF) using Doppler echocardiography.

Recently a new quantitative technique which uses spatio-temporal integration of digital colour Doppler velocity profile data has been developed for automated cardiac flow measurement (ACM). This method provides quick and accurate automated calculation of stroke volume and cardiac output. Recent studies have shown that it yields regurgitant volume and regurgitant fraction measurements that are equivalent to standard pulsed Doppler cross sectional echocardiography (PD-2D) in patients with mitral regurgitation. However, the only report of the use of ACM in the evaluation of aortic regurgitation was one animal study, some workers, therefore, have employed the ACM technique to patients with significant isolated aortic regurgitation to compare the ACM and the PD-2D methods for determining aortic regurgitant volume and regurgitant fraction.

Flow volume rate is obtained by spatial integration of the velocity profile throughout the systolic period. Flow volume is measured by the temporal integration of the flow volume rate obtained by spatial profile integration of the velocity profile throughout the diastolic period.

For mitral inflow volume measurements, colour Doppler image acquisition is obtained from both apical four chamber and two chamber views. Several beats of colour images were recorded sequentially on the image memory. A region of interest is set on the mitral annulus in the display to obtain the velocity profile. Flow volume is measured throughout the diastolic period by the temporal and spatial integration of measured velocity profile. Three measurements of each variable are averaged to determine flow volume in both four and two chamber views separately. Final mitral inflow volume is determined by averaging flow volume from the two views.

PD-2D Echocardiographic Analysis (Fig. 14.84)

Quantitative Doppler measurements and calculations were done at the time of the examination using an ultrasound imaging system with a 2.5 MHz transducer (Toshiba SSA-380A, Power Vision, Tochigi, Japan). The aortic outflow and mitral inflow volumes were calculated using the product of the pulsed Doppler time-velocity integral and the area of the annuli of the aortic and mitral valves. The diameter of the annulus in systole measured at the point of insertion of the leaflets. The diameter of the mitral annulus is measured at the time of maximum valvar opening from both four and two chamber views. Assuming an elliptic shape, cross-sectional annular area is calculated as ab, where "a" and "b" are halved diameters of the annulus in the four and two chamber views. The apical approach is used to record the pulsed wave Doppler signal at the aortic and mitral annuli, and integrals are obtained by manually tracing the Doppler spectrum. It therefore, traced the modal velocity of both the mitral inflow and the aortic outflow from the pulsed Doppler waveform. The average from the three measurements of each variable was recorded. The aortic regurgitant volume and percent regurgitant fraction (%RF) are calculated as follows:

Aortic regurgitant volume = Aortic outflow volume – Mitral inflow volume

Regurgitant fraction = Aortic regurgitant volume – Aortic outflow volume × 100

ACM method (Fig. 14.83)

The principle of the ACM method has been described previously. Colour Doppler echocardiography is undertaken with a Toshiba SSA-380A ultrasound imaging system equipped with prototype ACM software and a 2.5 MHz transducer. Frame rate is set at 27 frames/s with a 30° colour sector. The pulse repetition frequency is 4.5 kHz. The aliasing phenomenon is prevented by shifting the colour baseline (Doppler zero shift) velocity up to approximately 1.4 m/s. The cut-off frequency of the wall filter is set high enough to eliminate the clutter signals from the moving tissue (cut off frequency 900 Hz). An optimal gain setting is obtained without random colour noise in the nonflow areas by maximising the gain level.

ACM is done immediately after PD-2D by a single examiner who did not know the results of the PD-2D study. Colour Doppler image acquisition is obtained from the apical long-axis view for aortic outflow measurements. Several beats of colour images are recorded sequentially on the image memory. On the selected beat, the systolic period is manually defined by a trigger mark based on the ECG. A region of interest is set on the aortic annulus in the display to obtain the velocity profile. For each frame of the colour images, flow volume rate is calculated by rotational integration of the velocity profile in the region of interest. Stroke volume is measured by the temporal integration of the flow volume rate throughout the systolic period. Three measurements of each variable are averaged to determine aortic outflow volume.

It therefore, has shown that aortic regurgitant volume and regurgitant fraction assessed by the ACM method are closely correlated with the values obtained using the conventional PD-2D method. The time required for aortic regurgitant volume calculation by the ACM method is significantly shorter than by the PD-2D method. The ACM method would be clinically useful in the quantitative assessment of aortic regurgitant volume and regurgitant fraction in patients with isolated aortic regurgitation.

Tricuspid Valvular Disease (Figs 14.146–14.162)

It has been reported that about 25% of the patients with severe rheumatic heart lesions suffer from valvular disease but, clinically significant disease is found in approximately 5% to 10% of these patients. Severe tricuspid regurgitation can occur as a result of mitral and aortic valvular disease secondary to pulmonary hypertension due to these lesions.

Tricuspid Stenosis (TS) (Fig. 14.154)

Rheumatic fever is one of the topmost causes of tricuspid stenosis and only next to mitral and aortic valves. Other causes are congenital defects, systemic lupus erythematosus, and carcinoid tumors. The stenotic leaflets usually fuse, leaving a roundish hilum in the central area of the leaflets and some degree of insufficiency of the valve. Right atrial hypertrophy occurs, and cardiac output falls when the right ventricular filling is impaired because of further narrowing of the valve orifice.

Tricuspid Insufficiency (TR) (Figs 14.152–14.156)

Tricuspid regurgitation can be divided into two categories, such as functional and organic. Functional insufficiency is as a result of right ventricular failure, causing right ventricular dilation, which in turn can lead to dilation of valvular ring and finally producing tricuspid valve regurgitation. Organic regurgitation is caused by rheumatic disease but it can also be due to other causes such as Ebstein's disease and endocardial cushion defects, or bacterial endocarditis. The regurgitant flow leads to enlargement of right atrium causing hypertrophy and dilation. One can visualise the dilated right sided structures echocardiographically in a better way as compared to normal right atrium and ventricle.

Doppler Flow Evaluation of the Tricuspid Valve

Tricuspid regurgitation is commonly visualised by Doppler echo. The best window to record velocities from the tricuspid valve is the apical four-chamber window or the left parasternal long-axis window. Sometimes the velocities may be recorded from the parasternal short-axis window; as one demonstrates the aortic valve and right ventricular outflow tract, the transducer is angled slightly inferior to record the leaflets of the tricuspid valve with the right atrial chamber.

Tricuspid regurgitation can be categorised into mild, moderate, or severe. The mild form is seen just at the annulus level. The moderate form extends midways into the right atrial cavity, and the severe form extends to the base of the right atrium.

By the application of colour-flow mapping, one can learn that not all regurgitant jets flow from the tricuspid annulus to the medial wall of the interatrial septum. The path of the jet depends on the deformity of the valve and thus may dart in a lateral pathway, or even directly into the atrial cavity.

Systolic Pressure Gradient: With Doppler flow studies it is possible to calculate the systolic pressure gradient across the tricuspid valve by using the regurgitant velocity and the Bernoulli equation formula $(P_1 - P_2 = 4V^2)$ to accurately estimate the systolic pressure difference between the right ventricle and right atrium. By the addition of the estimated right atrial pressure to the calculated gradient gives right ventricle and pulmonary systolic pressure, values. In the presence of tricuspid regurgitation and normal pulmonary artery pressures, the calculated gradient across the tricuspid valve is less than 25 mm Hg (a maximum velocity of 2.5 m/sec). If pulmonary hypertension is present, higher gradient can be recorded. This gives us an indication whether tricuspid regurgitation is from a diseased tricuspid valve with normal pulmonary pressure or from pulmonary hypertension, secondary to mitral and aortic valvular disease.

Pulmonary Stenosis and Insufficiency

Pulmonary valve can also be affected by the rheumatic fever though very rarely by a similar inflammatory process as it happens with mitral aortic and tricuspid cusps. The other most common cause of pulmonic stenosis in the adult population is residual stenosis after surgical repair of tetralogy of Fallot (Figs 14.160–14.182).

The evaluation is performed through three conventional windows such as the apical five chamber view (this is the apical four-chamber view with the transducer directed slightly more anterior to record the left ventricular outflow tract, the aorta, and aortic cusps), the suprasternal notch to sample the ascending and descending aortic flow, and, the right parasternal long-axis view. Once the highest velocity is recorded, through any of the windows the modified, Bernoulli equation may be applied to calculate the transvalvular gradient, i.e.

Gradient: $4 (V_{max})^2$

For example, if a patient has a velocity of 3 m/sec. one would substitute V = 3; thus:

Gradient = $4(3)^2$
Gradient = 4(9)
Gradient = 36 m/s

The two-dimensional image and M-mode tracing usually reveals some thickening of the pulmonic cusp tissue narrowing of right ventricular outflow tract or the main pulmonary artery (subpulmonic stenosis or supra-pulmonic stenosis). The valves may show calcification, restricted movements, irregularity of orifice, doming of the valve, reduced E-F slope and loss of a wave on both M-mode and 2-D echocardiography.

Pulmonic insufficiency can be observed with the conventional two-dimensional and Doppler studies. The continuous wave probe should be used to record the maximum velocity. The modified Bernoulli equation (gradient $4 \times V^2$) may then be applied to calculate the gradient. $4 (V_{max})^2$ – Tricuspid regurgitation velocity

RVSP = RA + $4(V_{max})^2$
= 5 mm Hg + $4(3.3)^2$
= 5 mm Hg + 44 = 49 mm Hg

Table 14.4: *Echo-Doppler criteria in assessing severity of tricuspid valvular regurgitation*

Parameter	Mild	Moderate	Severe
Tricuspid valve	Usually Normal	Normal or Abnormal	Abnormal leaflet / poor coaptation
RV/RA/ Size	Normal	Normal or Dialated	Usually dialated
Jet area-central jets (cm²)	<5	<10	<10
VC width (cm)	Not defined	Not defined but <0.7	>0.7
PISA radius (cm²)	<0.5	<0.9	>0.9
Jet density and contour CW	Soft and parabolic	Dense, variable contour	Dense triangular with early peaking
Hepatic vein flow	Systolic dominance	Systolic blurting	Systolic reversal

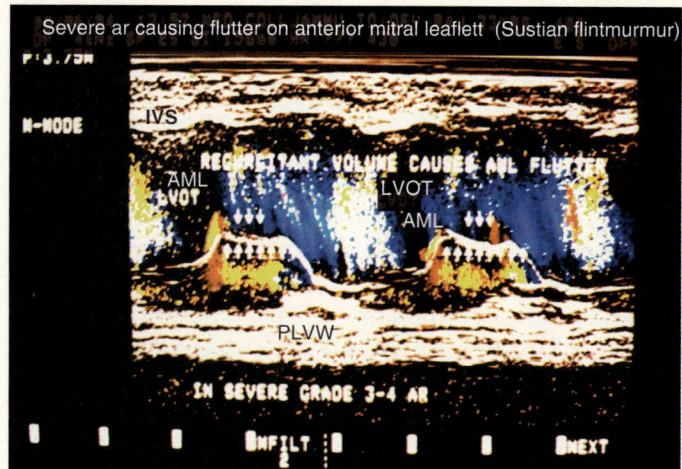

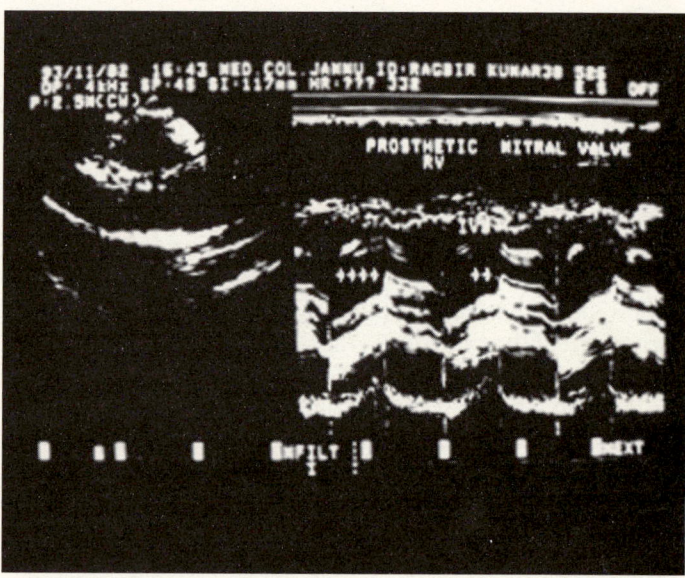

Fig. 14.94: M-Mode echocardiogram showing color flow jet of severe aortic regurgitation causing flutter of the anterior mitral leaflet (arrows). This regurgitant jet on anterior mitral leaflet causes mechanical obstruction during mid-diastole and hence is the genesis of clinical mid diastolic murmur (MDM) in the left parasternal region. This MDM is also called as Austian Flint murmur, after the name of the scientist

Fig. 14.95: M-Mode echocardiogram showing normally functioning Bjork shelly (arrow) prosthetic mitral valve in patient who had preoperative severe calcified mitral valvular stenosis with fixed cardiac decompensation

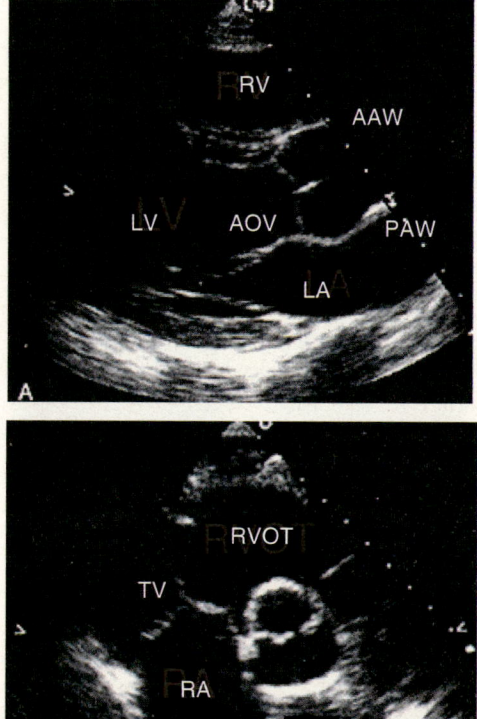

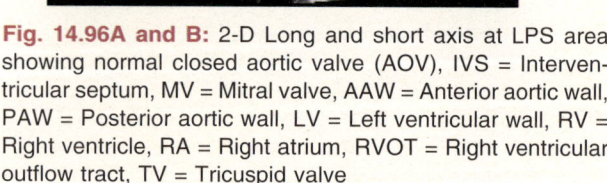

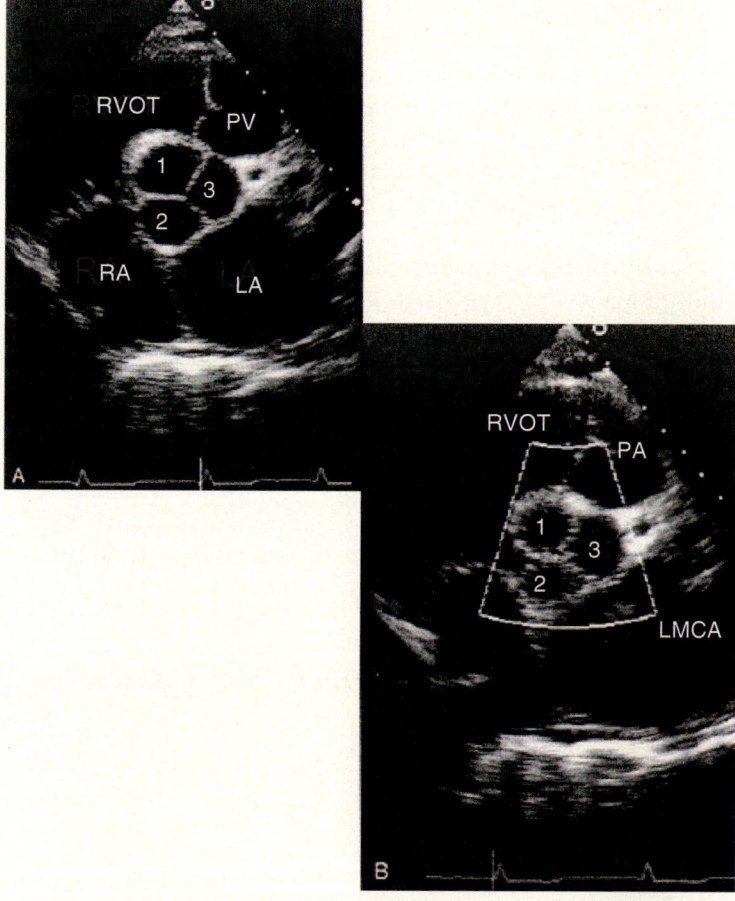

Fig. 14.96A and B: 2-D Long and short axis at LPS area showing normal closed aortic valve (AOV), IVS = Interventricular septum, MV = Mitral valve, AAW = Anterior aortic wall, PAW = Posterior aortic wall, LV = Left ventricular wall, RV = Right ventricle, RA = Right atrium, RVOT = Right ventricular outflow tract, TV = Tricuspid valve

Fig. 14.97A and B: Short axis view of aorta at higher LPS area showing tricuspid aortic valves along with their respective sinuses from where both right and left coronary arteries emerge (LMCA = Left main coronary artery) D

Anatomical Localization of Aortic Valve through Different Windows

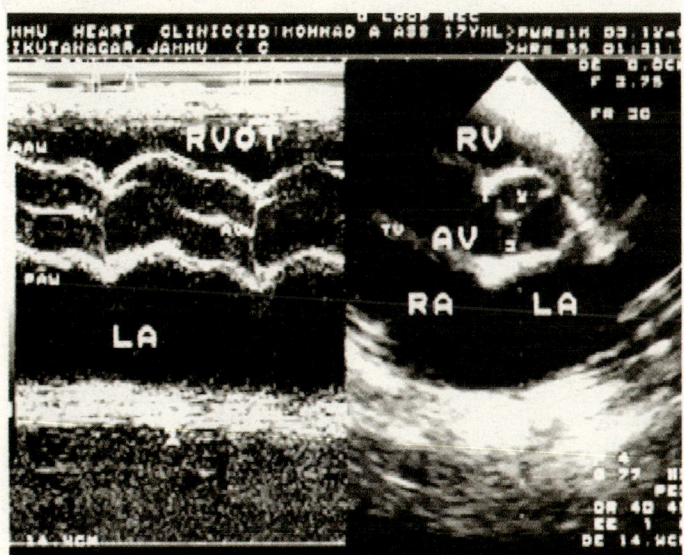

Fig. 14.98: M-Mode and short axis aorta showing location of aortic valve

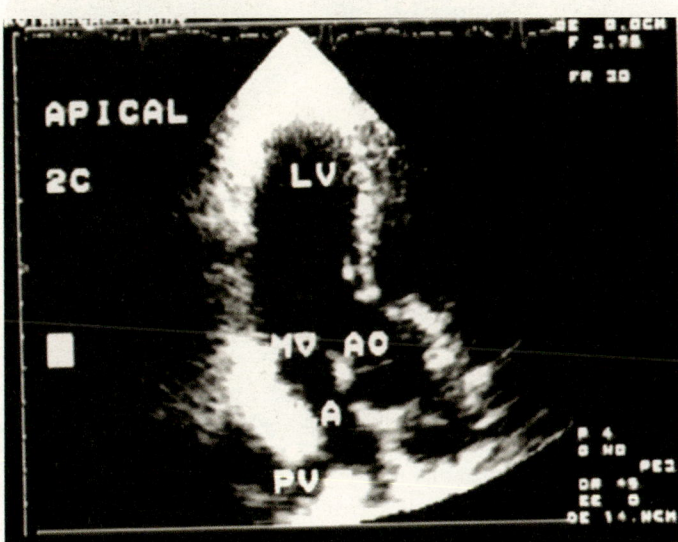

Fig. 14.99: Apical 5C view showing location of ascending aorta with aortic valve

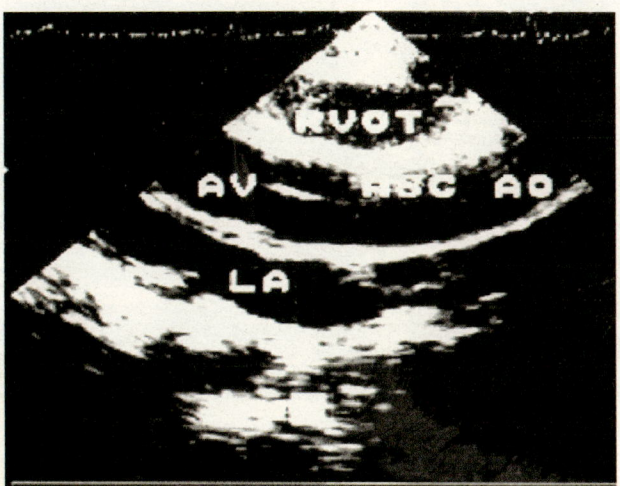

Fig. 14.100: Long axis aorta showing good length aorta along with aortic valve and aortic root

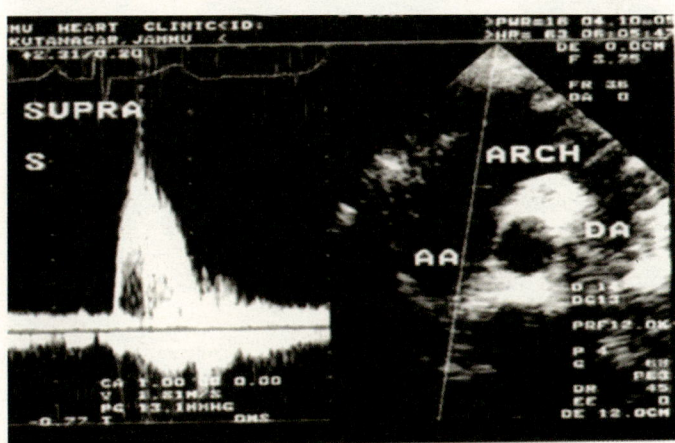

Fig. 14.101: Suprasternal approach showing ascending aorta arch and descending aorta (right) and Doppler flow velocity across ascending aorta

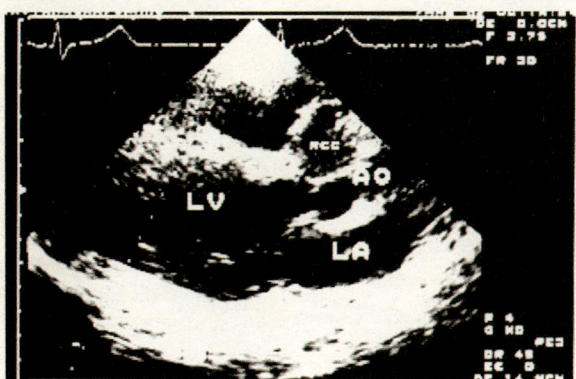

Fig. 14.102: Long axis LV showing aorta along with aortic valve and respective sinuses

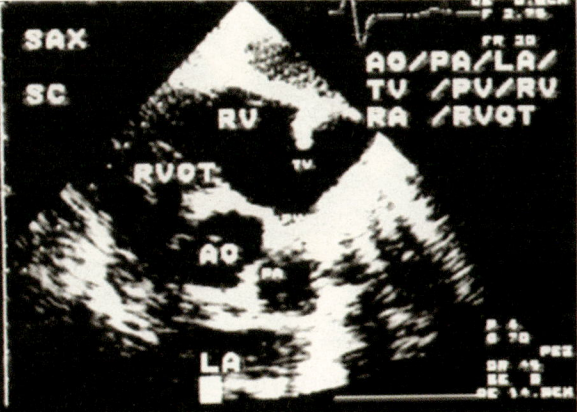

Fig. 14.103: Subcostal short axis view showing aorta and its valve

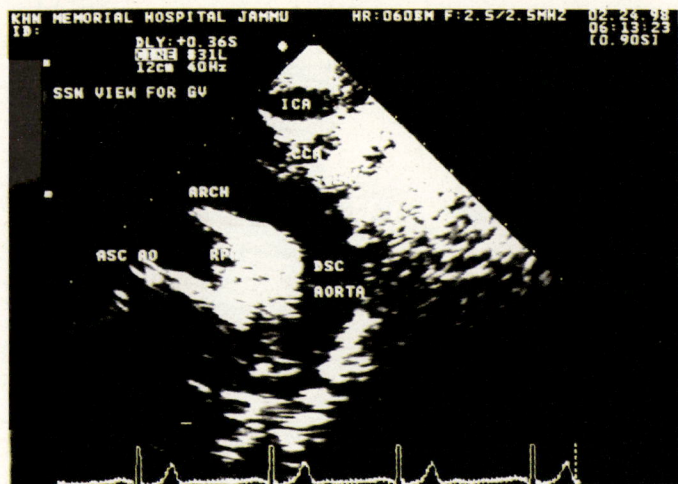

Fig. 14.104: Suprasternal notch window showing ascending aorta with its valve, arch and descending aorta along with centerally placed right pulmonary artery (RPA)

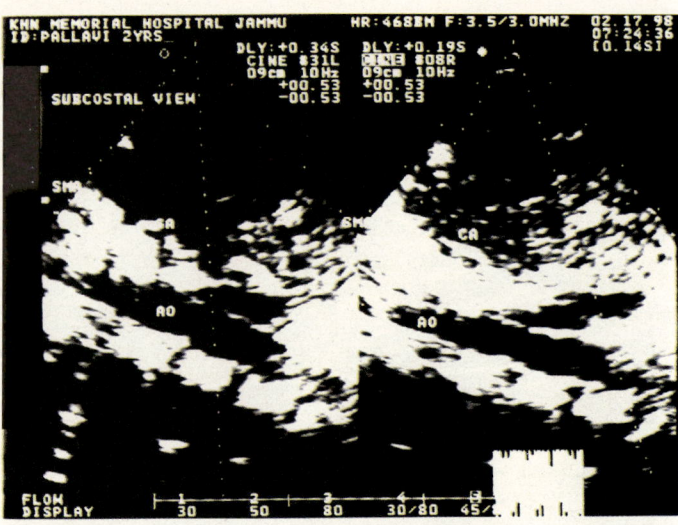

Fig. 14.105: Subcostal transverse view showing longitudinally placed abdominal aorta (AO)

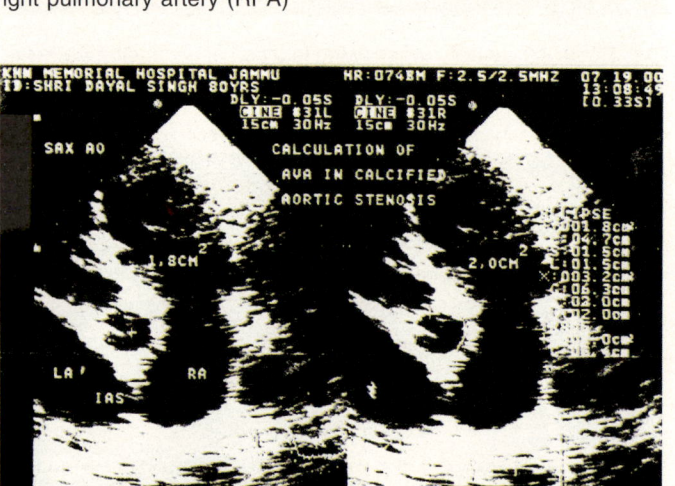

Fig. 14.106: Short axis views showing the method of calculating aortic valvular area in patient with calcified aortic valvular stenosis

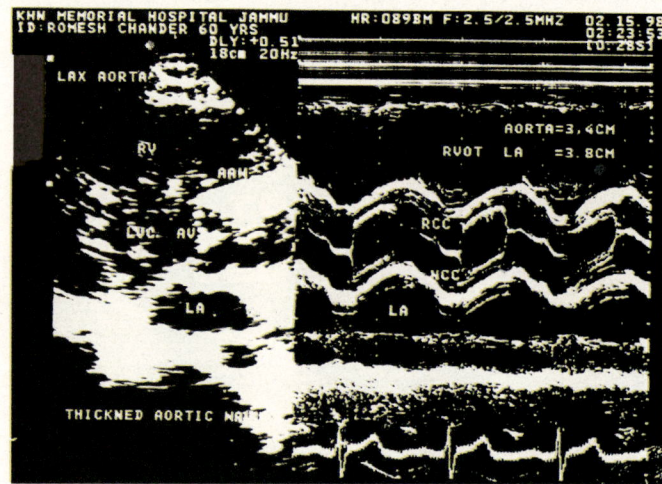

Fig. 14.107: M-Mode and 2D views showing measurements of aorta and left atrium (right) and long axis LV view (left) showing trileaflets aorta

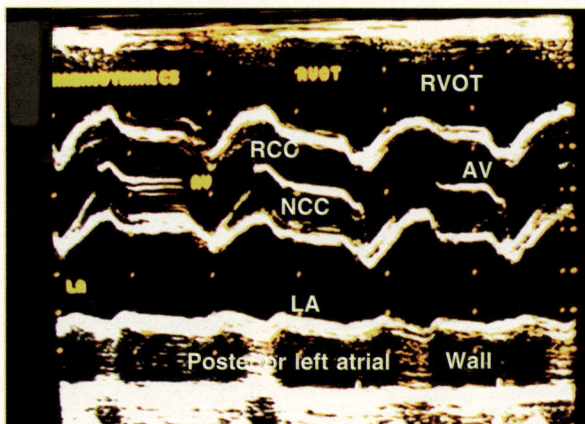

Fig. 14.108: M-Mode echogram showing anatomical relationship between right ventricular outflow tract, (RVOT) left atrium (LA) Aortic valve (AV), right (RCC) and non-coronary (NCC) cusps of aorta

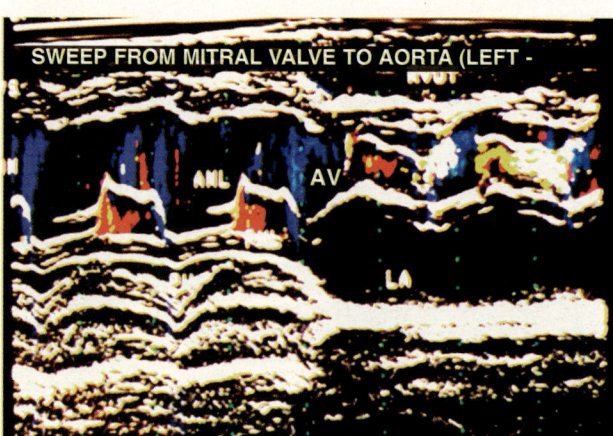

Fig. 14.109: M-Mode color echo scan showing sweep from normal mitral valve to stenosed aotic valve with mosaic color flow in aortic valve

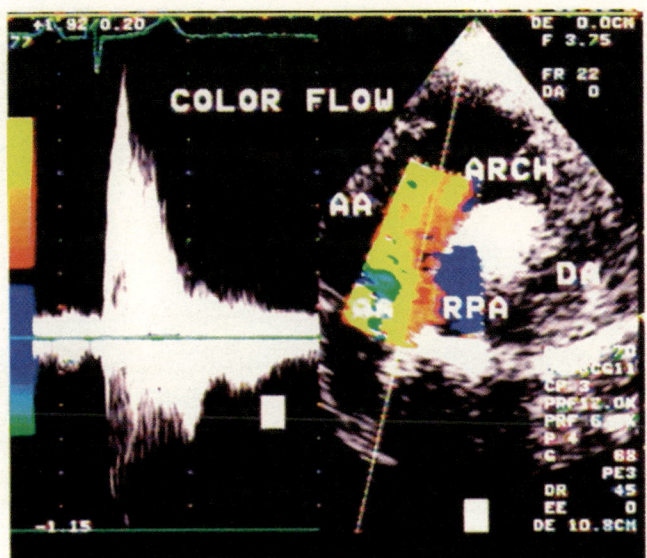

Fig. 14.110: Suprasternal great vessel view showing normal anatomical relationship between ascending aorta, arch, descending aorta and right pulmonary artery

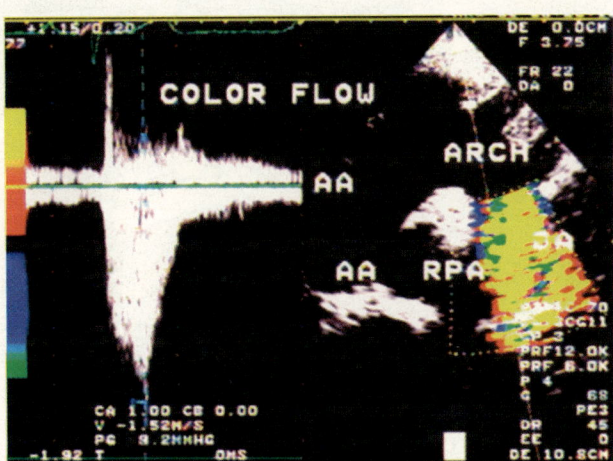

Fig. 14.111: Suprasternal great vessel view showing normal relationship between descending aorta, arch and right pulmonary artery

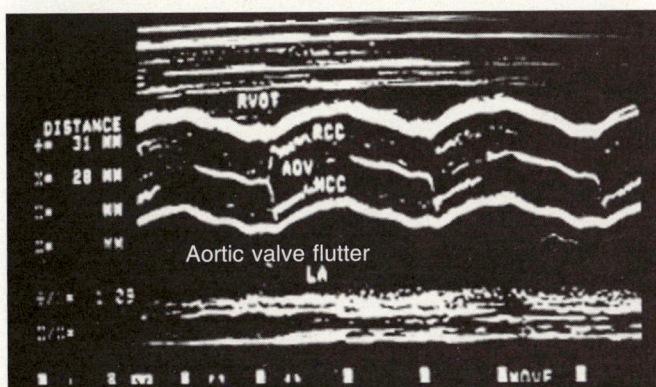

Fig. 14.112: M-Mode echo showing flutter of right and non-coronary cups in normal aortic valve

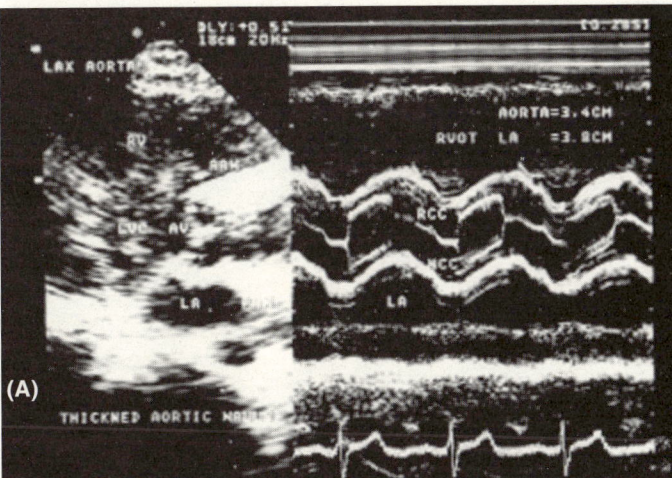

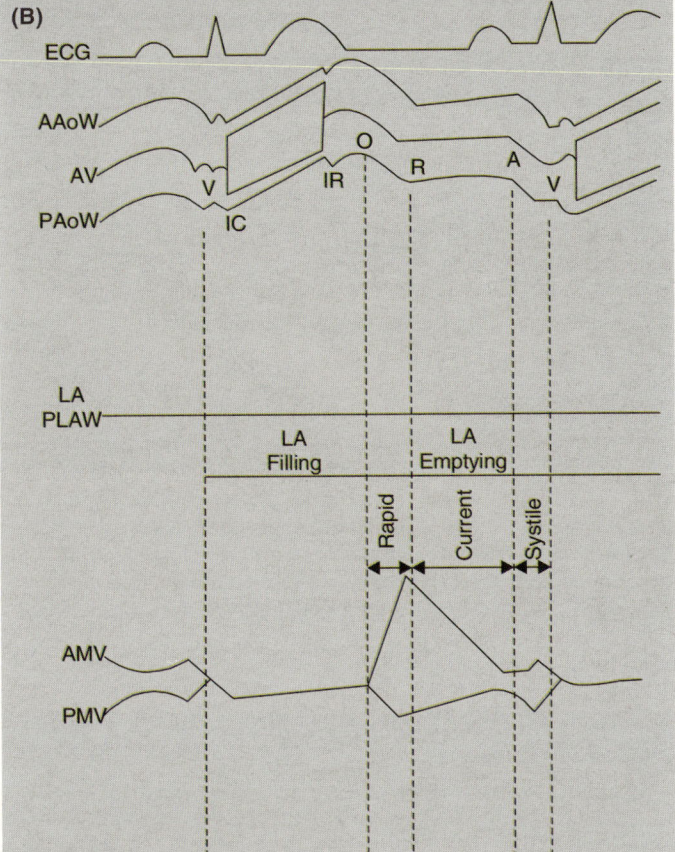

ECG—Electrocardiogram
AAoW—Anterior aortic wall
AV—Aortic valve
PAoW—Posterior aortic wall
PLAW—Posterior left atrial wall
AML—Anterior mitral leaflet
PML—Posterior mitral leaflet

Fig. 14.113A and B: (A) 2-D and M-Mode echocardiogram showing morphological features of aortic valve and its relationship with left atrium (LA) and right ventricular outflow tract (RVOT). **(B)** Diagrammatic representation of Fig. A. with additional features of various hemodynamic events such as filling and emptying of LA in relation to opening and closing of MV and aortic valves

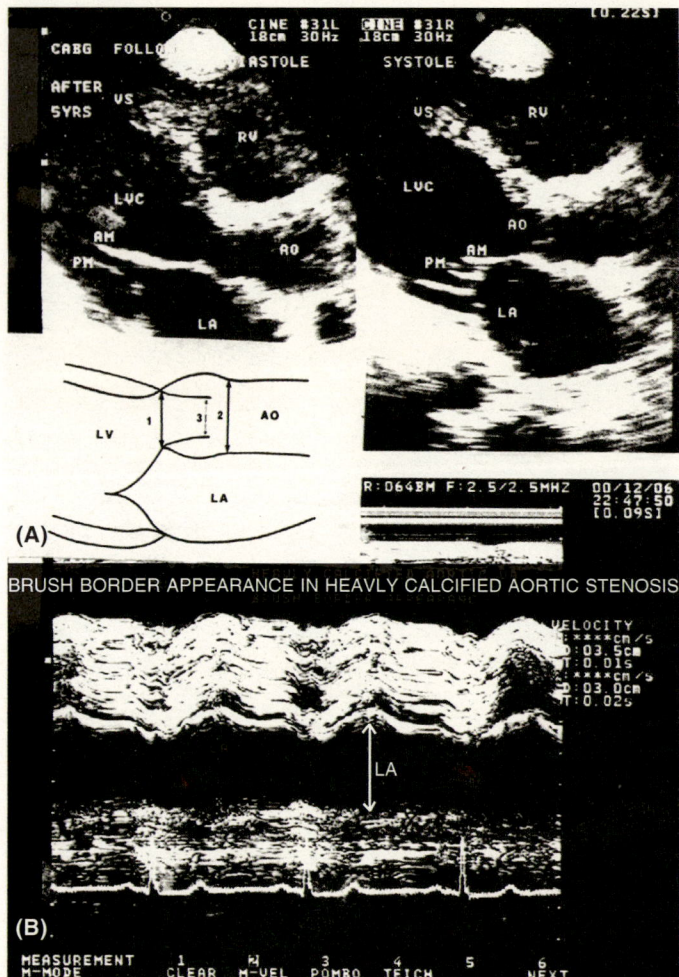

BRUSH BORDER APPEARANCE IN HEAVILY CALCIFIED AORTIC STENOSIS

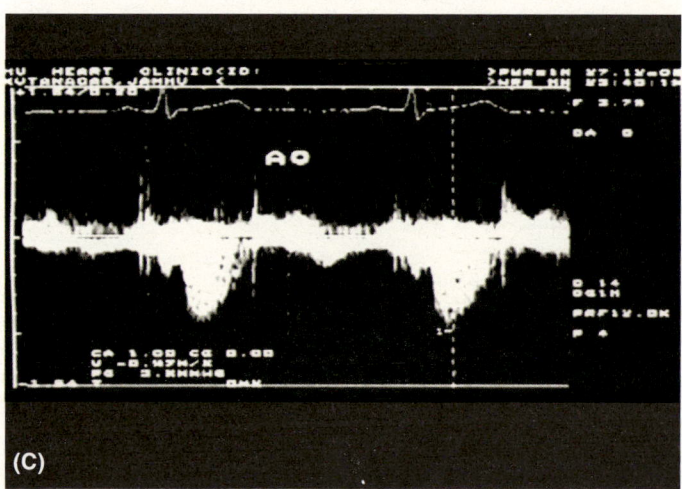

Fig. 14.114A and B: (A) 2-D Long axis view of aorta showing the method of calculating LVOT diameter for determining aortic flow in the final obtaining hemodynamic aortic flow volume. **(B)** M-Mode echocardiogram showing brush border appearance in calcified aortic valve including thickening both anterior and posterior aortic walls

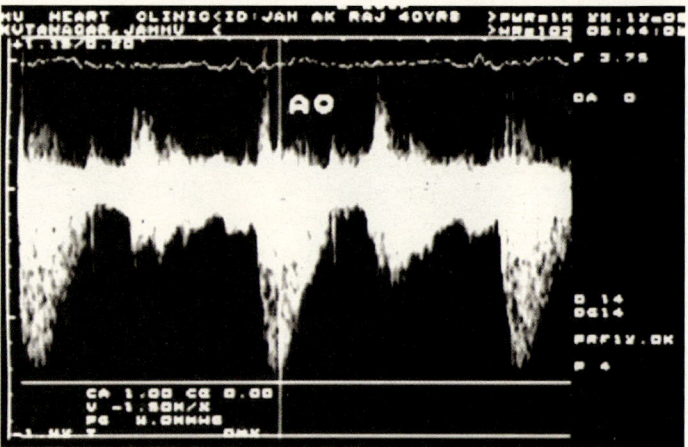

Fig. 14.115: Doppler flow velocity across aortic valve showing mild to moderate enhancement of aortic flow velocity in patient with rheumatic mild aortic valvular stenosis

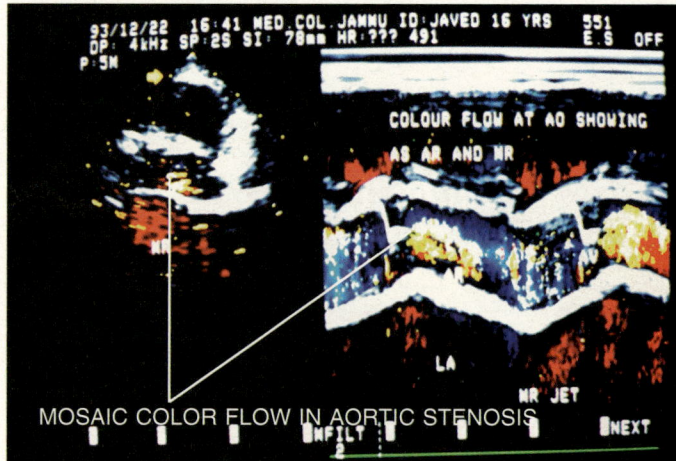

Fig. 14.116: 2D and M-Mode echocadiogram showing thickened aortic walls and mosaic color flow of aortic valvular stenosis

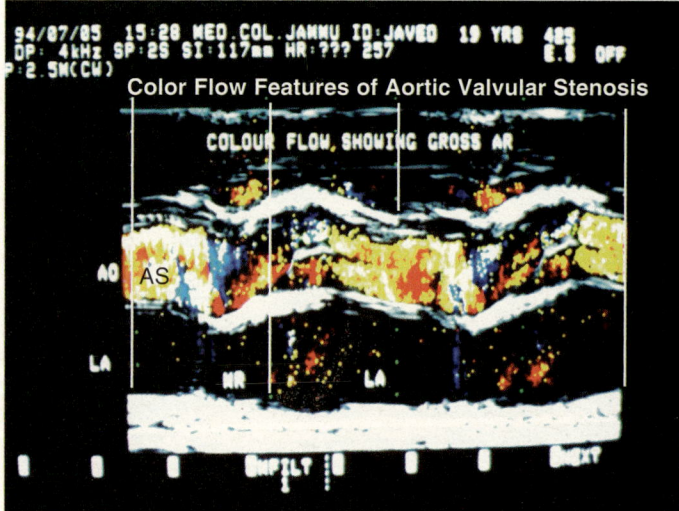

Fig. 14.117: Another example of color M-Mode echocardiographic features of aortic valvular stenosis

Fig. 14.114C: Doppler flow velocity across aortic valve showing mild enhancement of aortic velocity in patient with aortic valvulitis

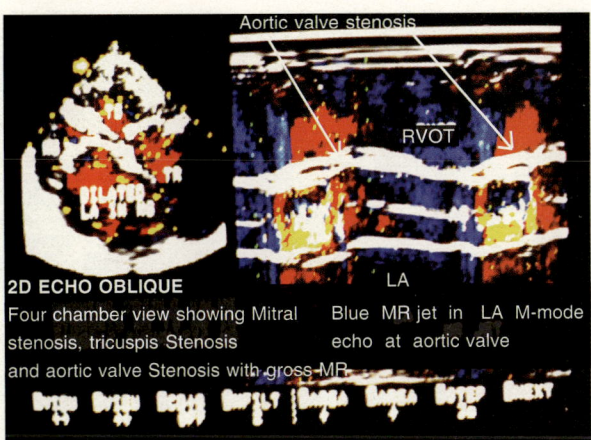

Fig. 14.118: 2-D and M-mode echocardiogram in color mode showing blue jet of mitral regurgitation in LA while studying aortic valvular pathology in patient with mitral stenosis with severe mitral regurgitation (MR) tricuspid stenosis with TR and aortic valvular stenosis with moderate regurgitation

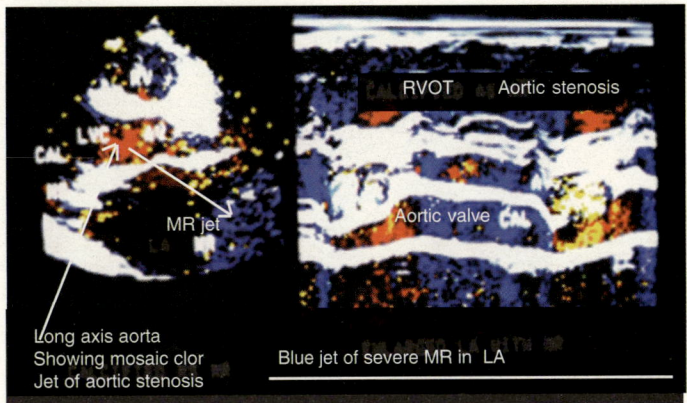

Fig. 14.119: Another example, 2-D and M-Mode echocardiogram in color mode showing blue jet of mitral regurgitation in LA while studying aortic valvular pathology in patient with mitral stenosis with severe mitral regurgitation (MR) and aortic valvular stenosis with moderate regurgitation

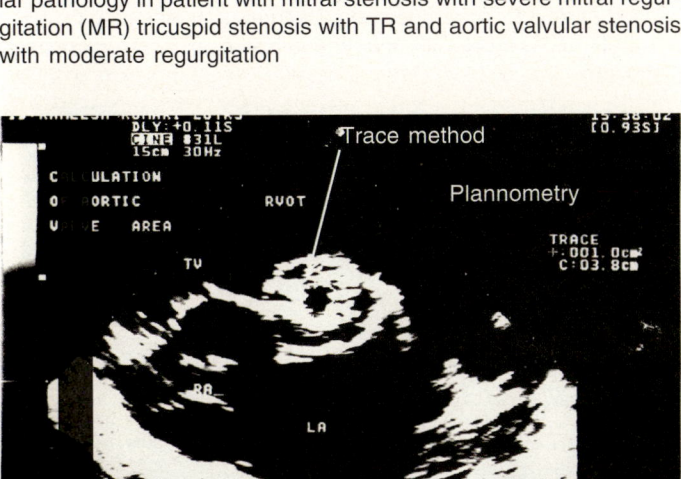

Fig. 14.120: 2-D Short axis view at aorta level showing the methods of obtaining aortic valvular area by trace and plannometry in the same patient with mitral valvular stenosis and aortic stenosis with enlagement of left atrium (LA)

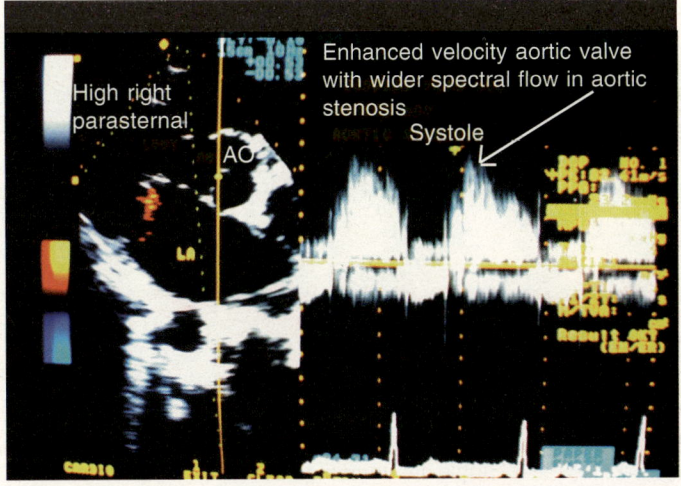

Fig. 14.121: 2-D Color Doppler dual echoscans showing Doppler flow velocity across the aortic valve which has been scanned in slightly oblique short axis plane from the high right parasternal region in patient with aortic valvular stenosis

The presence of pulmonary insufficiency may be considered if there is a flow disturbance in the right ventricular outflow tract below the pulmonic valve as seen with pulsed-wave probe. This pattern should be considered abnormal if it extends more than 1 cm into the right ventricular outflow tract during diastole.

Pattern of the coronary artery from that of insufficiency, the regurgitant jet is much harsher than normal coronary flow, and the time it occurs in the cardiac cycle. Yet in other method by using 2-D echo cardiography, one can place the Doppler beam away from the orifice of the coronary artery and thus may be able to separate the flow patterns more easily.

Colour-flow Doppler facilitates the visualisation of the coronary flow and the regurgitant jet pattern from pulmonic insufficiency very easily. The Doppler sample may then be placed in the jet stream to record the maximum flow patterns.

The use of combined Doppler and two-dimensional imaging techniques may prove very useful in the clinical assessment of the patient with heart disease. However, a number of factors are critical to performing an adequate Doppler examination, and these factors must be adhered to obtain the correct data.

The Doppler velocity recordings depend on the intercept angle between the direction of the sound beam and bloodflow. This angle is three-dimensional angle, and it cannot be determined completely even using two-dimensional colour-flow mapping techniques. The unpredictable direction of high-velocity jets, and the

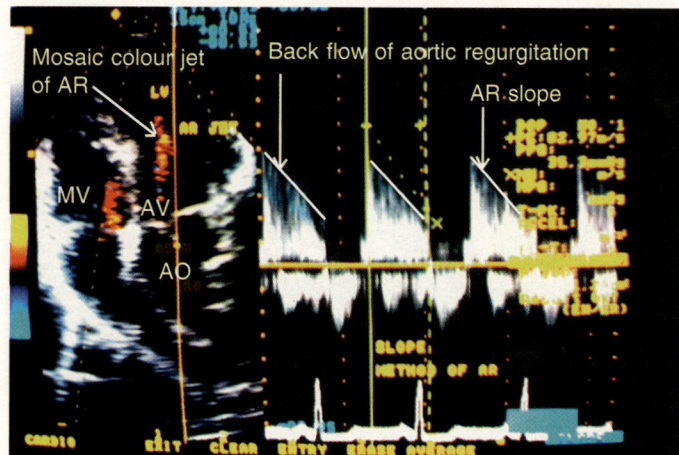

Fig. 14.122: 2-D Color Doppler dual scan taken in apical 5C View showing mosaic color jet of aortic regurgitation (left panel). Doppler flow showing forward flow of aortic stenosis below the line and backward flow of aortic regurgitation above the imaginary line (right panel). This scan also depicts as how to calculate severity of aortic regurgitation by slope method (see text for detail)

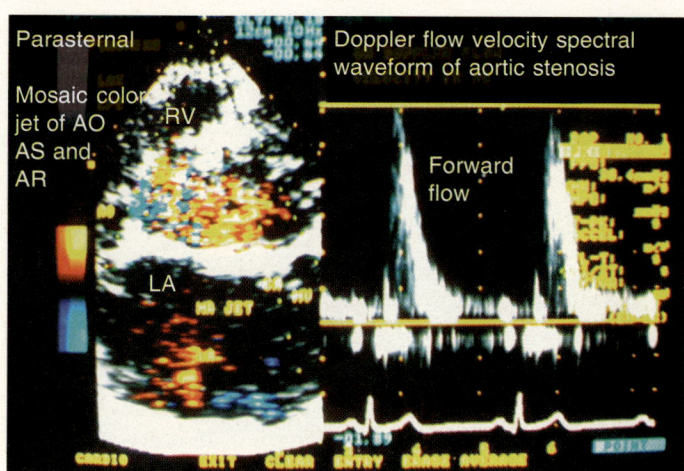

Fig. 14.123: 2-D Color Doppler study of aortic valve in high right parasternal region lying on the right lateral decubitus showing enhanced narrow Doppler spectral waveform of aortic stenosis (right scan) and mosaic color jet of both aortic stenosis and regurgitation (left scan)

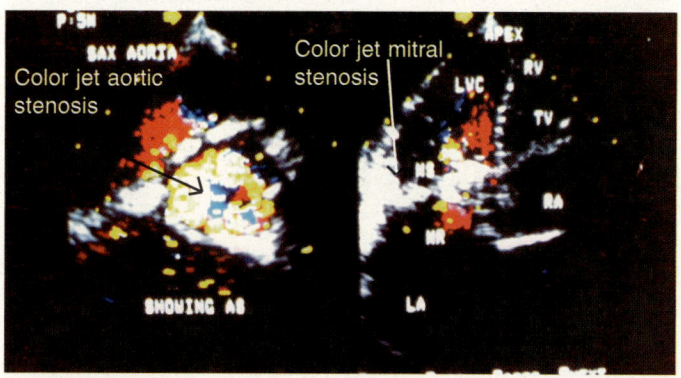

Fig. 14.124: 2-D Color flow short axis aorta (left scan) showing mosaic color jet of aortic stenosis and jet of mitral stenosis in apical 4C view (right scan) in the same patient with aortic and mitral valvular stenosis

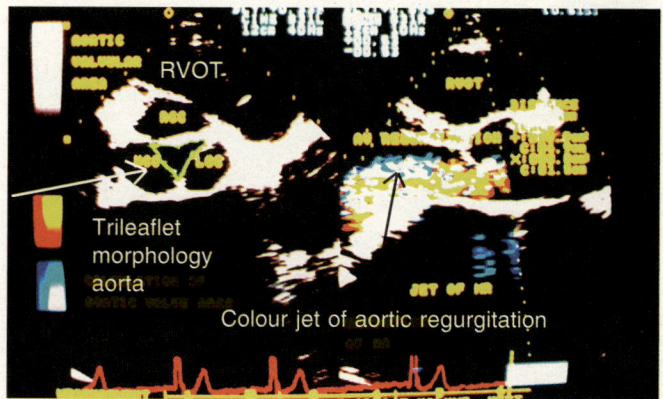

Fig. 14.125: 2-D Color flow short axis view at aorta showing mosaic color jet of aortic regurgitation (right scan) and normal trileaflet morphology of aorta (right scan)

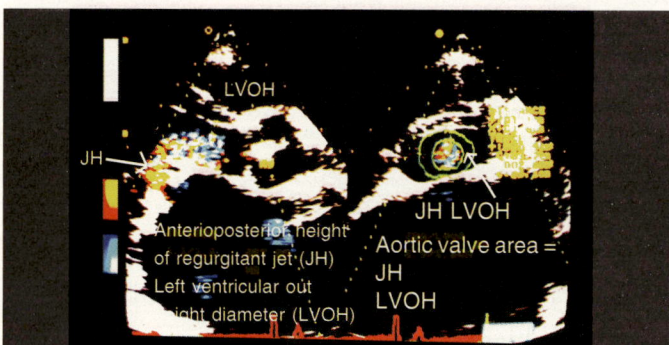

Fig. 14.126: Long and short axis dual color flow scans at aorta (L-R) showing the method of calculation of aortic flow area by the measurement of antero-posterior height of regurgitant jet at its initiation and diameter of LV outflow tract (LVOH) through which it traverses into LV cavity. Ratio of height of regurgitant jet (JH) and LVOH is determined. For calculation of flow area (see detail in text)

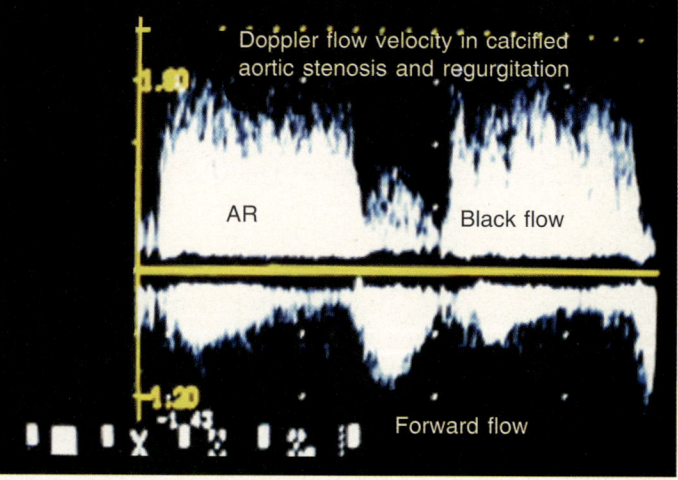

Fig. 14.127: Determination of Doppler flow velocity of aorta in grading severity of aortic regurgitation by slope method

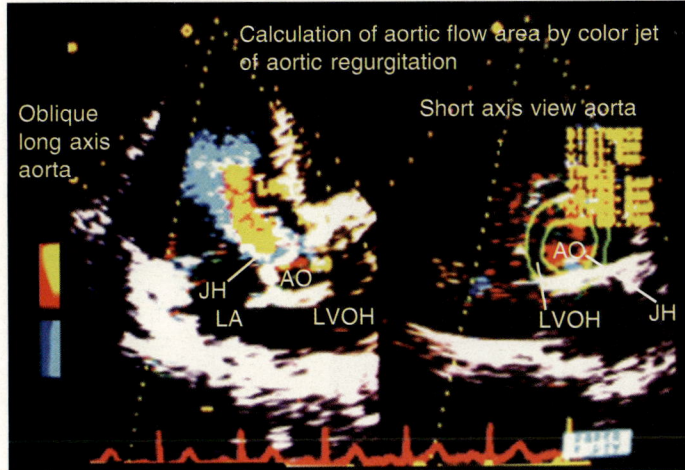

Fig. 14.128: Color 2-D oblique long axis aorta (left) and short axis aorta (right) showing another example of the technique of calculating aortic flow area by equation JH/LVOH as shown on scan(see text for detail)

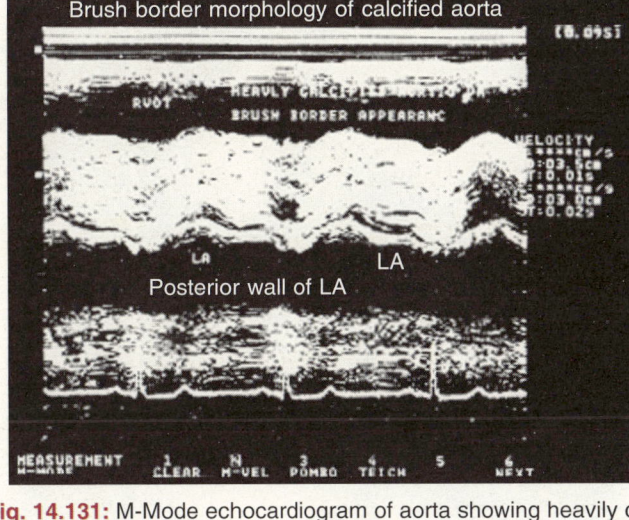

Fig. 14.131: M-Mode echocardiogram of aorta showing heavily calcified aorta resembling imprints of borders of paint brush, also called as brush border appearance of aorta

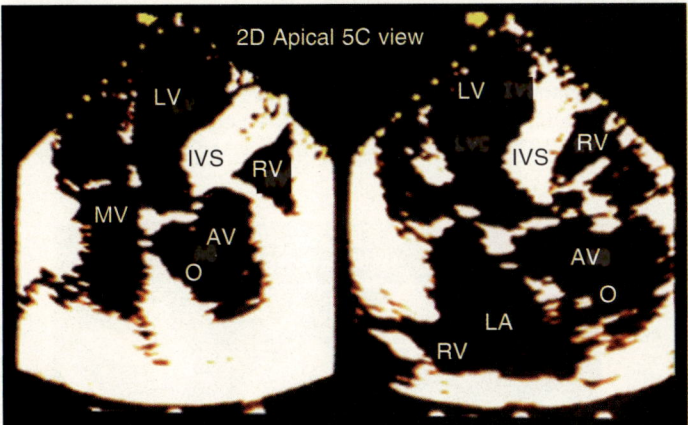

Fig. 14.129: 2-D Apical 5C showing aneurysmally dilated aorta with thickened aortic valves and aneurysm of LV with marked hypokinesia of interventricular septum (IVS) AO = Aorta, LV = Left ventricle

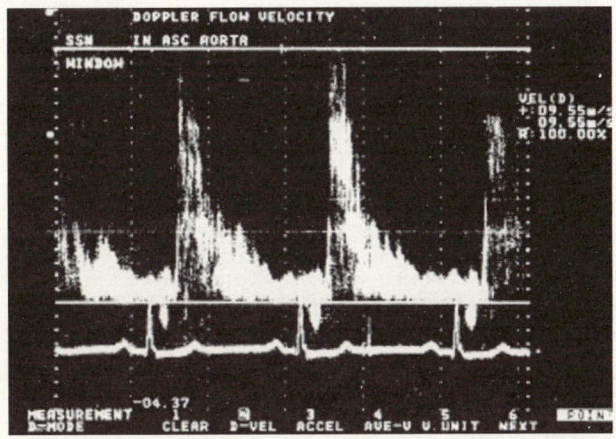

Fig. 14.132: Suprasternal notch window at ascending aorta showing doppler signatures of aortic valvular stenosis. Note high velocity jet exceeding 9.0 m/s with pressure

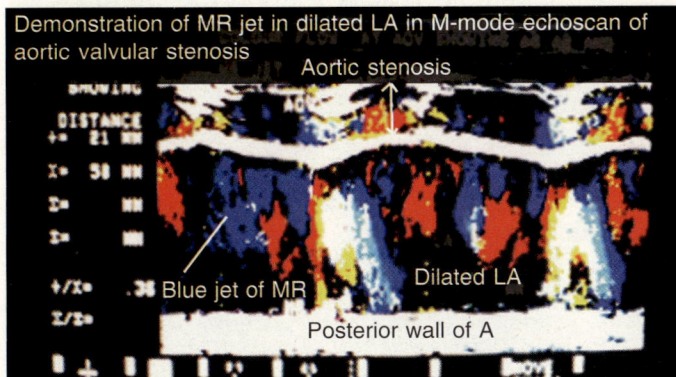

Fig. 14.130: M-Mode color flow aorta showing mosaic color jet coming out of stenosed aortic valve and appearance of blue color jet of gross mitral regurgitation in patient with rheumatic heart disease with mitral stenosis, aortic stenosis, aortic regurgitation and gross mitral regurgitation as depicted in this scan LA = left atrium

motion of regurgitant jets during the cardiac cycle, make angle correction based on the assumed direction of flow quite hazardous. Thus it is very important that the cardiac sonographer interrogate the flow velocity from several different cardiac windows to obtain the cleaned tracing with maximum velocity.

The second caution to be aware of is the use of pulsed Doppler range gating techniques. This probe is unable to record very high velocities without the alias pattern, and the sonographer should be aware of this limitation spatial resolution can also cause a number of problems in the Doppler evaluation.

For example, continuous-wave Doppler has adequate rates but has reduced spatial resolution. In the axial direction, multiple high-velocity flow fields may be interrogated by a single continuous-wave beam, and the sonographer needs to recognise clues that a second high-

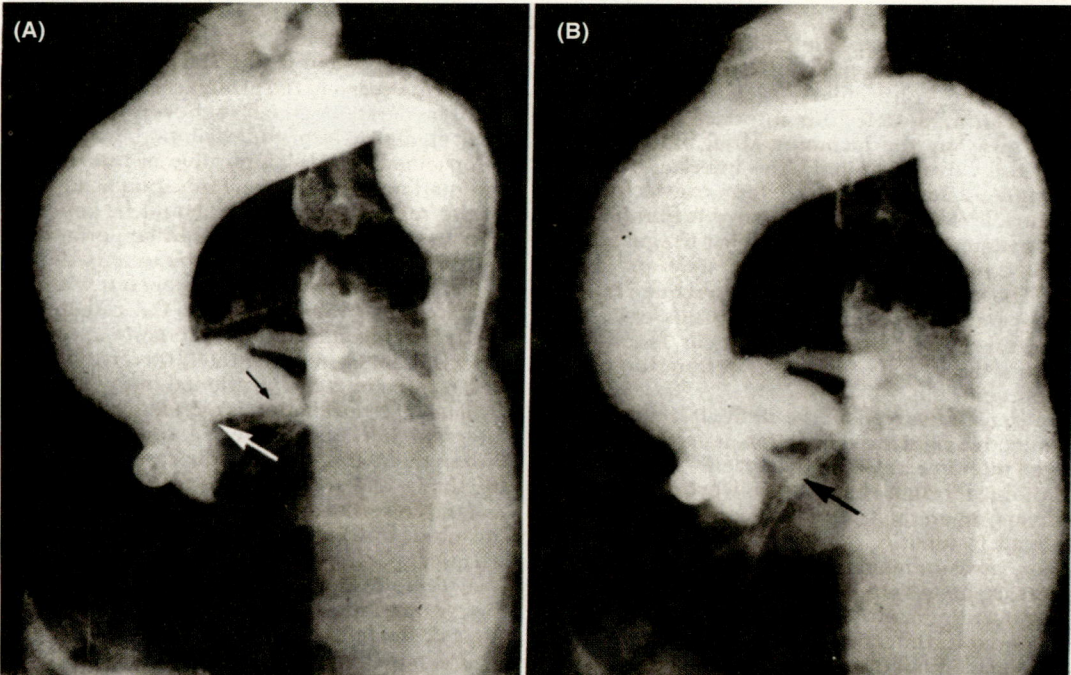

Fig. 14.133A and B: (A) In systole—Supravalvular aortogram showing radiological features of aortic stenosis. The aortic valve is rigid and cannot open the irrregular margins of the left coronary cusp (black arrow) is caused by a vegetation on the valve. There is post stenotic dilatation of the ascending aorta. **(B)** In diastole—The valve hardly moves at all, and there is a fine jet of aortic regurgitation (black arrow). White arrow represents radiolucent blood ejected from the left ventricle and indicates the diameter of the valve orifice

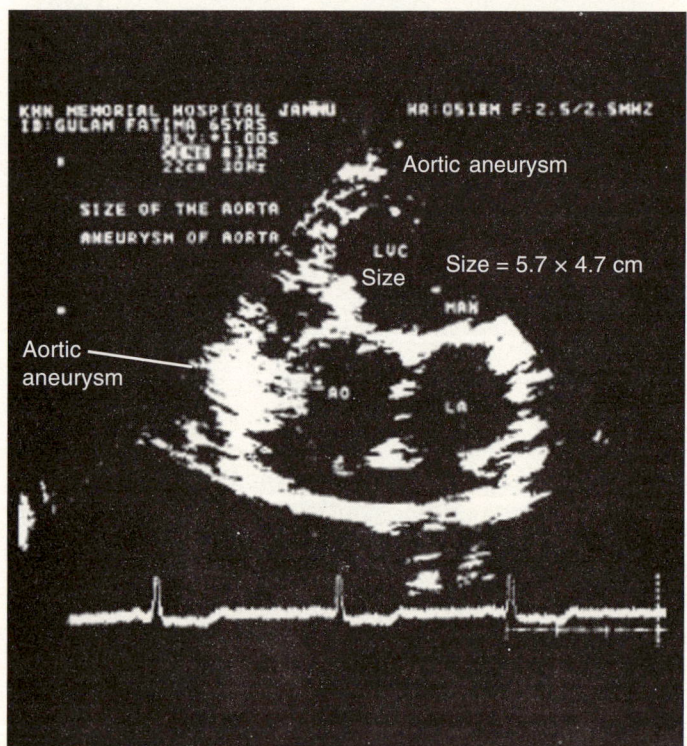

Fig. 14.134: 2D Apical 4C Views showing aneurysmal dilatation of ascending aorta with grade II-III aortic valvular regurgitation. There is also associated marked hypokinesia of interventricular septum in a patient with coronary artey disease, NIDDM and systemic hypertension

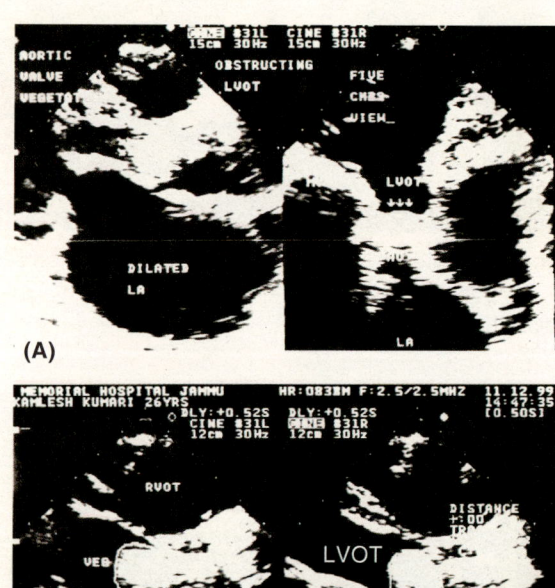

Fig. 14.135A and B: Long axis dual 2-D Scan showing a big vegetation on the aortic valve almost obstructing 3/4 of LVOT in patient with valvular aortic stenosis with regurgitation and mitral stenosis and MR. She also had prolonged pyrexia, anemia and other clinical signs of infective endocarditis

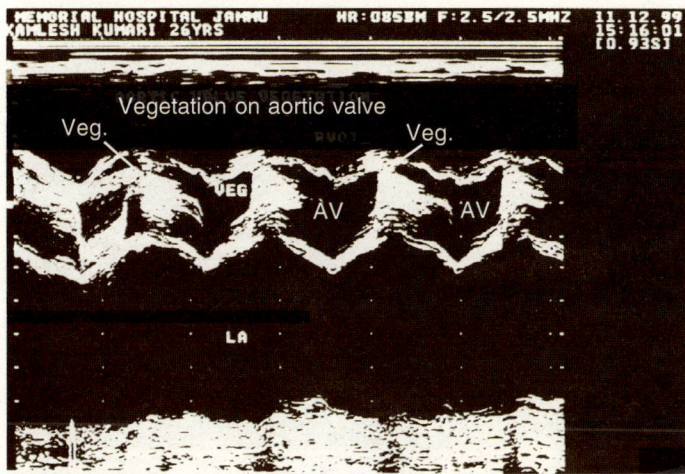

Fig. 14.136: M-Mode echocardiogram showing calcified aortic cusps with enlarged left atrium (LA) with vegetation on the valve (veg.)

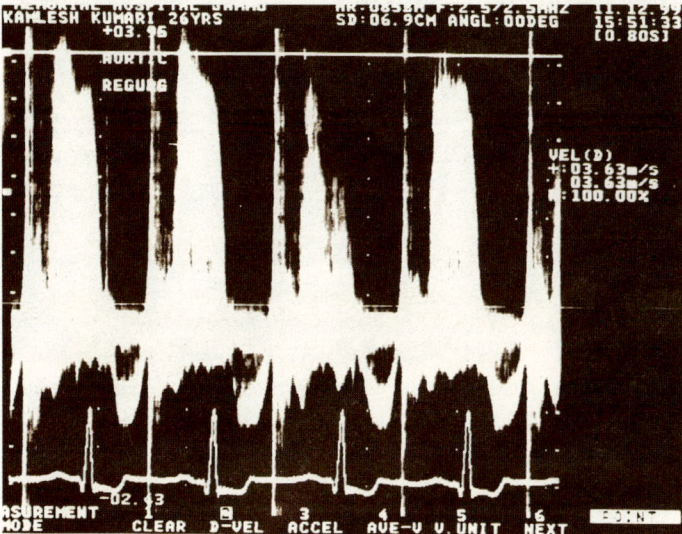

Fig. 14.137: Doppler flow velocity in the patient with aortic valve vegetation showing gross aortic valvular regurgitation with regurgitant velocity of > 3.50 m/s

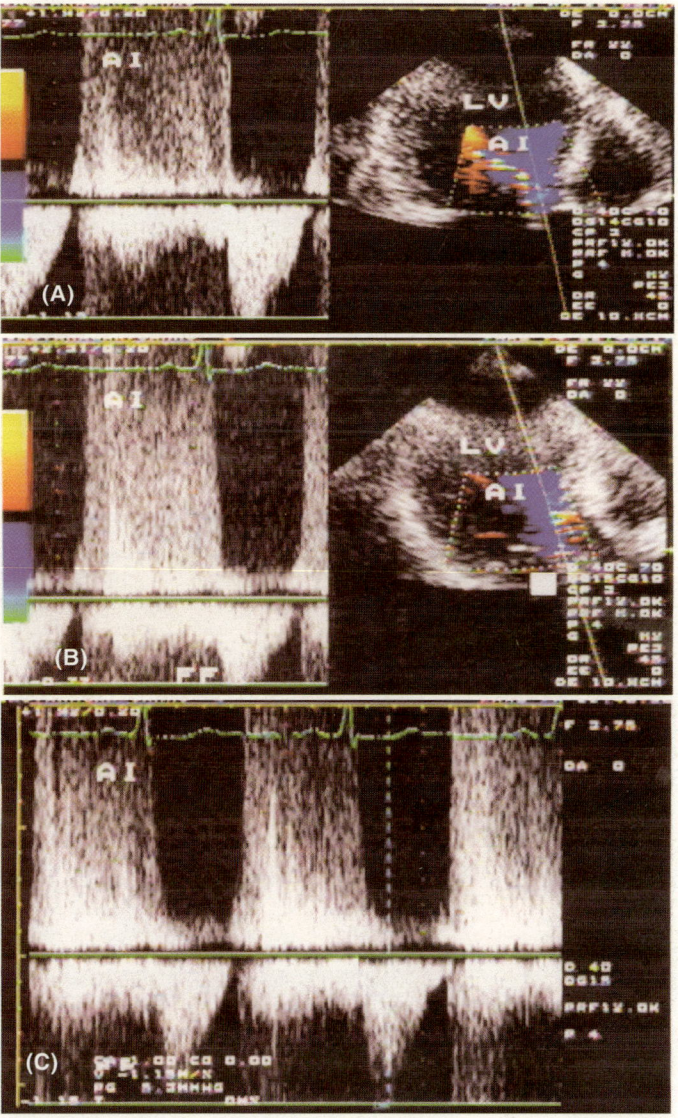

Fig. 14.138A to C: 2-D color Doppler flow velocity of aortic valve showing grade II-III aortic regurgitation in patient with rheumatic aortic valvulitis with thickening of both mitral and aortic valves

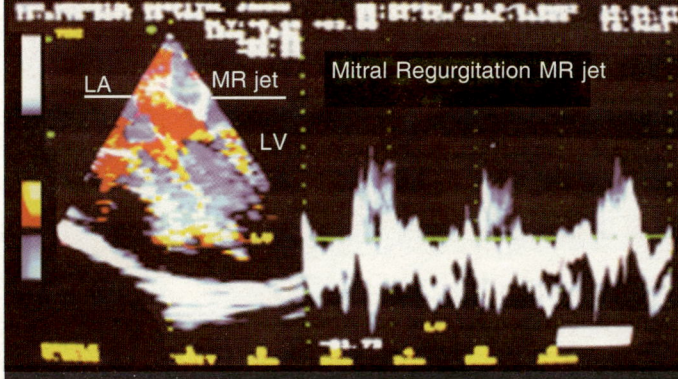

Fig. 14.139: 2-D TEE color Doppler showing mild to moderate mitral regurgitation (MR) in patient with mitral stenosis with MR and aortic regurgitation

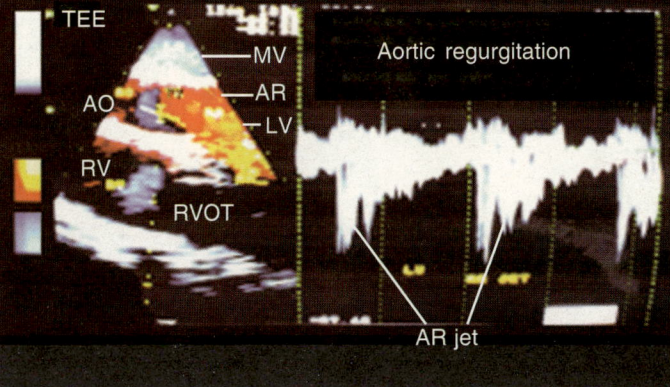

Fig. 14.140: 2-D TEE color Doppler showing aortic regurgitation (AR) in patient with rheumatic heart disease, mitral regurgitation (MR) with aortic regurgitation (AR)

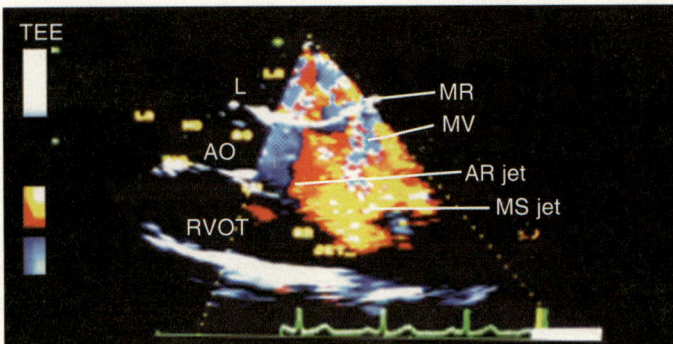

Fig. 14.141: 2-D Color aortic flow showing moderate aortic regurgitation in patient with rheumatic mitral stenosis, mitral regurgitation and aortic valvulitis

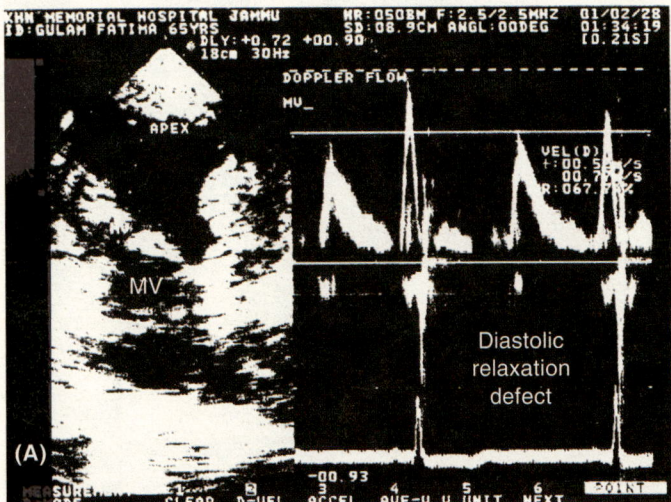

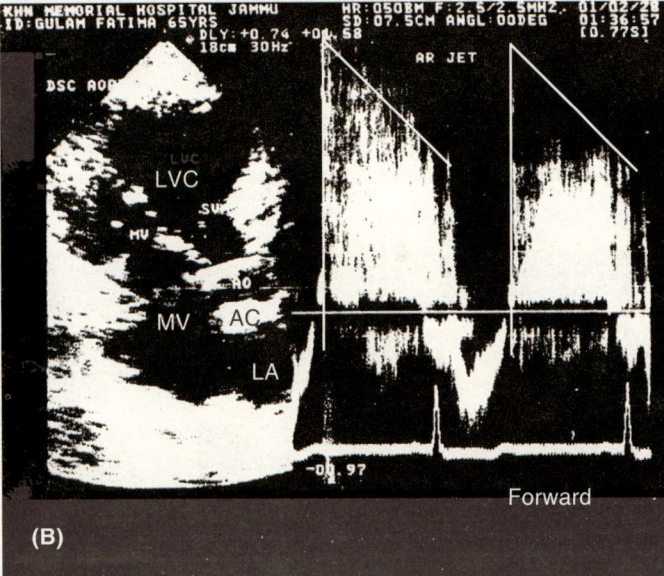

Fig. 14.142A and B: (A) Doppler flow velocity across mitral valve showing enhancement of A wave indicating defect in LV relaxation in patient with hypertension ischemic heart disease who had in addition aortic valvular regurgitation. **(B)** In the above said patient shows gross aortic regurgitation (AR) with significant deceleration AR slope

M-Mode echoscan showing eccentric opening of aortic value associated with coaraction of descending aorta

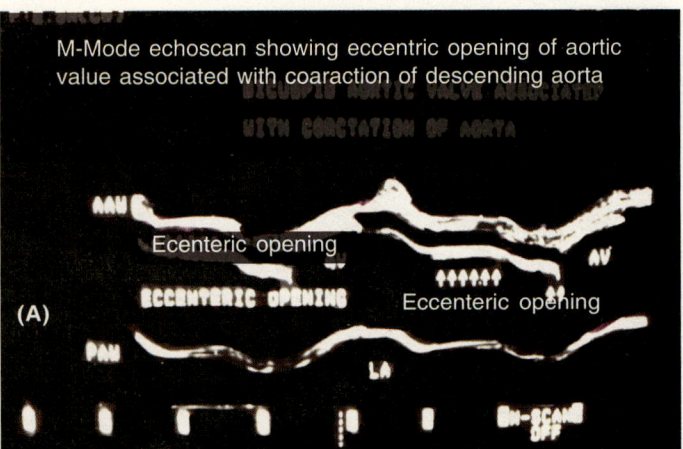

CW doppler flow velocity in coarctation of aorta associated with bicuspid aortic stenosis

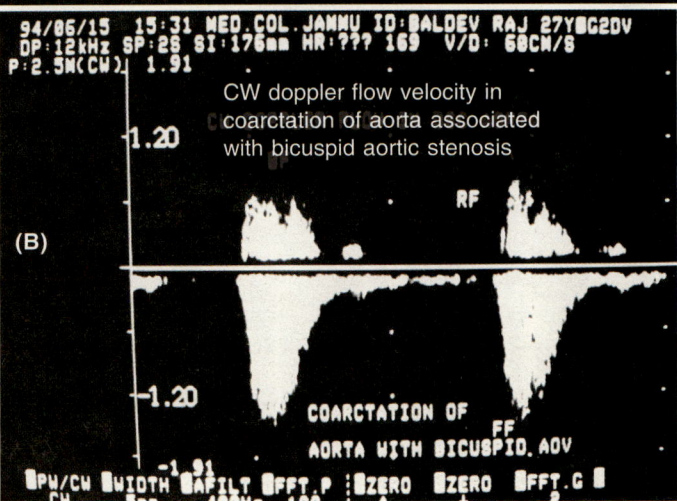

Fig. 14.143: (A) M-mode echocardiogram showing eccentric opening of aortic valve in bicuspid aortic valve stenosis. **(B)** Doppler flow velocity showing broad waveform jet in bicuspid aortic valve with coarctation of descending aorta

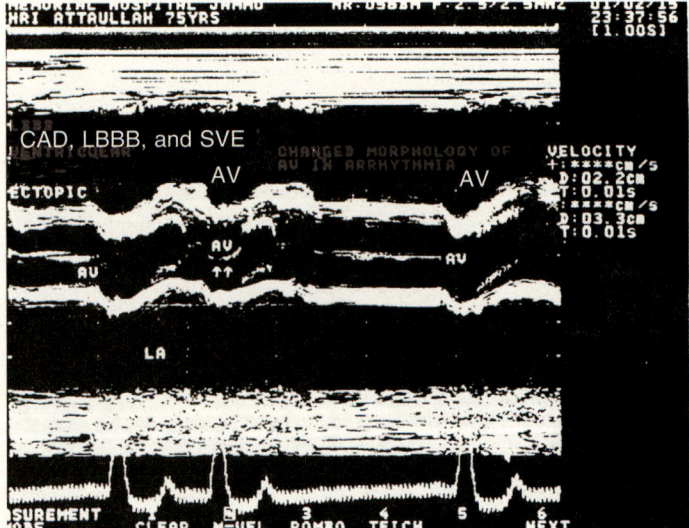

Fig. 14.144: M-Mode echocardiogram showing altred mitral valve morphology in supraventricular ectopic (SVE) along with left bundle branch block (LBBB) in patient with CAD, LBBB and SVE

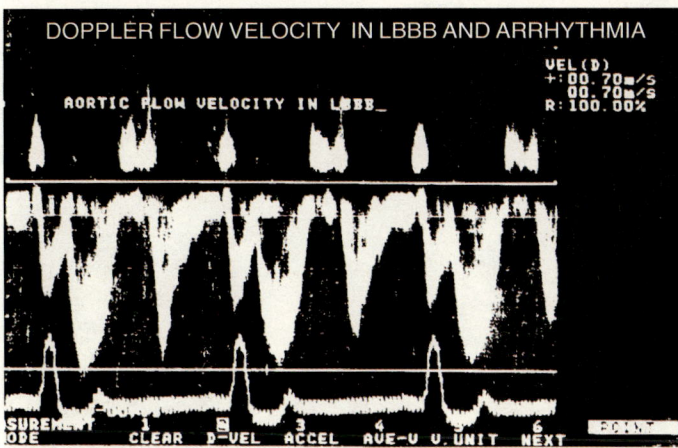

Fig. 14.145: Doppler flow velocity in aortic valve showing alternatively small flow along with major flow suffering from CAD, LBBB and cardiac arrhythmia m = major's = small

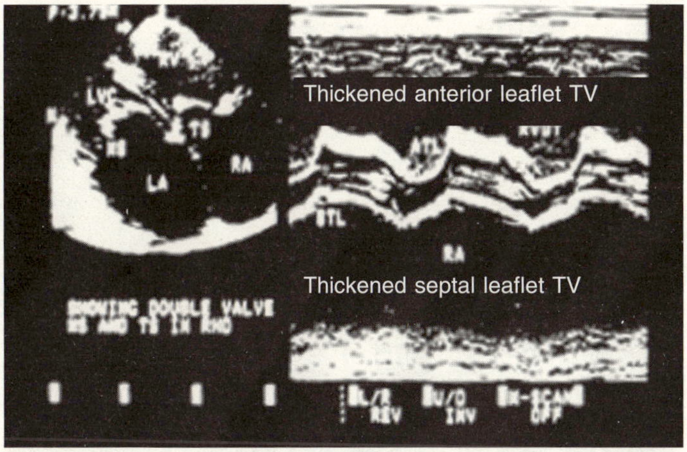

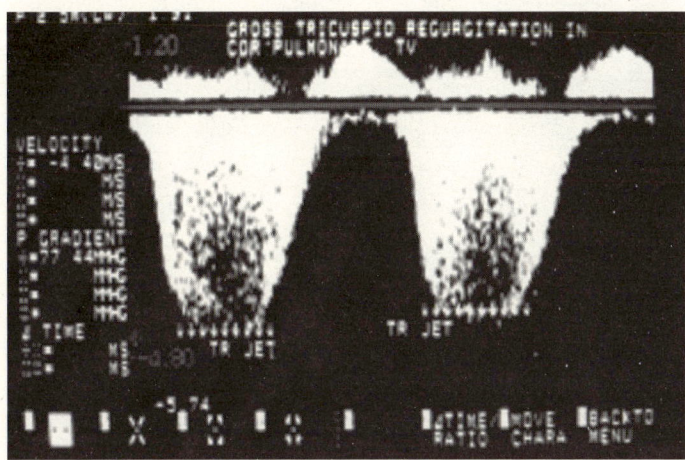

Fig. 14.148: 2-D Apical and M-Mode echocardiogram showing thickened both anterior and septal leaflets of tricuspid valve

Morphological and Anatomical Recognition of Tricuspid Valve

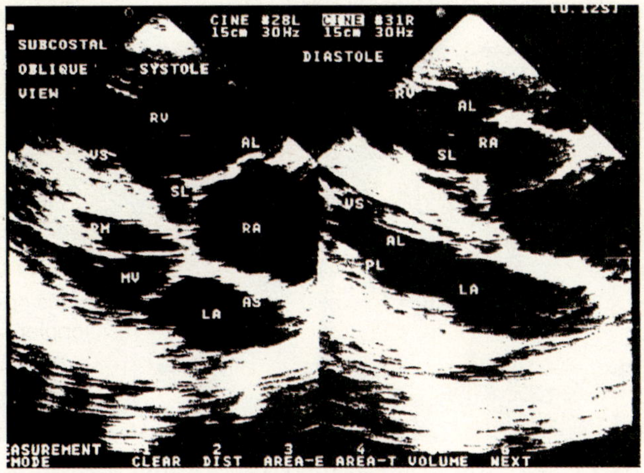

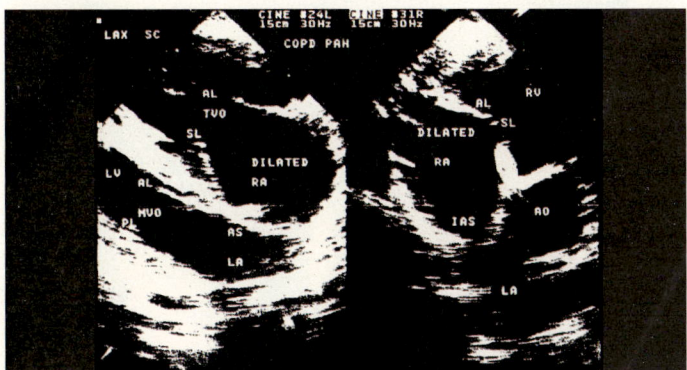

Fig. 14.146: Subcostal 4C view showing anterior and septal leaflets of tricuspid valve. SL = Septal leaflet, AL = Anterior leaflet

Fig. 14.149: Doppler flow velocity across tricuspid valve (TV) showing wide spectral envelope of tricuspid regurgitation (TR) with gradient of > 77.0 mm Hg in patient with cor-pulmonale (COPD)

Fig. 14.147: (L-R) 2-D Long axis aorta and short axis views at subcostal window showing anterior (AL) and septal leaflets (SL) in patient with chronic obstructive lung disease, interatrial septum (IAS) right atrium(RA), LA = Left atrium, LV = left ventricle, PL = Posterior leaflet of mitral valve, TVO = Tricuspid orifice

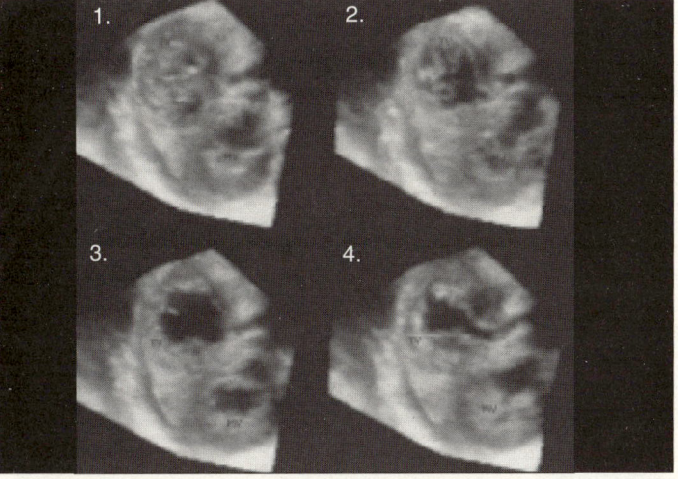

Fig. 14.150: 3DTTE view has been constructed using oblique plane to demonstrate enface view of all the three leaflets of the tricuspid valve in different diastolic phases 1. Closed 2. Early diastole 3. Mid diastole 4. Late diastole

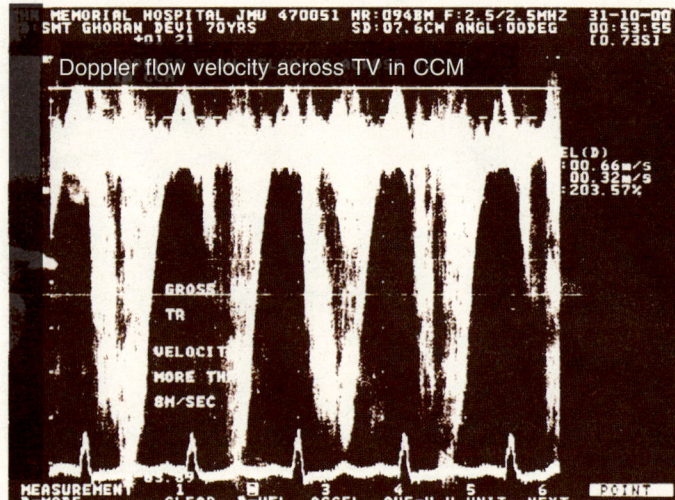

Fig. 14.151: Doppler flow velocity across tricuspid valve depicting gross tricuspid regurgitant jet in patient with dilated cardiomyopathy

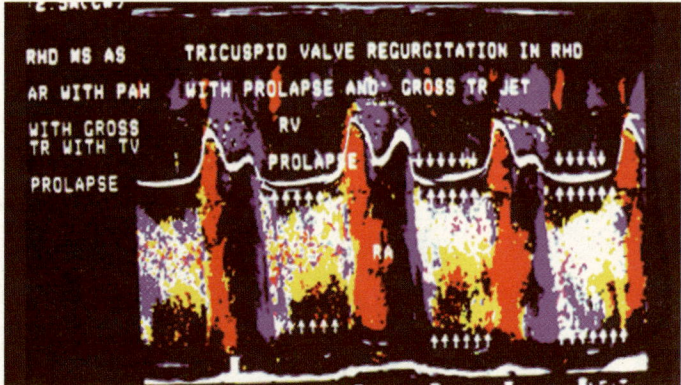

Fig. 14.152: M-Mode echocardiogram in color mode showing gross tricuspid regurgitation (arrows) in patient with rheumatic heart disease with mitral stenosis with MR tricuspid valvulitis with TR

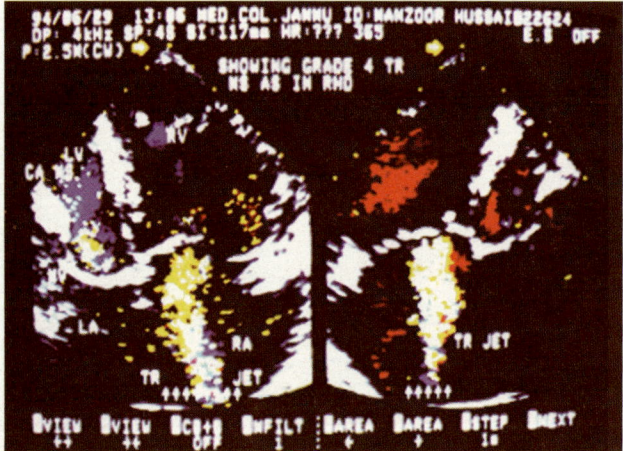

Fig. 14.153: 2-D Apical 4C dual scan view showing dilated RV and RA and gross mosaic colored tricuspid regurgitation jet (arrows) in patient with rheumatic mitral stenosis with MR, aortic stenosis with AR and severe type of both pulmonary venous and arterial hypertension

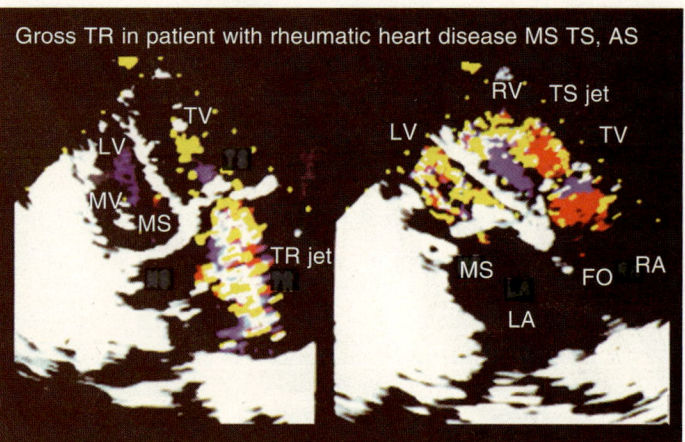

Fig. 14.154: 2-D Oblique 4C Dual scan views showing mosaic colored tricuspid regurgitation jet into right atrium in patient who had rheumatic heart disease with mitral stenosis, aortic stenosis tricuspid stenosis and pulmonary valvulitis with severe type of pulmonary venous and arterial hypertension

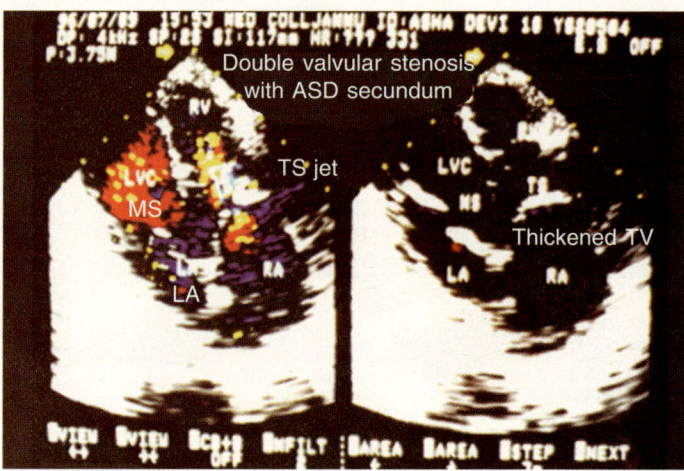

Fig. 14.155: 2-D color dual scan in modified apical 4C views showing blue jet of tricuspid regurgitation into right atrium and mosaic stenotic jet into right ventricle along with mitral regurgitation blue jet into left atrium and mosaic jet of mitral stenosis into left ventricle in patient with double valvular stenosis with ASD secundum

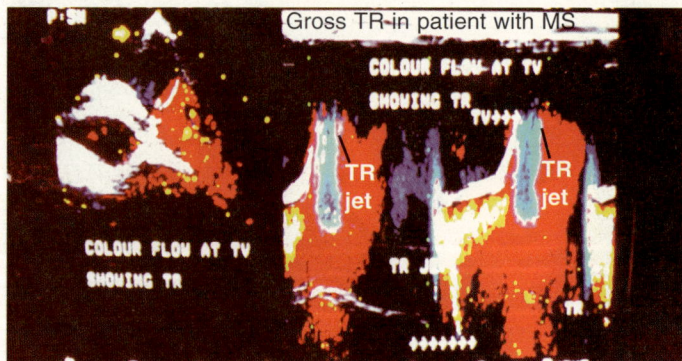

Fig. 14.156: 2-D Dual scan oblique 4C and M-Mode views showing tricuspid regurgitaton jet in patient with mitral stenosis and gross tricuspid regurgitation (TR)

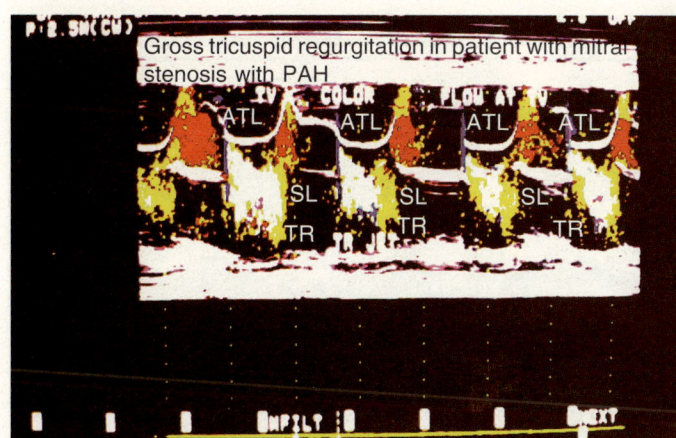

Fig. 14.157: M-Mode echocardiogram showing gross tricuspid regurgitation in patient with mitral stenosis with pulmonary arterial and venous hypertension. ATL = Anterior tricuspid leaflet, SL = Septal leaflet, TR = Tricuspid regurgitation

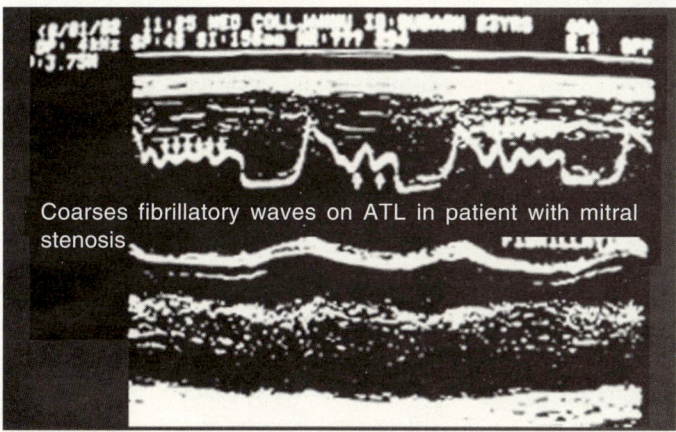

Fig. 14.158: M-Mode echocardiogram showing fibrillatory waves (arrows) on anterior tricuspid leaflet (ATL) in patient with mitral stenosis with atrial fibrillation, SL = Septal leaflet, RA = Right atrium

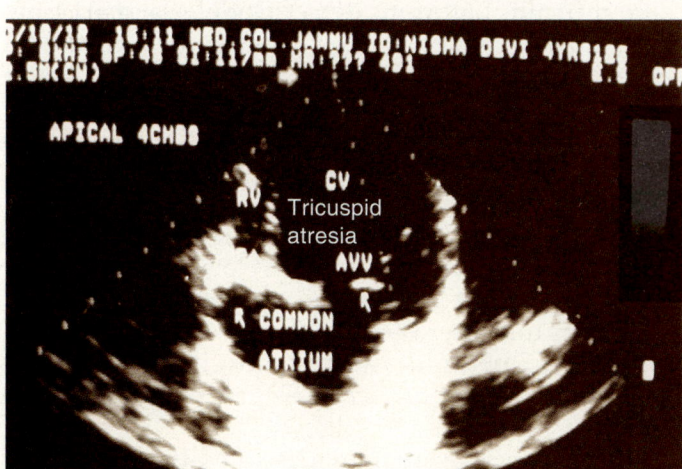

Fig. 14.159: 2-D View in apical 4C plane showing common ventricle (CV) common atrioventricular valve (AVV), common atrium with tricuspid atresia in a child with cyanotic heart disease, single ventricle with tricuspid atresia

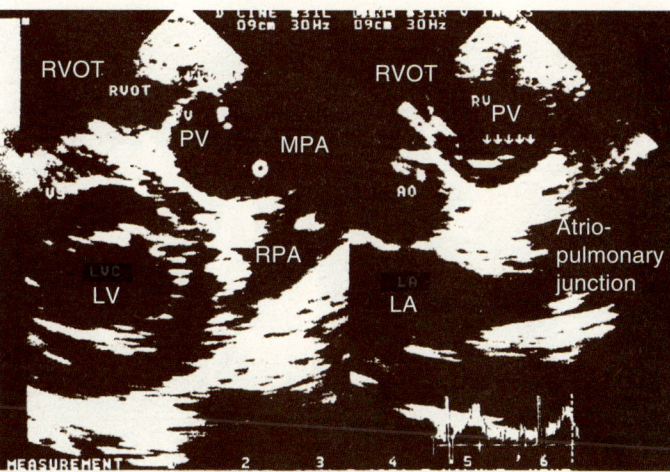

Fig. 14.160: 2-D Oblique short axis view of LV on dual scan showing the location of main pulmonary artery with its valve and LV cavity (left) and pulmonary valve (arrows) at short axis view at aorta for coronary vessels level at atrio-pulmonary junction (right)

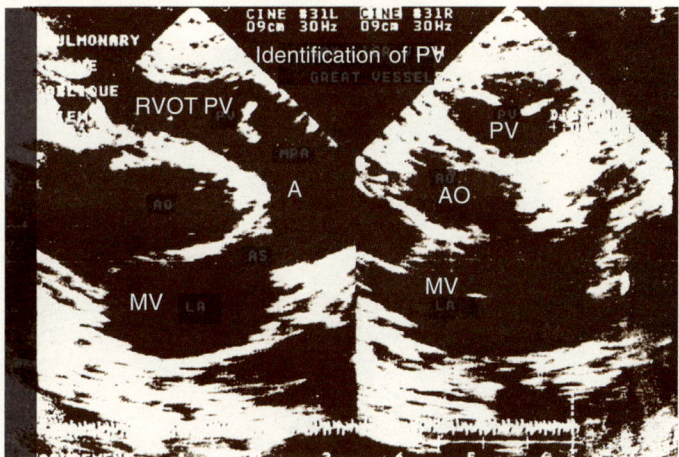

Fig. 14.161: Short axis oblique view in dual scan at aorta and short axis view of great vessels in the high left parasternal region showing identification of tricuspid morphology of pulmonary valve marked as 1, 2 and 3 and its relationship with surrounding structures. MPA = Main pulmonary artery, PV = Pulmonary valve

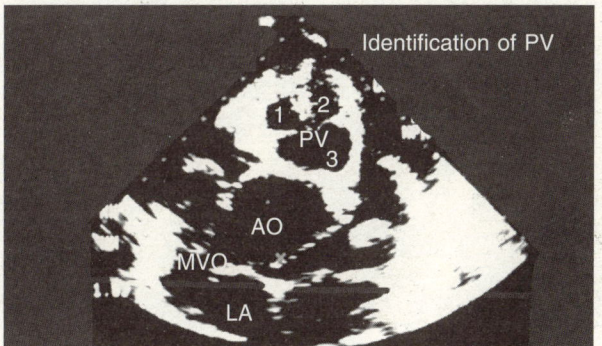

Fig. 14.162: 2-D Short axis view at great vessel level showing tricuspid (1, 2, 3) morphology of pulmonary valve and its relationship with surrounding structures. PV = Pulmonary valve, AO = Aorta, MVO = Mitral valve orifice, LA = Left atrium

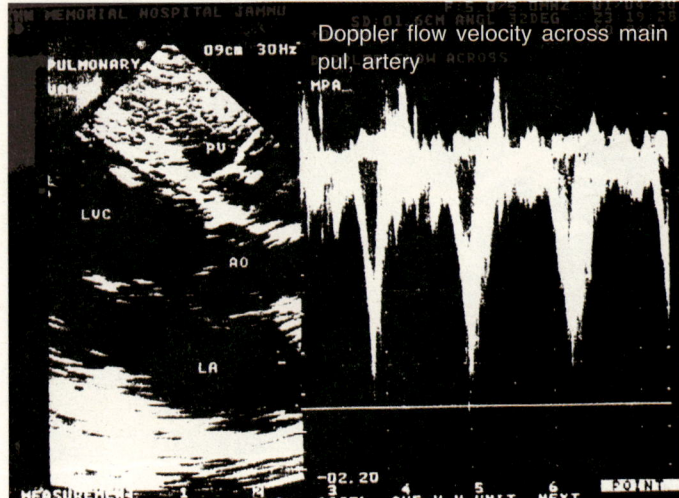

Fig. 14.163: 2-D Long axis view great vessel (left) and normal Doppler flow velocity in main pulmonary artery (right) along with mildly thickened tricuspid pulmonary valve morphology in patient with mild to moderate obstructive lung disease

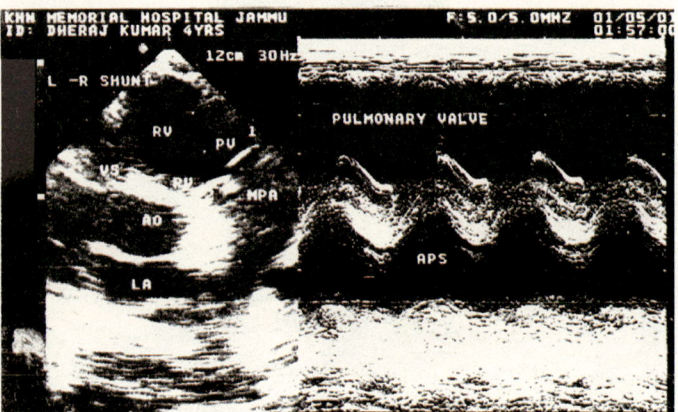

Fig. 14.164: 2-D Short axis view aorta (left) and M-Mode echoscan of pulmonary valve showing normal anatomical and morphological features of pulmonary valve

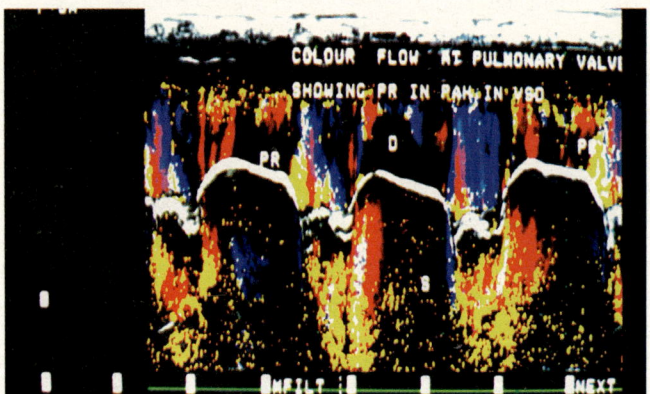

Fig. 14.165: Color M-Mode echoscan of pulmonary valve taken at atrio-pulmonary sulcus showing reduction in EF Slope and attenuation of A wave of pulmonary valve and PR jet in patient with pulmonary arterial hypertension in VSD along with pulmonary regurgitation

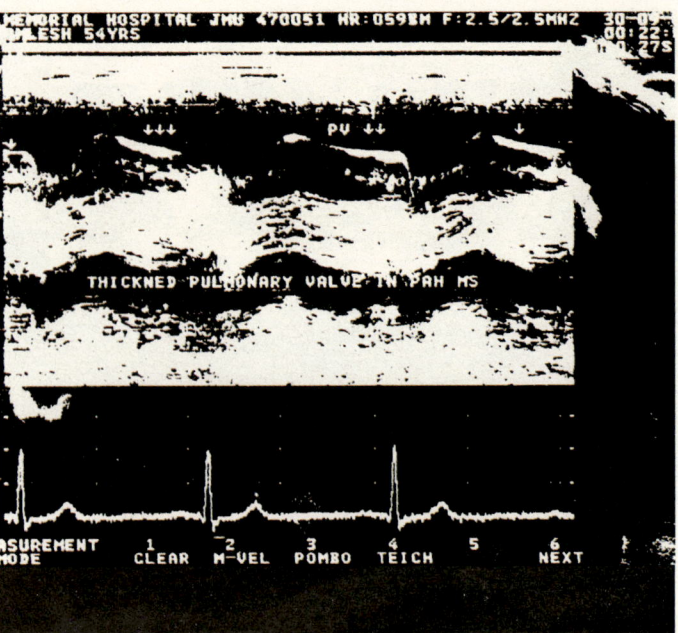

Fig. 14.166: M-Mode echoscan of pulmonary valve taken at atrio-pulmonary sulcus showing thickening of valve along with attenuation of (a) wave of pulmonary valve in patient with rheumatic mitral stenosis, aortic stenosis pulmonary arterial hypertension and pulmonary artery valvulitis

velocity lesion may be present, or else gradient over estimation may result. In the elevation directions, continuous wave beams are broader than range-gated pulsed wave beams, and so the possibility of detecting a high-velocity lesion with the lateral portions of the beams need also to be borne in mind.

Range-gated techniques are also subject to limitations in spatial resolution. When examining at increasing depths, loss of signal strength from background noise quite difficult; failure to detect Doppler signals from significant depths may be a function of attenuation rather than absence of flow abnormality. Doppler techniques are, to some extent, limited by their relative insensitivity to differences in flow profiles across regions of interest. Pulse techniques may be subject to sampling errors if flow profiles are not blunt, and continuous-wave techniques are best suited to showing the highest (rather than the spatial average) velocity.

Flow velocities depend on volume rates, so that conditions that alter volume rates, from normal (Ventricular dysfunction, valvular regurgitation, intracardiac shunting) may reduce or elevate the measure velocities.

Thus as one bears in mind these pitfalls and attempts to avoid them when performing the Doppler examination, the information obtained from a Doppler examination can be very useful in the clinical management of patients with valvular heart disease.

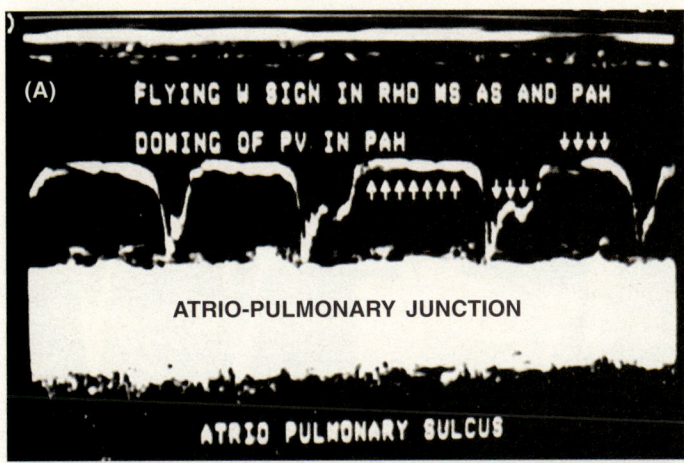

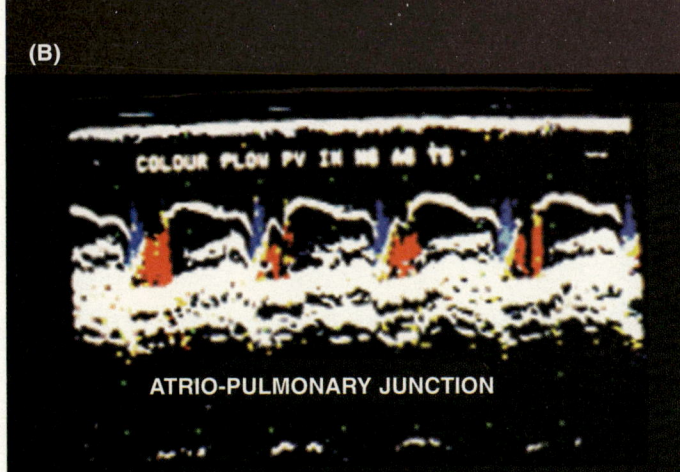

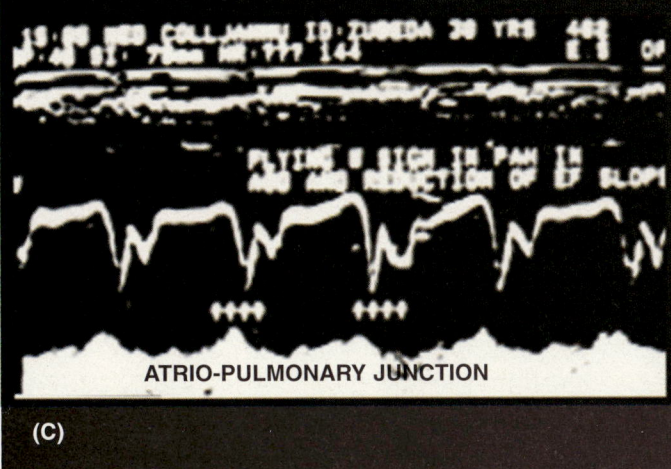

Fig. 14.167A to C: **(A)** and **(B)** M-Mode echoscan of pulmonary valve taken at atrio-pulmonary sulcus showing thickening of valve along with attenuation of (a) wave of pulmonary valve in two patients with rheumatic mitral stenosis, aortic stenosis pulmonary arterial hypertension and pulmonary artery valvulitis. **(C)** M-Mode echoscan of pulmonary valve taken at atrio-pulmonary sulcus showing thickening of valve along with attenuation of (a) wave and flying W sign equivalent to regression of systolic velocity on Doppler flow and angiographically severe pulmonary artery hypertension in patient with ASD. Secundum with isodirectional shunt in 38 years old female

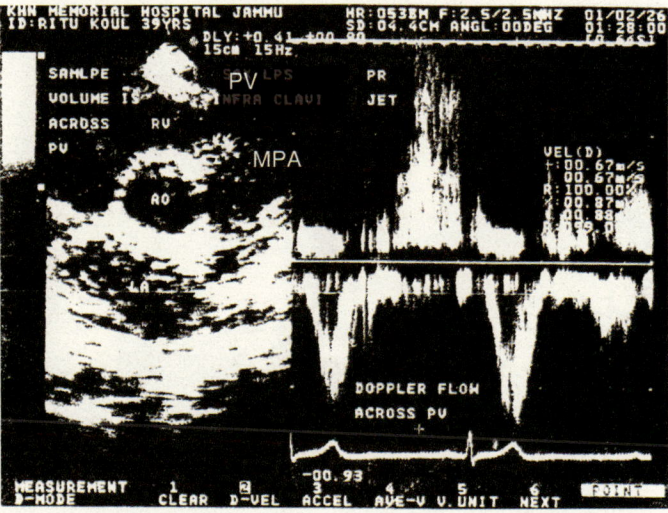

Fig. 14.168: Right infraclavicular region short axis (left) and Doppler flow velocity across main pulmonary artery (right) showing significant pulmonary artery regurgitation (PR JET) in patient with obstructive lung disease with pulmonary arterial hypertension

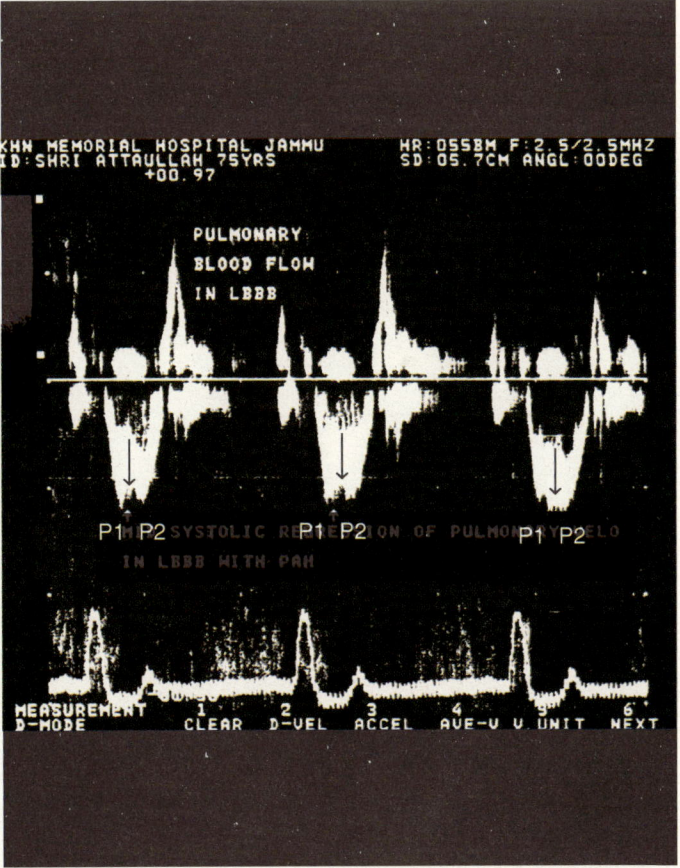

Fig. 14.169: Doppler flow velocity across pulmonary artery showing small systolic velocity (P1) at the beginning of the main flow velocity (P2) with systolic regression of main velocity (arrow) in patient with CAD, LBBB and pulmonary arterial hypertension. This small velocity (P1) at the initiation of main velocity could be explained due to the presence of conduction defect. (LBBB) and systolic regression of mian velocity is as a result of pulmonary arterial hypertension

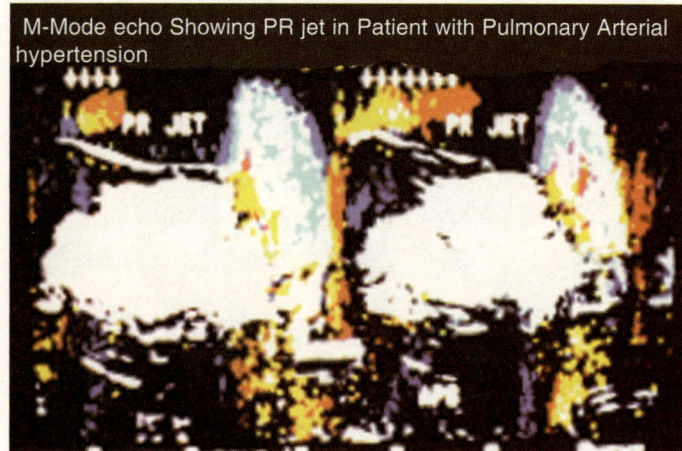

Fig. 14.170: M-Mode echocardiogram in color mode showing mosaic colored jet (arrows) of pulmonary regurgitation in patient with rheumatic mitral stenosis MR, aortic stenosis AR, and pulmonary venous and arterial hypertension. MR = Mitral regurgitation, AR = Aortic regurgitation, PR = Pulmonary regurgitation

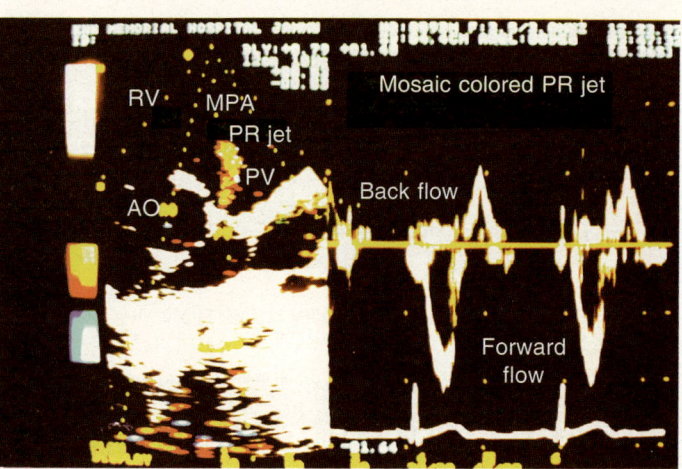

Fig. 14.171: 2-D Color in short axis view of great vessels level (left) and Doppler flow (right) showing mosaic colored pulmonary regurgitation jet (PR) and small signatures of PR jet on Doppler echocardiography in patient with pulmonary arterial hypertension

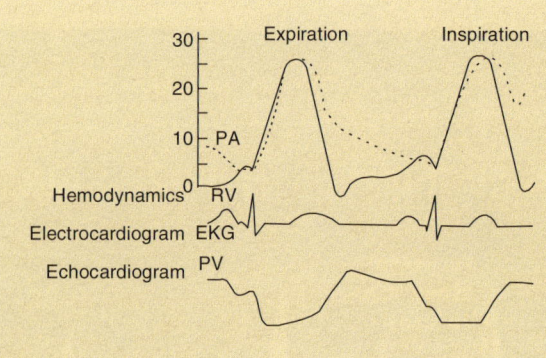

Fig. 14.172: Graphic representation of normal hemodynamics of pulmonary artery pressure in relation to M-mode echocardiogram and electrocardiogram

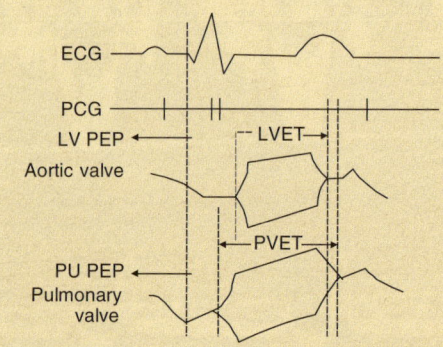

Fig. 14.173: Graphic representation of various time intervals employed for the calculation of hemodynamic information in respect to electrocardiogram, phonocardiogram, aortic and pulmonary valve echocardiogram.
LVET = Left ventricular ejection time
PV PET = Left ventricular pre-ejection time
PVET = Pulmonary valve ejection time
PV PEP = Pulmonary valve pre-ejection time

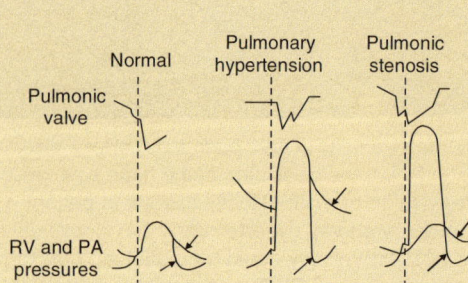

Fig. 14.174: Graphic representation of relationship of pulmonary echocardiogram and catheterization data in normal individual, patient with pulmonary hypertension and pulmonic stenosis. Pulmonary echocardiogram shows the Fig. of flying "W" sign in pulmonary hypertension (middle Fig.)

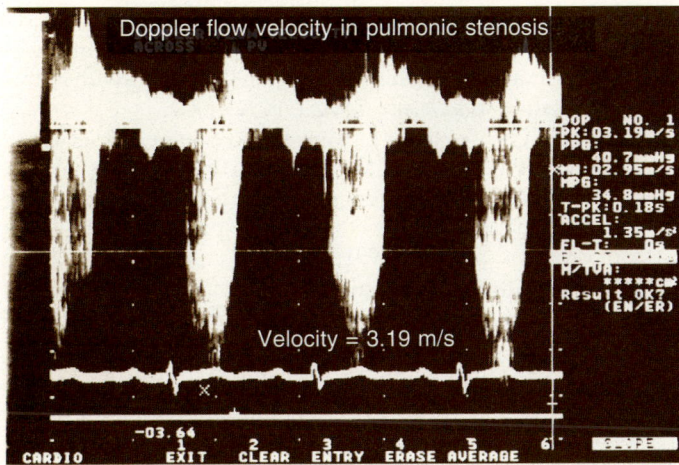

Fig. 14.175: Doppler flow velocity across pulmonary valve depicting wide spectral waveform with enhanced flow velocity in an adult patient with pulmonic valve stenosis

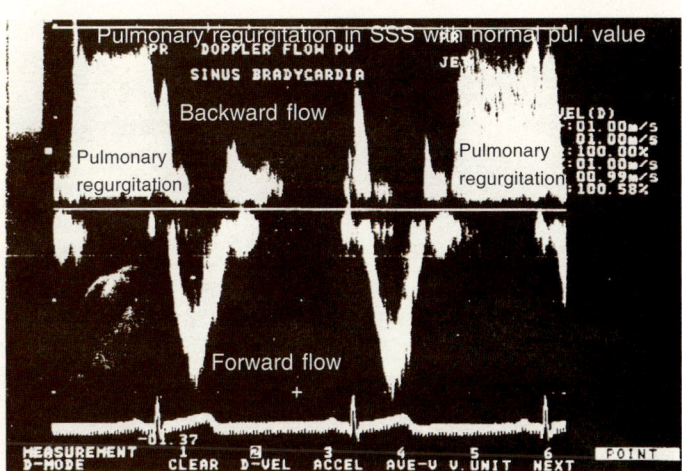

Fig. 14.176: Doppler flow velocity across main pulmonary artery showing pulmonary regurgitation in patient with sinus bradycardia as a part of sick sinus syndrome with normal pulmonary valve

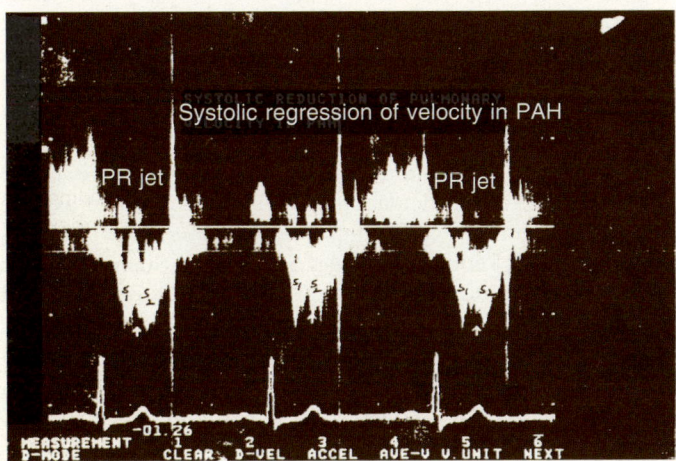

Fig. 14.177: Doppler flow velocity across pulmonary valve showing systolic regression of velocity (arrow) in patient with pulmonary arterial hypertension and mild regurgitation

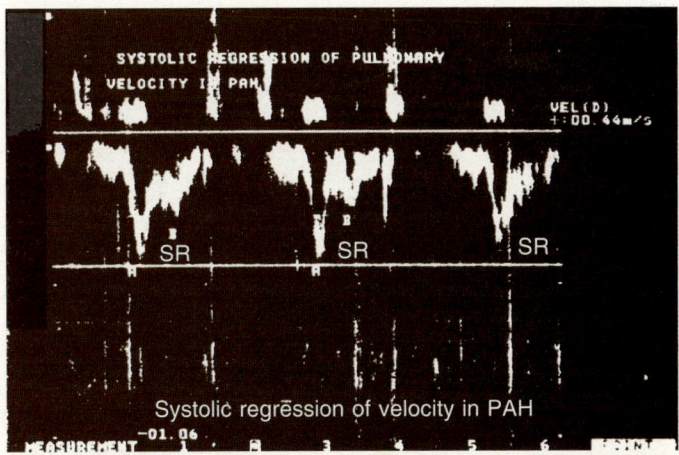

Fig. 14.178: Doppler flow velocity across pulmonary valve showing systolic regression of velocity (arrow) in another patient with rheumatic mitral stenosis and ASD secundum pulmonary arterial hypertension. SR = Systolic regression of velocity

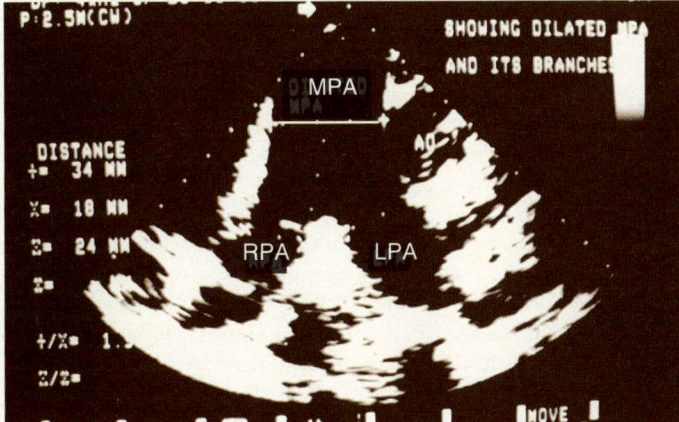

Fig. 14.179: 2-D View at great vessel level showing dilatation of main pulmonary artery along with its two left and right branches. RPA = Right pulmonary artery, LPA = Left pulmonary artery in patient with pulmonary arterial hypertension, MPA = Main pulmonary artery

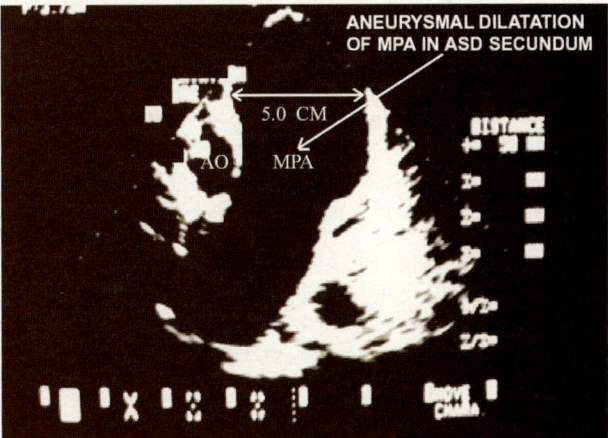

Fig. 14.180: There is aneurysmal dilatation of main pulmonary artery reaching upto 5.0 cm (normal size = 11–20 mm) in a patient with larger ASD secundum in in an adult patient

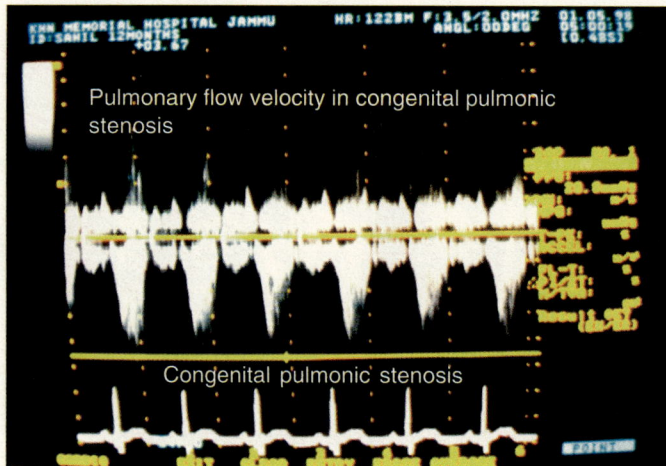

Fig. 14.181: Doppler flow velocity across pulmonary valve showing waveforms of congenital pulmonary valvular stenosis associated with atrial septal defect of secundum type

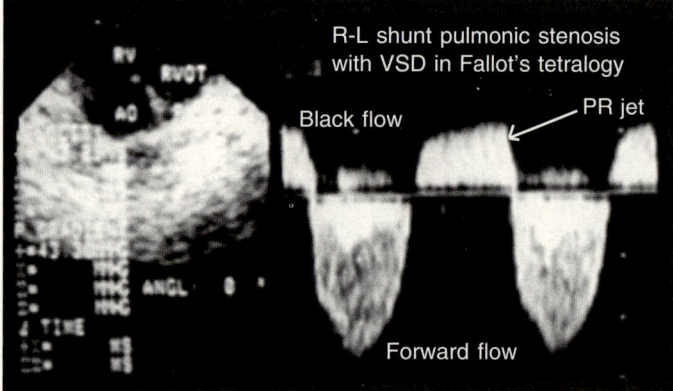

Fig. 14.182: Doppler flow velocity showing broad spectral waveform and enhanced systolic flow velocity with regurgitant flow in a patient with severe form of pulmonic stenosis, VSD and R-L shunt in Fallot's tetralogy

Bibliography

1. Abascal VM, Wilkins GT, Ghoong CY, Block PC, Palacios IF, and Weyman AE: Mitral regurgitation after percutaneous balloon mitral valvuloplasty in adults: Evaluation of pulsed Doppler echocardiography. *J Am Coll Cardiol* 1988; 11: 257.

2. Abbasi AS, Allen MW, DeCristofaroD, and Ungar I.: Detection and estimation of the degree of mitral regurgitation by range-gated pulsed Doppler echocardiography. *Circulation* 1980; 61:143.

3. Appleton CP, Hatle LK, Nellessen U, Schnittger I, Popp RL: Flow velocity acceleration in the left ventricle: A useful Doppler echocardiographic sign of hemodynamically significant mitral regurgitation. *J Am Soc Echocardiogr* 1990; 3: 35.

4. Application of the automated Bargiggia GS, Tronconi L, Sahn DJ, *et al.* A new method for quantitation of mitral regurgitation based on colour-flow Doppler imaging of flow convergence proximal to regurgitant orifice. *Circulation* 1991; 84:1481–9. Initial description of the proximal convergence method 113.

5. Bargiggia GS, Tronconi L, Raisaro A, Bertucci C, Bramucci E, Recusani F, Montemartini C: Colour Doppler analysis of the proximal flow convergence region in patients with mitral regurgitation. *Cardiovase. Imag* 1990; 2: 137.

6. Bargiggia GS, Tronconi L, Sahn DJ, Recusani F, Raisaro A, DeServi S, Valdes-Cruz LM, Montemartini C: A new method for quantitation of mitral regurgitation based on colour-flow Doppler imaging of flow convergence proximal to regurgitant orifice. *Circulation* 1991; 84: 1481.

7. Bland MJ, Atman DG. Stastical methods assessing agreement between two methods of clinical measurement. *Lancet* 1986; 1:306–310.

8. Bobkov VV, Danilchenko TA, Prelatov VA, Kuznetsova LM: Doppler echocardiographic study of patients with mitral insufficiency. *Kardiologiia* 1983; 23: 79.

9. Bouchard A, Yock P, Schiller NB Blumlein, S, Botvinick EH, Greenburg B, Cheitlin M, and Massie BM: Value of colour Doppler estimation of regurgitant volume in patients with chronic aortic insufficiency. *Am Heart J* 1989; 117:1099.

10. Braverman AC, Thomas JD, Lee RT. Doppler echocardiographic estimation of mitral valve area during changing hemodynamic conditions. *Am J Cardiol* 1991;68: 1485–1490.

11. Brenner JI, Baker KR, Berman MA: Prediction of left ventricular pressure in infants with aortic stenosis. *Br Heart J* 1980; 44:406.

12. Burwash IG, Blackmore GL, Koilpillai CJ: Usefulness of left atrial and left ventricular chamber sizes as predictors of the severity of mitral regurgitation. *Am J Cardiol* 1992; 70:774.

13. Caguioa ES, Reimold SC, Velez S, Lee RT: Influence of aortic pressure on effective regurgitant orifice area in aortic regurgitation. *Circulation*, 1992; 85: 1565.

14. Cannon SR, Richards KL, Crawford M. Hydraulic estimation of stenotic orifice area: a correction of the Gorlin formula. *Circulation* 1985; 71:1170–1178.

15. Casale PN, Palacios IF, Abascal VM, Harrell L, Davidoff R, Weyman AE, Fifer MA.: Effects on dobutamine on Gorlin and continuity equation valve area and valve resistance in valvular aortic stenosis. *Am J Cardiol* 1992; 70: 1175.

16. Castello R, Pearson AC, Lenzen P, Labovitz AJ: Effect of mitral regurgitation on pulmonary venous velocities derived from transesophageal echocardiography colour-guided pulsed Doppler imaging. *J Am Coll Cardiol* 1991;17: 1499.

17. Castello R, Fagan L, Lenzen JP, Pearson AC, Labovitz AJ: Comparison of transthoracic and transesophageal echocardiography for assessment of left side valvular regurgitation. *Am J Cardiol* 1991;68: 1677.

18. Castello R, Lenzen P, Aguirre F, Labovitz AJ: Quantitation of mitral regurgitation by transesophageal echocardiography with Doppler colour-flow mapping : Correlation with cardiac catheterization. *J Am Coll Cardiol* 1992;19: 1516.

19. Castello R, Lenzen P, Aguirre F, Labovitz, A: Variability in the quantitation of mitral regurgitation by Doppler colour-flow mapping: Comparison of transthoracic and transesophageal studies. *J Am Coll Cardiol* 1992;20: 433.

20. Castello R, Pearson AC, Lenzen P, *et al.* Effect of mitral regurgitation on pulmonary venous velocities derived from transesophageal echocardiography colour-guided pulsed Doppler imaging. *J Am Coll Cardiol* 1991;17:1499–506. Early

description of the utility of pulmonary venous flow reversal in identifying severe mitral regurgitation.

21. Chen C, KoschykD, Brockhoff C, Heik S, Hamm C, Bleifeld W, Kupper W: Non-invasive estimation of regurgitant flow rate and volume in patients with mitral regurgitation by Doppler colour mapping of accelerating flow field. *J Am Coll Cardiol* 1993;21: 374–383.

22. Chen CG, Thomas JD, Anconina J, *et al*. Impact of impinging wall jet on colour Doppler quantification of mitral regurgitation. A study demonstrating that wall jets are less than half the size of centrally directed jets for the same degree of regurgitation. *Circulation* 1991;84:712–20.

23. Chen WJ, Chen MF, Liau CS, Wu CC Lee YT: Safety of percutaneous transvenous balloon mitral commissurotomy in patients with mitral stenosis and thrombus in the left appendage. *Am J Cardiol* 1992;70: 117.

24. Chopra HK, Nanda NC, Fan P, Kapur KK, Goyal R, Daruwalla D, Pacifico A.: Can two-dimensional echocardiography and Doppler colour-flow maping identify the need for tricuspid valve repair *J Am Coll Cardiol* 1989;14:1255.

25. Ciobanu M, Abbasi AS, Allen M, Hermer A, Spellberg R.: Pulsed Doppler echocardiography in the diagnosis and estimation of severity of aortic insufficiency. *Am J Cardiol* 1982;49:339.

26. Come PC, Riley MF: M-mode and cross-sectional echocardiographic recognition of fibrosis and calcification of the mitral valve chordae and left ventricular papillary muscles. *Am J Cardiol* 1982;49:461.

27. Cooper JW, Nanda NC, Philpot EF, Fan P: Evaluation of valvular regurgitation by colour Doppler. *J Am Soc Echoardiogr*, 2:56, 1989.

28. Cooper JW, Nanda NC, Philpot EF, Fan P: Evaluation of valvular regurgitation by colour Doppler. *J Am Soc Echocardiogr* 1989;2: 56.

29. Dahan M, Paillole C, Martin D, Gourgon R: Determinants of stroke volume response to exercise in patients with mitral stenosis : a Doppler echocardiographic study. *J Am Coll Cardiol* 1993;21: 384.

30. DeMaria AN, Smith MD: Quantitation of Doppler colour-flow recordings: An oxymoron? *J Am Coll Cardiol* 1992; 20: 439.

31. Dent JM, Jayaweera AR, Glasheen WP, Nolan SP, Spotnitz WD, Villanueva FS, Kaul S: A mathematical model for the quantification of mitral regurgitation. *Circulation* 1992;86:553.

32. Derumeaux G, Remadi BF, Cribier A, Letac B. Non-invasive assessment of mitral stenosis before and after percutaneous balloon mitral valvotomy by Doppler continuity equation. *Eur Heart J* 1992; 13:1034–1039.

33. Desideri A, Vanderperren O, Serra A, Barraud P, Petitclerc R, Lesperance J, Dyrda I, Crepeau J, Bonan R: Long-term (9 to 33 months) echocardiographic follow-up after successful percutaneous mitral commissurotomy. *Am J Cardiol* 1992; 69: 1602.

34. Dev V, Singh LSK, Radhakrishnan S, Saxena A, Shrivastava S: Doppler echocardiographic assessment of transmitral gradients and mitral valve area before and after mitral valve balloon dilatation. *Clin Cardiol* 1988; 12:606.

35. Donner R, Black I, Spann JF, Carabello BA: Improved prediction of peak left ventricular pressure in infants with aortic stenosis. *Br Heart J* 1980; 44:406.

36. Dumesnil JG, Yoganathan AP. Theoretical and practical differences between the Gorlin formula and the continuity equation for calculating aortic and mitral valve areas. *Am J Cardiol* 1991; 67:1268–1272.

37. Enriquez-Sarano M, Bailey KR, Seward JB, *et al*. Quantitative Doppler assessment of valvular regurgitation. Summary and validation of the use of volumetric analysis in the quantification of valvar regurgitation. *Circulation* 1993; 87:841–8.

38. Esper RJ: Detection of mild aortic regurgitation by range-rated pulsed Doppler echocardiography. *Am J Cardiol* 1982; 50:1037.

39. Fisher EA, Goldman ME: Simple, rapid method for quantification of tricuspid regurgitation by two-dimensional quantification of tricuspid regurgitation by two-dimensional echocardiography. *Am J Cardiol* 1989; 63:1375.

40. Flachskampf FA, Weyman AE, Gillam L, ChunMing L, Abascal VM , Thomas JD: Aortic regurgitation shortens Doppler pressure half-time in mitral stenosis : Clinical evidence, in vitro simulation, and theoretic analysis. *J Am Coll Cardiol* 1990; 16: 396.

41. Fredman CS, Pearson AC, Labovitz AJ, Kern MJ: Comparison of hemodynamic pressure halftime method and Gorlin formula with Doppler and echocardiographic determinations of mitral valve area in patients with combined mitral stenosis and regurgitation. *Am Heart J*, 119: 121, 1990.

42. Galan A, Zoghbi WA, Quinones MA: Deter-mination of severity of valvular aortic stenosis by Doppler echocardiography and relation of findings to clinical outcome agreement with hemodynamic measurements determined at cardiac catheteri-zation. *Am J Cardiol* 67:1007, 1991.

43. Geibel A, Gornandt L, Kasper W, Buben-heimer P: Reproducibility of Doppler echocardiographic quantification of aortic and mitral valve stenosis: Comparison between two echocardiography centers. *Am J Cardiol* 1991; 67: 1013.

44. Giesler MO, Stauch M: Colour Doppler determination of regurgitant flow: From proximal isovelocity surface areas to proximal velocity profiles, *Echocardiography* 1992; 9: 51.

45. Griffin BP, Flachskampf FA, Reimold SC, *et al*. Relationship of aortic regurgitant velocity slope and pressure half-time to severity of aortic regurgitation under changing haemodynamic conditions. An animal study demonstrating the sensitivity of the aortic pressure half-time to changes in systemic vascular resistance. This limits its utility in following patients receiving vasodilator therapy. *Eur Heart J* 1994; 15:681–5.

46. Hall SA, Brickner ME, Willett DL, *et al*. Assessment of mitral regurgitation severity by Doppler colour-flow mapping of the vena contracta. Validation of the vena contracta method for assessing the severity of mitral regurgitation. *Circulation* 1997; 95:636–42.

47. Hatle L, Angelsen B: *Doppler Ultrasound in Cardiology: Physical Principles and Clinical Applications,* 2nd ed. Philadelphia, Lea & Febiger, 1985.

48. Hatle L, Brubakk A, Tromsdal A, Angelsen B.: Novinvasive assessment of pressure drop in mitral Stenosis by Doppler ultrasound. *Br Heart J* 40: 131, 1978.

49. Helmcke F, Nanda NC, Hsiung MC, *et al*. Colour Doppler assessment of mitral regurgitation with orthogonal planes. *Circulation* 1987; 75:175–83.

50. Holen J, Nanna M, Lockhart J, Waag R: Doppler colour-flow in echocardiography: Analytical and in vitro investigations of the quantitative relationship between orifice flow and colour jet dimensions. *Ultrasound Med Biol* 1990; 16:543.

51. Jain SK, Pechacek LW, DeCastro CM, Garcia E, Hall RJ: Non-invasive assessment of the stenotic mitral valve orifice by two-dimensional echocardiography. *Cardiovasc Dis* 1981; 8:29.

52. Jolly N, Arora R, Mohan JC, Khalilullah M: Pulmonary venous flow dynamics before and after balloon mitral valvuloplasty as determined by transesophageal Doppler echocardiography. *Am J Cardiol* 1992; 70:780.

53. Kai H, Koyanagi S, Takeshita A: Aortic valve prolapse with aortic regurgitation assessed by Doppler colour-flow echocardiography. *Am Heart J* 1992; 124:1297.

54. Kamp O, Eijkstra J-W, Huitink H, Van MJE, Werter CJPJ, Roos JP, Visser CA: Trans-esophageal colour-flow Doppler mapping in the assessment of native mitral valvular regurgitation: Comparison with left ventricular angiography. *J Am Soc Echocardiogr* 1991; 4: 598.

55. Kamp O, Huitink H, van Eenige MJ, Visser CA, Roos JP: Value of pulmonary venous flow characteristics in the assessment of severity of native mitral valve regurgitation: An angiographic correlated study. *J Am Soc Echocardiogr* 1992; 5: 239.

56. Karp K, Teien D, Bjerle P, Eriksson P: Reassessment of valve area determinations in mitral stenosis by the pressure half-time before and after balloon valvotomy in mitral stenosis. *Am J Cardiol* 1991; 67: 162.

57. Keren G, Pardes A, Miller HI, Scherez J, Laniado S: Pulmonary venous flow determined by Doppler echocardiography in mitral stenosis. *Am J Cardiol* 1990; 65: 246.

58. Khandheria BK, Tajik AJ, Reeder GS, Callahan MJ, Nishimura RA, Miller FA, Seward JB: Doppler colour-flow imaging: A new technique for visualization and characterization of the blood flow jet in mitral stenosis. *Mayo Clin Proc* 1986;61: 623.

59. Klein AL, Obarski TP, Stewart WJ, Casale PN, Pearce GL, Husbands K, Cosgrove DM, Salcedo EE.: Transesophageal Doppler imaging. *J Am Coll Cardiol* 1991;18:518.

60. Kulas A, Enriquez-Sarano L, Troley C, Acar J: Value of correction by receiving gains in the determination of mitral valve surface area by two-dimensional echocardiography. *Arch Mal Coeur* 1982;75: 757.

61. Kurokawa S, Takahashi M, Sugiyama T, Ikuri H, Kawano T, Tsukahara N, Abe W, Muramatsu J, Kikawada R, Nakazawa K, Ishii K: Noninvasive evaluation of the magnitude of aortic and mitral regurgitation by means of Doppler two-dimensional echocardiography, *Am Heart J*, 1990;120; 638.

62. Labovitz AJ, Ferrara RP, Kern MJ, Bryg RJ, Mrosek DG, Williams GA: Quantitative evaluation of aortic insufficiency by continuous wave Doppler echocardiography. *J Am Coll Cardiol* 1986;8:1341.

63. Leavitt JI, Coats MH, Falk RH: Effects of exercise on transmitral gradient and pulmonary artery pressure in patients with mitral stenosis or a prosthetic mitral valve: A Doppler echocardiographic study. *J Am Coll Cardiol* 1991;17: 1520.

64. Liddell NE, Stoddard MF, Talley JD, Guinn VL, Kupersmith J: Transesophageal echocardiographic diagnosis of isolated tricuspid valve prolapse with severe tricuspid regurgitation. *M Heart J*, 1992;123: 230.

65. Loyd D, Eng D, AskP, Wranne B.: Pressure half-time does not always predict mitral valve area correctly. *J Am Soc Echocardiogr* 1988;1: 313.

66. Manning WJ, Resis GJ, Douglas PS: Use of transesophageal echocardiography to detect left atrial thrombi before percutaneous balloon dilatation of the mitral valve: A prospective study. *Br Heart J* 1992;67: 170.

67. Marcus RH, Neumann A, Borow KM, Lang RM: Transmitral flow velocity in symptomatic severe aortic regurgitation: Utility of Doppler for determination of preclosure of the mitral valve. *Am Heart J*, 1990; 120:449.

68. Martin GR, Silverman NH, Soifer SJ, Lutin W, Scagnelli SA: Tricuspid regurgitation in children: A pulsed Doppler, contrast echocardiographic and angiographic comparison. *J Am Soc Echocardiogr* 1:257, 1988.

69. Martin R, Rakowski H, Kleiman JH, Beaver W, London E, Popp RL. Reliability and reproducibility of two-dimensional echocardiographic measurement of the stenotic mitral valve orifice area. *Am J Cardiol* 1979; 43:560–568.

70. Masuyama T, Sato H, Nanto S, Naka M, Taniura K, Hirayama A, Kodama K, Okamoto K, Morita K, Kitabatake A, Inoue M, Kamada T: Comparison of continuous wave and pulsed Doppler method in noninvasive evaluation of aortic regurgitation. *Jpn J Med Ultrasonics* 1986; 13:17.

71. Motro M, Schneeweiss A, Lehrer E, Rath S, Neufeld HN: Correlation between cardiac catheterization and echocardiography in assessing the severity of mitral stenosis. *Int J Cardiol* 1981; 1: 25.

72. Mugge A, Danile WG, Herrmann G, Simon R, Lichtlen PR: Quantification of tricuspid regurgitant by Doppler colour-flow mapping after cardiac transplantation. *Am J Cardiol* 1990; 66:884.

73. Nair M, Arora R, Mohan JC, Kalra GS, Sethi KK, NigamM, Khalilullah M. Assessment of mitral valver stenosis by echocardiography: utility of various methods before and after mitral valvotomy. *Int J Cardiol* 1991; 32:389–394.

74. Nakatani S, Masuyama T, Kodama K, Kitabatake A, Fuji K, Kamada T. Value and limitations of Doppler echocardiography in the quantification stenotic mitral valve area: comparison of the pressure half-time and the continuity equation methods. *Circulation* 1988; 77:78–85.

75. Natarajan D, Sharm VP, Chandra S, Dhar SK, Gaba M, Caroli B: Effects of percutaneous balloon mitral valvotomy on pulmonary venous flow in severe mitral stenosis. *Am J Cardiol* 1992; 69: 810.

76. Nishimura RA, Vonk GD, Rumberger JA, Tajik AJ: Semiquantitation of aortic regurgitation by different Doppler echocardiographic techniques and comparison with ultrafast computed tomography. *Am Heart J* 1992; 124:995.

77. Otto CM, Pearlman AS, Amsler LC: Doppler echocardiographic evaluation of left ventricular diastolic filling in isolated valvular aortic stenosis. *Am J Cardiol* 1989; 63: 313.

78. Otto CM, Pearlman AS, Gardner CL, Enmoto DM, Togo T, Tsuboi H, Ivey TD: Experimental validation of Doppler

echocardiographic measurement of volume flow through the stenotic aortic valve. *Circulation* 1988; 78:435.

79. Otto CM, Pearlman AS, Gardner CL, Kraft CD, Fujioka MC: Simplification of the Doppler continuity equation for calculating stenotic aortic valve area. *J Am Soc Echocardiogr* 1988; 1:155.

80. Parro A, Helmcke F, Mahan III E, Nanda NC, Kandath D, Dean LS: Value and limitations of colour Doppler echocardiography in the evaluation of percutaneous balloon mitral valvuloplasty for isolated mitral stenosis. *Am J Cardiol* 1991; 67: 1261.

81. Patel AK, Rowe GG, Thomsen JH, Dhanani SP, Kosolcharoen P, Lyle LEW: Detection and estimation of rheumatic mitral regurgitation in the presence of mitral stenosis by pulsed Doppler echocardiography. *Am J Cardiol* 1983; 51: 986.

82. Percy RF, Miller AB, Conetta DA: Usefulness of left ventricular wall stress at rest and after exercise for outcome prediction in asymptomatic aortic regurgitation. *Am Heart J* 1993; 125:151.

83. Perry GJ, Helmcke F, Nanda NC, *et al*. Evaluation of aortic insufficiency by Doppler colour-flow mapping. Initial description of the jet area within the left ventricular outflow tract as a measure of aortic regurgitant severity. *J Am Coll Cardiol* 1987;9:952–9.

84. Pu M, Griffin BP, Vandervoort PM, *et al*. The value of assessing pulmonary venous flow velocity for predicting severity of mitral regurgitation: a quantitative assessment integrating left ventricular function. A critical appraisal of the pulmonary venous approach to assessing valvar regurgitation, demonstrating that the blunted S wave is nonspecific with regards to regurgitant severity. *J Am Soc Echocardiogr* 1999;12:736–43.

85. Pu M, Prior DL, Fan X, *et al*. Calculation of mitral regurgitant orifice area with use of a simplified proximal convergence method: initial clinical application. Description and validation of a simplified method for applying the proximal convergence approach. *J Am Soc Echocardiogr* 2001;14:180–5.

86. Pu M, Vandervoort PM, Griffin BP, *et al*. Quantification of mitral regurgitation by the proximal convergence method using transesophageal echocardiography. Clinical validation of a geometric correction for proximal flow constraint. Analysis of flow overestimation due to constraint by proximal structures and a simple method for correcting this. *Circulation* 1995;92:2169–77.

87. Recusani F, Bargiggia GS, Yoganathan AP, Raisaro A, Valdes-Cruz LM, Sung HW, Bertucci C, Gallati M, Moises VA, Simpson IA, Tronconi L, Sahn DJ: A new method for quantification of regurgitant flow rate using colour Doppler flow imaging of the flow convergence region proximal to a discrete orifice. An *in vitro* study. *Circulation* 1991; 83: 594.

88. Reimold SC, Maier SE, Aggarwal K, *et al*. Aortic flow velocity patterns in chronic aortic regurgitation: implications for Doppler echocardiography. Demonstration of the utility of aortic flow reversal in identifying patients with hemodynamically significant aortic regurgitation. *J Am Soc Echocardiogr* 1996; 9:675–83.

89. Reimold SC, Thomas J, Lee RT: Relation between Doppler colour-flow variables and invasively determined jet variables in patients with aortic regurgitation. *J Am Coll Cardiol* 1992; 20: 1143.

90. Riggs TW, Lapin GD, Paul MH, Muster AJ measurement of mitral valve orifice area in infants and children by two-dimensional echocardiography. *J Am Coll Cardiol* 1983; 1: 873.

91. Rivera JM, Vandervoort PM, Thoreau DH, Levine RA, Weyman AE, Thomas JD: Quantification of mitral regurgitation with the proximal flow convergence method: A clinical study. *Am Heart J* 1992; 124: 1289.

92. Rodriguez L, Anconina J, Flachskampf FA, *et al*. Impact of finite orifice size on proximal flow convergence. Implications for Doppler quantification of valvular regurgitation. Analysis of flow underestimation due to contour flattening near the orifice and a simple method for correcting this. [Abstract]. *Circulation Res* 1992; 70:923–30.

93. Sadoshima J, Koyanagi S, Sugimachi M, Hirooka Y, Takeshita Evaluation of the severity of mitral regurgitation by transesophageal Doppler flow echocardiography. *Am Heart J* 1992; 123: 1245.

94. Samstad SO, Rossvoll O, Torp HG, Skjaerpe T, Hatle L: Cross-sectional early mitral flow velocity profiles from colour Doppler in patients with mitral valve disease. *Circulation* 1992; 86: 748.

95. Schwammenthal E, Chen C, Giesler M, *et al*. New method for accurate calculation of regurgitant flow rate based on analysis of Doppler colour-flow maps of the proximal flow field. Validation in a canine model of mitral regurgitation with initial application in patients. A proposed method to analyse the velocities along a colour M mode acquisition of the proximal convergence zone to adjust for variable regurgitant orifice areas. *J Am Coll Cardiol* 1996; 27:161–72.

96. Schweizer P, Bardos P, Krebs W, Erbel R, Minale C, Imm S, Massmer BJ, effert S: Morphometric investigations in mitral stenosis using two-dimensional echocardiography *Br Heart J* 1982; 48:54.

97. Sheikh KH, Bashore TM, Kitzman DW, Davidson CJ, Skeleton TN, Honan MB, Kisslo KB, Higginbotham MB, Kisslo J: Doppler left ventricular diastolic filling abnormalities in aortic stenosis and their relation of hemodynamic parameters. *Am J Cardiol* 1989; 63:1360.

98. Simpson IA, Sahn DJ. Quantification of valvular regurgitation by Doppler echocardiography. An excellent summary of instrumentation issues in visualisation of colour Doppler jets. *Circulation* 1991; 84(3 suppl): 1188–92.

99. Sitges M, Jones M, Shiota T, *et al*. Inter-aliasing distance of the flow convergence surface for determining mitral regurgitant volume: a validation study in a chronic animal model. A new method for avoiding the problem of localising the regurgitant orifice by measuring the distance between the first two aliasing contours Schwammenthal E, Chen C, Benning F, *et al*. Dynamics of mitral regurgitant flow and orifice area. Physiologic application of the proximal flow convergence method: clinical data and experimental testing. *J Am Coll Cardiol* 2001; 38:1195–202.

100. Smith MD, Grayburn PA, Spain MG, DeMaria AN, Kwan OL, Moffett CB: Observer variability in the quantitation of Doppler colour-flow jet areas for mitral and aortic regurgitation. *J Am Coll Cardiol* 11:579, 1988.

101. Smith MD, Harrison MR, Pinton R, Kandil H, Kwan OL, DeMaria AN: Regurgitant jet size by transesophageal compared with transthoracic Doppler colour-flow imaging. *Circulation* 1991; 83: 79.

102. Smith MD, Kwan OL, Spain MG, DeMaria AN.: Temporal variability of colour Doppler jet areas in patients with mitral and aortic regurgitation. *Am Heart J* 1992; 123: 953.

103. Spain MG, Smith MD, Grayburn PA, Harlamert EA, DeMaria AN, O'Brien M, Kwan OL: Quantitative assessment of mitral regurgitation by Doppler colour-flow imaging: Angiographic and hemodynamic correlations. *J Am Coll Cardiol* 1989; 13: 585.

104. Stamm RB, Martin RP: Quantification of pressure gradients across stenotic valves by Doppler ultrasound. *J Am Coll Cardiol* 1983; 2:707.

105. Stoddard MF, Arce J, Liddell NE, Peters G, Dillon S, Kupersmith J.: Two-dimensional transesophageal echocardiographic determination of aortic valve area in adults with aortic stenosis. *Am Heart J* 1991; 122:1415.

106. Sun JP, Pu M, Fouad FM, *et al.* Automated cardiac output measurement by spatiotemporal integration of colour Doppler data. In vitro and clinical validation. A validation study demonstrating that colour Doppler velocities can be integrated across the left ventricular outflow tract throughout space and time to yield stroke volume. *Circulation* 1997; 95:932–9.

107. Sun JP, Yang XS, Qin JX, *et al.* Quantification of mitral regurgitation by automated cardiac output measurement: experimental and clinical validation. *J Am Coll Cardiol* 1998; 32:1074–82.

108. Tabbalat RA, Haft JI. Effect of severe pulmonary hypertension on the calculation of mitral valve area in patients with mitral stenosis. *Am Heart J* 1991; 121:488–493.

109. Takao S, Miyatake K, Izumi S, Okamoto M, Kinoshita N, Nakagawa H, Yamamoto K, Sakakibara H, Nimura Y.: Clinical implications of pulmonary regurgitation in healthy individuals: Detection by cross-sectional pulsed Doppler echocardiography. *Br Heart J* 1988;59:542.

110. Teague SM, Heinsimer JA, Anderson JL, *et al.* Quantification of aortic regurgitation utilizing continuous wave Doppler ultrasound. Early description of the aortic pressure half-time method for assessing aortic regurgitant severity. *J Am Coll Cardiol* 1986; 8:592–9.

111. Thomas JD, Liu CM, Flachskampf FA, *et al.* Quantification of jet flow by momentum analysis. An in vitro colour Doppler flow study. An exposition on the physical and instrumentation determinants of colour jet area, demonstrating the importance of jet momentum (flow rate × velocity). *Circulation* 1990; 81:247–59.

112. Thuillez C, Theroux P, Bourassa MG, Blanchard D, Peronneau P, Guermonprez JL, DieboldB, Waters DD, Maurice P: Pulsed Doppler echocardiographic study of mitral stenosis. *Circulation* 1980; 61:381.

113. Trappe HJ, Daniel WG, Frank G, Lichtlen. PR: Comparisons between diastolic fluttering and reverse doming of anterior mitral leaflet in aortic regurgitation. *Am Heart J*, 1987; 114:1399.

114. Tribouilloy C, Avinee P, Shen WF, Rey JL, Slama M, Lesbre JP: End diastolic flow velocity just beneath the aortic isthmus assessed by pulsed Doppler echocardiography: A new predictor of the aortic regurgitant fraction. *Br Heart J* 1991; 65:37.

115. Tribouilloy C, Shen WF, Slama MA, Dufosses H, Choquet D, Marek A, Lesbre, JP: Non-invasive measurement of the regurgitant fraction by pulsed Doppler echocardiography in isolated pure mitral regurgitation. *Br Heart J* 1991; 66: 290.

116. Tribouilloy C, Shen WF, QuereJP: Assessment of severity of mitral regurgitation by measuring regurgitant jet width at its origin with transesophageal Doppler colour-flow imaging. *Circulation* 1992; 85: 1248.

117. Utsunomiya T, Ogawa T, Doshi R, Patel D, Quan M, Henry WL, Gardin JM: Doppler colour-flow: "Proximal isovelocity surface area" method for estimating volume flow rate: Effects of orifice shape and machine factors. *J Am Coll Cardiol* 1991; 17: 1103.

118. Utsunomiya T, Patel D, Doshi R, Quan M., Gardin JM: Can signal intensity of the continuous wave Doppler regurgitant jet estimate severity of mitral regurgitation. *Am Heart J* 1992; 123: 166.

119. Vandervoort PM, Rivera JM, Mele D, *et al.* Application of colour Doppler flow mapping to calculate effective regurgitant orifice area. An in vitro study and initial clinical observations. Application of the proximal convergence method for calculation of the regurgitant orifice area. *Circulation* 1993; 88:1150–6.

120. Vandervoort PM, Thoreau DH, Rivera JM, *et al.* Automated flow rate calculations based on digital analysis of flow convergence proximal to regurgitant orifices. Description of a computational method for analysing the full proximal flow field to automatically localise the regurgitant orifice and calculate the peak flow rate. *J Am Coll Cardiol* 1993;22:535.

121. Vasan RS, Shrivastava S, Kumar MV: Value and limitations of Doppler echocardiographic determination of mitral valve area in Lutembacher syndrome. *J Am Coll Cardiol* 1992; 20: 1362.
This early paper outlined the use of colour jet area in the assessment of mitral regurgitation, particularly as a proportion of left atrial area. Although it has many limitations, this method is still frequently used. *J Am Coll Cardiol* 1993; 22:535.

15

Echocardiographic Diagnosis of Infective Endocarditis

Infective endocarditis is a disease caused by microbial infection of the endothelial lining of the heart. The characteristic lesion is a vegetation, which usually develops on a heart valve. In the pathogenesis of infectious endocarditis, local turbulence is believed to promote a sterile network of fibrin and platelets on the endocardial surface which is colonized later by microorganisms entering the blood stream from a distant site. The infecting microorganisms are protected by the microthrombus from normal host defense mechanisms and from antibiotic penetration, requiring high dose parenteral antimicrobial agents over a long period. The result of colonization of previously damaged heart endothelium or infection of healthy tissues is a vegetation whose primary features are a heavy colonization of microorganisms, a stroma, consisting primarily of fibrin and a relative paucity of leukocytes. Suitable circumstances for infection include the following:

1. History of previous valvulitis (rheumatic, degenerative, idiopathic).
2. Congenital heart lesion (patent ductus arteriosus, ventricular septal defect with endocardial friction, bicuspid aortic valve).
3. Previous heart surgery (prosthetic valve, septal patch, in-dwelling catheter).
4. Immunosuppression (treatment of a malignant disease, prolonged use of steroids and antibiotics).
5. Drug addiction.

There are two types of infective endocarditis: acute and subacute. Acute bacterial endocarditis can occur during a septicemia from organisms such as *Staphylococcus aureus*, *Neisseria gonorrhoeae* or *Streptococcus pyogenes*. The cardiac valves may be invaded and destroyed by these bacteria. In subacute bacterial endocarditis, organisms of low-grade virulence invade a valve or an area of the endocardium that has been damaged by a previous acquired heart disease, such as rheumatic fever, or a congenital heart defect. The organism can enter the bloodstream as a result of one of several circumstances: dental extraction, apical tooth abscess diarrhea, osteomyelitis, cardiac surgery, or drug abuse. Most patients with bacterial endocarditis suffer left heart valvular disease involving aortic valve in 45%

Table 15.1: *Indications of echocardiography in patients with endocarditis*
1. Identifies predisposing heart disease
2. Pivotal role in diagnosis
3. Detects complications
4. Assesses hemodynamic consequences
5. Serial evaluation (assesses efficacy of therapy)
6. Prognosis (risk of complications)

Table 15.2: *Identification of vegetation by echocardiographic technique*	
Positive morphology	*Negative morphology*
Low reflectance Attached to valve location,	High echogenicity Non-valvular upstream side
Irregular shape amorphous	Smooth surface or fibrillar
Mobile oscillating	Non-mobile
Associated tissue changes valvular regurgitation	Absence of regurgitation

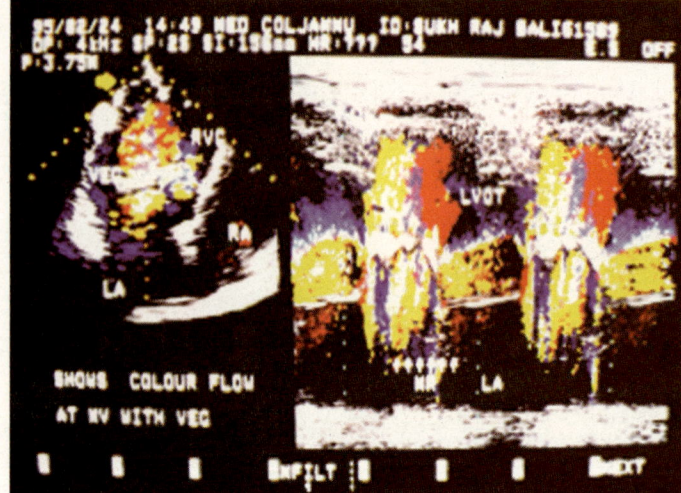

Fig. 15.1: Color 2-D apical 4C (left) and color M-mode echocardiogram showing vegetation on anterior mitral leaflet resulting into mosaic color jet of mitral regurgitation (arrows) in both views respectively. LVOT = Left ventricular outflow tract, LA = Left atrium, Veg = vegetation

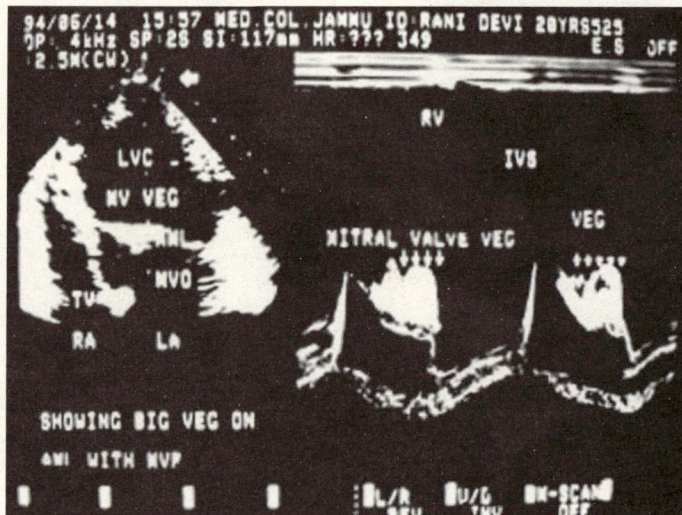

Fig. 15.3: 2-D and M-mode echocardiogram showing large vegetation located on the anterior mitral leaflet in patient with mild mitral valvular stenosis (see thickening of both anterior and posterior mitral leaflets). VEG = vegetation, MVO = mitral valve area, LVC = left ventricular cavity

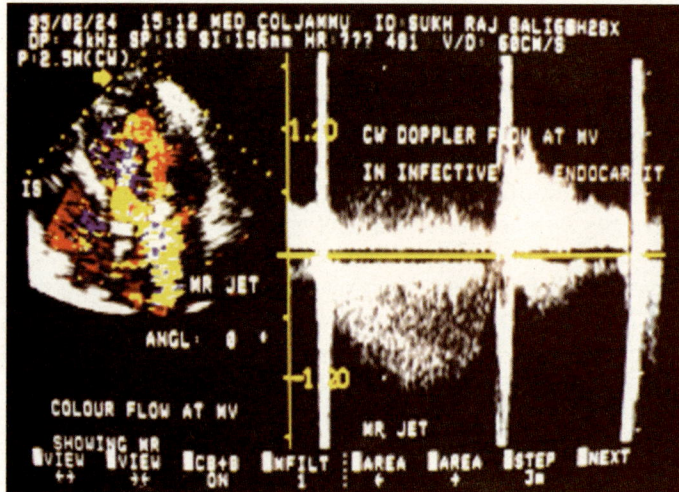

Fig. 15.2: (left panel) Color flow apical 4C left parasternal view and Doppler flow velocity across mitral valve showing mosaic jet of mitral regurgitation into left atrium (arrow) and regurgitant velocity flow on Doppler study (right panel) in patient with infective endocarditis of mitral valve with clinical mitral regurgitant murmur

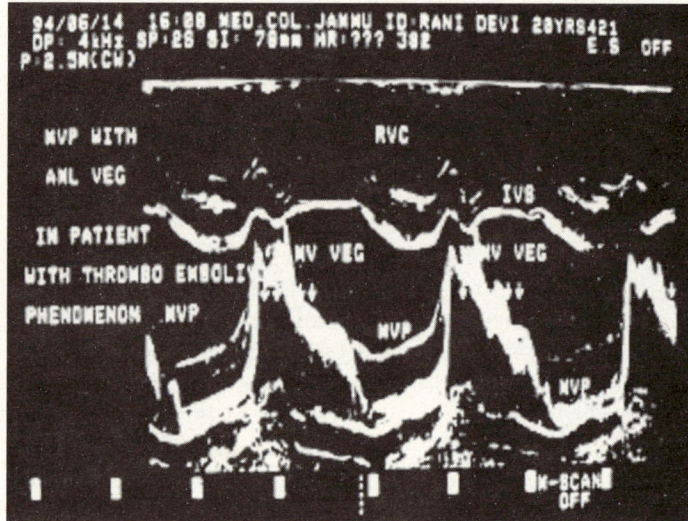

Fig. 15.4: M-Mode echocardiogram showing thickening of both anterior and posterior mitral leaflets in patient with mitral valve prolapse, vegetation on the anterior mitral leaflet and had cerebral thromboembolic phenomenon leading to hemipareis on the right side of the body. MVP = mitral valve prolapse, MV VEG = mitral valve vegetation

of patients, the mitral valve in 35%, and both valves in 19%. The right heart is affected less often, with the tricuspid valve affected more frequently than the pulmonary valve (<3–5%)(Figs 15.1–15.7).

Pathogenesis in Infective Endocarditis

The diagnosis of endocarditis is based on clinical findings, the history of predisposing factors, and sustained bacteremia. Sustained bacteremia refers to the positive blood cultures obtained from different venous channels over a short period, and it differentiates bacterial endocarditis from a transient bacteremia (e.g. after the brushing of teeth or a bowel movement).

Persistent circulation of microorganisms creates a favourable environment for organisms to be deposited on the damaged roughened valves. The organisms are enmeshed in deposits of fibrin and platelets on the endothelium of the valve to form irregular vegetations.

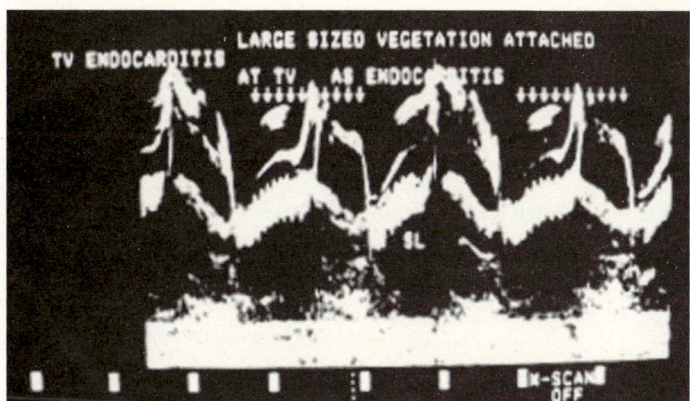

Fig. 15.5: M-Mode echocardiogram showing large-sized fluttering vegetation attached on the anterior tricuspid leaflet leading to infective endocarditis of the tricuspid valve. TV = tricuspid valve

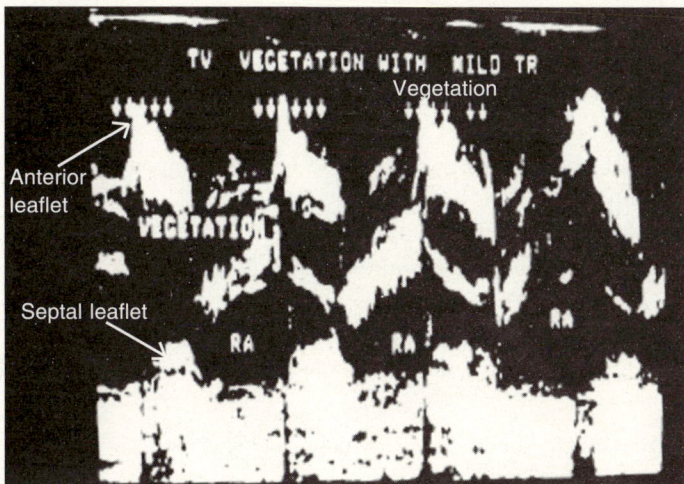

Fig. 15.6: M-Mode echocardiogram showing large sized vegetation on both anterior and septal leaflets of tricuspid valve (arrows) almost obstructing 50% of the valve area. TV = tricuspid valve, RA = right atrium

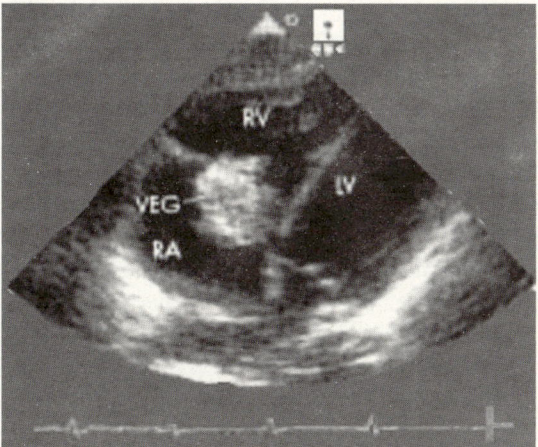

Fig. 15.7: Apical 4C view showing large vegetation attached to the tricuspid valve in patient with infective endocarditis of tricuspid valve who had been using intravenous narcotic drugs

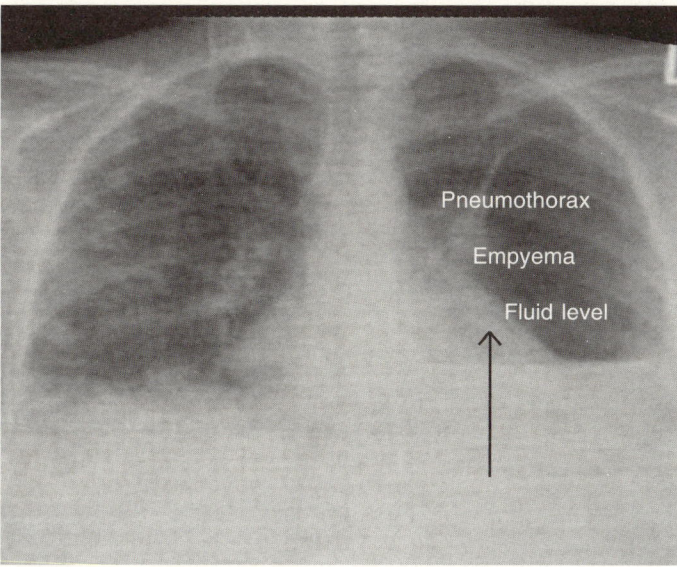

Fig. 15.8: X-ray chest PA view in the same patient (Fig. 15.7) showing multiple alveolar opacities in the right lung. Abscess formation in the left lung has caused a bronchopleural fistula, pneumothorax, and empyema

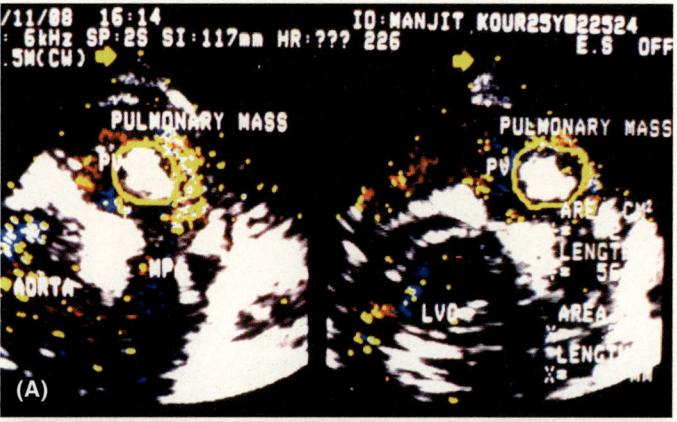

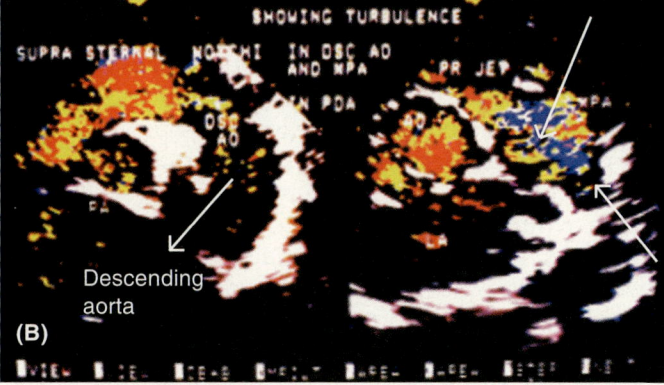

Fig. 15.9A and B: (A) 2D Color flow at great vessel level showing dilated pulmonary artery with pulmonary valvular endocardial vegetation (arrow). **(B)** (left panel) Showing descending aorta and short axis great vessel view (right panel) showing left to right shunt between descending aorta and pulmonary artery in patient with patent ductus arteriosus and ductal endarteritis in patient with persistent pyrexia and biventricular decompensation

Table 15.3: *Localization of organisms according to the condition and site of origin*

Condition	Location of stream
Coarctation (Figs 15.10 and 15.11)	Downstream wall
Patent ductus arterosus (Fig. 15.9A and B)	Pulmonary artery
A-V fistula (Fig. 15.13)	Veins
Aortic insufficiency (Fig. 15.11)	Ventricular surface of valves
Mitral insufficiency (Figs 15.1 and 15.2)	Atrial surface of mitral valve
Pulmonary insufficiency (Fig. 15.9A and B)	Ventricular surface of pulmonary valve
Tricuspid insufficiency (Fig. 15.7)	Atrial surface of tricuspid valve

Table 15.4: *Echocardiographic characteristics of infective endocarditis (Figs 15.3–15.19)*

Location	Findings
1. Aortic valve (Figs 15.10, 15.11 and 15.13)	Shaggy nonuniform thickening in systole or diastole with unrestricted leaflet motion.
	Dense shaggy echoes moving across valve and into LVOT
	Flail or ruptured cusps
	Fine diastolic fluttering on anterior mitral leaflet secondary to aortic insufficiency
2. Mitral valve (Figs 15.1–15.4)	Thick shaggy echoes attached to or moving behind leaflets demonstrating unrestricted motion.
	Systolic flutter of prolapsing segments of mitral valve
	Fuzzy leaflet echoes in left atrial cavity during systole (differentiate from myxoma)
3. TV and PV (Figs 15.5–15.7 and 15.9A and B)	Shaggy thickening of leaflets, demonstrating unrestrictive motion.
	Mass of echoes moving with leaflets (dependent motion rupture of tricuspid chord tendinae
4. Prosthetic valve	Thick shaggy collection located behind site of attachment of prosthesis to valve ring. Evidence of severe regurgitation.

These masses may vary in size and shape, and become quite large and friable in Candida infections. They occur on the downstream side of the damaged valve. The jet effect plays a significant role in the collection of bacteria on the valves and on the chordae tendineae. The effect is related to the insufficiency of one valve, causing a high-pressure source with a low-pressure sink. The infection usually occurs on the low-pressure side. Thus a patient with aortic insufficiency would have a jet stream from the aortic root into the left ventricle. The stream would flow directly into the chorda tendineae causing satellite regions of bacterial formation to develop on the chordae: Sink areas or areas just beyond the point of constriction where the forward velocity of the blood is highest and the lateral pressure is the lowest.

Complications of endocarditis may include an aneurysm, perforation, tear, or extensive destruction of the valve. The process may spread to the adjacent mitral endocardium or involve the chorda tendineae. The larger, more friable vegetations may obstruct the valve orifice or break off to cause dissemination of large emboli throughout the body.

Clinical Features

Clinical manifestations in a patient suffering from endocarditis include fever, anemia, cardiac murmur, embolic phenomena, splenomegaly, hematuria, nephritis or elevated rheumatoid factor. The sub-acute case may present as a fever of unknown origin with only a murmur of anemia. Cardiac findings include a changing murmur (usually over a short period of time because of the valvular destruction and subsequent regurgitation), cardiac failure, ventricular and muscular involvement (the infection on the aortic valve may spread to the interventricular septum, and an abscess may develop and rupture into the right heart or may interfere with the conduction of the cardiac impulse and cause heart block with or without syncope). In addition, there may be a septic abscess of the papillary muscle, with destruction of the mitral ring, or a flail mitral apparatus.

Echocardiographic Features

The vegetations usually seen are of varying size and shape often pedunculated and rather amorphous. They

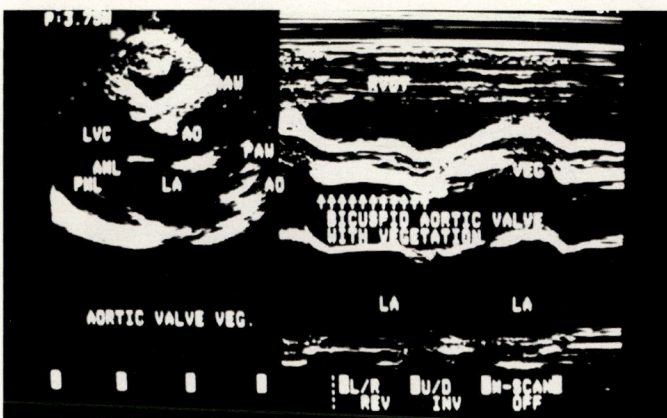

Fig. 15.10: 2-D and M-Mode echocardiogram showing thickening of right-coronary cusp of aortic valve due to vegetation in patient with bicuspid aortic valve (arrows)

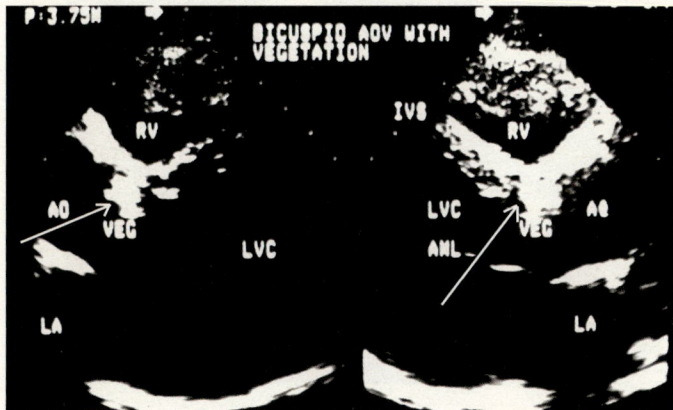

Fig. 15.11: 2-D Echocardiogram showing thickening of right-coronary cusp of aortic valve due to vegetation in the same patient as in Fig. 15.10 with bicuspid aortic valve (arrows) VEG = vegetation, LVC = left ventricular cavity, RV = right ventricle, AO = aorta, AML = anterior mitral leaflet, LA = left atrium

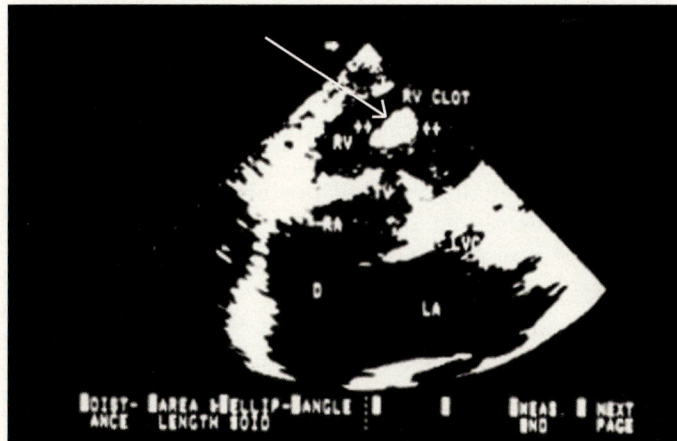

Fig. 15.12: Apical 4C view showing big mass in right ventricle arrow with dilated right atrium gross, tricuspid regurgitation and peak systolic pulmonary pressure more than 45 mm of Hg, in a patient with right heart failure, RV = right ventricle, RA = right atrium, LA = left atrium

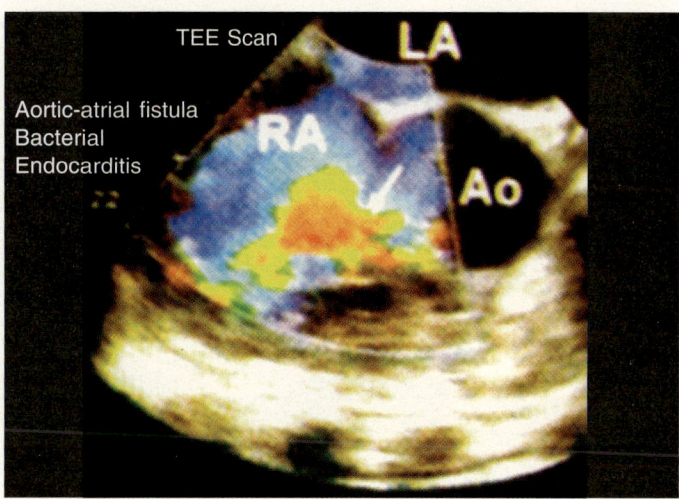

Fig. 15.13: Color TEE short axis transgastric view at aorta level showing blue and yellow jet traversing from aorta to right atrium in a young lady with persistent pyrexia lasting more than six weeks. Her echo-cardiographic examination revealed aorto-atrial fistula as a result of bacterial endocarditis

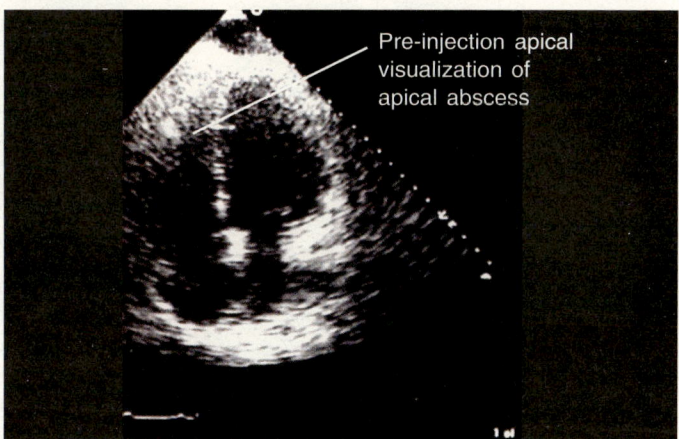

Fig. 15.14: Apical 4C view showing less distinct apical thrombosis in patient with dilated cardiomyopathy

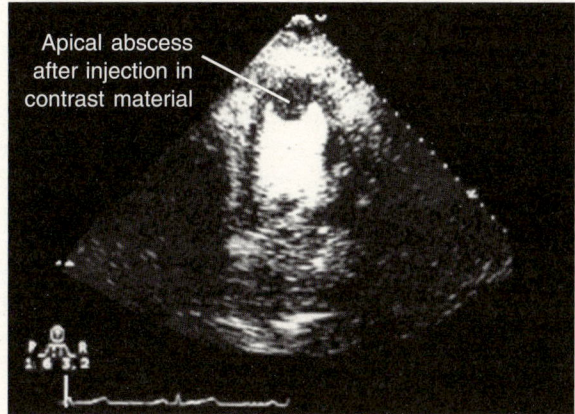

Fig. 15.15: Apical 4C view in the same patient as described above There is well distinct and prominent features of apical thrombosis after contrast injection

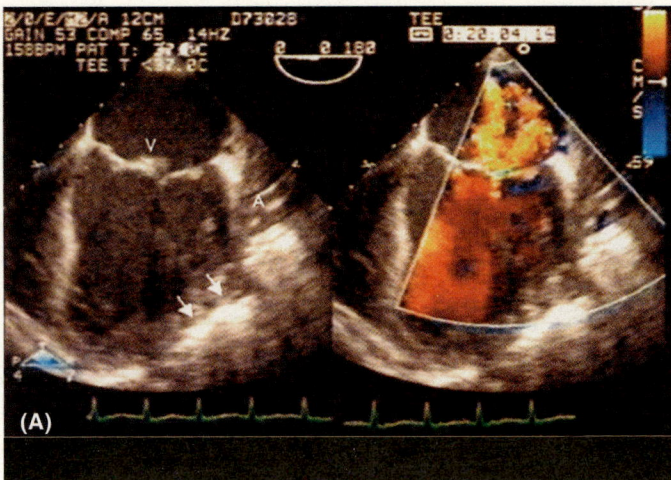

Fig. 15.16: Color flow TEE showing both mitral and aortic valvular regurgitation following metastatic emboli on the posterior mitral leaflet (PML) and almost disorganizing the aortic valve (AOV) due to pyogenic abscess on interventricular septum (MB)

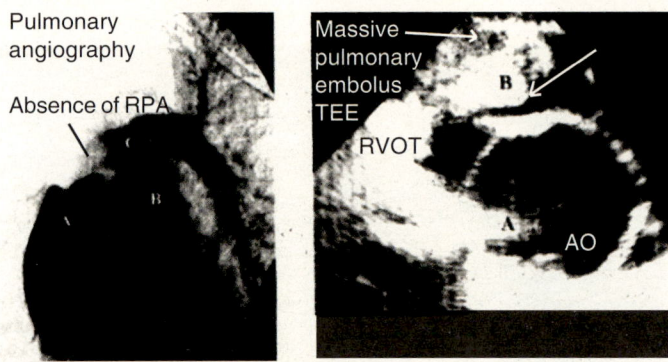

Fig. 15.17: Right panel transesophageal echocardiography shows massive pulmonary embolism almost total occlusion of the lumen of the pulmonary artery. Left panel shows angiographic features of not visualizing right pulmonary artery (RPA) but left pulmonary artery is very well seen

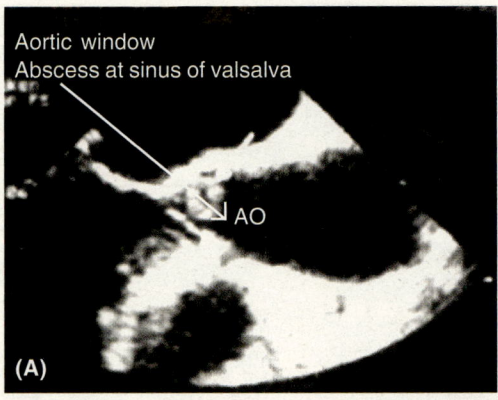

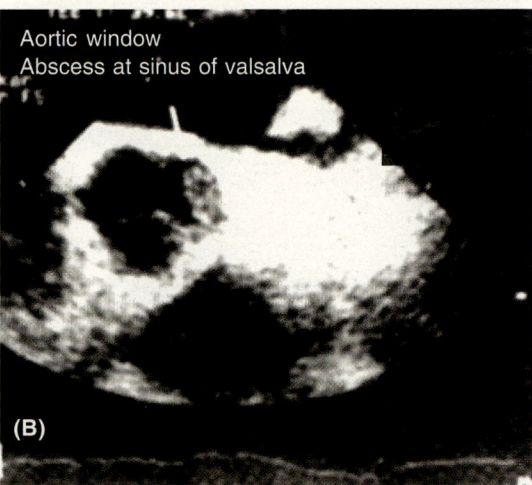

Fig. 15.18A and B: TEE at aorta level showing an echodense structure located in the left coronary sinus of valsalva, just proximal to the ostium of the left coronary artery (A) in patient with acute chest pain of short duration. Coronary artery angiogram revealed occlusion in left descending artery. Aortic root was found normal. Inspite of effective thrombolysis, this patients repeat scan did not improve (B) and died due to circulatory collapse

usually exhibit a distinct motion independent of valvular excursion. The lesions may be visualised on the leaflet tissue, the mitral or tricuspid chorda tendineae or on the atrial or ventricular endocardial surfaces.

M-mode echocardiography usually describes the lesions as shaggy, thick, irregular, bright echoes. Over the aortic valve they are better observed during both systole and diastole. The mitral valve may show vegetations originating from the atrial side of either the anterior or the posterior leaflet. Vegetations on the tricuspid valve are usually located over the anterior leaflet, often there is a mass of echoes somewhat attached to the posterior side of the anterior leaflet. One may encounter to see either systolic or diastolic flutter or both (Figs 15.3 to 15.18A and B).

Infective endocarditis may lead to rupture of the chordae tendineae to produce a flail leaflet. If it involves

chordae tendineae of posterior mitral leaflet, an early systolic plunge of the leaflet to the posterior left atrial wall would be visualised during systole followed by an anterior motion at the onset of diastole, and the posterior leaflet may be recorded in the left atrium behind the aorta. Occasionally the flail posterior leaflet produces multiple diastolic echoes posterior to the anterior leaflet, and these may mimic an atrial myxoma.

Other associated abnormalities that can develop during endocarditis are premature closure of mitral valve secondary to acute aortic insufficiency, diastolic flutter of the mitral valve secondary to aortic insufficiency, coarse systolic flutter of aortic valve leaflets, localized thickening of the aortic wall secondary to abscess formation, or left ventricular volume overload and hypercontractility. Abnormal echo findings may need exhaustive review in order to differentiate vegetations from another disease process that may be mimicking the vegetations and various kinds of artifacts produced by incorrect gain settings. The various valvular involvement due to rheumatic process leading to thickening, fibrosis and valve calcification, myxomatous degeneration of the valve or cardiac mass due to neoplastic growth, need critical evaluation and differentiation by clinical history, examination with echocardiographic study and other relevant tests of the presenting disease (Figs 15.12–15.18).

Transthoracic, M-mode and 2-dimensional echocardiography permits assessment of the location, size, and morphology of the vegetation, the examination of both the right and left sides of the heart for valvular and other endocardial involvement. It should be very clear that the absence of vegetative mass by echo does not rule out bacterial endocarditis. Lesions smaller than 2.0 mm are difficult to detect by echography and previous rheumatic heart disease lesions may leave the valves somewhat thickened and thus make it difficult to judge whether the thickening has resulted from the rheumatic disease or the presence of vegetations on the valves.

It is also difficult to assess the presence of vegetations on prosthetic valves since the bright reflection from the prosthesis make it difficult to isolate increased thickness resulting from vegetative lesions. Doppler evaluation may be useful on a serial basis to follow the course of regurgitation and to see if the leakage increases in intensity over a ashort period of time. Transesophageal echocardiography carries most sensitivity and specificity in detecting vegetations on different valves including prosthetic valves even if these are less than 2.0 mm in size (Figs 15.16–15.18).

Bibliography

1. Abramson MA, Sexton DJ: Nosocomial methicillin-resistant and methicillin-susceptible *Staphylococcus aureus* primary bacteremia: at what costs? *Infect Control Hosp Epidemiol* 1999; 20:408.
2. ACOG Practice Bulletin. Prophylactic antibiotics in labor and delivery. Number 47, October 2003. American College of Obstetricians and Gynecologists: *Obstet Gynecol* 2003; 102:875.
3. Antibiotic prophylaxis for gastrointestinal endoscopy. American Society for Gastrointestinal Endoscopy: *Gastrointest Endosc* 1995; 42:630.
4. Appelbe AF, Olson D, Mixon R, Craver JM, Martin RP: Libman-Sacks endocarditis mimicking intracardiac tumor. *Am J Cardiol* 1991; 68: 817.
5. Aragam JR, Keroack MA, Kemper AJ: Doppler echocardiographic diagnosis of aortopulmonary fistula following aortic valve replacement for endocarditis. *Am Heart J*, 1989; 117: 1392.
6. Arvan S, Cagin N, Levitt B, Kleid JJ: Echocardiographic findings in a patient with Candida endocarditis of the aortic valve. *Chest,* 1976; 70: 300.
7. Baltimore RS: Infective endocarditis in children, *Pediatr Infect Dis J*. 1992; 11: 907
8. Bamford J, Hodges J, Warlow C: Late rupture of a mycotic aneurysm after "cure" of bacterial endocarditis. *J Neurol* 1986; 233:51.
9. Bansal RC, Wangnes KM, and Bailey L: Right aortic sinus of Valsalva-to-right ventricle fistula complicating bacterial endocarditis of membranous ventricular septal defect: evaluation by two-dimesional colour-flow, and Doppler echocardiography. *Am Soc Echocardiogr* 1993; 6: 308.
10. Bayer AS, Bolger AF, Taubert KA, *et al*. Diagnosis and management of infective endocarditis and its complications. *Circulation* 1998; 98:2936.
11. Benn M, Hagelskjaer LH, Tvede M: Infective endocarditis, 1984 through 1993: A clinical and microbiological survey. *J Intern Med* 1997; 242:15
12. Blanchard DG, Ross RS, Dittrich HC: Non-bacterial thrombotic endocarditis. Assessment by transesophageal echocardiography. *Chest* 1992; 102:954.
13. Blumberg EA, Karalis DA, Chandrasekaran K, *et al*. Endocarditis-associated paravalvular abscesses: do clinical parameters predict the presence of abscess? *Chest* 1995; 107:898.
14. Blumberg EA, Robbins N, Adimora A, *et al*. Persistent fever in association with infective endocarditis. *Clin Infect Dis* 1992; 15:983.
15. Bouvet A: Human endocarditis due to nutritionally variant streptococci: *Streptococcus adjacens* and *Streptococcus defectivus*. *Eur Heart J* 1995; 16(suppl B):24.
16. Brust JCM, Dickinson PCT, Hughes JEO, *et al*. The diagnosis and treatment of cerebral mycotic aneurysms. *Ann Neurol* 1990; 27:238.
17. Bullock R, Van Dellen JR, Van Den Heever CM: Intracranial mycotic aneurysms: a review of 9 cases. *S Afr Med J* 1981; 60:970.
18. Calderwood SB, Swinski LA, Waternaux CM, *et al*. Risk factors for the development of prosthetic valve endocarditis. *Circulation* 1985; 72:31.
19. Camarata PJ, Latchaw RE, Rufenacht DA, *et al*. Intracranial aneurysms. *Invest Radiol* 1993; 28:373.
20. Come PC, Isaacs RE, Riley MF: Diagnostic accuracy of M-mode echocardiography in active infective endocarditis and prognostic implications of ultrasound-detectable vegetations. *Am Heart J* 1982; 103:839.
21. Conlon PJ, Jefferies F, Krigman HR, *et al*. Predictors of prognosis and risk of acute renal failure in bacterial endocarditis. *Clin Nephrol* 1998; 49:96.
22. Cunha BA, Gill MV, Lazar JM: Acute infective endocarditis: diagnostic and therapeutic approach. *Infect Dis Clin North Am* 1996; 10:811.
23. D'Agostino RS, Miller DC, Stinson EB, *et al*. Valve replacement in patients with native valve endocarditis: what really determines operative outcome? *Ann Thorac Surg* 1985; 40:429.
24. Dajani AS, Taubert KA, Wilson W, *et al*. Prevention of bacterial endocarditis: recommendations by the American Heart Association. *Circulation* 1997; 96:358.
25. Dajani AS, Taubert KA, Wilson WR, *et al*. Prevention of bacterial endocarditis: recommendations by the American Heart Association. *Circulation* 1997; 96:358.

26. Daniel WG, Mugge A, Grote J, *et al.* Comparison of transthoracic and transesophageal echocardiography for detection of abnormalities of prosthetic and bioprosthetic valves in the mitral and aortic positions. *Am J Cardiol* 1993; 71:210.

27. Daniel WG, Mugge A, Martin RP, *et al.* Improvement in the diagnosis of abscesses associated with endocarditis by transesophageal echocardiography. *N Engl J Med* 1991; 324:795.

28. Dankert J, Krijgsveld J, van Der WJ, *et al.* Platelet microbicidal activity is an important defense factor against viridans streptococcal endocarditis. *J Infect Dis* 2001; 184:597.

29. Davis RS, Strom JA, Frishman W, Becker R, Matsumoto M, Lejemtel TH, Sonnenblick EH, Frater RWM: The demonstration of vegetations by echocardiography in bacterial endocarditis. An indication for early surgical intervention. *Am J Med* 1980; 69:57.

30. Dhawan VK, Bayer AS, Yeaman MR: In vitro resistance to thrombin-induced platelet microbicidal protein is associated with enhanced progression and hematogenous dissemination in experimental *Staphylococcus aureus* infective endocarditis. *Infect Immun* 1998; 66:3476.

31. Dodds GA, Sexton DJ, Durack DT, *et al.* Negative predictive value of the Duke criteria for infective endocarditis. *Am J Cardiol* 1996; 77:403.

32. Doern GV, Ferraro MJ, Brueggmann AB, *et al.* Emergence of high rates of antimicrobial resistance among viridans group streptococci in the United States. *Antimicrob Agents Chemother* 1996; 40:891.

33. Drancourt M, Mainardi JL, Brouqui P, *et al. Bartonella (Rochalimaea) quintana* endocarditis in three homeless men. *N Engl J Med* 1996; 332:419.

34. Durack DT, Beeson PB: *Pathogenesis of infective endocarditis. Infective Endocarditis* Rahimtoola SH, Ed. Grune & Stratton, New York, 1978.

35. Durack DT, Bright DK, Lukes AS, *et al.* New criteria for diagnosis of infective endocarditis: utilization of specific echocardiographic findings. *Am J Med* 1994; 96:200.

36. Durack DT: Evaluating and optimizing outcomes of surgery for endocarditis. *JAMA* 2003; 290:3250.

37. Durack DT: Prevention of infective endocarditis. *N Engl J Med* 1995; 332:38.

38. Durack DT: Prophylaxis of infective endocarditis. Mandell, *Douglas and Bennett's Principles and Practice of Infectious Diseases,* 6th ed. Mandell GL, Bennett JE, Dolin R, Eds. Elsevier, Philadelphia, 2004.

39. Eishi K, Kawazoe K, Kuriyama Y, *et al.* Surgical management of infective endocarditis associated with cerebral complications: multicentre retrospective study in Japan. *J Thorac Cardiovasc Surg* 1995; 110:1745.

40. Eliopoulos GM: Aminoglycoside resistant enterococcal endocarditis. *Infect Dis Clin North Am* 1993; 7:117.

41. Ellis ME, Al-Abdely H, Sandridge A, *et al.* Fungal endocarditis: evidence in the world literature, 1965–1995. *Clin Infect Dis* 2001; 32:50.

42. Fang G, Keys TF, Gentry LO, *et al.* Prosthetic valve endocarditis resulting from nosocomial bacteremia: a prospective, multicenter study. *Ann Intern Med* 1993; 119:560.

43. Fernandez-Guerrero ML, Verdejo C, Azofra J, *et al.* Hospital-acquired infectious endocarditis not associated with cardiac surgery: an emerging problem. *Clin Infect Dis* 1995; 20:16.

44. Fournier PE, Casalta JP, Habib G, *et al.* Modification of the diagnostic criteria proposed by the Duke Endocarditis Service to permit improved diagnosis of Q fever endocarditis. *Am J Med* 1996; 100:629.

45. Gagliardi JP, Nettles RE, McCarty DE, *et al.* Native valve infective endocarditis in elderly and younger adult patients: comparison of clinical features and outcomes with use of the Duke criteria and the Duke Endocarditis Database. *Clin Infect Dis* 1998; 26:1165.

46. Goldenberger D, Kunzli A, Vogt P, *et al.* Molecular diagnosis of bacterial endocarditis by broad-range PCR amplification and direct sequencing. *J Clin Microbiol* 1997; 35:2733.

47. Gomes JA, Calderon J, Lajam F, *et al.* Echocardiographic detection of fungal vegetations in *Candida parasilopsis* endocarditis. *Am J Med* 1976; 61: 273.

48. Gordon SM, Serkey JM, Longworth DL, *et al.* Early onset prosthetic valve endocarditis: the Cleveland Clinic experience 1992–1997. *Ann Thorac Surg* 2000; 69:1388.

49. Gouello JP, Asfar P, Brenet O, *et al.* Nosocomial endocarditis in the intensive care unit: an analysis of 22 cases. *Crit Care Med* 2000; 28:377

50. Grover FL, Cohen DJ, Oprian C, *et al.* Determinants of the occurrence of and survival from prosthetic valve endocarditis: experience of the Veterans Affairs Cooperative Study on Valvular Heart Disease. *J Thorac Cardiovasc Surg* 1994; 108:207.

51. Hamed KA, Dormitzer PR, Su CK, *et al. Haemophilus parainfluenzae* endocarditis: application of a molecular approach for identification of pathogenic bacterial species. *Clin Infect Dis* 1994; 19:677.

52. Hasbun R, Vikram HR, Barakat LA, *et al.* Complicated left-sided native valve endocarditis in adults: risk classification for mortality. *JAMA* 2003; 289:1933.

53. Heiro M: Extensive analysis of the utility of serum C-reactive protein, erythrocyte sedimentation rate and white blood cell count in assessing the outcome of infective endocarditis. (Personal communication, 2004).

54. Hickey AJ, Wolfers J, Wilcken DEL: Reliability and clinical relevance of detection of vegetations by echocardiography in bacterial endocarditis. *Br Heart J* 1981; 46:624.

55. Hoen B, Alla F, Beguinot I, *et al.* Changing profile of infective endocarditis: results of a one-year survey in France in 1999. *JAMA* 2002; 288:75.

56. Hoen B, Beguinot I, Rabaud C, *et al.* The Duke criteria for diagnosing infective endocarditis are specific: analysis of 100 patients with acute fever or fever of unknown origin. *Clin Infect Dis* 1996; 23:298.

57. Hoen B, Selton-Suty C, Danchin N, *et al.* Evaluation of the Duke criteria versus the Beth Israel criteria for the diagnosis of infective endocarditis. *Clin Infect Dis* 1995; 21:905.

58. Hoen B, Selton-Suty C, Lacassin F, *et al.* Infective endocarditis in patients with negative blood cultures: analysis of 88 cases from a one-year nationwide survey in France. *Clin Infect Dis* 1995; 20:501

59. Houpikian P, Raoult D: Diagnostic methods: current best practices and guidelines for identification of difficult-to-

culture pathogens in infective endocarditis. *Cardiol Clin* 2003; 21:207.

60. Huston J, Nichols DA, Luetmer PH, *et al.* Blinded prospective evaluation of sensitivity of MR angiography to known intracranial aneurysms: importance of aneurysm size. *AJNR Am J Neuroradiol* 1994; 15:1607.

61. Infective endocarditis caused by beta-hemolytic streptococci. The Infectious Diseases Society of America's Emerging Infections Network: *Clin Infect Dis* 1998; 26:66.

62. Jaffe WM, Morgan DE, Pearlman AS, Otto CM: Infective endocarditis, 1983-1988: Echocardiographic findings and factors influencing morbidity and mortality. *J Am Coll Cardiol* 1990; 15:1227.

63. Jault F, Gandjbakhch I, Chastre JC, *et al.* Prosthetic valve endocarditis with ring abscesses: surgical management and long-term results. *J Thorac Cardiovasc Surg* 105:1106, 1993 96.

64. John MD, Hibberd PL, Karchmer AW, *et al.* Staphylococcus aureus prosthetic valve endocarditis: optimal management and risk factors for death. *Clin Infect Dis* 1998; 26:1302.

65. Karalis DG, Bansal RC, Hauck AJ, *et al.* Transesophageal echocardiographic recognition of subaortic complications in aortic valve endocarditis: clinical and surgical implications. *Circulation* 1992; 86:353.

66. Karchmer AW, Gibbons DW: Infections of prosthetic heart valves and vascular grafts. *Infections Associated with Indwelling Medical Devices*. Bisno AL, Waldvogel FA, Eds. American Society for Microbiology, Washington DC, 1994.

67. Karchmer AW: Infective endocarditis. *Heart Disease: A Textbook of Cardiovascular Medicine* Braunwald E, Ed. WB Saunders Co, Philadelphia, 1996.

68. Kavey RE, Frank DM, Byrum CJ, Blackman MS, Sandheimer HM, Bove EL: Two-dimensional echocardiographic assessment of infective endocarditis in children. *Am J Dis Child* 1983; 137: 851.

69. Kazanjian PH: Infective endocarditis: review of 60 cases treated in community hospitals. *Infect Dis Clin Pract* 1993; 2:41.

70. Kronzon I, Winer HE, Cohen ML: Sterile, caseous mitral annular abscess. *J Am Coll Cardiol* 1983; 2:186.

71. Lancellotti P, Galiuto L, Albert A, *et al.* Relative value of clinical and transesophageal echocardiographic variables for risk stratification in patients with infective endocarditis. *Clin Cardiol* 1998; 21:572

72. Larbalestier RI, Kinchla NM, Aranki SF, *et al.* Acute bacterial endocarditis: optimizing surgical results. *Circulation* 1992; 86(5 suppl):II68.

73. Lederman MM, Sprague L, Wallis RS, *et al.* Duration of fever during treatment of infective endocarditis. *Medicine* (Baltimore) 1992; 71:52.

74. Lee KS, Topol EJ, Stewart WJ: Atypical presentation of papillary fibroelastoma mimicking multiple vegetations in suspected subacute bacterial endocarditis. *Am Heart J* 1993; 125: 1443.

75. Levine DP, Fromm BS, Reddy BR: Slow response to vancomycin or vancomycin plus rifampin in methicillin-resistant *Staphylococcus aureus* endocarditis. *Ann Intern Med* 1991; 115:674.

76. Li JS, Sexton DJ, Mick N, *et al.* Proposed modifications to the Duke criteria for the diagnosis of infective endocarditis. *Clin Infect Dis* 2000; 30:633.

77. Lisby G, Gutschik E, Durack DT: Molecular methods for diagnosis of infective endocarditis. *Infect Dis Clin North Am* 2002; 16:393.

78. Lukes AS, Bright DK, Durack DT: Diagnosis of infective endocarditis, Infect Dis. *Clin North Am.* 7: 1, 1993.

79. Mansur AJ, Grinberg M, da Luz PL, *et al.* The complications of infective endocarditis: a reappraisal in the 1980s. *Arch Intern Med* 1992; 152:2428.

80. Mansur AJ, Grinberg M, Leao PP, *et al.* Extracranial mycotic aneurysms in infective endocarditis. *Clin Cardiol* 1986; 9:65.

81. Martin RP, Meltzer RS, Chia BL, Stinson EB, Rakowski H, Popp RL: Clinical utility of two-dimensional echocardiography in infective endocarditis. *Am J Cardiol* 1980; 46: 379.

82. Martinez E, Miro JM, Almirante B, *et al.* Effect of penicillin resistance of *Streptococcus pneumoniae* on the presentation, prognosis, and treatment of pneumococcal endocarditis in adults. *Clin Infect Dis* 2002; 35:130.

83. Meine TJ, Nettles RE, Anderson DJ, *et al.* Cardiac conduction abnormalities in endocarditis defined by the Duke criteria. *Am Heart J* 2001;142:280.

84. Melgar GR, Nasser RM, Gordon SM, *et al.* Fungal prosthetic valve endocarditis in 16 patients: an 11-year experience in a tertiary care hospital. Medicine (Baltimore) 1997; 76:94.

85. Millaire A, Leroy O, Gaday V, *et al.* Incidence and prognosis of embolic events and metastatic infections in infective endocarditis. *Eur Heart J* 1997; 18:677.

86. Miro JM, del Rio A, Mestres CA: Infective endocarditis and cardiac surgery in intravenous drug abusers and HIV-1 infected patients. *Cardiol Clin* 2003; 21:167

87. Moreillon P, Entenza JM, Francioli P, *et al.* Role of *Staphylococcus aureus* coagulase and clumping factor in pathogenesis of experimental endocarditis. *Infect Immun* 1995; 63:4738.

88. Moreillon P, Que YA, Bayer AS: Pathogenesis of streptococcal and staphylococcal endocarditis. *Infect Dis Clin North Am* 2002; 16:297.

89. Morris AJ, Drinkovic D, Pottumarthy S, *et al.* Gram stain, culture, and histopathological examination findings for heart valves removed because of infective endocarditis. *Clin Infect Dis* 2003; 36:697.

90. Morris CD, Reller MD, Menashe VD: Thirty-year incidence of infective endocarditis after surgery for congenital heart defect. *JAMA* 1998; 279:599.

91. Moskowitz MA, Rosenbaum AE, Tyler HR: Angiographically monitored resolution of cerebral mycotic aneurysms. *Neurology* 1974; 24:1103.

92. Mugge A, Daniel WG, Frank G, *et al.* Echocardiography in infective endocarditis: reassessment of prognostic implications of vegetation size determined by the transthoracic and transesophageal approach. *J Am Coll Cardiol* 1989; 14:631.

93. Mugge A, Daniel WG, Frank G, Lichtlen PR: Echocardiography in infective endocarditis: Reassessment of prognostic implications of vegetation size determined by the transthoracic and the transesophageal approach. *J Am Coll Cardiol* 1989; 14:631.

94. Nettles RE, McCarty DE, Corey GR, *et al.* An evaluation of the Duke criteria in 25 pathologically confirmed cases of prosthetic valve endocarditis. *Clin Infect Dis* 1997; 25:1401.

95. Olaison L, Pettersson G: Current best practices and guidelines: indications for surgical intervention in infective endocarditis. *Cardiol Clin* 2003; 21:235.

96. Perivalvular abscesses associated with endocarditis: clinical features and prognostic factors of overall survival in a series of 233 cases. Perivalvular Abscesses French Multicentre Study: *Eur Heart J* 1999; 20:232.

97. Pierrotti LC, Baddour LM: Fungal endocarditis, 1995–2000. *Chest* 2002; 122:302.

98. Piper C, Korfer R, Horstkotte D: Prosthetic valve endocarditis. *Heart* 2001; 85:590.

99. Piper C, Wiemer M, Schulte HD, *et al.* Stroke is not a contraindication for urgent valve replacement in acute infective endocarditis. *J Heart Valve Dis* 2001; 10:703.

100. Que YA, Francois P, Haefliger JA, *et al.* Reassessing the role of *Staphylococcus aureus* clumping factor and fibronectin-binding protein by expression in *Lactococcus lactis*. *Infect Immun* 2001; 69:6296.

101. Raoult D, Fournier PE, Drancourt M, *et al.* Diagnosis of 22 new cases of *Bartonella* endocarditis. *Ann Intern Med* 125:646, 1996.

102. Rice LB, Calderwood SB, Eliopoulos GM, *et al.* Enterococcal endocarditis: a comparison of prosthetic and native valve disease. *Rev Infect Dis* 1991; 13:1.

103. Roe MT, Abramson MA, Li J, *et al.* Clinical information determines the impact of transesophageal echocardiography on the diagnosis of infective endocarditis by the Duke criteria. *Am Heart J* 2000; 139:945.

104. Rohmann S, Erbel R, Gorge G, *et al.* Clinical relevance of vegetation localization by transoesophageal echocardiography in infective endocarditis. *Eur Heart J* 1992; 12:446.

105. Rosoff MH, Cohen MV, Jacquette G: Pulmonary valve gonococcal endocarditis. A forgotten disease. *Br Heart J* 1983; 50: 290.

106. Ruoff KL, Miller SI, Garner CV, *et al.* Bacteremia with *Streptococcus bovis* and *Streptococcus salivarius:* clinical correlates of more accurate identification of isolates. *J Clin Microbiol* 1989; 27:305.

107. Sachdev M, Peterson GE, Jollis JG: Imaging techniques for diagnosis of infective endocarditis. *Cardiol Clin* 2003; 21:185.

108. Sande MA, Lee BL, Mills J, *et al. Endocarditis in intravenous drug users. Infective Endocarditis.* Kaye D, Ed. Raven Press, New York, 1992.

109. Sandre RM, Shafran SD: Infective endocarditis: Review of 135 cases over 9 years. *Clin Infect Dis* 1996; 22:276.

110. Sanfilippo AJ, Picard MH, Newell JB, *et al.* Echocardiographic assessment of patients with infectious endocarditis: prediction of risk for complications. *J Am Coll Cardiol* 1991; 18:1191.

111. Sekeres MA, Abrutyn E, Berlin JA, *et al.* An assessment of the usefulness of the Duke criteria for diagnosing active infective endocarditis. *Clin Infect Dis* 1997; 24:1185.

112. Sett SS, Hudson MP, Jamieson WR, *et al.* Prosthetic valve endocarditis: experience with porcine. *J Thorac Cardiovasc Surg* 1993; 105:428.

113. Shapiro DS, Kenney SC, Johnson M, *et al.* Brief report: *Chlamydia psittaci* endocarditis diagnosed by blood culture. *N Engl J Med* 1992; 326:1192.

114. Shapiro SM, Young E, De Guzman S, *et al.* Transesophageal echocardiography in diagnosis of infective endocarditis. *Chest* 1994; 105:377.

115. Sharma R, Prakash R, Kaushik VS, Oparah SS, Mandal, A.: Reliability of two-dimensional echocardiography in diagnosing fungal endocarditis. *Clin Cardiol* 1983; 6:37.

116. Shively BK, Gurule FT, Roldan CA, *et al.* Diagnostic value of transesophageal compared with transthoracic echocardiography in infective endocarditis. *J Am Coll Cardiol* 1991; 18:391.

117. Simmons NA: Recommendations for endocarditis prophylaxis. *J Antimicrob Chemother* 1993; 31:437.

118. Sochowski RA, Chan KL: Implication of negative results on a monoplane transesophageal echocardiographic study in patients with suspected infective endocarditis. *J Am Coll Cardiol* 1993; 21:216.

119. Spach DH, Koehler JE: *Bartonella*-associated infections. *Infect Dis Clin North Am* 1998; 12:137

120. Steckelberg JM, Murphy JG, Ballard D, *et al.* Emboli in infective endocarditis: the prognostic value of echocardiography. *Ann Intern Med* 2001; 114:635.

121. Stein A, Raoult D: Q fever endocarditis. *Eur Heart J* 16(suppl B):1995; 19.

122. Strom BL, Abrutyn E, Berlin JA, *et al.* Dental and cardiac risk factors for infective endocarditis: a population-based case-control study. *Ann Intern Med* 1998; 129:761.

123. Thompson KR, Nanda NC, Gramiak R: The reliability of echocardiography in the diagnosis of infective endocarditis. *Radiology*, 1977; 125: 373.

124. Tornos P, Sanz E, Permanyer-Miralda G, *et al.* Late prosthetic valve endocarditis: immediate and long-term prognosis. *Chest* 1992; 1:37.

125. Torres-Tortosa M, de Cueto M, Vergara A, *et al.* Prospective evaluation of a two-week course of intravenous antibiotics in intravenous drug addicts with infective endocarditis. Grupo de Estudio de Enfermedades Infecciosas de la Provincia de Cadiz. *Eur J Clin Microbiol Infect Dis* 1994; 13:559.

126. Towns ML, Reller LB: Diagnostic methods: current best practices and guidelines for isolation of bacteria and fungi in infective endocarditis. *Cardiol Clin* 2003; 21:197.

127. Tunick PA, Lefkow P, Kronzon I.: Aorta to right atrium fistula caused by endocarditis: Diagnosis by colour Doppler echocardiography. *J Am Soc Echocardiogr* 1989; 2:53.

128. Tunkel AR, Kaye D: Endocarditis with negative blood cultures. *N Engl J Med* 1992; 326:1215.

129. Veltrop MH, Langermans JA, Thompson J, *et al.* Interleukin-10 regulates the tissue factor activity of monocytes in an in vitro model of bacterial endocarditis. *Infect Immuno* 2001; 69:3197.

130. Vered Z, Mossinson D, Peleg E, *et al.* Echocardiographic assessment of prosthetic valve endocarditis. *Eur Heart J* 1995; 16(suppl B):63.

131. Verhagen DW, van der Feltz M, Plokker HW, *et al.* Optimisation of the antibiotic guidelines in the Netherlands. VII. SWAB guidelines for antimicrobial therapy in adult

patients with infectious endocarditis. *Neth J Med* 2003; 61:421.

132. Vlessis AA, Hovaguimian H, Jaggers J, *et al.* Infective endocarditis: ten year review of medical and surgical therapy. *Ann Thorac Surg* 1996; 61:1217.

133. Vlessis AA, Khaki A, Grunkemeier GL, *et al.* Risk, diagnosis and management of prosthetic valve endocarditis: a review. *J Heart Valve Dis* 1997; 6:443.

134. Watanakunakorn C: Increasing importance of intravascular device-associated *Staphylococcus aureus* endocarditis. *Clin Infect Dis* 1999; 28:115.

135. Weyman AE, Rankin R, King H.: Loeffler's endocarditis presenting as mitral and tricuspid stenosis. *Am J Cardiol* 1977; 40:438.

136. Wilson WR, Geraci JE, Danielson GK, *et al.* Anticoagulant therapy and central nervous system complications in patients with prosthetic valve endocarditis. *Circulation* 1978; 57:1004.

137. Wilson WR, Karchmer AW, Dajani AS, *et al.* Antibiotic treatment of adults with infective endocarditis due to viridans streptococci, enterococci, staphylococci and HACEK microorganisms. *JAMA* 274:1706, 1995.

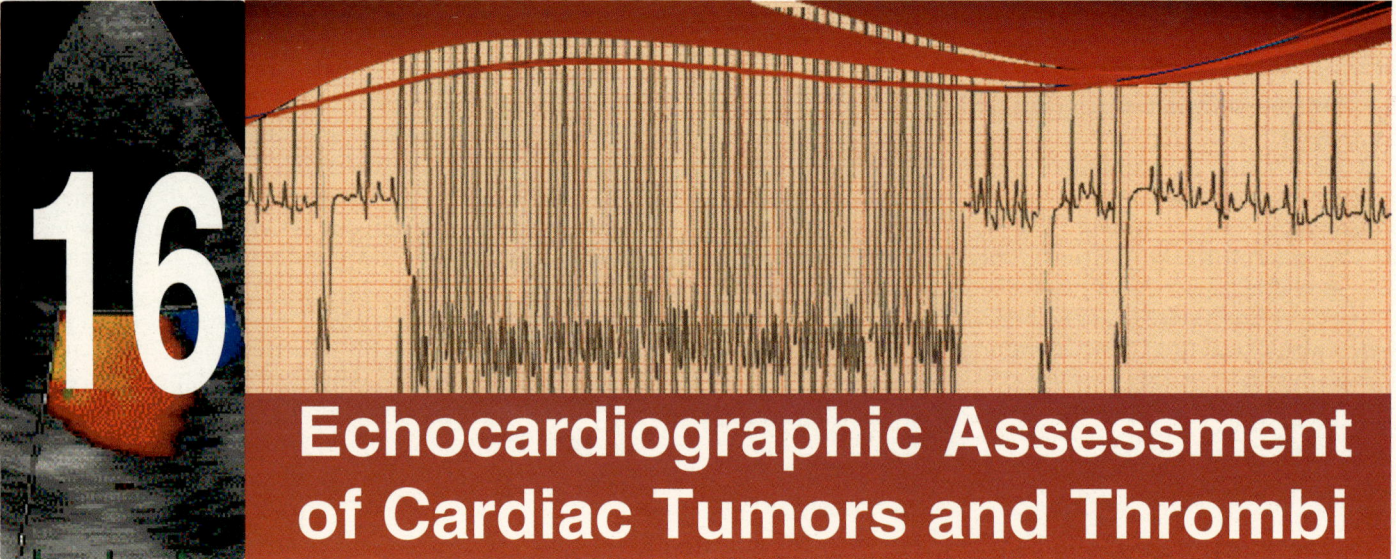

16

Echocardiographic Assessment of Cardiac Tumors and Thrombi

Tumor masses originating from the cardiac structure may be categorized as benign or malignant. They are either from a primary source or metastatic in origin. Metastatic type of cardiac tumors are generally common than the primary neoplastic tissue of the heart.

Primary Tumor

Lungs or the breast tissue is often seen as the cause of primary tumor thereby indicating that the tumor is likely to spread locally to involve the heart or pericardium. Metastases seldom affect left ventricular function, although large collections of pericardial fluid may show manifestations of cardiac temponade.

The commonly encountered primary malignant tumors involving the heart are sarcomas of various types. These account for 20% of primary cardiac tumors. The tumor usually grows in the right atrium, and leads high mortality from extension through the wall of the heart into the pericardium rather than from herniation into the chambers just like an atrial myxoma.

Clinically sarcoma tumor manifests as a malignant pericardial disease leading to retrosternal pain, tachycardia, pulsus paradoxicus and raised jugular venous pressure, due to cardiac temponade or cardiac rupture. Other primary cardiac tumors include rhabdomyoma, fibroma, lipoma, teratoma, and angioma (Figs 16.7 and 16.8).

Myxoma (Figs 16.1–16.6 and 16.12)

It is considered as the most common benign tumor of the heart and comprises about 50% of all benign tumor affecting the cardiac structure. The myxoma is a polypoid mass of gelatinous tissue usually found in the left atrial cavity, although it has been reported in all the four cardiac chambers. The tumor is usually pedunculated and attached to the area of the fossa ovalis, atrial appendage, or origin of a pulmonary vein. Patients with this tumor have a high risk of embolization to the peripheral system because the tumor is generally of such a size that it is very mobile within the cardiac chamber.

Table 16.1: *Indications of echocardiography in cardiac masses and tumors*

Indications	Class
1. Evaluation of patients with clinical syndromes and events suggesting an underlying cardiac mass.	I
2. Evaluation of patients with underlying cardiac disease known to predispose to mass formation for whom a therapeutic decision regarding surgery or anticoagulation will depend on the results of echocardiography.	I
3. Follow-up or surveillance studies after surgical removal of masses known to have a high likelihood of recurrence (i.e. myxoma).	I
4. Patients with known primary malignancies when echocardiographic surveillance for cardiac involvement is part of the disease staging process.	I
5. Screening persons with disease states likely to result in mass formation but for whom no clinical evidence for the mass exists.	IIb
6. Patients for whom the results of echocardiography will have no impact on diagnosis or clinical decision making.	III

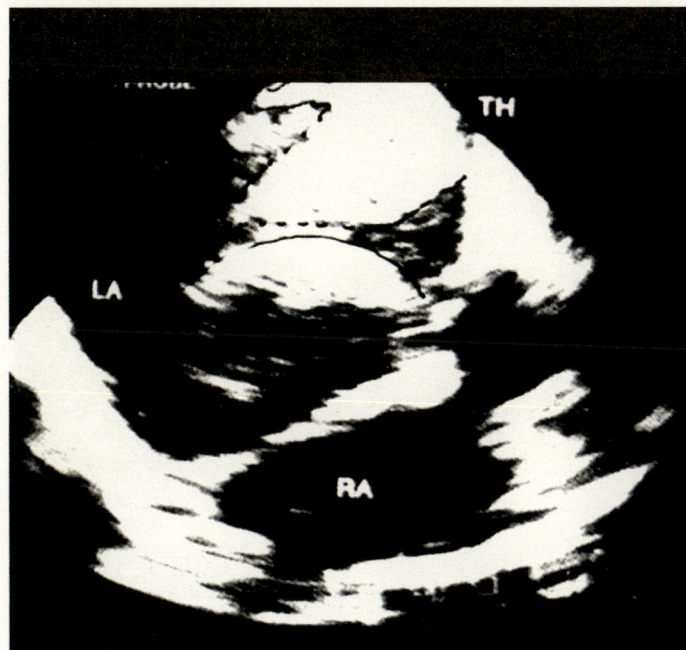

Fig. 16.1: TEE echocardiographic scan in biatrial plane showing a big tumor mass (T) in left atrium (LA)

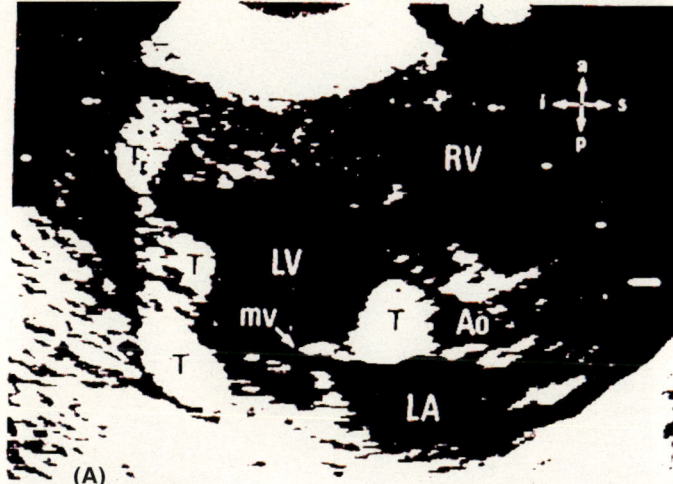

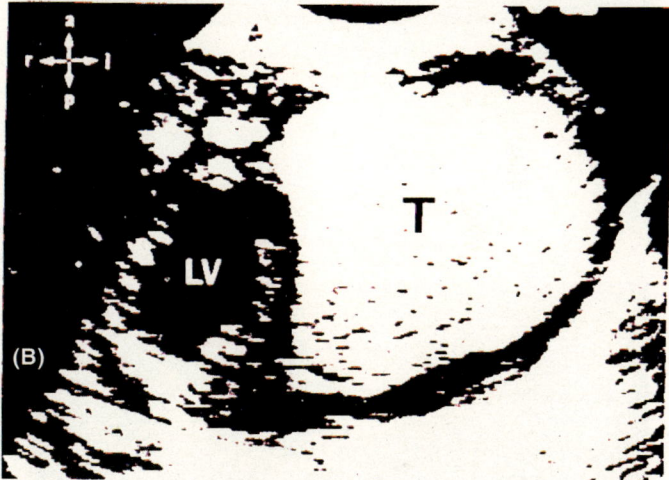

Fig. 16.3: Long axis (A) and short axis (B) echocardiographic views in a newborn with multiple myocardial tumors (T) who clinically had recurrent episodes of ventricular tachycardia

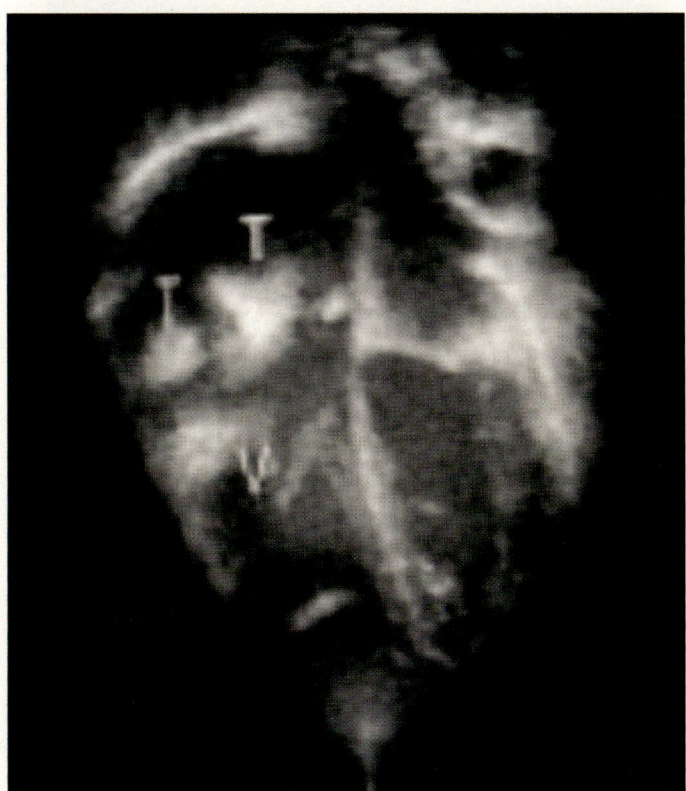

Fig. 16.2: Apical 4C view reverse plane showing multiple tumor massess (T) in right atrium in patient with beta-thalassaemia. Histologically, these masses were found to be calcified thrombus with no signs of iron deposition. This case was concluded to be a dystrophic calcification of multiple atrial thrombi caused by long-term insertion of a Hickman line

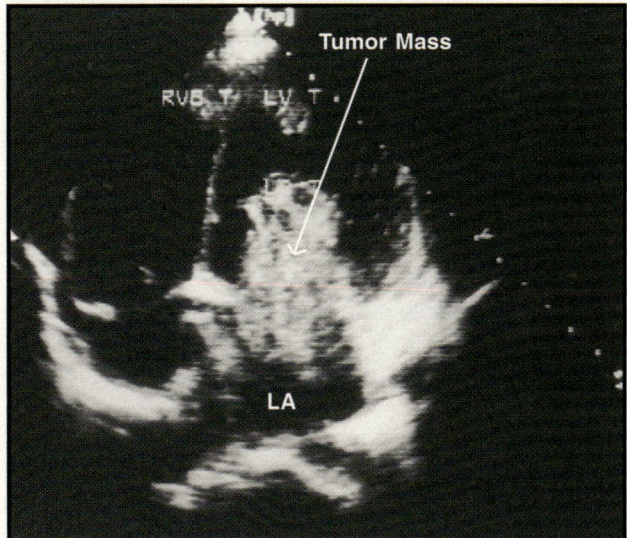

Fig. 16.4: Apical four chamber view showing tumor mass in left ventricle (LV) protruding into LA cavity through mitral valve orifice

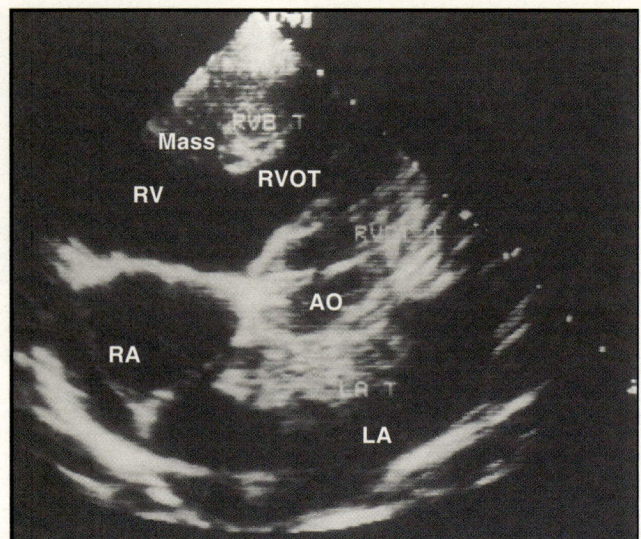

Fig. 16.5: Short axis view at aorta and right ventricle (RV) showing tumor mass in right ventricular cavity (arrow)

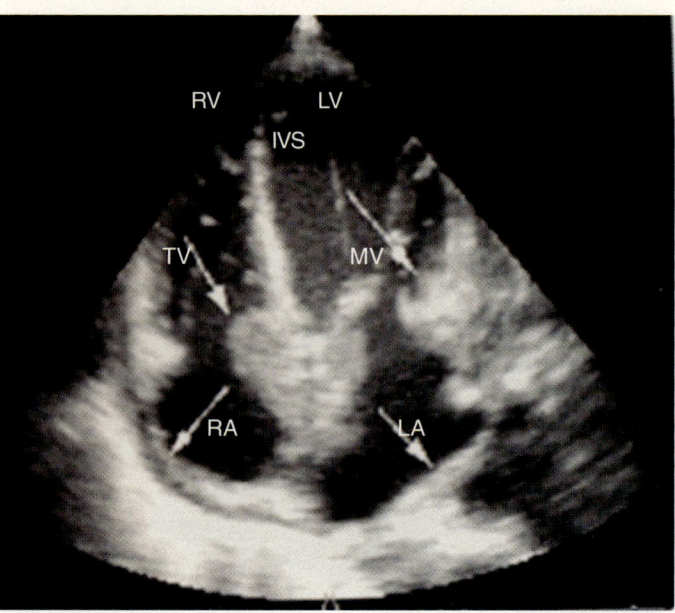

Fig. 16.7: Apical 4C view showing larger tumor mass eroding both atria (arrows) in patient with large beta B cell lymphoma

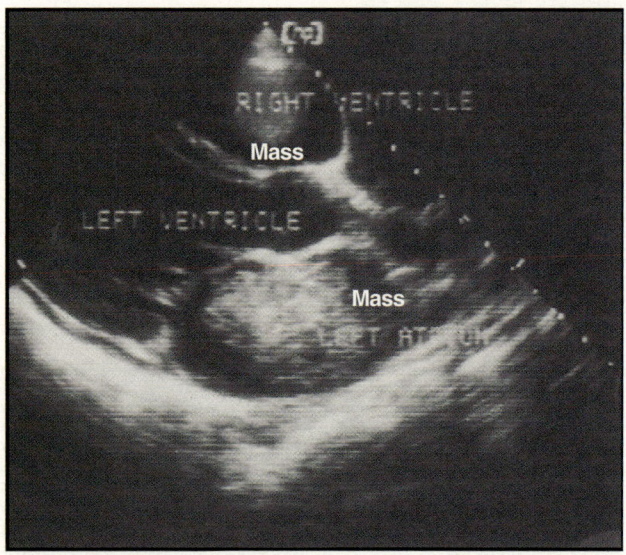

Fig. 16.6: Long axis view showing a big tumor mass in left atrium (LA) and body of right ventricle (RV)

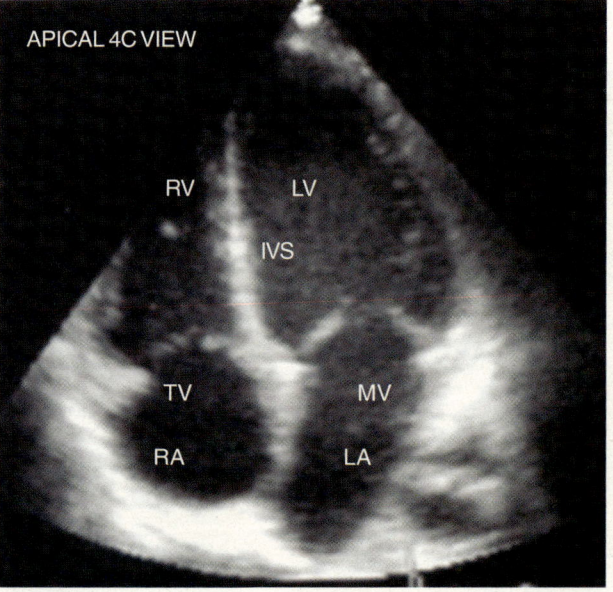

Fig. 16.8: Apical 4C view after 2 weeks of chemotherapy, there is complete remission and no complications noted in her follow up period

If the myxoma is not completely removed surgically, it may recur in the same area. Death may result if fragments of the tumor break off to become systemic or pulmonary emboli.

The main signs and symptoms of myoxma are as a result of obstruction created by a tumor mass while prolapsing into mitral or tricuspid valves, systemic embolism with possible tumor fragments, chest pain, syncope, and constitutional disturbances (i.e. weakness, fatigue, weight loss). One can also hear the changing cardiac murmur in cases of cardiac myxoma and the tumor plop may be confused with the diastolic rumble of mitral stenosis.

Since the tumor is often pedunculated and mobile, the degree of obstruction to bloodflow varies with posture and with hemodynamic events. In such cases one may also encounter changing diastolic murmur in one particular body position, while absent in another one.

Table 16.2: *Some lesions which may mimick like tumour/mass thrombus/clot*

Left atrium	*Right atrium*	*Left ventricle*	*Aorta*	*Right ventricle*
Suture line following transplant	Chiari network	False chords	Brachiocephalic vein	Moderator band
Fossa ovalis Calcified mitral annulus	Eustachian valve Crista terminalis	Papillary muscles	Innominate vein	Muscle bundle/ trabeculations
Coronary sinus	Catheters/pacemaker leads	LV trabeculations	Pleural effusion	Catheters and pacemaker leads
Ridge between LUPV and LAA	Lipomatous hypertrophy of interatrial septum pectinate muscles			
Lipomatous hypertrophy of interatrial septum pectinate muscles Transverse sinus	Fatty materials surrounding the TV annulus			

LAA = Left atrial appendage; LUPV = Left upper pulmonary vein; LV = Left ventricle

Table 16.3: *The patients in whom echocardiography is needed before cardioversion*

	Indications	*Class*
1.	Patients requiring urgent (not emergent) cardioversion for whom extended precardioversion anticoagulation is not desirable.	I
2.	Patients who have had prior cardioembolic events thought to be related to intraatrial thrombus.	I
3.	Patients for whom anticoagulation is contraindicated and for whom a decision about cardioversion will be influenced by TEE results.	I
4.	Patients for whom intraatrial thrombus has been demonstrated in previous TEE.	I
5.	Evaluation of patient for whom a decision concerning cardioversion will be impacted by knowledge of prognostic factors (such as LV function, coexistent mitral valve disease, etc.).	I
6.	Patients with atrial fibrillation of <48 hours duration and other heart disease.	IIa
7.	Patients with atrial fibrillation of <48 hours duration and no other heart disease.	IIb
8.	Patients with mitral valve disease or hypertrophic cardiomyopathy who have been on long-term anticoagulation at therapeutic levels before cardioversion unless there are other reasons for anticoagulation (e.g. prior embolus or known thrombus on previous TEE).	IIb
9.	Patients undergoing cardioversion from atrial flutter.	IIb
10.	Patients requiring emergent cardioversion.	III
11.	Patients who have been on long-term anticoagulation at therapeutic levels and who do not have mitral valve disease or hypertrophic cardiomyopathy before cardioversion unless there are other reasons for anticoagulation (e.g. prior embolus or known thrombus on previous TEE)	III
12.	Precardioversion evaluation of patients who have undergone previous TEE and with no clinical suspicion of a significant interval change.	III

Echocardiographic Evaluation of a Cardiac Mass
(Figs 16.3–7, 16.11, 16.12, 16.15, 16.19, 16.20, and 16.22)

Two-dimensional echocardiography is the best means of diagnosis and has its proven value to be effective in detecting, characterizing, and locating masses in any of the four cardiac chambers. These tumor masses can be visualized by 2-D imaging from various planes and views such as parasternal, long-and short-axis, apical four-chamber, and subxiphoid views. The cardiac sonographer must be able to differentiate true lesions from artifacts produced by the instrumentation ("side lobes" by off-axis beam direction) or from incorrect gain settings. Real mass lesions remain in the same anatomic position when imaged from different transducer positions, whereas artifacts disappear.

Both inferior and superior vena cava and right atrial cavity may be carefully evaluated for the presence of extension from a primary tumor elsewhere in the body, especially from the kidney. The best view to visualise the inferior vena cava is a long-axis or "sagittal" abdominal view. The patient should be instructed to hold his or her breath for a short period, since this forces the Valsalva maneuver, which helps to dilate inferior vena cava. Careful sweeping of the transducer in a medial to lateral direction allows a maximal visual-isation of the inferior vena cava to look for low-level echo formation, which reflected from the invading tumor. The superior vena cava is best evaluated with the suprasternal or deep subxiphoid approach (Figs 16.21, 16.25, 16.26, 16.27 and 16.28A and B).

Thrombi

A thrombosis is the formation of a blood clot in the blood vessels or in any of the cardiac chambers. After the thrombus forms, part or all of it may break loose to create an embolus that travels downstream to lodge at peripheral site. The potential danger of a thrombosis or embolism is the ischemic necrosis of these lodging sites causing crippling infarction or gangrene. Mural thrombi can occur either in the cavity of the heart or aorta and attach to one of the walls, usually in the area of infarction. Other sites for mural thrombi are the atrial appendages and left ventricular walls juxtaposed to myocardial infarcts. In the aorta, they usually are found attached to previously damaged areas as a result of atherosclerotic invasion of the aortic wall (Figs 16.9, 16.10, 13A–C, 16.23 and 16.24).

Emboli

An embolism is the occlusion of some part of the cardiovascular system by the impaction of a foreign mass transported through the bloodstream. Throm-bo-embolism is the term used for an embolus that is part or a whole thrombus that has become dislodged and carried downstream to occlude a smaller vessel (Fig. 16.10).

Evaluation of Thrombi by Echocardiography
(Figs16.23 and 16.28)

Apical and subxiphoid four chamber approaches are the best ways of diagnosing thrombi located in either of atrium or ventricular cavities as a result either myocardial infarction or calcified rheumatic valvular heart disease.

Ventricular thrombi are usually visualised at the cardiac apex, therefore this region must be carefully assessed for abnormal masses and separated from large papillary muscles or artifactual masses resulting from side lobes. It is more difficult to detect all left atrial thrombi; possibly the pressure to which the left atrial thrombi are subjected causes the organizing ventricular thrombi to be firmer and better reflective targets than the left atrial thrombi, which are not subjected to the same type of pressure.

According to study by Martin, *et al.* five points must be taken into consideration while searching for left ventricular thrombi:

1. Left ventricular thrombi are often closely adherent to the endocardial surfaces of the ventricle but have a margin or site of origin distinct from the surrounding endocardial echoes.
2. Whereas the myocardium often appear as a dark structure with bright endocardial surfaces. Left ventricular thrombi frequently have a granular appearance quite different from that of the surrounding myocardium.
3. The site of the mass lesion is often near the cardiac apex, so the apical and subxiphoid transducer positions are best for detecting ventricular thrombi.
4. Mural thrombi appear to have a motion synchronous with that of the adjacent ventricular walls.
5. Left ventricular thrombi can arise on a short stalk (adjacent to the akinetic-dyskinetic area) or appear as a large, firmly adherent mass of echoes.

Thus echo may prove to be a valuable procedure in the detection of intracardiac masses and thrombi. Care must be taken to separate artifacts produced by sidelobes or large papillary muscles from the real intracardiac mass echoes. Investigation into tissue characterization of echoes within the cardiac chambers is currently being performed in several laboratories, with the objective of making echocardiography an even more specific and sensitive technique.

Echinococcosis (Hydatid Cyst Disease) (Fig. 16.29)

This is a well-known disease affecting pericardium, myocardium and ventricular lumen. It is caused by the

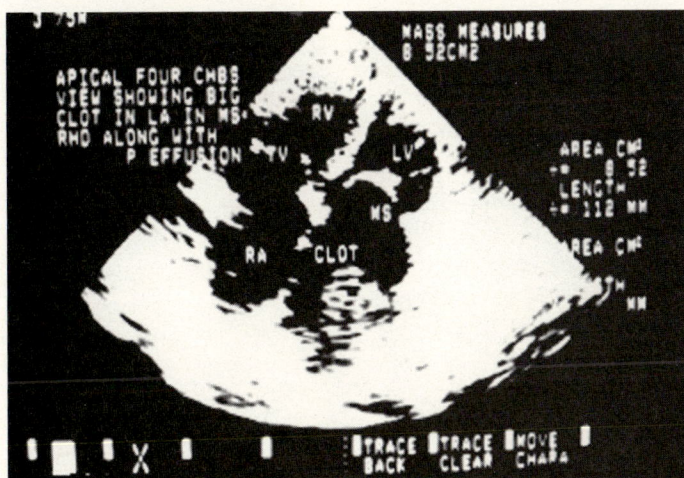

Fig. 16.9: Apical 4C view showing a big clot attached to the left atrial wall in patient with rheumatic heart disease with mitral stenosis. MS = mitral stenosis, LA = left atrium, RV = right ventricle

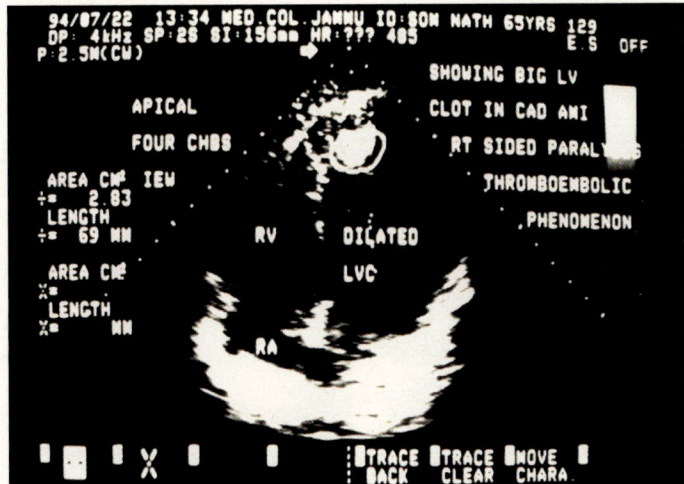

Fig. 16.10: Apical 4C view showing dense thrombosis in apical position in patient with coronary artery disease and right sided hemiparesis due to thromboembolic phenomenon

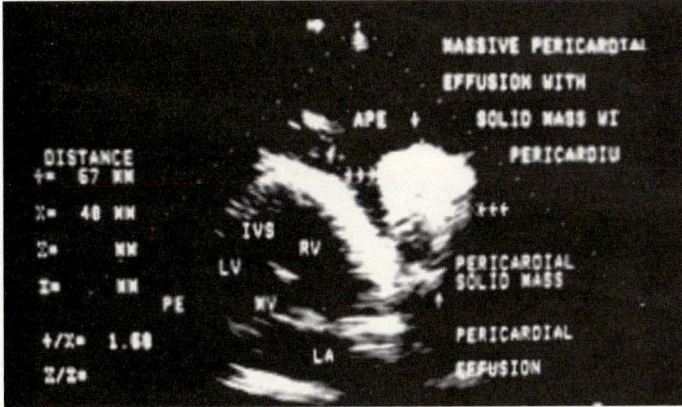

Fig. 16.11: Oblique 4C view. Transthoracic echocardiography showing a large pericardial mass (arrows) in patient with breathlessness on exertion and signs of cardiac decompensation

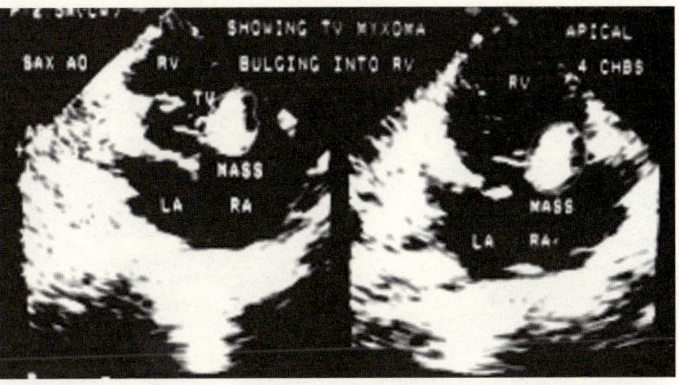

Fig. 16.12: Apical 4C view showing solid mass attached to the tricuspid valve in patient with dyspnoea on exertion, chest pain and intermittent prolonged pyrexia and poor weight gain

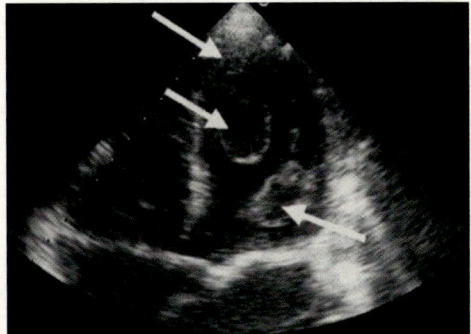

A. Apical 4C LV view

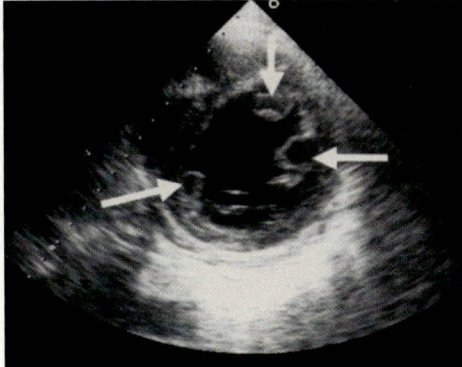

B. Short axis LV view

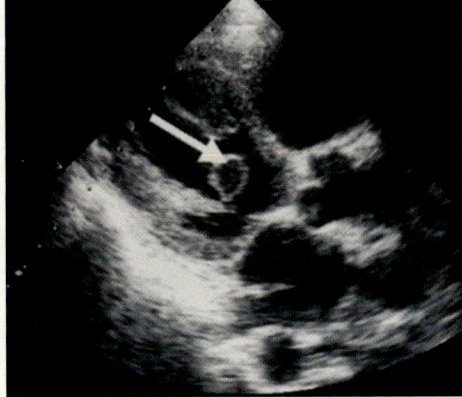

C. Long axis LV view

Fig. 16.13A to C: Transthoracic echocardiogram showing multiple blood cysts (arrows) which were well circumscribed and thin wall in patient with dyspnoea on exertion and cardiac decompensation

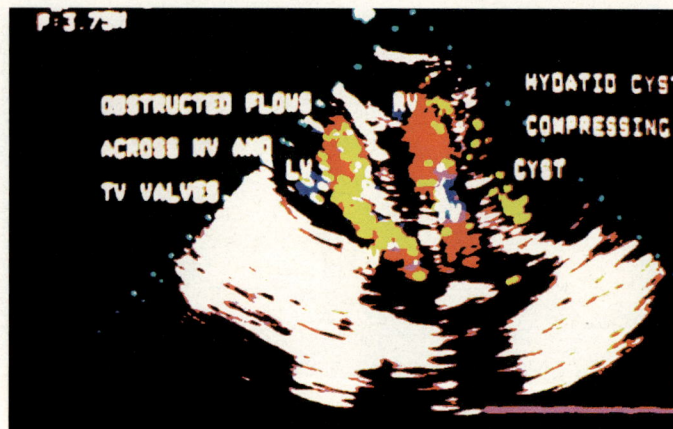

Fig. 16.14: Apical 4C view showing obstructive flow pattern through tricuspid valve (TV) and MV due to compression of hydatid cyst

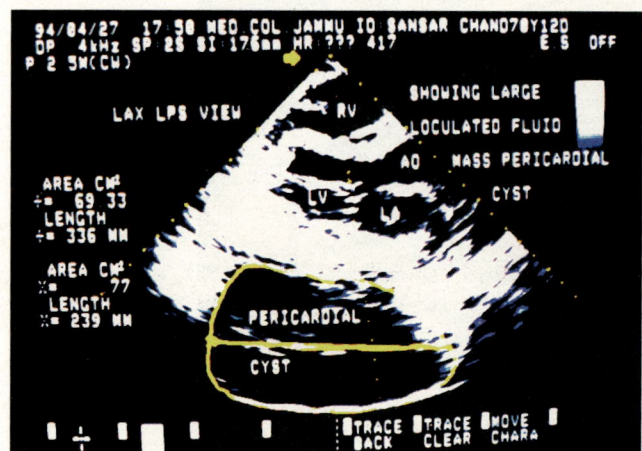

Fig. 16.15: Long axis view LV showing a big pericardial mass compressing posterior LV wall disturbing its relaxation in patient with dyspnoea on exertion of longer duration

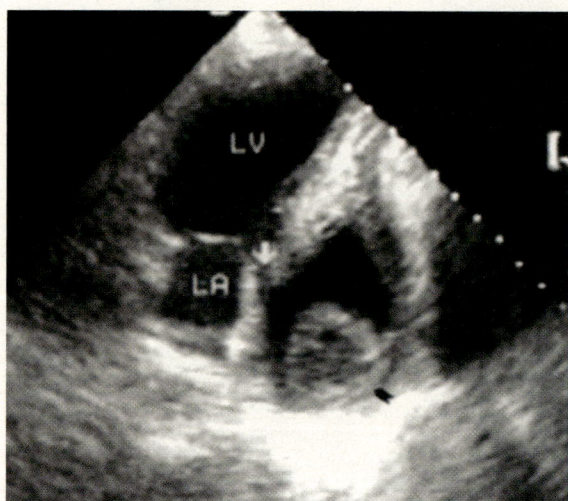

Fig. 16.16: Apical 2C view showing hydatid cyst of pericardium (arrow) very close to left atrium (LA)

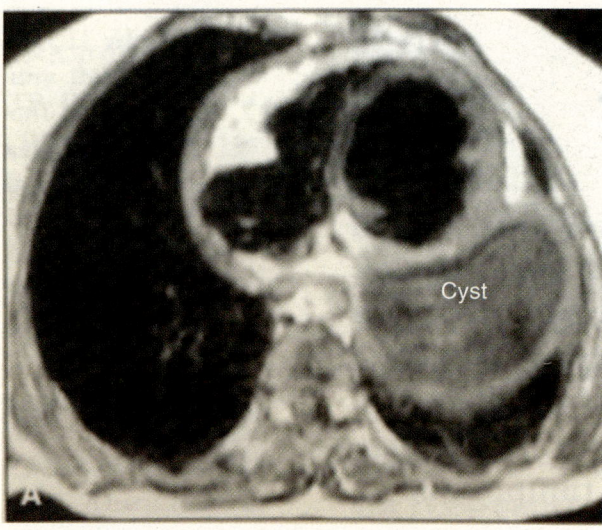

Fig. 16.17: Spin echo T1 weighted showing characters of a hydatid cyst and excluding the tumor mass or thrombosis

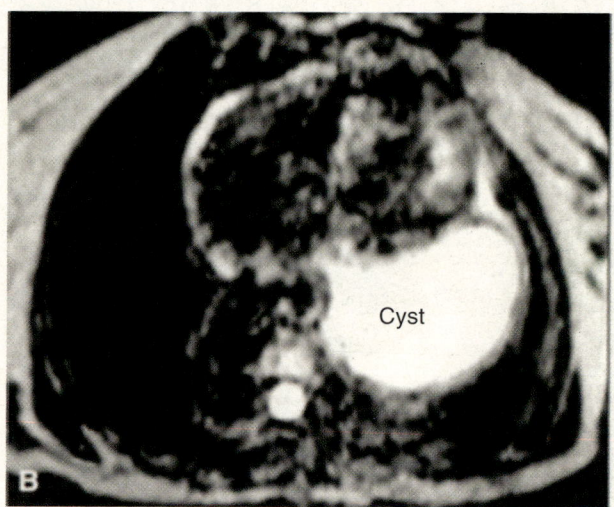

Fig. 16.18: Spin echo T2 weighted showing characters of a hydatid cyst and excluding the tumor mass or thrombosis

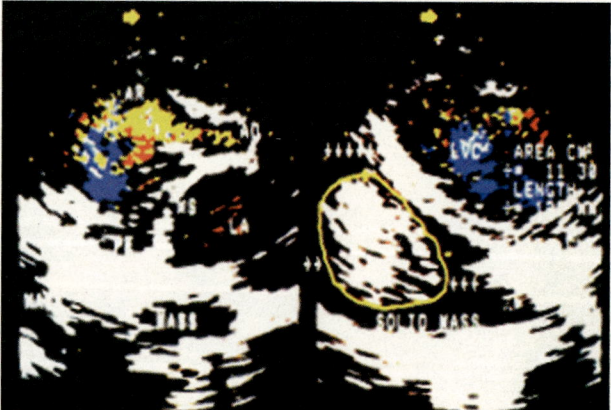

Fig. 16.19: Long axis LV showing solid mass (encircled) below the LV posterior wall compressing the left ventricular cavity in patient with rheumatic mitral stenosis and valvular regurgitation

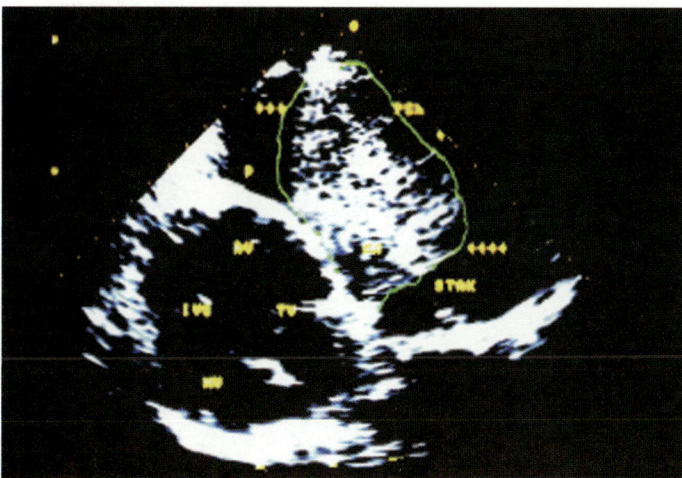

Fig. 16.20: Apical 4C view showing a big mass (encircled) attached to pericardium with compression on the anterior wall of the left ventricle

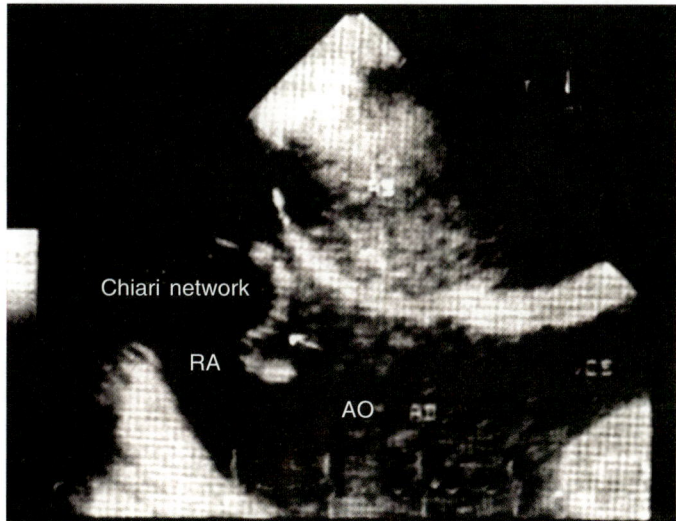

Fig. 16.21: TEE AO and biatrial view showing a worm like clot in right atrium (RA) simulating chiari network in right atrium

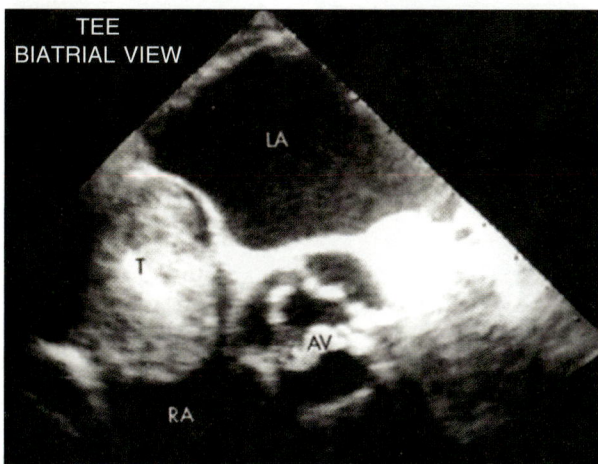

Fig. 16.22: TEE view showing big tumor mass (T) in right atrium

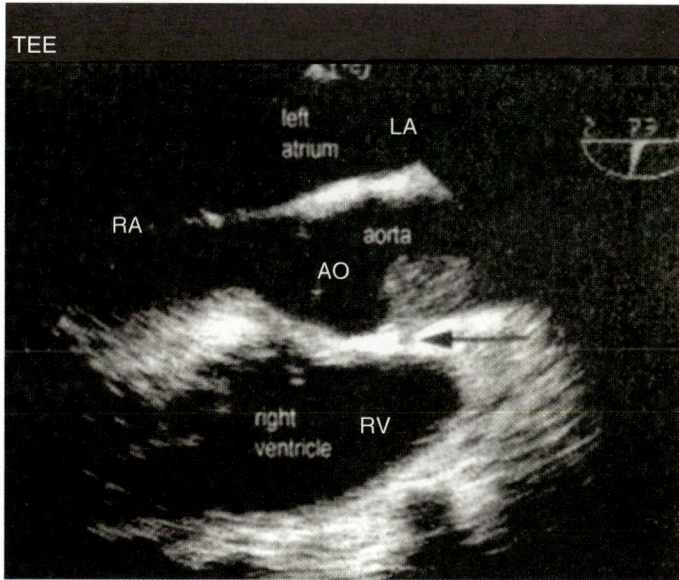

Fig. 16.23: TEE showing a thrombus like free floating tumour (T) was seen in the proximal ascending aorta, originating in the proximal right coronary artery in a patient who had an acute chest pain and found to have acute myocardial infarction by ECG and raised myocardial enzymes and infarct markers. However, aortic valve endocarditis was excluded histologically

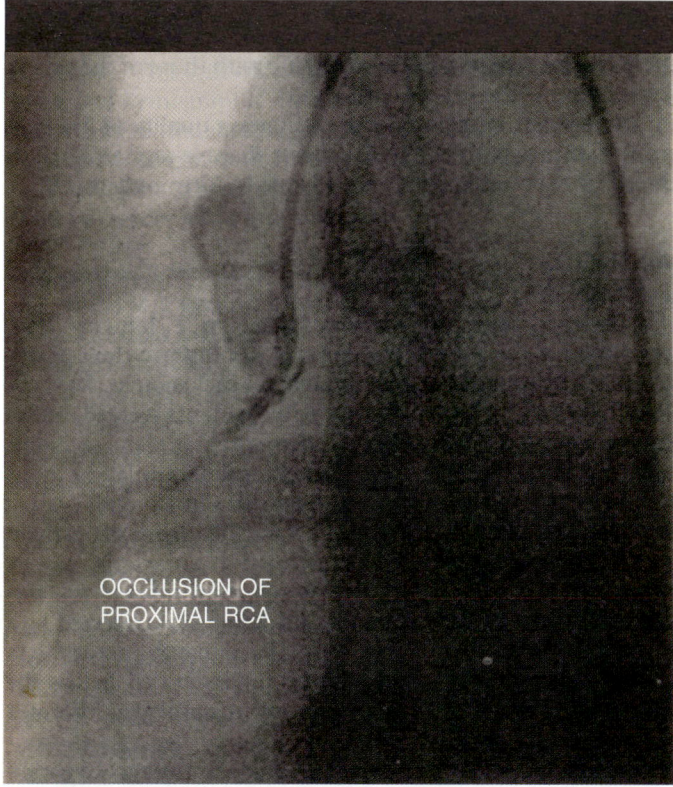

Fig. 16.24: In the same patient as in Fig. 16.23 coronary angiogram showed a proximal occlusion of the right coronary artery due to pressure of the coronary thrombus (proved histologically) in a patient who had an acute chest pain and found to have acute myocardial infarction by ECG and raised myocardial enzymes and infarct markers

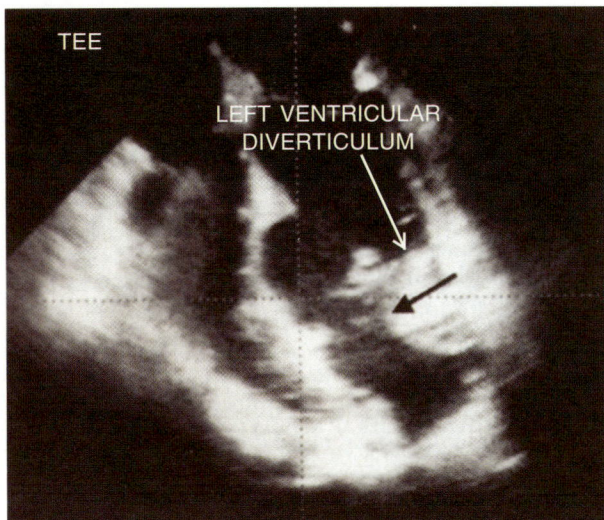

Fig. 16.25: TEE showing the left ventricular diverticulum connected with the main left ventricular chamber through narrow neck

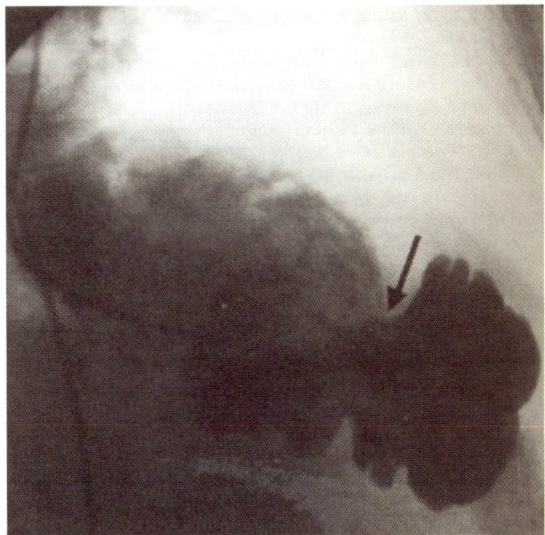

Fig. 16.26: Left ventriculogram in right anterior oblique projection showing the diverticulum depicting good contractions during diastole (arrow)

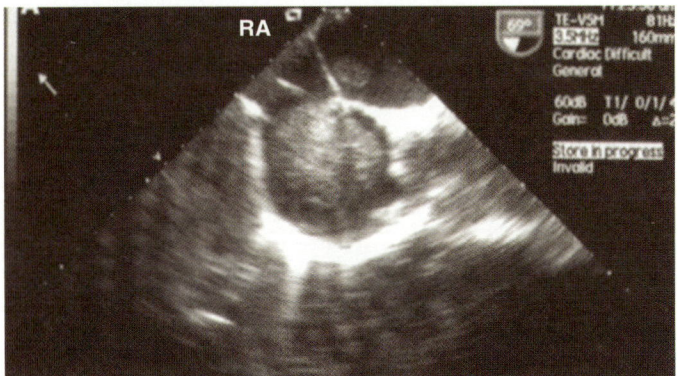

Fig. 16.27: TEE shows a large echogenic mass in the right atrium and ASD secundum in a patient with angina pectoris and coronary artery disease

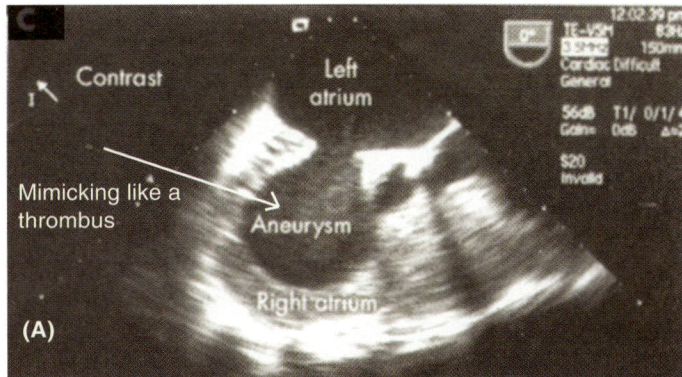

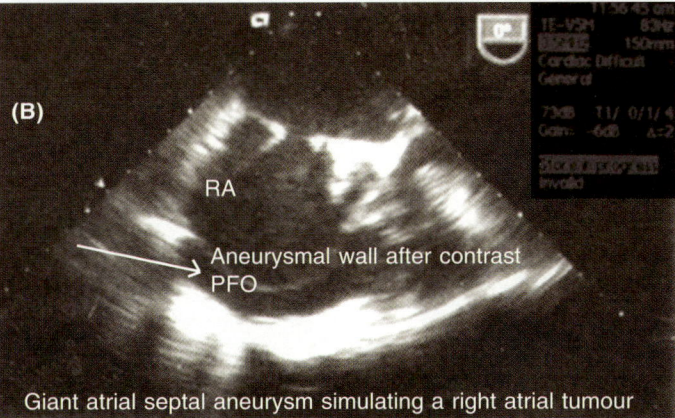

Giant atrial septal aneurysm simulating a right atrial tumour

Fig. 16.28A and B: **(A)** In the same patient contrast injection was administred and it was thought to be a large thrombus or myxoma attached to the atrial septum.After bolus injection of normal saline in the right jugular vein, intra-atrial shunt was ruled out and a giant atrial septal aneurysm with automated contrast and low flow through the patent foramen ovale was visualized. The diagnosis was subsequently confirmed when the patient condition deteriorated and presented with clinical picture of shock. The automatic contrast disappeared and the aneurysm wall was clearly delineated. **(B)** The patient was managed with resection of atrial septal aneurysm and CABG

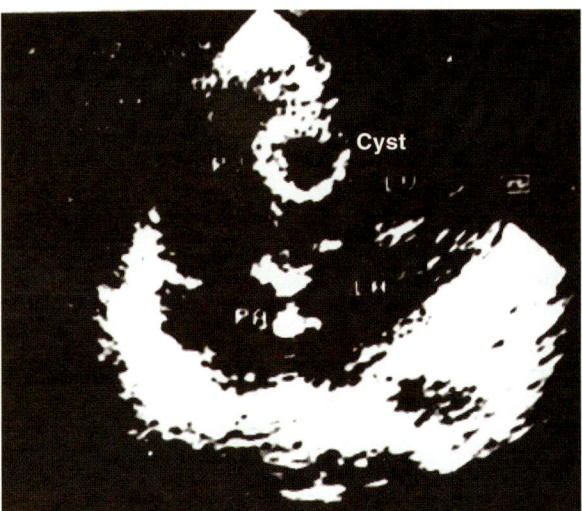

Fig. 16.29: Apical 4C view showing a big hydatid cyst in the region of apical septum in patient with complete heart block

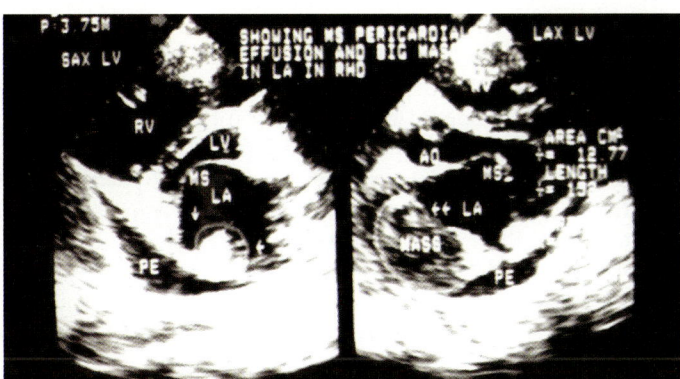

Fig. 16.30: Short and long axis views LV showing a big clot in LA (arrow) in patient with mitral stenosis, MR and pericardial effusion

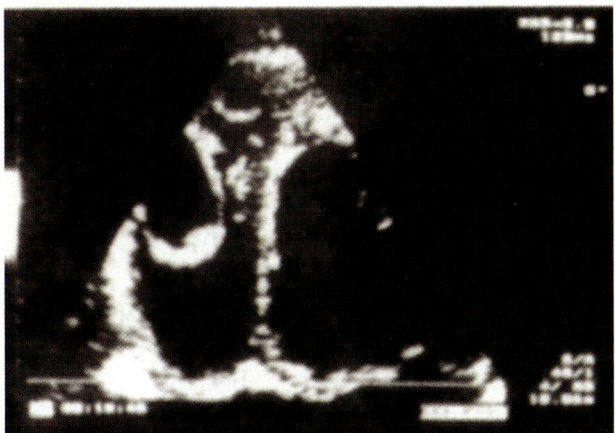

Fig. 16.31: Apical four chamber view showing cystic masses attached along the free wall of the right ventricle in patient with SIRS

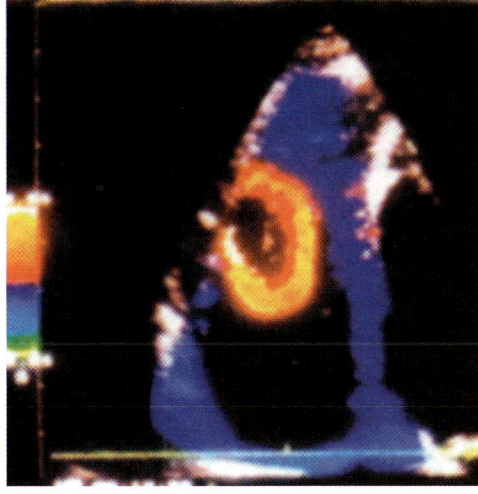

Fig. 16.32: Myocardial tissue Doppler echocardiography showing ring like cystic mass in LV in patient with systemic inflammatory response syndrome (SIRS)

tapeworm; *Taenia echinococcus*. Hydatid cyst are at first embedded in the myocardium, usually of the ventricles. As the cyst enlarges, it may project into the pericardium or into one of the cardiac chambers. There is a great danger of the cysts or daughter cysts rupturing into the lumen of the heart or into the pericardium. Intracardiac rupture may result in embolic phenomenon or anaphylactic/allergic reactions; while intrapericardial rupture causes an acute or subacute pericarditis. The diagnosis is suspected by 2-dimensional echocardiography as it may reveal, cystic mass, pericardial effusion/cardiac tamponade or ventricular dysfunctions as a result of its spontaneous rupture in one of the cardiac chambers. Several workers are still engaged in making this technique of echocardiography even more specific and sensitive by tissue characterization of echoes well within the cardiac chambers, so that intracardiac tumors and thrombi are detected easily and aetiological diagnosis of a particular mass is made more frequently by mere visualising the mass right into its respective cavity of the heart. (Figs 16.13(A-C), 16.14, 16.16, 16.17, 16.18, 16.29, 16.31 and 16.32).

Bibliography

1. Acebo E, Val-Bernal JF, Gomez-Roman JJ, *et al.* Clinicopathologic study and DNA analysis of 37 cardiac myxomas: a 28-year experience. *Chest* 123:1379, 2003.
2. Alam M. Pitfalls in the echocardiographic diagnosis of intracardiac and extracardiac masses. *Echocardiography* 1993;10:181–191.
3. Bhan A, Mehrotra R, Choudhary SK, *et al.* Surgical experience with intracardiac myxomas: long-term follow-up. *Ann Thorac Surg* 66:810, 1998.
4. Cheitlin MD, Alpen IS, Armstrong WF, *et al.* ACCIAHA Guidelines for the Clinical Application of Echocardiography: a report of the American College of Cardiology/American Heart Association Task Force on Practice Guidelines (Committee on Clinical Application of Echocardiography) developed in collaboration with the American Society of Echocardiography. *Circulation* 1997; 95:1686–1744.
5. Colucci WS, Schoen FJ, Braunwald E. Primary cardiac tumors of the heart. *In Heart disease: A textbook of cardiovascular medicine.* Braunwald E, 5th edn. 1997. Bangalore: Prism Books.
6. Come PC, Riley MF, Blvas NK. Roles of echocardiography and antithymia monitoring in the evaluation of patients with suspected systemic embolism. *Ann Neurol* 1983;13:527–531.
7. Comess KA, DeRook FA, Beach KW, *et al.* Transesophageal echocardiography and carotid ultrasound in patients with cerebral ischemia: prevalence of findings and recurrent stroke risk. *J Am Coll Cardiol* 1994;23:1598–603.
8. Cujec B, Polasek P, Voll C, *et al.* Transesophagical echocardiography in the detection of potential cardiac source of embolism in stroke patients. *Stroke* 1991 ;22:727–733.
9. Dc Rook FA, Comess KA, Albers GW, *et al.* Transesophageal echocardiography in the evaluation of stroke. *Ann Intern Med* 1992;117:922–932.
10. de Belder MA, Tourikis L, *et al.* Limitations of transoesophageal echocardiography in patients with focal cerebral ischaemic events. *Br Heart J* 1992;67:297–303.

11. Ezekowitz MD, Wilson DA, Smith EO, *et al.* Comparison of Indium-III platelet scintigraphy and two-dimensional echocardiography in the diagnosis of left ventricular thrombi. *N Engl J Med* 1982;306: 1509–1513.

12. Farfel I, Shechter M, Vered I, *et al.* Review of echocardiographically diagnosed right heart entrapment of pulmonary embolism. In-trans emphasis on management. *Am Heart J* 1987;113:171–178.

13. Fatkin D, Kelly RP, Feneley MP. Relations between left atrial appendage bloodflow velocity, spontaneous echocardiographic contrast and thromboembolic risk *in vivo. J Am Coll Cardiol* 1994; 23:961–969.

14. Fisher DC. Fisher EA, Budd JH. *et al.* The incidence of patent foramen ovale in 1,000 consecutive patients. A contrast transesophageal echocardiography study. *Chest* 1995;107:1504–1509.

15. Fisher J. Cardiac myxoma. *Cardiovasc Rev Rep* 1983; 9 1195.

16. Fowle RE, Miller DC, Egbert SM, *et al.* Systemic embolization from a mitral valve papillary endocardial fibroma detected by two-dimensional echocardiography. *Am Heart J* 1981;102:128–130.

17. Freedberg RS, Kronzon I, Rumaneik W, Lieleskind D. The contribution of magnetic resonance imaging to evaluation of intracardiac tumours diagnosed by echocardiography. *Circulation* 1988;77:96–103.

18. Fyke FE III, Tajik AJ, Edwards WD, *et al.* Diagnosis of lipomatous hypertrophy of the atrial septum by two-dimensional echocardiography. *J Am Coll Cardiol* 1983; 1:1352–1357.

19. Fyke FE, Segard JB, Edwards WD. Primary cardiac tumour: experience with 30 conservative patients since the introduction of two dimensional echocardiography. *J Am Coll Cardiol* 1985;5: 1465–1469.

20. Fyke III FE, Seward JB, Edwards WD, *et al.* Primary cardiac tumors: Experience with 30 consecutive patients since the introduction of two-dimensional echocardiography. *J Am Coll Cardiol* 1985; 5: 1465–1473.

21. Goldman M, Kronzon I. Goldstein M, *et al.* Value of Transesophageal Echo (VOTE): results in 3001 patients. *Circulation* 1994;90:1–20.

22. Gomez FP, Devan H, Tamames S, Perrote JL, Blames A. Cardiac echinococcosis: Clinical picture and complications. *Br Heart J* 1973; 35: 1326–1331.

23. Gowda RM. Khan IA, Nair CK, *et al.* Cardiac papillary fibroelastoma: a comprehensive analysis of 725 cases. *Am Heart J* 2003; 146:404–41.

24. Grenadier E, Lima CO, Barron N. *et al.* Two-dimensional echocardiography for evaluation of metastatic cardiac tumors in pediatric patients. *Am Heart J* 1984;107:122–126.

25. Grimm RA, Stewart WJ, Black IW, *et al.* Should all patients undergo transesophageal echocardiography before electrical cardioversion of atrial fibrillation? *J Am Coll Cardiol* 1994;23:533–541.

26. Hofman T, Kasper W, Meinertz T, *et al.* Echocardiographic evaluation of patients with clinically suspected arterial emboli. *Lancet* 1990;336:1421–1424.

27. Hwang JJ, Chen JJ, Lin SC, *et al.* Diagnostic accuracy of transesophageal echocardiography for detecting left atrial thrombi in patients with rheumatic heart disease having undergone mitral valve operations. *Am J Cardiol* 1993;72:677–681.

28. Johnson MH, Soulen RL. Echocardiography of cardiac metastasis. *Am J Roentgenol* 1983;141:677–681.

29. Khandheria BK, Seward JB, Tajik AJ. Critical appraisal of transesophageal echocardiography: limitations and pitfalls. *Crit Care Clin* 1996; 12:235–251.

30. Kindman LA. Wright A, *et al.* Lipomatous hypertrophy of the interatrial septum: characterization by transesophageal and transthoracic echocardiography, magnetic resonance imaging, and computed tomography. *J Am Soc Echocardiogr* 1988;1:450–454.

31. Klarich KW, Enriquez–Sarano M, Gura GM, *et al.* Papillary fibroelastoma echocardiographic characteristics for diagnosis and pathologic correlation. *J Am Coll Cardiol* 1997;30:784–790.

32. Klein AL, Grimm RA, Black IW, *et al.* Cardioversion guided by transesophageal echocardiography: the Acute Pilot Study. A randomized controlled trial. Assessment of cardioversion using transesophageal echocardiography. *Ann Intern Med* 1997;126: 200–209.

33. Klein AL, Grimm RA, Murray RD, *et al.* Use of transesophageal echocardiography to guide cardioversion in patients with atria fibrillation. *N Engl J Med* 2001;344:1411–1420.

34. Labovitz AJ. Bransford TL. Evolving role of echocardiography in the management of atrial fibrillation. *Am Heart J* 2001;141:518–527.

35. Laupacis A, Albers G, Dalen J, *et al.* Antithrombotic therapy in atrial fibrillation. *Chest* 1995; 108:3525–3595.

36. Lee RJ, Bartzokis T, Yeoh TK, *et al.* Enhanced detection of intracardiac sources of cerebral emboli by transesophageal echocardiography *Stroke* 1991; 22:734–739.

37. Leung DY, Black IW, Cranney GB, *et al.* Prognostic implications of left atrial spontaneous echo contrast in nonvalvular atrial librillation. *J Am Coll Cardiol* 1994;24:755–762.

38. Levisman JA, MacAlpin RN, Abbasi AS, Ellis N, Eber LM. Echocardiographic diagnosis of a mobile, pedunculated tumor in the left ventricular cavity. *Am J Cardiol* 1975; 36: 957–959.

39. Llmng DY, Davidson PM, Cranney GB, et al. Thromboembolic risks of left atrial thrombus detected by transesophageal echocardiogram. *Am J Cardiol* 1997;79:626–629.

40. Manning WJ, Silverman W, Katz SE, *et al.* Impaired left atrial mechanical function after cardioversion: relation to the duration of atrial fibrillation. *J Am Coll Cardiol* 1994;23:1535–1540.

41. Manning WJ, Silverman DI. Gordon SP. *et al.* Cardioversion of atrial fibrillation without prolonged anticoagulation with use of transesophageal echocardiography to exclude the presence of atrial thrombi. *N Engl J Med* 1993;328:750–755.

42. Manning WJ, Weintraub RM, Waksmonski CA, *et al.* Accuracy of transesophageal echocardiography for identifying left atrial thrombi. A prospective intraoperative study. *Ann Intern Med* 1995; 123:817–822.

43. Meng Q, Lai H, Lima J, *et al.* Echocardiographic and pathologic characteristics of primary cardiac tumors: a study of 149 cases. *Int J Card* 84:69, 2002.

44. Muggae A, Daniel G, Haverich A, Litchlen PR. Diagnosis of noninfectious cardiac mass lesion by two-dimensional echocardiography. *Circulation* 1991; 83:70–73.

45. O'Neil M Jr, Grehl, T, Hurley E. Cardiac myxomas: a clinical and diagnostic challenge. *Am J Surg* 1979; 138: 68–73.

46. Obeid AI, Marvasti M, Parker F, Rosenberg J. Comparison of transthoracic and transoesophageal echocardiography in diagnosis of left atrial myxoma. *Am J Cardiol* 1989;63: 1006–1010.

47. Pinede L, Duhaut P, Loire R: Clinical presentation of left atrial cardiac myxoma: a series of 112 consecutive cases. *Medicine* (Baltimore) 80:159, 2001.

48. Rahilly GJ Jr, Nand NC. Two dimensional echocardiographic identification of tumor haemorrhages in atrial myxomas. *Am Heart J* 1981; 101: 237–239.

49. Rolla G, Bertero MT, Pastena G, *et al.* Primary lymphoma of the heart. A case report and review of the literature. Leuk Res 26:117, 2002 view of 3314 consecutive autopsies. *Am J Cardiovasc Pathol* 1990;3: 195–198.

50. Shapiro LM: Cardiac tumours: diagnosis and management. *Heart* 85:218, 2001.

51. Siwach SB, Dua Abha, Sharma Deepak. Multichamber intra-cardiac thrombi in a patient without any predisposing cardiac or non-cardiac disease. *Intern J Cardiol* 1992; 37: 263–265.

52. Siwach SB, Fraser AG. LV Myxoma-An echocardiographic diagnosis. *Indian Heart J* 1987; 39: 249–250.

53. Siwach SB, Katyal VK, Jagdish. Cardiac echinococcosis—A rare echocardiographic diagnosis. *Heart* 1997; 77: 378–379.

54. Siwach SB, Singh HP, Saini BK. Intracardiac thrombosis following acute myocardial infarction. *Indian Practitioners* 1998; 58: 195–198.

55. Stern MJ, Cohen MV, Fish B, Rosenthal R. Clinical presentation and noninvasive diagnosis of right heart masses. *Br Heart* 1981; 46: 552–558.

56. Stiller BB, Hetzer R, Meyer R, *et al.* Primary cardiac tumours: when is surgery necessary? *Eur J Cardiovasc Surg* 20:1002, 2001.

57. Sun JP, Asher CR, Yang XS, *et al.* Clinical and echocardio-graphic characteristics of papillary fibroelastomas: a retrospective and prospective study in 162 patients. *Circulation* 103:2687, 2001.

58. Transchenberg W, Schluter M, Kremer P, *et al.* Transesoph-ageal two-dimensional echocardiography for the detection of left atrial appendage thrombus. *Am J Cardiol* 1986;7:163–166.

59. Wiseman MN, Giles MS, Camm AJ. Unusual echocardio-graphic appearance on intracardiac thrombi in a patient with endomyocardial fibrosis. *Br Heart J* 1986; 56: 179–181.

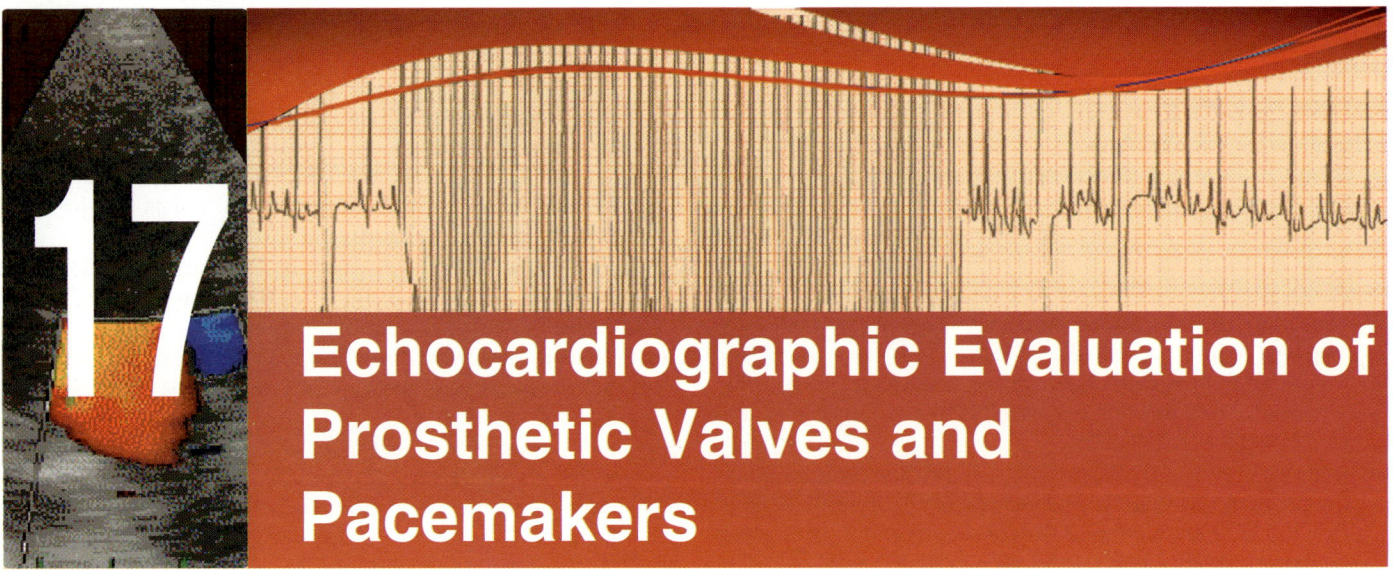

17
Echocardiographic Evaluation of Prosthetic Valves and Pacemakers

When a patient develops rheumatic heart disease, progressive degeneration and calcification of the valvular structures causes heart failure. To relieve the narrowing of these valves, it is necessary to replace the damaged tissue with a prosthetic heart valve. There are several types of prosthetic valves; caged-ball, caged-disk, tilting disk, and bioprosthesis (Figs 17.28 and 17.29). It is important for the sonographer to know the type of prosthetic valve, the patient has implanted for adequate recording (Figs 17.1–17.4).

There are three basic parts of each type of mechanical valve, the disk or ball, the strut or cage, and the sewing ring or seating of the valve, the upper and lower round attachment of the valve. All of these components are subject to changes. The Starr-Edwards ball is composed of silicon and is subject to ball variance or a grooving irregularity. This ball variance is not seen in the Teflon disk valves. Some of the valves are cloth covered and not subject to thrombus formation (Figs 17.7 and 17.17A and B).

The incidence of thrombosis with good anticoagulation is 30%. The upper and lower seating is frequently subject to thrombus, which in turn narrows the valve. The lower seating thrombosis interferes with closure of the valve and eventually can lead to regurgitation. In addition to these problems with thrombosis, the sutures around the area of the valve can become loose, causing regurgitation (Fig. 17.32A–D).

The evaluation of defects in the valve is sometimes difficult. Most patients are asymptomatic. Some demonstrate signs of fatigue. Some go into congestive heart failure because of sticking poppet. Embolism to various organs may be seen as a result of thrombus formation on the valve. Bacterial endocarditis is one complication of prosthetic valves because the malfunctioning valve is seedbed for bacteria (Figs 17.33 and 17.34).

The disk and hinge valve can be used interchangeably in the aorta and mitral valve by reversing their positions. During auscultation, the valves should make two noises during one cycle. At the onset of systole the mitral valve should have closing click, whereas the aortic valve should have a opening click. Likewise, during diastole the mitral valve should have an opening click and the arotic valve a closing click. With the valve in the aortic area there is normally a slight gradient. In the mitral area, there is a small gradient as the blood flows from low pressure to high pressure, giving rise to the mid-diastolic murmur. For example, a Bjork-Shiley prosthesis has a soft opening and a loud closing (Figs 17.9 and 17.11).

The presence of a systolic murmur in the mitral valve area is abnormal and is frequently attributed to a paravalvular leak. If there is a clot inside the cage, it causes the valve to close improperly, and regurgitation is the inevitable result. Diagnostic studies useful in assessing prosthetic function are chest radiography, fluoroscopy, angiography, and echocardiography (Fig. 17.8).

Chest radiography can determine cardiac enlargement or the position of the prosthesis. Fluoroscopy is helpful if there is a detachment of the valve or a paravalvular leak, causing the valve to tilt in the mitral position (i.e. into the left atrium). In the aortic valves, the situation can change very dramatically and side to side flapping movements of the valve can be recorded in a dysfunctional valve. Angiography can detect leakage, but since there is a slight degree of regurgitation with the prosthesis, it may be physiological regurgitation. In pathologic regurgitation, the dye is seen going into the ventricle during systole.

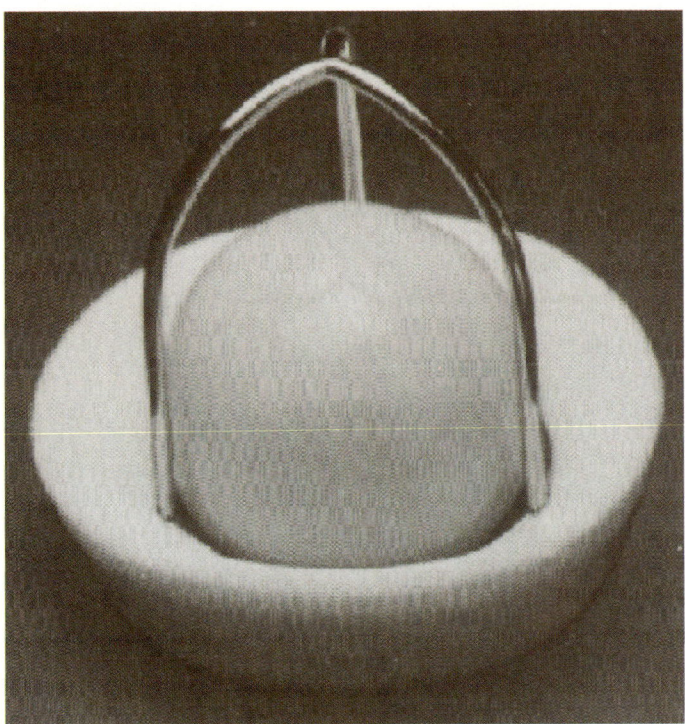

Fig. 17.1: Aortic mechanical prosthesis Starr-Edward ball in cage prosthesis

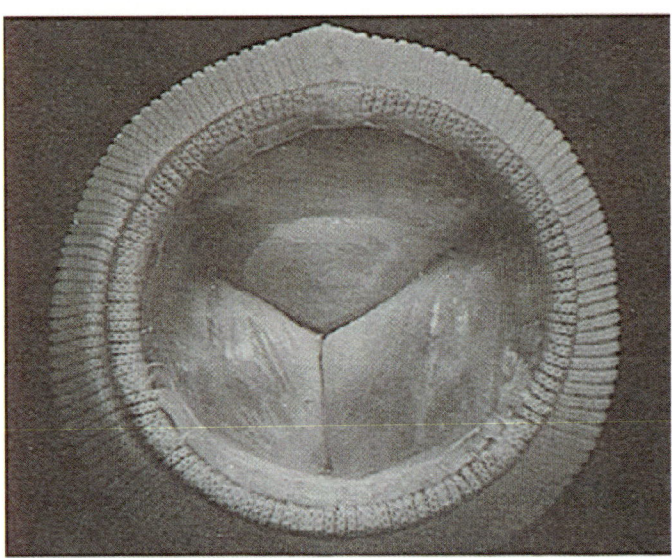

Fig. 17.3: Top view of an aortic porcine xenograft that has been mounted on a flexible plastic stent

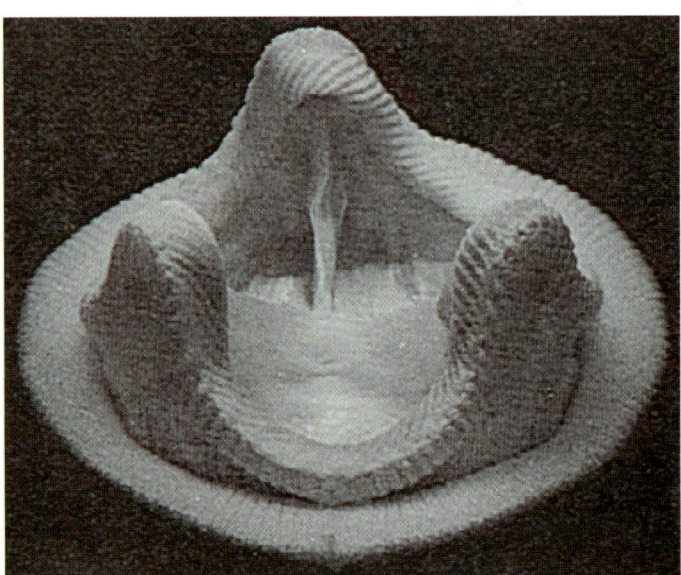

Fig. 17.4: Bottom view of aortic porcine xenograft that has been mounted on a flexible plastic stent

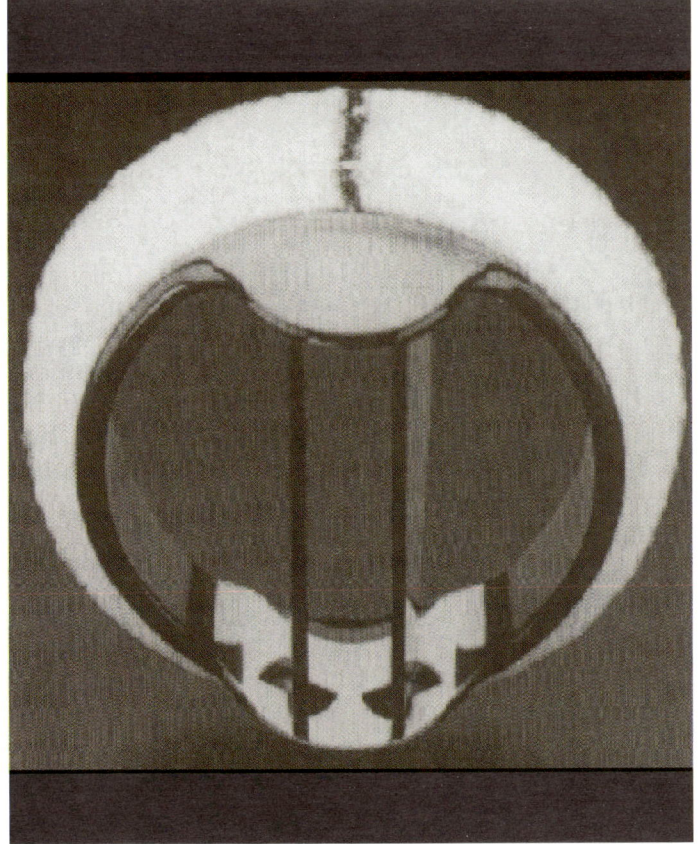

Fig. 17.2: Aortic mechanical prosthesis St.Jude bileaflet tilting disc prosthesis

Echocardiography has proved useful in assessing valve function because of the strong reflecting interface between the artificial valve and the surrounding structures. The exact model and size of the prosthesis are noted before recording the valve movement. If the examiner is not careful, only the supporting structures of the cage may be recorded without disk or ball movement. By angling the transducer in such a direction that beam is perpendicular to the prosthesis, the proper echoes can be recorded. This transducer angle is critical in assessing valvular motion and excursion. The motion of the prosthesis is determined by valve characteristics and the entire cardiac structure. To provide the most

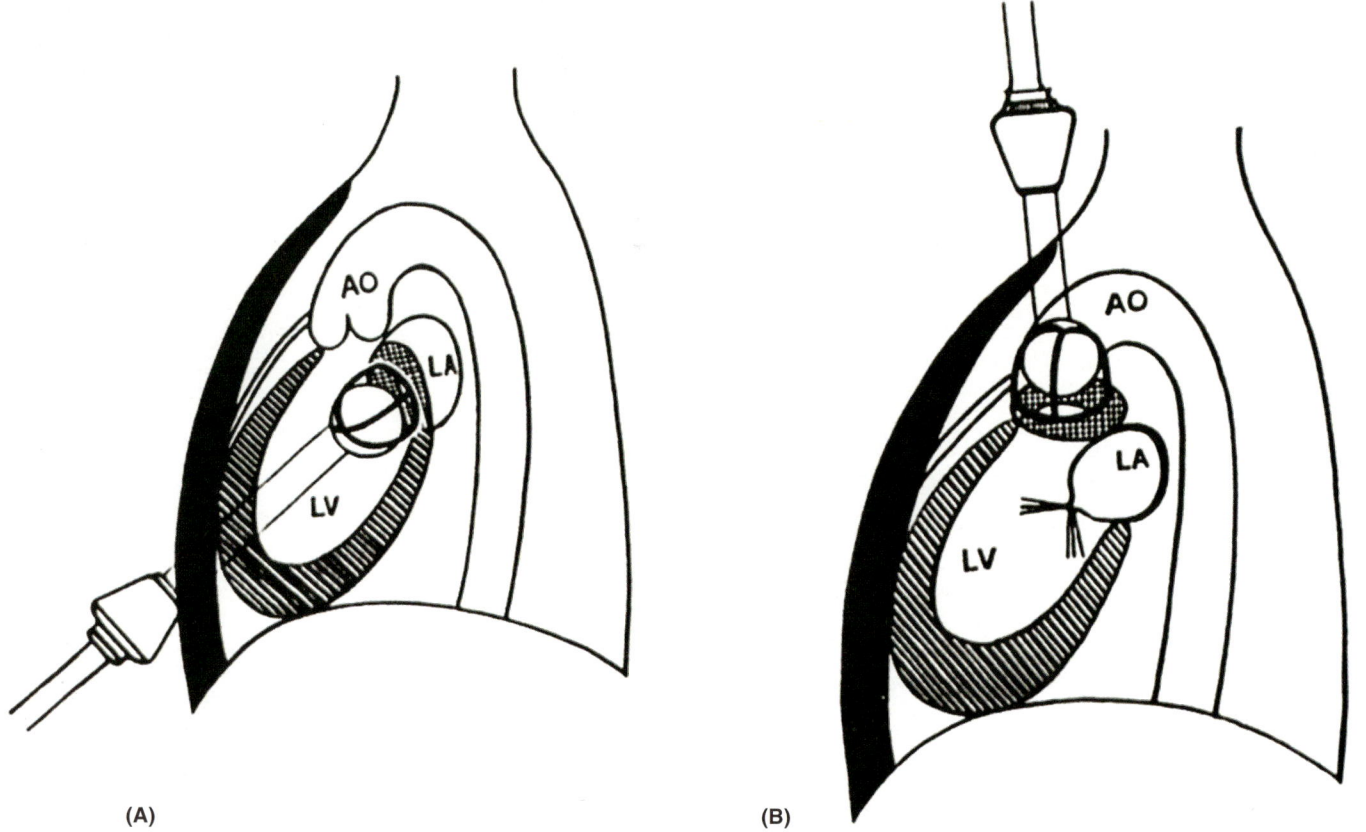

(A)   (B)

Fig. 17.5A and B: **(A)** Diagrammatic representation of prosthetic valve in anatomical mitral area. **(B)** Diagrammatic representation of prosthetic valve in anatomical aortic area

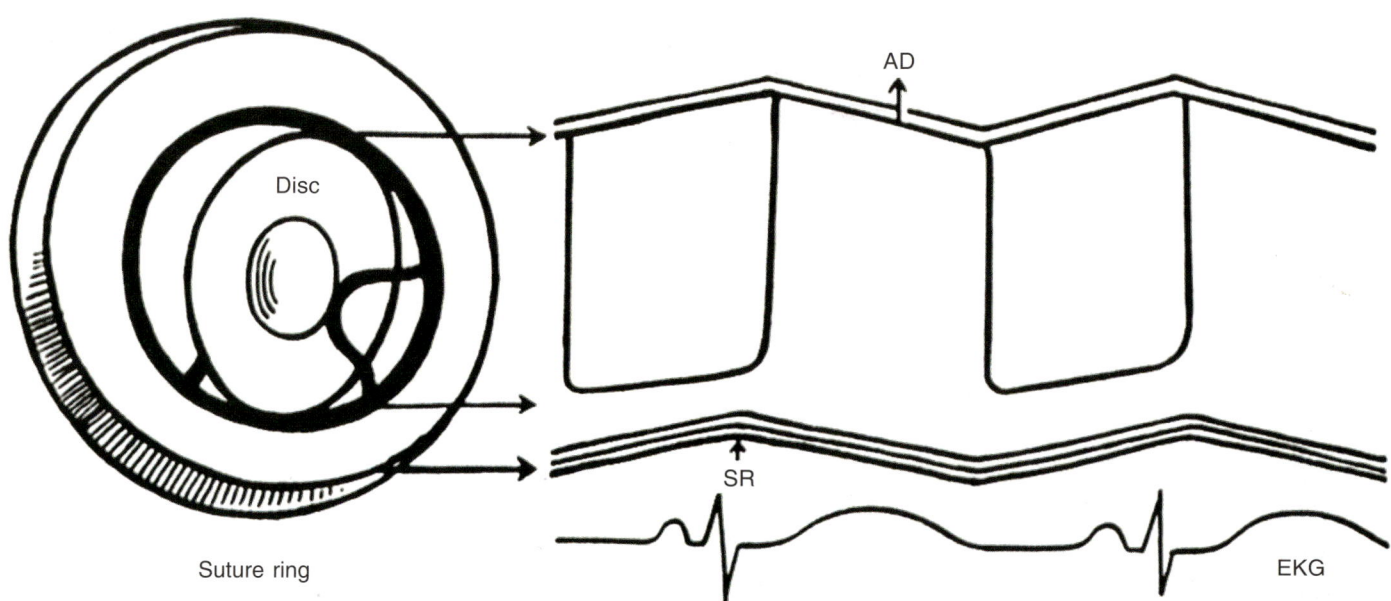

Fig. 17.6: Diagrammatic representation of configuration of tilting disc type of prosthetic valve (left) along with its M-Mode echo signatures (right), AD = Anterior disc, SR = Suture ring, EKG = Electrocardiogram

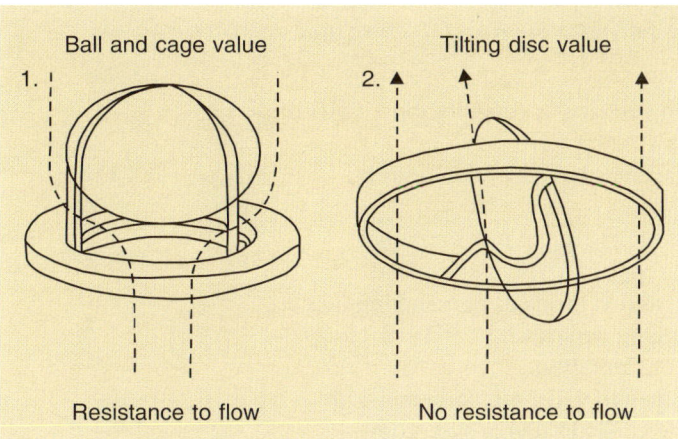

Fig. 17.7: Diagrammatic configuration of two types of prosthetic valves: 1. Ball and cage and 2. Tilting disc with difference in flow resistance

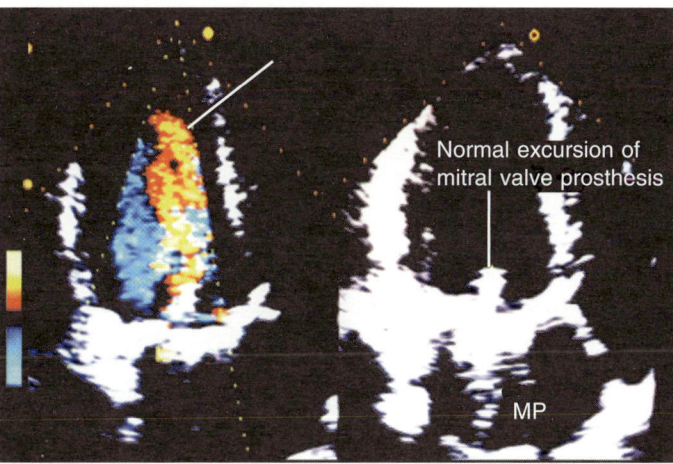

Fig. 17.10: Apical 4C on dual scan showing normal up and down movement of a prosthetic valve (right)and normal mosaic color jet from mitral valve orifice into the left ventricular cavity (left) in patient with normally functioning mitral valve prosthesis (MP)

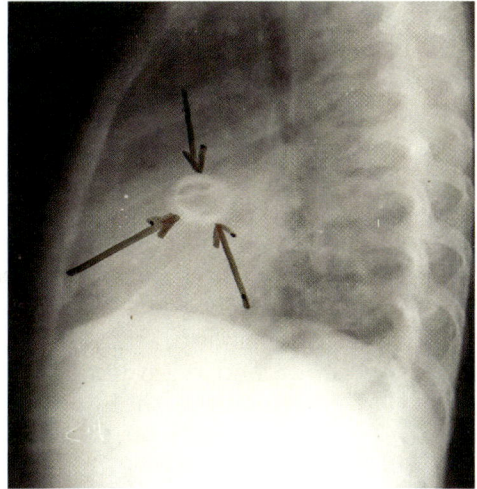

Fig. 17.8: Anatomical location of Bjork Shiley mitral valve as visualized in lateral position of X-ray chest PA view in patient with mitral valve replacement suffering from calcified native mitral valve disease

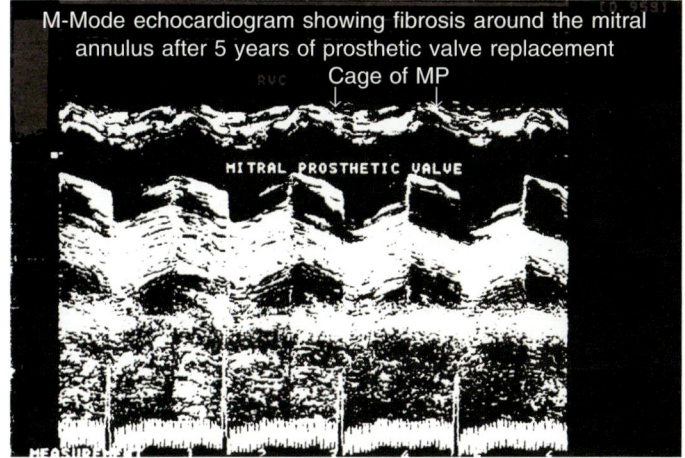

Fig. 17.11: M-Mode echoscan of prosthetic mitral valve (Bjork Shiley) showing fibrosis around the place of sutures and mitral annulus

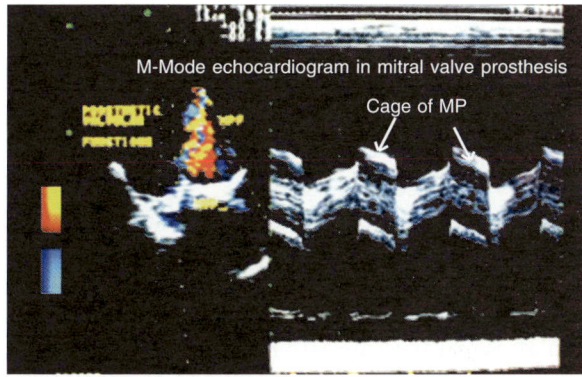

Fig. 17.9: Apical 4C and M-Mode (L-R) in color mode showing normal functioning of Bjork Shiley mitral prosthetic valve (MP). Mosaic color jet is due to functional stenosis which normally can happen in prosthetic valves if other parameters of evaluation are normal

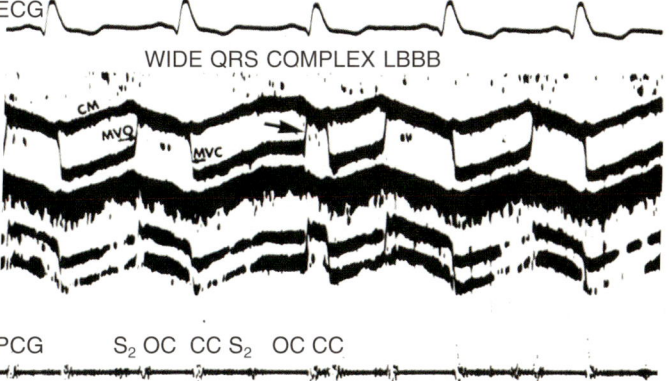

Fig. 17.12: M-Mode echocardiogram showing a delayed mitral valve opening (MVO) in the third cardiac complex (arrow) in patient with malfunctioning mitral prosthetic valve CM = cage of mitral valve, MVC = Mitral valve closing, S2 = Second heart sound, OC = Opening click CC = Closing click

Table 17.1: *Indications for echocardiography in interventions for valvular heart disease and prosthetic valves*

Indications	Class
1. Assessment of the timing of valvular intervention based on ventricular compensation, function, and/or severity of primary and secondary lesions.	I
2. Selection of alternative therapies for mitral valve disease (such as balloon valvuloplasty, operative valve repair, valve replacement).	I
3. Use of echocardiography (especially TEE) in guiding the performance of interventional techniques and surgery (e.g. balloon valvotomy and valve repair) for valvular disease.	I
4. Postintervention baseline studies for valve function (early) and ventricular remodelling (late)	1
5. Reevaluation of patients with valve replacement with changing clinical signs and symptoms; suspected prosthetic dysfunction (stenosis, regurgitation) or thrombosis.	1
6. Routine reevaluation study after baseline studies of patients with valve replacements with mild to moderate ventricular dysfunction without changing clinical signs or symptoms.	IIa
7. Routine reevaluation at the time of increased failure rate of a bioprosthesis without clinical evidence of prosthetic dysfunction.	IIb
8. Routine reevaluation of patients with valve replacements without suspicion of valvular dysfunction and unchanged clinical signs and symptoms.	III
9. Patients whose clinical status precludes therapeutic interventions.	III

accurate assessment of valve function, recordings should be made after surgery and followed at specific time intervals.

Mitral Valve Prosthesis (Figs 17.9–23)

The best mitral recording clearly records the valve opening and closure and most closely approximates the valve's normal excursion. Disk or hinge valves can generally be recorded in their usual mitral position. However, it may be necessary to locate the Starr-Edwards valve position on the radiographic film for proper transducer angulation. Often the echographer must move to the apex of the heart and angle the transducer cephalad to record the valve at its most perpendicular angle.

The actual thrombus formation is difficult to distinguish by echo, but the altered valve motion may be recorded. Sometimes there is a delay in the valve opening, or there is no opening at all during some cycles. Decreased amplitude of valve opening must be assessed with the transducer in various angles to ascertain the maximum excursion. Because of the intense echo reflection of the valve apparatus, there often appears to be large clumps or 'ring-down' echoes behind the opened valve. This should not be confused with thrombus and usually can be eliminated by slight transducer angulation or a reduction in the sensitivity of the equipment.

Johnson describes the actual measurement of the older type of ball valves by echo and has multiple charts available for analysis of individual tracings. He also discovered that the Starr-Edwards ball was made of Silastic rubber, a slower sound conduction material. Thus when recordings are made from such a valve, it appears that the posterior edge of the ball is actually

beyond its posterior cage. A correction factor of 0.64 can be applied to the measurement of the ball diameter to adjust for this factor.

Doppler Assessment of Mitral Valve Dysfunction

Most prosthetic valves result in a slight-to-moderate obstruction of flow, which results in increased velocity across the prosthetic valve. The velocity and pressure drop depend on the valve area, heart rate, flow across the valve, cardiac output, and regurgitant flow. Hatle states that pressure halftimes are slightly longer than across normal valves (i.e. wider 60 m sec), usually between 70 and 120 m sec, varying with the type and size of prosthesis (Fig. 17.23).

It is difficult to record regurgitant flow velocity with the disk-type prosthesis. If there is leakage around the valve (paravalvular), it may be easier to record by Doppler and is certainly much easier to record with colour-flow Doppler. If the valve is a tissue valve, the Doppler recordings can be made as with a native valve.

Aortic Valve Prosthesis (Figs 17.24 to 17.26)

Because of its anatomical position, the aortic valve is usually more difficult to assess.

The poppet motion of the value can be record in perpendicular path.

Various angles of the transducer are used to record its greatest amplitude. As in the mitral valve, a loss of motion may represent thrombus formation. Many prostheses are associated with aortic regurgitation. In this case the echographic changes are shown on the anterior leaflet of the mitral valve as fine flutter during diastole.

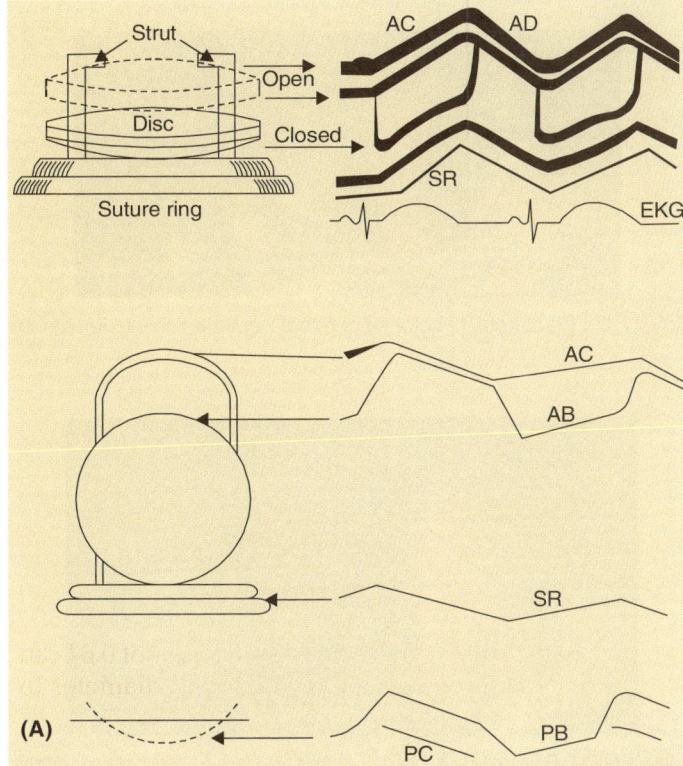

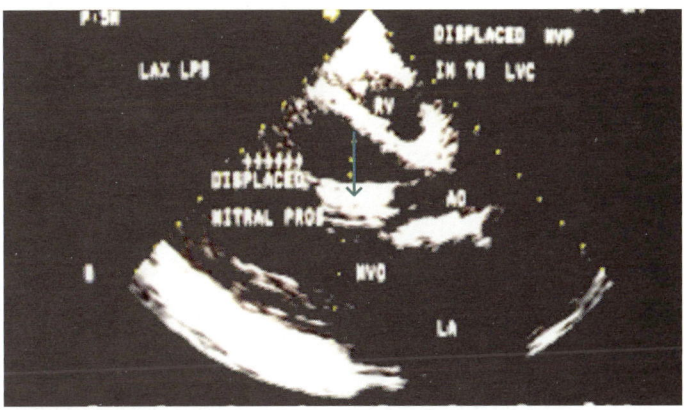

Fig. 17.14: Long axis LV x LPS showing displacement of partly fibrosed mitral prosthesis into left ventricular outflow tract after 10 years of replacement causing disturbance in flow pattern in patient with dyspnoea and cardiac arrhythmia

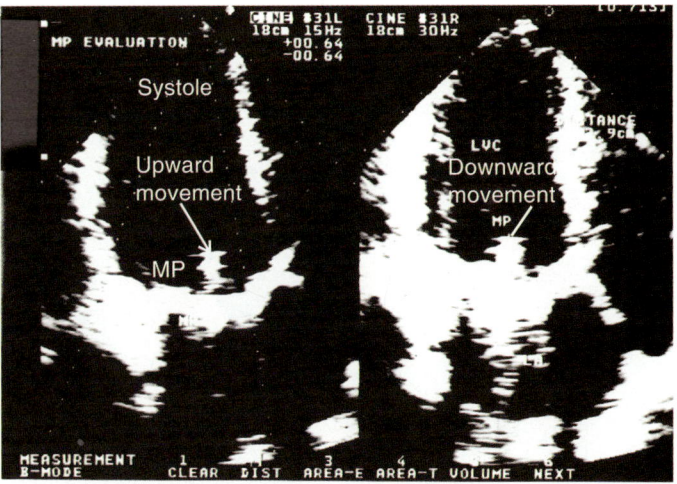

Fig. 17.15: Apical 4C dual scan views showing normal excursion of mitral prosthetic valve (MP) during systole and diastole

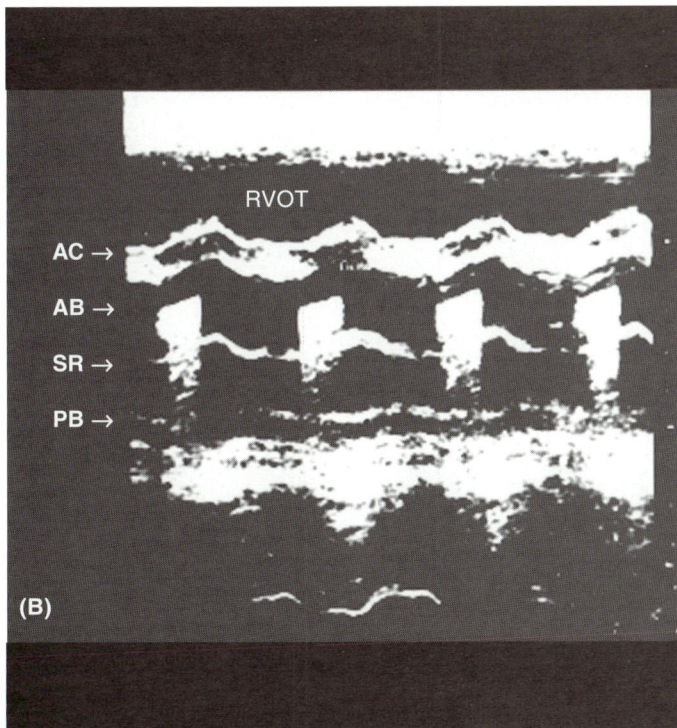

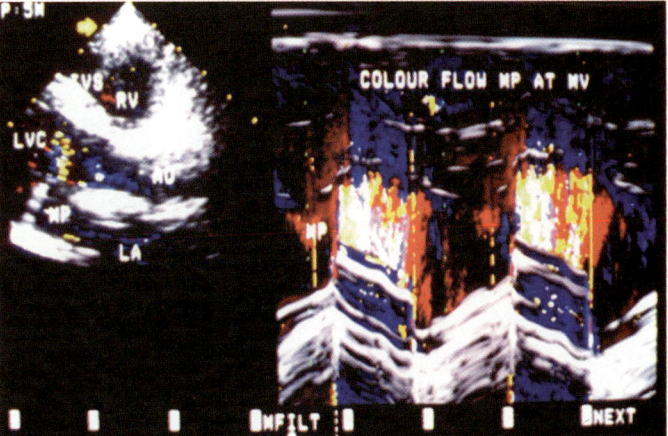

Fig. 17.13A and B: (A) Showing diagrammatic representation of mitral disc prosthesis in M-Mode simulation of ball in cage prosthesis. AC = Anterior cage, AD = Anterior disc, SR = Sewing ring, AB = Anterior ball, PB = Posterior ball, **(B)** M-Mode echocardiogram at prosthetic aortic valve showing different parts of the artificial valve in patient with replacement of prosthetic valve who had critical calcified aortic stenosis

Fig. 17.16: 2-D Long axis and M-mode echocardiogram in color mode showing mosaic color jet into LV cavity in patient with mild obstructive mitral prosthetic flow pattern in patient in whom Bjork Shiley valve was replaced more than 15 years back

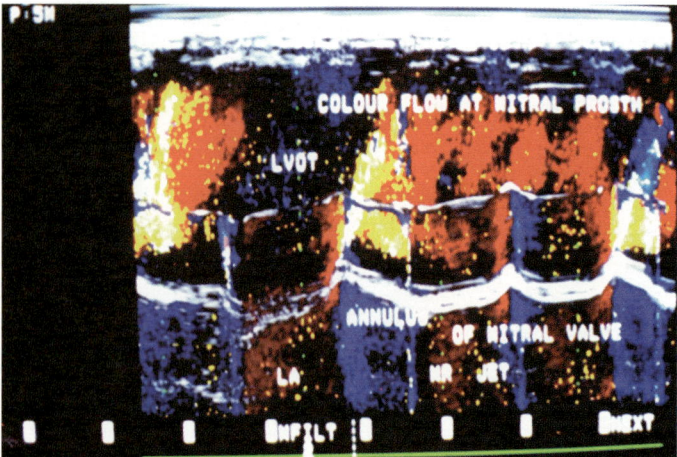

Fig. 17.17: M-Mode echocardiogram showing multiple red flow jets of paravalvular leakage and blue jet of mitral regurgitation into LA cavity in patient with tissue valve replaced 10 years back

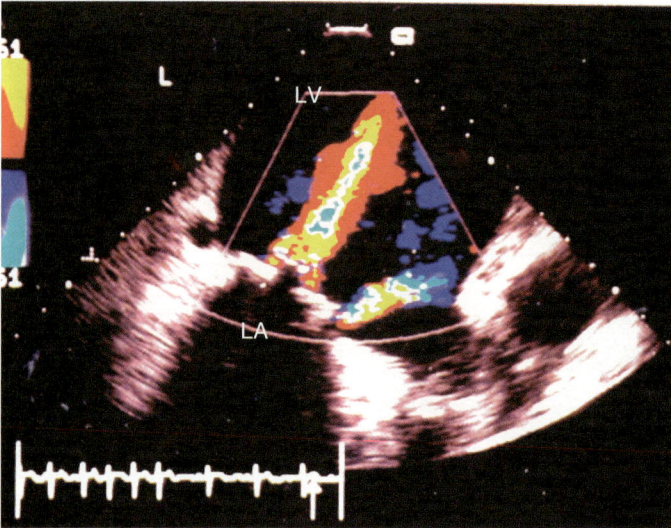

Fig. 17.18: 2-D color scan showing color flow jets through mitral prosthesis (MP) and native aortic valve (AO)

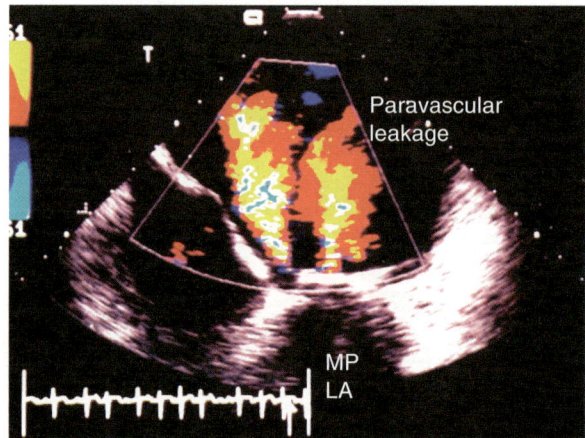

Fig. 16.19: 2-D Apical 4C showing two jets of flow into LV cavity in patient with mitral prosthetic paravalvular leakage

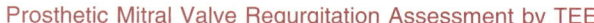

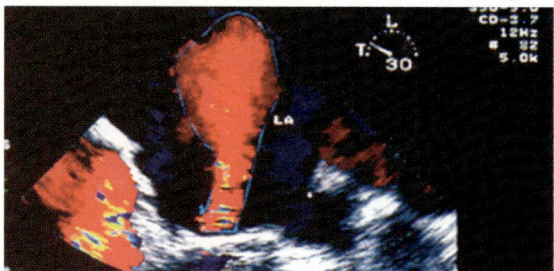

Fig. 17.20: Planimetry of color jet of mitral regurgitation into left atrium

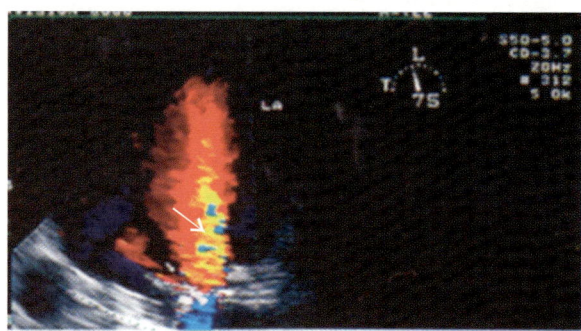

Fig. 17.21: Regurgitant color jet measured at its origin (arrow indicates PJD)

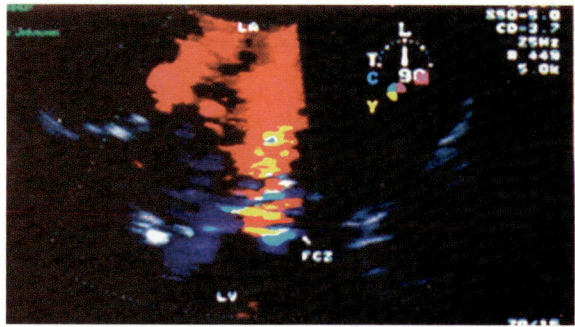

Fig. 17.22: FCZ visualized as a blue flow pattern of increasing brightness with a yellow-red central region (aliased velocities)

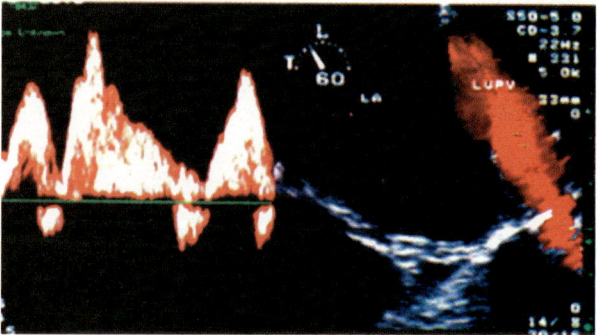

Fig. 17.23: Left upper PVF velocity pattern in systole and diastole LA = Left atrium LUPV = Left upper pulmonary vein, LV = Left ventricle, TEE Color jet mitral regurgitation area (MRA), proximal jet diameter (PJD). Flow convergence zone (FCZ) and pulmonary vein flow (PVF) velocities in patient with mitral valve prosthesis

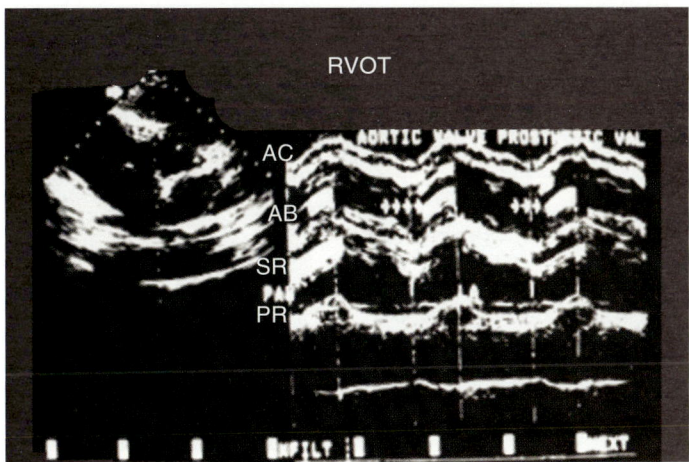

Fig. 17.24: M-Mode and 2D (L-R) echocardiogram at prosthetic aortic valve showing different parts of the artificial valve and fibrosis along the posterior ball after 10 years of follow up in patient with replacement of prosthetic valve who had critical calcified aortic stenosis AC = Anterior cage, AD = Anterior disc, SR = Sewing ring, AB = Anterior ball, PB = Posterior ball

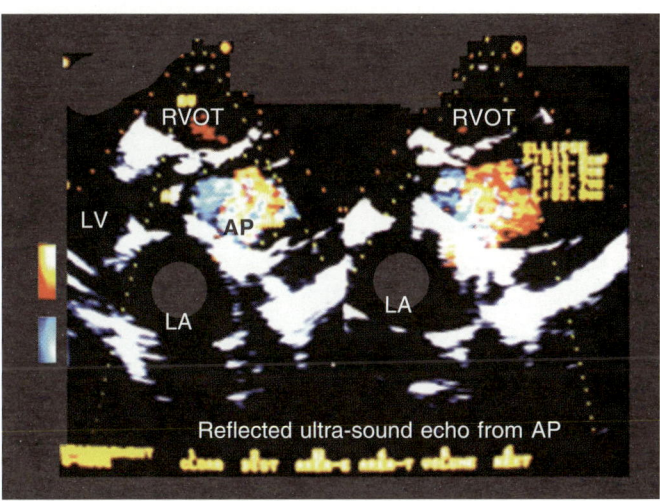

Fig. 17.25: Long and short axis view (L-R) at aortic valve plane showing mosaic colored jet of normally functoning prosthetic aortic valve in patient who had critical calcified aortic valvular stenosis. AP = Aortic prosthetic valve. LA = Left atrium RVOT = Right ventricular out flow tract

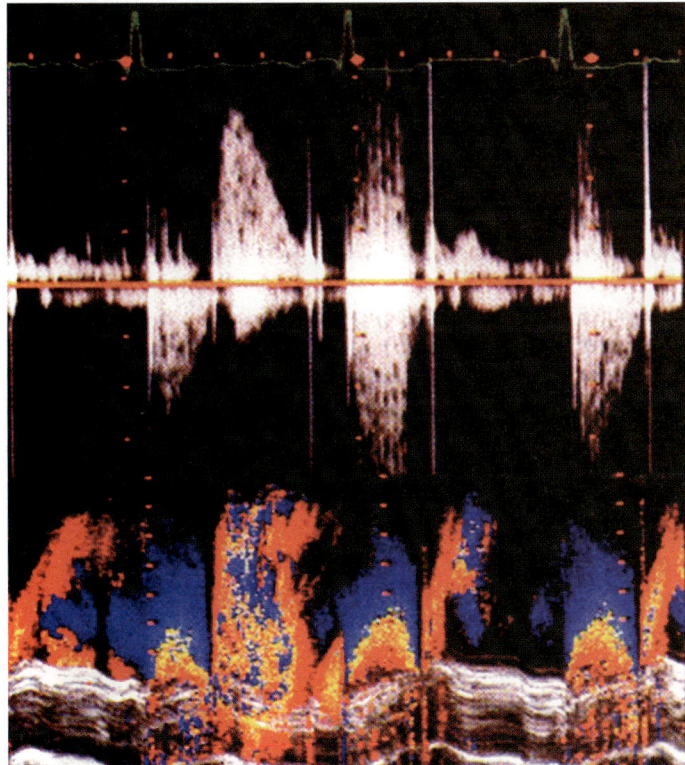

Fig. 17.26: Dopper flow and colorflow through malfunctioning Carpentier-Edward prosthetic aortic valve showing a cyclic (every 30–60 beats) failure in closure of a leaflet resulting in acute massive aortic regurgitation. In these sporodic cycles continuous wave Doppler (upper panel) showed the absence of closing click, followed by the signal of acute massive regurgitation (slope of the diastolic regurgitant jet > 3 m/s) with an increase in the velocity of forward aortic flow in subsequent systole. Color flow showed a two dimensional display of the aortic regurgitation jet (mid panel) in patient with acute severe breathlessness and intermittent syncopal episodes

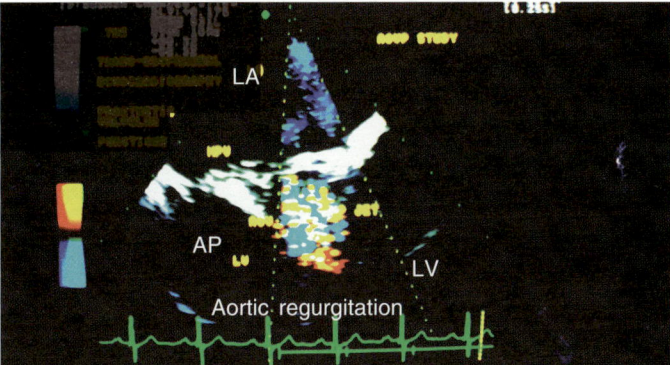

Fig. 17.27: TEE view in color mode showing mosaic color jet of mild aortic regurgitation, AP = Aortic prosthetic valve, LA = Left atrium, LV = Left ventricle

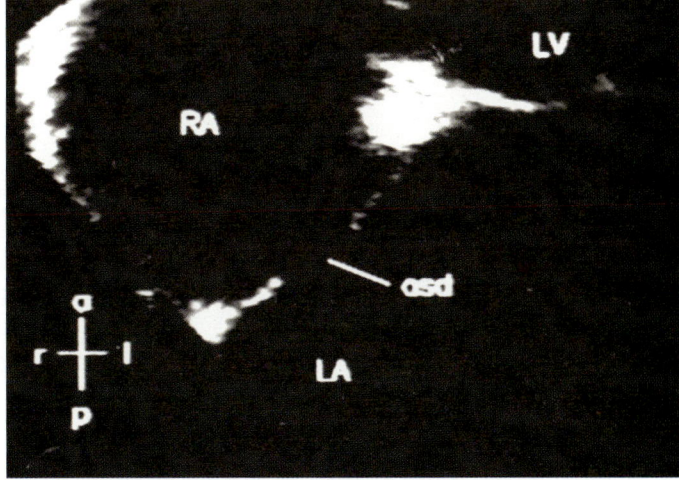

Fig. 17.28: A big atrial septal defect of secundum (ASD) type with dilated right atrium. RA = Right atrium, LA = Left atrium

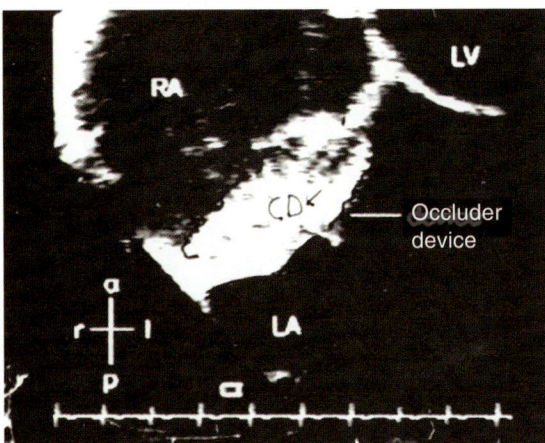

Fig. 17.29: Showing ASD Occluder device in position at the location of defect completely covering the defect in the management of congenital atrial septal defect

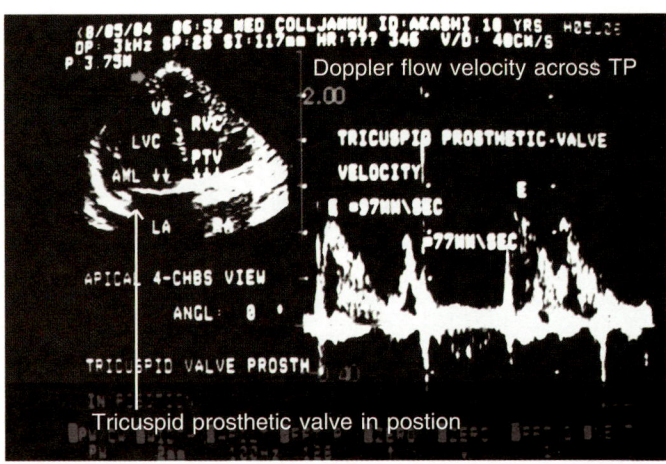

Fig. 17.30: Doppler flow velocity across prosthetic tricuspid valve in young girl with congenital tricuspid regurgitation with progressive right heart failure

Tricuspid Valve Prosthesis in PrimaryTricuspid Regurgitation along with Epicardial Pacemakers in a Young Child

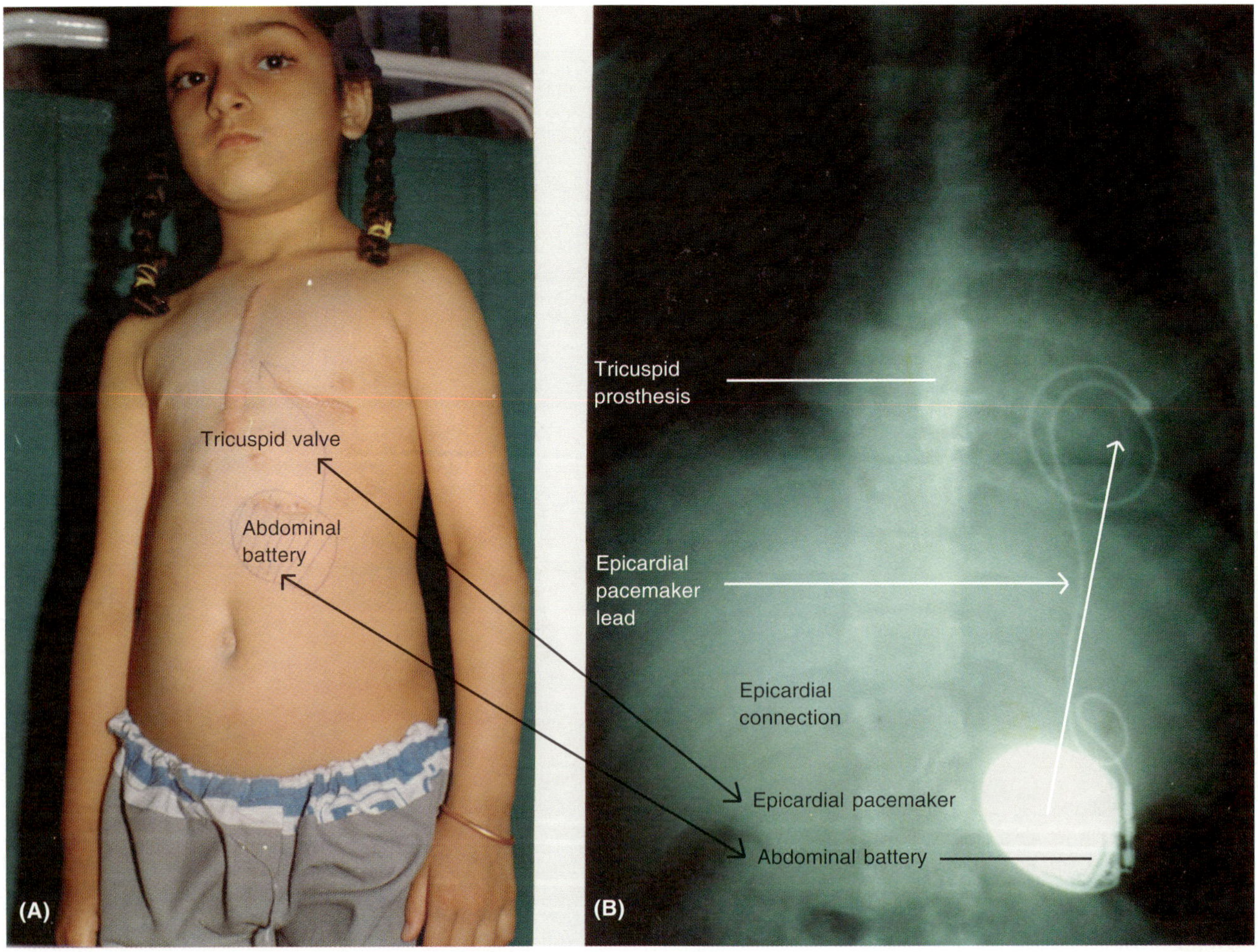

Fig. 17.31A and B: (A) 10 years old girl was suffering from progressive severe form of primary tricuspid regurgitation with CCF with dyspnoea on exertion since her childhood. She was fully investigated and decided to replace tricuspid prosthetic valve but during operation she developed complete heart block for which epicardial pacemaker was installed. **(B)** X-ray photograph showing epicardial connection with heart and battery has been placed in the abdominal cavity as indicated with long arrow. She is now 22 yrs old and is found normal on cardiovascular follow up

Interatrial Aneuryrsm Presenting as Halo Sign in the Middle of Left Atrium

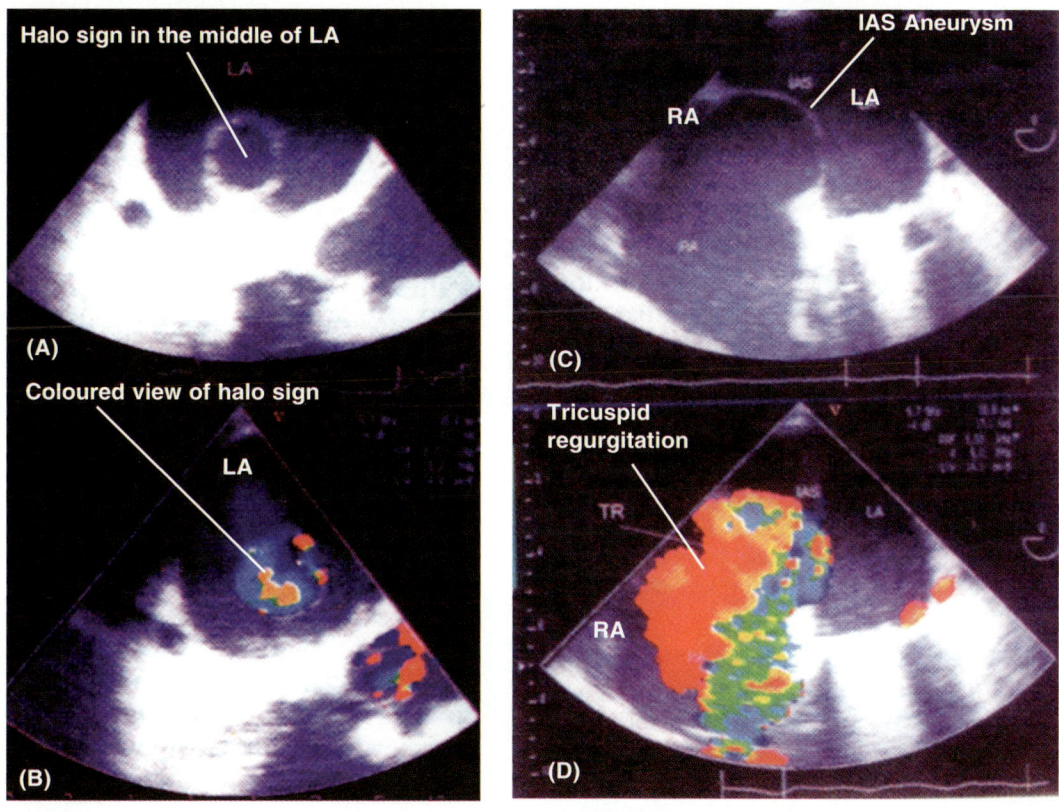

Fig. 17.32 A to D: TEE Views showing halo sign in the middle of the left atrium on the proximal view. Color Doppler imaging showed a isolated colored halo image and there was no communication between this image and the left atrial wall of prosthetic mitral valve. This colored image was only be found during systolic period and would disappear during diastole. Decremental rotation of the probe angle revealed a large interatrial aneurysm type II and moderate tricuspid regurgitation which was eccentrically positioned toward the aneurysmatic pouch. None of the paravalvar prosthetic mitral regurgitation was detected in a middle aged person suffering from rheumatic heart disease with severe mitral valve stenosis, mitral regurgitation and moderate tricuspid regurgitation and in whom St. Jude prosthetic mitral valve had been replaced

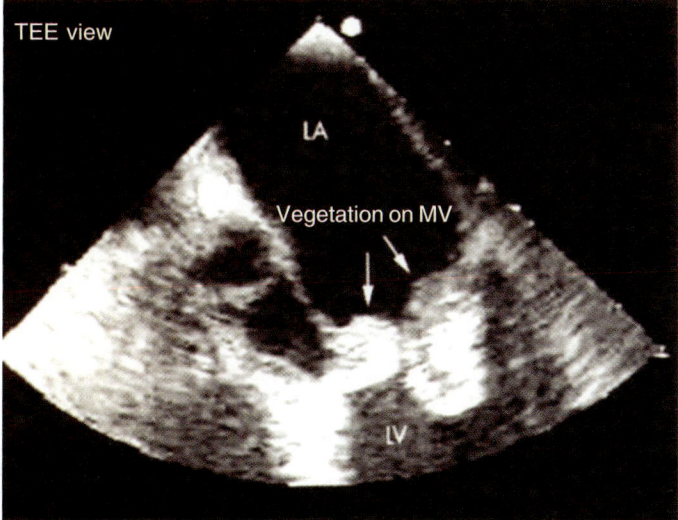

Fig. 17.33: TEE View showing large vegetation (arrow) in the prosthetic mitral valve secondary to fungal endocarditis

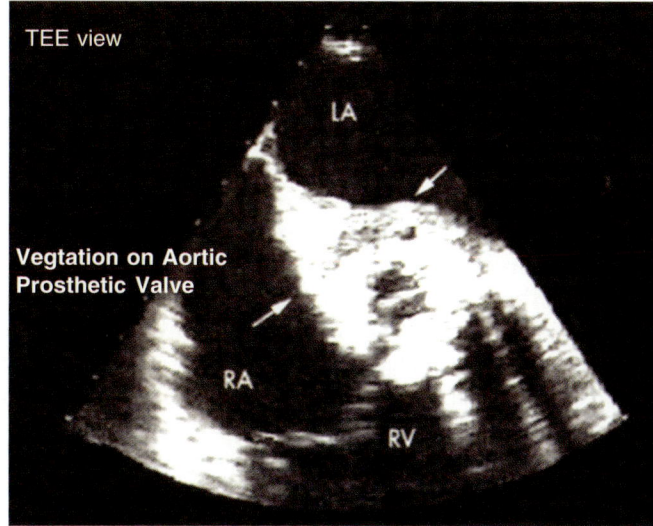

Fig. 17.34: TEE View showing periannular abscess (arrows) in a prosthetic valve endocarditis

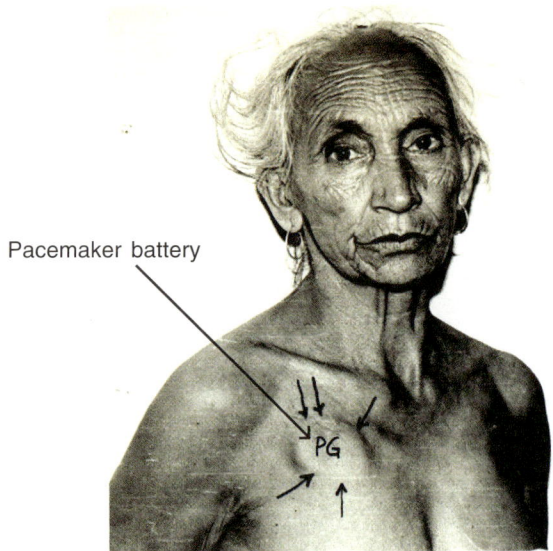

Fig. 17.35: Permanent transvenous pacemaker was implanted in this elderly women with atherosclerotic coronary heart disease and complete A-V dissociation at JMC hospital by the author

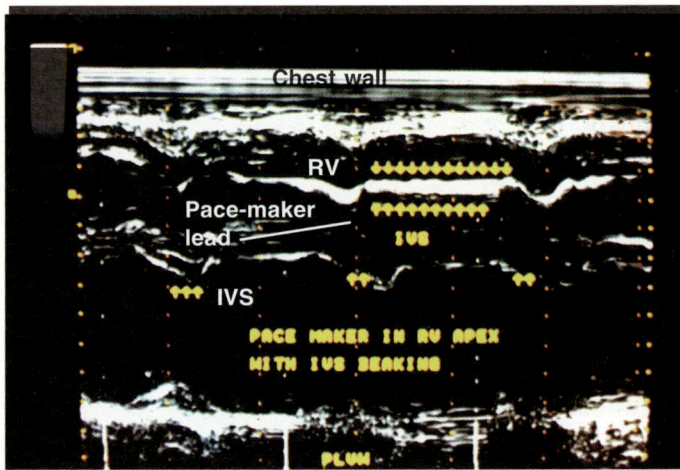

Fig. 17.36: M-Mode echocardiogram showing an organized pacemaker lead in the right ventricle cavity (arrows) with beaking of interventricular septum (arrows) in patient with complete heart block in whom permanent pacemaker was installed by the author

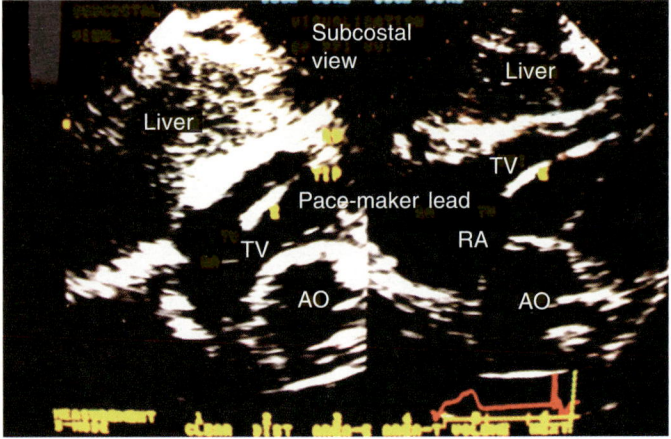

Fig. 17.37: Subcostal plane in short axis at aorta in dual scan view showing tracking of pacemaker lead entering from right atrium to right ventricle

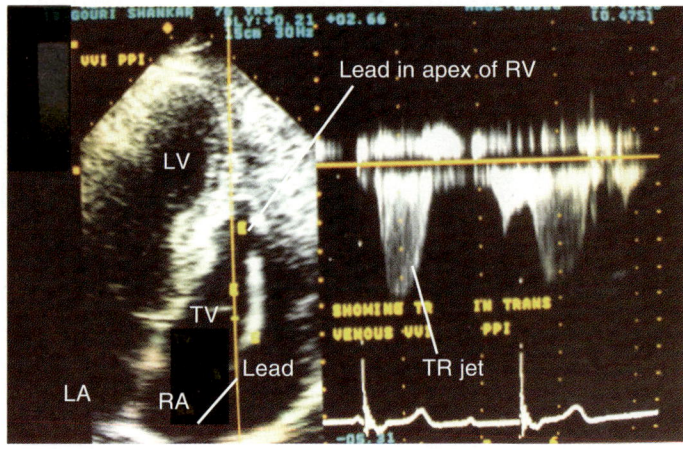

Fig. 17.38: (left) 2D Apical 4C views and Doppler echocardiography showing pacemaker (VV1) lead entering from right atrium to right ventricular apex as marked on the scan. Right panel showing mild to moderate tricuspid regurgitation 3 months after the implantation of permanent pacemaker

Doppler Assessment of Aortic Valve Function
(Fig. 17.26)

The ability to record insufficiency is usually quite good with the aortic valve prosthesis; the sample volume is placed in the left ventricular outflow tract, beneath the aortic prosthesis. In addition to the apical four-chamber view, the suprastenal approach should be used to record the regugitant jet in the ascending aorta.

Tricuspid Valve (Figs 17.30 and 17.31A and B)

It is often confusing to evaluate a patient with two or three prosthetic valves, and careful examination must be done to separate each of the valves. With routine cardiac sweeps, the transducer may record the individual valves to help the sonographer to evaluate the most perpendicular axis. Then the transducer can be moved to the tricuspid area or to of the heart to record the maximum amplitude of the valves.

Doppler Assessment of Tricuspid Valve Function
(Figs 17.31A and B and 17.38)

The Doppler evaluation of tricuspid prosthetic valve dysfunction would be approached in a manner similar to that for the mitral valve evaluation. Care must be taken to avoid the reflections from the prosthetic device so that they do not interfere with the Doppler reflections.

Evaluation of Pacemakers (Figs 17.35–17.38)

Echocardiography can also evaluate the pacing lead, and its placement in the cardiac chamber. It can also assess its functioning with respect to fracture and thrombosis formation.

Bibliography

1. Bansal RC, Morrison DL, Jacobson JG. Echocardiography of porcine aortic prosthesis with flail leaflets due to degeneration and calcification *Am Heart J* 1984;107:591–593.

2. Barratt-Boyes BG, Roche AH, Subramanyan R, Pemberton JR, Whitlock RM. Long-term follow-up of patients with the antibiotic-sterilized aortic homograft valve inserted freehand in the aortic position. *Circulation* 1987;75:768–777.

3. Baumgartner H, Khan S, DeRobertis M, Czer L, Marer G. Effect of prosthetic aortic valve design on the Doppler – catheter gradient correlation: An in vitro study of normal, St. Jude, Medtronic-Hall, Starr-Edwards and Hancock valves. *J Am Coll Cardiol* 1992;19:324–332.

4. Baumgartner H, Schima H. Kuhn P. Effect of prosthetic valve malfunction on the Doppler- catheter gradient relation for bileaflet aortic valve prostheses. *Circulation* 1993;87:1320–1327.

5. Bjork VO. A new tilting disc valve prosthesis. *Scand J Thorac Cardiovac Surg* 1969;3: 1–10.

6. Cannegieter SC, Rosendaal FR, Briet E. Thromboembolic and bleeding complications in patients with mechanical heart valve prostheses. *Circulation* 1994;89:635–641.

7. Chastre J, Trouillet JL. Early infective endocarditis on prosthetic valves. *Eur Heart J* 1995 (SupplB);16:32.

8. Garcia MJ, Vandervoort P, Stewart W, Lytle B, Cosgrove D, Thomas J, Griffin BP. Mechanisms of hemolysis with mitral prosthetic regurgitation: A study using transesophageal echo and fluid dynamic simulation. *J Am Coll Cardiol* 1996;27: 399–406.

9. Garcia MJ. Prosthetic valve disease. In: *Textbook of Cardiovascular Medicine. Topol Ej. Lippincott Raven*. Philadelphia 1997;579–606.

10. Gueret P, Vignon P, Fournier P, Chabernaud JM, Gomez M, La Croix P, Bensaid J. Transesophageal echocardiography for the diagnosis and management of nonstructive thrombosis of mechanical mitral valve prosthesis. *Circulation* 1995;91:103–110.

11. Hanania G, Thomas D, Michel PL, Garbarz E, Age C, Millaire A, Acar, J. Pregnancy and prosthetic heart valves. A French cooperative retrospective study of 155 cases. *Eur Heart J* 1994;15:1651–1658.

12. Heras M, Chesebro JH, Fuster V, *et al*. High risk of thromboemboli early after bioprosthetic cardiac valve replacement. *J Am Coll Cardiol* 1995;25:1111–1119.

13. Kolter MN, Goldman A, Parry WR. Noninvasive evaluation of cardiac valve prostheses. *Cardiovasc Clin* 1986;17:201–241.

14. Ledain LD. Ohayon JP. Colle JP, *et al*. Acute thrombotic obstruction with disc valve prostheses: diagnostic considerations and fibrinolytic treatment. *J Am Coll Cardiol* 1986;7:743–751.

15. Levine RA. Jimoh A. Cape EG, *et al*. Pressure recovery distal to a stenosis: potential cause of gradient "overestimation" by Doppler echocardiography. *J Am Coll Cardiol* 1989;1306–715.

16. Linden PA. Cohn LH. Medium-term follow up of pulmonary autograft aortic valve replacement: technical advances and echocardiographic follow up. *J Heart Valve Dis* 2001;10:35–42.

17. Lowry RW, Zoghbi WA, Baker WB, Wray RA, Quinones MA. Clinical impact of transesophageal echocardiography in the diagnosis and management of infective endocarditis. *Am J Cardiol* 1994; 73:1089–1091.

18. Magilligan DJ Jr, Lewis JW Jr, Stein P, Alam M. The porcine bioprosthetic heart valve: Experience at 15 years. *Ann Thorac Surg* 1989;48:324–329.

19. McHenry MM. Smeloff EA. Fong WY. *et al*. Critical obstruction of prosthetic heart valves due to lipid absorption by Silastic. *J Thorne Cardiovasc Surg* 1970;59:413–425.

20. Mohr-Kahaly S. Kupferwasser T. Erbel R, *et al*. Regurgitant flow in apparently normal valve prostheses: improved detection and semiquantitative analysis by transesophageal two-dimensional colour coded Doppler echocardiography. *J Am Echocardiogr* 1990;3:187–195.

21. Morguet AJ. Werner GS. Andreas S. *et al*. Diagnostic value of transesophageal compared with transthoracic echocardiography in suspected prosthetic valve endocarditis. *Heart* 1995;20:390–398.

22. Morton MJ, Rahimtgoola SH. How to follow patients with prosthetic heart valves. *J Cardiovasc Med* 1980;5:475–495.

23. Nellessen U. Masuyama T. Appleton CPO *et al*. Mitral prosthesis malfunction. Comparative Doppler echocardiographic studies of mitral prostheses before and after replacement. *Circulation* 1989; 79:330–336.

24. Nettles RE. McCarty DE. Corey GR. *et al*. An evaluation of the Duke criteria in 25 pathologically confirmed cases of prosthetic valve endocarditis. *Clin Infect Dis* 1997; 25:1401–1403.

25. Onoda K, Yasuda F, Takao M, *et al*. Long-term follow-up after Carpentier-Edwards ring annuloplasty for tricuspid regurgitation. *Ann Thorac Surg* 2000;70:796–799.

26. Otto CM, Yoganathan AP, Brandon T. Fluid dynamics of prosthetic valves. In: Otto CM. ed. *The Practice of Clinical Echocardiography*. 2nd Ed. Philadelphia: WB Saunders. 2002:514–518.

27. Panldis P, Ross J, Mintz GS, Normal and abnormal prosthetic valve function as assessed by Doppler echocardiography. *J Am Coll Cardiol* 1986;8:317–326.

28. Puleo JA, Fontanet HL, Schocken DD. The role of prolonged thrombolytic infusion and transesophageal echocardiography in thrombosed prosthetic heart valves: Case report and review of the literature. *Clin Cardiol* 1995;18:679–684.

29. Rahimtoola SH. The problem of valve prosthesis-patient mismatch. *Circulation* 1978:58:20–24.

30. Rosenhek R. Binder T. Maurer G. Baumgartner H. Normal values (or Doppler echocardiographic assessment of heart valve prostheses. *J Am Soc Echocardiogr* 2003;16:1116–1127.

31. Ross DN. Replacement of aortic and mitral valve stenosis with a pulmonary autograft. *Lancet* 1967:2:956–958.

32. Rothbart RM, Castriz JL, Harding LV, *et al*. Determination of aortic valve area by two-dimensional and Doppler echocardiography in patients with normal and stenotic bioprosthetic valves. *J Am Coll Cardiol* 1990;15:817.

33. Sand RM, Barbetseas J. Olmos L, *et al.* Application of the continuity equation and valve resistance to the evaluation of St. Jude Medical prosthetic aortic valve dysfunction. *Am J Cardiol* 1977;80: 1239–1242.

34. Shively BK, Gurule FT, Roldan CA. *et al.* Diagnostic value of transesophageal compared with transthoracic echocardiography in infective endocarditis. *J Am Coll Cardiol* 1991;18:391–397.

35. Tischler MD, Cooper KA, Rowen M, *et al.* Mitral valve replacement mitral valve repair. A Doppler and quantitative stress echocardiographic study. *Circulation* 1994; 89:132–137.

36. Tong AT. Roudaut R. Ozkan M, *et al.* Transesophageal echocardiography improves risk assessment of thrombolysis of prosthetic valve thrombosis: results of the international PRO. *J Am Coll Cardiol* 2004;43:77–84.

37. Vanden Brink RB, Visser CA, Basart DC, Duren DR, de Jong AP, Dunning AJ. Comparison of transthoracic and transesophageal colour Doppler flow imaging in patients with mechanical prostheses in the mitral valve position. *Am J Cardiol* 1989;63:1471–1474

38. Vandervoort PM, Greenberg NL, Powell KA. *et al.* Pressure recovery in bileaflet heart valve prostheses. Localized high velocities and gradients in central and side orifices with implications for Doppler catheter gradient relation in aortic and mitral position. *Circulation* 1995;92:3464–3472.

39. Watarida S. Shirnishi S, Nishi T, *et al.* Strut fracture of Bjork.Shiley convexo-concave valve in Japan risk of small valve size. *Ann Thorne Cardiovasc Surg* 2001;7:246–249.

40. Weyman AE. Principles of flow. In: *Principles and practice of Echocardiography.* Weyman, AE. 2nd edn., Lea and Febiger. Philadelphia, 184–200.

41. Wilkes HS. Berger M. Gallerstein PE, *et al.* Left ventricular outflow obstruction after aortic valve replacement: detection with continuous wave Doppler ultrasound recording. *J Am Coli Cardiol* 1983;1: 550–553.

42. Wilkins GT. Gillam LD, Kritzer GL, *et al.* Validation of continuous wave Ryan T, Armstrong WF, Dillon JC, *et al.* Doppler echocardiographic measurements of mitral and tricuspid prosthetic valve gradients: a simultaneous Doppler-catheter study. *Circulation* 1986;4:786–795.

43. Williams GA, Labovitz AJ. Doppler hemodynamic evaluation of prosthetic (Starr-Edwards and Bjork-Shiley) and bioprosthetic (Hancock and Carpentier-Edwards) cardiac valves. *Am J Cardiol* 1985;56:325–332.

44. Xie GY. Bhakta D, Smith MD. Echocardiographic follow up study of the Ross procedure in various younger patients. *Am Heart J* 2001 142:331–335.

45. Yoganathan AP. Flow characteristics of prosthetic heart valves. *Int J Cardiovasc Imaging* 1989;4:5–8.

46. Young E. Shapiro SM, French WJ, *et al.* Use of transesophageal echocardiography during thrombolysis with tissue plasminogen activator of a thrombosed prosthetic mitral valve. *J Am Sue Echocardiogr* 1992;5:153–15.

47. Zoghbi WA. Desir RM. Rosen L, *et al.* Doppler echocardiography: application to the assessment of successful thrombolysis of prosthetic valve thrombosis. *J Am Sue Echocardiogr* 1989;2:98–101.

18

Echocardiographic Evaluation of Conduction Defects and Cardiac Arrhythmias

M-Mode and Doppler echocardiographic approach can be of great help in evaluating and understanding abnormalities of electrical activation. It would help in providing knowledge as to how changes in cardiac electrical activity can influence the echocardiogram.

Conduction Blocks

Left Bundle Block (Figs 18.1, 18.4–18.6 and 18.10)

Patients with left bundle branch block (LBBB) serve as an excellent example of how altered electrical depolarization can influence cardiac motion. The echocardiography in patients with left bundle branch block usually reveals abnormal motion of the interventricular septum (IVS), during ventricular ejection which may be considered as an important hemodynamic consequence of this electrical abnormality. This abnormal septal motion during ejection bring significant hemodynamic changes in ventricular functions, particularly during diastole. Although septal motion is usually paradoxic during ventricular ejection in LBBB but it may not be found in all the patients. The early systolic dip or beaking immediately following electrical depolarization is considered as a diagnostic sign on echocardiography in LBBB. It has also been seen that in RBBB when septal motion is paradoxical during ventricular ejection, the patient usually has a more severe form of the disease with a wider QRS large left ventricle and reduced ejection fraction. This abnormality on echocardiography has been linked to the altered path of depolarization, which has been further verified by noticing almost identical abnormality on both ECG and echocardiography in right ventricular pacing. The abnormal early systolic septal motion is also seen secondary to an early rise in the right ventricular pressure due to the development of pressure difference in left and right ventricles

consequence to the abnormal depolarization in LBBB. However, smaller and an early septal beaking can be considered as a variant of normal in certain individuals even in the absence of LBBB on echocardiographic scans.

Right Bundle Branch Block

Right bundle branch block (RBBB) when compared to LBBB usually does not show any echocardiographic abnormality in region of septum. However, one may find certain changes in intervals between closure of the mitral, tricuspid and pulmonary valves. This difference in intervals of closure of valves in RBBB has been used in the localization of block in the upper or in the lower part of the conduction system. When the delay is found in the closure of mitral and tricuspid valves (MVc-TVc) the block is usually considered in the proximal portion of the right bundle and when there is increase in interval between closure of tricuspid and pulmonary valves; is in the distal portion of the right bundle (Fig. 18.34).

Pre-Excitation Syndrome
(Wolff-Parkinson-White Syndrome)

In type A W-P-W syndrome, one may find abnormal motion of the posterior left ventricular wall. It is a brief anterior displacement of the posterior left ventricular wall following the onset of electrical depolarization. Whereas in type B W-P-W syndrome a sharp and brief downward or posterior dip of the interventricular septum may appear after the electrical depolarization as it happens in the case of LBBB (Figs 18.8 and 18.9).

Conduction Abnormalities (Heart Block)

In case of prolonged atrioventricular conduction or heart block, there is:

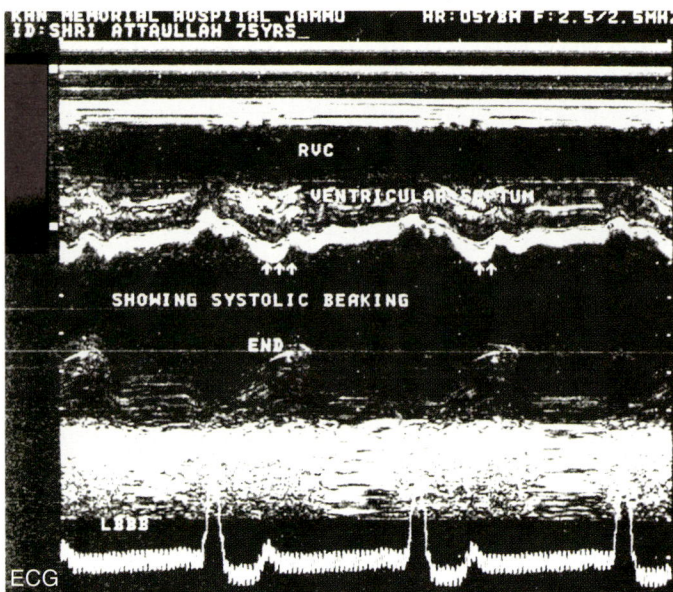

Fig. 18.1: M-Mode echocardiogram showing an early systolic beaking (arrow) in left bundle branch block (LBBB) in patient with coronary artery disease and hypertension

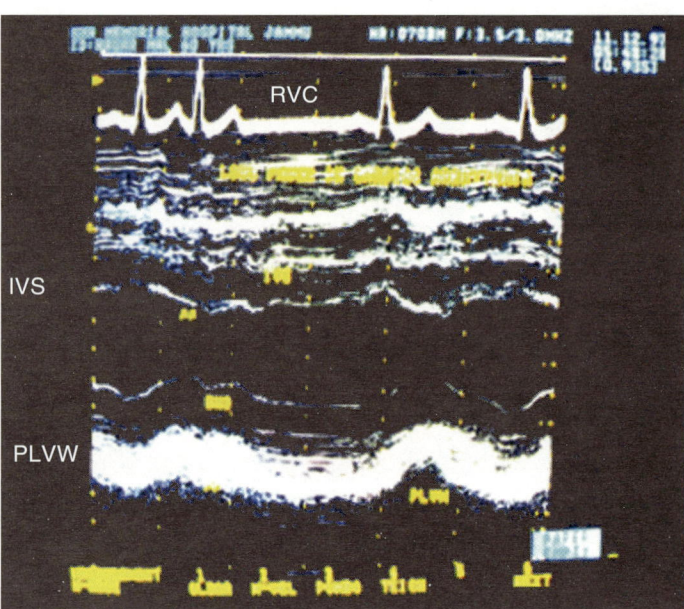

Fig. 18.3: M-Mode echocardiogram at LV cavity showing normal IVS and PLVW movements

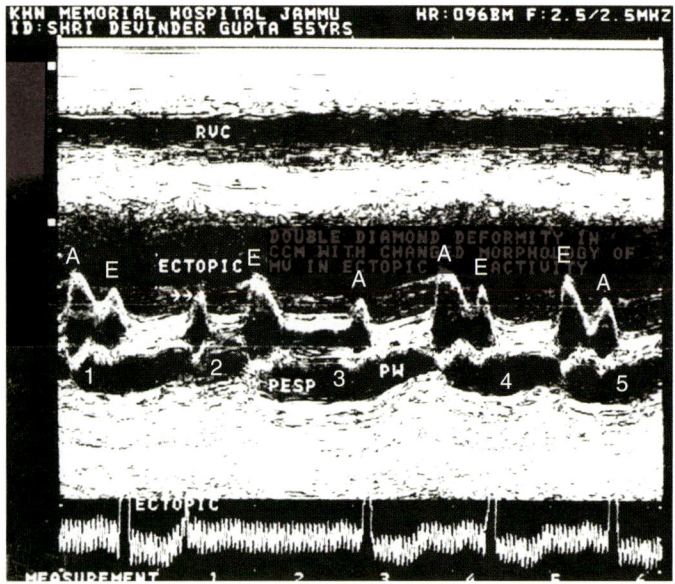

Fig. 18.2: M-Mode echocardiogram showing incomplete (opening) configuration of mitral valve echo in isolated SVE followed by complete echo of mitral valve but with increased duration between E and A points without any alteration in MV morphology in five beats scan 1 = N, 2 = APC, (atrial premature contraction) 3. Post-extra systolic period MV morphology 4 = N 5 = N, i.e. N = Normal)

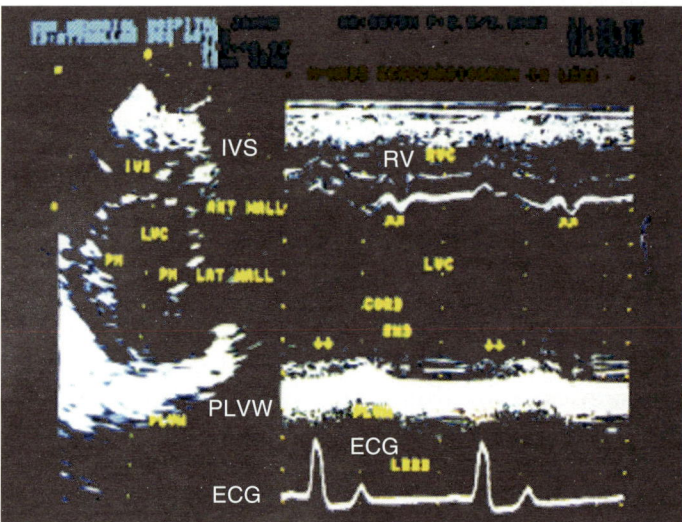

Fig. 18.4: 2-D Short-axis LV (left) and M-mode echocardiogram (right) showing downward early systolic contraction (systolic beaking) along interventricular septum in left bundle branch block in patient with CAD, HT, LBBB with poor LV function

1. Premature closure of the mitral valve due the fact that mitral valve closes before the onset of ventricular systole in a patient with first degree A-V block and a prolonged P-R interval. This echocardiographic event is in turn, dependent on atrial systole which is not synchronous with ventricular contraction in prolonged A-V conduction or heart block.

2. A dip of the pulmonary valve follow each P wave on the electrocardiogram. The C point which represents opening of the valve following ventricular systole remains related to ventricular depolarization. Thus echocardiogram may be helpful in identifying P wave when it is not possible to trace on routine electrocardiographic study in complete heart block with atrial fibrillation or other type of arrhythmias.

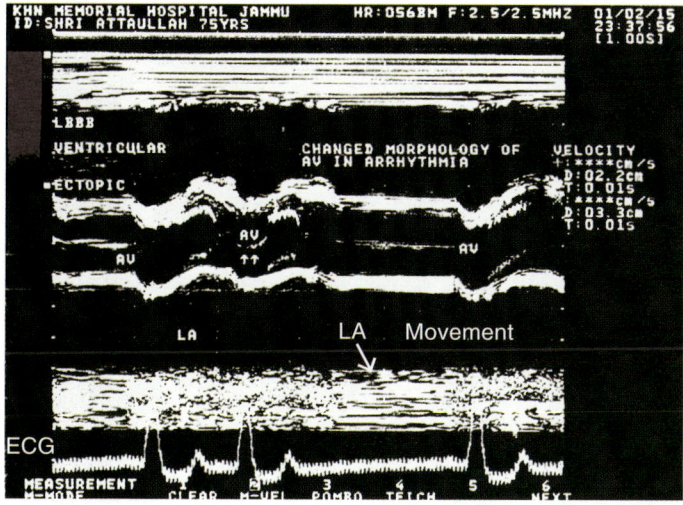

Fig. 18.5: M-Mode echocardiogram showing brief (ejection period) opening of aortic valve followed by no flow in post-extrasystolic period, minimal contraction of anterior LA wall and then by vigorous opening of aortic valve after premature contraction in patient with CAD, LBBB and premature contraction

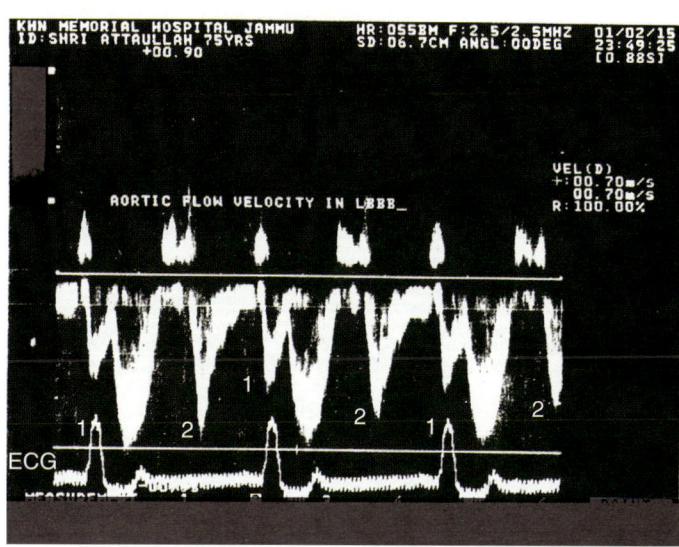

Fig. 18.6: Doppler flow velocity across aortic valve in patient with wide QRS LBBB showing double stroke morphology of aortic flow. 1 = normal is being followed by 2 = smaller ejection flow in patient with CAD, LBBB and poor LV functions

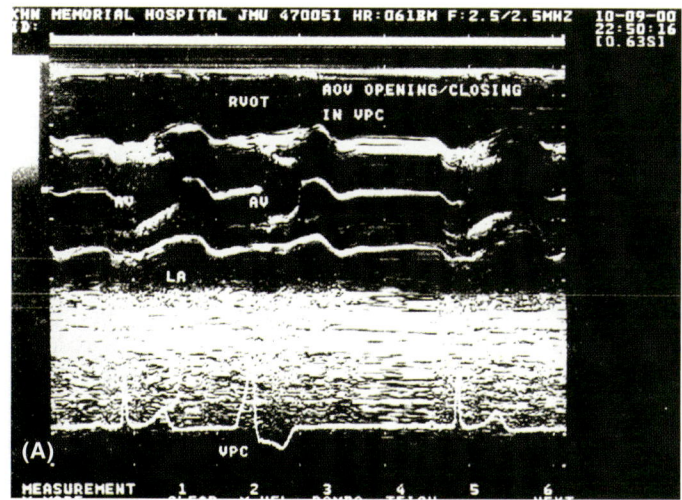

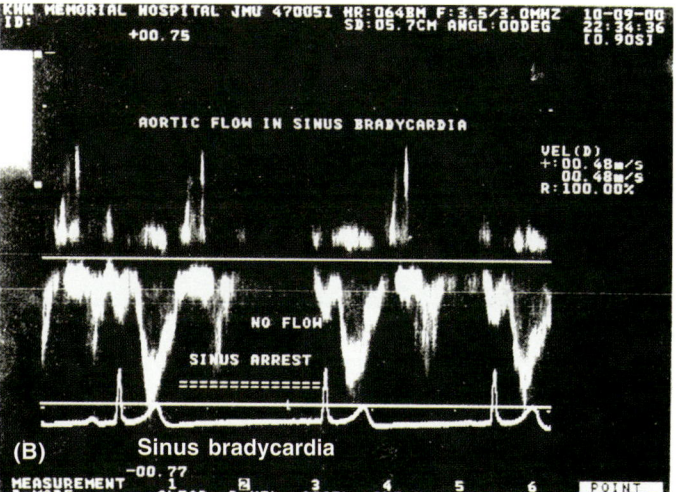

Fig. 18.7A and B: (A) M-Mode echocardiogram showing premature opening of aortic valve with short ejection time during episode of isolated premature ventricular contraction. **(B)** Normal flow velocity across aortic valve during normal beats but negligible or no flow during sinus arrest with at times smaller flows in sinus bradycardia in patient with sick sinus syndrome

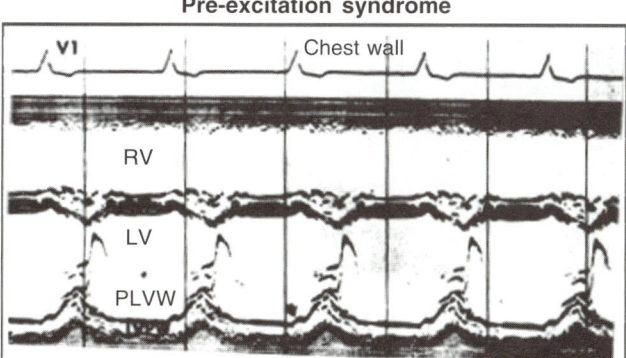

Fig. 18.8: M-Mode echoardiogram at the level of LV cavity showing premature contraction or anterior motion (arrow) along the posterior left ventricular wall in patient with Wolff-Parkinson-White syndrome type A

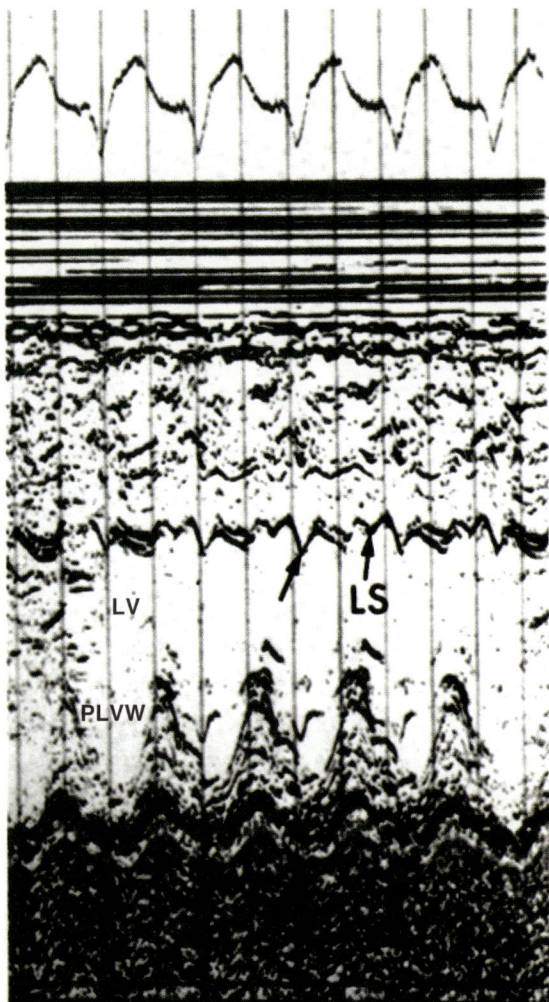

Fig. 18.9: M-Mode echocardiogram showing an early systolic downward beaking (arrow) in patient with type B Wolff-Parkinson-White syndrome

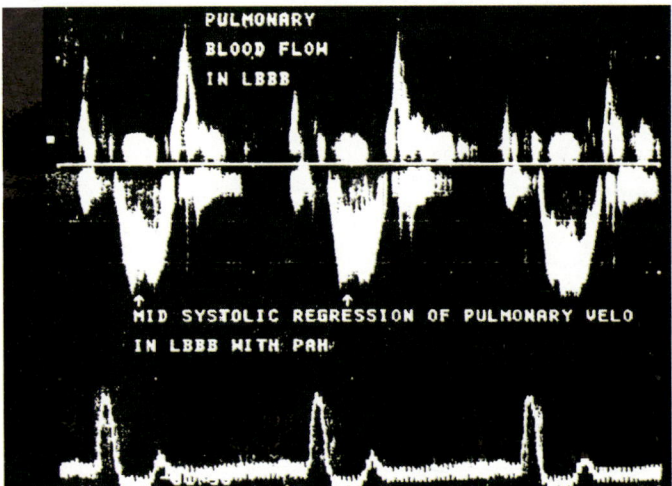

Fig. 18.10: Doppler flow across pulmonary valve showing systolic regression in LBBB as it happens with pulmonary arterial hypertension which was associated in this patient with hypertension with poor LV function

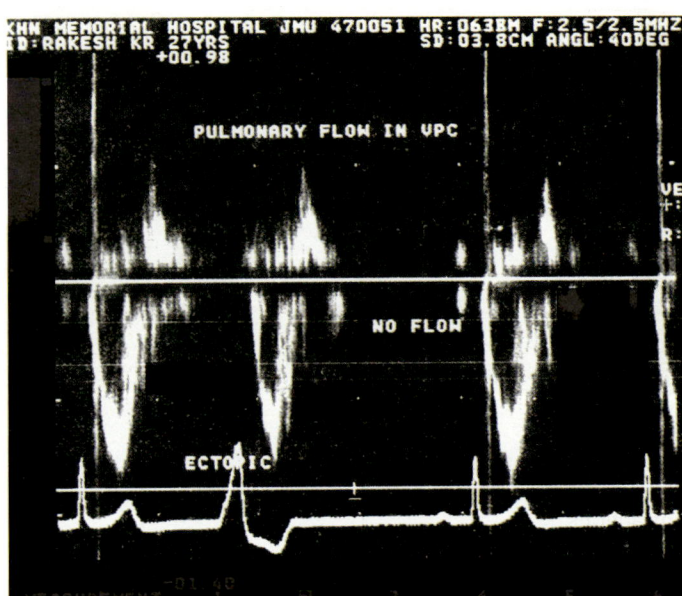

Fig. 18.11: Doppler flow velocity across pulmonary valve showing slightly lesser velocity flow at ventricular premature contraction (beat 2) followed by a vigorous velocity flow after accumulation of good volume during post-extrasystolic period (beat 3). Beats 1 and 4 are normal beats

3. Echocardiogram may show diastolic mitral regurgitation (dMR) in prolonged P-R interval, second degree A-V heart block and in third degree heart block. (Figs 18.16A and B, 18.17, 18.18, 18.20 and 18.28).

Accessary Pathways

Echocardiography has been employed for the localization of accessory pathways with the help of a sensitive phased digital imaging technique. This method incorporates finding out of minimal and mean phased angles of various left ventricular wall segments. Thereafter a comprehensive histogram is generated to determine the homogeneity of segmental contraction. Later the phase angle sequence is calculated to estimate the contraction sequence. The angles are displayed in colour format and these regional specific colours therefore determine the premature segmental mobility in the type of accessory pathway under study.

Cardiac Arrhythmias (Figs 18.2 and 18.5)

Premature Beat

It has been shown that premature beat does bring hemodynamic alterations by virtue of premature systole, it therefore, also affects the motion of either interventricular septum (IVS) or the posterior ventricular wall. These alterations are attributed to the abnormal path of depolarization as it occurs in conditions such as LBBB; W-P-W syndrome or electrical pacing. Echocardiographically, a wave of the mitral

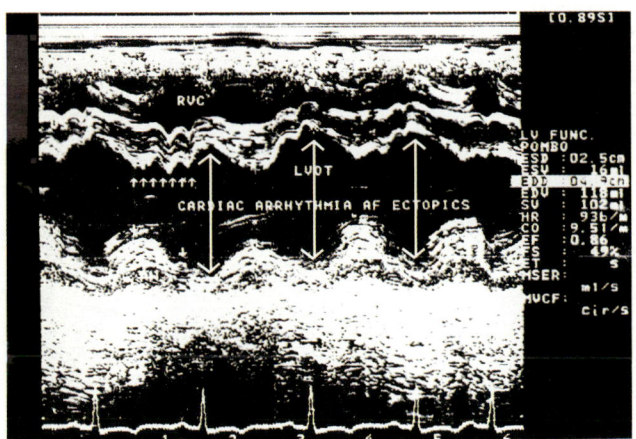

Fig. 18.12: M-Mode echocardiogram showing variations in cardiac volumes (vertical lines/dimensions) and irregular septal wall contractions (arrows) in patient with supraventricular cardiac arrhythmia

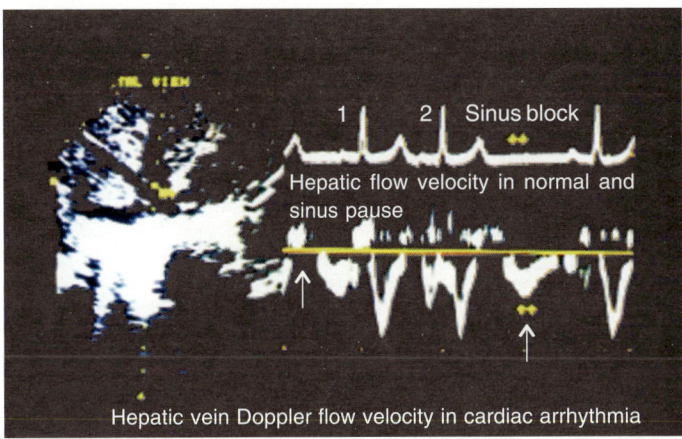

Fig. 18.15: Subcostal transhepatic view of visualization of hepatic venous system showing normal pulsed Doppler flow velocity in hepatic vein during two normal beats and minimal flow during sinus pause (arrows) in patient with sinus block

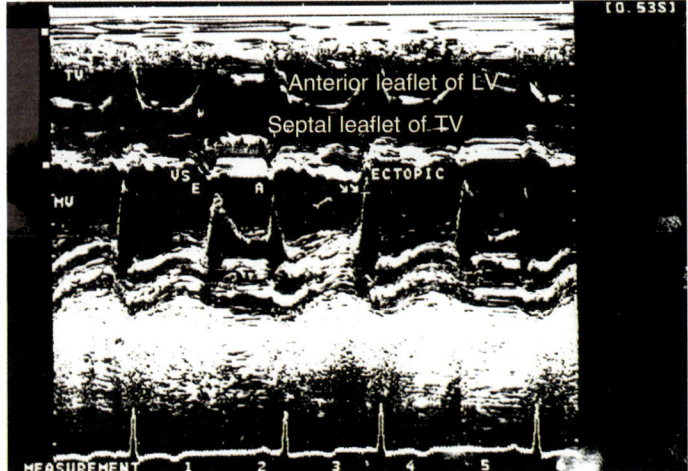

Fig. 18.13: M-Mode echocardiogram at mitral valve motion during premature atrial contraction showing incomplete opening morphology of mitral valve with almost negligible E-A point separation. Beat 1 = Premature atrial contraction. Beat 2 = Normal beat. Beat 3 = Premature atrial contraction. Beat 4 = Premature atrial contraction. Similar changes are being seen on TV simultaneously

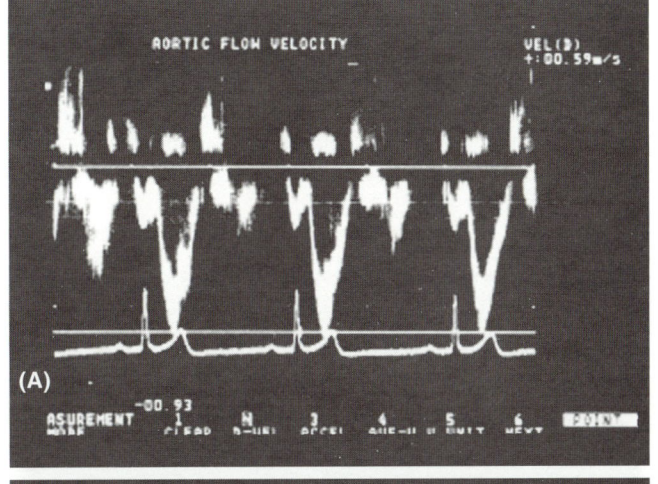

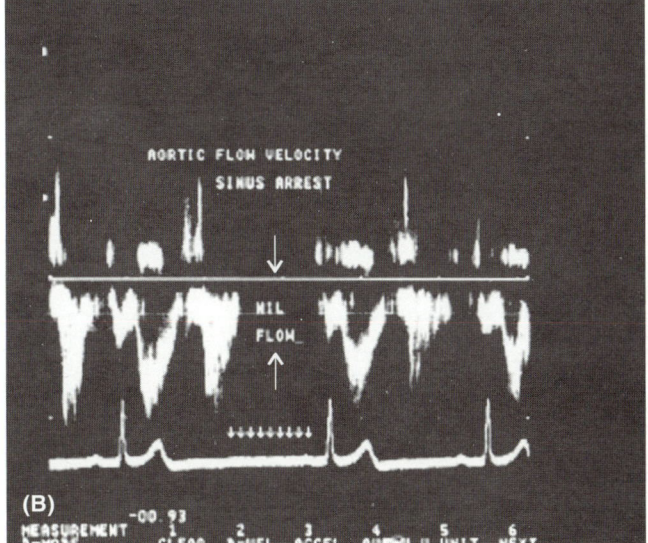

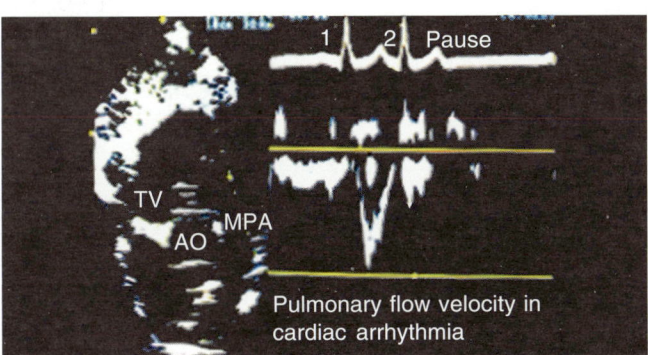

Fig. 18.14: Subcostal great vessels view and short axis at aorta showing normal flow in pulmonary artery during first beat minimal flow in second and absent flow in sinus pause

Fig. 18.16A and B: **(A)** Doppler flow velocity at aorta showing normal flow. **(B)** Minimal and nil flow (arrows) during prolonged sinus arrest in patient with sick sinus syndrome

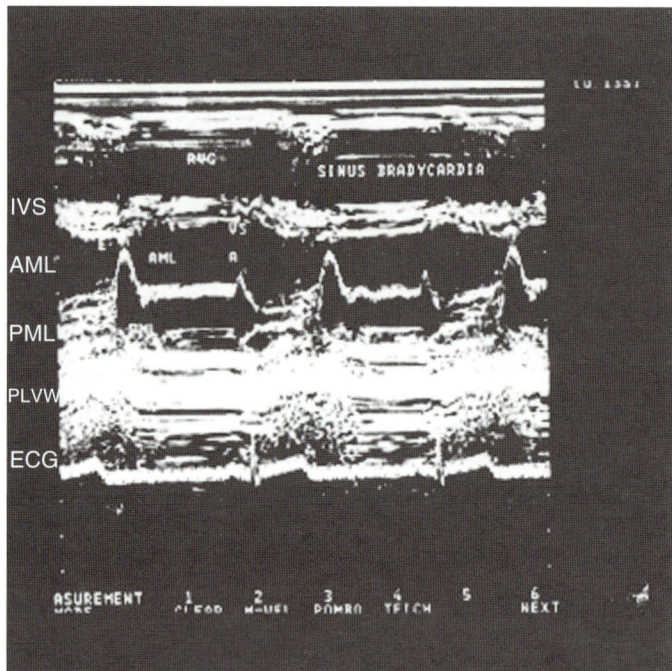

Fig. 18.17: M-Mode echocardiogram showing the effect of brady-cardia on mitral valve. There is widening of interval between points E and A retaining the normal configuration of mitral valve. It also depicts flat movements of both interventricular and posterior left ventricular wall

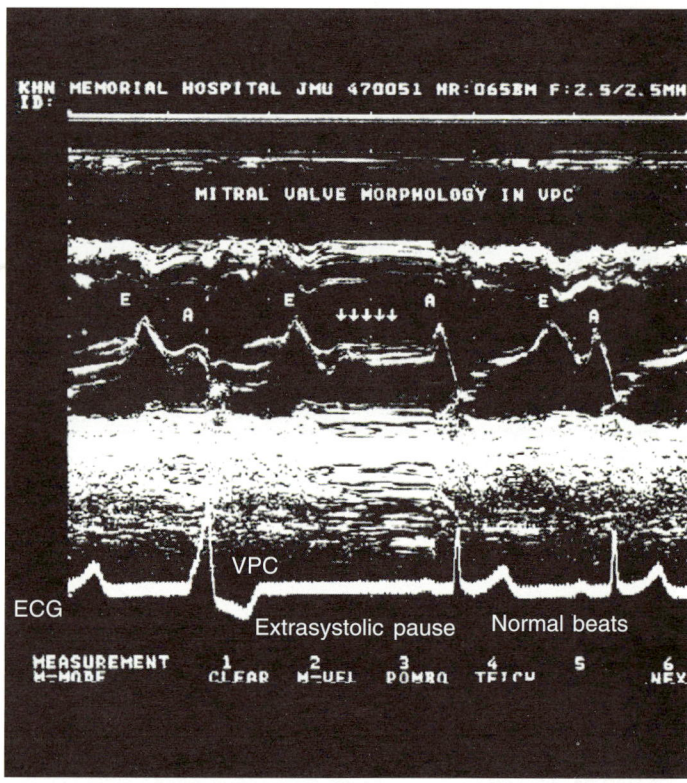

Fig. 18.19: M-Mode echocardiogram showing short DE amplitude of mitral valve opening with wider apart E–A duration during extrasystolic pause (arrows)in patient with isolated ventricular premature contraction

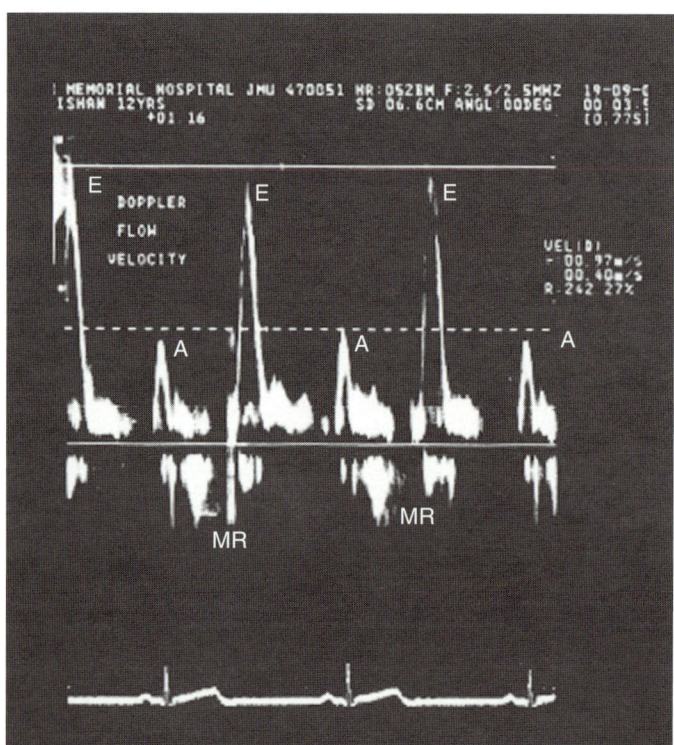

Fig. 18.18: Doppler flow velocity showing the effect of bradycardia on mitral valve velocity. It shows widening the interval of E and A velocities with trace mitral regurgitation along with reduction in LV diastolic velocity (A wave amplitude)

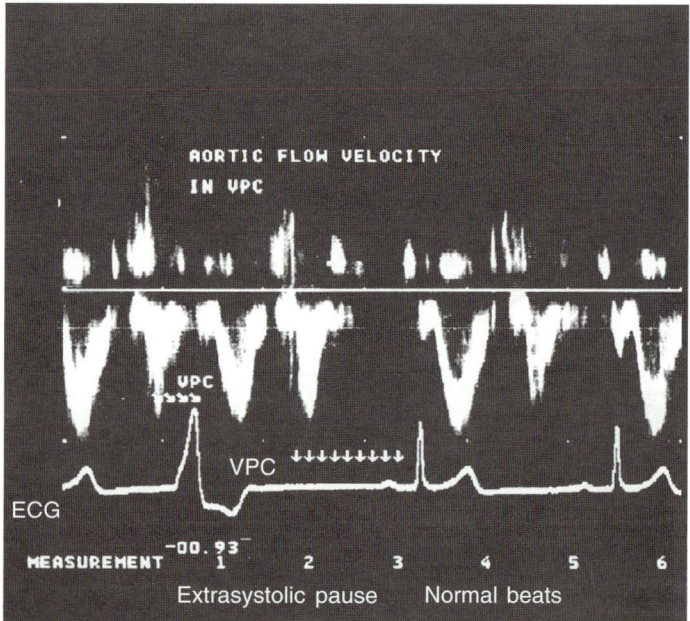

Fig. 18.20: Doppler flow velocity in aorta showing smaller flow velocities during diastole in sinus bradycardia (vertical arrow) and good flow during ventricular premature contraction and nil flow during late post extrasystolic period or prediastolic period prior to the origin of normal sinus beat (arrows) in patient with isolated ventricular premature contraction and sinus bradycardia in sick sinus syndrome

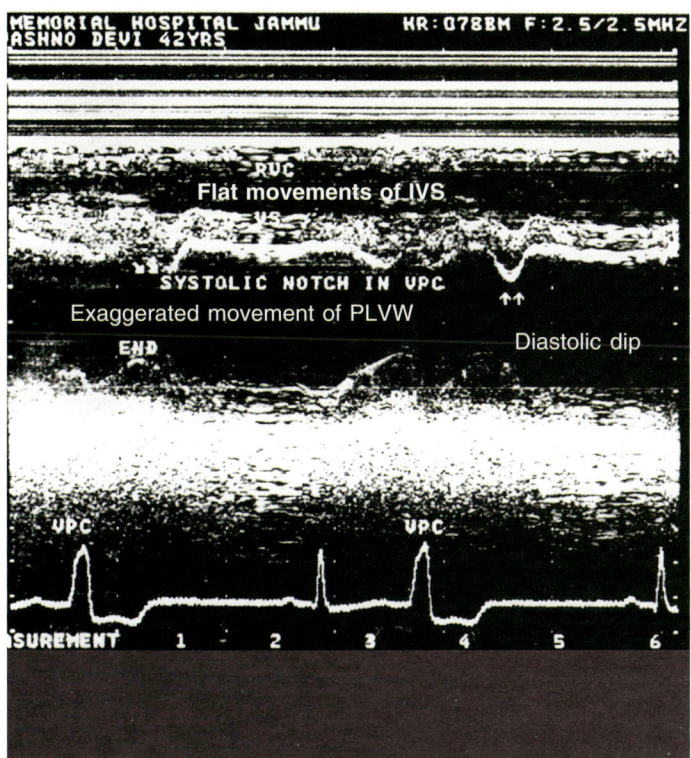

Fig. 18.21: M-Mode echocardiogram showing an early systolic downward beaking of septum in broad QRS ventricular premature contraction (arrows) along with exaggerated diastolic septal dip (arrow) due to flat to absent systolic motion of the septum following ventricular ejection

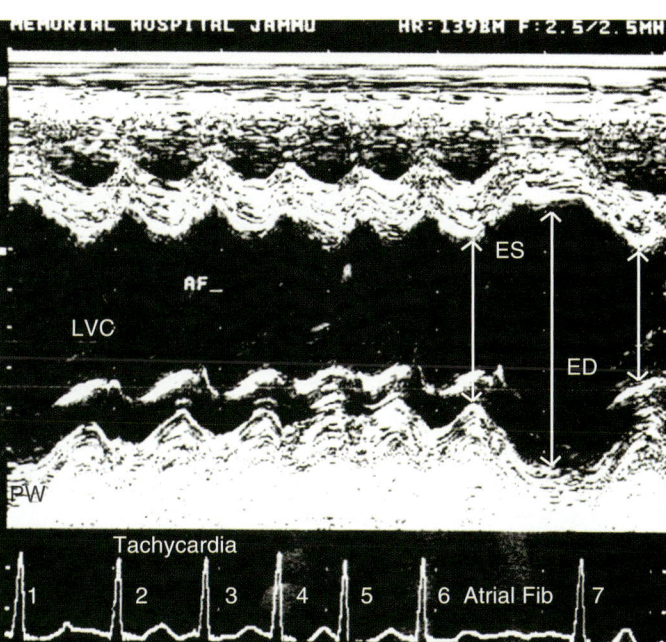

Fig. 18.23: M-Mode echocardiogram showing almost constant endsystolic and enddiastolic volumes along with exaggerated movements of both interventricular septum (IVS) and posterior LV wall (PLVW) (verticle lines) during episode of supraventricular tachycardia but there is increase in both endsystolic and enddiastolic volumes with the onset of atrial fibrillation with slow ventricular response. Note also the absence of IVS and PLVW movements due to lack of ventricular excitation during period of atrial fibrillation (Beat 6–Beat 7) but there is further exaggerated movements of IVS and PLVW with subsequent normal endsystolic and enddiastolic volumes following beat 7

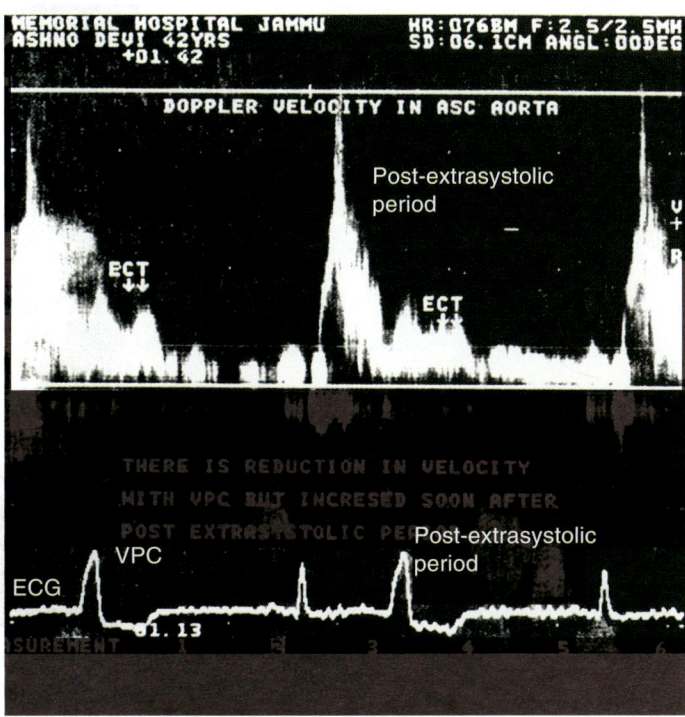

Fig. 18.22: Doppler flow velocity in ascending aorta through suprasternal notch showing minimal aortic flow following premature ventricular contraction (arrows)

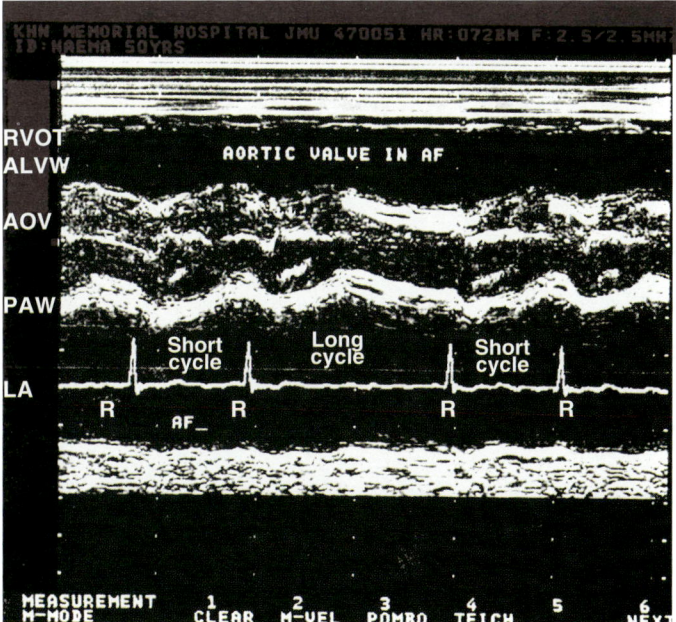

Fig. 18.24: M-Mode echocardiogram showing variable opening of aortic cusps in patient with atrial fibrillation but during periods of long ventricular cycle (arrows) there is hardly any opening of aortic valve (bold line on aortic echo)

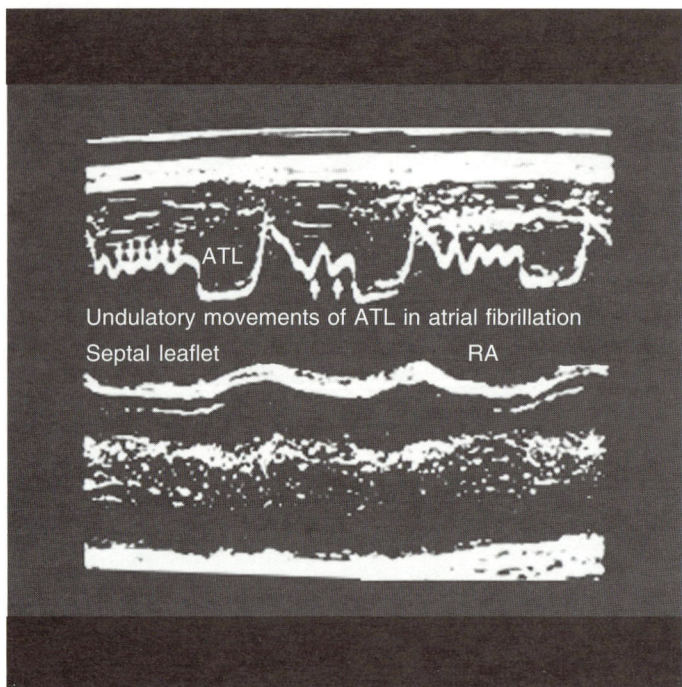

Fig. 18.25: M-Mode echocardiogram showing undulatory waves (arrows) on anterior tricuspid leaflet (ATL) in patient with mitral stenosis with atrial fibrillation SL = Septal leaflet, RA = Right atrium

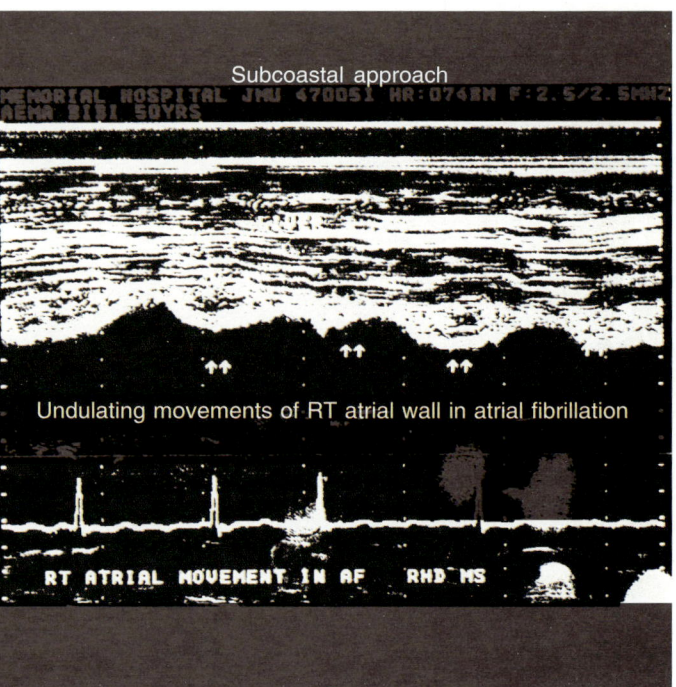

Fig. 18.27: Subcostal approach. M-Mode echocardiography showing undulating movements of right atrial wall in patient with atrial fibrillation (arrows)

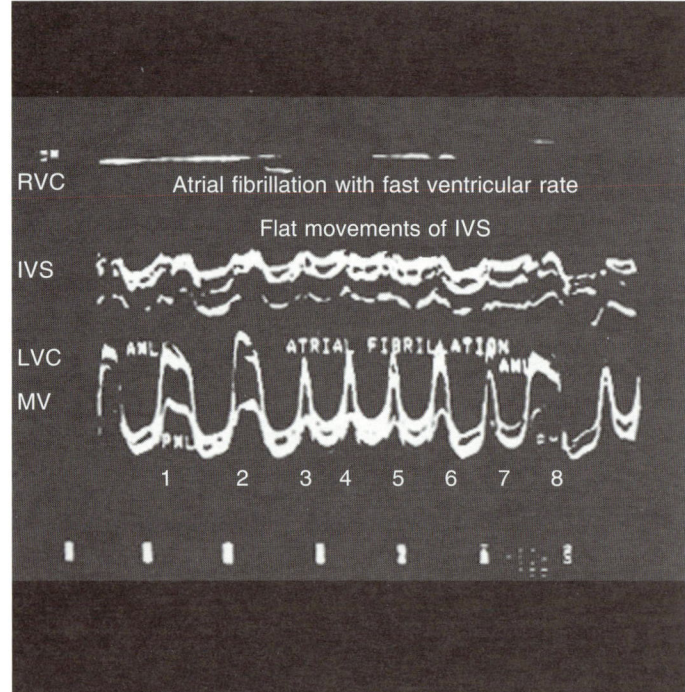

Fig. 18.26: M-Mode echocardiogram showing incomplete opening of mitral valve(almost atrial A waves only) with fast ventricular response (beats 3–7) in patient with rheumatic mitral valvular stenosis with atrial fibrillation. Note also the minimal to flat movements of interventricular septum (IVS) from beats 3–7 followed by normal thickening of IVS in cycle 1 and 8 which showed restricted opening of valve due to mitral stenosis

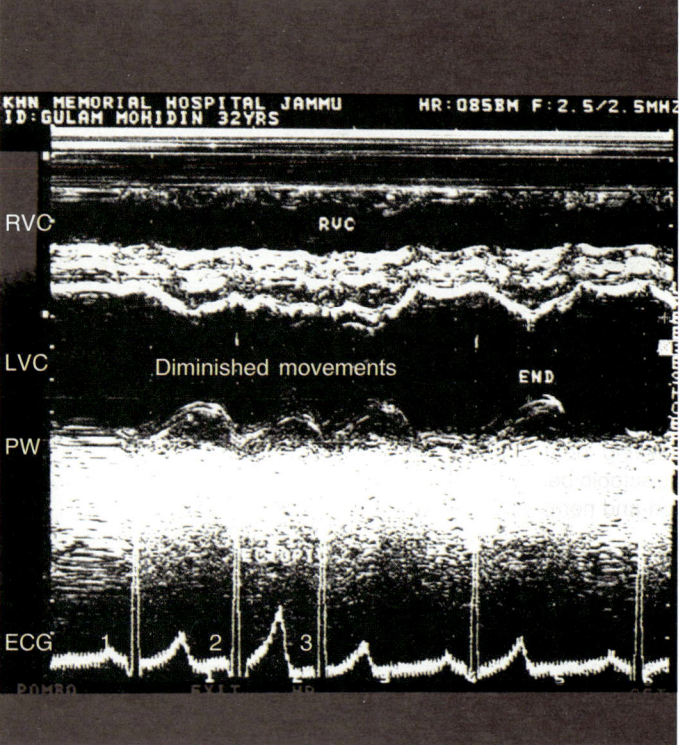

Fig. 18.28: M-Mode echocardiogram showing diminished septal wall and posterior left ventricular wall movements (beats 1–3) along with lower cardiac volumes during an episode of supraventricular tachycardia followed by normal movements during normal sinus rhythm (beats 4–5)

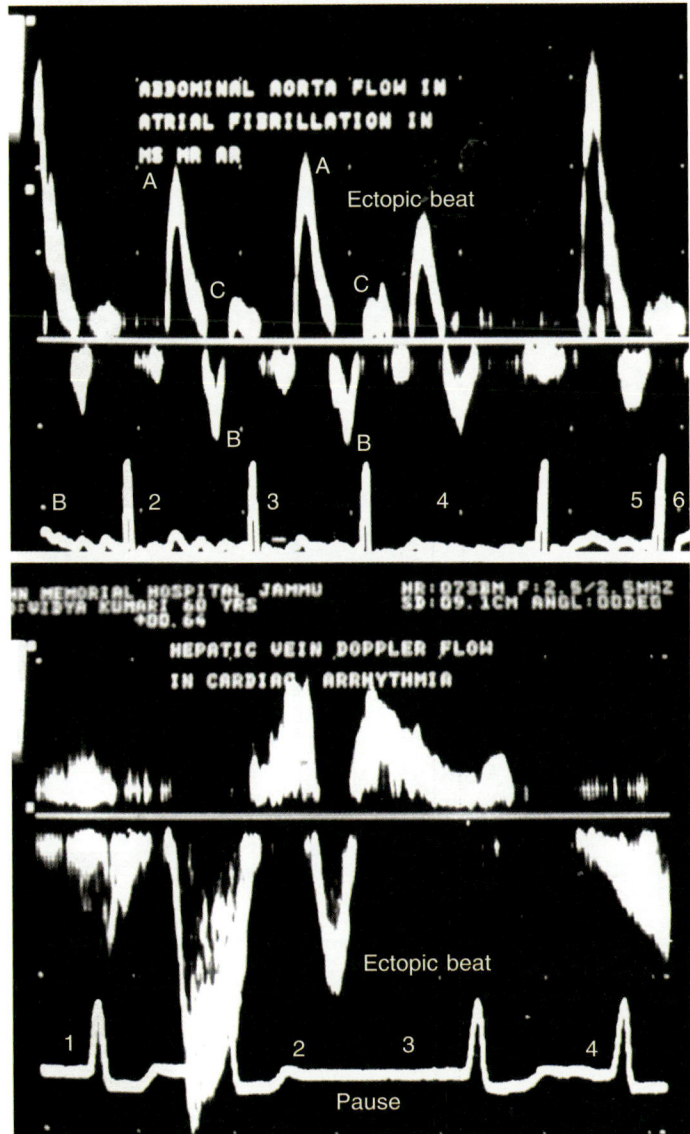

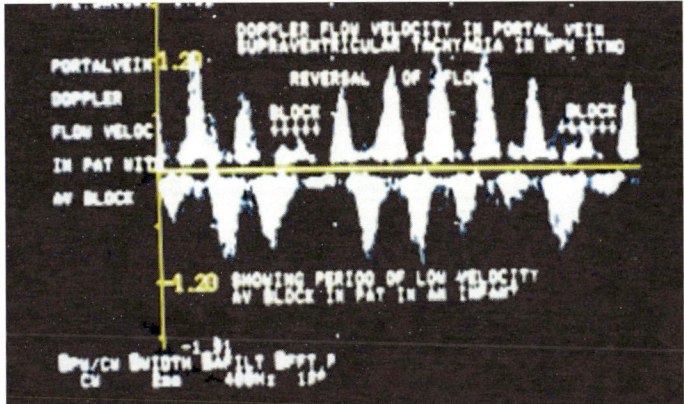

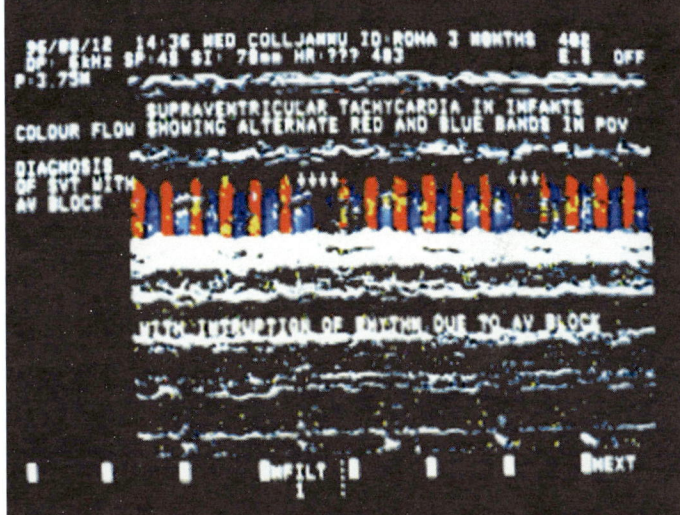

Fig. 18.30A and B: (A) Doppler flow velocity across portal vein showing reversal of flow in tachycardia beats and almost nil flow during A-V block (arrows). **(B)** Color M-Mode echocardiogram at portal vein showing alternate blue and red signatures of flow except missing this link during A-V block (arrows) in 3 months old child with proxysmal atrial tachycardia with block

Fig. 18.29A and B: (A) Pulsed Doppler flow velocity across abdominal aorta showing typical triphasic signatures of one cycle (A, B and C) but velocities are seen diminished (beats 2, 3) and lowest (4th) in patient with rheumatic mitral stenosis, MR, AR and atrial fibrillation. **(B)** Pulsed Doppler flow velocity across hepatic vein showing normal flow in beat 1 exaggerated flow following ventricular ectopic beat 2 and reversal of flow during post-extrasystolic period and normal flow in beats 3 and 4.

valve is aborted in that cardiac cycle as premature beat occurs before atrial depolarization. Systolic motion of the IVS and posterior left ventricular wall (PLVW) is diminished. Diastolic filling in mitral valve echogram is reduced and the ventricular dimension between IVS and PLVW increases because the ventricle is inadequately emptied with the premature beat. Aortic valve opening is reduced in both amplitude and duration. Pulmonary valve is also influenced by the premature beat to the extent that no A wave is seen on pulmonary valve on M-mode echocardiogram with single premature beat but in the presence of two consecutive premature beats a prominent A wave is observed on the pulmonary valve echocardiogram. Appearance of A wave on account of two premature beats is attributed to a change in hemodynamics that has occurred during the premature beats. The premature beats and the long diastolic interval allowed fall in the diastolic pulmonary artery pressure enough to elevate the pressure in the right ventricle to force open the pulmonary valve and thus generate A wave on pulmonary echogram in case of two consecutive premature beats. Motion of IVS and the PLVW is also influenced by the premature beat. Following a ventricular premature beat however, there is downward or posterior displacement of the IVS followed by anterior motion of the septum during ventricular systole almost similar to the LBBB due to abnormal depolarization.

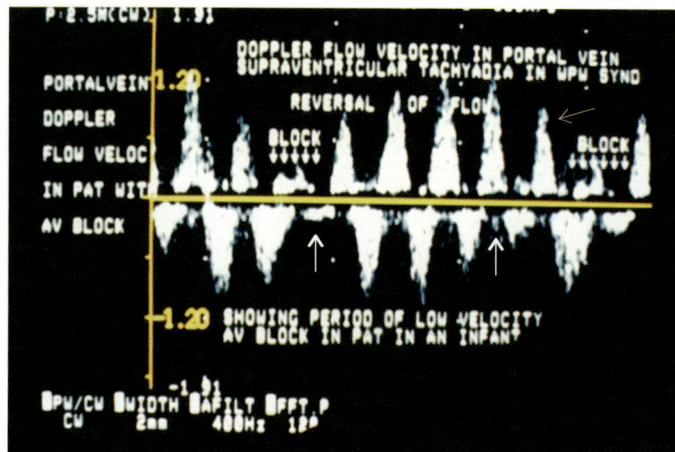

Fig. 18.31: Doppler flow velocity across portal vein showing reversal of flow in tachycardia beats and almost nil flow during A-V block (arrows)

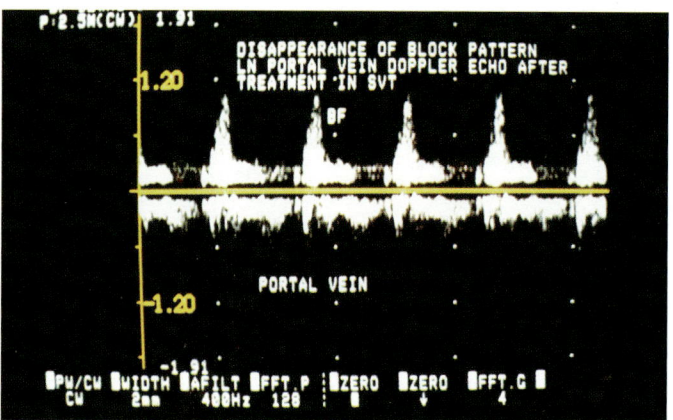

Fig. 18.32: Disappearance of A-V block and nomalization heart rate and portal vein flow after treatment of tachycardia

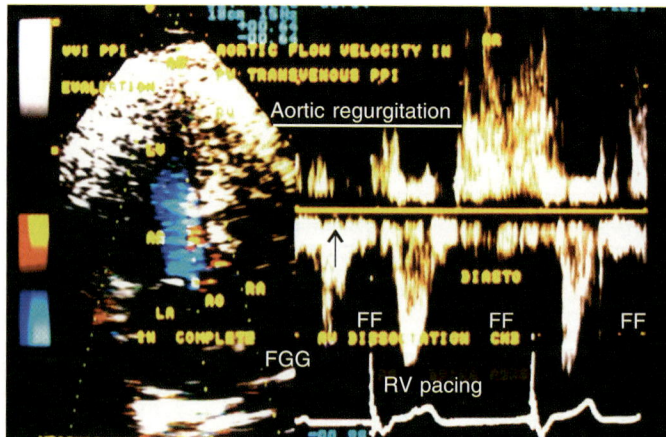

Fig. 18.33: Apical 4C (left) and Doppler flow at aorta (right) in right ventricular pacing in patient with complete heart block showing early systolic forward velocity close to the paced ventricular depolarization (white arrow) prior to true ventricular polarization and mild to moderate aortic valvular regurgitation (blue jet) and Doppler flow study (right)

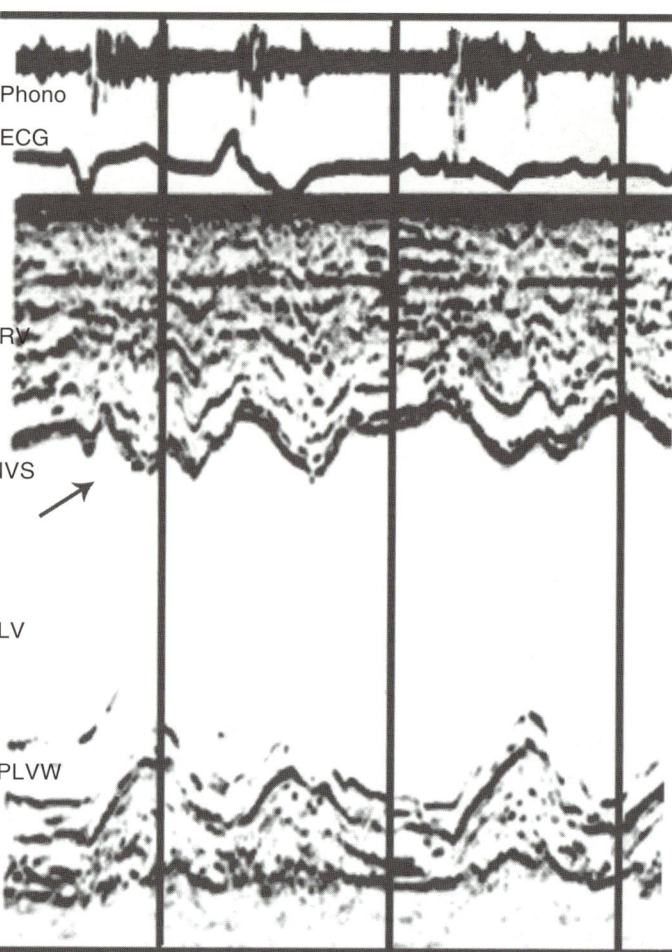

Fig. 18.34: M-Mode echocardiogram showing an early beaking similar to the beaking of LBBB. The first paced beat produces an aberrant depolarization in RV pacemaker implantation

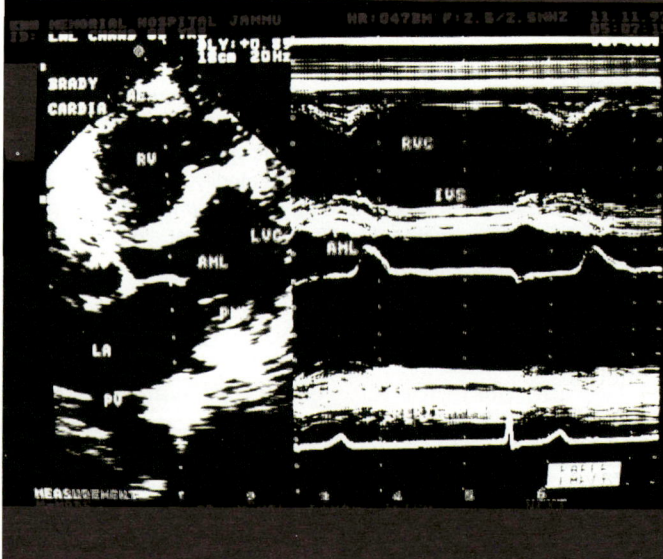

Fig. 18.35: Long axis and M-mode echocardiogram showing an early opening of the mitral valve as seen on M-Mode echogram in prolonged sinus bradycardia in patient with sick sinus syndrome

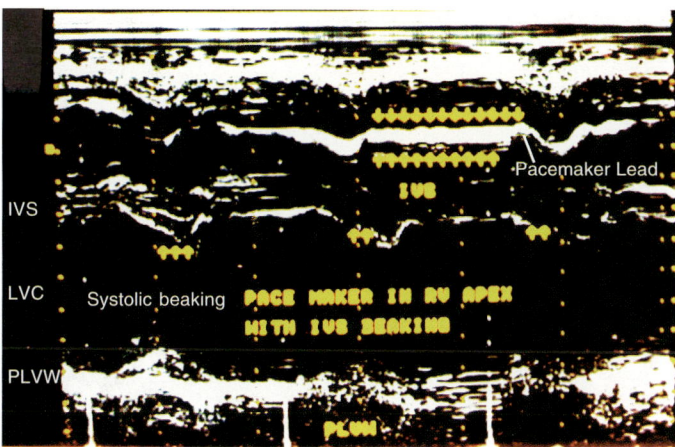

Fig. 18.36: M-Mode echocardiogram showing pacemaker lead traversing through RV (arrows) and creating an early systolic beaking on IVS similar to LBBB during the contraction of interventricular septum (IVS) in RV pacing mode in patient with complete heart block

Supraventricular Arrhythmias (Figs 18.30–18.32)

Sinus Arrhythmia: Changes in mitral valve motion occurs due to varying R-R intervals. The main difference lies in the length of the mid-diastolic filling period. The mitral valve motion in early diastole and late diastole is unchanged by the varying diastolic intervals. The height of the E and A on mitral valve echogram are almost equal in all cardiac cycles (Fig. 18.28).

Premature Atrial Contractions: These have identical effect on echocardiogram as seen in premature ventricular systoles. In *atrial premature beat* there is rapid downward motion of the right atrial wall and the patients with *atrial-fibrillation or flutter* frequently reveal, prominent oscillations of the anterior mitral leaflet and posterior mitral leaflet also moves with the same frequency in its opposite direction as its counterpart anterior mitral leaflet. It has been noticed that with the onset of atrial fibrillation there is often reduction in motion of both IVS and PLVW and decrease in the left ventricular diastolic dimension (Figs 18.23–18.29).

Echocardiographic Evaluation of Different Pacemakers (Figs 18.33–18.36)

The following are the various ways by which echocardiography can be of some help in evaluating functions of different types of pacemakers (Figs 18.34–18.37)

1. Echocardiography can identify atrial mechanical systole after implantation of a dual-chamber pacemaker even without an electrocardiographic P wave.
2. In patients with a ventricular pacemaker Doppler venous flow patterns can differentiate sinus node dysfunction from atrioventricular block.
3. Echocardiography can also differentiate between VVI pacemaker and dual chamber pacemaker by the application of aortic Doppler flow velocities. The flow velocity integral (FVI) is lowest with a VVI pacemaker which stimulates only the ventricles and atrial contractions are asynchronous, on the other hand in dual chamber's pacing (VDD and DVI) where ventricular and atrial contractions are synchronous, the aortic flow is increased.
4. Doppler echocardiography is quite helpful in studying diastolic mitral regurgitation with atrioventricular conduction abnormality. While observing simultaneous Doppler recording of mitral flow velocity and left atrial and left ventricular pressures in patients with heart block, after each of the P waves on mitral echogram; there appears diastolic regurgitation and after the non-conducted P wave this diastolic regurgitation becomes longer.
5. Echocardiography has also the potential of studying the influence of left atrial systolic emptying on left ventricular early filling dynamics by Doppler in patients with sequential atrial ventricular pacemakers. Prolongation of atrioventricular period from 75 to 150 m sec decreases the E wave and increases the A wave of the mitral flow.

Bibliography

1. De Maria AN, Mason DT: Echocardiographic evaluation of disturbances of cardiac rhythm and conduction. *Chest* 1977;71:439.
2. DeMaria AN, Vismara LA, Vera Z, Miller RR, Amsterdam EA, Mason DT: Hemodynamic effects of cardiac arrhythmias. *Angiology*, 1977;28:427.
3. Dillion JC, Chang S, Feigenbaum H: Echocardiographic manifestations of left bundle branch block. *Circulation* 1974;49:876.
4. Drinkovic N: Use of echocardiography in the diagnosis of cardiac arrhythmias. *Pract. Cardiol* 1985; 11:124.
5. Fujii J, Watanabe H, Watanabe T, Takahashi N, Ohta A, Kato K:M-mode and cross-sectional echocardiographic study of the left ventricular wall motions in complete left bundle branch block. *Br Heart J*, 1979;42:255.
6. McDonald, IG: Echocardiographic demonstration of abnormal motion of the interventricular septum in left bundle branch block. *Circulation* 1973;48:272.
7. Wish, M, *et al.* M-mode echocardiogram for determination of optical left atrial timing in patients with dual chamber pacemakers. *Am J Cardiol* 1988;61:319.
8. Xiao HB, Lee CH, Gibson DG: Effect of left bundle branch block on diastolic function in dilated cardiomyopathy. *Br Heart J* 1991;66:443.

19

Echocardiographic Evaluation of Right Heart Diseases

Right Heart Dimensions

There are a few difficulties which may arise in the assessment of dimensions of right ventricle because of its triangular shape as compared to its counterpart left ventricle which almost attains a circular configuration when observed through short-axis view. Right ventricular dimensions are dependent upon the position, transducer placement respiratory phases and proper gain settings (Figs 19.1–19.3).

It has also been seen that the position of the patient affects the observed dimensions of the right ventricular chamber. When the patient lies in a left decubitus position, the right ventricle measures slightly large. In addition, the position of the transducer affects the right ventricular chamber dimensions. Dimensions taken from a low parasternal window are smaller than those obtained from a higher window because of the triangular shape of the right ventricle. It has also been remarked significantly that respiration affects the right ventricular size and function in children. It is, therefore, emphasised that one should be very careful about above-said factors affecting apparent right ventricular dimensions when doing serial comparisons by M-mode echocardiography. One may encounter another difficulty in measuring the right ventricular dimensions in defining the right ventricular anterior wall. Since the right ventricular wall is just behind the chest wall, hence the gain settings of the equipment at the "near field" must be brought lower in order to delineate the anterior free wall of the right ventricular for both M-mode and two-dimensional echocardiography.

While employing multiple views with the help of 2-dimensional echo, one can generate three-dimensional configuration of right ventricle for obtaining appropriate dimensions. The right ventricle is distinguished from the left ventricle by the presence of the moderator band near the apex, and the slight apical displacement of the tricuspid valve compared with mitral valve. However, a few workers have advocated measuring the maximum short-axis dimension of the right ventricle at end diastole and obtaining the area of the right ventricle chamber at end-diastole by planimetry.

Yet another method has been described by Koul, *et al.* to estimate right ventricular function by using the tricuspid valve annular plane. From the apical four-chamber view, a line is drawn from the apex to the tricuspid annular plane. The excursion of the tricuspid valve annular plane from end-diastole to endsystolic is then measured. The resultant tricuspid annular plane systolic excursion has been correlated well with the right ventricular ejection fraction. With the application of 2-dimensional echocardiography automatic border detection (ABD) has been developed in order to obtain instantaneous continuous automatic measurement of areas and volumes. This technique promises to be a useful application in the assessment of right ventricular dimensions but needs further refinement to be adopted finally.

Right Ventricular Volume and Pressure Overload
(Figs 19.4–19.10, 19.14, 19.32, and 19.33)

It has been observed that ASD secundum is the commonest cause of right ventricular overload; is usually with left-to-right shunt. In atrial septal defects with left-to-right shunt of 2:1 or greater, there is usually paradoxical septal motion in addition to right ventricular enlargement. Right ventricular chamber enlargement can be readily demonstrated on two-dimensional echocardiogram from parasternal, apical four-chamber, and subcostal views. However, with its

Anatomical Recognition of Right Heart Structures

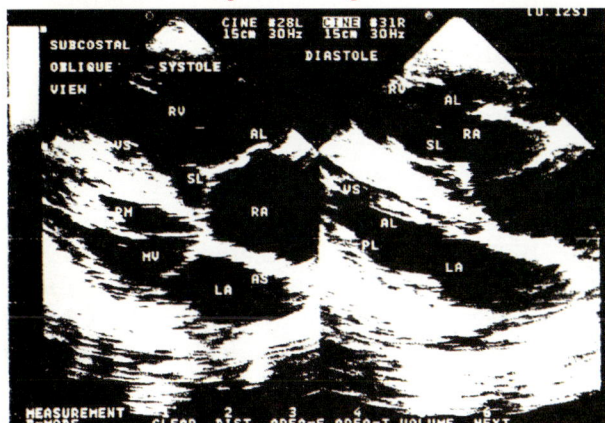

Fig. 19.1: Long axis 4C view through subcostal window showing normal anatomical relationship between chambers and connecting valves of the right heart. RA = Right atrium, RV = Right ventricle, AL = Anterior tricuspid leaflet, SL = Septal leaflet, IVS = Interventricular septum, IAS = Interatrial septum

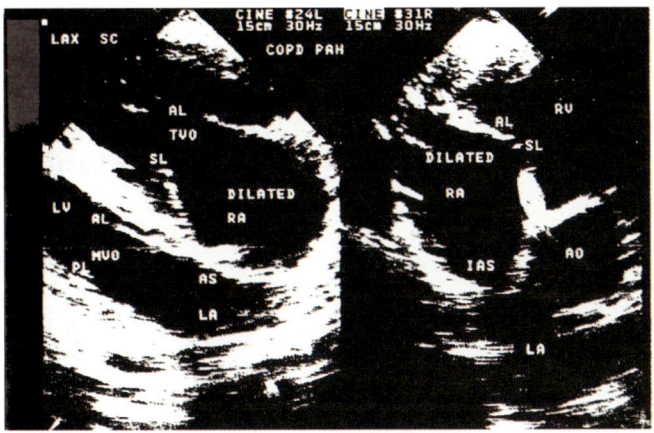

Fig. 19.2: (L-R) 2D. Long axis aorta and short axis views at subcostal window showing anatomical localization of structures of right heart. Anterior (AL) and septal leaflets (SL) of tricuspid valve interatrial septum (IAS). right atrium (RA), tricuspid orifice (TVO), and interventricular septum (IVS)

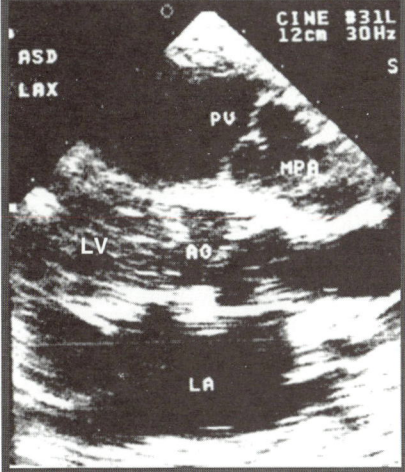

Fig. 19.3: 2-D Short axis view at great vessel level showing anatomical localization of main pulmonary artery (MPA) and its valve (PV) connecting to right ventricle (RV) as constituents of right heart

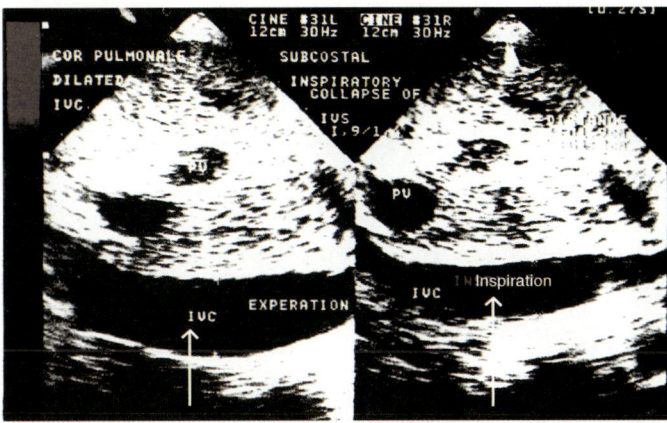

Fig. 19.4: Subcostal approach transverse view through liver showing dilatation of inferior vena cava (left) in elevated right atrial and right ventricular diastolic pressure in right heart failure

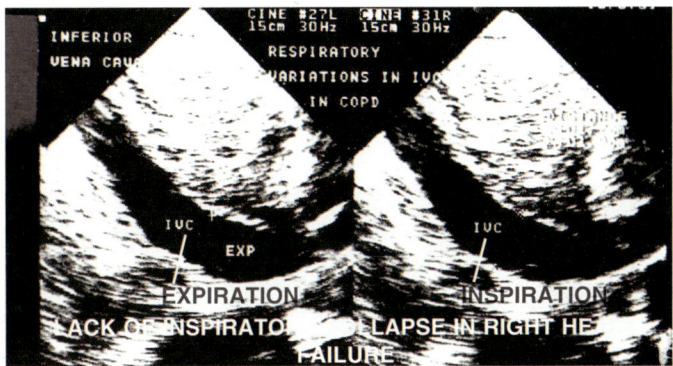

Fig. 19.5: Subcostal approach inferior vena caval view showing distended inferior vena cava and absence of inspiratory collapse during respiration in patient with pulmonary arterial hypertension with right heart failure (Note: There is always >50% reduction of inferior vena caval size during inspiration in normal individual, i.e. inspiratory collapse and lack of this sign therefore, suggests the presence of elevated right atrial and right ventricular diastolic pressure as it usually happens in right heart failure syndrome)

faster sampling rate, M-mode is better suited for the timing of events. In paradoxical septal motion the septum moves anteriorly with onset of systole (i.e. the septum moves in the same direction as the posterior wall). The systolic thickening of the septum is preserved in paradoxical septal motion which distinguished it from left ventricular dysfunction involving the septum.

It is also true to understand that right ventricular dilation may also be seen in right ventricular pressure overload, the interventricular septum is the key to separating right ventricular volume and pressure overload. Some of the workers have categorically shown that the progressive systolic flattening of the septum to convex bulging into the left ventricle at end systole is associated with severe pulmonary hypertension and right ventricular hypertrophy.

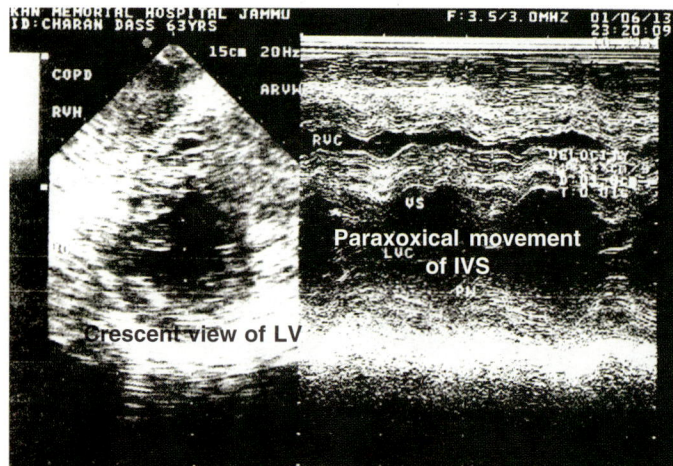

Fig. 19.6: 2-D Subcostal biventricular view (left) and M-mode echocardiogram (right) showing dilatation and hypertrophy of right ventricle with concave configuration of interventricular septum (crescent) and small left ventricular cavity (left panel). Right panel shows paradoxical movement of IVS in patient with chronic obstructive lung disease with pulmonary arterial hypertension

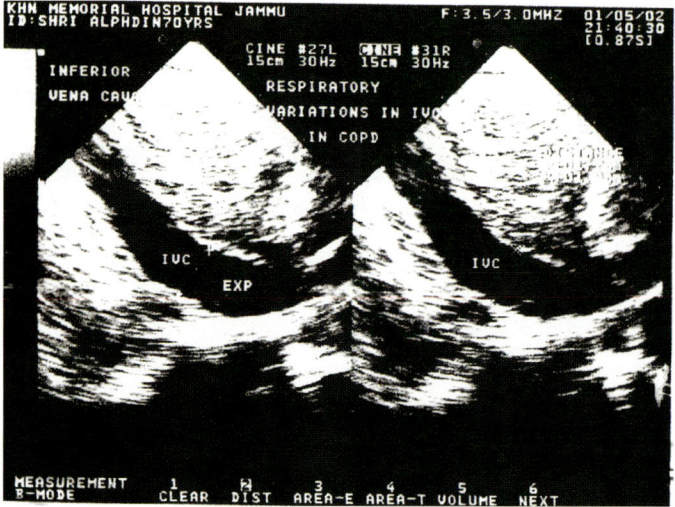

Fig. 19.7: Subcostal 4C long axis view showing dilatation of both right atrium and right ventricle in patient with moderate chronic obstructive lung disease with moderate pulmonary arterial hypertension

Tricuspid Valve (TV)

With the help of M-mode and 2-D and Doppler echocardiography one can visualise the thickening, movements, vegetations and regurgitations of tricuspid valve (Fig. 19.8A).

Prolapse of TV (Figs 19.19 and 19.20)

While employing, 2-dimensional echocardiography one can visualise an elongated redundant tricuspid valve. Diagnosis of tricuspid prolapse is even more difficult than diagnosis of mitral valve prolapse due to the lack of standardised parameters. An isolated occurrence of tricuspid valve prolapse is rare, even though concomitant tricuspid valve prolapse in patients with mitral valve prolapse of up to 48% has been reported.

Stenosis of TV (Figs 19.9 and 19.11)

An average tricuspid valve area is approximately 7.0 cm^2. In tricuspid stenosis, leaflets appear thickened with restricted motion on both M-mode and two dimensional echocardiography. Tricuspid stenosis may occur accompanying other complex congenital defects, such as pulmonary atresia or severe stenosis where the ventricular septum is intact.

In terms of priority, rheumatic fever affects the mitral, aortic and tricuspid valves, but it seldom leads to severe type of tricuspid stenosis, as it happens with mitral valve. In tricuspid stenosis valve area is reduced to 1.5 cm^2. Besides tricuspid valve being affected by rheumatic process, other conditions which may involve the valves are carcinoid syndrome, thrombotic occlusion, and right atrial neoplastic or myxoma invasion, leading to obstruction of bloodflow from right atrium to right ventricle and consequently, right atrial enlargement with pressure overload.

Infective Endocarditis (Fig. 19.37)

This condition involving tricuspid valve is commonly seen among the intravenous drug-users. Vegetations are seen as shaggy, pedunculated masses that attach to the valve leaflet without restriction of movement of the leaflet. Vegetations are usually seen on the flowside of the valves where circulating blood first contacts the valve. Transesophageal echocardiography has been shown to be superior to precordial echo in the diagnosis of valvular vegetations. Although echocardiography is the method of choice in diagnosing valvular vegetations, the treatment of bacterial endocarditis with antibiotics should not be solely based on demonstration of vegetations on echocardiography, as it may misguide at times the treating physician and hence clinical judgement is still the best.

Ebstein's Anomaly

Apical displacement of tricuspid valve in Ebstein anomaly is an isolated congenital malformation and the extent of displacement may vary. The result is an atrialized portion of the right ventricle from the annulus to the insertion of the tricuspid valve leaflets in the right ventricle. This malformation is usually accompanied by tricuspid regurgitation but one may encounter though rarely tricuspid stenosis. Although Ebstein's anomaly is a congenital condition, it can be well tolerated and most patients reach adolescence or even adulthood. This

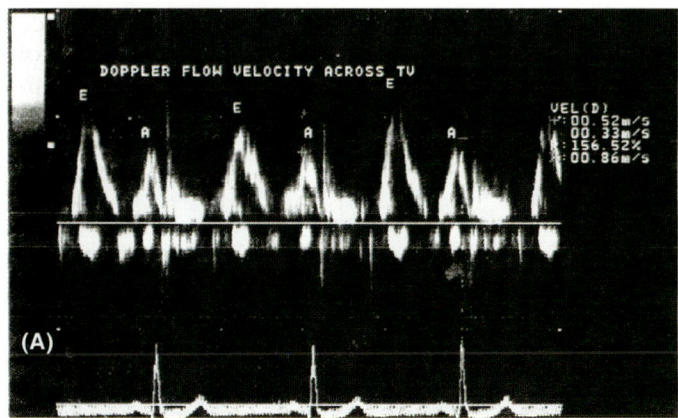

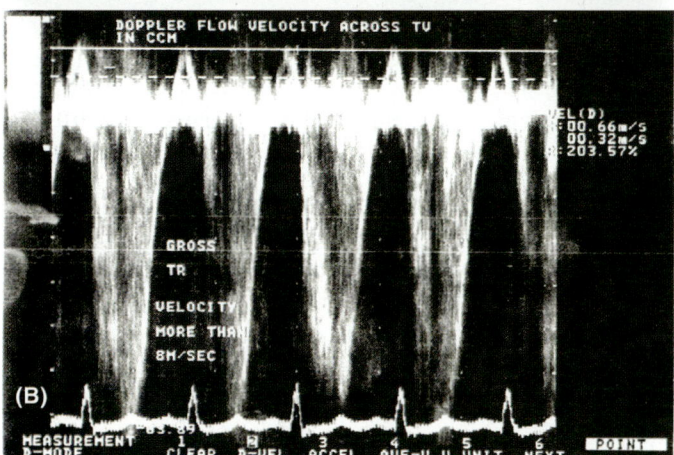

Fig. 19.8A and B: (A) Doppler flow velocity across tricuspid valve showing normal morphology of the valve. **(B)** Doppler flow velocity across tricuspid valve showing severe type of tricuspid valvular regurgitation (>8.0 m/s with pressure gradient of = 25.0 mmHg in patient with critical type of rheumatic mitral stenosis associated with severe pulmonary arterial hypertension

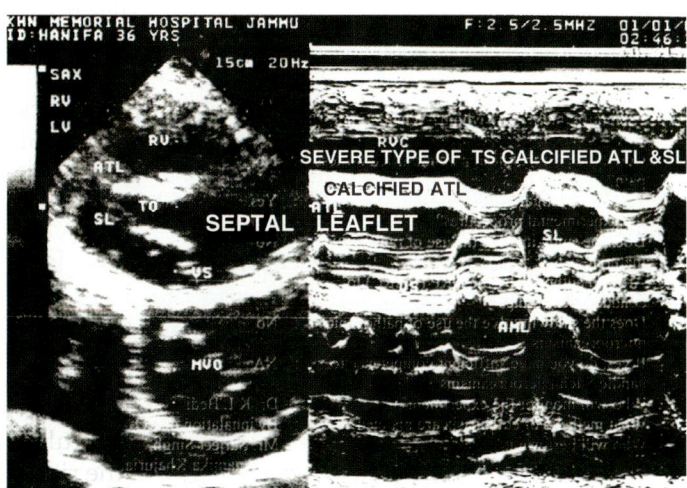

Fig. 19.9: 2-D long and short axis biventricular view LV and RV (left) and M-mode echoscan visualization of both mitral and tricuspid valves showing marked thickening and calcification of tricuspid valve with thickening of mitral valve in patient with rheumatic severe type of tricuspid valvular stenosis with mitral valvulitis

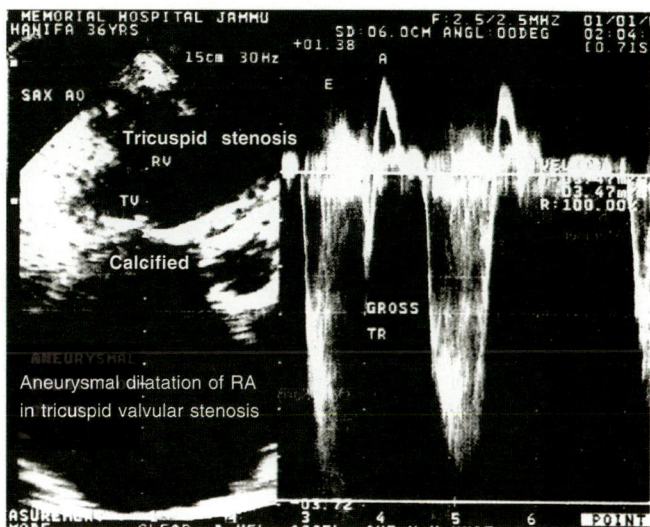

Fig. 19.10: 2-D right-sided two chamber view (left) and Doppler flow velocity across TV (right) showing marked thickening and calcification of both leaflets of tricuspid valve, aneurysmal dilatation of right atrium and moderate dilatation of RV (left). It also depicts gross tricuspid regurgitation (right) in patient with rheumatic severe tricuspid valvular stenosis and regurgitation and mitral valvulitis

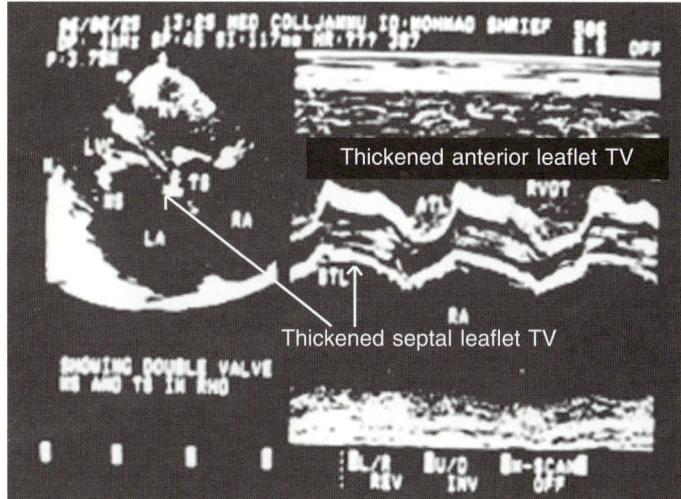

Fig. 19.11: 2D Apical and M-mode echocardiogram showing thickened both anterior and septal leaflets of tricuspid valve in patient with tricuspid valvular stenosis

condition can lead to heart failure and paroxysmal supraventricular tachyarrhythmia and hence, the patient with Ebstein anomaly may first manifest clinically with either of the two (Figs 19.30, 19.31 and 19.35).

Tricuspid Regurgitation (TR)

CW Doppler and colour B-flow echocardiography are the most sensitive methods for detecting tricuspid valve regurgitation. The systolic flow from right ventricle to right atrium can be recorded as the result of tricuspid

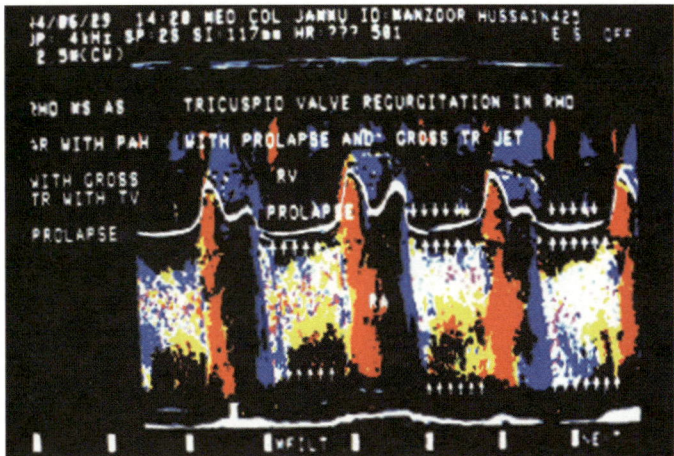

Fig. 19.12: M-Mode echocardiogram in color mode showing gross tricuspid regurgitation (arrows) in patient with rheumatic heart disease with mitral stenosis with MR tricuspid valvulitis with TR

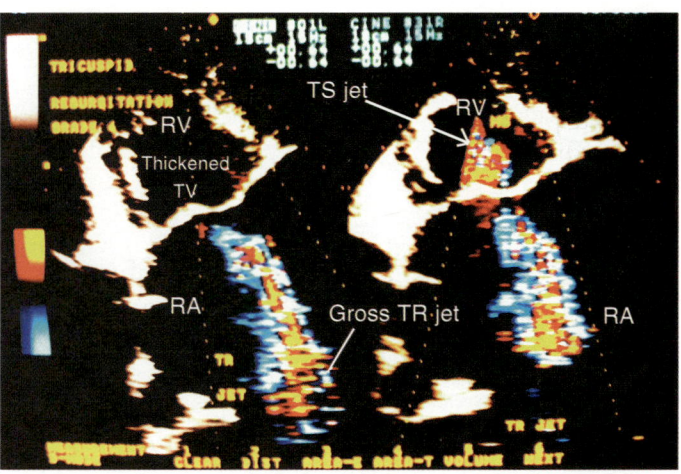

Fig. 19.13: Dual scan 2-D color flow in two chamber view showing gross degree of tricuspid valvular regurgitation jet and thickening of tricuspid valve in patient with MS, tricuspid stenosis and tricuspid regurgitation

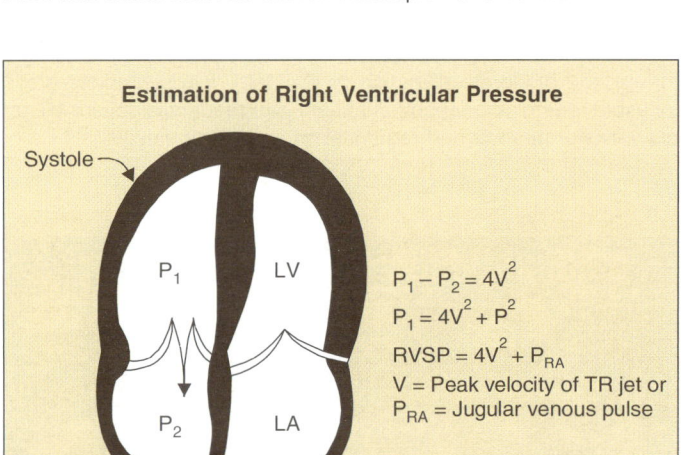

Fig. 19.14A and B: Calculation of RV pressure by echocardiography, For example take first the regurgitant velocity across tricuspid valve; i.e. 4.40 m/s in this case, convert it into pressure by Bernoullis formula as $4 \times V^2 = 77.44$ mm Hg and add jugular venous pressure/inferior vena cava pressure as 10 mm Hg. Hence RVSP = 87.44 mm Hg

pulse wave, continuous wave, or colour-flow imaging techniques. Before the advent of Doppler, peripheral injections of contrast agents into the right atrium were used in conjunction with two dimensional echocardiography for noninvasive assessment of tricuspid regurgitation.

The incidence of Doppler detected tricuspid regurgitation in the normal population may vary from 68% to 95%. Pulse Doppler mode has been employed to estimate the severity of the tricuspid regurgitation and to map the extent of the regurgitation in the right atrium. Hepatic vein scanning has also been used to assess regurgitation. By the application of multiple windows of colour Doppler imaging, one may be able to quantitate regurgitant flow. One should always keep in mind as how to optimise the equipment for detection of maximal lesion and the factors which may influence the jet size including rapid heart rate and the Coanda effect, both of which may cause underestimation of the severity. The Coanda effect indicate that when a jet is adjacent to a wall, the apparent size of the jet is smaller than when that jet is directed centrally and free from any walls. Therefore, when assessing the severity of tricuspid regurgitation in the presence of jets that are hugging the right atrial wall, increase the severity of the regurgitation by at least one grade.

Physiological or minimal tricuspid valve regurgitation in anatomically normal is also very common to observe. Pathologically, it is usually secondary to right ventricular dilation, which could be as the result of other diseases, such as pulmonary hypertension resulting from mitral stenosis or cor pulmonale or dilated cardiomyopathy and myocardial infarction.

The other causes of pathological TR include bacterial endocarditis, prolapse, papillary muscle dysfunction, rheumatic disease. Ebstein's anomaly, and laceration of the tricuspid apparatus from traumatic injury. Doppler echocardiography is very useful technique in obtaining hemodynamic information by employing tricuspid regurgitation to calculate right ventricular systolic pressure noninvasively with continuous-wave Doppler (Figs 19.8, 19.10, 19.12–19.14).

Pulmonic Valve

High left parasternal and subcostal views on 2-dimensional echo are best suited for evaluation of main pulmonary artery and its respective valve. Most occurrences of pulmonic valve diseases are of congenital nature, although the presence of carcinoid tumor may produce varying grades of pulmonary dysfunctions. Pulmonic valve stenosis and insufficiency may be detected and quantitated by Doppler echocardiography.

Pulmonic Stenosis (Figs 19.15 and 19.16)

Like aortic valvular stenosis, pulmonary stenosis is divided into three types, depending on the location of the stenosis: valvular, supravalvular, or subvalvular.

In congenital valvular stenosis which is more common than the other forms described. The pulmonic valve is a dome-shaped structure with a small opening. The doming of the pulmonic valve can be better visualised in parasternal short-axis view on 2-D echocardiogram in systole. It is often associated with poststenotic dilation of the pulmonary artery. Using continuous-wave Doppler transversing the pulmonic valve, a high velocity may be observed in systole. Applying the modified Bernoulli equation, the systolic pressure gradient between the right ventricle and the pulmonary artery can be obtained to determine the severity of the stenosis.

In the other form of pulmonic valve stenosis the pulmonic valve is dysplastic with immobile cusps from thickened myxomatous tissue. The pulmonary arteries in these congenital cases are usually hypoplastic or underdeveloped.

In patients with supravalvular pulmonic stenosis which may be seen along any part of the main pulmonary artery and its peripheral branches, 2-D Doppler echocardiography is the best means of recording high velocities in such cases. However, for establishing a peripheral pulmonary artery stenosis, transesophageal echocardiography has been found better than transthoracic approach.

In the rarest type of acquired pulmonic valve stenosis as seen in carcinoid syndrome, the restricted cusp motion usually results from the proliferation of connective tissue on the arterial side of cusps.

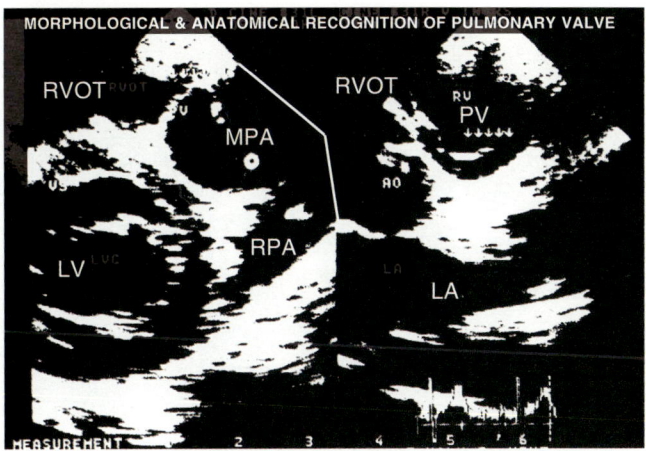

Fig. 19.15: 2D oblique short axis view of LV on dual scan showing the location of main pulmonary artery with its valve and LV cavity (left) and pulmonary valve (arrows) at short axis view at aorta for coronary vessels level at atrio-pulmonary junction (right)

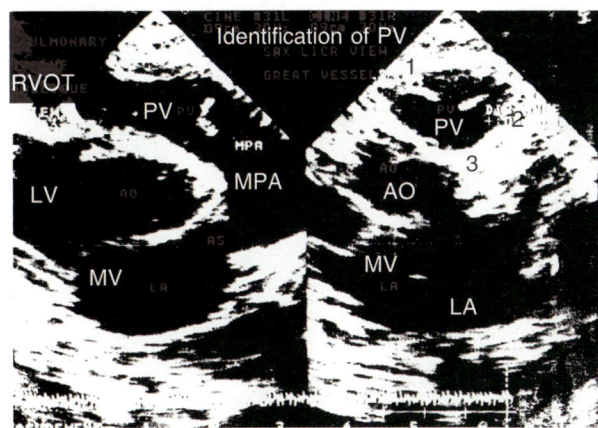

Fig. 19.16: Short axis oblique view in dual scan at aorta and short axis view of great vessels in the high left parasternal region showing identification of tricuspid morphology of pulmonary valve marked as 1, 2 and 3 and its relationship with surrounding structures. MPA = Main pulmonary artery, PV = Pulmonary valve

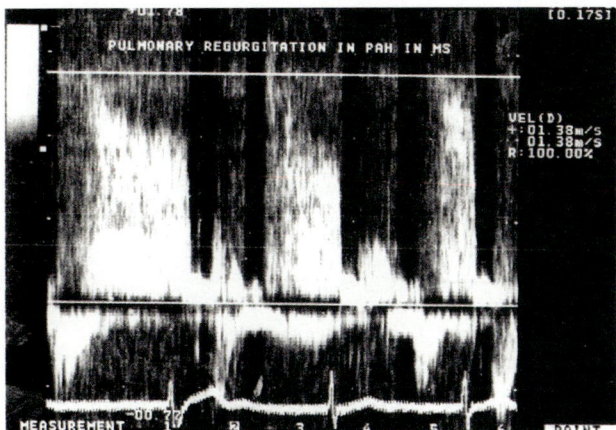

Fig. 19.17: Doppler flow velocity showing moderate type of pulmonary regurgitation in patient with rheumatic mitral stenosis with pulmonary arterial hypertension

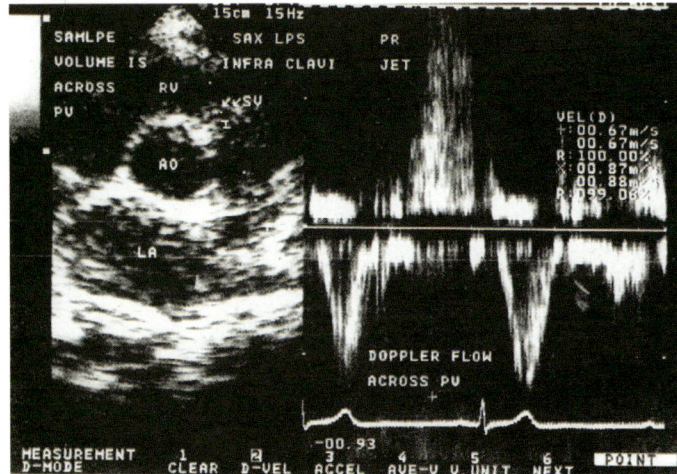

Fig. 19.18: 2-D Doppler flow showing normal pulmonary flow velocity and mild pulmonary regurgitation in patient with sinus bradycardia with normal valve and pulmonary pressure

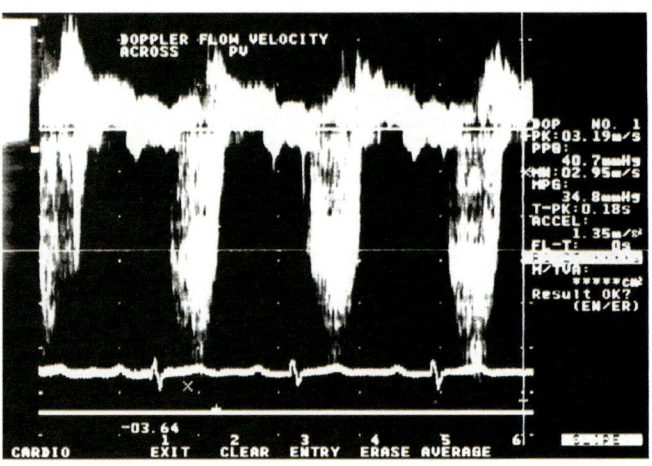

Fig. 19.21: Doppler flow velocity across pulmonary valve depicting wide spectral waveform with enhanced flow velocity in an adult patient with pulmonic valve stenosis

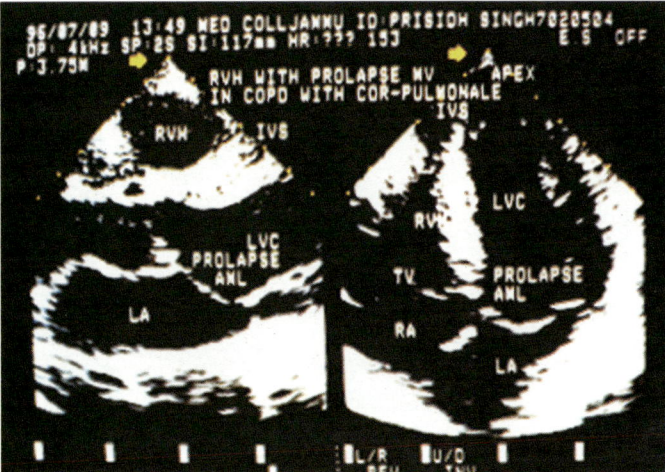

Fig. 19.19: 2-D Long and apical 4C dual scan views showing mitral valve prolapse into LA (left) and mitral and tricuspid prolapse into their respective LA and RA chambers (right)

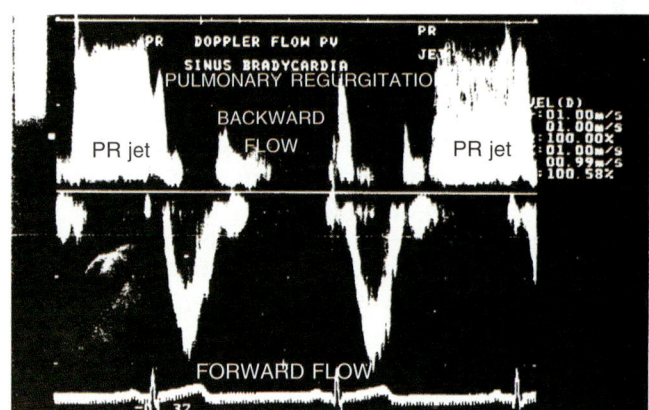

Fig. 19.22: Doppler flow velocity across main pulmonary artery showing pulmonary regurgitation in patient with sinus bradycardia as a part of sick sinus syndrome with normal pulmonary valve

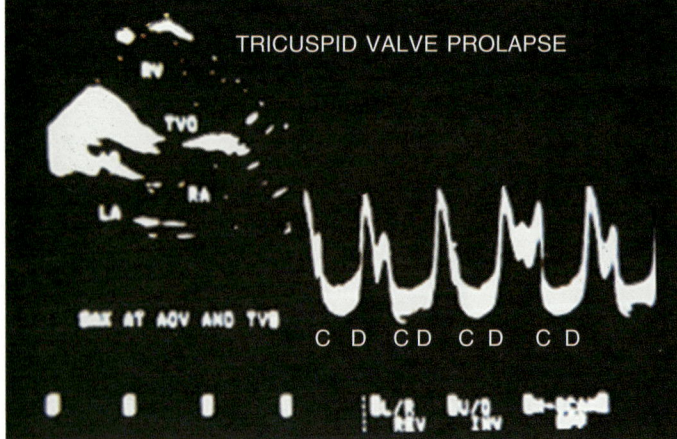

Fig. 19.20: 2-D and M-mode echocardiogram of anterior tricuspid leaflet(L-R) showing mid-systolic sagging of anterior tricuspid leaflet from an imaginary line connecting C-D points in patient with rheumatic mitral and tricuspid valvulitis with bivalvular prolapse due to associated myocarditis

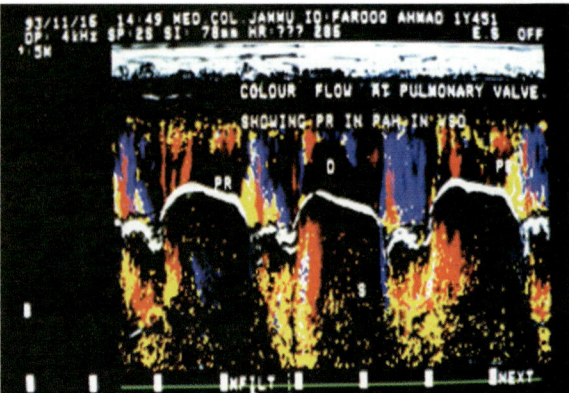

Fig. 19.23: M-Mode echoscan of posterior valve showing attenuation of A wave with color regurgitant jet in patient with primary pulmonary aterial hypertension

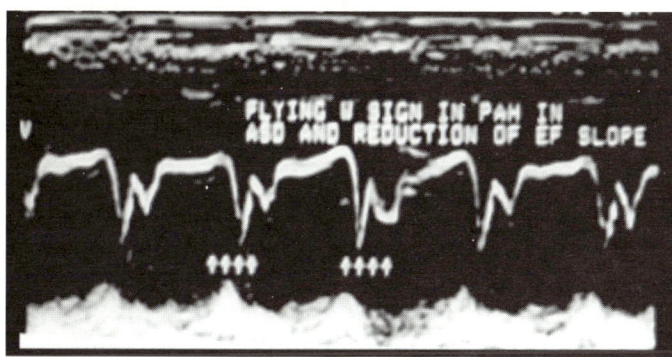

Fig. 19.24: M-Mode of posterior pulmonary valve showing absence of A (a) wave negative E-F slope and mid systolic notching (n) of the leaflet in patient with pulmonary arterial hypertension. It is also called flying W sign

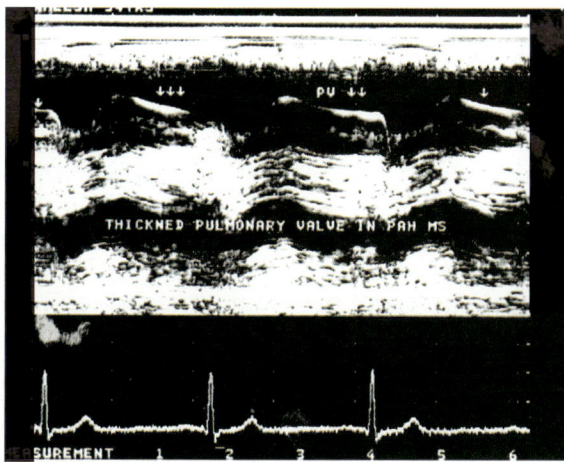

Fig. 19.25: M-Mode echocardiogram showing thickening of posterior pulmonary leaflet and attenuation of A wave in patient with mitral, tricuspid and aortic stenosis with regurgitation and pulmonary arterial hypertension

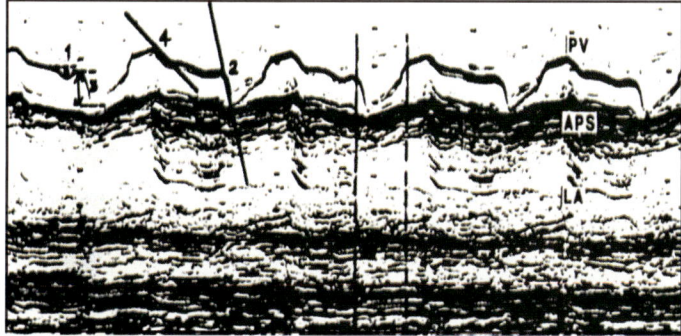

Fig. 19.26: M-Mode echocardiogram taken at atrio-pulmonary sulcus showing various hemodynamic points and slopes to be employed in the gradation of severity and nature of pulmonary valvular disease. 1. a-max = maximum depth of a-wave which is recorded during quite respiration. (n = 3–7mm) 2. b-c slope = It is the opening velocity of pulmonary valve (n = <300 mm/sec). 3. b-c amplitude = The opening amplitude from b-c points (n = 10–14 mm) 4. e-f slope = This is the diastolic slope of the pulmonary valve measured by drawing the diagonal over the e-f portion of the pulmonary valve. (n = 6–115 mm/sec)

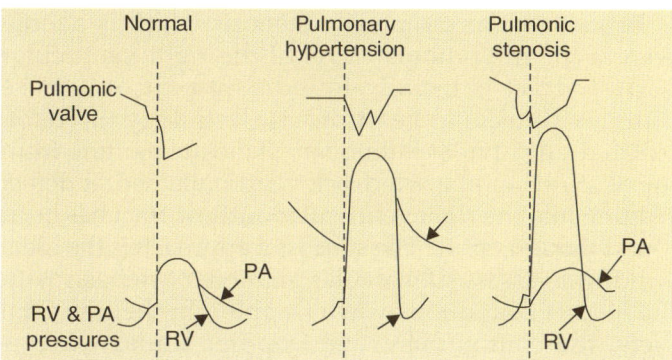

Fig. 19.27: Graphic representation of relationship between M-Mode echocardiographic signatures of normal pulmonary valve, pulmonary arterial hypertension and congenital pulmonic stenosis and their corresponding hemodynamic pressure changes in RV and RA thereby stressing the need of non-invasive echocardiographic evaluation of these disorders

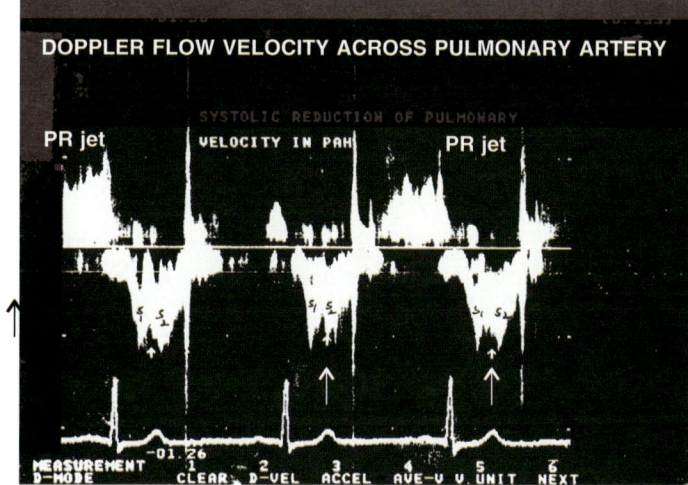

Fig. 19.28: Doppler flow velocity across pulmonary valve showing systolic regression of velocity (arrow) in patient with pulmonary arterial hypertension and mild regurgitation

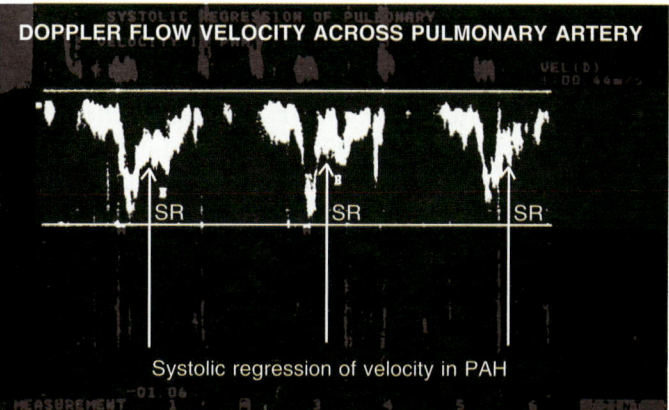

Fig. 19.29: Doppler flow velocity across pulmonary valve showing systolic regression of velocity (arrow) in another patient with rheumatic mitral stenosis and ASD Secundum pulmonary arterial hypertension, SR = Systolic regression of velocity

In subvalvular pulmonary stenosis which is oftenly seen at the infundibular level of the right ventricular outflow tract is usually found as a part of a more complex congenital heart disease, tetralogy of Fallot. Isolated subvalvular Pulmonary stenosis resulting from the obstruction of a windsock ventricular septal defect bulging into the right ventricular outflow tract has been found though rarely. The subcostal approach is the ideal window to assess subvalvular pulmonary stenosis with the help of continuous-wave Doppler. In the subcostal view, the continuous-wave Doppler sound wave is parallel to the right ventricular outflow tract.

Pulmonic Regurgitation

Congenital pulmonary valve stenosis or pulmonary hypertension has been observed as the most common cause of pulmonic regurgitation. Doppler is the most sensitive noninvasive method for detecting pulmonic valve regurgitation. It is possible to calculate the pulmonary end diastolic pressure by finding out pulmonary regurgitation by Doppler velocity and applying the modified Bernoulli's equation (Figs 19.17, 19.18 and 19.22).

Pulmonary Arterial Hypertension (PAH)

The vascular resistance of pulmonary arteries is much lower than that of systemic arteries due to their thin structure and low resting muscular tone. The normal mean pulmonary arterial pressure is about 12 to 17 mmHg. Pulmonary hypertension can occur as a primary disease or secondary to other heart disease. The cause of primary pulmonary hypertension is unknown. The main cause of secondary pulmonale hypertension is mitral stenosis due to elevated left atrial pressure followed by heart failure with elevated left ventricular end-diastolic pressure, cor pulmonal, thrombotic emboli to the lungs, or congenital heart disease with a left-to-right shunt.

The patients with PAH when evaluated with M-mode echocardiograph, typically shows a midsystolic closure of the pulmonic valve, mimicking flying-W sign. Although it is not very sensitive method but it is quite specific for echocardiographic evaluation of PAH.

Right ventricular systolic time-interval measurements have also been used from M-mode to assess pulmonary hypertension. In children the ratio of the pulmonic valve preejection period, PVPEP, to ejection time, PVET is 0.30 or less, can predict a pulmonary arterial end-diastolic pressure of less than 30 mm Hg.

Doppler echocardiography can reliably determine pulmonary artery pressure.

1. It is most reliable and most often used method in tricuspid regurgitation with the modified Bernoulli equation.
2. It measures pulmonary flow velocity indices.
3. It measures the right ventricular isovolumic relaxation time.

In the absence of pulmonic stenosis the use of tricuspid regurgitation to calculate right ventricular systolic pressure noninvasively is further dependant upon the presence of sufficient tricuspid regurgitation to produce an adequate Doppler envelope. In the absence of pulmonary stenosis, pulmonary systolic pressure is equivalent to right ventricular systolic pressure. Tricuspid regurgitation represents the instantaneous systolic pressure gradient between the right ventricle and the right atrium. With the help of CW Doppler mode, the maximum velocity of the tricuspid regurgitation can be ascertained from the parasternal, apical, or occasionally the subcostal window. By the application of colour Doppler, one is able to see alignment of the Doppler beam to the regurgitant jet. Once the Doppler spectral envelop is optimized, peak velocity measurement is obtained. Then the modified Bernoulli equation, $P = 4V^2$, where P is the pressure gradient and V is the peak velocity measure from the tricuspid regurgitation, is applied to calculate the pressure gradient. Once the systolic pressure gradient is calculated, add the right atrial pressure to obtain the right ventricular systolic pressure. The former can be estimated from the jugular venous pressure. Often a standard figure of 10 mm of mercury is used where there is severe tricuspid regurgitation, 15 or even 20 mm of mercury for the right atrial pressure may be used. A high right atrial pressure can be sensed by examining the inferior vena cava, which is usually dilated and does not collapse with inspiration or if the tricuspid regurgitation can be visualised as systolic backflow into the inferior vena cava. These are the parameters of high right atrial pressure. The right atrium is usually dilated in these cases. Normal pulmonary systolic pressure exceeding 40 mm Hg is considered significant.

Secondly PAH can be assessed by the application of Doppler flow velocity indices. In this method a pulsed-wave Doppler sample volume is interrogated just distal to the pulmonic valve, in the centre of the pulmonary artery. Different indices that are employed, are the acceleration time (AcT) and the ratio of acceleration time to right ventricular ejection time (RVET) (AcT/RVET). To minimize the degree of error faster speed should be adjusted (100 mm/sec). In most equipment, this means using the 100 mm/sec chart speed. The acceleration time is measured on the pulmonary Doppler spectral display from the onset of systolic flow to the peak of the velocity. The normal value of AcT is 100 msec or more. An acceleration time of 80 msec or less usually indicated significant pulmonary hypertension. The ratio is expressed as the acceleration time divided by the

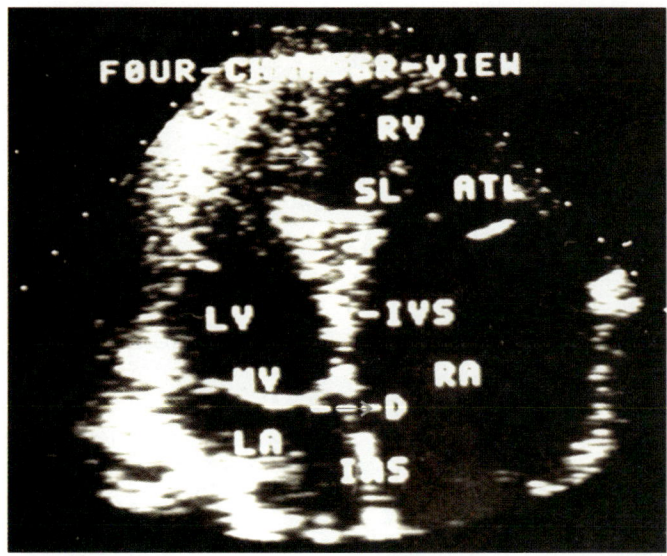

Fig. 19.30: Apical 4C view showing displacement of incompetent tricuspid valve and atrialization of RV with reference to proximally positioned MV. There is also associated septum primum (D) and apical VSD (arrow) in a patient with Ebstein anomaly of TV

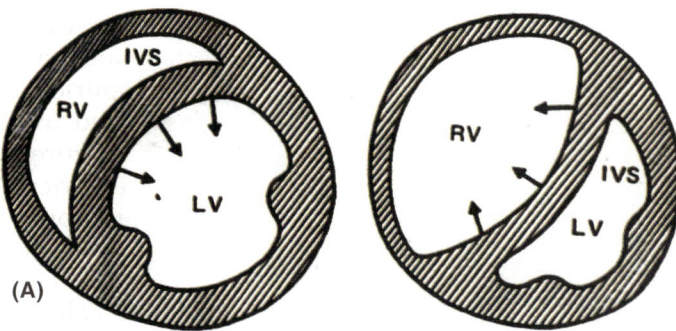

1. Normal LV Shape   2. Crescent shape (half moon) LV in high RV pressure

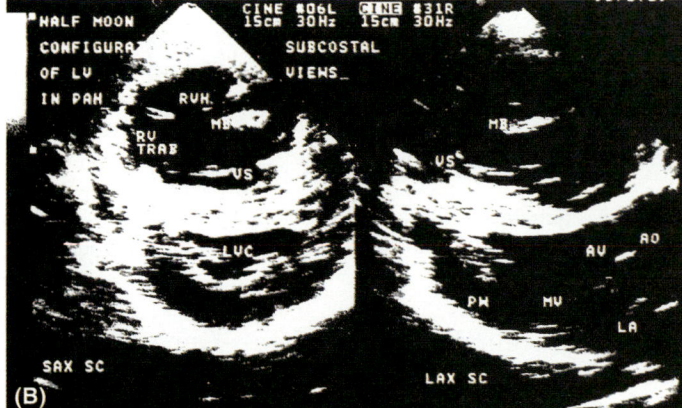

Fig. 19.32A and B: (A) 1. Diagrammatic representation of normal LV configuration 2. Half moon configuration of LV in high RV pressure. **(B)** 2-D Short and long axis views showing half moon shaped (crescent) LV. There is also dilated and hypertrophied RV in patient with chronic obstructive lung disease with severe pulmonary arterial hypertension with structurally normal pulmonary valve

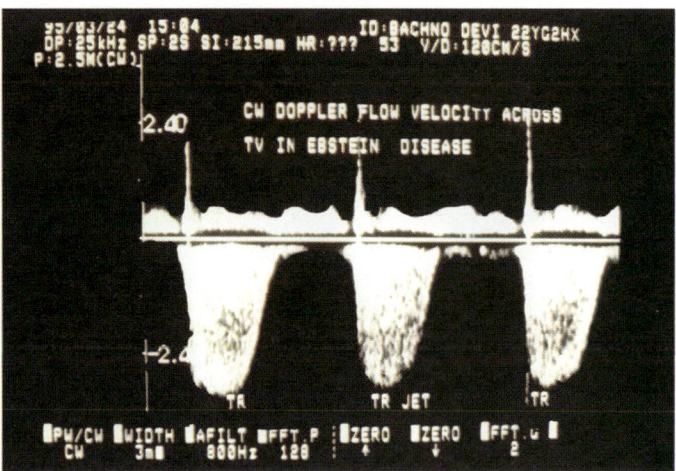

Fig. 19.31: 2-D Doppler flow velocity across tricuspid valve showing enhanced velocity >3.0 cm/s in a child with single ventricle common AV valve and Ebstein disease of TV

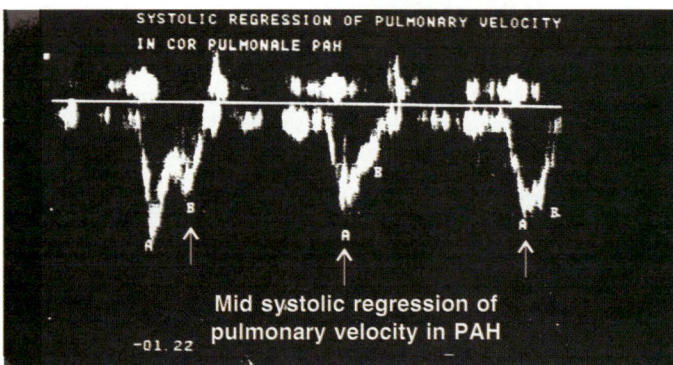

Fig. 19.33: Doppler flow velocity across pulmonary valve showing mid systolic regression (arrow) of velocity in pulmonary arterial hypertension and is equavalent to mid-systolic notch and flying W sign as seen on M-mode echocardiogram of pulmonary valve in severe pulmonary arterial hypertension

ejection time. In normal subjects, this ratio is 0.45. In patients with significant pulmonary hypertension, this ratio is reduced to 0.25. Incorporating the ejection time into the measurement minimizes the effect of heart rate variations.

Thirdly it can be assessed by using the right ventricular isovolumic relaxation time. This isovolumic relaxation time is the interval from the closure of the pulmonic valve (Pc) to the opening of the tricuspid valve (To). In order to record the opening and closing movements of the pulmonic valve Doppler sample volume is usually placed at the valve orifice as the pulmonic and tricuspid valves are not recorded simultaneously by this method, phonocardiography is facilitated by the addition of the Doppler recordings to help with the timing. The Pc to To interval in normal subjects is very short. This interval is directly related to

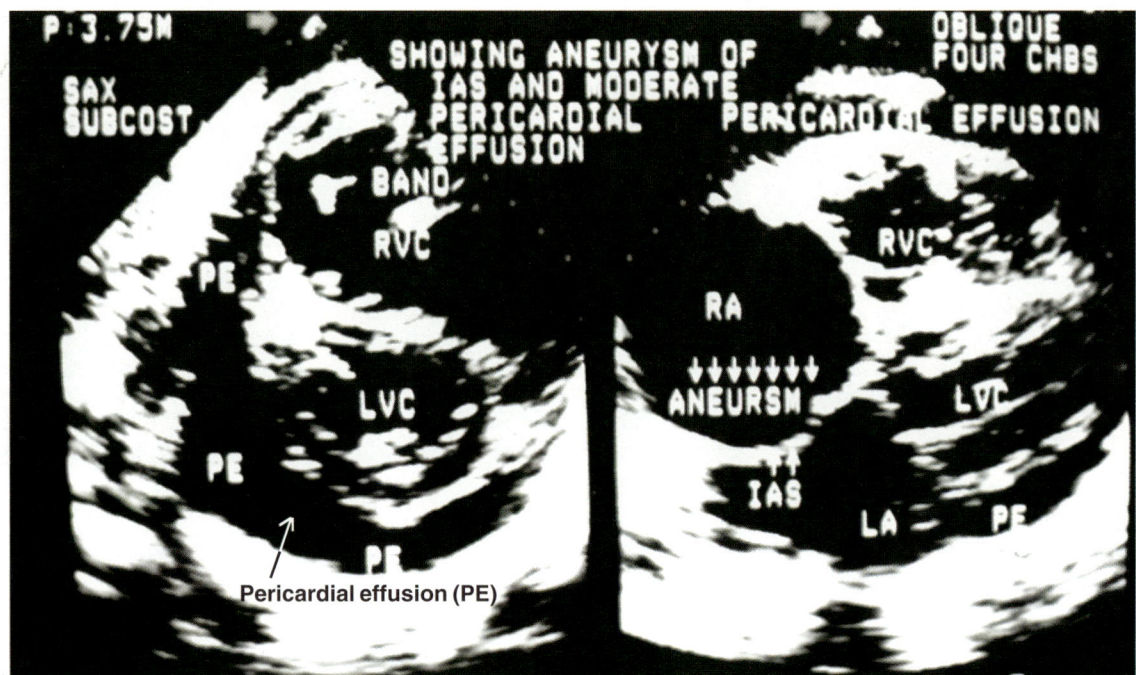

Fig. 19.34: Subcostal short axis and 4C dual scan views (L-R) showing dilated RV with posterior pericardial effusion (left) and hypertrophied RV, dilated RA, greatly distended interatrial septum (IAS) almost attaining concave contour and simulating aneurysmal configuration in patient with rheumatic mitral stenosis MR, TR and severe pulmonary arterial hypertension with RV failure

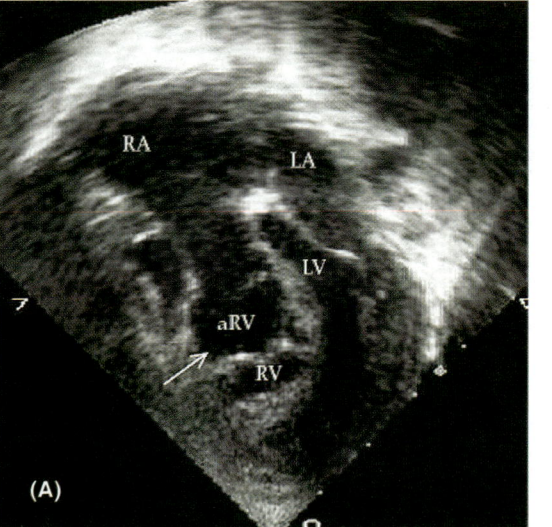
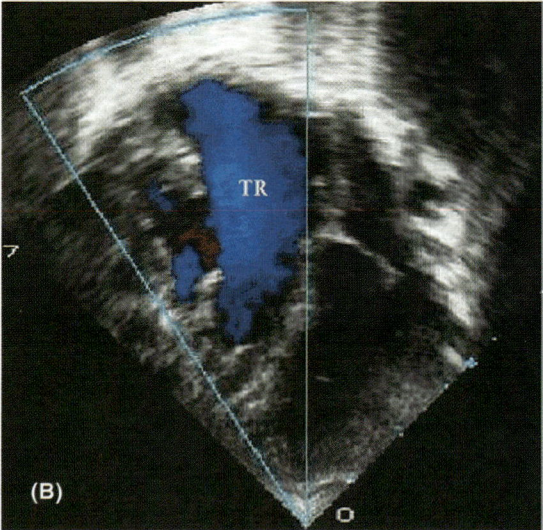

Fig. 19.35A and B: Atrialization of tricuspid valve (A) and blue jet of tricuspid regurgitation due to incompetent TV (B) in a patient with Ebstein disease of TV. aRV = Atrialized RV, LA = Left atrium, RA = Right atrium, LV = Left ventricle, TR = Tricuspid regurgitation, ATL = Anterior tricuspid leaflet, SL = Septal leaflet of tricuspid leaflet

the pulmonary systolic pressure in the absence of severe tricuspid regurgitation or elevated right atrial pressure (Figs 19.23–19.29, 19.32 and 19.33).

Right Atrial and Right Ventricular Masses

When examining diseases of the right heart, one must be able to distinguish normal variant, artifact, and pathology. Some of the masses more commonly seen, include pacemaker wires, Swan-Ganz catheters, eustachian valve, Chiari network, and prominent moderator band (Figs 19.34 and 19.36).

Pathologic masses seen in the right atrium include myxoma, thrombus, and carcinoid growth. All modalities of echocardiography such as M-mode, 2-D, 2D Doppler, colour flow Doppler through both transthoracic and transesophageal windows can be used in

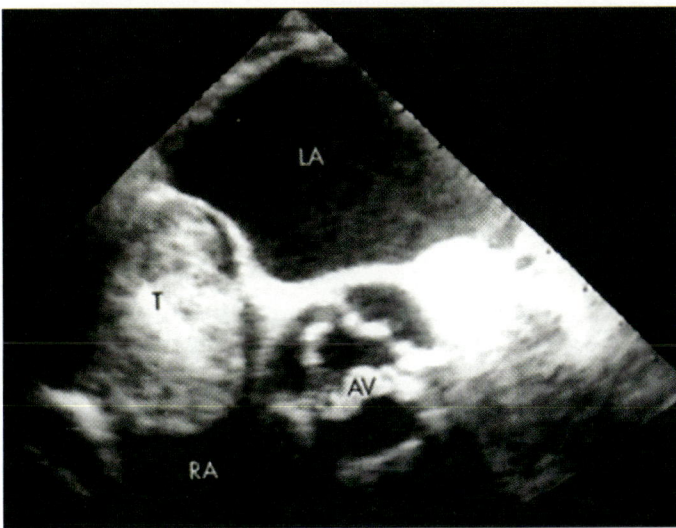

Fig. 19.36: TEE view showing big tumor mass (T) in right atrium

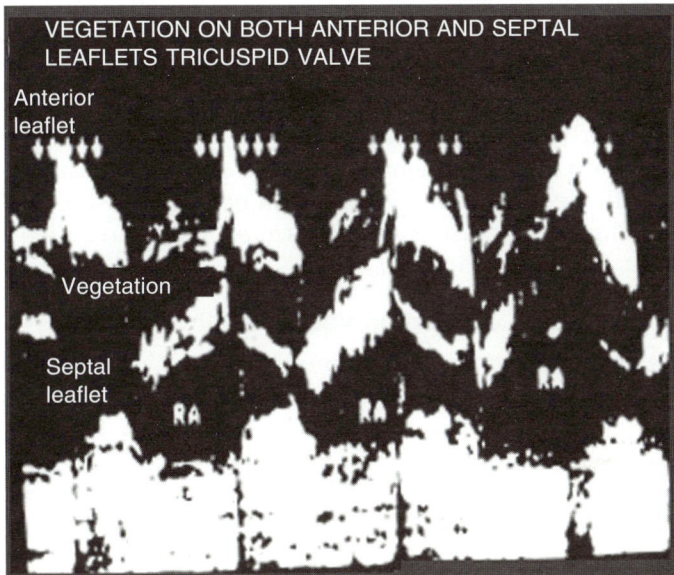

Fig. 19.37: M-Mode echocardiogram showing large-sized vegetation on both anterior and septal leaflets of tricuspid valve (arrows) almost obstructing 50% of the valve area TV = Tricuspid valve, RA = Right atrium

different views and planes to achieve the best and clear picture of an above said conditions affecting right atrium and right ventricular cavities.

Bibliography

1. Bommer W, Weinert L, Neumann A, *et al.* Determination of right atrial and right ventricular size by two-dimensional echocardiography, *Circulation* 1979;60:91.
2. Cape EG, Yoganathan AP, and Levine RA: Increased heart rate can cause underestimation of regurgitant jet size by Doppler colour flow mapping. *J Am Coll Cardiol* 1993;21:1029.
3. Gibson TC, Miller SW, Aretz T, *et al.* Method for estimating right ventricular volume by planes applicable to cross-sectional echocardiography: correlation with angiographic formulas. *Am J Cardiol* 1985;55: 1584.
4. Hagan AD, Francis GS, Sahn D, *et al.* Ultrasound evaluation of systolic anterior septal motion in patients with and without right ventricular volume overload. *Circulation* 1974;50: 248.
5. Kaul S, Tei C, Hopkins JM, *et al.* Assessment of right ventricular function using two-dimensional echocardiography. *Am Heart J* 1984;107:526.
6. Kaul S, Tei C, Hopkins JM, *et al.* Ultrasound evaluation of systolic anterior septal motion in patients with and without right ventricular volume overload. *Circulation* 1974;50:248.
7. King ME, Braun H, Goldblatt A, *et al.* Interventricular septal configuration as a predictor of right ventricular systolic hypertension in children: a cross-sectional echocardiography study. *Circulation* 1983;68:68.
8. Lavie CJ, Hebert K, and Cassidy M: Prevalence and severity of Doppler-detected valvular regurgitation and estimation of right-sided cardiac pressures in patients with normal two-dimensional echocardiograms. *Chest* 1993;103:226.
9. Levine RA, Gibson TC, Aretz T, *et al.* Tricuspid valve prolapse diagnosed by cross-sectional echocardiography. *Chest* 1981;79: 201.
10. Sakai K, Nakamura K, Satomi G, *et al.* Evaluation of tricuspid regurgitation by blood flow pattern in the hepatic vein using pulsed Doppler technique. *Am Heart J* 1984;108: 516.
11. Waggoner AD, Perez JE, Miller JG, *et al.* Differentiation of normal and ischemic right ventricular myocardium with quantitative two-dimensional integrated backscatter imaging. *Ultrasound Med Biol* 1992;18:249.
12. Watanabe T, Katsume H, Matsukubo H, *et al.* Estimation of right ventricular volume with two-dimensional echocardiography. *Am J Cardiol* 1982;49: 1946.

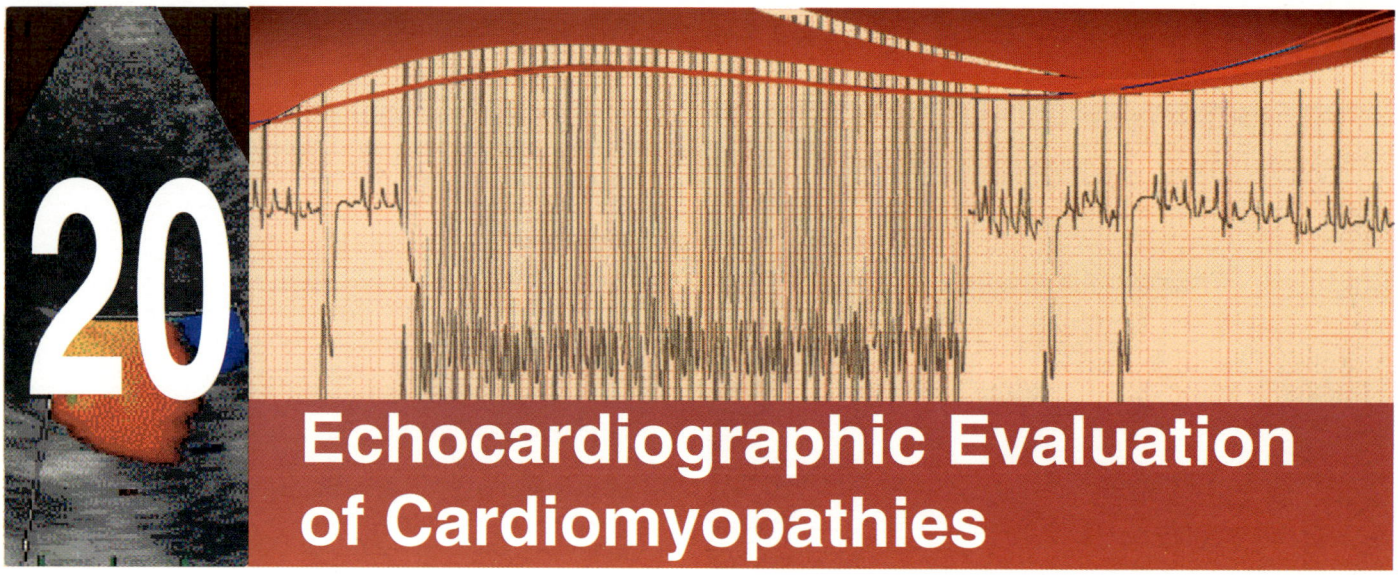

20

Echocardiographic Evaluation of Cardiomyopathies

Cardiomyopathies and their resultant systolic and diastolic heart failure remain a major cause of cardiovascular morbidity and mortality. The prevalence of heart failure continues to increase and it remains a major public health threat, particularly in the elderly. The overall annual healthcare expenditure for heart failure continues to increase. While a new diagnosis of heart failure is associated with substantial risk of death within one year, the institution of appropriately guided pharmacologic treatment has led to substantial reductions in cardiovascular mortality. Identification of potential candidates for such treatment can be facilitated through use of echocardiography.

In many patients the diagnosis of a cardiomyopathy is made after the onset of heart failure symptoms, atrial or ventricular arrhythmias, or a stroke. These complications of the underlying cardiomyopathy represent major causes of cardiovascular morbidity and mortality and frequently result in referral for echocardiography. Echocardiography provides an assessment of systolic and diastolic function as well as an estimation of left and right heart filling pressures. In addition, specific echocardiographic features allow the clinician to determine more accurately the aetiology of the cardiomyopathy. Integration of clinical and echocardiographic features now allows for a better assessment of both immediate risk and long term prognosis in patients with a cardiomyopathy.

Classification of Cardiomyopathies (Table 20.1)

Cardiomyopathies are defined by the World Health Organization as diseases of the myocardium which

Table 20.1: *Aetiological classification of cardiomyopathy*

Dilated cardiomyopathy	High-output cardiomyopathy	Hypertrophic cardiomyopathy	Restrictive cardiomyopathy	Other
Idiopathic cardiomyopathy	Tachycardia-mediated	Asymmetric septal	Idiopathic	Friedreich
Familial cardiomyopathy	cardiomyopathy	hypertrophy (idiopathic	Infiltrative	ataxia
Noncompacted myocardium	Thyrotoxicosis	hypertrophic	Amyloidosis	Muscular
Postpartum cardiomyopathy	Nutritional (beriberi,	cardiomyopathy)	Glycogen storage	dystrophies
Hemachromatosis	thiamine deficiency)	Obstructive vs.	diseases	
Infectious	Peripheral left-to-right	nonobstructive	Hemachromatosis	
Postviral myocarditis	shunt lesions	Concentric hypertrophic	Post-radiation	
Human immunodeficiency	Anemia	cardiomyopathy	therapy	
virus related		Isolated apical	Endocardial	
Legionella infection		cardiomyopathy	fibroelastosis	
Sepsis (gram negative)		Atypical hypertrophic		
Toxic cardiomyopathy		cardiomyopathy		
Adriamycin				
Alcohol				
Carbon monoxide poisoning				
Other chemotherapy				

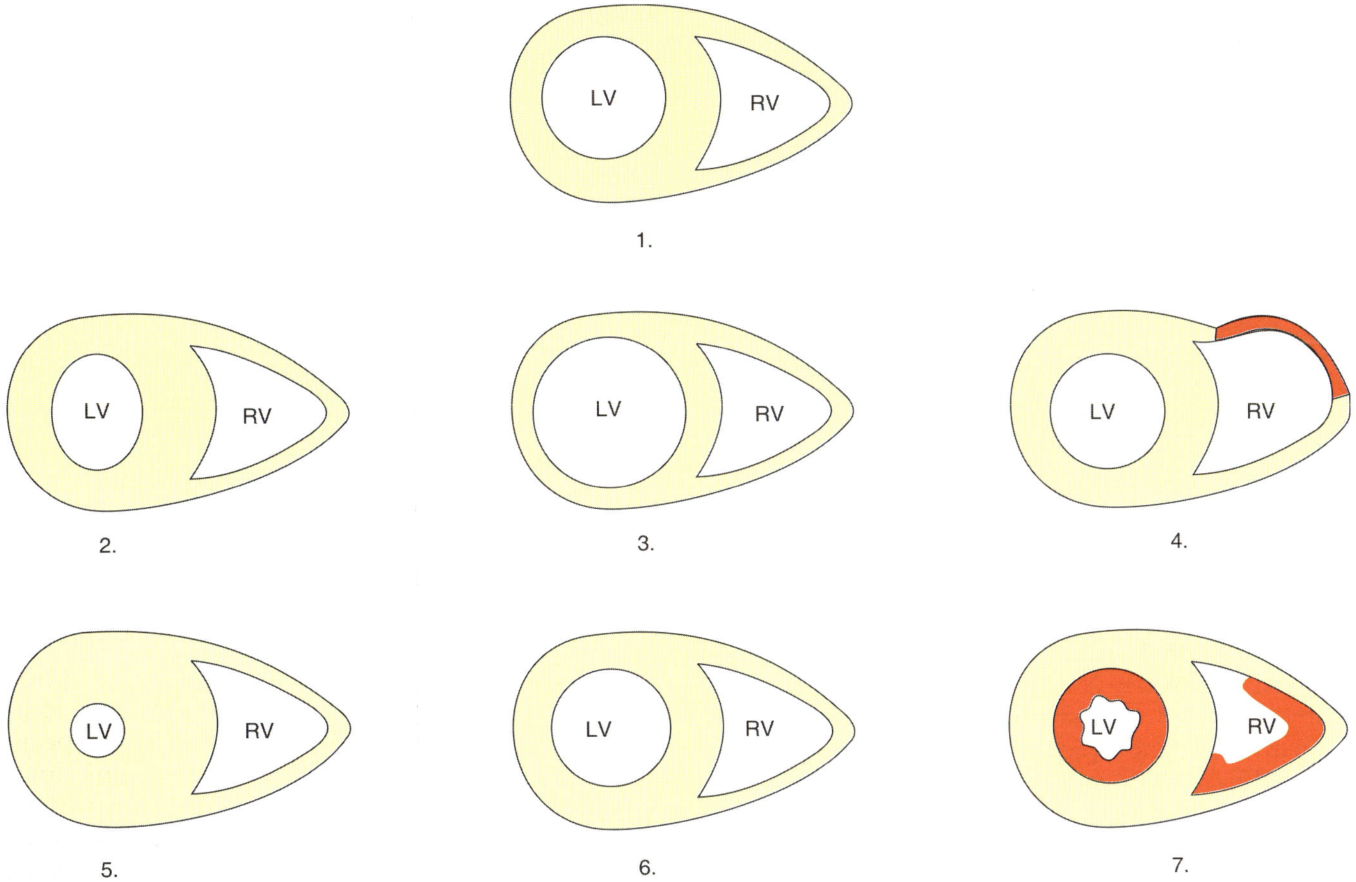

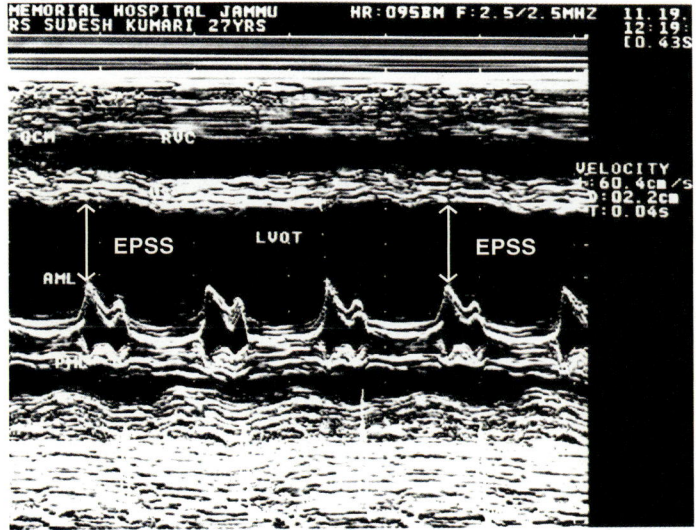

Fig. 20.1: Diagrammatic representation of different types of cardiomyopathies at short axis views of right and left ventricles at mid septal levels 1. = Normal 2. HCM = Hypertrophic cardiomyopathy. 3. DCM = Dilated cardiomyopathy. 4. ARVD = Arrhythmogenic right ventricular dysplasia. 5. HCM = Hypertrophic cardiomyopathy. 6. RCM = Restrictive cardiomyopathy. 7. EMF (OCM) = Endomyocardial fibrosis (obliterative cardiomyopathy)

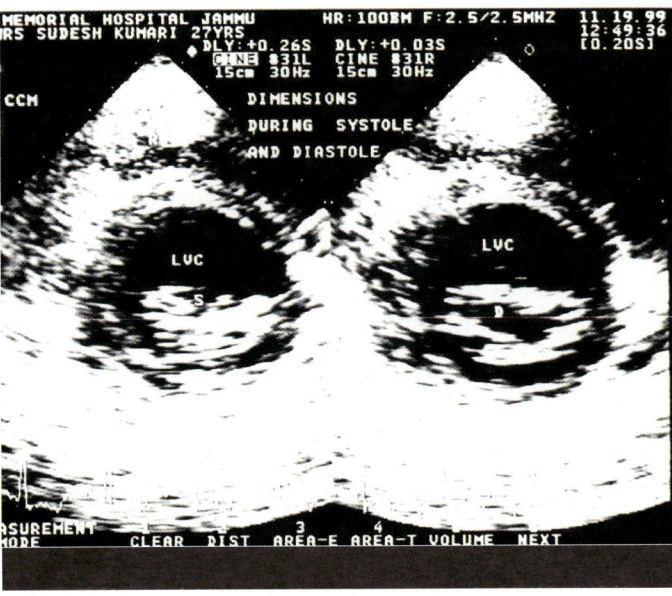

Fig. 20.2: M-Mode echocardiogram showing dilated RV, dilated LV, thinned and hypokinetic interventricular septum. There is also increased distance between septum and E point of mitral valve (EPSS) and double diamond type of MV configuration in patient with dilated cardiomyopathy

Fig. 20.3: 2D Short axis dual scan at LV showing poor LV contractions during systole and diastole in patient with dilated cardiomyopathy

result in cardiac dysfunction. The WHO classification of cardiomyopathies includes: hypertrophic, dilated, restrictive, and arrhythmogenic right ventricular cardiomyopathies. Although isolated noncompaction of the ventricular myocardium has not yet been identified as a distinct cardiomyopathy by WHO, it will also be discussed in this review. It is a rare but important cardiomyopathy with distinctive echocardiographic features. The echocardiographic features of specific cardiomyopathies are presented (Fig. 20.1).

The distinguishing features of the various forms of cardiomyopathies are easily identified by echocardiography. In the case of dilated and hypertrophic cardiomyopathies—the most common forms of cardiomyopathy—the definitions reflect the underlying ventricular function, wall thickness, and chamber size. In hypertrophic cardiomyopathy the ventricular walls are hypertrophied, the cavity is small, and ventricular function is normal or hyperkinetic.

In dilated cardiomyopathy the cavity is enlarged, wall thickness is normal or thin, and ventricular function is depressed. Restrictive cardiomyopathies are characterised by impaired or restricted ventricular filling as demonstrated by the typical transmitral Doppler profile (increased E/A ratio, rapid E-wave deceleration time). The wall thickness, cavity size, and ventricular function can vary depending on the underlying aetiology and duration of the restrictive cardiomyopathy. Echocardiographic features of arrhythmic right ventricular dysplasia include focal dilatation, thinning, and hypokinesis of the right ventricle (Table 20.3).

Principles of Echocardiography in Patients with Cardiomyopathy

Systolic Function (Fig. 20.30)

When using echocardiography to measure indices of global systolic function it is important to remember that most of the measures commonly assessed by echocardiography are load dependent.

These measures include left ventricular (LV) ejection fraction, dp/dt, and stroke volume. The change in pressure over change in time or dp/dt can be measured by quantifying the slope of the Doppler profile of the mitral regurgitant jet. This is accomplished by measuring the time required for the mitral regurgitant profile to increase from 1 m/s to 3 m/s.

There are several less load dependent measures of global systolic function now in clinical use that allow a more comprehensive, less load dependent assessment of ventricular function. These include measurement of elastance (emax), which can be derived from the end systolic pressure-volume or pressure-dimension relationships, cyclic variation of integrated backscatter, and LV strain/strain rate. Myocardial strain is measured

using data obtained through colour Doppler myocardial imaging and provides non-invasive quantification of myocardial deformation. Strain and strain rate (which represents the velocity of deformation) appear to be less affected by cardiac motion and segmental myocardial tethering.

Though it has recognised limitations, the most common measure of systolic function derived from echocardiography is the LV ejection fraction. There are numerous approaches to measuring ventricular volumes and most make assumptions about the geometry of the ventricle. The biplane Simpson's method utilising two apical echocardiographic views incorporates much of the shape of the ventricle in its calculation of volume; this is particularly important in the myopathic heart with its alterations in shape.

Diastolic Function (Fig. 20.53)

The transmitral and pulmonary venous spectral Doppler and mitral annular tissue velocity. Doppler profiles can be used to identify patterns of impaired ventricular relaxation and restriction to filling. The propagation of bloodflow in the LV cavity can be quantified by colour M-mode imaging. The flow propagation velocity is inversely proportional to time constant of isovolumic relaxation.

Mitral annular Doppler velocity is a relatively new method for quantifying the base to apical longitudinal motion of the ventricle through the cardiac cycle. The ratio of transmitral E velocity to mitral annular E velocity (E/Ea) is related to left atrial pressure.

Impaired ventricular relaxation is characterised by a decreased transmitral Doppler E/A ratio, a prolonged transmitral Doppler E-wave deceleration time (>240 ms), and a pulmonary venous Doppler systolic/diastolic velocity ratio >1. A progressive increase in the LV end diastolic pressure can alter this pattern of delayed relaxation and such a "pseudonormal" transmitral Doppler pattern will have a normal E/A ratio, a pulmonary venous Doppler systolic/diastolic wave velocity ratio <1, but a reduced tissue Doppler (TDI) annular E-wave (Ea) velocity (<10 cm/s). With further increases in left atrial pressure, the transmitral E-wave deceleration time decreases and the E/A ratio increases resulting in a restrictive pattern with E-wave deceleration time <150 ms, E/A ratio >2, and mitral annular TDI Ea velocity <10 cm/s (Tables 20.2 and 20.4).

Valvular Regurgitation (Figs 20.7 and 20.30)

Tricuspid and mitral regurgitation are common findings in the heart failure patients. In some patients, these volume overload lesions along with aortic insufficiency, are the aetiology for a dilated cardiomyopathy and can be quantified with echocardiography and Doppler. However, in those with dilated and ischaemic cardio-

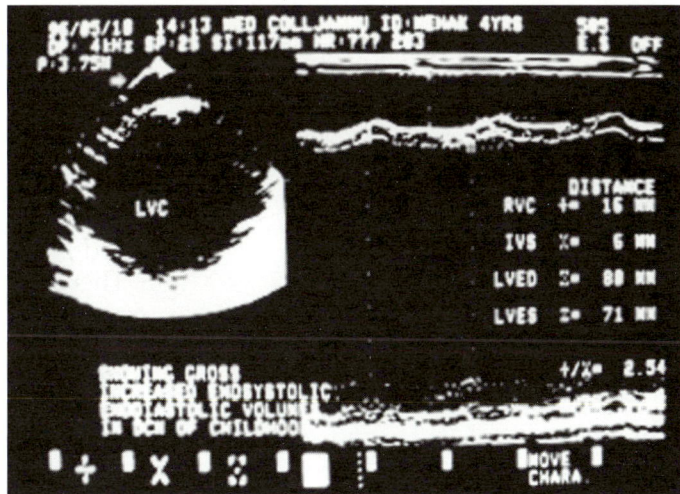

Fig. 20.4: M-Mode and 2-D echocardiogram showing dilated RV, dilated LV, thinned and hypokinetic interventricular septum in a very young patient with dilated cardiomyopathy

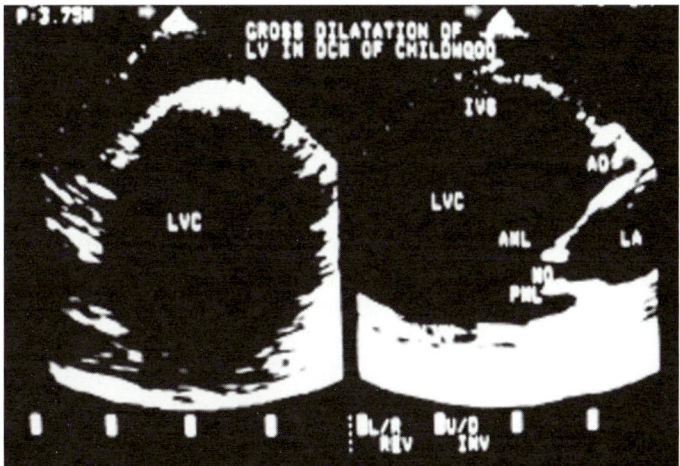

Fig. 20.5: 2-D short axis and modified long axis views of LV showing gross dilatation of LV and thinned wall with poor contractions in a young girl with dilated cardiomyopathy

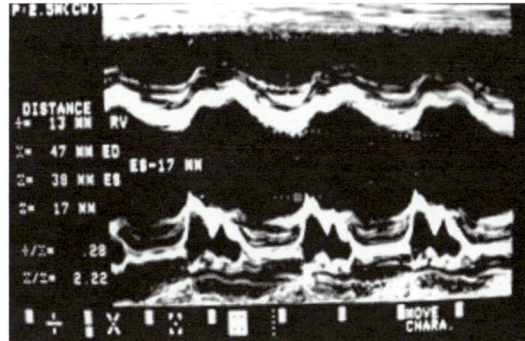

Fig. 20.6: M-Mode echocardiogram showing dilated RV, dilated LV, thinned and hypokinetic interventricular septum. There is also increased distance between septum and E point of mitral valve and double diamond type of MV configuration in patient with dilated cardiomyopathy

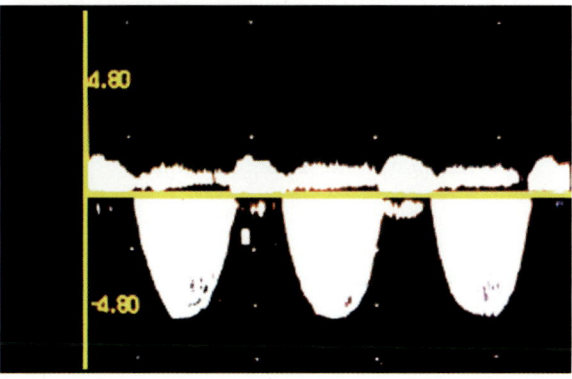

Fig. 20.7: Doppler flow velocity across MV showing gross mitral regurgitaton in patient with dilated cardiomyopathy

myopathy, the atrioventricular valve incompetence is typically "functional" and reflects geometric distortions of the chambers, which displace the normal valvar and subvalvar closing mechanisms. The closure of the valve leaflets tends to be displaced into the ventricle and is known as incomplete valve closure. This functional mitral regurgitation is typically a marker of adverse LV remodelling and increased sphericity of the chamber, while functional tricuspid regurgitation is a marker of both primary right ventricular (RV) systolic dysfunction, RV dilation, and pulmonary hypertension. Since LV remodelling and pulmonary hypertension have prognostic value in heart failure patients it is easy to see that the presence of functional mitral and tricuspid regurgitation assessed by echocardiography also has additive prognostic value.

Dilated Cardiomyopathy (Figs 20.2–20.14)

Dilated cardiomyopathy is characterised with echocardiography by the presence of a dilated left ventricle with impaired ventricular systolic function. The aetiology of this form of cardiomyopathy may be idiopathic, familial, viral, ischaemic or immunological. Echocardiography may be utilised to determine the degree of impairment of LV systolic function and to characterise diastolic function. Specific echocardiographic features, when present, are helpful in identifying the aetiology of the dilated cardiomyopathy. The presence of isolated wall motion abnormalities which correlate with a specific coronary artery distribution suggests the presence of underlying coronary artery disease.

RV function is an important predictor of prognosis in individuals with a dilated cardiomyopathy. Not only do individuals with biventricular dysfunction have a lower New York Heart Association (NYHA) functional class, they also have more severe LV dysfunction and worse long-term prognosis.

Table 20.2: *Echocardiographic evaluation of systolic and diastolic functions*

Dependent factors	*Less dependent factors*
Systolic function LVEF	Cyclic variation of integrated
LVV (left ventricular volume)	backscatter (CVIB)
Left ventricular systolic strain/ strain rate	Systolic mitral annular longitudinal shortening
Diastolic function	Elastance
Colour M-Mode flow propagation velocities	Peak transmitral E and A Velocities (Vp)
E/A ratio	E deceleration time
Pulmonary venous systolic and	Mitral annular tissue Doppler (Ea)
diastolic Doppler velocities	
LVEF = left ventricular ejection fraction; **LVV** = left ventricular volume	

Layered Concept of Interventricular Septum

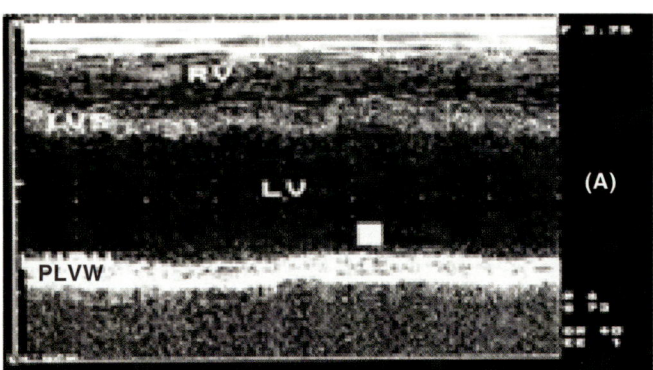

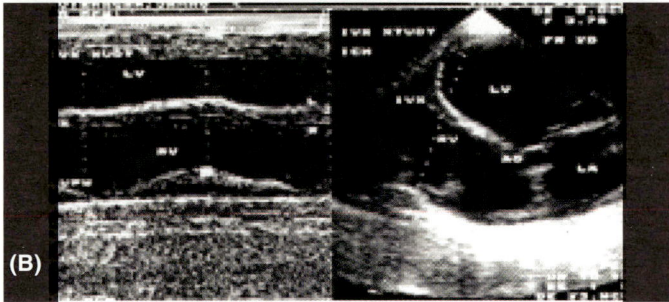

Fig. 20.8A and B: M-Mode and 2-D echoscan in modified 4C in plane from apex cutting through mid septum and posterior left ventricular wall showing layered interventricular septum depicting almost loss of myocardium on left aspect (L) and normal to reduced thickness of IVS on the right side (R) of IVS in patient with 3-vessel coronary artery disease and clinically presenting as dilated cardiomyopathy

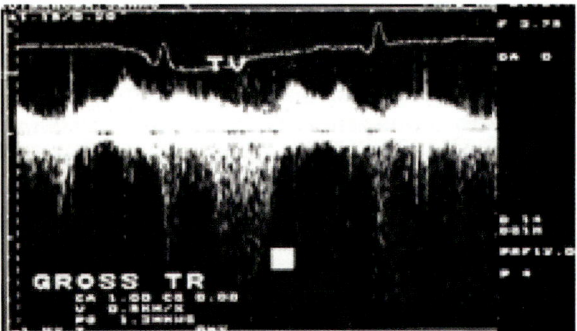

Fig. 20.9: Doppler flow velocity across tricuspid valve with gross tricuspid regurgitation in the same patient as described above

In addition to LV size and systolic function, specific features of dilated cardiomyopathy which can be assessed by echocardiography include the degree, if any, of RV dilatation and systolic dysfunction, an estimation of RV systolic pressures derived from the tricuspid regurgitation Doppler velocities, the presence of LV thrombus and an assessment of left atrial (LA) and LV end diastolic pressure (LVEDP). In the presence of adequate aortic and mitral regurgitant Doppler velocity profiles, and assuming there is no obstruction to left heart inflow or outflow, left atrial and LV end diastolic pressures can be estimated using the simultaneous systolic and diastolic blood pressures with simplified Bernoulli equation: $P = 4V^2$, where P represents the instantaneous pressure gradient in mmHg, and V represents the instantaneous velocity in m/s. LA pressure = (systolic blood pressure) – (peak LV to LA pressure gradient from mitral regurgitation. LVEDP = (diastolic blood pressure) – (maximal AV to LV gradient at end diastole from the aortic regurgitant velocity). The presence of a restrictive LV Doppler filling pattern results in a tripling of the mortality rate compared to patients with a non-ischaemic dilated cardiomyopathy without the marker of increased risk.

Hypertrophic Cardiomyopathy (Figs 20.35–20.56)

Hypertrophic cardiomyopathy is an autosomal dominant disorder associated with a high risk of sudden death in otherwise healthy young individuals, particularly athletes. It is characterised by variable degrees of LV hypertrophy and diastolic dysfunction. While genetic screening studies can be useful in predicting risk of sudden cardiac death, echocardiography remains the most useful diagnostic method. Characteristic echocardiographic features of hypertrophic cardiomyopathy include variable degrees of RV and/or LV hypertrophy. Several forms of the disease are seen with echocardiography: hypertrophic non-obstructive cardiomyopathy, hypertrophic obstructive cardiomyopathy (HOCM), and apical variant of hypertrophic cardiomyopathy. In those with HOCM, systolic anterior motion of the mitral valve and the presence of left ventricular outflow tract (LVOT) obstruction are noted on echocardiography. LV wall thickness in excess of 13 mm without apparent cause, or a ratio of the septal to posterior wall thickness of >1.3, is diagnostic of HOCM. Systolic anterior motion of the mitral valve and LVOT obstruction occurs in approximately 25% of individuals with hypertrophic cardiomyopathy. This obstruction occurs as anterior motion of the anterior mitral leaflet during systole results in a narrowing of the LVOT. The presence of a resting LVOT gradient of >30 mmHg in individuals with hypertrophic cardiomyopathy is predictive of an increased risk of death related to the hypertrophic cardiomyopathy, progression to NYHA class III or IV heart failure, or death from heart failure or stroke. Right ventricular outflow tract obstruction occurs less frequently. Echocardiography can be utilised to tailor treatment for individuals with hypertrophic cardio-myopathy. The response to medical treatment for hypertrophic cardiomyopathy, including a decrease in an outflow tract gradient or improvement in diastolic function, can be evaluated by serial echocardiographic studies. The decision to proceed with nonmedical therapeutic options, including surgical septal reduction, percutaneous alcohol septal reduction, or DDD pacing, can also be guided by echocardiography. The presence and degree of LVOT obstruction detected by echocardiography aids the clinician in determining whether or not to perform septal reduction. Surgical septal reduction is recommended in individuals with symptoms refractory to medical treatment in the presence of a resting gradient of >50 mm Hg. Indications for percutaneous alcohol septal reduction include a septal thickness >18 mm Hg, the presence of a resting LVOT gradient of >30 mm Hg, or an inducible gradient of >60 mm Hg in the presence of NYHA functional class III or IV symptoms unrelieved by maximal medical treatment. Echocardiographic guidance during alcohol septal ablation, using intravenous contrast selectively into septal coronary vessels, allows the operator to identify the correct vessel supplying the appropriate myocardial territory, thus decreasing the likelihood of infarction of other portions of the heart and reducing the need for permanent pacing.

In addition to characterising the degree of ventricular hypertrophy in affected individuals, echocardiography can also be used to screen asymptomatic relatives of affected individuals. Most recently, tissue Doppler imaging has been used to identify abnormal diastolic function in individuals with genotypes for hypertrophic cardiomyopathy before the development of significant ventricular hypertrophy. The sensitivity and specificity of the mitral annular early diastolic (Ea) velocity varies in the different reports and this may relate to the genotype studied.

Table 20.3: *Echocardiographic abnormalities in cardiomyopathy*

Left ventricular dilation
Increasing sphericity of left ventricular geometry
Apical and lateral displacement of papillary muscles
Functional mitral regurgitation
Left ventricular thrombus
Left atrial dilation
Atrial fibrillation
Left atrial thrombosis/stasis of blood
Pulmonary hypertension
Tricuspid regurgitation
Right ventricular dilation

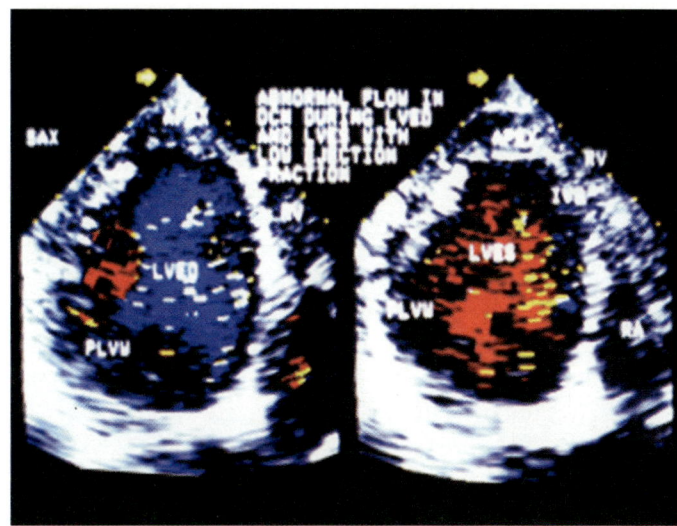

Fig. 20.10: Color 2-D short axis dual scan LV views showing gross dilation of left ventricular cavity during systole and diastole and churning of blood with abnormal flow motion patterns in dilated cardiomyopathy

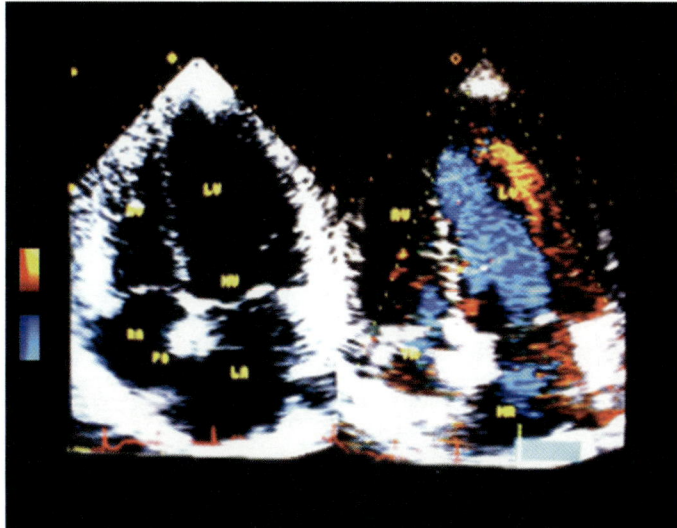

Fig. 20.11: Color flow in 2-D apical 4C dual scan views showing gross dilatation of all four chambers of the heart along with abnormal color flow motions in patient with dilated cardiomyopathy

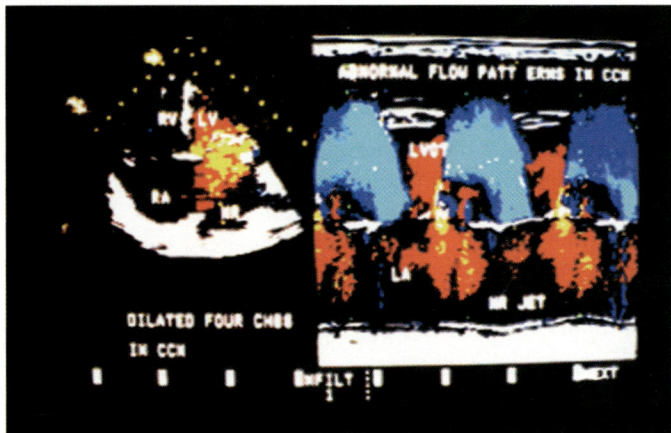

Fig. 20.12: 2-D Apical 4C and color flow at mitral valve showing mitral regurgitation as blue jet into LA and red and blue color flows in LVOT in patient with dilated cardiomyopathy

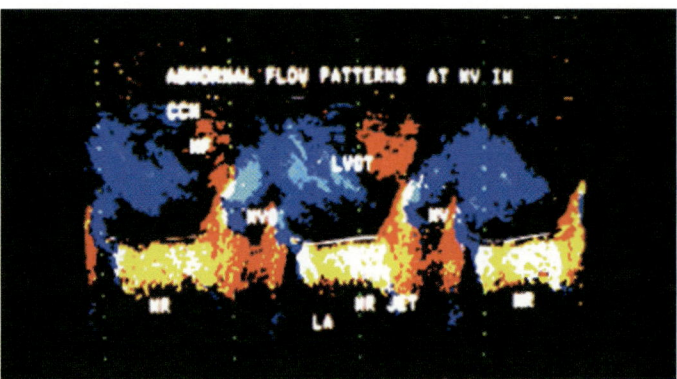

Fig. 20.15: Abnormal flow patterns as disorganized blue and red like clouds in patient with dilated cardiomyopathy

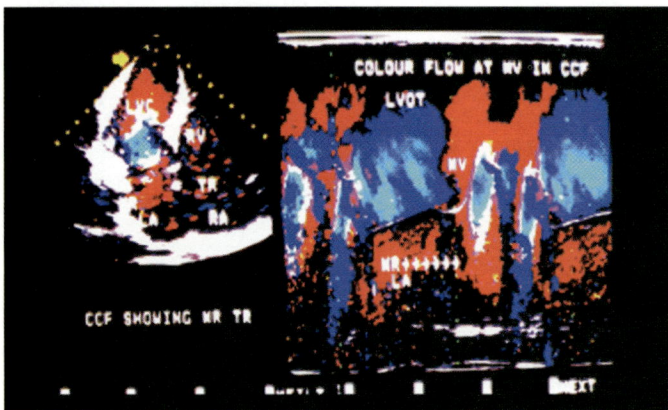

Fig. 20.13: 2-D Apical 4C and color flow at mitral valve showing mitral regurgitation as blue jet into LA and TR (left) and red and blue color flow as disorganized clouds in LVOT in patient with dilated cardiomyopathy (right)

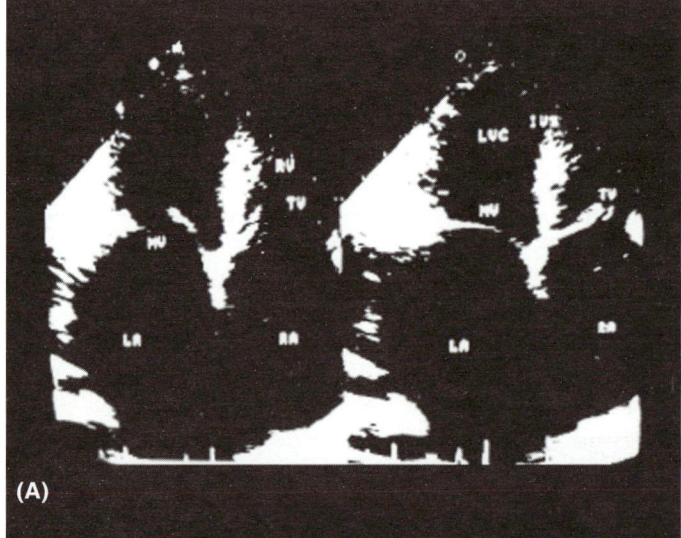

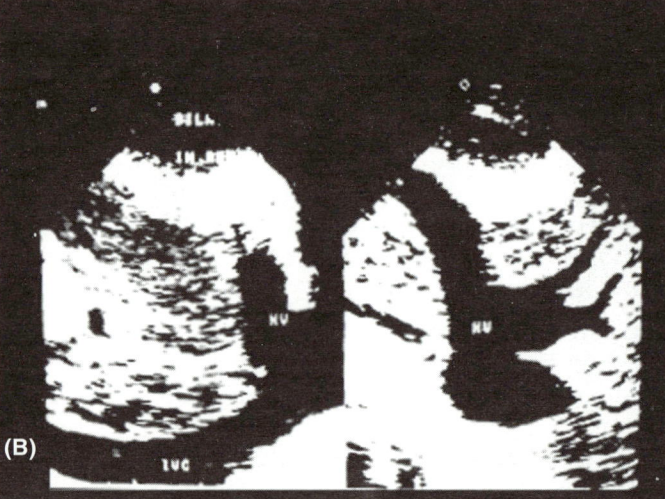

Fig. 20.16: (A) Apical 4C dual scan views (upper panel) showing marked dilatation of all four chambers of the heart in patient with restrictive cardiomyopathy **(B)** (lower panel) showing grossely dilated inferior vena cava and portal venous system in patient with restrictive cardiomyopathy

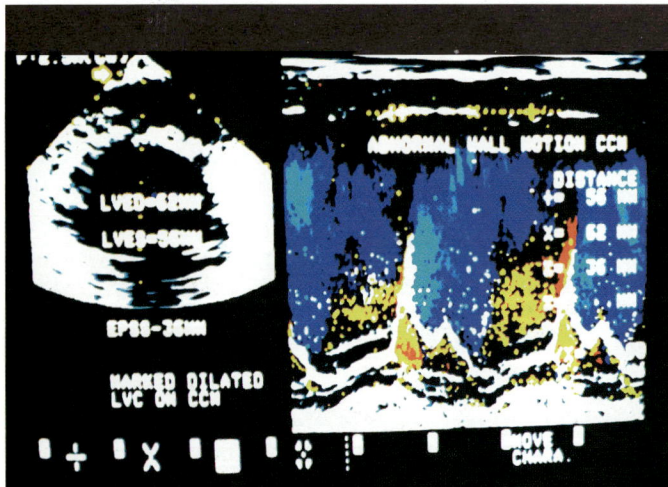

Fig. 20.14: 2-D short axis view at LV and color M-Mode echocardiography showing color flows in LVOT area as blue clouds due to poor LV functions in patient with congestive cardiomyopathy

Restrictive Cardiomyopathy

While restrictive cardiomyopathies are less common than dilated and hypertrophic cardiomyopathies, they are associated with greater morbidity and mortality. As the name implies, restrictive cardiomyopathies are associated with impaired ventricular filling and increased LV end diastolic pressure. Echocardiographic features include biatrial dilatation, hypertrophied ventricles with decreased compliance, initially small LV cavities, and normal to depressed systolic function. Infiltrative processes and metabolic storage diseases including amyloidosis, haemochromatosis, sarcoidosis, Fabry's disease, and glycogen storage diseases are the most frequent causes of restrictive cardiomyopathies. Less common forms of restrictive cardiomyopathies include endocardial fibrosis associated with the hypereosinophilic syndrome (Loeffler's cardiomyopathy) and idiopathic restrictive cardiomyopathy. The echocardiographic features of endocardial fibrosis associated with hypereosinophilia (Fig. 20.17) include haemodynamic evidence of restriction and obliteration of the ventricular apices caused by deposition of thrombus and eosinophilic cationic protein. The regional myocardial motion adjacent to this deposition remains normal (Figs 20.17 to 20.24).

While the clinical distinction between a restrictive cardiomyopathy and pericardial constriction in a patient with symptoms of systemic congestion can be challenging, echocardiography can noninvasively separate these two distinct entities. This distinction is extremely important since the treatments are dramatically different; pericardial constriction can be successfully treated with pericardial stripping while the treatment of restrictive cardiomyopathy is largely aimed at improvement in symptoms. The constraining effect of a thickened pericardium leads to rapid early diastolic filling characterised by a tall transmitral Doppler E-wave with rapid deceleration phase (<150 ms), >30% increase in the mitral inflow peak velocity with exhalation, hepatic venous dilation and flow reversal, and two distinct septal motions which are unrelated to contraction. One of these septal motions is high amplitude and low frequency, and reflects differential filling of the ventricles during the phases of the respiratory cycle which is due to ventricular interdependence. The second is a low amplitude, high frequency diastolic septal motion which reflects differences in timing of the filling of the ventricles (the "septal bounce"). While the restrictive pattern of the transmitral E wave is similar in both constriction and restriction, there is no significant respiratory change in the transmitral inflow pattern associated with restrictive cardiomyopathy. Restrictive processes are also much more likely to be associated with pulmonary hypertension and the presence of diastolic mitral regurgitation. Tissue Doppler imaging can also distinguish between constriction and restriction. While the early mitral annular velocity (Ea) is notably decreased in restriction reflecting a myocardial abnormality, it remains normal in the presence of pericardial constriction since in this disease the myocardium typically remains normal.

Idiopathic restrictive cardiomyopathy is a rare entity distinguished from the other forms of restrictive cardiomyopathy by the presence of normal ventricular wall thickness. This disease is seen in individuals where other aetiologies for cardiomyopathy have been excluded such as connective tissue disease, carcinoid syndrome, amyloidosis, haemochromatosis, eosinophilic syndrome, malignancy, radiation exposure, cardiotoxic drug exposure, or history of alcohol abuse. In addition these individuals do not have a history of ischaemic heart disease, treated hypertension for more than five years, or organic valvar, pericardial or congenital diseases.

Cardiac Amyloidosis (Figs 20.23 and 20.24)

Myocardial infiltration by amyloid fibrils can occur in primary, familial, secondary, and senile amyloidosis. The degree of involvement is variable depending upon the type of amyloidosis. Two-dimensional echocardiography remains the ideal method for identifying and following individuals with cardiac amyloidosis.

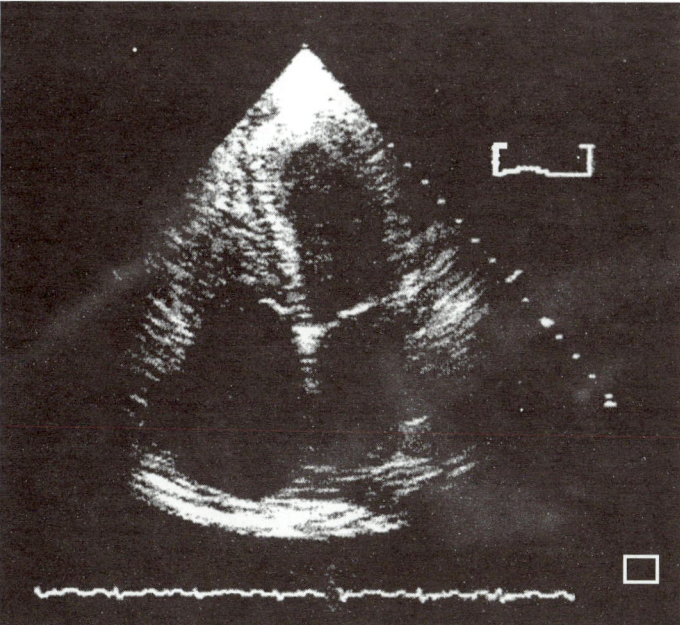

Fig. 20.17: Apical four-chamber echocardiographic image from an individual with cardiomyopathy associated with hypereosinophilic syndrome showing soft tissue thrombus deposition within the left and right ventricular apices. Right atrial deposition is also present

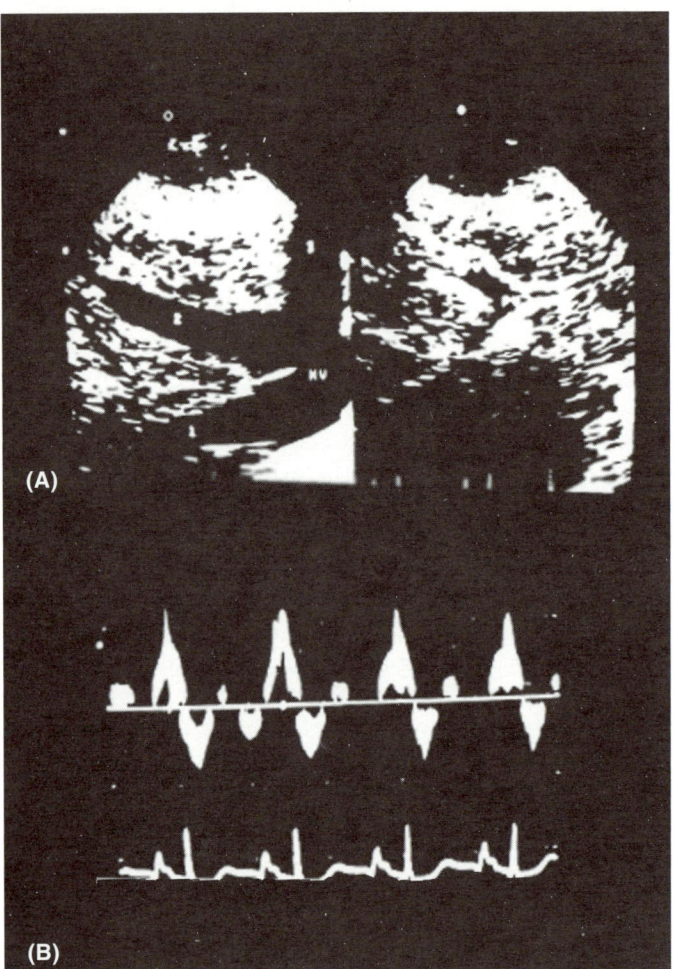

Fig. 20.18A and B: **(A)** (upper) subcostal approach transhepatic view showing markedly dilated three branches of main hepatic vein in patient with restrictive cardiomyopathy. **(B)** Doppler flow velocity across main hepatic vein showing reversal of flow in patient with restrictive cardiomyopathy (lower panel)

Characteristic two-dimensional and Doppler echocardiographic features have been described in individuals with cardiac amyloidosis. Two-dimensional features include thickening of the LV walls, increased reflectivity of these walls (the "speckled" or "granular" myocardium), biatrial enlargement, thickening of the interatrial septum, thickening and regurgitation of the mitral and tricuspid valves, and the presence of a small pericardial effusion. Transmitral Doppler flow patterns in patients with amyloidosis exhibit evidence of diastolic dysfunction. Characteristic transmitral. Doppler patterns representative of early impaired relaxation and later restrictive filling have been demonstrated in this population. An increase in both the pulmonary venous Doppler atrial reversal duration and the ratio of this atrial reversal duration to the transmitral A-wave duration have been observed in these patients and reflect increased LA pressure.

Cardiac amyloidosis should be considered in individuals in whom several of these echocardiographic features are observed. The coexistence of increased thickening of the LV walls on echocardiography and low voltage on electrocardiography is highly suggestive of amyloid infiltration of the myocardium.

Differentiating cardiac amyloidosis from hypertrophic cardiomyopathy can be difficult on echocardiography. Asymmetric septal thickening can result from focal amyloid deposition and can mimic hypertrophic cardiomyopathy. The presence of decreased LV function would argue strongly against hypertrophic cardiomyopathy.

The presence of highly reflective myocardium can also be seen in individuals with primary and secondary causes of LV hypertrophy, ventricular fibrosis, and other infiltrative processes. The integration of clinical, echocardiographic, and electrocardiographic data is essential when making the diagnosis of cardiac amyloidosis.

While the long-term prognosis is substantially worse in patients with primary amyloidosis, the echocardiographic distinction between familial, primary, and secondary amyloidosis can be difficult. Impaired LV systolic function is more common in primary amyloidosis than in the other forms.

Doppler tissue echocardiography is helpful in differentiating amyloid patients from those with similar two-dimensional echocardiographic features but without amyloidosis. Abnormally low tissue Doppler diastolic velocities are present in individuals with cardiac amyloid compared with control patients.

Arrhythmic Right Ventricular Dysplasia

Arrhythmic right ventricular dysplasia (ARVD), also known as arrhythmic right ventricular cardiomyopathy, is an idiopathic cardiomyopathy that appears to be genetically transmitted. ARVD is associated with RV fibrosis, fatty infiltration, and dysfunction. It can be complicated by symptoms of heart failure, heart block, and ventricular arrhythmias, and is associated with an increased risk of sudden cardiac death. Pathologic features include loss of RV myocardium, fibrofatty tissue replacement, and resultant aneurysmal dilation of the "triangle of dysplasia" (diaphragmatic, infundibular, and apical RV regions). While RV involvement is universal, the left ventricle is involved less frequently and the degree of involvement is less severe.

The diagnostic criteria for ARVD include a family history of ARVD or sudden cardiac death, imaging (echocardiographic, magnetic resonance imaging, or ventriculography), evidence of characteristic RV dysfunction, typical electrocardiographic features (electrocardiographic depolarisation and repolarisation

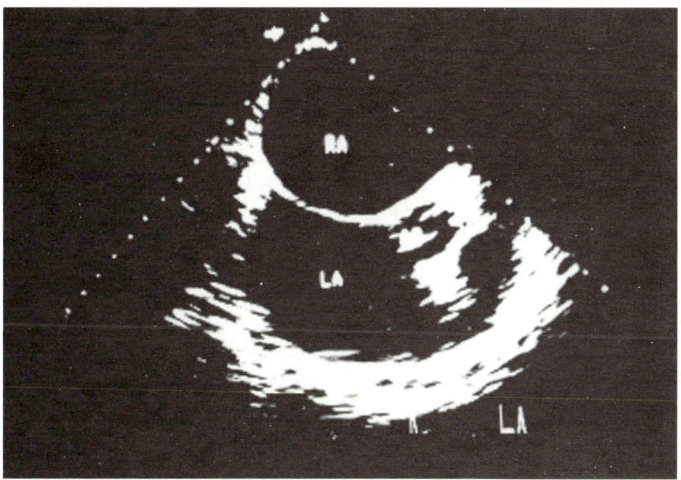

Fig. 20.19: Subcostal biatrial view showing dilated RA and LA with concave shaped intact interatrial septum (IAS) due to raised intracavitary pressure in patient with restrictive cardiomyopathy

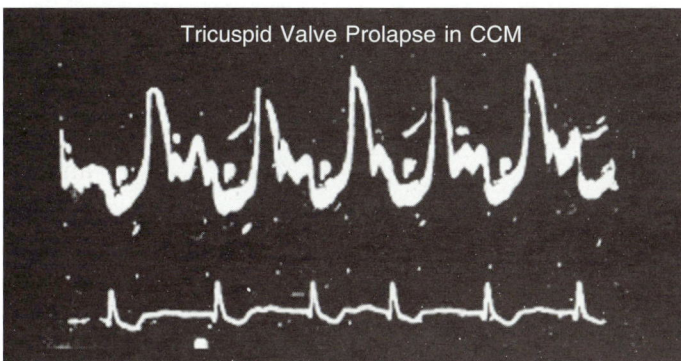

Fig. 20.20: Doppler flow velocity across tricuspid valve (TV) showing prolapse (P) of anterior leaflet of TV in patient with dilated cardiomyopathy

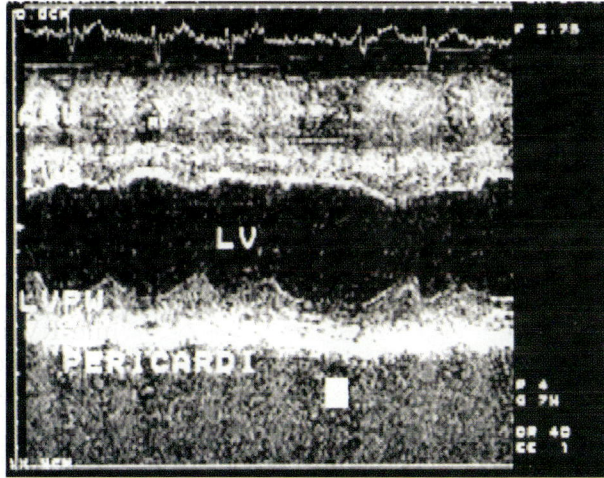

Fig. 20.21: M-Mode echocardiogram showing hypertrophic anterior free wall of right ventricle with hypokinesia of interventricular septum (IVS), dilated LV, irregular movements of IVS and posterior left ventricular wall due to atrial fibrillation in patient with restrictive type of cardiomyopathy syndrome

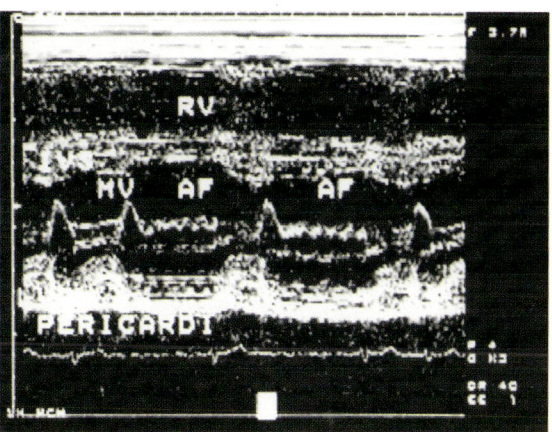

Fig. 20.22: M-Mode echoscan showing dilated RV, irregular thickening of IVS and PLVW and prominent fibrillatory waves of both anterior and posterior mitral leaflets due to atrial fibrillation with restrictive cardiomyopathy

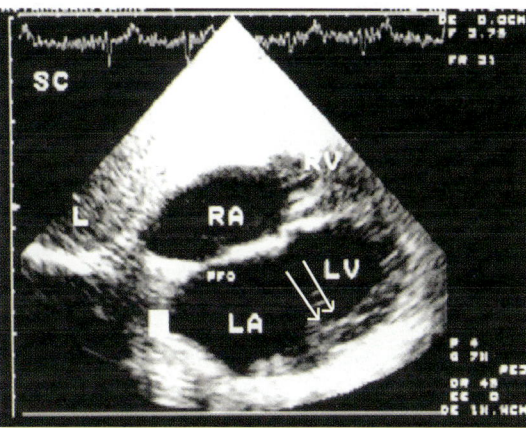

Fig. 20.23: Subcostal approach through biatrial plane showing markedly dilated both right and left atrium, dilated LV and irregularily thickened LA and LV endocardium (arrows) in patient with restrictive cardiomyopathy

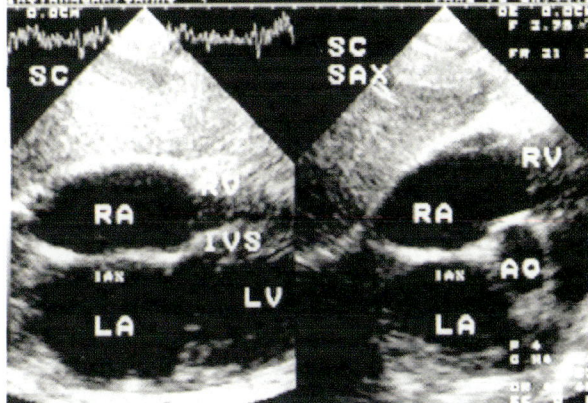

Fig. 20.24: Subcostal approach biatrial view (left) and short axis view at aorta (right) showing equally dilated right and left atria with well preserved thickness of interatrial septum along with irregular thickening of endocardial surface in patient with restrictive cardiomyopathy syndrome

Table 20.4: *Echocardiographic differences between constrictive pericarditis and restrictive cardiomyopathy*

Structural change	Constriction	Restriction
Atrial size	Normal	Dilated
Pericardial appearance	Thick/bright	Normal
Septal motion	Abnormal	Normal
Septal position	Varies with respiration	Normal
Mitral E/A	Increased (>2.0)	Increased (>2.0)
Deceleration time	Short (<160 ms)	Short (<160 ms)
Annular E.	Normal	Reduced (<10 cm/s)
Pulmonary hypertension	Rare	Frequent
Left ventricular size/function	Normal	Normal
Mitral/tricuspid regurgitation	Infrequent	Frequent (TR > MR)
Isovolumic relaxation time	Varies with respiration	Stable with respiration
Respiratory variation of mitral E velocity	Exaggerated (>25%)	Normal

MR = mitral regurgitation; **TR**= tricuspid regurgitation

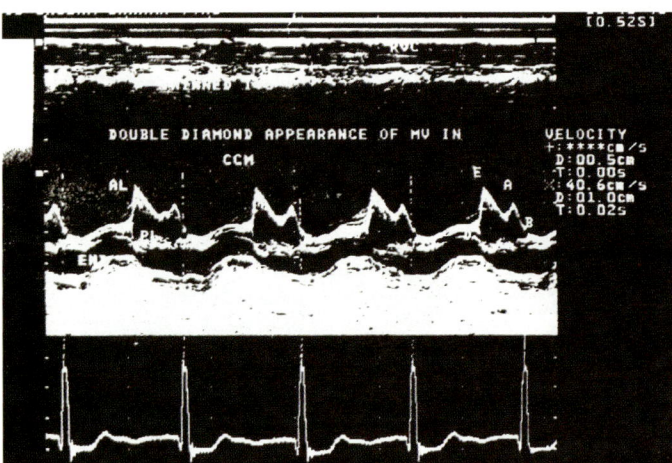

Fig. 20.25: M-Mode echocardiogram showing dilated LV cavity with increased dimension of septal-mitral separation with an early closure of mitral valve in patient with dilated cardiomyopathy

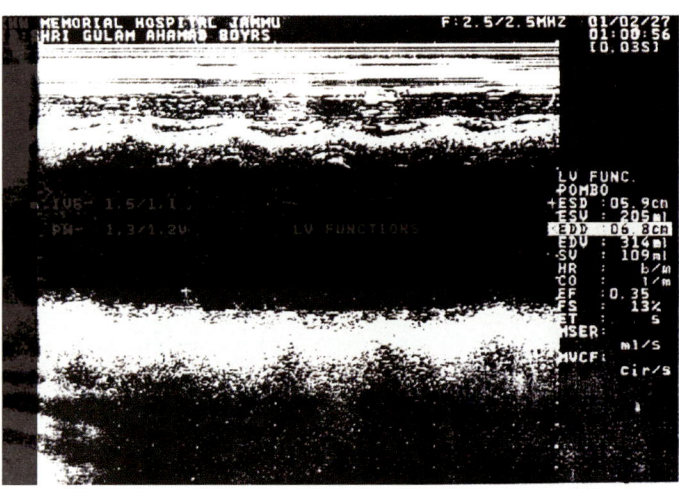

Fig. 20.27: M-Mode echocardiogram across mid cavity showing dilated LV cavity in patient with dilated cardiomyopathy

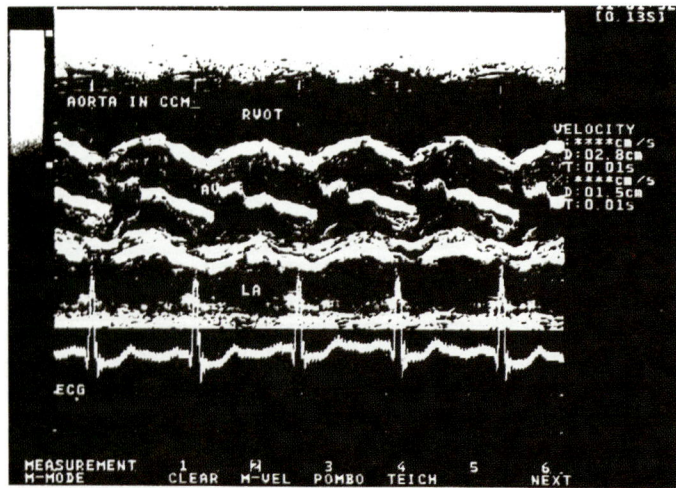

Fig. 20.26: M-Mode echocardiogram showing an early closure of aortic valve in patient with dilated cardiomyopathy

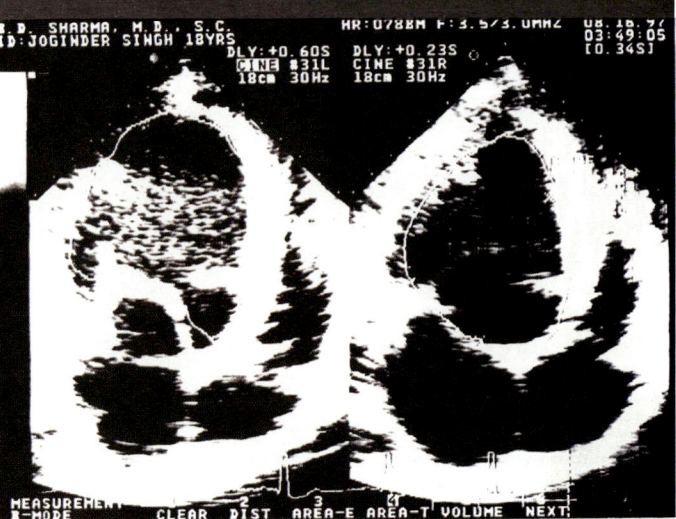

Fig. 20.28: Apical 4C dual scan views at LV showing grossly dilated LV cavity and spontaneous contrast in LV cavity (left) in patient with dilated cardiomyopathy

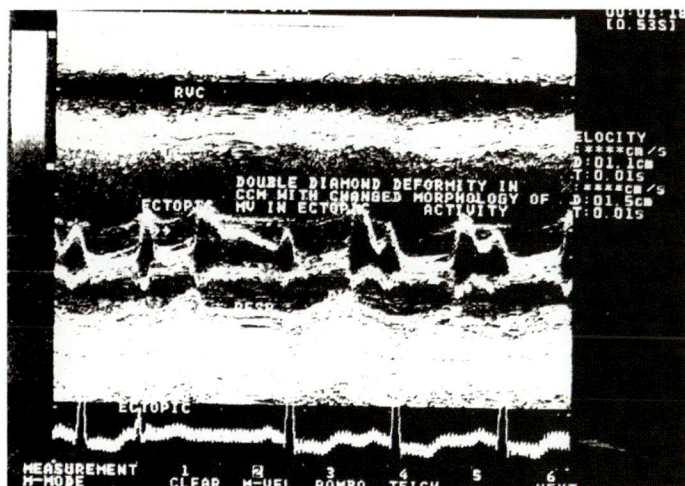

Fig. 20.29: M-Mode echocardiogram showing marked thinning and hypokinetic apical septum, dilated LV cavity along with hypokinesia of posteroinferior wall of LV associated with ventricular ectopics in patient with cardiac sarcoidosis

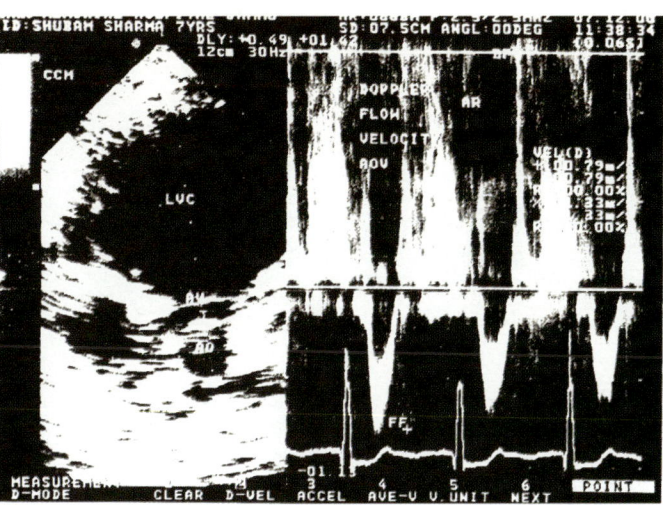

Fig. 20.32: Doppler flow velocity across aortic valve showing gross aortic regurgitation in patient with dilated cardiomyopathy

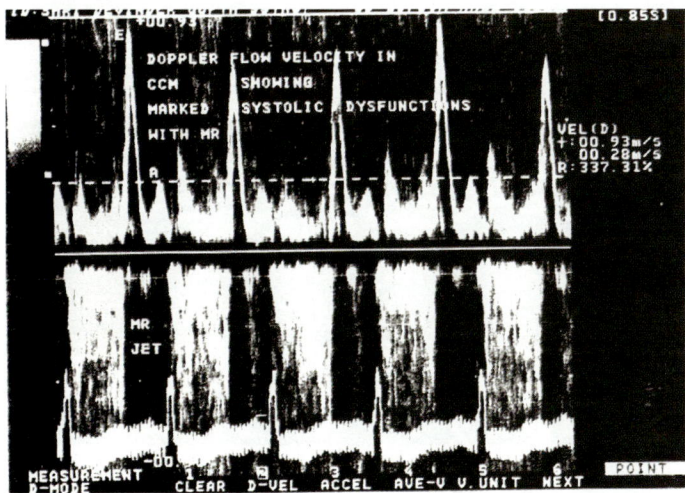

Fig. 20.30: Doppler flow velocity across MV showing gross MR in patient with cardiac sarcoidosis type of dilated cardiomyopathy

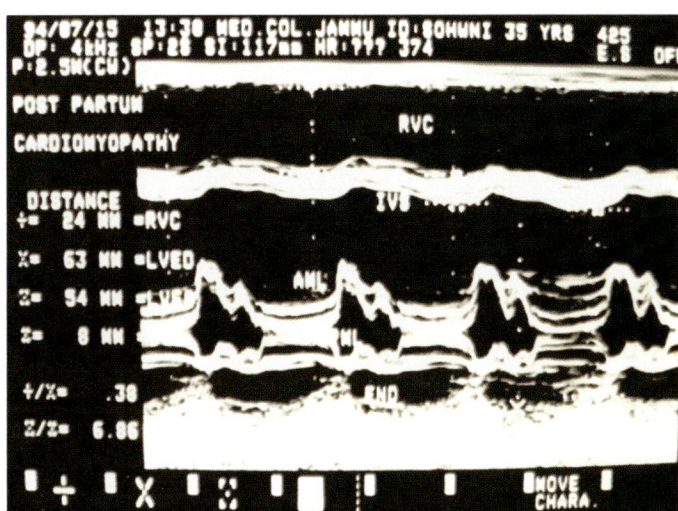

Fig. 20.33: M-Mode echocardiogram showing all the characteristics of dilated cardiomyopathy in patient with post-partum dilated cardiomyopathy

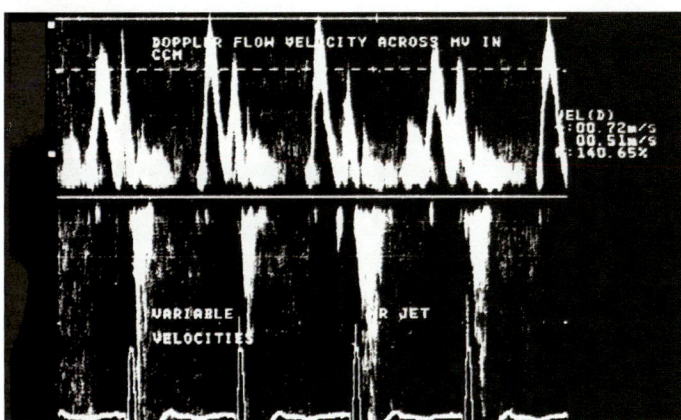

Fig. 20.31: Doppler flow velocity across MV showing mild form of mitral regurgitation and pseudo stabilization of diastolic LV dysfunction in patient with dilated cardiomyopathy

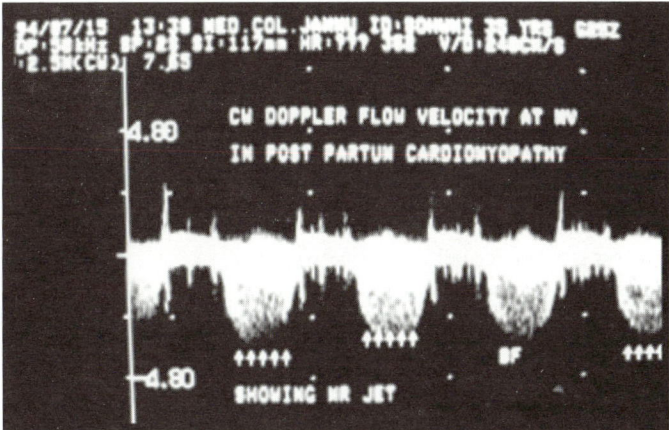

Fig. 20.34: Doppler flow velocity across MV showing gross mitral regurgitation (MR) in patient with postpartum cardiomyopathy

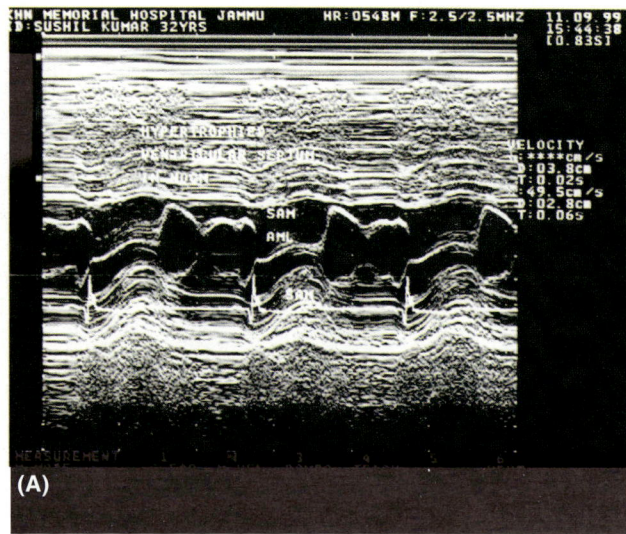

Diagrammatic representation of systolic anterior motion in hypertrophic cardiomyopathy

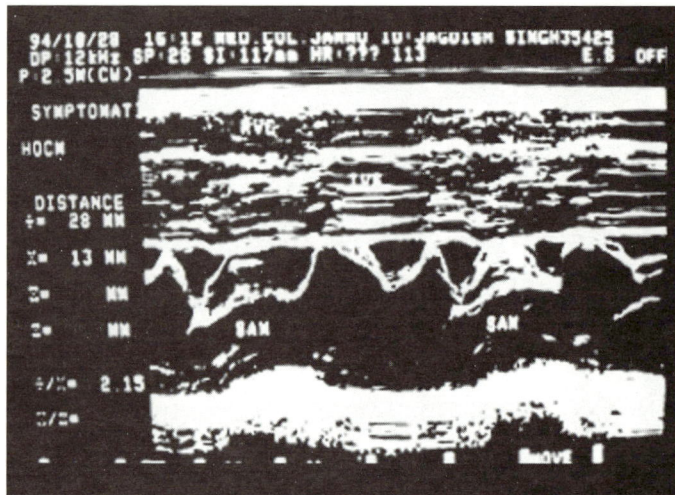

Fig. 20.36: M-Mode echocardiogram showing marked hypertrophy of IVS and systolic anterior motion (SAM) with hypertrophic cardiomyopathy

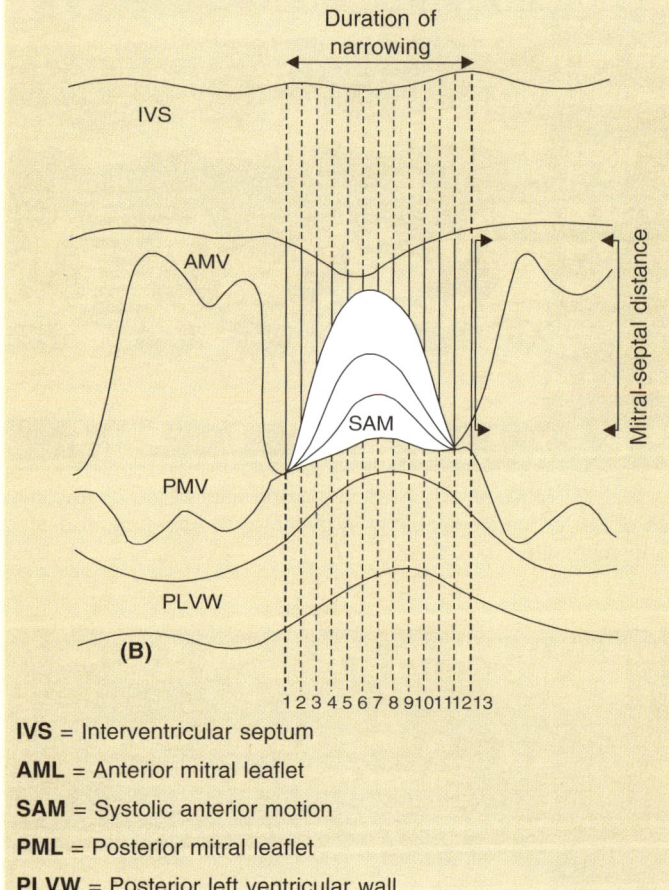

IVS = Interventricular septum

AML = Anterior mitral leaflet

SAM = Systolic anterior motion

PML = Posterior mitral leaflet

PLVW = Posterior left ventricular wall

Fig. 20.35A and B: (A) (upper panel) M-Mode echocardiogram showing marked hypertrophy of interventricular septum (IVS) and systolic anterior motion (SAM) of mitral valve (MV) towards left ventricular outflow tract (LVOT) in patient with hypertrophic cardiomyopathy. **(B)** (lower panel) Diagrammatic representation showing anatomical location and different grades of anterior motion of mitral valve (SAM) in hypertrophic cardiomyopathy (HOCM)

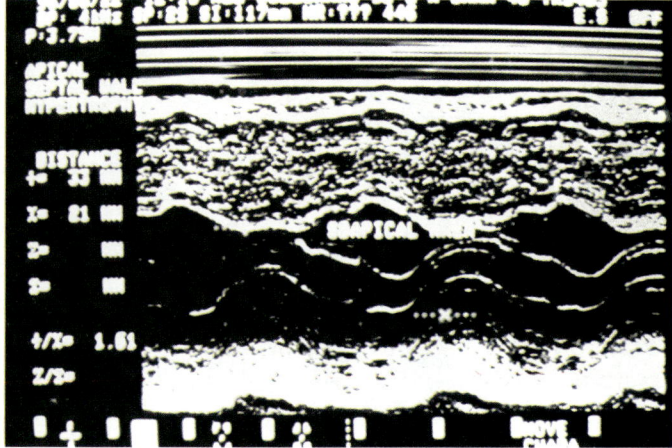

Fig. 20.37: M-Mode echoscan showing asymmetrical septal wall hypertrophy in patient with systemic hypertension

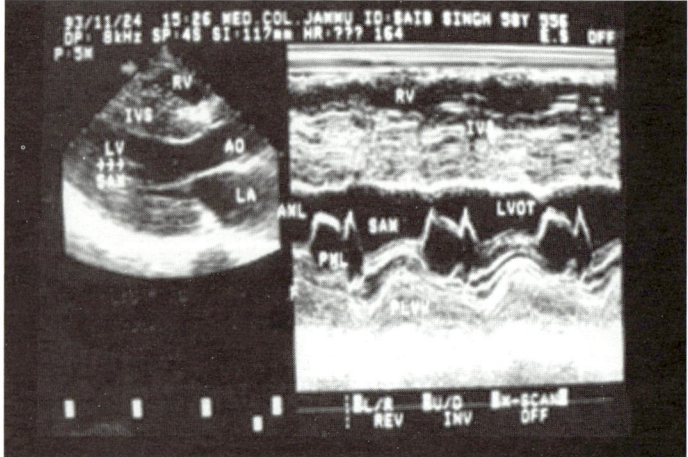

Fig. 20.38: M-Mode (right) and 2-D long axis (left) echo scans showing hypertrophic and hypokinetic IVS normal LVOT, thickening of posterior LV wall in patient with cardiac amyloidosis

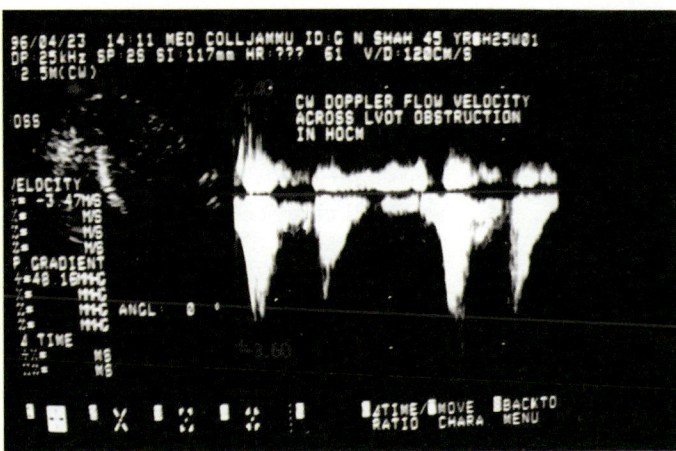

Fig. 20.39: Doppler flow velocity across LVOT showing increased flow velocity in patient with hypertrophic obstructive cardiomyopathy with amyloid disease with chronic renal failure

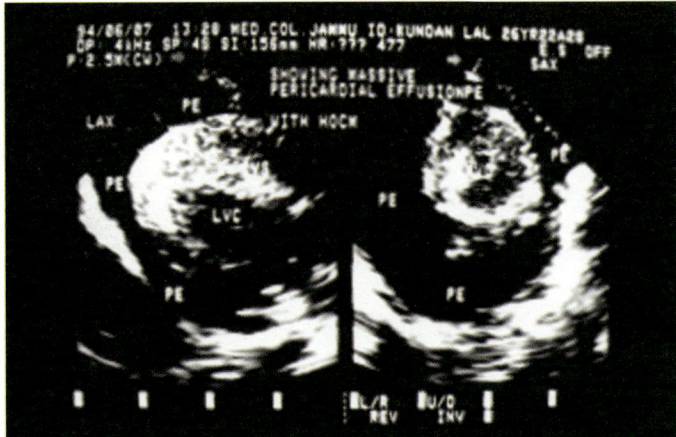

Fig. 20.40: Oblique 4C (left) and short axis LV (right) showing massive pericardial effusion (PE) localised both anteriorly and posteriorly in patient with hypertrophic obstructive cardiomyopathy, amyloid disease and chronic renal failure

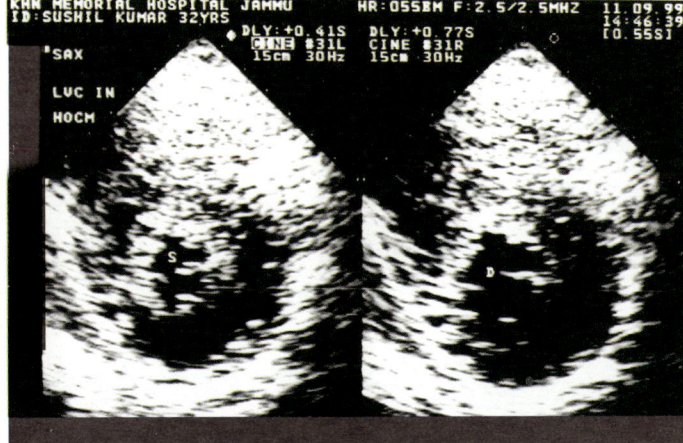

Fig. 20.41: 2D Short axis LV during systole and diastole showing marked hypertrophy of walls of LV and reduced dimension of LVOT in patient with hypertrophic cardiomyopathy

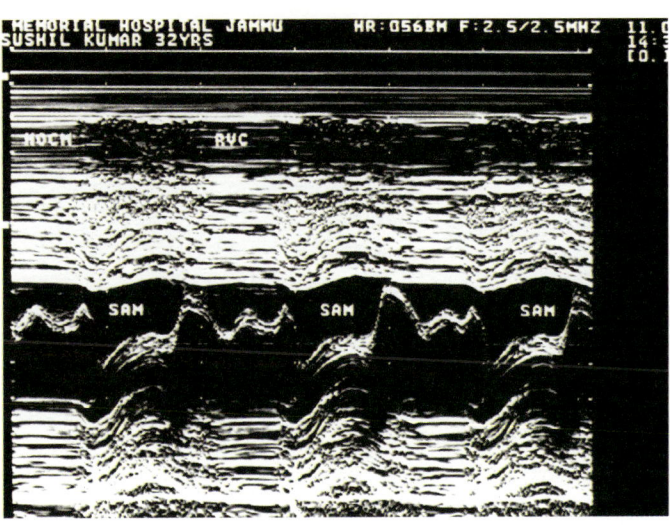

Fig. 20.42: M-Mode echocardiogram showing marked hypertrophy of interventricular septum (IVS) and anterior systolic motion of mitral valve in patient as another example of hypertrophic cardiomyopathy

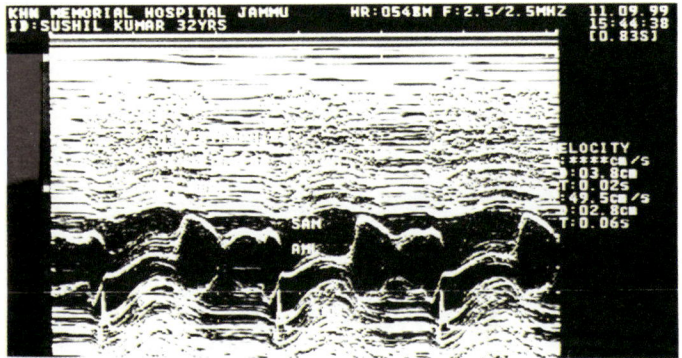

Fig. 20.43: M-Mode echocardiogram showing marked hypertrophy of interventricular septum (IVS) with systolic anterior motion of mitral valve in hypertrophic cardiomyopathy

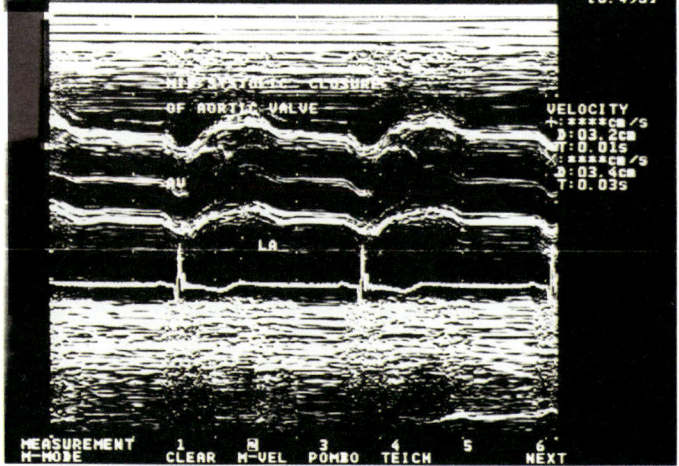

Fig. 20.44: M-Mode echocardiogram showing midsystolic closure of aortic valve in patient with hypertrophic cardiomyopathy

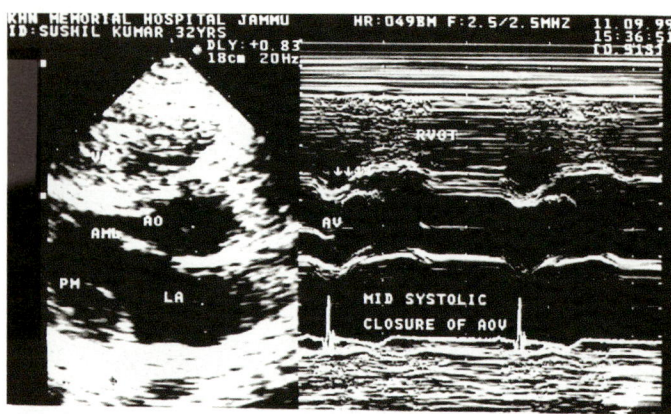

Fig. 20.45: 2-D Long axis (left) and M-Mode echocardiogram showing midsystolic closure of aortic valve (right) in patient with hypertrophic cardiomyopathy

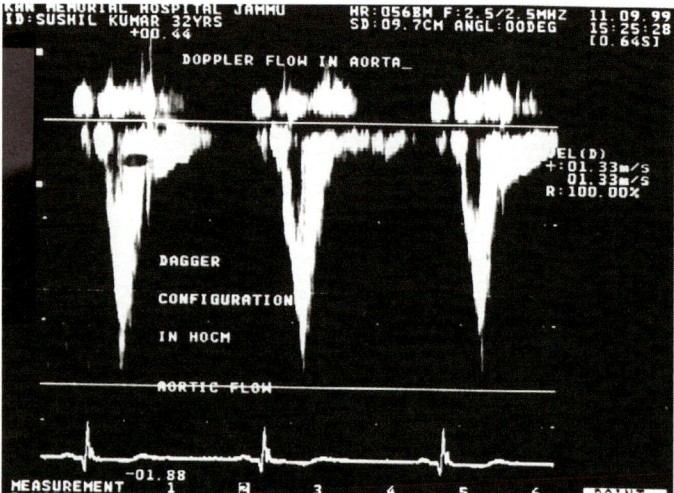

Fig. 20.46: Doppler flow velocity across LVOT showing typical dagger configuration of velocity in patient with hypertrophic cardiomyopathy

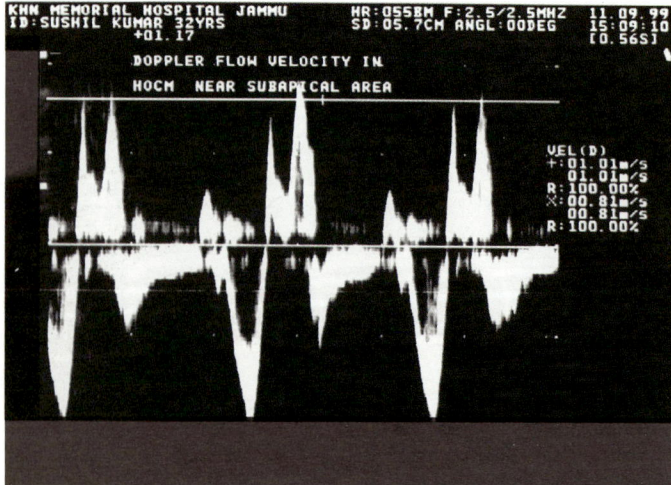

Fig. 20.47: Doppler flow velocity in subapical area showing both forward and backward velocities in patient with hypertrophic cardiomyopathy

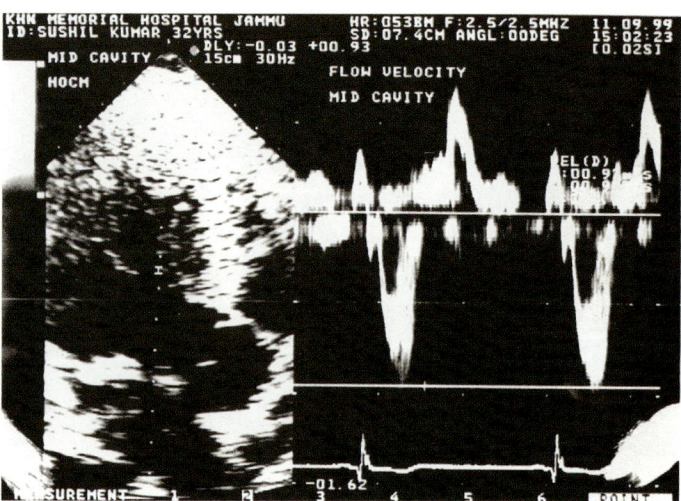

Fig. 20.48: 2D LV Mid cavity (left) and Doppler flow velocity in mid cavity showing late peaking of forward velocity in patient with hypertrophic cardiomyopathy

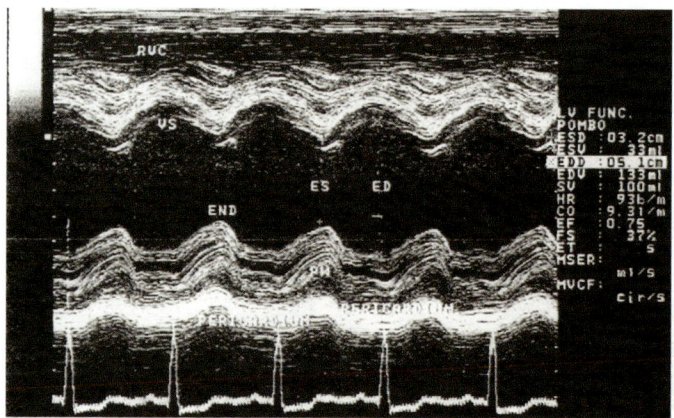

Fig. 20.49: M-Mode echocardiogram showing non-obstructive concentric left ventricular hypertrophy in patient with chronic systemic hypertension

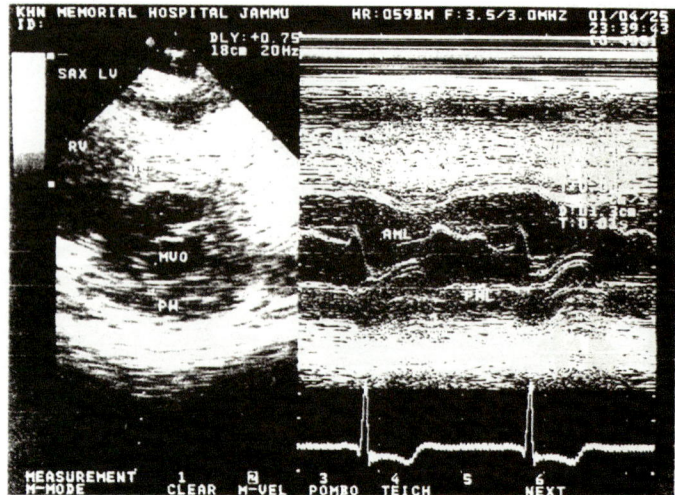

Fig. 20.50: 2D short axis LV and M-Mode echocardiogram showing another example of non-obstructive type of LV hypertrophy

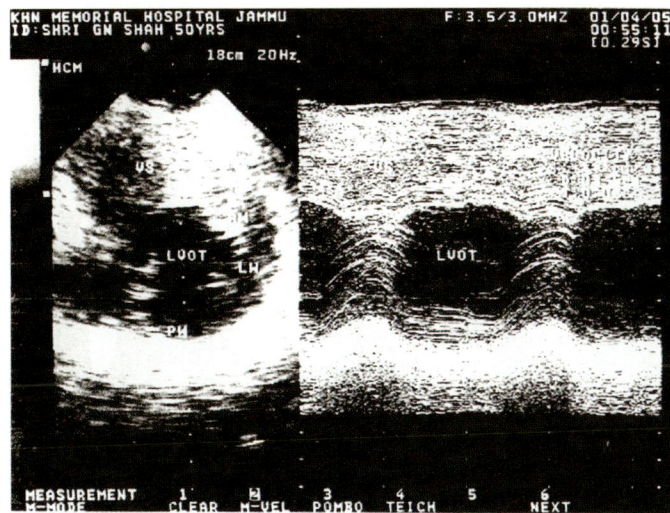

Fig. 20.51: 2-D Short axis LV and M-mode echocardiogram showing another example of non-obstructive hypertrophic cardiomyopathy in patient with uncontrolled systemic hypertension

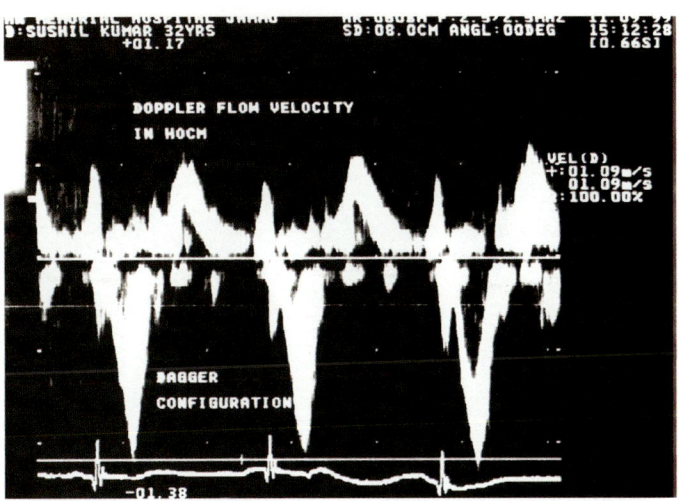

Fig. 20.54: Doppler flow velocity across LVOT showing midsystolic peaking of forward velocity giving an impression of dagger configuration in patient with hypertrophic obstructive cardiomyopathy

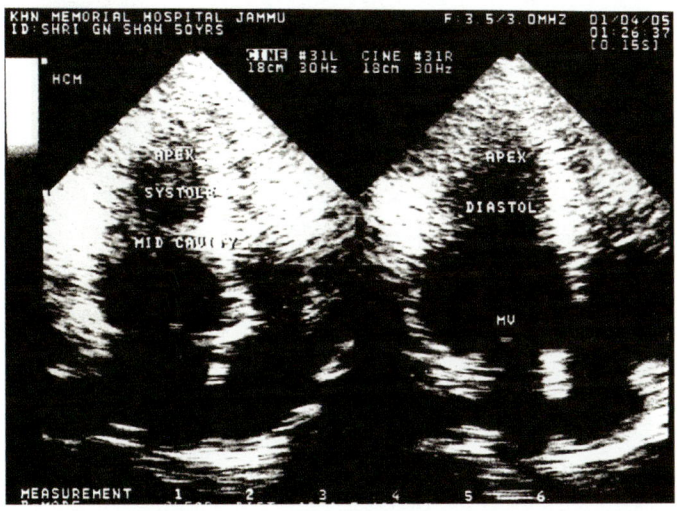

Fig. 20.52: 2-D Apical 4C dual scan views showing apical and right ventricular mid cavity hypertrophy in patient with hypertension and NIDDM

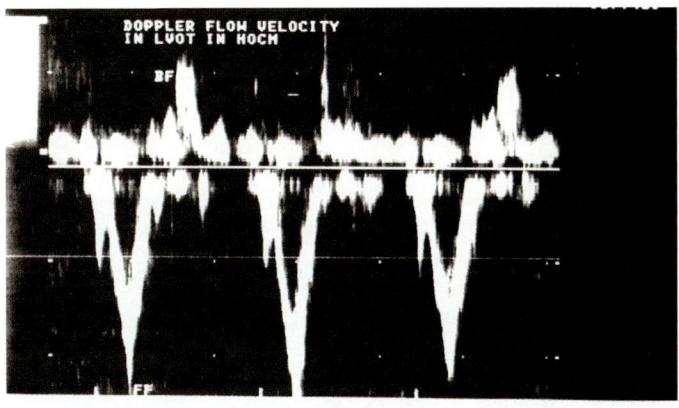

Fig. 20.55: Doppler flow velocity across LVOT showing very sharp flow velocity in mid systole with narrow spectral waveform in subaortic obstruction in patient with hypertrophic obstructive cardiomyopathy

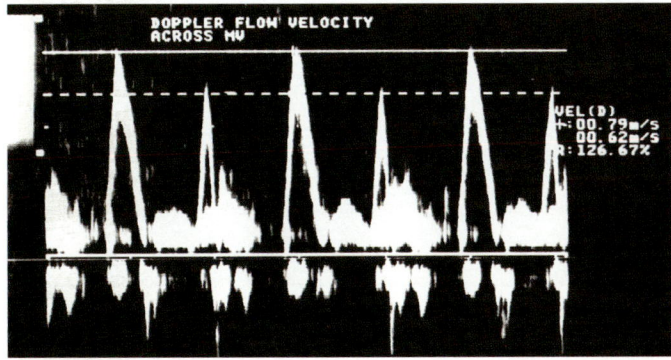

Fig. 20.53: Doppler flow velocity across mitral valve showing delayed E and A velocities in patient with hypertrophic obstructive cardiomyopathy

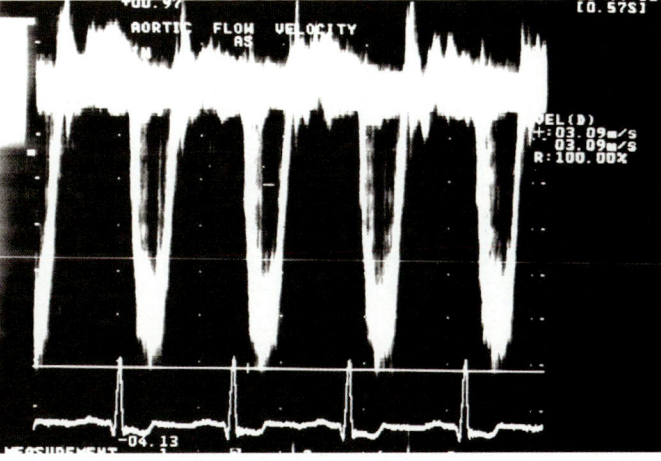

Fig. 20.56: Doppler flow velocity across aortic valve showing enhanced flow velocity with wide spectral waveform in patient with rheumatic aortic valvular stenosis when compared with subaortic obstruction (Fig. 20.55)

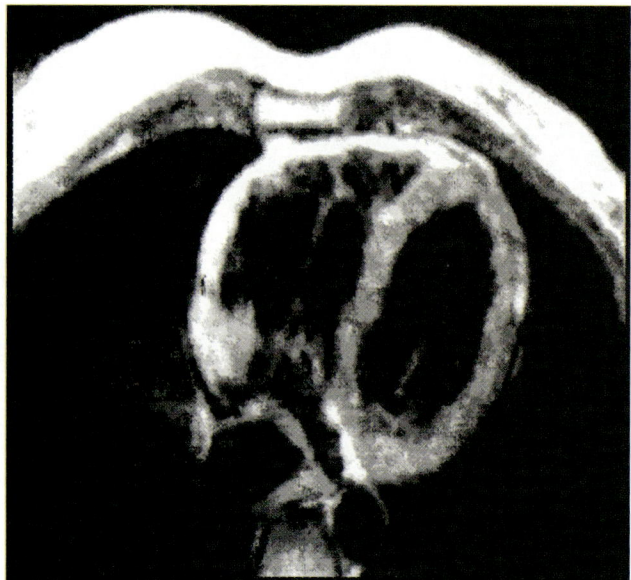

Fig. 20.57: MRI findings in a 22 year old woman with a history of dizziness and sustained ventricular tachycardia with an LBBB pattern. Short axis view showing a dilated right ventricle with a brighter signal from a thin anterior free wall. Spin-echonuclear magnetic resonance for tissue characterisation in arrhythmogenic right ventricular cardiomyopathy

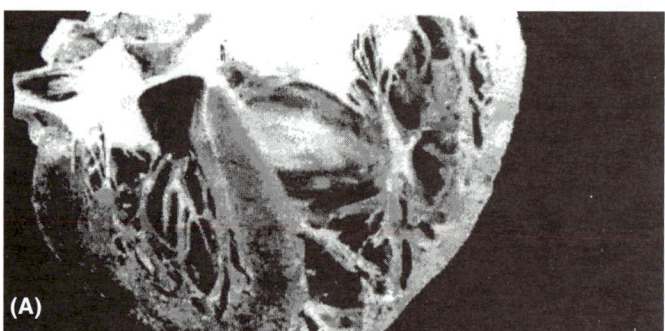

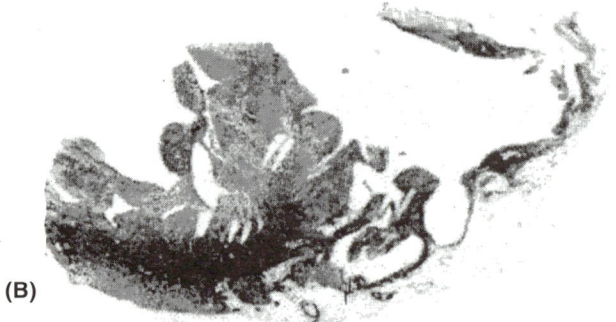

Fig. 20.58: Morphologic features in a 25 year old man who died suddenly from arrhythmogenic right ventricular cardiomyopathy. **(A)** Four chamber view cut of the heart specimen showing the transmural fatty replacement of the right ventricular free wall and the translucent infundibulum. **(B)** Panoramic histologic view of the same heart confirming that the myocardial atrophy is confined to the right ventricle and substantially spares the interventricular septum as well as the left ventricular free wall in arrhythmogenic right ventricular cardiomyopathy dysplasia

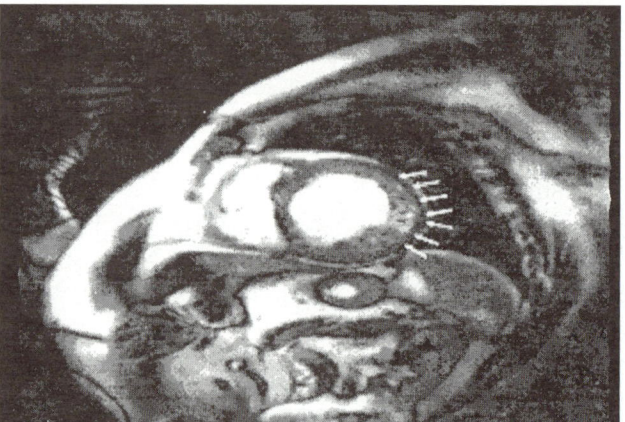

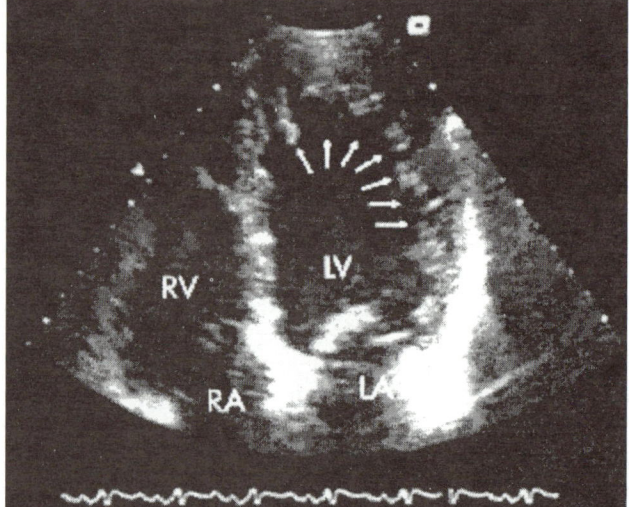

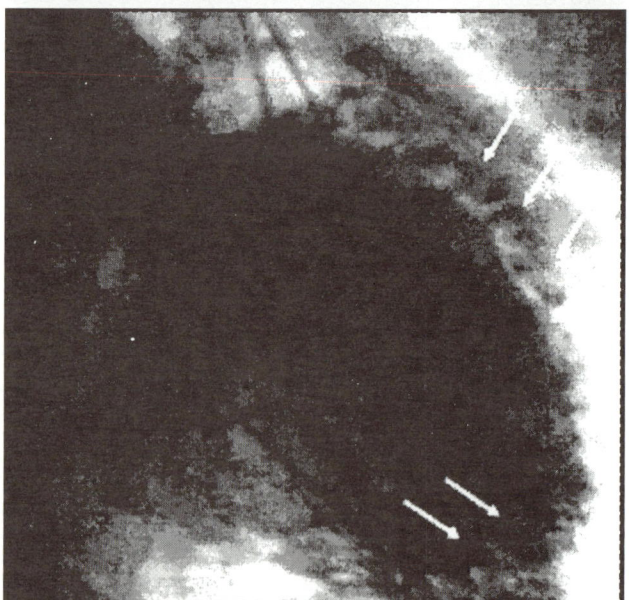

Fig. 20.59: (upper) MRI (middle) Echoscan 4C view of LV and (lower) LV angiography reveal a dilated hypocontractile left ventricle with a two tailored wall; the inner zones of heavily spongious, trabecularised endocardial layers with deep intertrabecular recesses can be distinguished from thin outer zones of compacted myocardium in patient with non-compaction of LV

abnormalities), and pathologic evidence of fibrofatty replacement of myocardium on tissue obtained by endomyocardial biopsy (Figs 20.57 and 20.58).

The electrocardiographic abnormalities include right precordial T-wave inversion, the presence of an epsilon wave (small amplitude potential occurring after the QRS complex), and prolonged QRS duration.

Echocardiographic features are variably present and include RV and RV outflow tract dilation, RV wall thinning, aneurysms of the posterior RV wall or RV free wall, and highly reflective moderator band and trabecular disarray. The relative value of various echocardiographic features is currently being examined in the multicentre study of arrhythmogenic RV dysplasia.

Isolated Ventricular Noncompaction (Fig. 20.59)

While isolated ventricular non-compaction (IVNC) remains an "unclassified" form of cardiomyopathy, its echocardiographic and clinical features have recently been characterised and IVNC is now being recognised with increasing frequency. This disease, which results from an interruption of the normal process of embryologic myocardial compaction, is associated with a high risk of systolic dysfunction, systemic embolisation, and ventricular arrhythmias. Accurate recognition requires knowledge of the echocardiographic features which include the presence of a thin (compacted) epicardium and a thick, spongy endocardial (noncompacted) surface with extensive trabeculation and sinusoid formation. Communication between the deep intertrabecular spaces and the ventricular cavity can be demonstrated by colour Doppler imaging. In the majority of cases the noncompacted myocardium involves the mid lateral, apical, or inferior walls. A ratio of noncompacted to compacted myocardium of > 2:1 is diagnostic of this entity. Additionally, both regional and generalised LV hypokinesis has been observed in this condition. RV involvement has been described in some patients with this condition. The hypokinetic segments can occur in both the affected area and the surrounding normally compacted myocardial segments.

Numerous studies have been performed demonstrating the prognostic value of echocardiographic indices of cardiac size and function in heart failure patients. Regardless of the aetiology of the heart failure, the findings suggest that these echocardiographic measures provide prognostic value and should be integrated in the assessment of these patients. Echocardiographic measures with documented prognostic value in heart failure patients include LV systolic function, RV systolic function, LV diastolic function, LV size, RV size, LA size, severity of mitral regurgitation, severity of tricuspid regurgitation, RV systolic pressure, ventricular synchrony, and measures of contractile reserve.

LV ejection fraction has long been the primary index used as a marker of risk in heart failure and recently the strength of this marker has been demonstrated even in the elderly.

While most studies have focused on ejection fraction as a marker of prognosis in chronic heart failure, the same relation holds in acute heart failure and cardiogenic shock. Particularly in cardiogenic shock, the value of ejection fraction has been shown to remain present regardless of type of treatment.

While initial measures of diastolic filling and function by echocardiography were shown to be of value in patients with symptoms of heart failure but preserved systolic function, the prognostic value of these diastolic indices remain even when the ejection fraction is low. These measures appear to be additive in value to the ejection fraction and may even be stronger measures of prognosis than LV ejection fraction. The transmitral pulse wave Doppler deceleration time has been shown to be a powerful predictor of functional capacity and correlates with maximum oxygen consumption. Thus it is no surprise that measures of diastolic filling have prognostic value in heart failure patients.

For example, in symptomatic congestive heart failure patients, the restrictive filling pattern of transmitral Doppler, especially a deceleration time 140 ms, has been shown to be the single best predictor of cardiac death in patients with ischaemic and dilated cardiomyopathy. For those with cardiac amyloid diastolic function it has been shown to be a stronger predictor of cardiac death than LV wall thickness or systolic function regardless of symptom status.

The pattern of transmitral Doppler velocity profiles are highly dependent on preload and, as described above, pseudonormal patterns can be produced. Since the diastolic measures with prognostic value are indirect measures of LA and LV diastolic pressure and the pseudonormal patterns are a response to increased diastolic pressures, it is logical to ask if pseudonormal patterns have prognostic value in heart failure patients. In fact the pseudonormal transmitral Doppler filling pattern has been shown to identify patients with an intermediate prognosis. Specifically those with abnormal relaxation patterns appear to have the lowest of all cause of death and rehospitalisation for congestive heart failure compared to those with pseudonormal filling or restrictive filling.

In both ischaemic and idiopathic dilated cardiomyopathy, the prognostic value of tricuspid regurgitation has been demonstrated. Additionally for patients with impaired systolic function increasing degrees of mitral regurgitation have a direct impact on survival. While the majority of investigations have focused on the value of valvar regurgitation in assessing prognosis in chronic heart failure, similar relations are seen with acute heart failure shock, where the one-year survival has been shown to depend on the extent of mitral regurgitation assessed at presentation with shock.

Contractile reserve and myocardial viability are important prognostic factors in ischaemic cardiomyopathy. Viable myocardium identified by dobutamine echocardiography identifies the subset of ischaemic cardiomyopathy patients who benefit most from revascularisation. Specifically those with myocardial viability who undergo revascularisation have a three-fold lower long term mortality than those ischaemic cardiomyopathy patients without viability or those with viability who do not undergo revascularisation.

Recently investigators have focused on LV synchrony as a marker of prognosis and shown that those with widened QRS duration have a poorer long term survival than those with coordinated wall motion and dilated cardiomyopathy.

Summary

Echocardiography is a powerful tool for assessing systolic and diastolic heart failure, the specific aetiology of the cardiomyopathy, assessing response to treatment, and categorising prognosis. It is noninvasive, relatively low cost, does not expose patients to ionising radiation, and serial studies can be done at the bedside. Thus echocardiography continues to have advantages over competing technologies.

Bibliography

1. Afridi I, Grayburn PA, Panza JA, *et al.* Myocardial viability during dobutamine echocardiography predicts survival in patients with coronary artery disease and severe left ventricular systolic dysfunction. *J Am Coll Cardiol* 1998; 32:921–6.

2. Agmon Y, Connouy HM, Olson U. *et al.* Noncompaction of the ventricular myocardium. *J Am Soc Echocardiogr* 1999;12:859–863.

3. Ajizad A, Seward JB. Echocardiographic features of genetic diseases: Part 1. Cardiomyopathy. *J Am Sac Echocardiogr* 2000;13:73–86.

4. Ammash NM, Seward JB. Bailey KR, *et al.* Clinical profile and outcome of idiopathic restrictive cardiomyopathy. *Circulation* 2000;101:2490–2496.

5. Aurigemma GP, Gottdiener JS, Shemanski L, *et al.* Predictive value of systolic and diastolic function for incident congestive heart failure in the elderly: the cardiovascular health study. *J Am Coll Cardiol* 2001;37:1042–1048.

6. Bargiggia GS, Bertucci C, Recusani F. *et al.* A new method for estimating left ventricular dP/dt by continuous wave Doppler-echocardiography. Validation studies at cardiac catheterization. *Circulation* 1989;80:1287–1292.

7. Beithardt OA, Sinha AM, Schwammenthal E, *et al.* Acute effects of cardiac resynchronization therapy on functional mitral regurgitation in advanced systolic heart failure. *J Am Coll Cardiol* 2003:41:765–770.

8. Braunwald E, Seidman CE, Sigwart U. Contemporary evaluation and management of hypertrophic cardiomyopathy. *Circulation* 2002; 106:1312–16.

9. Chen C. Rodriguez L, Lethor JP, *et al.* Continuous wave Doppler echocardiography for noninvasive assessment of left ventricular dP/dt and relaxation time constant from mitral regurgitant spectra in patients. *J Am Coll Cardiol* 1994;23:970–976.

10. Dujardin KS, Tei C, Yeo Te. *et al.* Prognostic value of a Doppler index combining systolic and diastolic performance in idiopathic-dilated cardiomyopathy. *Am J Cardiol* 1998;82:1071–1076.

11. Faber L, Seggewiss H, Gleichmann U. Percutaneous transluminal septal myocardial ablation in hypertrophic obstructive cardiomyopathy: results with respect to intra-procedural myocardial contrast echocardiography. *Circulation* 1998;998:2415–21.

12. Fans R, Coats AJ, Henein MY. Echocardiography-derived variables predict outcome in patients with nonischemic dilated cardiomyopathy with or without a restrictive filling pattern. *Am Heart J* 2002;144: 343–350.

13. Faris R, Coats AJ, Henein MY. Echocardiography-derived variables predict outcome in patients with nonischemic dilated cardiomyopathy with or without a restrictive filling pattern. *Am Heart J* 2002;144:343–50.

14. Felker GM, Boehmer JP, Hruban RH, *et al.* Echocardiographic findings in fulminant and acute myocarditis. *J Am Coll Cardiol* 2000:36: 227–232.

15. Garcia MJ, Palac RT, Malenka DJ, *et al.* Color M-mode Doppler flow propagation velocity is a relatively preload-independent indent of left ventricular filling. *J Am Soc Echocardiogr* 1999;12:129–137.

16. Garcia MJ, Thomas RO. Klein AL. New Doppler echocardiographic applications for the study of diastolic function. *J Am Coll Cardiol* 1998;32:865–875.

17. Garcia MJ. Smedira NG, Greenberg NL, *et al.* Color M-mode Doppler flow propagation velocity is preload insensitive indent of left ventricular relaxation: animal and human validation. *J Am Coll Cardiol* 2000;35:201–208.

18. Gottdiener JS, McClelland RL, Marshall R, *et al.* Outcome of congestive heart failure in elderly persons: influence of left ventricular systolic function: the cardiovascular health study. *Ann Intern Med* 2002;147:631–9.

19. Hatle LK, Appleton CP, Popp RL. Differential of constrictive pericarditis and restrictive cardiomyopathy by Doppler echocardiography. *Circulation* 1989;79:357–70.

20. Heimdal A, Stoylen A, Torp H, *et al.* Real-time strain rate imaging of the left ventricle by ultrasound. *J Am Soc Echocardiography* 1998;11:1013–9.

21. Ho CY, Sweitzer NK, McDonough B, *et al.* Assessment of diastolic function with Doppler tissue imaging to predict genotype in preclinical hypertrophic cardiomyopathy. *Circulation* 2002;105:2992–7.

22. Hung J, Koelling T, Semigran MJ, *et al.* Usefulness of echocardiographically determined tricuspid regurgitation in predicting event-free survival in severe heart failure secondary to idiopathic-dilated cardiomyopathy or to ischemic cardiomyopathy. *Am J Cardiol* 1998;82:1201–3, A10.

23. Jenni R, Oechslin E, Schnieder J, *et al.* Echocardiographic and pathoanatomical characteristics of isolated left ventricular non-compaction: a step towards classification as a distinct cardiomyopathy. *Heart* 2001;86:666–71.

24. Key reference describing the nomenclature and classification of cardiomyopathies. Denault AY, Gorcsan J 3rd, Mandarin WA, *et al.* Left ventricular performance assessed by echocardiographic automated border detection and arterial pressure. *Am J Physiol* 1997; 272(1 Pt 2):H138–47.

25. Klein AL' Hade UK. Taliercio CP. *et al.* Prognostic significance of Doppler measures of diastolic function in cardiac amyloidosis. A Doppler echocardiography study. *Circulation* 1991; 83:808–816.

26. Klein AL, Hatle LK, Taliercio CP, *et al.* Prognostic significance of Doppler measures of diastolic function in cardiac amyloidosis. A Doppler echocardiographic study. *Circulation* 1991;83:808–16.

27. Koelling TM, Aaronson KD, Cody RJ, *et al.* Prognostic significance of mitral regurgitation and tricuspid regurgitation in patients with left ventricular systolic dysfunction. *Am Heart J* 2002;144:524–9.

28. Koelling TM, Aaronson KD, Cody RJ. *et al.* Prognostic significance of mitral regurgitation and tricuspid regurgitation in patients with left ventricular systolic dysfunction. *Am Heart J* 2002:144:524–529.

29. La Vecchia L, Paccanaro M, Bonanno C, *et al.* Left ventricular versus biventricular dysfunction in idiopathic dilated cardiomyopathy. *Am J Cardiol* 1999;83:120–2.

30. Maron MS, Olivotto I, Betocchi S, *et al.* Effect of left ventricular outflow tract obstruction on clinical outcome in hypertrophic cardiomyopathy. *N Engl J Med* 2003;348:295–303.

31. Morales FJ, Asencia MC, Oneto J, *et al.* Deceleration time of early filling in patients with left ventricular systolic dysfunction: functional and prognostic independent value. *Am Heart J* 2002;143:1101–6.

32. Moyssakis I, Triposkiadis F, Rallidid L, *et al.* Echocardiographic features of primary, secondary and familial amyloidosis. *Eur J Clin Invest* 1999; 29:484–9.

33. Murray JJ, Stewart S. Epidemiology, aetiology, and prognosis of heart failure. *Heart* 2000;83:596–602.

34. Palka P, Lange A, Donnelly JE, *et al.* Doppler tissue echocardiographic features of cardiac amyloidosis. *J Am Soc Echocardiogr* 2002; 15:1353–60.

35. Picard MH, Davidoff R, Sleeper LA, *et al.* SHOCK trial. Should we emergently revascularize occluded coronaries for cardiogenic shock. *Circulation* 2003;107:279–84.

36. Portner PM, Oyer PE, Pennington DG, *et al.* Implantable electrical left ventricular assist system: bridge to transplantation and the future. *Ann Thorac Surg* 1989; 47:142–50.

37. Richardson P, McKenna W, Bristow M, *et al.* Reports of the 1995 World Health Organization/International Society and Federation of Cardiology task force on the definition and classification of cardiomyopathies. *Circulation* 1996;93:841–2.

38. Towbin JA, Roberts R. Cardiovascular diseases due to genetic abnormalities. In: Schlant RC, Alexander RW, eds. *The heart arteries and veins.* 8th ed. New York: McGraw-Hill, 1994:1725–59.

39. Whalley GA, Doughty RN, Gamble GD, *et al.* Pseudonormal mitral filling pattern predicts hospital readmission in patients with congestive heart failure. *J Am Coll Cardiol* 2002;39:1787–95

40. Xie GY, Berk MR, Smith MD, *et al.* Prognostic value of Doppler transmitral flow patterns in patients with congestive heart failure. *J Am Coll Cardiol* 1994; 24:132–9.

41. Yang SS, Bentiboglio LG, Maranhao V, *et al.* Cardiac volumes. In: From Cardiac Catheterization to Hemodynamic parameters. Philadelphia: FA Davis, 1978.

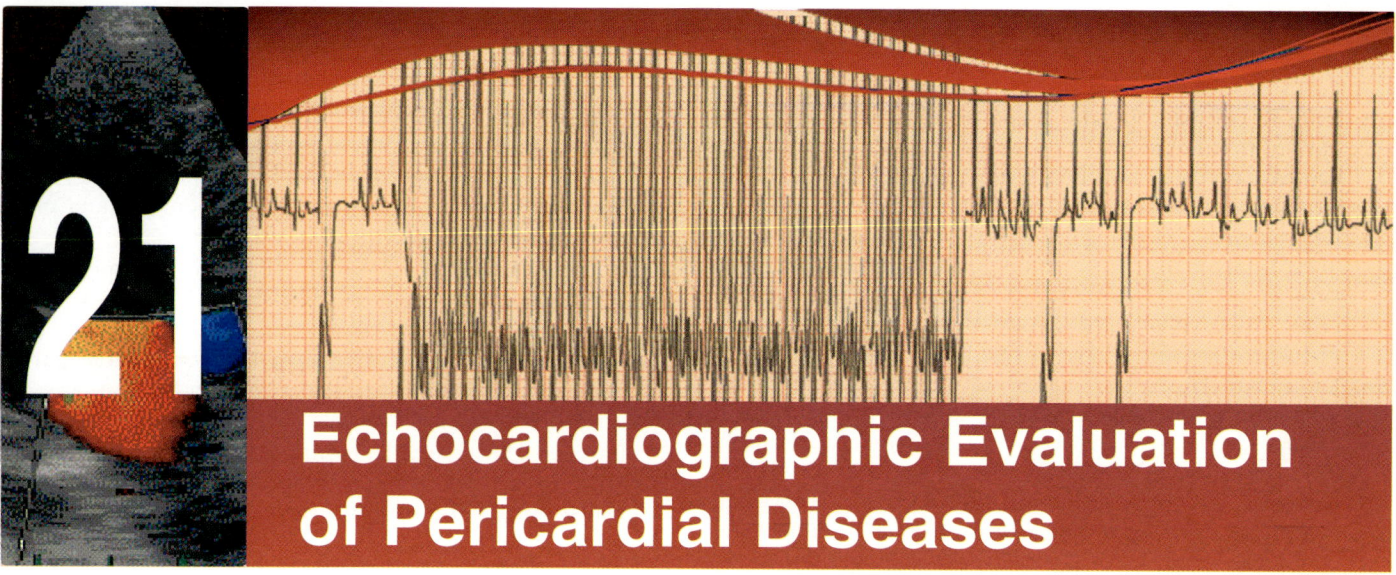

Echocardiographic Evaluation of Pericardial Diseases

Morbid anatomy of the heart, has revealed that in normal human being, pericardium has two layers, the inner; visceral and the outer parietal. In between the two layers is a small amount of lubricating pericardial fluid amounting less than 5.0 ml. Only the lower one-third of the pericardium is sensitive to pain. Pericardial diseases can be categorized into three forms:

1. Acute pericarditis,
2. Pericardial effusion with or without tamponade and
3. Chronic constrictive pericarditis.

There are numerous aetiological factors which can directly or indirectly involve the pericardium such as bacterial infection, including tuberculosis, myocardial infarction, renal disease, radiation therapy, heart failure, Neoplasm aortic dissection, myxedema, hypersensitivity and cardiomyopathies (Table 21.1).

Acute Pericarditis

The classical clinical symptoms of acute pericarditis is pain (sometimes mimicking that of myocardial infarction). Other symptoms, such as chills, fever, and sweating, depend on the etiology of the pericarditis. The major sign is cardiac enlargement with a possible pericardial friction rub, which is a scraping sound heard over the heart in the presence of pericardial effusion. This friction rub is produced from the inflamed pericardial layers grating on each other with to and fro character, is heard both in systole and diastole. A fibrinous or dry pericarditis usually occurs in the presence of a viral infection or rheumatic fever. Deposits of serum and fibrin are seen in the pericardial cavity.

Echocardiographic Features of Pericardial Effusion
(Figs 21.1–21.6, 21.13–21.36)

Echocardiography is the best and highly sensitive and specific modality of evaluating pericardial effusion. If effusion is present, then serial examinations of the

patient may be made with echo to follow the decrease or increase in the fluid accumulation.

A patient with pericardial effusion should be evaluated carefully and systematically. A routine

Table. 21.1 *Various etiological factors in different types of pericardial diseases*

Idiopathic

Acute idiopathic pericarditis
Chronic idiopathic effusion
Infectious
Viral
Bacterial
Tuberculosis
Spread from contiguous infection (e.g. pneumonia)
Fungal

Inflammatory

Associated with connective tissue disease, rheumatoid arthritis
Systemic lupus erythematosus

Other

Post-myocardial infarction
Acute after transmural infract
Partial V complete free wall rupture
Delaye-Dressler syndrome
Associated with systemic disease
Uremia
Hypothyroidism
Pregnancy
Cirrhosis
Malignancy
Direct tumor involvement
Effusion due to lymphatic obstruction

Miscellaneous

Post-trauma
Post-surgical
Congestive heart failure
Severe pulmonary hypertension, right heart failure

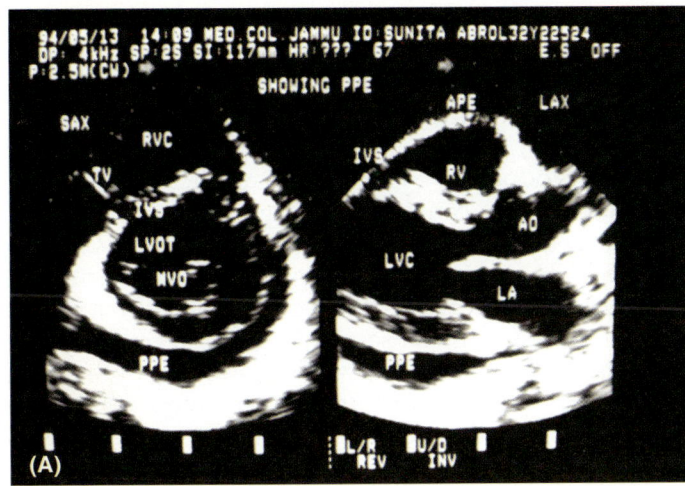

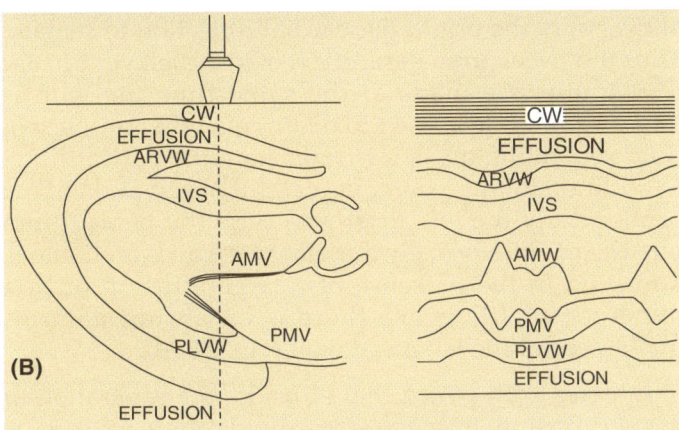

Fig. 21.1A and B: (A) (upper panel) Short axis (left) and long axis (right) dual scan views of LV showing mild to moderate anterior and posterior pericardial effusion in patient with hypertension and chronic renal failure. (B) (lower panel) Showing diagrammatic representation of various anatomical relationship of pericardial sac and other surroundiing structures explaining the location of effusion in Fig. (A)

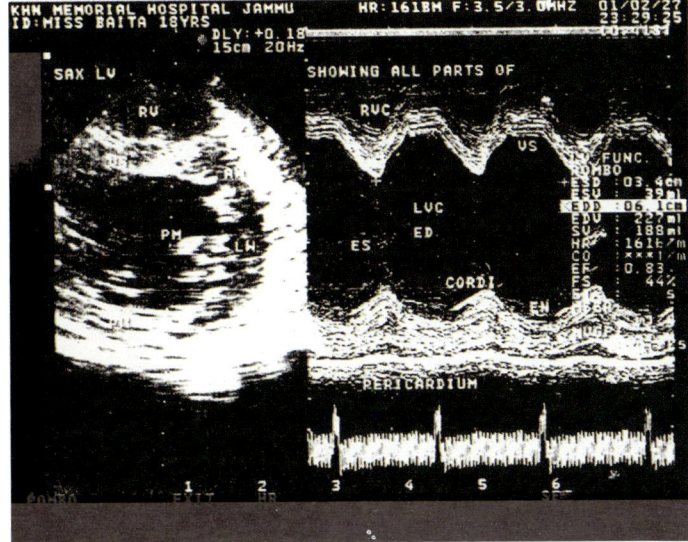

Fig. 21.2: Short axis (left) and M-Mode echocardiogram (right) showing minimal pericardial effusion localized to posterior sac only

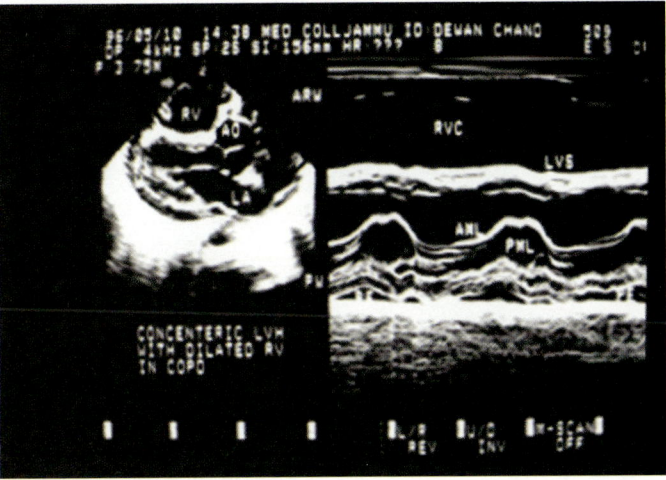

Fig. 21.3: Mild pericardial effusion localized to posterior sac only but more than in patient cited Fig 21.2

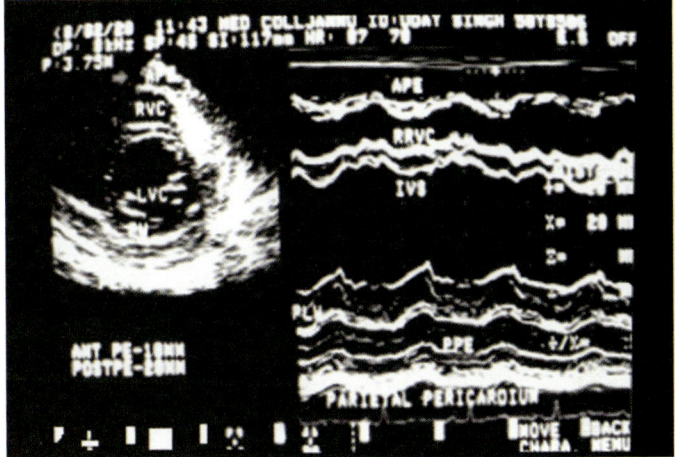

Fig. 21.4: Short axis (left) and M-mode echocardiogram (right) showing moderately severe pericardial effusion localized to both anterior (APE) and posterior pericardial sacs (PPE)

parasternal long axis scan is made to locate the aorta, left atrium and mitral apparatus. The transducer is then directed inferiorly and slightly lateral towards the left hip of the patient. The contractility of the ventricle should be followed throughout the cardiac cycle for any compensation or decompensation factors that may result from the rapid accumulation of fluid. The pericardial echo reflection is the strongest reflection in the normal heart and thus is easily recognised on the M-mode and two-dimensional recordings as the brightest echo reflector. The three layers of the posterior wall (endocardium, myocardium, and epicardium) must be defined so that echoes can be separated from the pericardial echo. Various gain settings are used to define these. Occasionally a small pericardial effusion contains pus. The accumulation of such inflammatory products

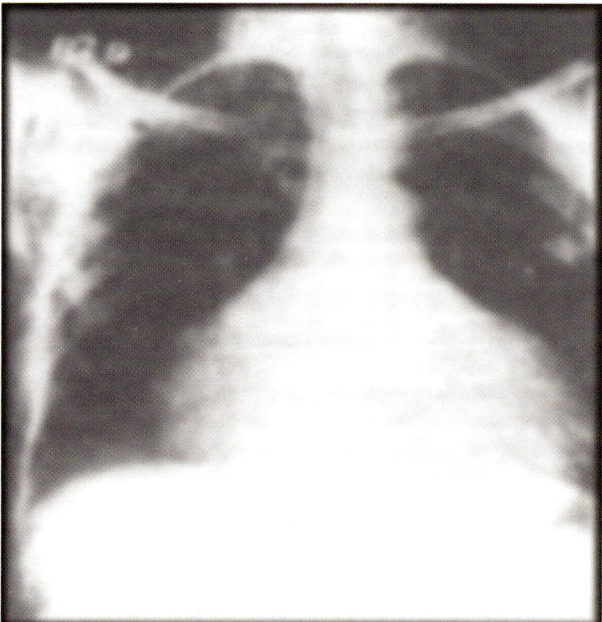

Fig. 21.5: X-Ray chest showing money bag appearance of cardiac silhoute in patient with moderate pericardial effusion

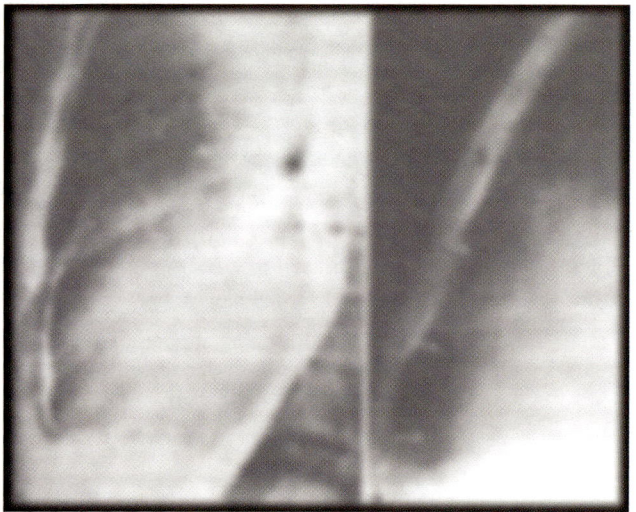

Fig. 21.6: X-Ray chest lateral view showing calcification of pericardium in patient with constrictive pericarditis

eventually leads to constrictive pericarditis. A haemorrhagic pericarditis is usually caused by a malignancy or injury to the pericardium, and blood is mixed with the inflammatory fluid.

Pericardial Effusion

Clinically pericardial effusion is characterised by an enlarged shadow of the heart and may be mistaken with cardiac dilation as it occurs in valvular heart disease or cardiomyopathy. Clinical signs of pericardial effusion are the distant heart sound (muffled by the fluid accumulation) and a low-voltage electrocardiogram

(ECG). The speed with which the fluid accumulates largely determines the subsequent clinical manifestations: a rapid accumulation of 200 to 300 ml may lead to tamponade and shock from acute cardiac insufficiency, whereas a slower accumulation of 1000 ml may produce no evidence of cardiac insufficiency. The pericardium can adapt to large collections of fluid if permitted to do so over a long period of time. Cardiac temponade may result from trauma, a ruptured aneurysm, or pericarditis. With tamponade, the systemic venous pressure increases while the arterial pressure decreases. A high gain allows visualisation, of the right ventricular wall, septum, posterior layers of the left ventricular wall, and pericardium. As the gain is reduced, the finer, less dense echoes of the chordae and endocardium are recorded. Further reduction in gain allows only the bright pericardial reflection to remain. Thus the sweep from the aortic root to the left ventricular cavity must be made at the same time the gain is increased and decreased to distinguish the presence of fluid separating the epicardium from the pericardium. In addition to this technique, careful observation of the continuity of the left atrial wall with the pericardium must be made. Normally the left atrial wall is motionless, however, in the presence of a large effusion or in a hypercontractile heart, there is an abrupt anterior movement of the left atrial wall (Fig. 21.20).

In cases with pericardial effusion, the separation of the pericardium from the epicardium causes the cardiac pulsation to be dampened by the time they reach the pericardium. Thus one of the more obvious features of an effusion is a nonmobile pericardium, separated from the posterior heart wall by fluid. In a limited small amount of fluid is so small that these pulsations are transmitted slightly to the pericardium, in which case the sonographer sees diminished motion of the pericardium (Figs 21.1 and 21.2).

Mild to moderate pericardial effusion tends to accumulate in the most posterior dependent area of the heart, accounting for the visualisation of a posterior effusion before any anterior effusion is seen. Small effusions may produce an echo-free space behind the epicardium in systole but disappear in diastole. Many echocardiographer prefer to see the separation in diastole before they report a small effusion. A systolic separation of 5 to 10 mm may indicate a small effusion of approximately 100 ml.

Moderate effusions produce an echo-free space in systole and diastole in the anterior and posterior pericardial space. Usually a separation of 10 mm systole means the patient has a moderate-sized effusion of approximately 200 to 300 ml. A large effusion of 500 ml or greater exhibits wide spaces anteriorly and posteriorly with a systolic separation to extend posterior to the left atrium (in the area of the oblique sinus). One may visualise erratic motion of the heart leading to the problem of cardiac tamponade (Fig. 21.5).

Several efforts have been made to employ both M-mode and two-dimensional echocardiography to quantitate pericardial effusion. The techniques basically attempt to calculate the volume of the pericardial sac and subtract the volume of the heart. By obtaining major and minor dimensions of the pericardium in the apical four chamber and short-axis views and then deriving cardiac dimension in the same view, one can calculate volume of the pericardium and subtract the volume of the heart to determine the volume of the pericardial fluid. The M-mode technique is similar except that one uses single linear pericardial and cardiac dimension to make the volume calculations (Figs 21.7–21.12).

As reported by Nanda and Gramiak, the heart may "swing" in the pericardial effusion space, with a resultant change in the pattern of wall motion. Normally the right ventricular wall moves posteriorly in systole and anteriorly in diastole. When the heart "swings," it may move posteriorly in one cardiac cycle and anteriorly in the next, so that it is physically nearer the chest wall with every other beat. This form of cardiac- "swinging" is associated with the phenomenon of electrical alterations as seen in patients with cardiac temponade. Temponade occurs when the intrapericardial pressure reaches a sufficient level to compromise the filling of the heart. An emergency periardiocentesis, with or without ultrasound guidance, must be performed to relieve the intrapericardial pressure (Fig. 21.21).

Pericardiocentesis (See Appendix)

Aspiration of pericardial effusion is called as pericardiocentesis. It may be carried out either therapeutically or diagnostically to save the patient from ensuing cardiac tamponade. The aspiration is best performed in a semi-upright position, since the fluid tends to gravitate anteriorly and inferolaterally. The apical or subxiphoid approach is generally used. The cardiac sonographer may locate the position of maximum fluid accumulation and guide the clinician as the fluid is withdrawn from the pericardial cavity. The needle may be followed with two-dimensional image under ECG monitoring in order to avoid damage to the myocardium.

The parastenal short-axis view can be used to locate the descending thoracic aorta to differentiate pericardial from pleural effusion. It has been shown that patients with an isolated pericardial effusion has an echo-free space between the descending thoracic aorta and the left ventricular posterior wall. Patients with isolated pleural effusion has an echo-free space posterior to the descending aorta. The other group of patients have both

a pericardial and a pleural effusion and have echo-free spaces between the descending thoracic aorta and the left ventricular wall and also posterior to the descending aorta. Thus the descending aorta serves as a valuable landmark differentiating pericardial from pleural effusions (Fig. 21.36).

Other Structures

Other structures near the atrioventricular groove such as aorta, pulmonary veins, coronary sulcus can produce a posterior echo-free space and thus may be differentiated from an effusion by a careful sweep from the left atrium to the apex of the ventricle. When such structures appear and disappear quickly as one sweeps to the left ventricular apex.

Anterior separation of the heart wall from the pericardium may result from subepicardial fat. As one scans towards the apex, the space decreases in size; however, with pericardial effusion, the space tends to increase towards the apex (Fig. 21.20).

Mass Lesions (Figs 21.41–21.43)

Other lesions such as a pericardial cyst or a tumor mass may lie along the anterior heart wall or posterior heart wall and mimic an effusion. With increased gain, the tumor mass may fill in with low-level echoes if the mass is heterogeneous; however, the cyst would remain echo-free. Careful evaluation with two-dimensional tracing may help to separate the mass from the presence of pericardial effusion. X-ray studies would also help to differentiate the two diagnoses (Figs 21.5 and 21.6).

Calcification

Calcification of the chordal structures or mitral annulus can be mistaken with pericardial effusion. However, the two-dimensional parasternal long and short axis, along with the apical four-chamber view, can permit easy assessment for the presence of pericardial effusion.

Constrictive Pericarditis (Figs 21.33–21.38)

This entity usually results from chronic pericardial inflammation and fibrosis caused by an infectious process, neoplasm, or uremia. The disease interferes with cardiac filling and contraction (reduced cardiac output) and leads to chronic congestion in the venous system supplying the right heart. The cardiac rate is increased, with a decreased pulse pressure and paradoxical pulse. Signs of congestive heart failure are present with edema and dyspnea.

Tuberculosis is a common cause of constrictive pericarditis, in which the pericardium becomes shaggy and thickened, with resultant fibrosis and calcification, and fibrosis may lead to constriction around the normal heart. (Figs 21.6, 21.9 and 21.36).

Till recently a new *Traffic jam sign* on echocardiography has been observed to differentiate between right-

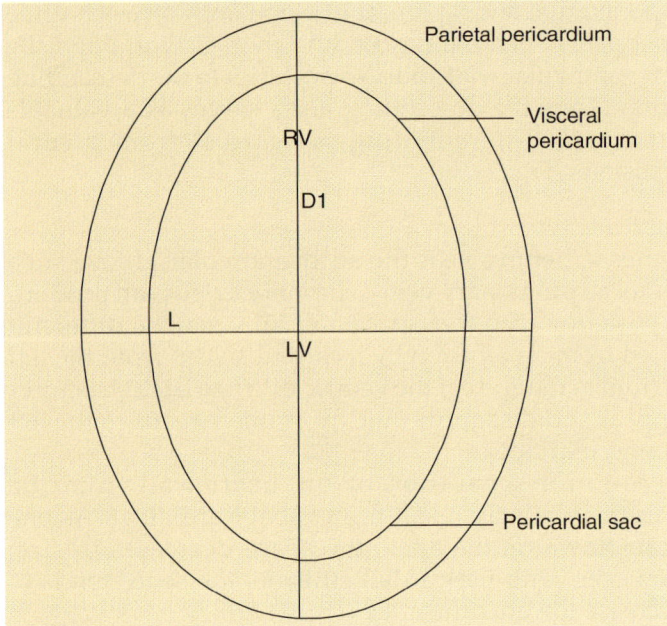

Fig. 21.7: Diagrammatic apical 4C view to determine interpericardial dimensions (D_1)

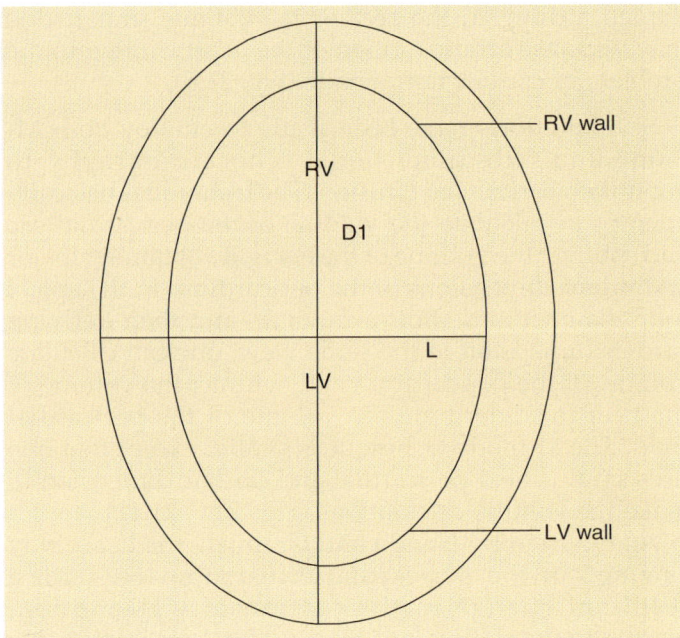

Fig. 21.8: Diagrammatic apical 4C view to determine interpericardium dimension (D_1)

Quantitative calculation of pericardial fluid

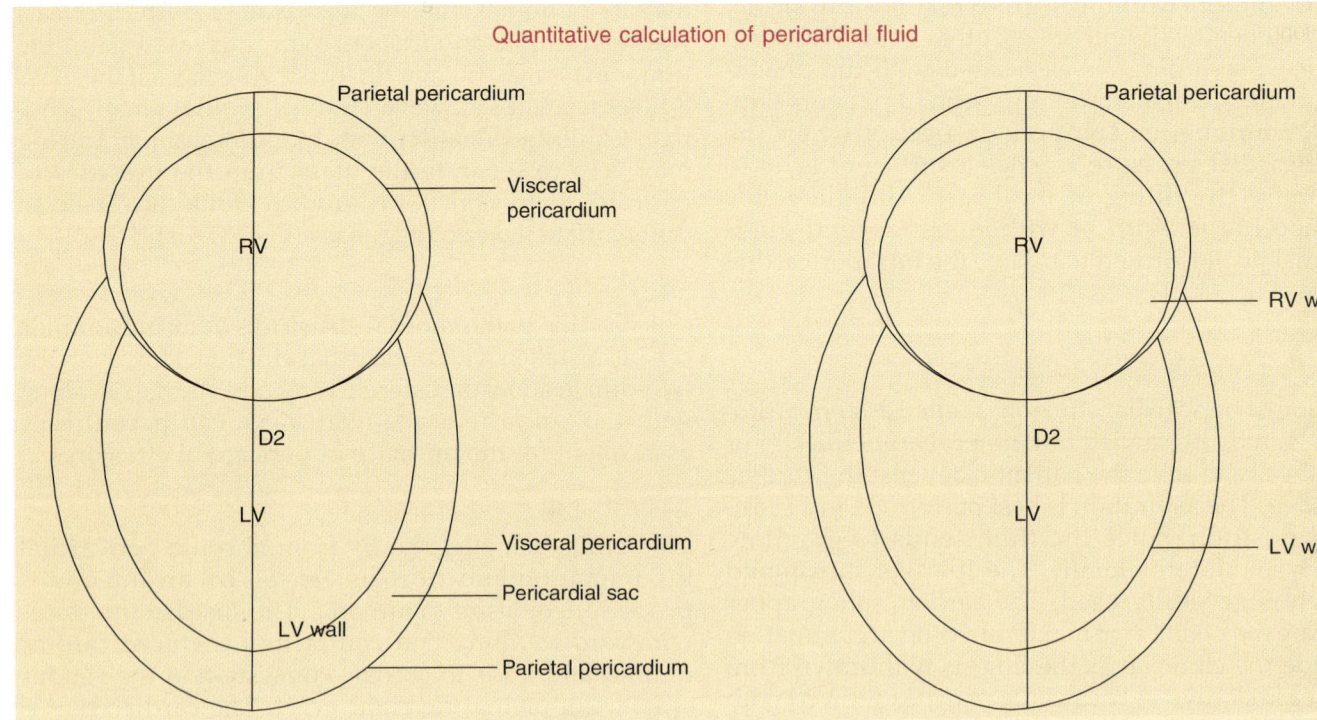

Fig. 21.9: Short axis view to determine longitudinal intrapericardial dimension (D_2)

Fig. 21.10: Short axis view to determine longitudinal intracardiac dimension (D_2)

sided endomyocardial fibrosis and constrictive pericarditis. On subcostal 4-chamber view including the inferior vena cava and hepatic veins draining into the right atrium, spontaneous contrast of moving blood column has been seen in the dilated inferior vena cava and hepatic veins. These have characteristic movement

pattern. When the tricuspid valve opens, this column moves forward into the right atrium from the inferior vena cava and hepatic veins. As the early diastolic filling stops due to the restriction imposed by the thickened, constricting pericardium, the traffic jam occurs and this column stops at inferior vena cava with a slight

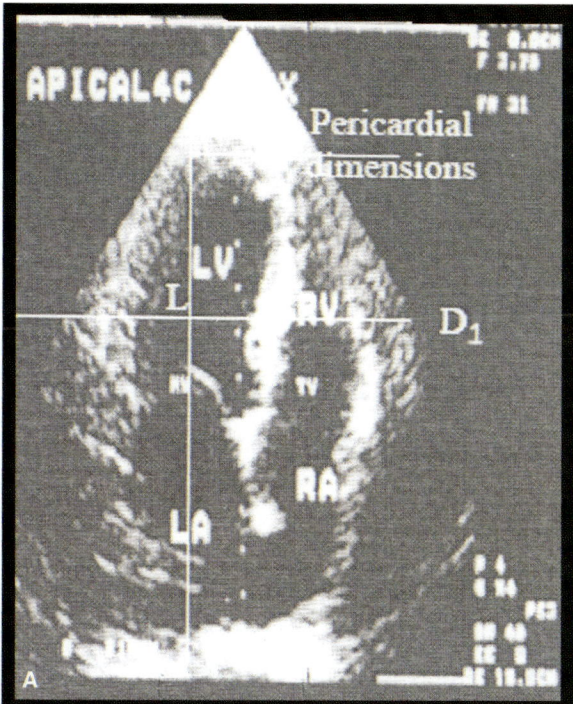
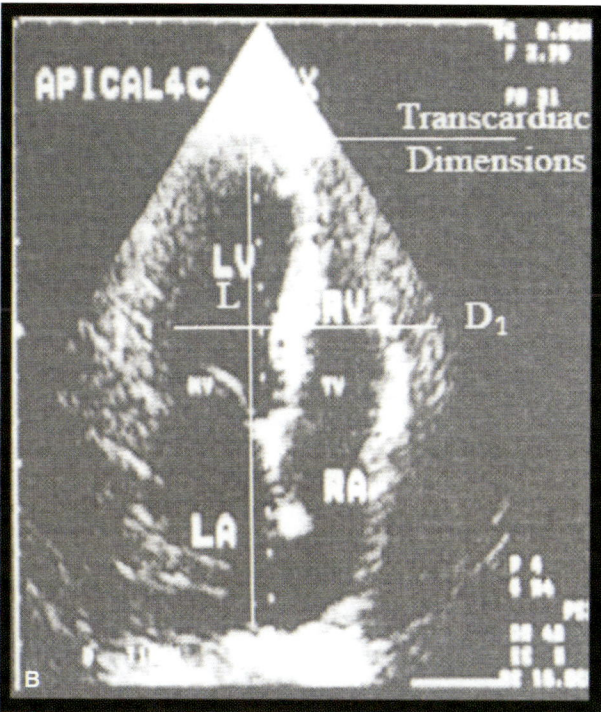

Figs 21.11A and B: Apical 4C view longitudinal interpericardial dimension (L) and transverse interpericardial dimension (D₁) Fig. B. Showing longitudinal intracardiac dimension (L) and transverse intracardiac transverse dimension (D₁)

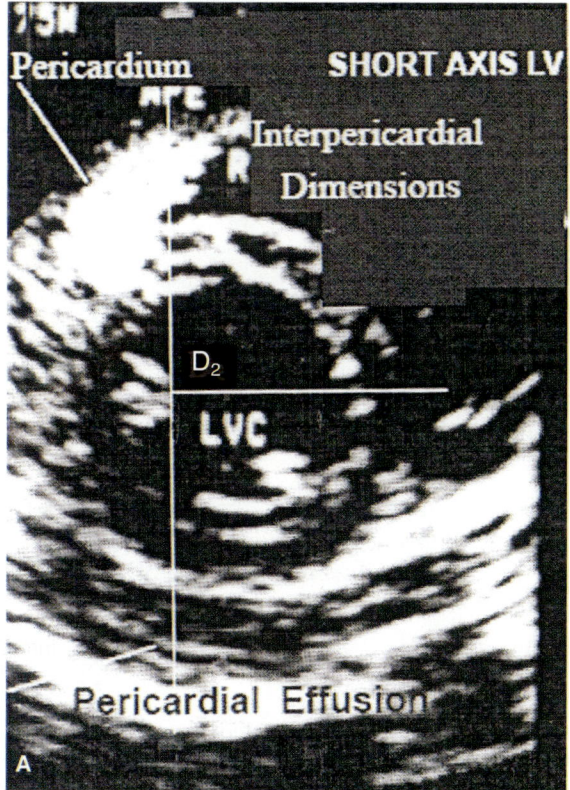
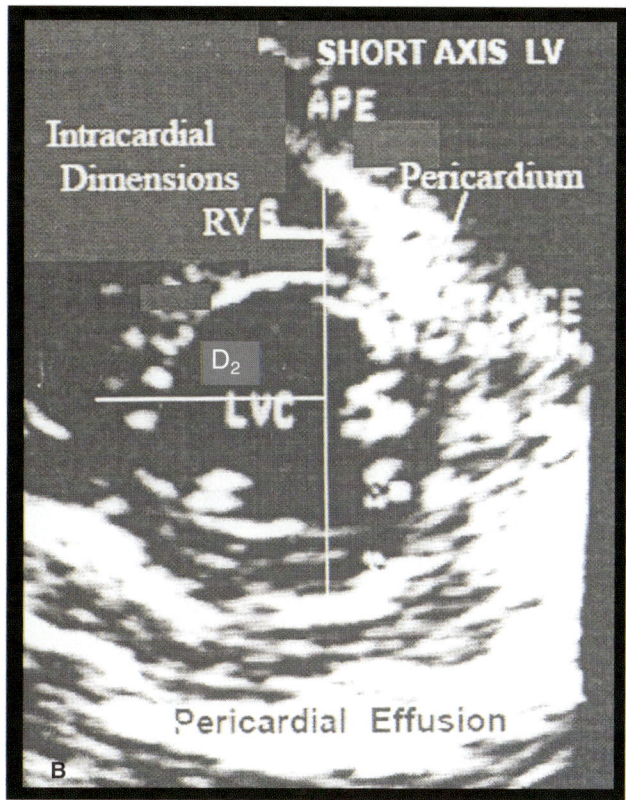

Fig. 21.12A and B: Short axis view; longitudinal interpericardial dimension (D₂) and Fig. B showing longitudinal intracardiac dimension (D₂). These dimensions are to be converted into volumes automatically by computer. After having calculated pericardial volume and cardiac volumes by converting dimensions into volumes by the computer, the amount of pericardial fluid can be determined by simply subtracting the volume of the heart, i.e. (total pericardial volume minus cardiac volume = pericardial fluid in ml.)

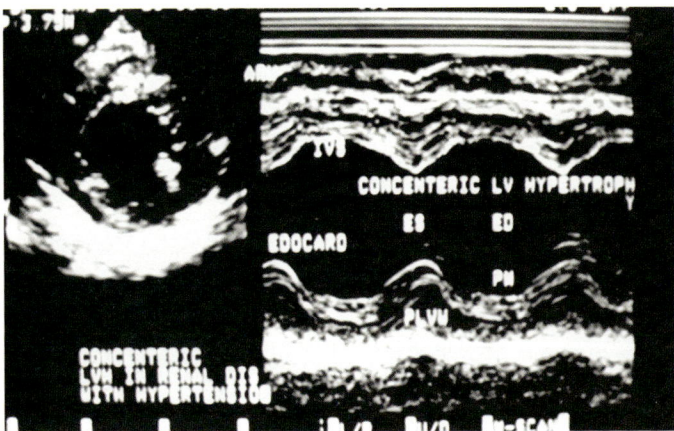

Fig. 21.13: Short axis and M-mode echoscans at LV cavity level showing moderate pericardial effusion localized posteriorly only with marked thickening of posterior pericardial sac in patients with tubercular pericarditis with effusion

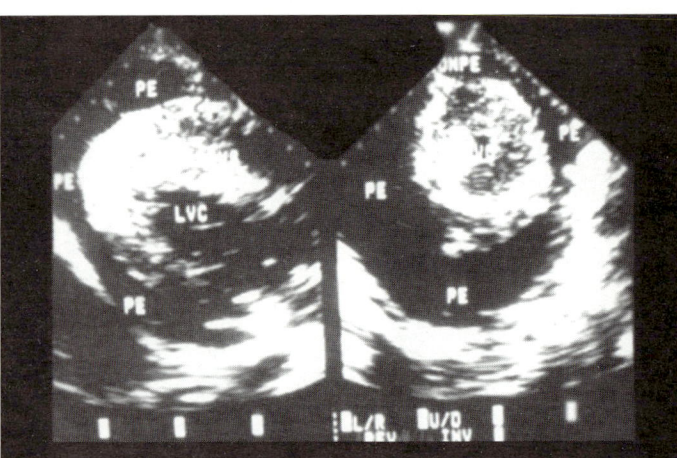

Fig. 21.15: Oblique and short axis views(L-R) showing hypertrophic cardiomyopathy with massive pericardial effusion (PE) encircling the heart

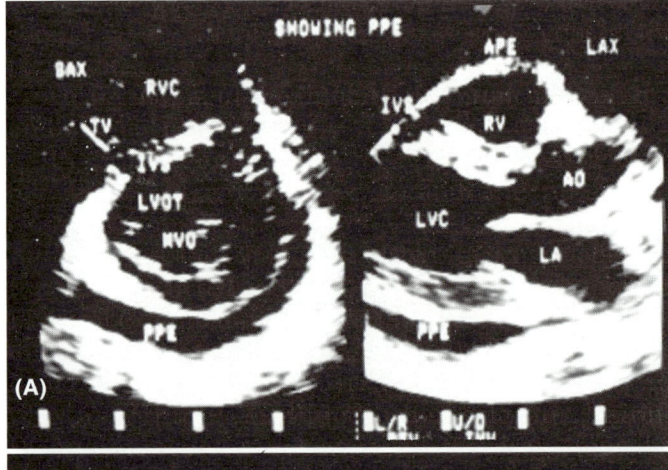

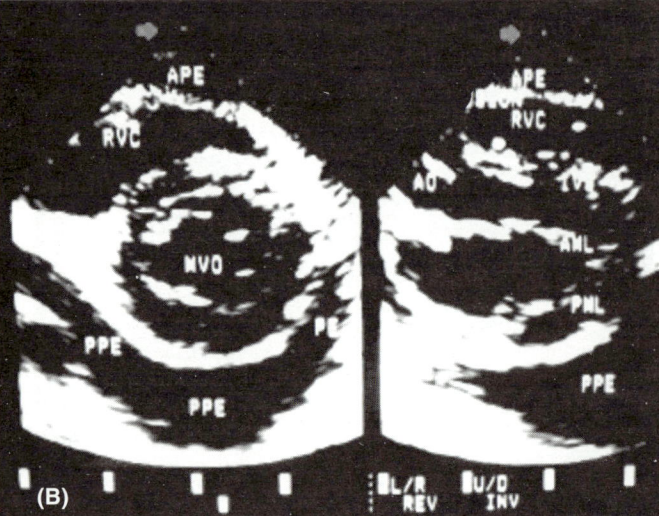

Fig. 21.14A and B: **(A)** Apical 4C dual scan showing dilated all four chambers of the heart finding suggestive of congestive cardiomyopathy with posteriorly localized pericardial effusion in patient with goitrous hypothyroidism. **(B)** Short and long axis LV views showing echo-free space in the regions of anterior (APE) and posterior pericardial spaces (PPE) in patient with moderate pericardial effusion

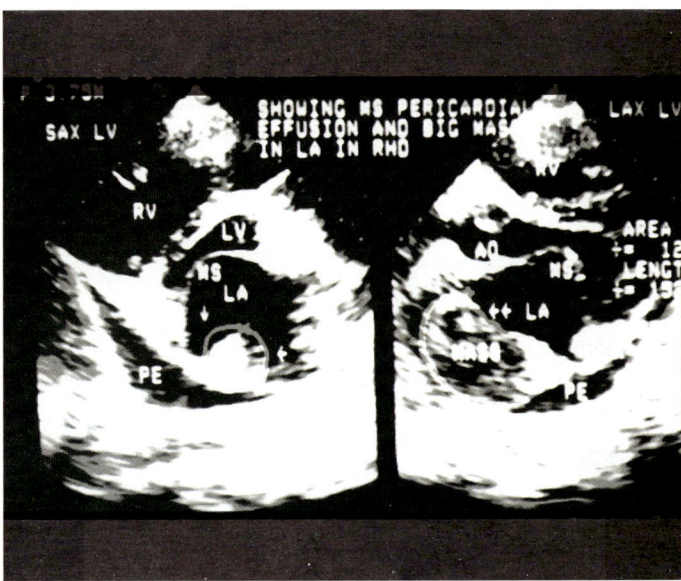

Fig. 21.16: Short and long axis views LV showing posteriorly located pericardial effusion (PE) and a big thrombosis in LA (arrows) in patient with rheumatic mitral stenosis with MR and effusive pericarditis

reflux into the hepatic veins. This sign is consistent with severe haemodynamic findings of constrictive pericarditis and usually not found so frequently in restrictive cardiomyopathy. Distinction between constrictive pericarditis and other forms of restrictive heart disease is often difficult by simple mitral inflow Doppler.

Tissue Doppler Imaging (Fig. 20.44)

Reviewing of the patterns, constrictive pericarditis has a smaller S height, Et, At and Et/At is similar to normal. The Et/At ratio and ET/At × E/A are significantly higher in restrictive heart disease as compared to constrictive pericarditis and controls. This suggests that in constrictive pericarditis, there is diastolic dysfunction

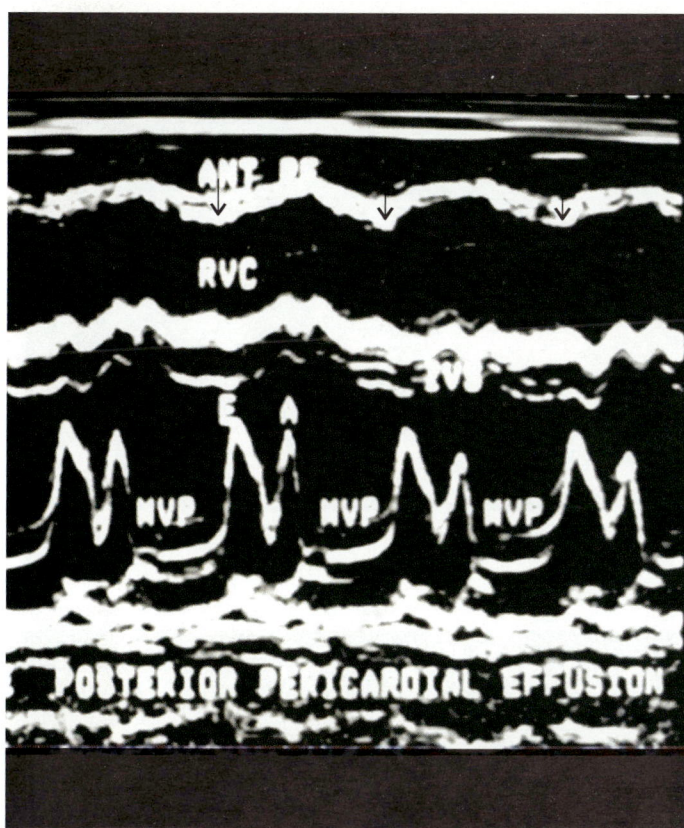

Fig. 21.17: M-Mode echocardiogram showing diastolic invagination of free wall of RV into RV cavity (arrows) and systolic sagging of mitral valve called pseudo prolapse of mitral valve (MVP) in patient with anterior and posterior massive pericardial effusion

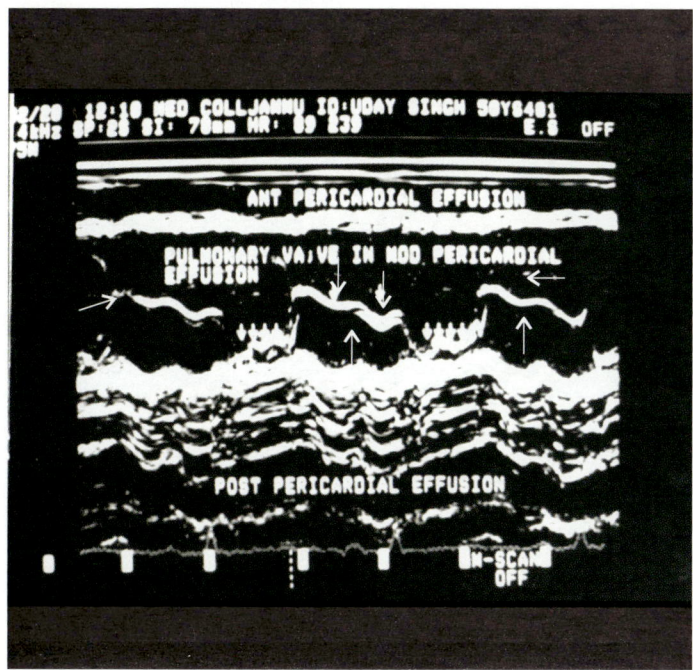

Fig. 21.18: M-Mode echocardiogram showing premature opening of pulmonary valve in moderately severe pericardial effusion (arrows)

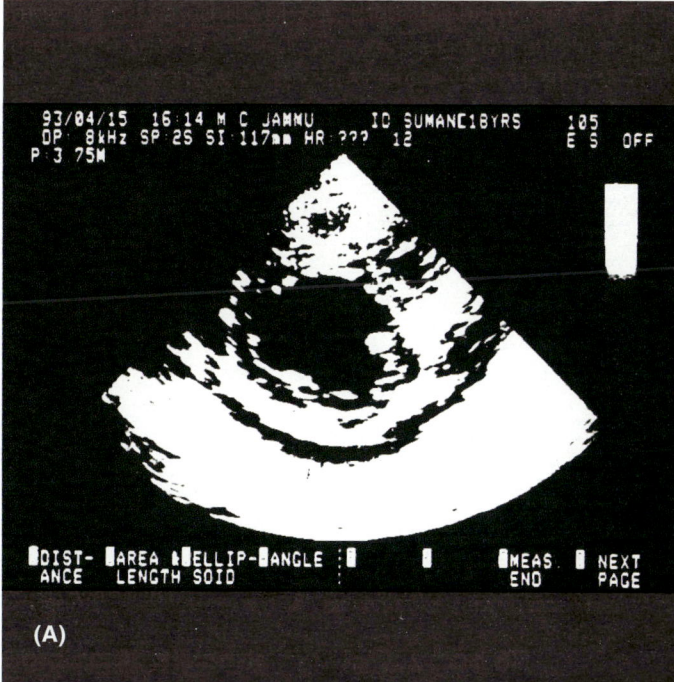

(A)

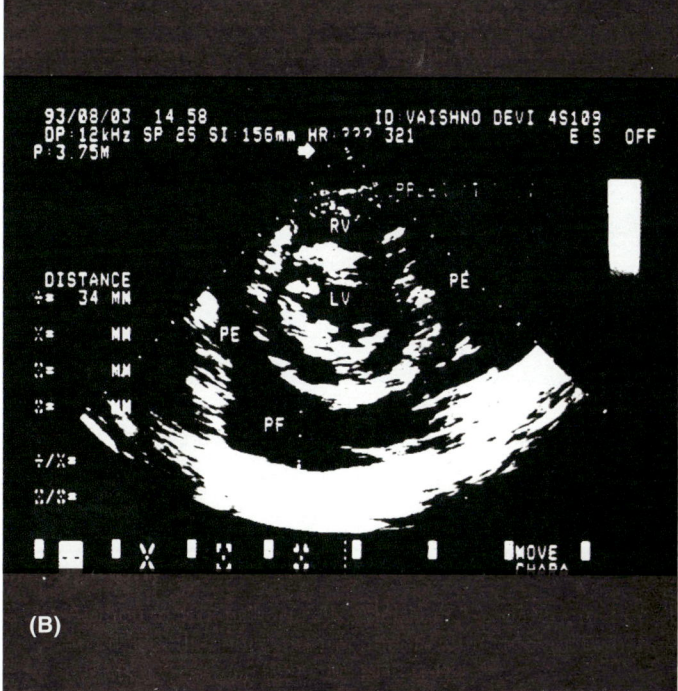

(B)

Fig. 21.19A and B: Mild (upper panel) and moderate (lower) pericardial effusion (PE) in patient with pulmonary tuberculosis

manifested only by a sharp E deceleration slope. In restrictive heart disease, the atrial contribution is reduced, which could be, because these patients have some variety of endomyocardial fibrosis, where atrial dysfunction is also there.

Tissue Doppler imaging may therefore be helpful in distinguishing between constrictive pericarditis and restrictive heart disease.

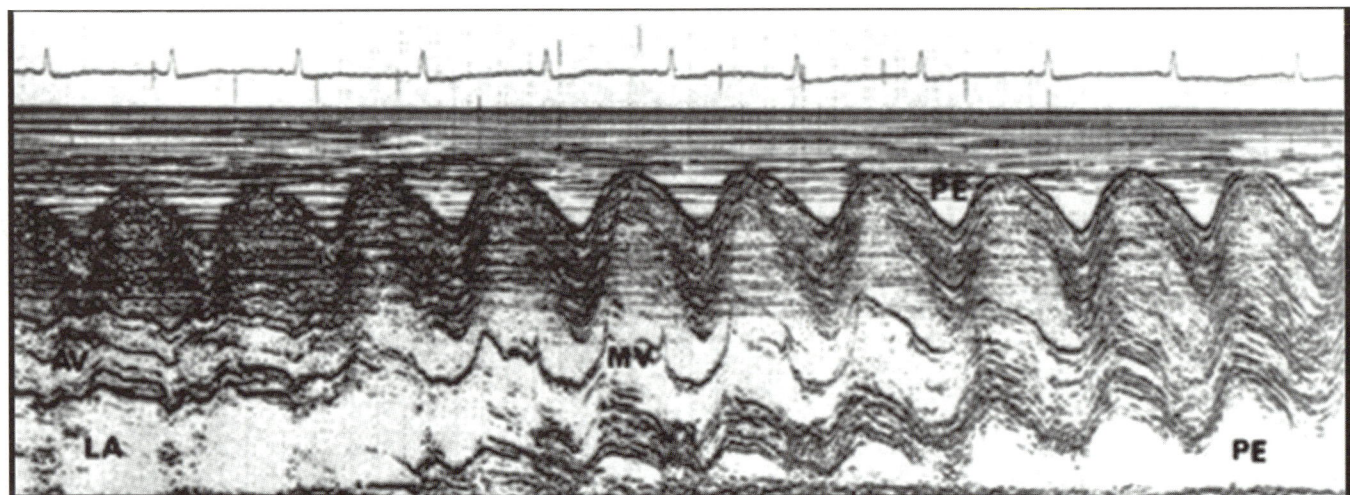

Fig. 21.20: M-Mode echocardiogram showing the increase in posterior echo-free space (PE) as the sweep marches from LA towards the cardiac apex and distorting the cardiac echos in rapid motion

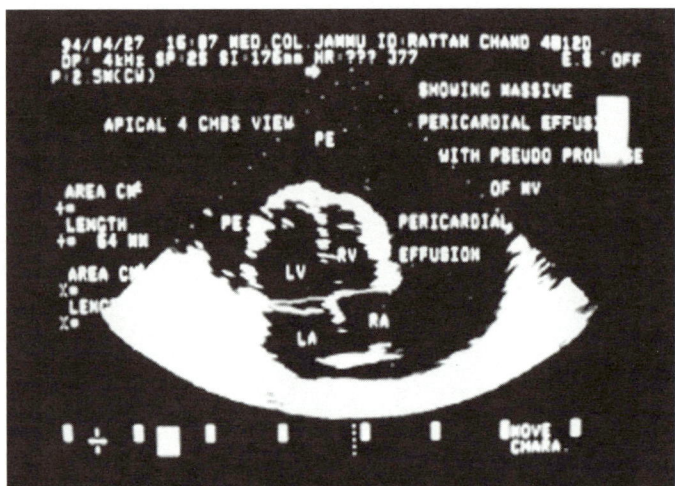

Fig. 21.21: Apical 4C view showing massive pericardial effusion and compressed small heart moving like a pendulum in the centre of the fluid

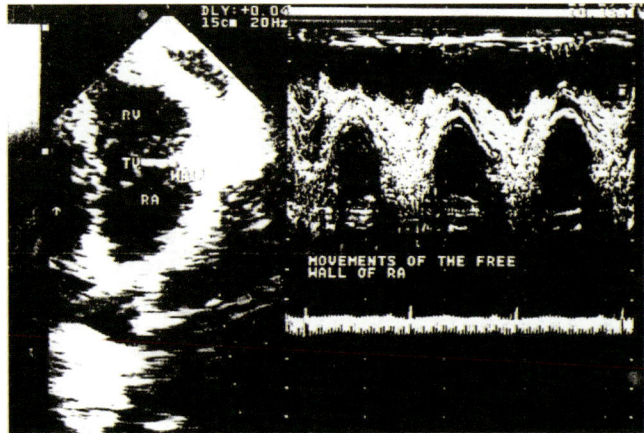

Fig. 21.22: Subcostal approach at RV showing diastolic invagination of free wall of RV in patient with massive pericardial effusion

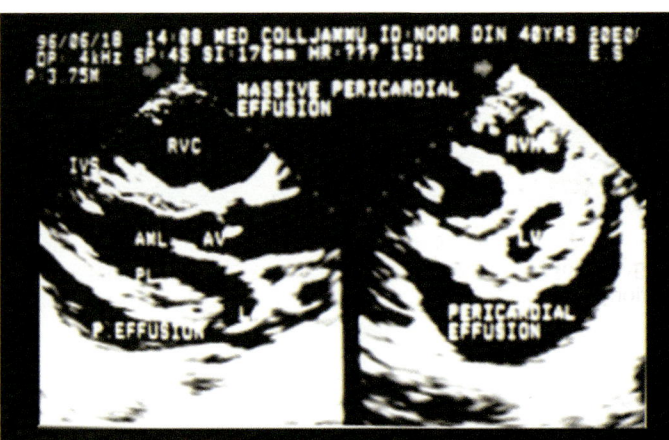

Fig. 21.23: Long and short axis dual scan views showing echo-free space around the heart in patient with massive pericardial effusion

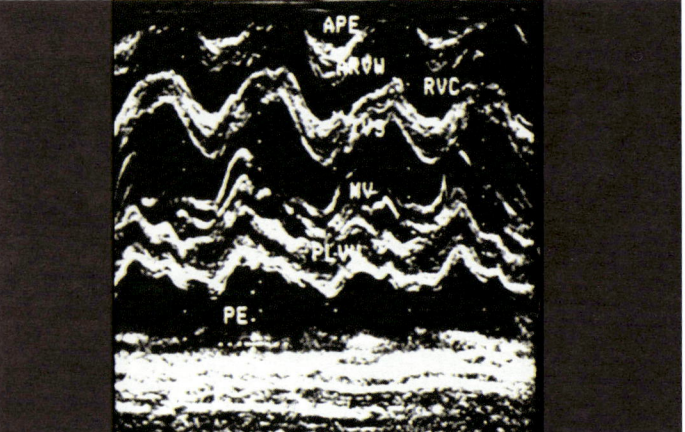

Fig. 21.24: M-Mode echocardiogram showing vigorous movements of interventricular septum (IVS) during inspiration and expiration with posterior movement, diastolic collapse of free wall of RV and diminished amplitude of MV in patient with massive pericardial effusion (APE and PE)

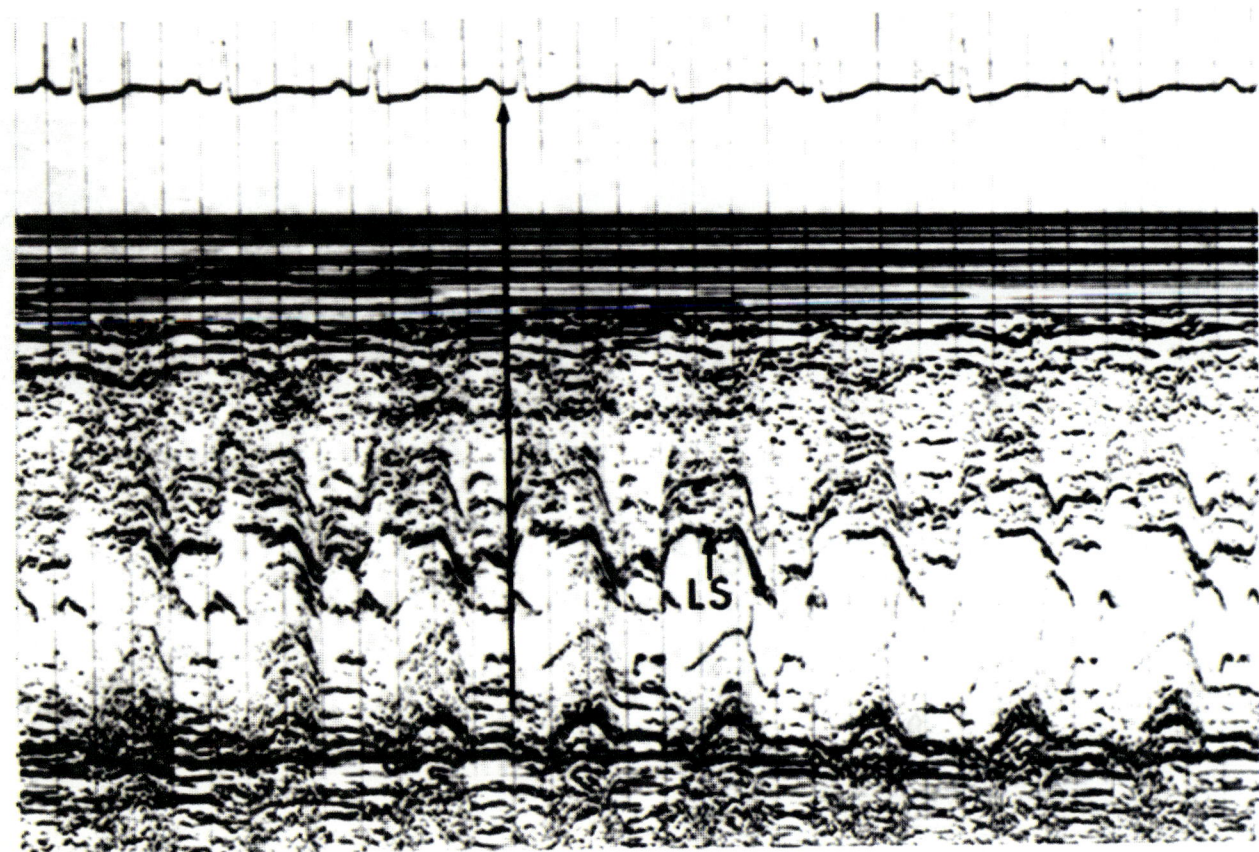

Fig. 21.25: M-Mode echocardiogram showing brisk anterior motion of interventricular septum during ventricular ejection and moves posteriorly during ventricular relaxation in patient with constrictive pericarditis

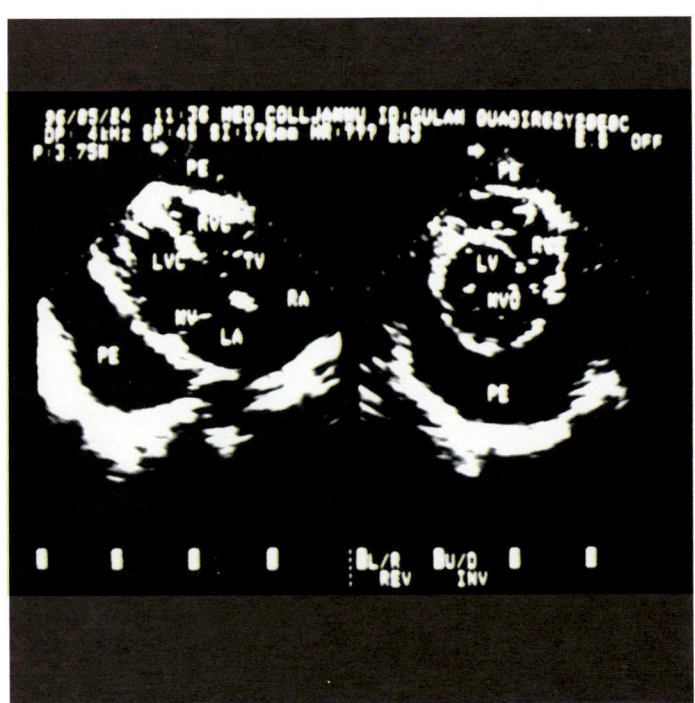

Fig. 21.26: Apical 4C and short axis views (L-R) showing diastolic collapse of left atrium (LA) in patient with massive pericardial effusion

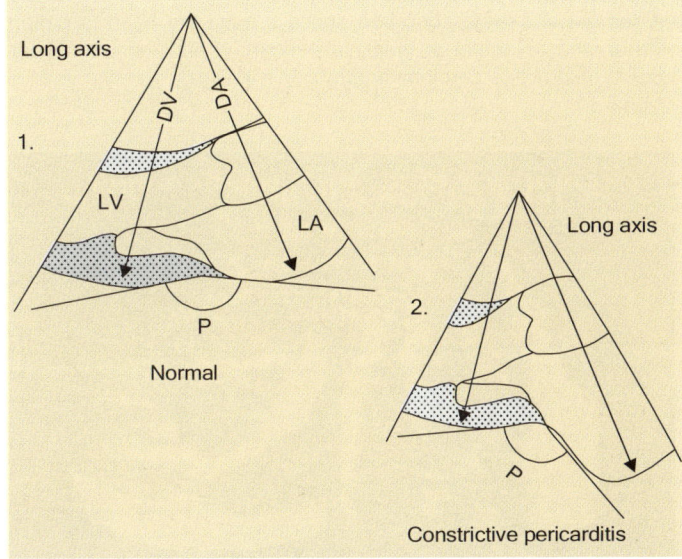

Fig. 21.27: (1) Showing how the angle (P) and the distances from the transducer to the posterior left atrial wall DA and the left ventricular wall DV can be used to differentiate the normal relationship of the posterior left ventricular and the left atrial walls from that with percardial constriction. With pericardial constriction (2), the angle P is smaller and the difference between DA and DV is greater than in normal subject

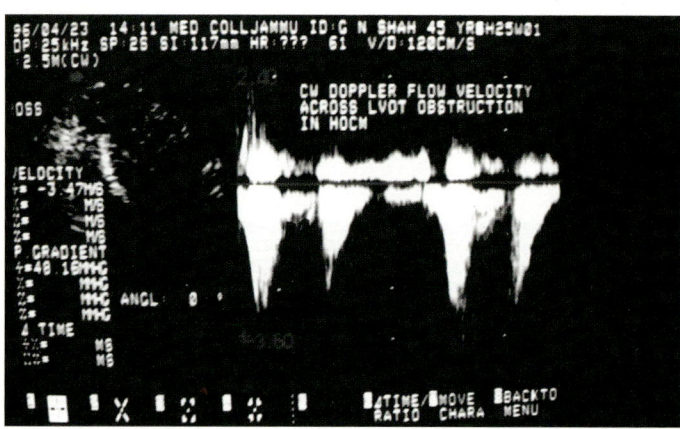

Fig. 20.28: Doppler flow velocity across LVOT showing enhanced velocity in patient with hypertrophic obstructive cardiomyopathy

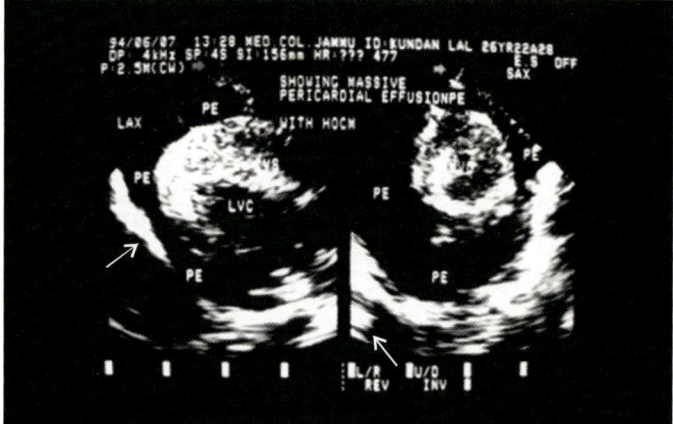

Fig. 21.29: Long and short axis views showing diastolic collapse of LA (arrow) and large echo-free space around the heart in patient with another example of massive pericardial effusion with hypertrophic obstructive cardiomyopathy

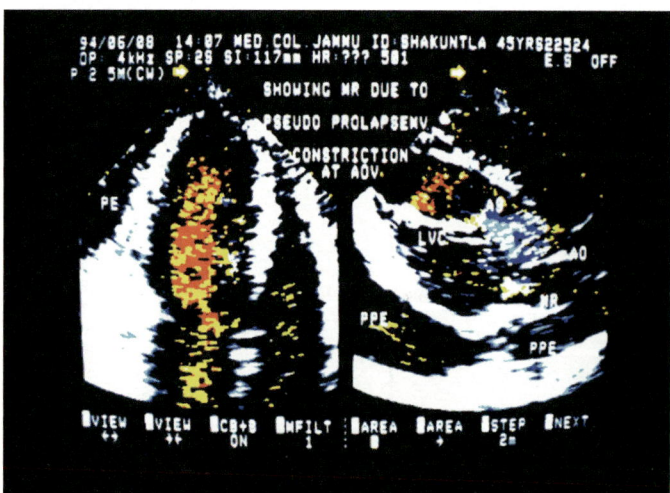

Fig. 21.30: Apical 4C and Doppler flow velocity across MV in color mode showing diastolic collapse of LA and pseudoprolapse of MV with MR due to compression caused by encircled massive pericardial effusion

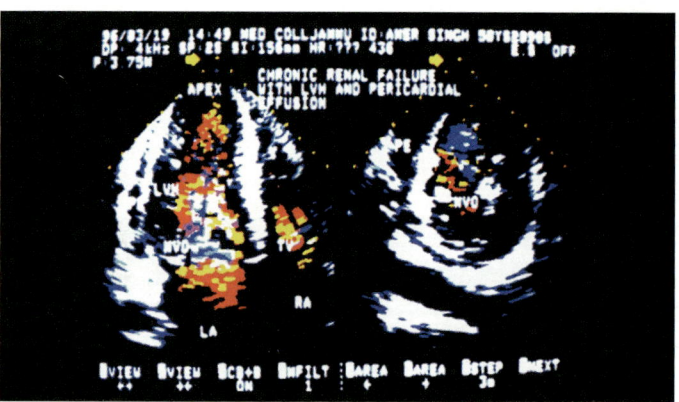

Fig. 21.31: Apical 4C and short axis views on dual scans showing mosaic colored MR jet into LA and mitral jet into LV almost up to the apex of LV due to pseudoprolapse of mitral valve due to compression of massive pericardial effusion

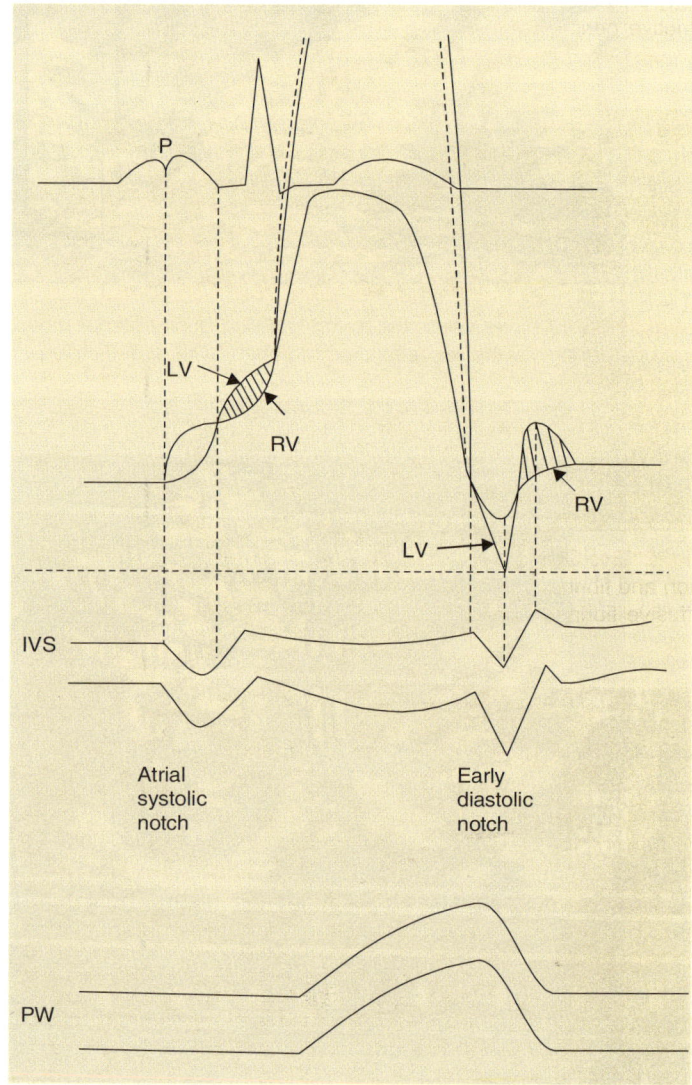

Fig. 21.32: Diagrammatic representation demonstrating systolic and early diastolic notches on interventricular septum (IVS) and its relationship with pressure alterations in LV and RV in cases with constrictive pericarditis

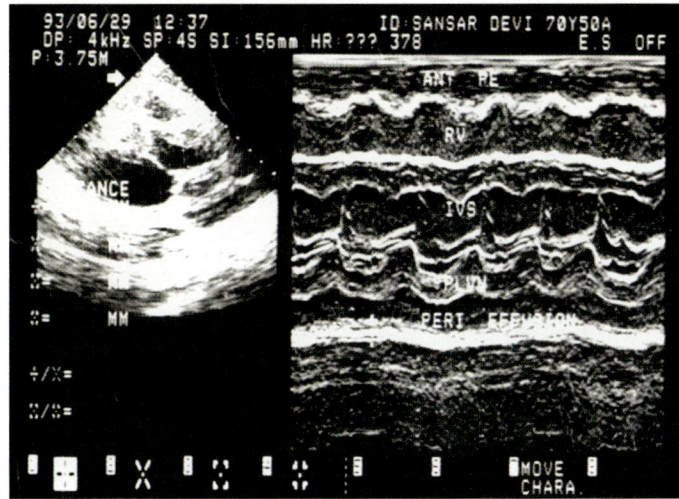

Fig. 21.33: 2D and M-mode echocardiogram showing systolic and early diastolic notches on IVS (arrows) in patient with effusive constrictive pericarditis

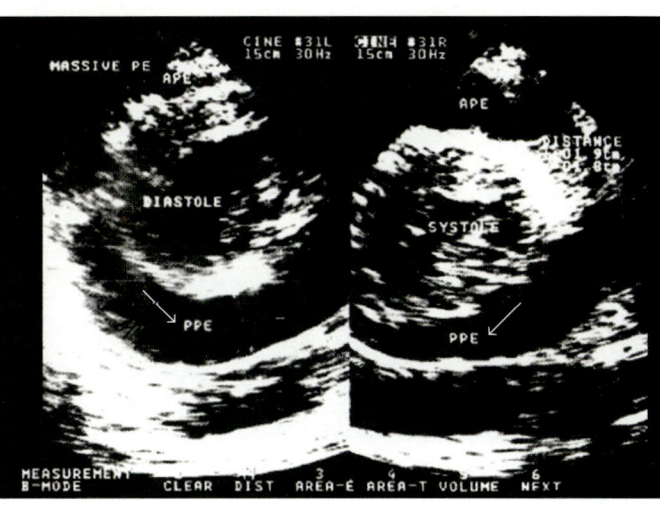

Fig. 21.36: SAX LV in systole and diastole showing massive pericardial (PPE) and pleural effusion (PLE) in patient with chronic pulmonary tuberculosis

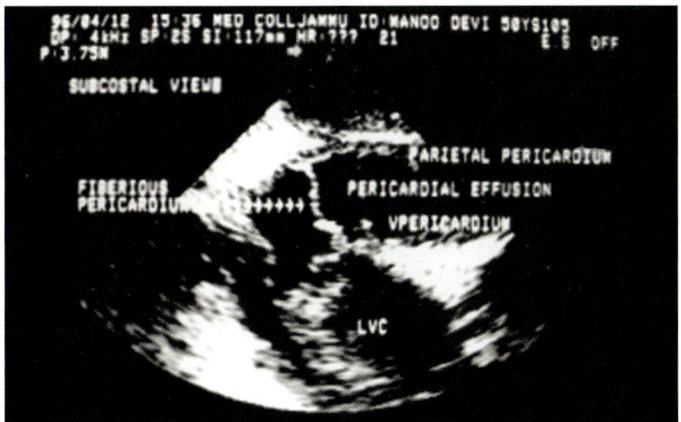

Fig. 21.34: Oblique 4C view showing thickened pericardium, effusion and fibrinous strands (arrows) in pericardial sac in patient with effusive fibrinous constrictive pericarditis

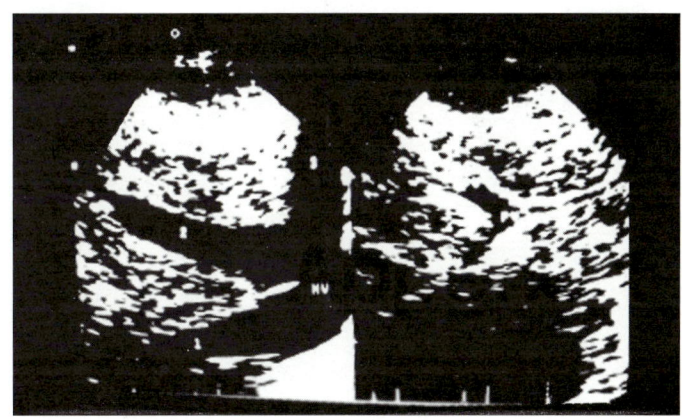

Fig. 21.37: Subcostal transverse transhepatic view showing gross distension of hepatic venous system in patient with constrictive pericarditis

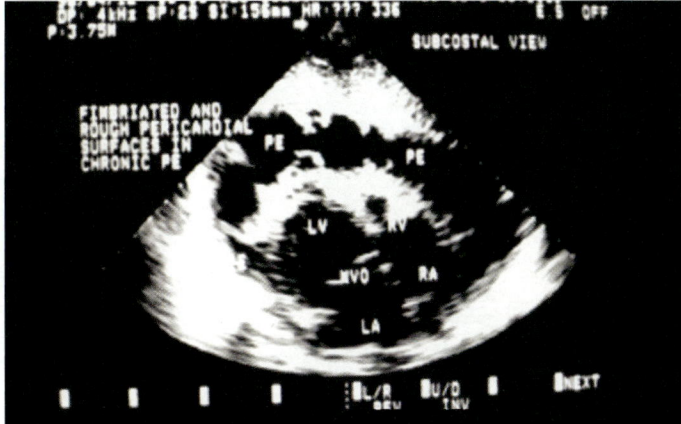

Fig. 21.35: Short axis view LV showing markedly thickened pericardium with irregular and shaggy margins of visceral pericardium in patient with effusive constrictive pericarditis of rheumatic aetiology

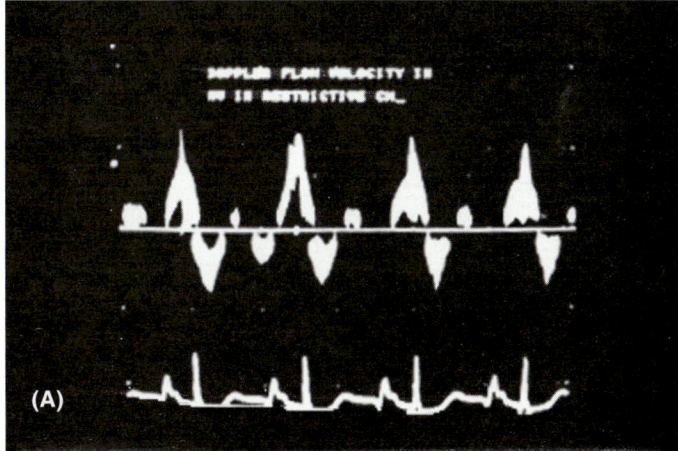

Fig. 21.38A: Doppler flow velocity across hepatic vein showing marked reversal of flow

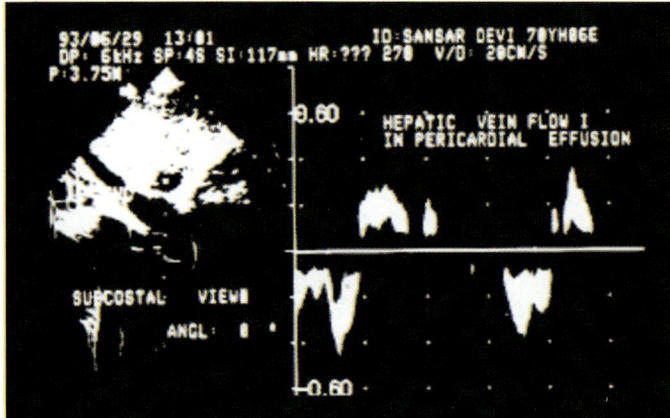

Fig. 21.38B: Doppler flow velocity across hepatic vein showing mild reversal of flow in patient with constructive pericarditis

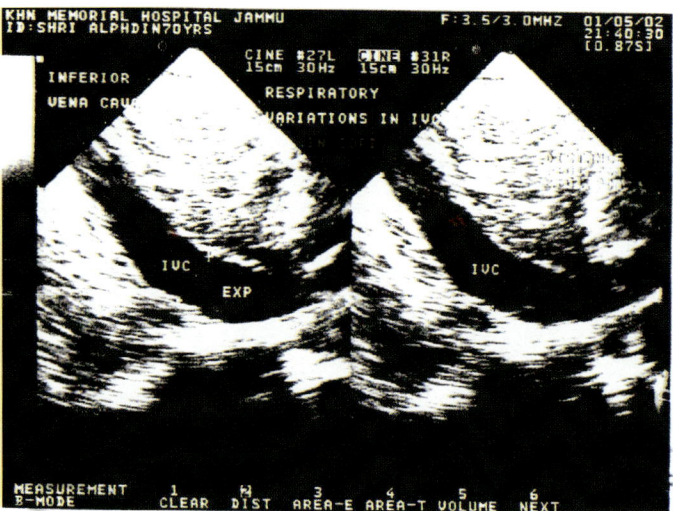

Fig. 21.39: Subcostal approach inferior vena caval view showing distended inferior vena cava and absence of inspiratory collapse during respiration in patient with constrictive pericarditis

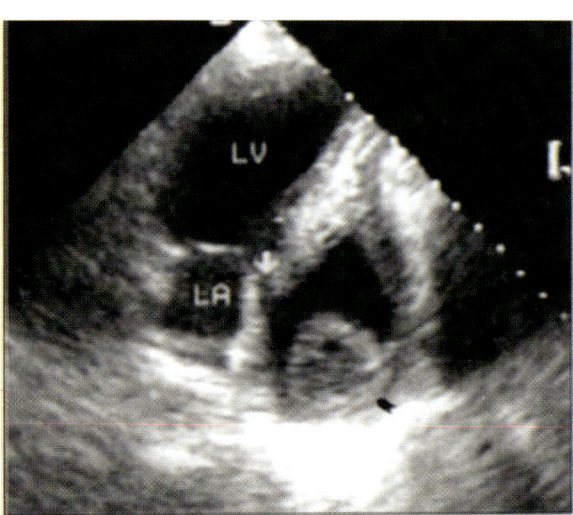

Fig. 21.40: Apical 2C view showing hydatid cyst of pericardium (arrow) very close to left atrium (LA)

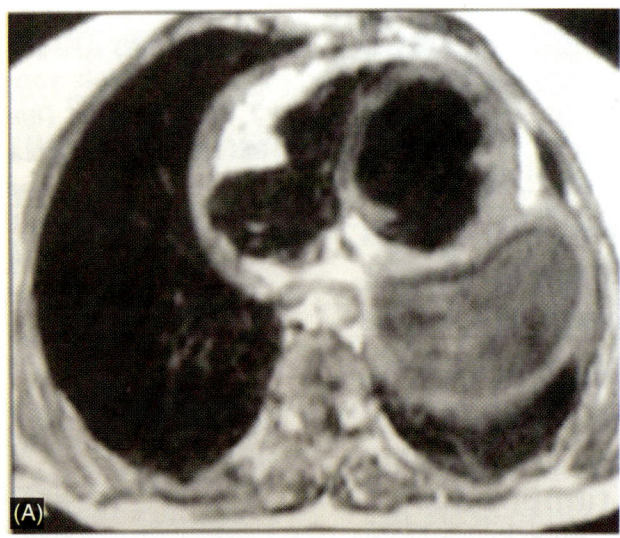

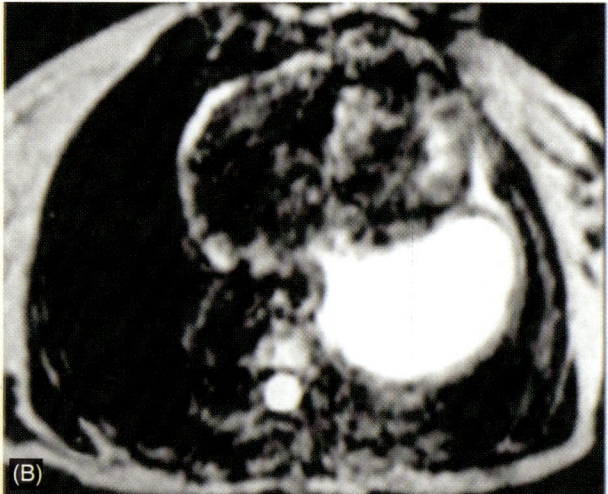

Fig. 21.41A and B: Spin echo T1 and T2 weighted showing characters of a hydatid cyst and excluding the tumor mass or thrombosis from that of pericardial effusion

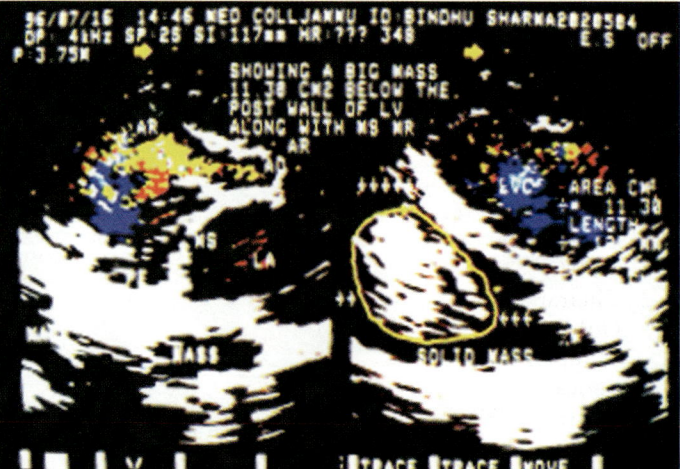

Fig. 21.42: Long axis LV showing solid mass (encircled) in pericardial sac. compressing the left ventricular cavity in patient with rheumatic mitral stenosis and valvular regurgitation

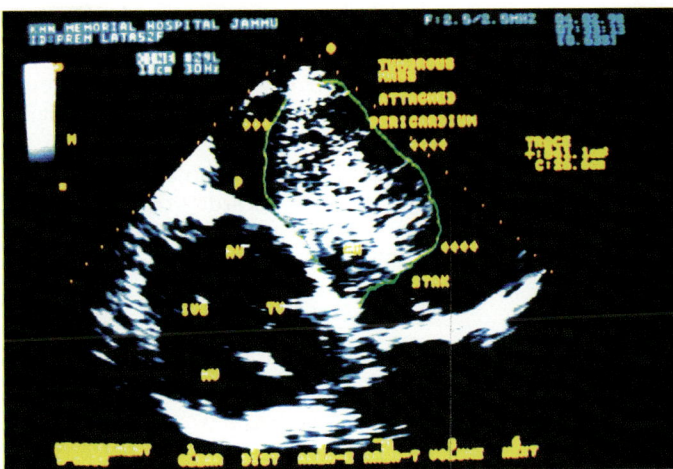

Fig. 21.43: Apical 4C view showing a big mass (encircled) with pericardial effusion attached to pericardium with compression on the anterior wall of the left ventricle

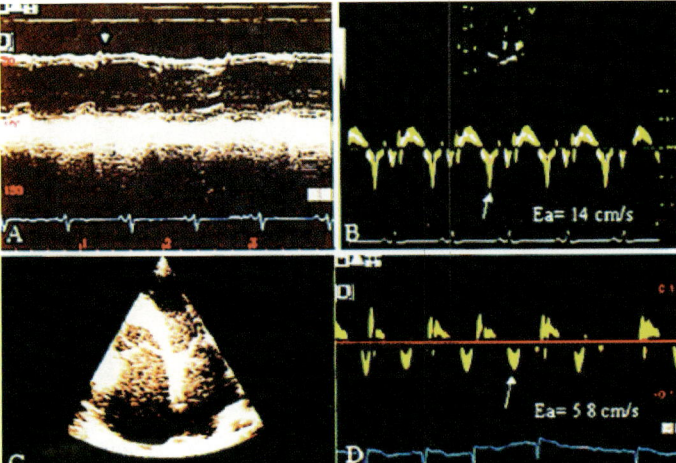

Fig. 21.44A to D: TDI Scans showing typical septal bounce (arrow) and pericardial thickening (arrow) in patient with constrictive pericarditis (A) Early diastolic longitudinal annular velocity (Ea) recorded by the pulsed Doppler are found normal and helps differentiating this condition from that of restrictive cardiomyopaty (C) where it is markedly diminished (D)

Bibliography

1. Byrd BF, Linden RW: Superior vena cava Doppler flow velocity patterns in pericardial disease. *Am J Cardiol* 1990;65:1464.
2. Chiaramida SA, Goldman MA, Zema MJ, Pizzarello RA, Goldberg HM: Echocardiographic identification of intrapericardial fibrous strands in acute pericarditis with pericardial effusion. *Chest,* 1980;77: 85.
3. D'Cruz, I. A. and Hoffman, P.K.: A new cross sectional echocardiographic method for estimating the volume of large pericardial effusions. *Br Heart J* 1991;66: 448.
4. Eisenberg MJ, Oken K, Guerrero S, Saniei MA, Schiller NB: Prognostic value of echocardiography in hospitalized patients with pericardial effusion. *Am J Cardiol* 1992;70: 934.
5. Feigenbaum H: Echocardiographic diagnosis of pericardial effusion. *Am J Cardiol* 1970;26: 475.
6. Hancock EW: Subacute effusive-constrictive pericarditis, *Circulation* 1971;43: 183.
7. Hatle LK, Appleton CP, Popp RL: Differentiation of constrictive pericarditis and restrictive cardiomyopathy by Doppler echocardiography. *Circulation* 1989;79: 357.
8. Hayes SN, Freeman WK, Gersh BJ: Low pressure cardiac tamponade: Diagnosis facilitated by Doppler echocardiography. *Br Heart J,* 1990;63: 136.
9. Himelman RB, Kircher B, Rockey DC, Schiller NB: Inferior vena cava plethora with blunted respiratory response: A sensitive echocardiographic sign of cardiac tamponade. *J Am Coll Cardiol* 1988;12:1470.
10. Hoit BD, Ramrakhyani K: Pulmonary venous flow in cardiac tamponade; Influence of left ventricular dysfunction and the relation to pulsus paradoxus. *J Am Soc Echocardiogr;* 4;559,1991
11. Horowitz MS, Schultz CS, Stinson EB, *et al.* Sensitivity and specificity of echocardiographic diagnosis of pericardial effusion, *Circulation* 50: 239,1974.
12. Hynes JK, Tajik AJ, Osborn MJ, Orszulak TA, Seward JB: Two-dimensional echocardiographic diagnosis of pericardial cyst, *Mayo Clin Proc* 1983;58;60.
13. Kirkland LL and Taylor RW: Pericardiocentesis. *Crit Care Clin* 1992;8: 699.
14. Klopbestein HS, *et al.* The relative merits of pulsus paradoxus and right ventricular diastolic collapse in the early detection of cardiac tamponade: An experimental echocardiographic study, *Circulation* 1985;71: 829.
15. Lam D, Rapaport E: Two-dimensional echocardiographic demonstration of intrapericardial fibrinous strands in rheumatoid pericarditis. *Am Heart J* 1987;114: 442.
16. Lemire F, Tajik AJ, Giuliani ER, *et al.* Further echocardiographic observations in pericardial effusions. *Mayo Clin Proc* 1976;51:13.
17. Lin TK, Stech SM, Eekert WG, *et al.* Pericardial angiosarcoma simulating pericardial effusion by echocardiography. *Chest* 1978;73: 881.
18. Mantana A, Marvric Z, Vukas D, Beg-Zec Z: Spontaneous contrast echoes in pericardial effusion: Sign of gas-producing infection. *Am. Heart J.,* 1992;124: 521.
19. Millman A, Meller J, Motro M, *et al.* Pericardial tumor or fibrosis mimicking pericardial effusion by echocardiography, *Am Intern Med* 1977;86: 434.
20. Payvandi MN, Kerber RE: Echocardiography in congenital and acquired absence of pericardium. *Circulation* 1976;53: 86.
21. Reydel B, Spodick DH: Frequency and signification of chamber collapses during cardiac tamponade. *Am Heart J* 1990;119:1160.
22. Schiavone WA, Calafiore PA, Currie PJ, Lytle BW: Doppler echocardiographic demonstration constrictive pericarditis before and after pericardiectomy. *Am J Cardiol* 1989;63: 145.
23. Schiavone WA, Calafiore PA, Salcedo EE: Transesophageal Doppler echocardiographic demonstration of pulmonary venous flow velocity in restrictive cardiomyopathy and constrictive pericarditis. *Am J Cardiol* 1989;63: 1286.

24. Tajik AJ: Echocardiography in pericardial effusion. *Am J Med* 1977;63: 29.

25. Torelli J, Marwick TH, Salcedo EE: Left atrial tamponade: Diagnosis by transesophageal echocardiography. *J Am Soc Echocardiogr* 1991;4: 413.

26. Torelli J, Marwick TH, Salcedo EE: Left atrial tamponade: Diagnosis by transesophageal echocardiography. *J Am Soc Echocardiogr* 1991;4: 413.

27. Vaitkus PT, Kussmaul WG: Constrictive pericarditis versus restrictive cardiomyopathy: A reappraisal and update of diagnostic criteria. *Am J Cardiol* 1989; 63: 1286.

28. Vaska K, Wann LS, Sagar K, Klopfenstein HS: Pleural effusion as a cause of right ventricular diastolic collapse. *Circulation* 1992; 86:609.

29. Weintraub AR, Schwartz SL, Smith J, Hsu T-L, Pandian NG: Intracardiac two-dimensional echocardiography in patients with pericardial effusion and cardiac tamponade. *J Am Soc Echocardiogr* 1991; 4: 571.

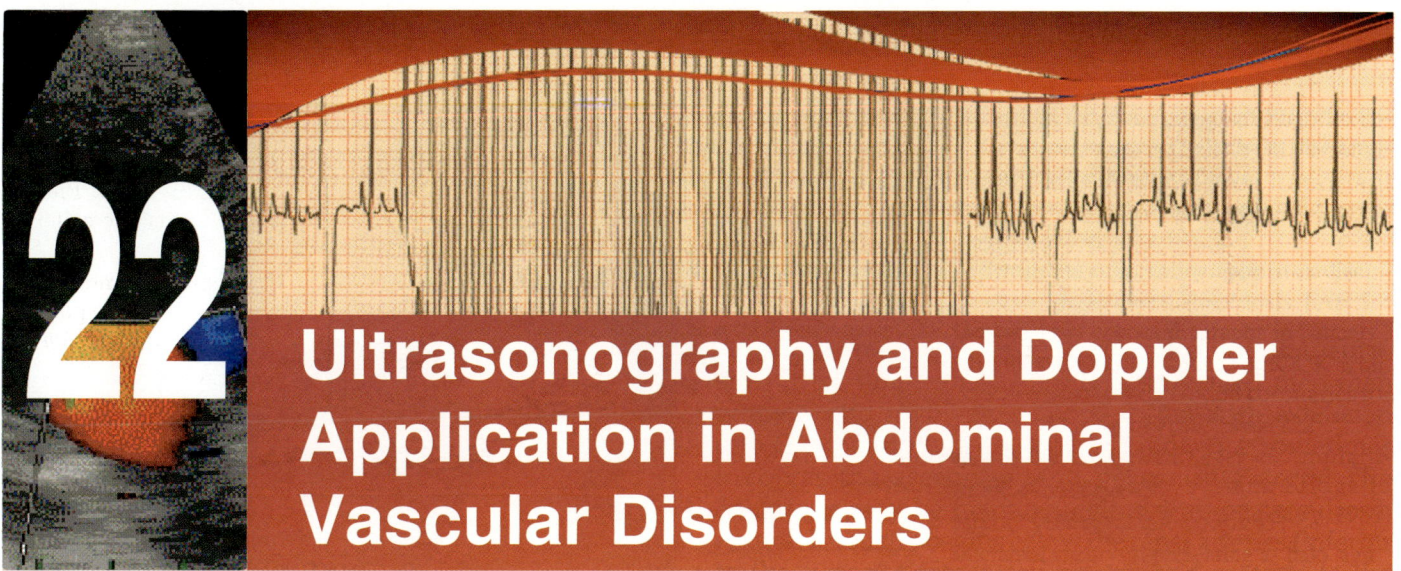

22

Ultrasonography and Doppler Application in Abdominal Vascular Disorders

Historical Background

Many diseases and conditions in the human body have led investigators to discover a vascular etiology where a completely different diagnosis was expected. Unfortunately the source often has not been found in time to save a diseased organ or limb or has been discovered only after the patient's death.

The introduction of radiographic imaging of the arterial system in 1923 made possible accurate vascular diagnosis and greatly enhanced the potential for surgical repair of vascular lesions. The first carotid arteriogram was performed in 1927, and the first translumbar aortogram in 1929. Many years were required to perfect angiographic equipment and techniques, but angiography has become the standard method for assessing vascular anatomy.

Angiography also has numerous drawbacks. There are risks resulting from reactions to the iodine based contrast media. Furthermore, the examination is performed with the patient in an immobile position; needle punctures or cutdowns and rapid injections of contrast are required, all of which contribute to patient anxiety and occasionally result in patients refusing the examination.

Digital subtraction angiography was introduced later as a breakthrough in technology. It was intravenous as opposed to intraarterial and could be performed on an outpatient basis. Various studies undertaken since its introduction, however, have shown as little as a 65% overall accuracy when compared with ultrasonic noninvasive methodology. Intravenous Digital Subtraction Angiography has been supplemented by arterial injections in most institutions now. This imaging procedure had the same risks found with conventional arteriography.

Many of the pitfalls of arteriography, venography, and DSA stem from the fact that these procedures are capable only of showing those structures that can be actively utilized by the radiographic contrast material, thus, only filling defects can be interpreted as suspect. The images are in two dimensions only and lack the ability to show the vessel from more angles without reinjection and running another film series. The contrast agents can often mask underlying anatomy, or "sneak by" low-density soft plaques that do not obstruct flow.

In addition to invasive procedures, many other noninvasive and nonangiographic methods are available, including ultrasonic techniques. The ideal noninvasive vascular diagnostic method is truly noninvasive, has a high overall accuracy, is comfortable to the patient, can be performed quickly, and does not require bulky equipment or long setup procedures.

Doppler and high-resolution duplex ultrasonic techniques fulfil all the requirements. Doppler and duplex techniques have come a long way since their inception. Doppler techniques were first used for vascular purposes during the late 1960s and early 1970s, and commercial duplex scanners were developed and made available in the late 1970s. Initial physicians gave way to widespread acceptance as numerous papers and presentations began to document the accuracy and usefulness of these techniques. Among the pioneers in the vascular field are Eugene Strandness, Robert Barnes, and David Sumner, whose techniques and diagnostic criteria are still in use today. Hundreds of clinical and laboratory studies have been performed comparing noninvasive techniques to angiography and surgical findings, and high degrees of sensitivity, specificity, and overall accuracy have been reported over

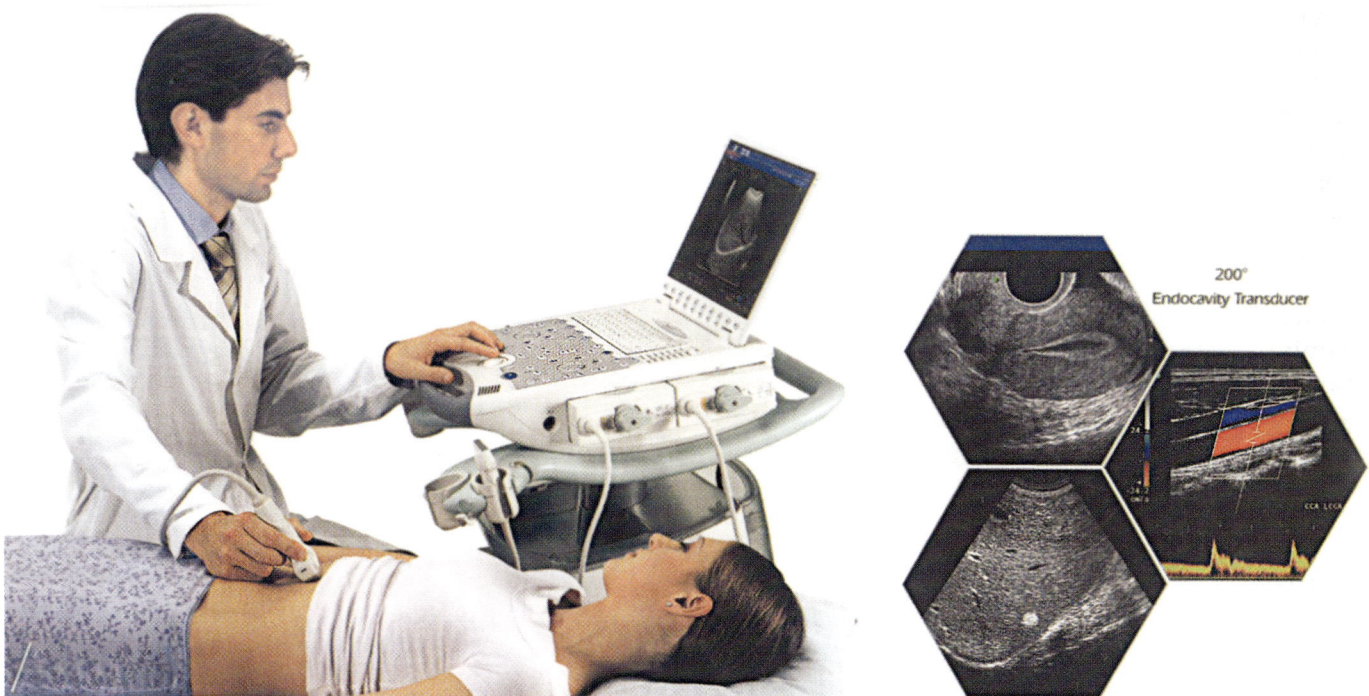

Fig. 22.1: Showing both operator and the patient (left) and echoscans on monitor of the machine (right) in performing abdominal ultrasonography in the laboratory

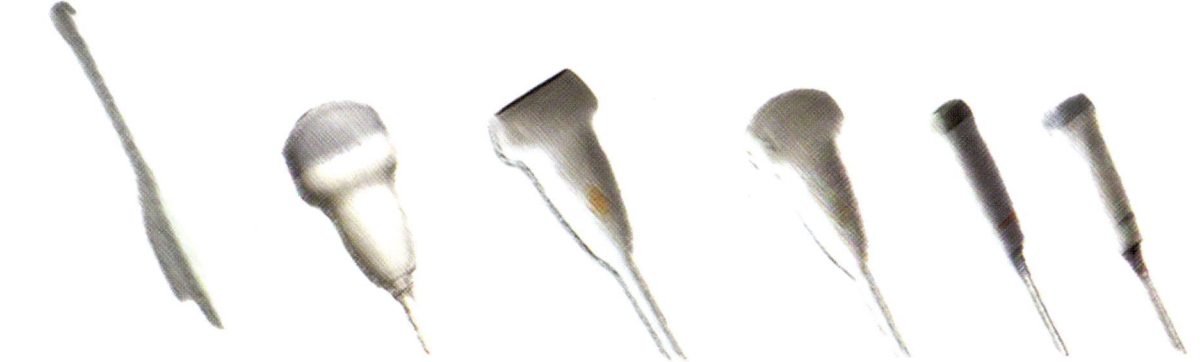

Fig. 22.2: Different types and sizes of ultrasonographic transducers used in performing abdominal sonography

the years with colour-imaging, and other noninvasive techniques for arterial and venous evaluation (Figs 22.1 and 22.2), including evaluation of the extremity vessels and the cerebrovascular system.

The Doppler ultrasound apparatus makes use of the Doppler effect, which was described by the Austrian physicist Johann Doppler, who first described this phenomenon in relation to reflection of light waves from planets and other celestial bodies. He observed that the frequency of sound waves varied depending on the speed of the sound transmitter relative to the listener, about 2 years after Doppler's equation was developed to express the phenomenon.

The Vascular System

Anatomic Composition of Vascular Structures

Blood is carried away from the heart by the arteries and returned from the tissues to the heart by the veins. Arteries divide into smaller and smaller branches, the smallest of which are the arterioles. These lead into the capillaries, which are minute vessels that branch and form a network where the exchange of materials between blood and tissue fluid takes place. After the blood passes through the capillaries, it is collected in the small veins or venules. These small vessels unite to form larger vessels that eventually return the blood to the heart for recirculation.

A typical artery in cross-section consists of the following three layers (Figs 22.3 and 22.4):

1. Tunica intima (inner layer), which itself consists of the following three layers: a layer of endothelial cells lining the arterial passage (lumen), a layer of delicate connective tissue, and an elastic layer made up of a network of elastic fibres.
2. Tunica media (middle layer), which consists of smooth muscle fibers with elastic and collagenous tissue.
3. Tunica adventitia (external layer), which is composed of loose connective tissue with bundles of smooth muscle fibers and elastic tissue.

Specific differences exists between the arteries and the veins. The arteries are hollow elastic tubes that carry blood away from the heart. They are enclosed within a sheath that includes a vein and nerve. The smaller arteries contain less elastic tissue and more smooth muscles than the larger arteries. The elasticity of the larger arteries is important in maintaining a steady blood-flow.

The veins are hollow collapsible tubes with diminished tunica media that carry blood toward the heart. The veins appear collapsed because they have little elastic tissue or muscle within their walls. Veins have a larger total diameter than the arteries, and they move blood more slowly. The veins contain special valves that prevent backflow and permit blood to flow only in one direction towards the heart. Numerous valves are found within the extremities, especially the lower extremities, because flow must work against gravity. Venous return is also aided by muscle contraction, overflow from capillary beds, gravity, and suction from negative thoracic pressure.

The capillaries are minute, hair-size vessels connecting the arterial and venous systems. Their walls have only one layer. The cells and tissues of the body receive their nutrients from the fluids passing through the capillary walls; at the same time, waste products from the cells pass into the capillaries. Arteries do not always end in capillary beds; some end in anastomoses, which are end-to-end grafts between different vessels that equalize over vessel length and also provide alternate flow channels.

Major Vessels

Aorta (Fig. 22.6)

The aorta is the largest principal artery of the body. It divides into the following five sections:

1. Root of the aorta,
2. Ascending aorta,
3. Descending aorta,
4. Abdominal aorta, and
5. The bifurcation of the aorta into iliac arteries.

Root of the Aorta: The systemic circulation leaves the left ventricle of the heart by way of the aorta. The root of the aorta arises from the left ventricular outflow tract in the heart. It is comprised of three semilunar cusps that prevent blood from flowing back into the left ventricle. The cusps open with ventricular systole to allow blood to be ejected into the ascending aorta; the cusps are closed during ventricular diastole. The coronary arteries arise superiorly from the right and left coronary cusps to form the right and left coronary arteries, respectively. These coronary arteries further bifurcate to supply the vasculature of the cardiac structures. After the aorta arises from the left ventricle, it ascends posterior to the main pulmonary artery to form the ascending aorta.

Ascending Aorta: The ascending aorta arises a short distance from the ventricle and arches superior to form the aortic arch. Three arterial branches arise from the superior border of the aortic arch to supply the head, neck, and upper extremities: the right innominate, left common carotid, and left subclavian arteries.

Descending Aorta: From the aortic arch, the aorta descends posteriorly along the back wall of the heart through the thoracic cavity, where it pierces the diaphragm. The descending aorta enters the abdomen through the aortic opening of the diaphragm in front of the twelfth thoracic vertebra in the retroperitoneal space.

Abdominal Aorta: The aorta then continues to flow anterior to the vertebral column to the level of the fourth lumber vertebra, where it bifurcates into the right and left common iliac arteries. At this point the aorta

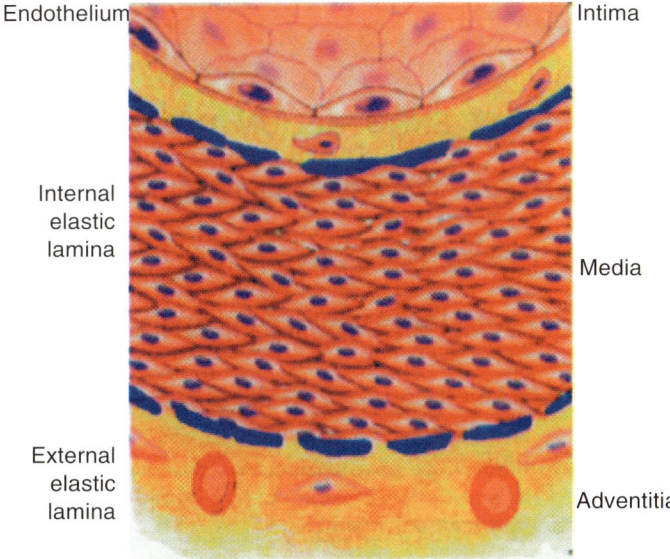

Endothelium   Intima

Internal elastic lamina

Media

External elastic lamina

Adventitia

Fig. 22.3: Histological features of three layers of peripheral artery

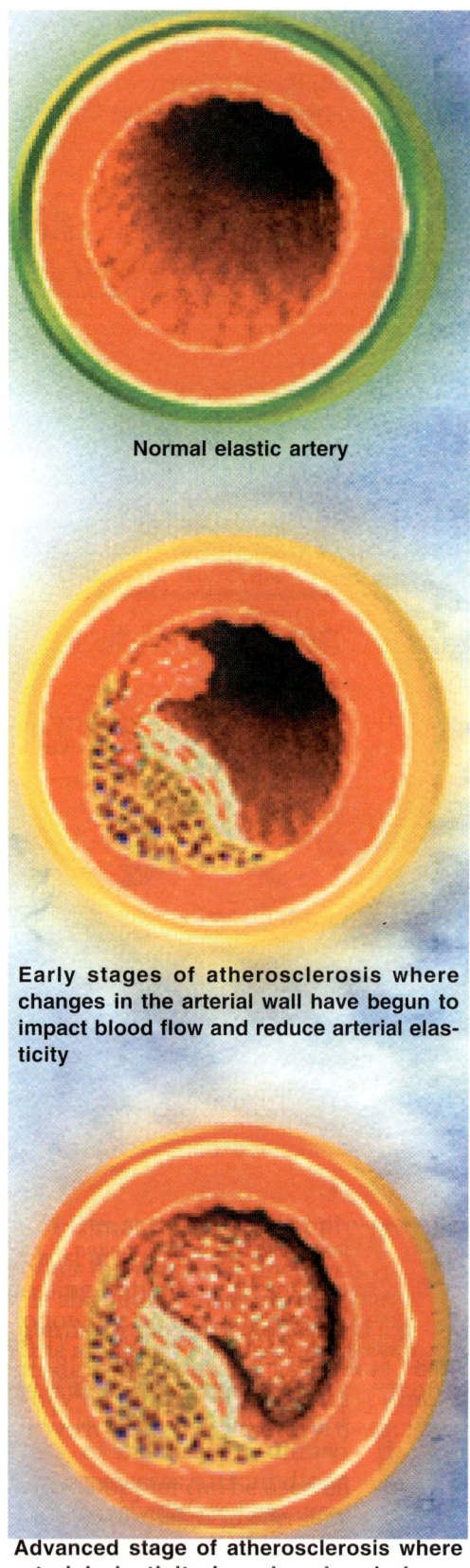

Normal elastic artery

Early stages of atherosclerosis where changes in the arterial wall have begun to impact blood flow and reduce arterial elasticity

Advanced stage of atherosclerosis where arterial elasticity is reduced and plaque formation has restricted blood flow

Fig. 22.4: Progressive thickening and formation of thrombosis in peripheral artery

measures 2 to 3 cm in diameter. The aorta has four branches that supply other visceral organs and the mesentery; the celiac trunk, the superior and inferior mesenteric arteries, and the renal arteries.

Abdominal Aortic Branches: The celiac trunk is the first anterior branch of the aorta, arising to 2 cm from the diaphragm. The celiac trunk gives rise to three smaller vessels; the splenic, hepatic, and left gastric arteries. The superior mesenteric artery is the second anterior branch, arising approximately 2 cm from the celiac trunk. The right and left renal arteries are lateral branches arising just inferior to the superior mesenteric artery. The small inferior mesenteric artery arises anteriorly near the bifurcation. The distribution of these branch arteries is to the visceral organs and the mesentery.

Common Iliac Arteries: The common iliac arteries arise at the bifurcation of the abdominal aorta at the fourth lumber vertebra. These vessels divide into the internal and external iliac arteries. The internal iliac artery enters the pelvis anterior to the sacroiliac joint, at which point it is crossed anteriorly by the ureter. It divides into anterior and posterior branches to supply the pelvic viscera, peritoneum, buttocks, and sacral canal. The external iliac artery runs along the medical border of the psoas muscle following the pelvic brim. The inferior epigastric and deep circumflex iliac branches branch off before they pass under the inguinal ligament to become the femoral artery. The portion of the femoral artery posterior to the knee is the popliteal artery. This artery further divides into the anterior and posterior tibial arteries (Fig. 22.5).

Ultrasound Characteristics

The abdominal aorta is usually one of the easiest abdominal structures to visualise by ultrasound because of the marked change in acoustic impedance between its elastic walls and its blood-filled lumen. Sonography provides the diagnostic information needed to provide an image of the entire abdominal aorta, to assess its diameter, and to visualise the presence of thrombus, calcification, or dissection within the walls (Figs 22.7 and 22.8).

The patient is routinely scanned in the supine position. Gas-filled or barium-filled loops of bowel may prevent adequate visualisation of the aorta, but this can sometimes be overcome by applying gentle pressure with the transducer or by changing the angle of the transducer to move the gas out of the way.

Sagittal scans should be made beginning in the midline with a slight angulation of the transducer to the left, from the xiphoid to well below the level of bifurcation. In the normal individual the luminal dimension of the aorta gradually tapers as it proceeds distally in the abdomen. A low to medium gain should be used to demonstrate the walls of the aorta without

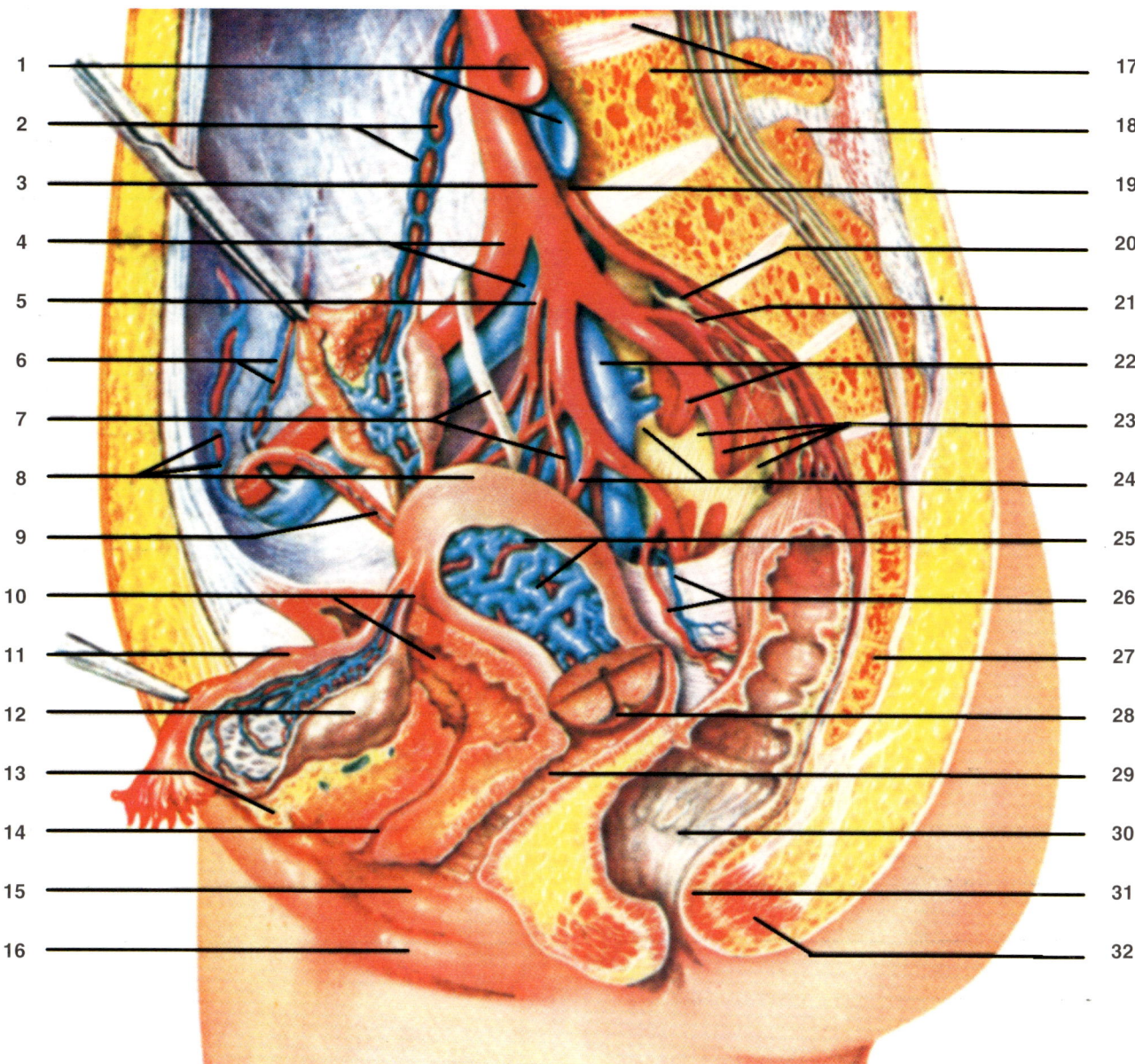

1. Common iliac artery and vein
2. Ovarian artery and vein
3. Internal iliac (hypogastric) artery
4. External iliac artery and vein
5. Umbilical artery
6. Deep iliac circumflex artery and vein
7. Ureter; uterine artery
8. Inferior epigastric artery and vein; uterus
9. Round ligament of uterus
10. Ovarian ligament; urinary bladder
11. Fallopian tube
12. Ovary
13. Clitoris
14. Urethra
15. Labium minus
16. Labium majus
17. Intervertebral fibrocartilage; fifth lumbar vertebra
18. Middle sacral crest
19. Middle sacral artery
20. Ganglion of sympathetic trunk
21. Lateral sacral artery
22. Internal iliac vein; superior gluteal artery
23. Sacral nerves; inferior gluteal artery
24. Inferior vesical artery; lumbosacral trunk
25. Uterine artery and vein
26. Middle hemorrhoidal artery and vein
27. Coccyx
28. Cervix of uterus
29. Vagina
30. Rectum
31. Sphincter ani internus muscle
32. Spinchter ani externus muscle

Fig. 22.5A: The female pelvic organs

POSTERIOR ASPECT

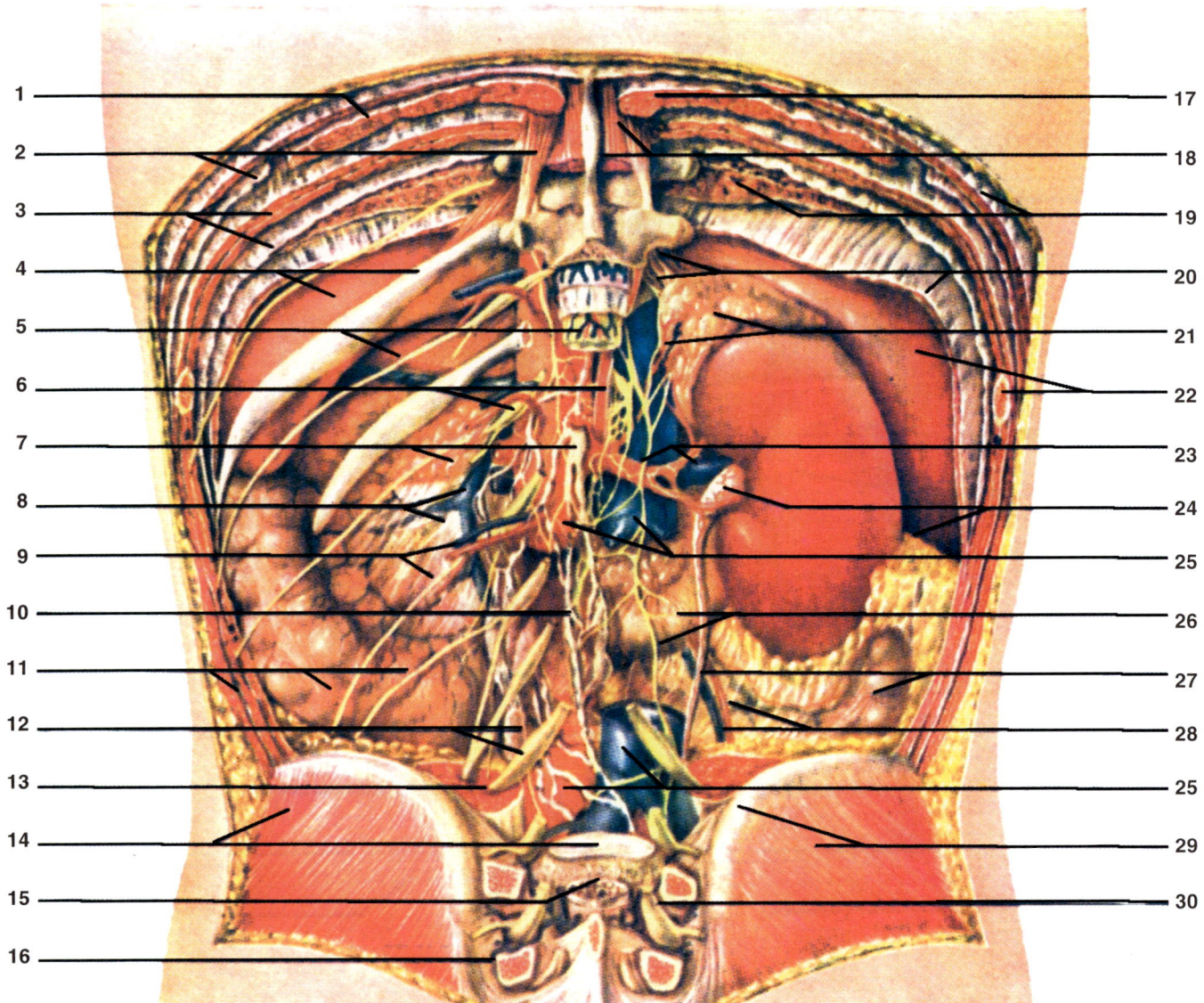

1. Iliocostalis lumborum muscle
2. Intertransversari muscle and lumbodorsal fascia
3. Internal and external intercostal muscles and pleura
4. Spleen and eleventh rib
5. Spinal cord and eleventh thoracic nerve
6. Crus of diaphragm and twelfth thoracic ganglion
7. Cisterna chyli and pancreas
8. Mesocolon and inferior mesenteric vein
9. Dorsal branches of first lumbar artery and vein, and iliohypogastric nerve
10. Right lumbar lymphatic trunk
11. Obliquus abdominis externus muscle, descending colon and ilioinguinal nerve
12. Lumbar lymph node and forth lumbar ganglion
13. Psoas major muscle
14. Intervertebral fibrocartilage and gluteus medius muscle
15. Cauda equina
16. Interosseous sacroiliac ligament
17. Longissimus dorsi muscle
18. Supraspinal ligament and multifidus muscle
19. Lung and latissimus dorsi muscle
20. Diaphragm and superior suprarenal arteries, veins and nerves
21. Right suprarenal gland and inferior suprarenal artery and vein
22. Liver and tenth rib
23. Renal artery and vein
24. Renal pelvis and perirenal fat
25. Abdominal aorta and inferior vena cava
26. Duodenum and sympathetic trunk
27. Ureter and ascending colon
28. Internal spermatic artery and vein
29. Crest of ilium and gluteus maximus muscle
30. First sacral ganglion

Fig. 22.5B: Diagrammatic picture showing anatomical placement of structures including vascular supply to the kidneys and in the region of pelvis which is most essential for any operator to know before pertaining lower abdominal ultrasonography

"noisy" artifactual internal echoes. These weak echoes may result from increased gain, reverberation from the anterior abdominal wall, or poor lateral resolution. These factors result in echoes being recorded at the same level as those from soft tissues that surround the vessel lumen, particularly if the vessels are smaller in diameter than the transducer.

Since the aorta follows the anterior course of the vertebral column, it is important that the transducer also follow a perpendicular path along the entire curvature of the spine. The anterior and posterior walls of the aorta should be easily seen as two thin lines. This facilitates measuring the anteroposterior diameter of the aorta, which in most institutions is done from the leading outer edge of the anterior wall to the leading inner edge of the posterior wall.

In the transverse plane, the aorta is imaged as a circular structure anterior to the spine and slightly to the left of the midline. In some cases the transverse diameter of the aorta differs from that found in longitudinal measurements; thus it is important to identify the vessel in two dimensions. Multiple scans should be made from the xiphoid to the bifurcation.

If the patient has a very tortuous aorta, scans may be difficult to obtain in a single plane. As one scans in the longitudinal plane, the upper portion of the abdominal aorta may be well visualised, but the lower portion may be out of the plane of view. In this case the sonographer should obtain a complete scan of the upper segment and then concentrate fully on the lower segment. In some patients, it has been seen that the aorta stretch from the far right of the abdomen to the far left.

To better visualise the aortic bifurcation, use the lateral decubitus position. The patient should be examined in deep inspiration, which projects the liver and diaphragm into the abdominal cavity and provides an acoustic window to image the vascular structures. The patient should be rotated 5 to 10 degrees from the true lateral position. Slight medial to lateral angulation may be needed to image the bifurcation in the longitudinal plane. In this oblique plane the inferior vena cava is visualised anterior to the aorta.

Inferior Vena Cava

The inferior vena cava is formed by the union of the common iliac veins posterior to the right common iliac artery. The inferior vena cava ascends vertically through the retroperitoneal space on the right side of this aorta posterior to the liver, piercing the central tendon of the diaphragm at the level of the eighth thoracic vertebra to enter the right atrium of the heart. Its entrance into the lesser sac separates it from the postal vein. Caudal to the renal vein entrance, the inferior vena cava shows posterior "ammocking" through the bare area of liver.

The tributaries of the inferior vena cava are the

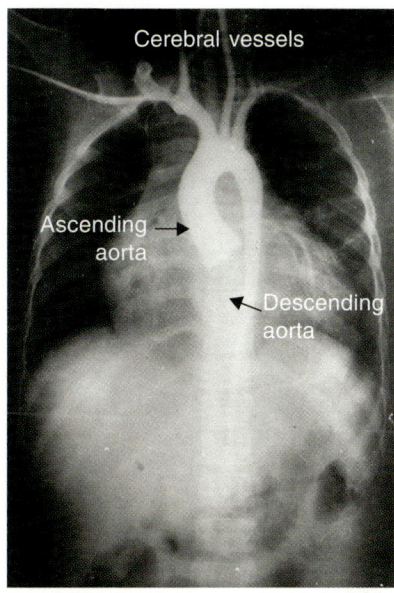

Fig. 22.6: Aortogram showing cerebral vessels, ascending and descending aorta

hepatic veins, the right adrenal vein, the renal veins, the right testicular or ovarian vein, the inferior phrenic vein, the four lumbar veins, the two common iliac veins, and the median sacral vein. The distribution of the venous system is such that blood drains from all organs and structures into the upper and lower abdomen through the system's major tributaries.

Ultrasound Findings (Figs 22.9–22.17)

The inferior vena cava serves as a landmark for many other abdominal structures and should be routinely visualised on all examinations. On the sagittal image, the distended inferior vena cava can be seen with the patient in full inspiration from the diaphragm to its bifurcation. The aorta is easily differentiated from the vena cava since the latter has horizontal course, its proximal portion curving slightly anterior as it empties into the right atrial cavity; the aorta follows the curvature of the spine, its distal portion moving more posterior before bifurcating into the iliac vessels.

On transverse scan, the almond-shaped inferior vena cava serves as a landmark for localizing the superior mesenteric vein, which is generally found anterior and slightly to the right of or just medial to the cava. On sagittal scans, it serves as landmark for the portal vein, which is located just anterior to or midway down the anterior wall of the cava. It is also useful in identifying the pancreas and common bile duct. The head of the pancreas is seen just inferior to the portal vein and anterior to the inferior vena cava as it makes a slight impression or indentation on the anterior wall of the cava. The common duct is seen anterior to the portal vein as it dips posterior to enter the head of the pancreas.

The inferior vena cava is first imaged on a sagittal

scan beginning at the midline, the transducer being angled slightly to the right with a slight oblique tilt, until the entire vessel is seen. The patient should be instructed to hold their breath; this causes the patient to perform a slight Valsalva maneuver towards the end of inspiration, which dilates the inferior vena cava and other venous structures. The inferior vena cava may expand to as such as 3 to 4 cm in diameter with this maneuver (Figs 22.22 and 22.24).

Dilation of the inferior vena cava is noted in several pathologic conditions, including right ventricular heart failure, congestive heart disease, constrictive pericarditis, tricuspid disease, and right heart obstructive tumours. In patients with hepatomegaly the hepatic veins are dilated and increased pressure is transmitted through the sinusoids, resulting in portal vein distension. If severe cirrhosis is present, the sinusoids may be unable to transmit pressure, and the portal veins will not distend. The presence of thrombus within the vessel should be evaluated, especially in patients with a known renal tumour. Other distortions of the inferior vena cava may be caused by an extrinsic retroperitoneal mass, hepatic neoplasm, or pancreatic mass (Fig. 22.21).

Branches of the Abdominal Aorta

Celiac Trunk (Fig. 21.13)

The celiac trunk originates within the first 2 cm from the diaphragm. It is surrounded by the liver, spleen, inferior vena cava, and pancreas. After arising from the anterior wall it immediately branches into the following three vessels: the common hepatic, left gastric, and splenic arteries.

Common Hepatic Artery (Fig. 22.5)

The common hepatic artery arises from the celiac trunk and courses to the right of the abdomen at almost a 90° angle. It courses along the upper border of the head of the pancreas, behind the posterior layer of the peritoneal omental bursa, to the upper margin of the superior part of the duodenum, which forms the lower boundary of the epiploic foramen. The head of the pancreas, the duodenum, and parts of the stomach are supplied by the gastroduodenal artery and the right gastric artery. Along with the hepatic artery duct and the portal vein, the common hepatic artery then ascends into the liver, where it divides into two branches, the right and left hepatic arteries.

Left Hepatic Artery (Fig. 22.5)

The left hepatic artery is a small branch supplying the caudate and left lobes of the liver.

Right Hepatic Artery (Fig. 22.5)

The right hepatic artery supplies the gallbladder via the cystic artery.

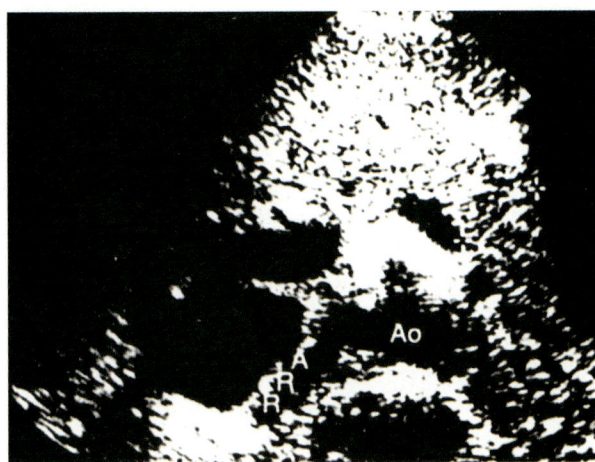

Fig. 22.7: Transvere scan of the right renal artery (RRA) as it extends from the posterior lateral wall of the aorta to enter the central sinus

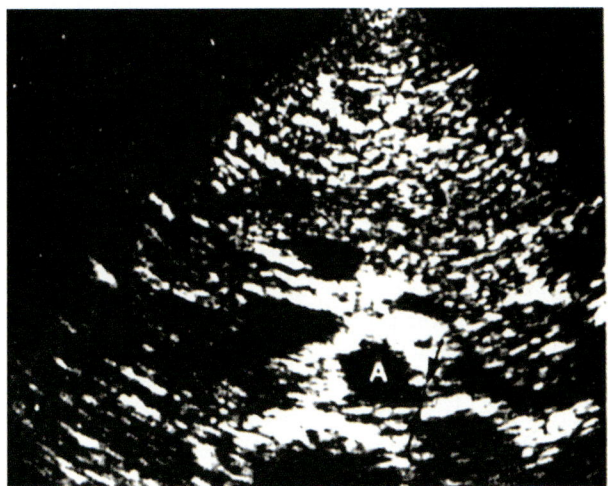

Fig. 22.8: The left renal artery (arrow) runs from the posterior lateral wall of the aorta (A) the central renal sinus

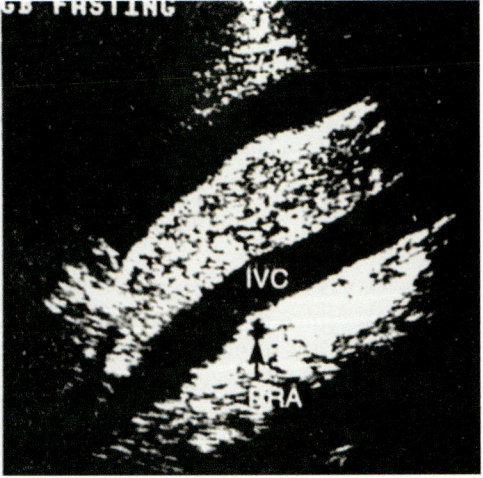

Fig. 22.9: Longitudinal scan showing right renal artery RRA (arrow) as a circular structure posterior to the inferior vena cava (IVC)

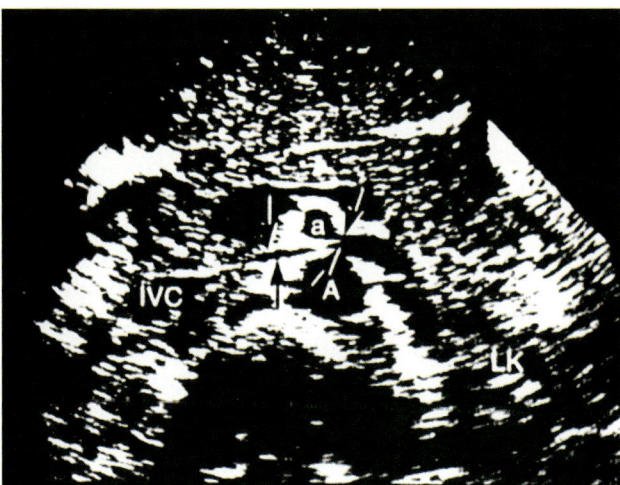

Fig. 22.10: Anterior to aorta (A) and posterior to the superior mesenteric artery (a) it is the left renal vein that can be seen flowing from the central sinus to join the inferior vena cava (IVC)

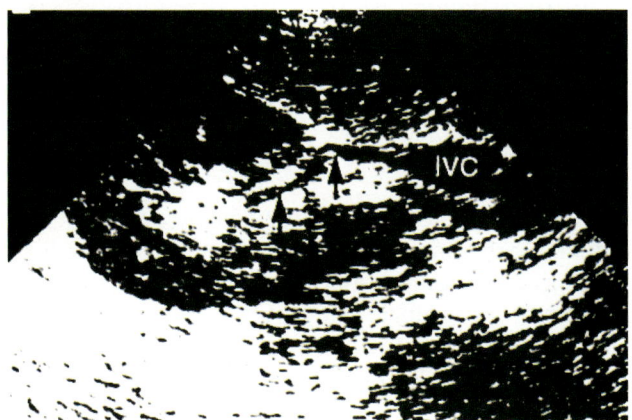

Fig. 22.11: Right renal vein (arrow) extends from the central renal sinus directly into the inferior vena cava (IVC)

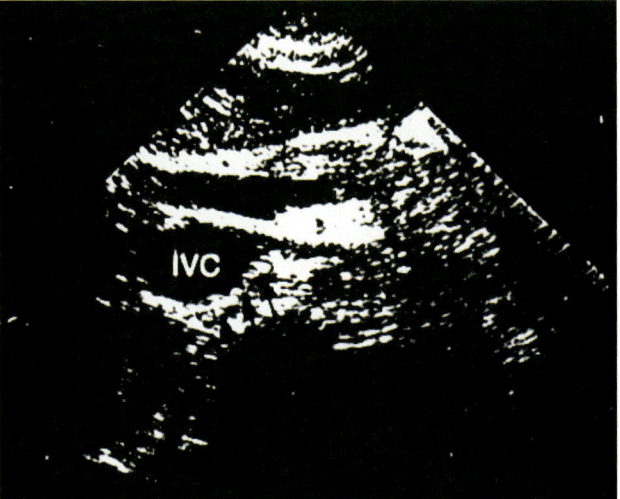

Fig. 22.12: The crura of the diaphragm lie posterior to the renal arteries and should be identified by their absence of pulsations and Doppler flow

Left Gastric Artery (Fig. 22.5)

The left gastric artery is a small branch of the celiac trunk, passing anterior, cephalic, and left to reach the esophagus and then descending along the lesser curvature of the stomach. It supplies the lower third of the esophagus and the upper right of the stomach.

Splenic Artery (Fig. 22.5)

The splenic artery is the largest of the three branches of the celiac trunk. From its origin, the artery takes a somewhat tortuous course horizontally to the left, as it forms the superior border of the pancreas. At a variable distance from the spleen, it divides into two branches. One of these branches, the left gastroepiploic, runs caudally into the greater momentum towards the right gastroepiploic artery. The other courses in a cephalic direction and divides into the short gastric artery, which supplies the fundus of the stomach, and a number of splenic branches, which supply the spleen.

Several smaller arterial branches originate at the splenic artery, as it courses through the upper border of the pancreas: the dorsal pancreatic, great pancreatic, and caudal pancreatic arteries. The dorsal or superior pancreatic artery originates from the beginning of the splenic artery or from the hepatic artery, celiac trunk, or aorta. It runs behind and in the substance of the pancreas, dividing into right and left branches. The left branch is the transverse pancreatic artery. The right branch constitutes an anastomotic vessel to the anterior pancreatic arch and also a branch to the uncinate process. The great pancreatic artery originates from the splenic artery further to the left and passes downward, dividing into branches that anastomose with the transverse or inferior pancreatic artery. The caudal pancreatic artery supplies the tail of the pancreas and divides into branches that anastomose with terminal branches of the transverse pancreatic artery. The transverse pancreatic artery courses behind the body and tail of the pancreas close to the lower pancreatic border. It may originate from or communicate with the superior mesenteric artery.

The distribution of the celiac trunk vessels is to the liver spleen, stomach, pancreas and duodenum.

Ultrasound Findings

The celiac trunk is best visualised sonographically on the longitudinal scan. It is usually seen as a small vascular structure arising anteriorly from the abdominal aorta just below the diaphragm. Since it is only 1 to 2 cm long, it is sometimes difficult to record unless the area near the midline of the aorta is carefully evaluated. Sometimes the celiac trunk can be seen to extend in a cephalic rather than a caudal presentation. The superior mesenteric artery is usually just inferior to the origin of the celiac trunk and may be used as a landmark in locating the celiac trunk. Transversely, one can

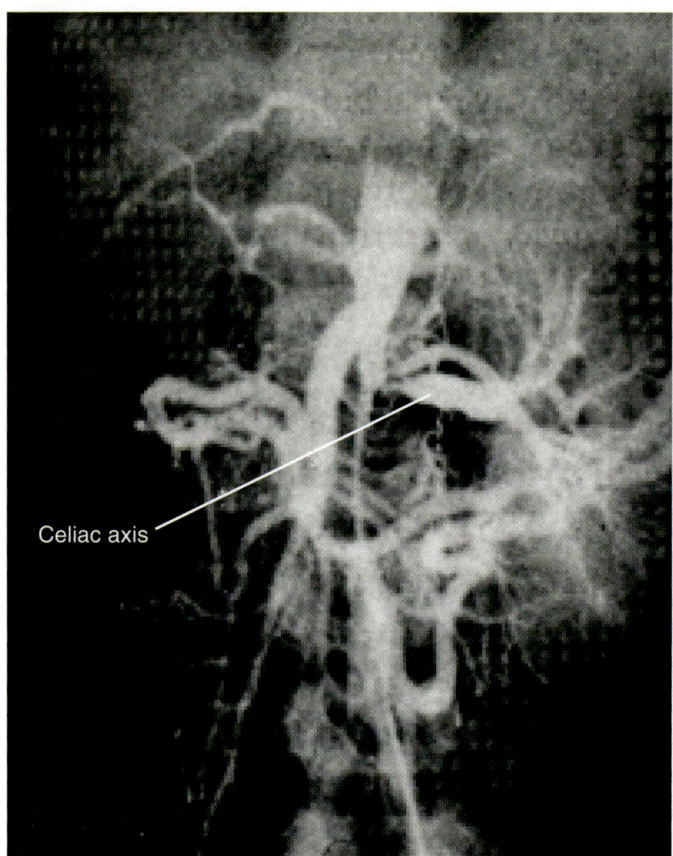

Celiac axis

Fig. 22.13: Abdominal aortogram showing different branches of celiac axis

differentiate the celiac trunk as the wings of the seagull arising directly anterior from the abdominal aorta.

The splenic artery may be seen to flow from the celiac trunk towards the spleen. Since it is so tortuous, it may be difficult to follow on the transverse scan. Generally small pieces of the splenic artery are visible as the artery weaves in and out of the left upper quadrant.

The hepatic artery can be seen to flow anterior and to the right of the celiac trunk, where it then divides into the right and left hepatic arteries.

The left gastric artery is of very small diameter and often is difficult to visualise by ultrasound. It becomes difficult to separate from the splenic artery, unless distinct structures are seen in the area of the celiac trunk branching to the left of the abdominal aorta.

Superior Mesenteric Artery (Fig. 22.5)

The superior mesenteric artery arises from the anterior abdominal aortic wall approximately 1 cm inferior to the celiac trunk. It runs posterior to the neck of the pancreas and anterior to the uncinate process, which is anterior to the third part of the duodenum; it then branches into the mesentery and colon. The right hepatic artery is sometimes seen to arise from the superior mesenteric artery.

The superior mesenteric artery has the following five main branches (Fig. 22.5):
1. Inferior pancreatic artery
2. Duodenal artery
3. Colic artery
4. Iliocolic artery
5. Intestinal artery.

These branch arteries supply the small bowel; each consists of 10 to 16 branches arising from the left side of the superior mesenteric trunk. They extend into the mesentery, where adjacent arteries unite with them to form loops or arcades. Their distribution is to the proximal half of the colon (cecum, ascending, and transverse) and the small intestine.

Inferior Mesenteric Artery

The inferior mesenteric artery arises from the anterior abdominal aorta approximately at the level of the third or fourth lumbar vertebra. It proceeds to the left to distribute arterial blood to the descending colon, sigmoid colon, and rectum. It has the following three main branches: the left colic, sigmoid, and superior rectal arteries. The distribution is to the left transverse colon, descending colon, sigmoid colon and rectum.

Ultrasound Findings

The inferior mesenteric artery is more difficult to visualise by ultrasound; when it is seen, it is generally on a longitudinal scan. It is small structure inferior to the superior mesenteric artery. On transverse scans it is difficult to separate from small loops of bowel within the abdomen (Fig. 22.14A and B).

Lateral Branches of the Abdominal Aorta
Phrenic Artery

The phrenic artery is small vessel that clings to the underface of the diaphragms which it supplies.

Renal Arteries

The renal arteries arises anterior to the first lumbar vertebra and inferior to the superior mesenteric artery. Both vessels divide into the anterior and inferior suprarenal arteries.

Right Renal Artery (Fig. 22.4)

The right renal artery is a longer vessel than the left; it courses along the aorta posterior to the inferior vena cava and anterior to the vertebral column in a posterior and slightly caudal direction to enter the hilus of the right kidney. The artery passes posterior to the renal vein before entering the renal hilus.

Left Renal Artery

The left renal artery courses aorta directly into the hilus of the left kidney.

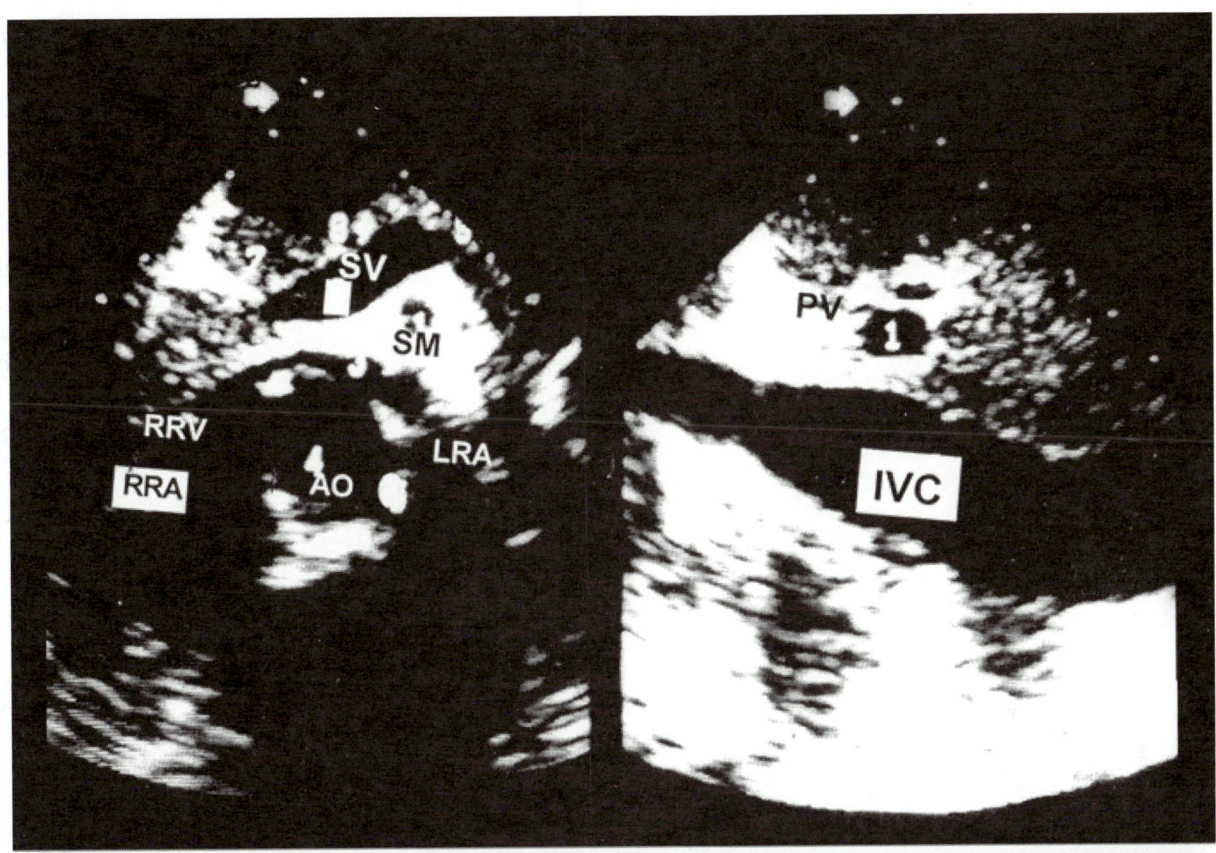

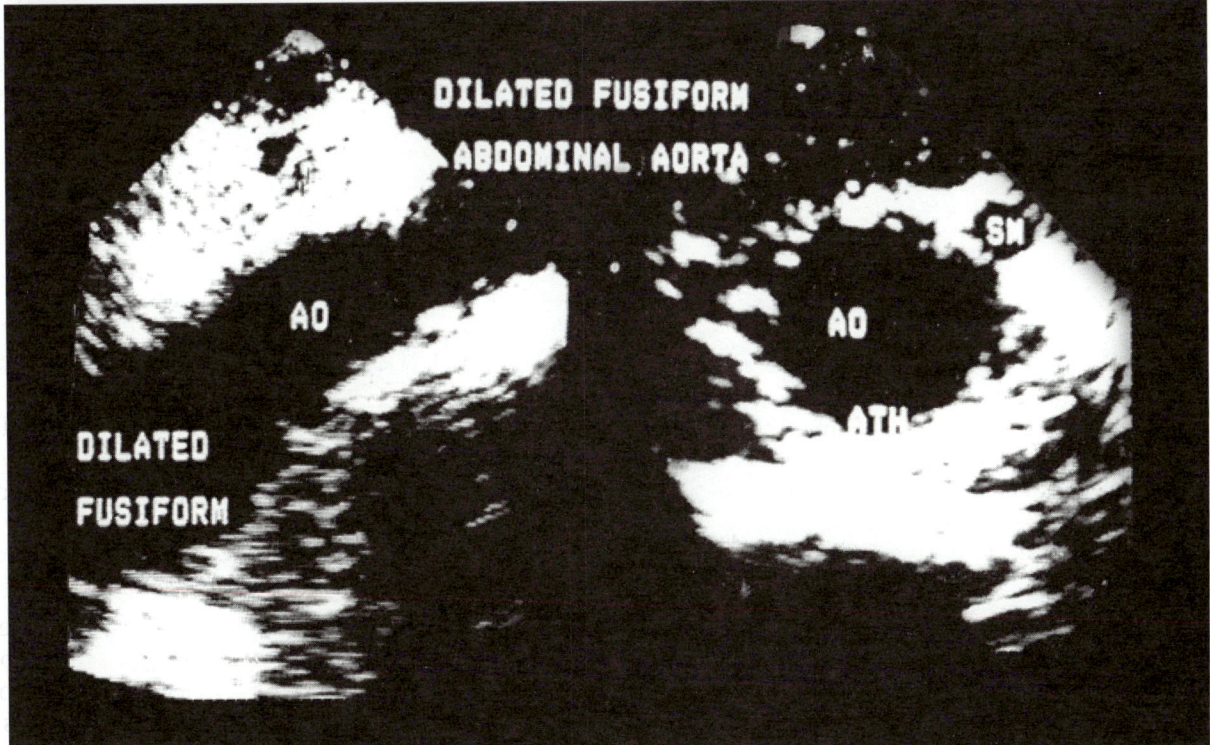

Fig. 22.14A and B: (A) Short axis and transverse view from subcostal approach showing abdominal aorta (AO) and its different branches such as RRA = Right renal artery, LRA = Left renal artery. RRV = Right renal vein, SM = Superior mesenteric artery and SV = Superior mesenteric vein (left). Right scan showing portal venous system. PV = Portal vein, IVC = Inferior vena cava. **(B)** Longitudinal subcostal view showing fusiform and dilated atherosclerotic aorta (left) and short axis view of atherosclerotic aorta with posteriorly located superior mesenteric artery (SM)

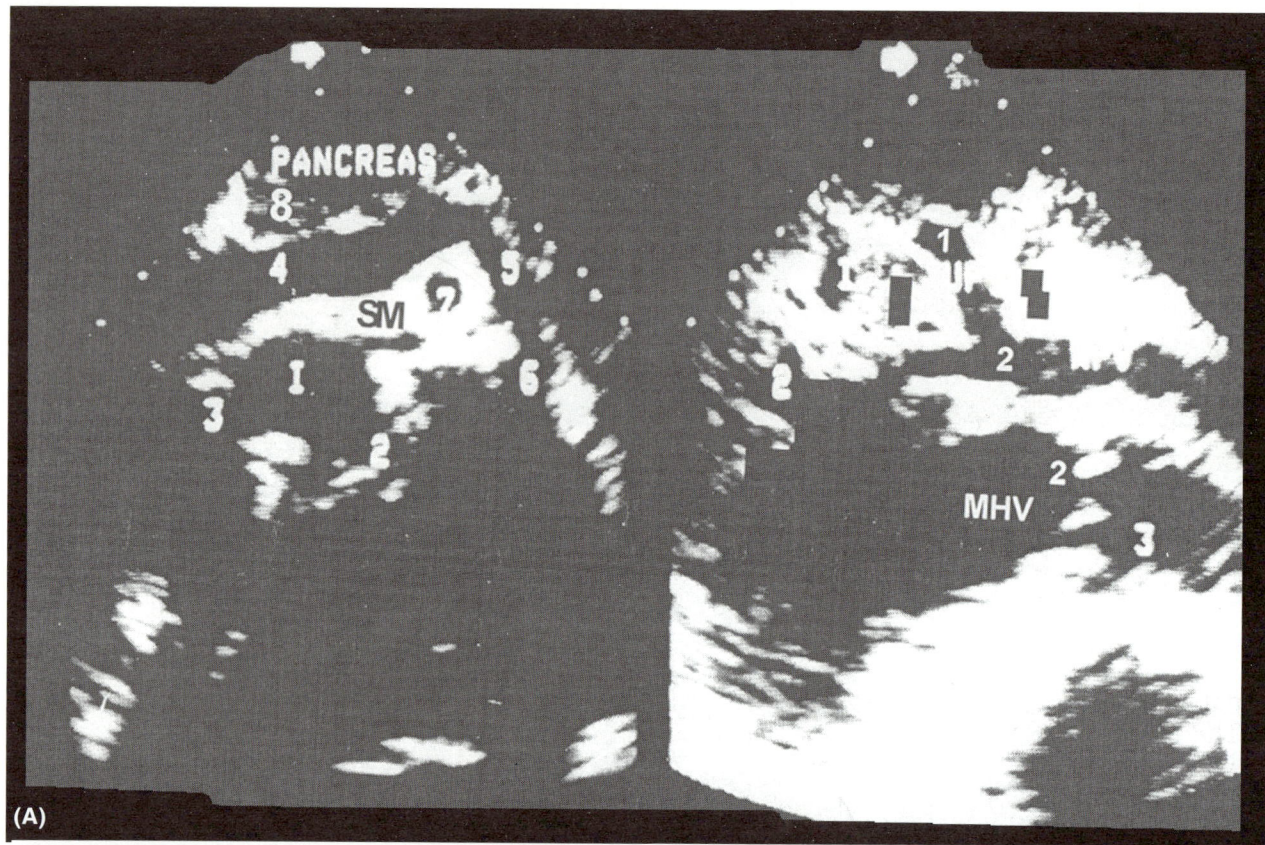

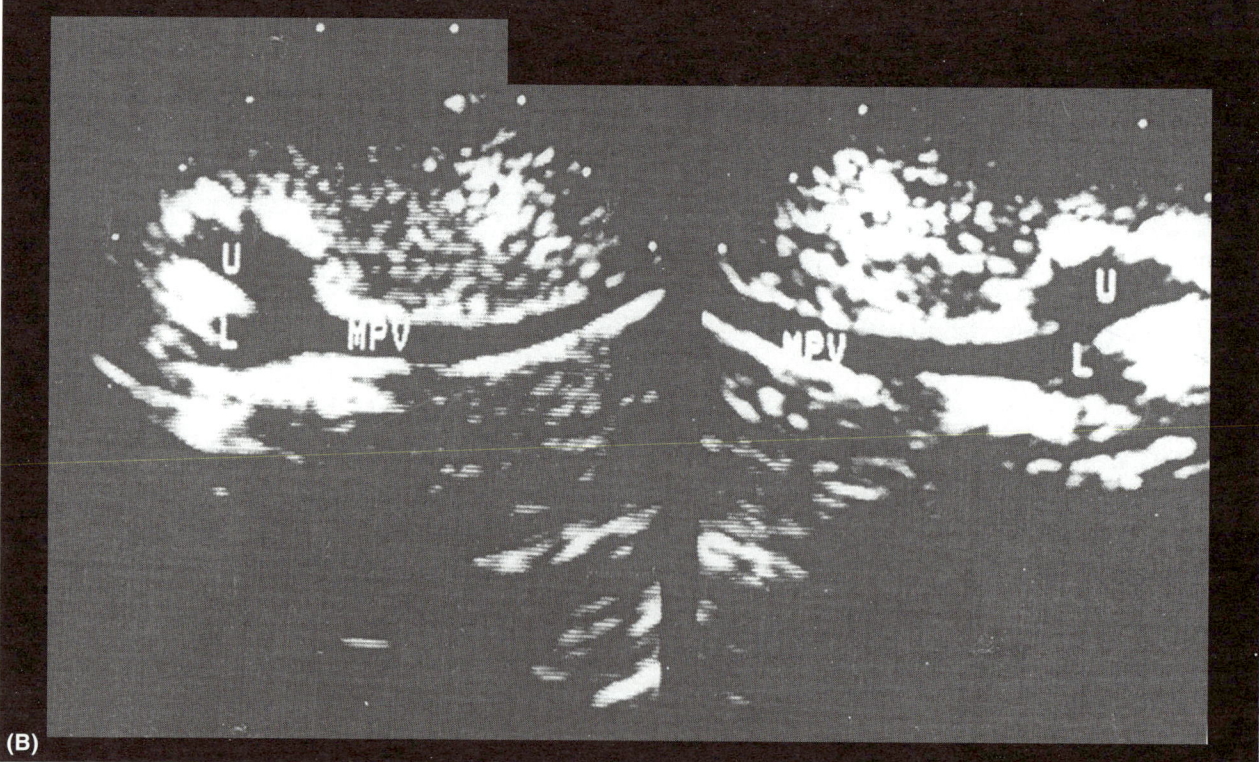

Fig. 22.15A and B: (A) Subcostal transhepatic approach showing anatomical localization of different abdominal aorta such as 1. Aorta, 2. left renal artery, 3. Right renal artery, 4. Superior mesenteric vein, 5. Renal sinus, 6. Splenic vein, 7. Superior mesenteric artery, 8. Pancreas. Right scan showing portal venous system and its branches as 1. left hepatic vein, 2. Right hepatic vein, 3. Inferior vena cava. **(B)** Subcostal transhepatic portal venous system showing main portal vein (MPV) and its two upper (U) and lower branches (L)

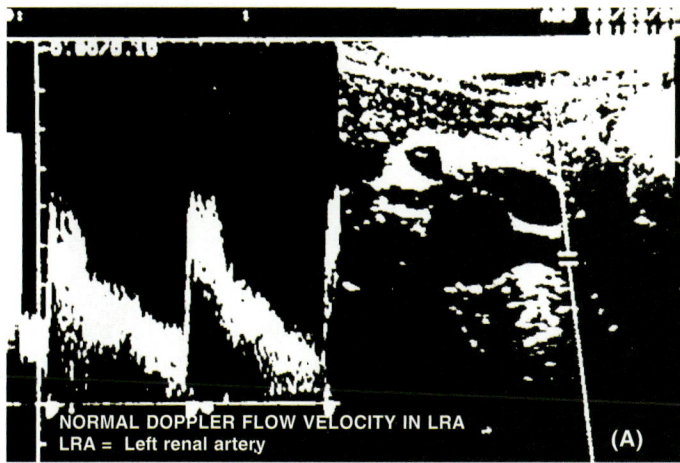 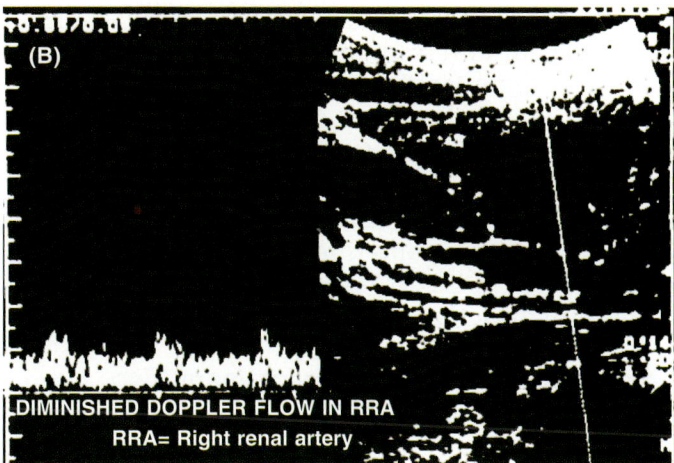

Fig. 22.16A and B: (A) Transverse scan of the left renal artery. The main renal artery has a low impedance (non-resistive) pattern with significant diastolic flow usually 30–50% of peak systole. **(B)** Transverse scans of the right renal artery in which there is always difficulty in obtaining adequate Doppler flow because the ultrasonic beam is perpendicular in the flow pattern resulting into decreasing of blood flow velocity

Ultrasound Findings

Both renal arteries are best seen on transverse sonograms. The right renal artery passes posterior to the inferior vena cava and anterior to the vertebral column in a posterior and slightly caudal direction. Occasionally on longitudinal scans at slight angle to the anterior wall of the aorta and then follow a parallel course. If the angle is severe (greater than 15°), adenopathy should be considered (Figs 22.15A and B 22.16A and B).

Transversely the artery can be seen as a separate small circular structure anterior to the abdominal aorta and posterior to the pancreas. Characteristically it is surrounded by highly reflective echoes from the retroperitoneal fascia. The left renal artery takes direct course from the aorta anterior to the psoas muscle to enter the renal sinus.

The coronal oblique scan of the aorta and inferior vena cava is excellent for demonstrating the origin of the renal arteries and veins. The patient is rolled into a steep decubitus position. The transducer is directed longitudinally with its axis across the inferior vena cava and aorta in efforts to see the origin of the renal vessels. The patient should be in full inspiration to dilate the venous structures for better visualisation.

Gonadal Artery (Fig. 22.5)

The gonadal artery arises inferior to the renal arteries and courses along the psoas muscle to the respective gonadal area.

Dorsal Aortic Branches (Fig. 22.5)

Lumbar Artery

There are usually four lumber arteries on each side of the aorta. The vessels travel lateral and posterior to

supply muscle, skin, bone, and spinal cord. The mid sacral artery supplies the sacrum and rectum.

Minor Venous Vessels (Fig. 22.5)

Lateral Tributaries to the Inferior Vena Cava

Renal Veins (Fig. 22.14A)

Five or six branches of the renal vein unite to form the main renal vein. The vessels arise anterior to the renal arteries at their respective sides of the inferior vena cava at the level of L_2.

Left Renal Vein

The left renal vein arises medially to exit from the hilus of the kidney. It flows from the left kidney posterior to the superior mesenteric artery and anterior to the aorta to enter the lateral wall of the inferior vena cava. Above the entry of the renal veins, the inferior vena cava enlarges because of the increased volumes of blood returning from the kidneys. The left vein is larger than the right renal vein. It accepts branches from the left adrenal, left gonadal, and lumbar veins.

Right Renal Vein

The right renal vein is seen best on transverse images as it flows directly from the right kidney into the posterolateral aspects of the inferior vena cava. It seldom accepts tributaries—the right adrenal and right gonadal enter the vena cava directly.

Gonadal Veins

The gonadal veins (testicular and ovarian) course anterior to the external and internal iliac veins and continue cranially and retroperitoneally along the psoas muscle until their terminus. The left gonadal vein usually enters the left renal vein or the left adrenal vein, which empties into the inferior vena cava. The right gonadal vein enters the inferior vena cava on the anterolateral border above the entrance of the lumbar veins.

Suprarenal Veins

The right suprarenal vein arises from the suprarenal gland and usually grains directly into the inferior vena cava. The left arises from the suprarenal gland and drains into the left renal vein.

Anterior Tributaries to the Inferior Vena Cava

Hepatic Veins

The hepatic veins are the largest visceral tributaries of the inferior vena cava. They originate in the liver and drain into the inferior vena cava at the level of the diaphragm. The hepatic veins return unoxygenated blood from the liver. The veins collect blood from the three minor tributaries within the liver: the right hepatic vein drains the right lobe of the liver, the middle hepatic drains the caudate lobe, and the left hepatic drains the left lobe of the liver.

Ultrasound Findings (Fig. 22.30)

The hepatic veins are best visualized on longitudinal scans of the liver as they drain into the inferior vena cava at the level of the diaphragm. Transverse scans obtained with a cephalic angle of the transducer at the level of the xiphoid often show at least two of the three veins draining into the inferior vena cava. The hepatic veins resemble the "playboy" bunny or "reindeer" sign on the sonogram (Fig. 22.15B).

To distinguish hepatic veins from other vascular structures requires recognition of their anatomic patterns. Hepatic veins drain cephalad towards the diaphragm and then dorsomedially towards the inferior vena cava. Hepatic veins increase in caliber as they approach the diaphragm. Unlike portal veins, they are not surrounded by bright acoustic reflections, although a slight amount of acoustic enhancement may be seen along their posterior border.

Portal Veins

The portal vein is formed posterior to the pancreas by the union of the superior mesenteric and splenic veins at the level of L_2. Its trunk is 5 to 6 cm in length. The portal vein courses posterior to the first portion of the duodenum and then flows between the layers of the lesser omentum to the porta hepatis where it bifurcates into its hepatic upper ends to the anal canal, pancreas, gallbladder, bile ducts, and spleen. It has an important anastomosis with the esophageal veins, rectal venous plexus, and superficial abdominal veins. The portal

venous blood traverses the liver and drains into the inferior vena cava via the hepatic veins.

Ultrasound Findings (Figs 22.17, 22.18, 22.21 and 22.24)

The portal vein is clearly seen on both transverse and sagittal scans. On transverse scans the main portal vein is a thin-walled circular structure, generally lateral and somewhat anterior to the inferior vena cava. It is often possible to record the splenic vein as it crosses the midline of the abdomen to join the superior mesenteric vein to form the main portal trunk. Thus a long section of the splenic vein can be visualised. Often the right or left portal vein can be seen branching from the portal trunk to enter the hilum of the liver.

Portal veins become smaller as they progress into the liver from the porta hepatis. Large radicles situated near or approaching the porta hepatis are portal veins, not hepatic veins. The portal veins are characterised by high-amplitude acoustic reflections that presumably arise from the fibrous tissues surrounding the portal triad as it courses through the liver substance.

The right and left portal veins course transversely through the liver. Thus transverse scans display their longest extent. The right portal vein is most consistently demonstrated on the sonogram. Anatomically any intraparenchymal segment of the portal venous system lying to the right of the lateral aspect of the inferior vena cava is a branch of the right portal system. The left portal vein has a narrow-caliber trunk and may be seen coursing transversely through the left hepatic lobe from posterior to an anterior position.

Since the portal radicle may have many different variations, it is important to become familiar with their patterns to be able to distinguish them from dilated biliary radicles.

Splenic Vein (Fig. 22.15A)

The splenic vein is a tributary of the portal circulation. It begins at the hilum of the spleen, where it is formed by the union of several veins. It is subsequently joined by the short gastric and left gastroepiploic veins. The portal vein passes to the right within the ileorenal ligament and runs along the posteromedial border of the pancreas. It joins the superior mesenteric vein posterior to the neck of the pancreas to form the portal vein. Additional veins from the pancreas and inferior mesenteric vein join the splenic vein. It drains blood from the stomach, spleen, and pancreas.

Ultrasound Findings

The splenic vein is best visualised in the transverse plane as it crosses the upper abdomen from the hilum of the spleen to join the superior mesenteric to form the portal vein slightly to the right of midline. The splenic vein crosses anteriorly to the aorta and the inferior vena cava and generally relates to the medial

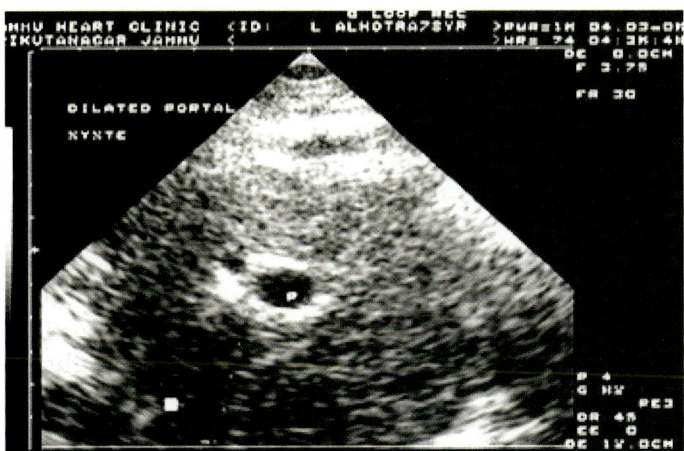

Fig. 22.17: Subcostal approach liver showing hugely dilated and thickened wall portal vein in patient with known case of chronic liver disease (cirrhosis of liver) with portal hypertension along with bleeding esophageal varices and hemorrhoids and severe anemia (Hb = 4, 5 Gm%)

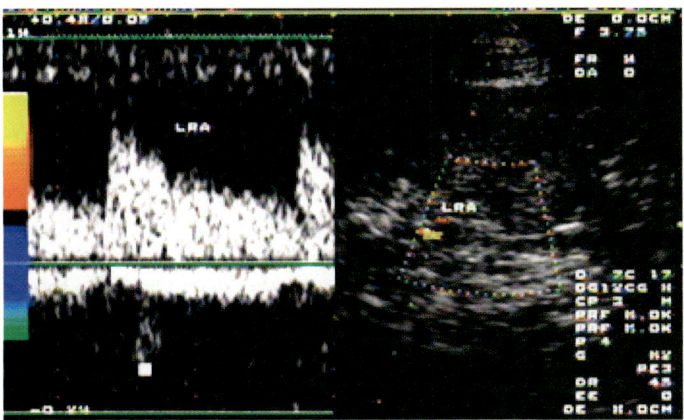

Fig. 22.18: Subcostal approach liver showing enhanced Doppler flow velocity in portal vein in patient with known case of chronic liver disease (cirrhosis of liver) with portal hypertension along with bleeding esophageal varices and hemorrhoids and severe anemia (Hb = 4, 5 Gm%)

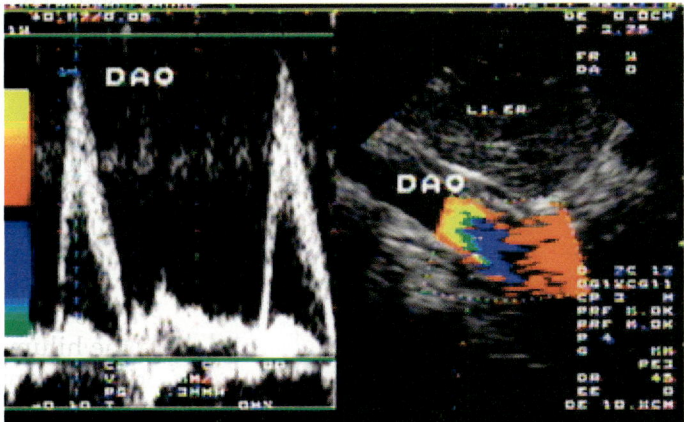

Fig. 22.19: Subcostal approach showing color (right) Doppler flow velocity (left) across abdominal aorta in normal healthy individual

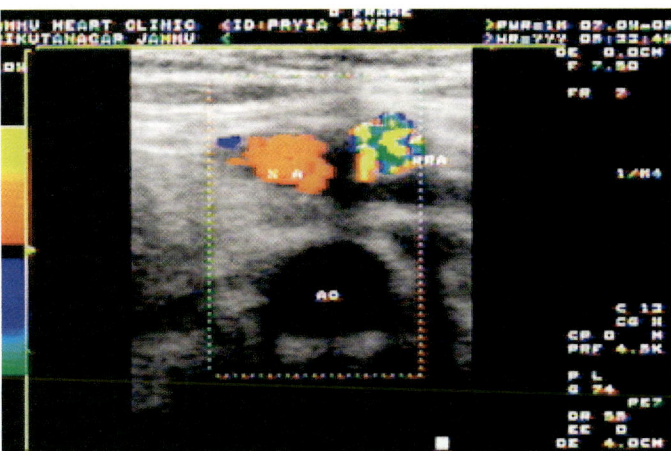

Fig. 22.20: Subcostal approach short axis view of abdominal aorta showing normal colour flow in normal individual

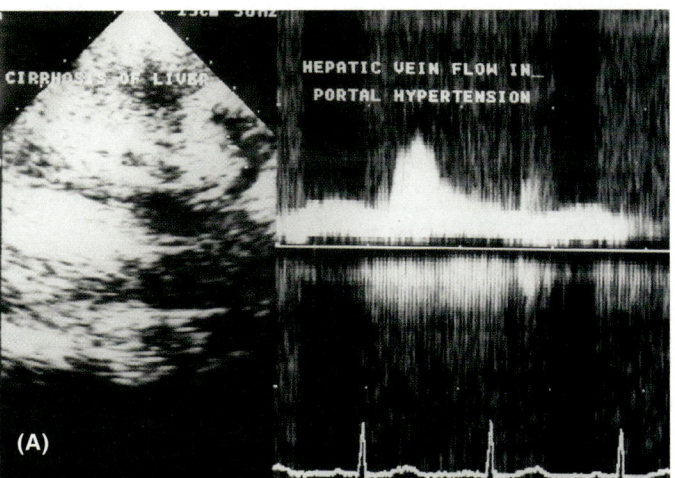

(A)

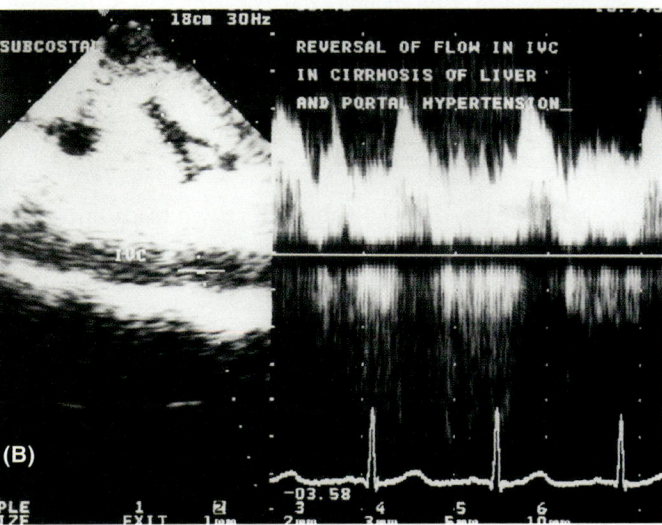

(B)

Fig. 22.21A and B: **(A)** Subcostal transhepatic scan showing reversal of blood flow in hepatic vein in portal hypertension in patient with cirrhosis of liver. **(B)** Scan showing reversal of blood flow in inferior vena cava (IVC) in portal hypertension in a patient with chronic liver disorder

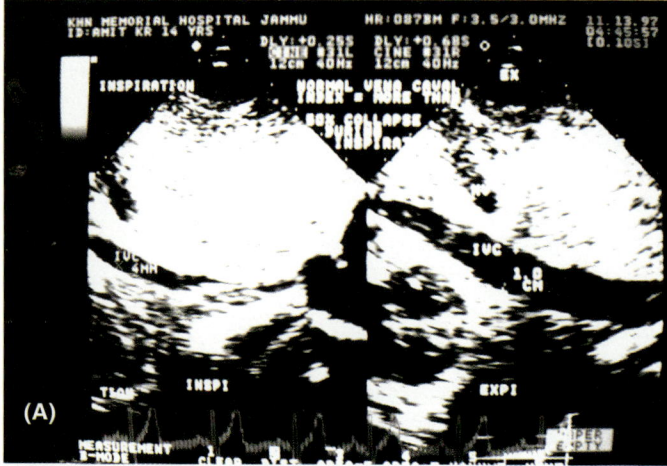

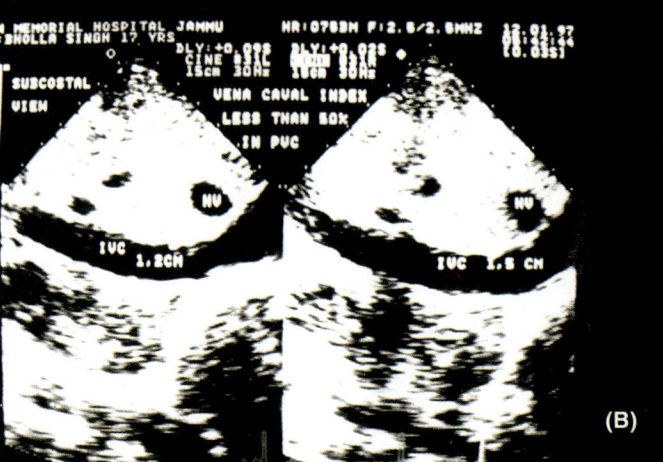

Fig. 22.22A and B: (A) Subcostal horizontal scan showing inspiratory collapse of inferior vena cava (IVC) on left side and normal opening of IVC during expiration in calculation of normal vena caval index which is derived as IVC Index = size of IVC during inspiration(cm)/size of IVC during expiration (cm) = <50%. **(B)** Showing failure of inspiratory collapse during inspiration in comparison to opening of IVC during expiration in a patient with chronic obstructive lung disease having severe form of pulmonary arterial hypertension with IVC Index more than 80%

and posterior borders of the pancreatic body and tail. Its course is variable, so small degrees of obliquity may be necessary to image the vein entirely. It is usually smaller than the superior mesenteric vein and the main portal vein.

On sagittal scans the splenic vein can be visualised posterior to the left lobe of the liver and anterior to the major vascular structures. The pancreas may be seen inferior and slightly anterior to the vein. The larger diameter of the portal vein is the result of the influx of blood from the superior mesenteric vein. An obvious widening is demonstrated at the junction of the portal and splenic veins. When splenomegaly is present, it is often possible to identify the origin of the splenic vein at the splenic hilum.

Superior Mesenteric Vein (Fig. 22.15A)

The superior mesenteric vein is also a tributary to the portal vein. It begins at the ileocolic junction and runs cephalad along the posterior abdominal wall within the root of the mesentery of the small intestine to the right of the superior mesenteric artery. The superior mesenteric vein passes anterior to the third part of the duodenum and posterior to the neck of the pancreas, where it joins the splenic vein to form the main portal vein. It also receives tributaries that correspond to the branches of the superior mesenteric artery, where it is joined by the inferior pancreaticoduodenal vein to the right gastroepiploic vein from the right aspect of the greater curvature of the stomach. The superior mesenteric vein drains blood from several smaller veins: the middle colic vein (transverse colon), right, colic vein (ascending colon), and pancreatic duodenal vein.

Ultrasound Findings

The superior mesenteric vein is somewhat variable in its anatomic location. Generally it is anterior to the inferior vena cava and to the right of the superior mesenteric artery. The superior mesenteric vein drains into the main portal vein (with the splenic vein), therefore the sonographer should not be able to demonstrate these three structures together on a single transverse scan. The superior mesenteric vein is the posterior border of the neck of the pancreas and the anterior border of the uncinate process of the pancreatic head.

On sagittal scan, the vein is seen as a long tubular structure anterior to the inferior vena cava. With correct oblique angulation of the transducer, the path of the superior mesenteric vein can be followed, as it enters the portal system.

The following points help to distinguish the superior mesenteric artery from the vein:
1. The superior mesenteric vein is of larger caliber than the artery (Fig. 22.15A).
2. Respiratory variations are seen in the vein.
3. On sagittal scans the superior mesenteric artery angles away from the aorta, whereas the vein tends to parallel the aorta or course anteriorly away from the aorta near the portal-splenic confluence.
4. Real time identification of the confluence of the superior mesenteric vein—portal vein or superior mesenteric artery is possible as the superior mesenteric artery originates from the aorta.

Inferior Mesenteric Vein

The inferior mesenteric vein arises from the left third of colon and upper colon and ascends retroperitoneally along the left psoas muscle. It begins midway down the anal canal as the superior rectal vein. It runs cranial in

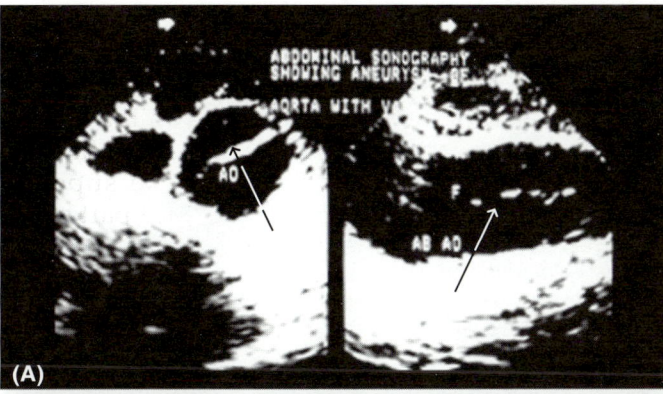

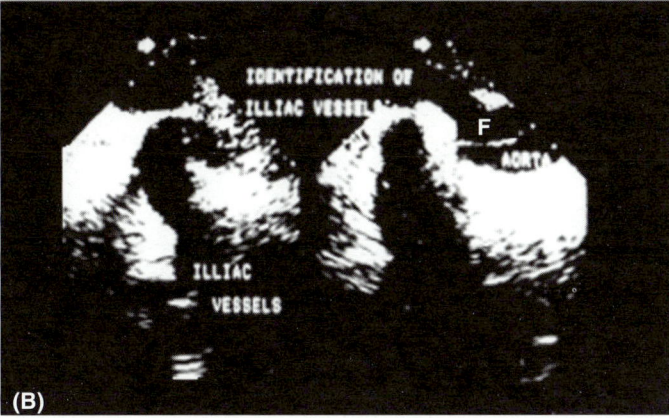

Fig. 22.23A and B: (A) Dual scan subcostal short axis and transverse plane for abdominal aorta showing aneurysmally dilated atherosclerotic abdominal aorta with a big intra-aortic false lumen of dissociation (F) (arrow) on left side and same abnormality has been depicted in horizontal scan on the right side. **(B)** Dual scan showing fusiform dilated illiac arteries in the same patient with atherosclerotic disease of the heart and peripheral vessels

the posterior abdominal wall on the left side of the inferior mesenteric artery and duodenojejunal junction to join the splenic vein posterior to the pancreas. It receives many tributaries along its way, including the left colic vein. The inferior mesenteric vein drains several tributaries: the left colic vein (descending colon), sigmoid vein (sigmoid colon), and superior rectal vein (upper rectum).

Ultrasound Findings

The inferior mesenteric vein is difficult to recognize with ultrasound because of its anatomic location and small diameter. It is generally covered by small bowel and has no major vascular structures posterior to it to aid in its recognition (Fig. 22.15A).

Pathophysiology of Vascular Disease
Aortic Abnormalities
Aortic Aneurysm (Fig. 22.23)
The visualisation of the abdominal aorta has traditionally been an asset in diagnosing the clinical problem. Ultrasound is very capable of demonstrating abnormal-

ities in the diameter, length, and extent of the abdominal aortic aneurysm. An aneurysm is defined as a localized abnormal dilation of any vessel. Three important factors predispose to aneurysms formation: arteriosclerosis, syphilis, and cystic medial necrosis.

Arteriosclerosis
Arteriosclerosis is the most common cause of aneurysms. It is found more often in middle-aged men than women, and involves the aorta, often with extension into the common iliac arteries. The disease sometimes involves the ascending and descending aorta. The aneurysm may be fusiform, cylindrical, or saccular in nature. It usually begins below the renal arteries (inferior to the superior mesenteric artery) and extends to the bifurcation (Fig. 22.14B).

Classifications of Aneurysms
The most common presentation of an atherosclerotic aneurysm is as a fusiform dilation of the distal aorta at the aortic bifurcation. Saccular aneurysms are somewhat spherical and larger (5–10 cm) than the fusiform aneurysm. This type of aneurysm is connected to vascular lumen by a mouth that varies in size but may be as large as an aneurysm. It may be partially or completely filled with thrombus. The sonographer must carefully follow the course of such an aneurysm to separate it from a retroperitoneal mass or lymphadenopathy. Pulsations are usually diminished secondary to clot formation.

The aneurysm may extend into the iliac arteries. The sonographer should examine both iliac arteries in at least two planes. At the level of the bifurcation the iliac vessel may be seen as circular, pulsatile vessel just anterior to the spine. The oblique longitudinal scan is used to produce an image of the vessel in its entire length. Normal iliac arteries do not measure over 1 cm in diameter. If the artery becomes so enlarged, it has an increased chance of rupture.

Ultrasound Findings (Figs 22.14B, 22.19, 22.20 and 22.23)
The aorta is thought to be aneurysmal when the diameter is increased to over 3 cm in an anteroposterior measurement. This measurement should be made from leading edge. The sonographer should search for focal dilation of the abdominal aorta or lack of normal tapering distally. When an aneurysm is present, the presence of thrombus should be evaluated. Thrombus usually occurs along an anterior or anterolateral wall. Old clot is easier to see because of calcification that appears as thick, echogenic, sometimes with posterior shadowing.

If an aneurysm extends beyond the diaphragm into the thoracic aorta, it may be difficult to tract with ultrasound because of lung interference in the beam. Several attempts may be necessary to demonstrate this thoracic aneurysm. The transducer can be sharply angled from the xiphoid towards the sternal notch to visualise the lower extent of the aorta. Another technique allows the sonographer to make a longitudinal parasternal scan over the long axis of the heart. The thoracic aorta should be seen posterior to the cardiac structures. A third alternative is to scan along the patient's back with the patient sitting upright or prone. The transducer should be angled slightly medially and placed in a sagittal plane along the left intercostal space. This is very effective if the thoracic aorta is deviated slightly to the left of the spine. Scalloped reverberations from the ribs will be recorded, with the luminal echoes of the thoracic aorta directly posterior. Thrombus within an aneurysm is shown ultrasonically as medium to low-level echoes. Generally increased sensitivity is likely to highlight the thrombus echoes. Echoes should be seen in both planes on more than one scan to be separated from low level reverberation echoes. Thrombus formation is usually more frequent along the anterior and lateral wall than along the posterior wall of the aorta.

Aortic Dissection

A dissecting aneurysm may be detected by ultrasound, usually displays one or more clinical signs and symptoms. Sonographer should look for a dissection flap or recent channel with or without frank aneurysmal dilation. The dissection of blood is along the laminar planes of the aortic media with formation of blood-filled channel within the aortic wall. Most aneurysms enlarge fairly symmetrically in the anteroposterior and lateral dimensions; therefore an irregular enlargement with scattered internal echoes may represent an aneurysm with clot.

The typical patients are 40 to 60 years old and hypertensive males predominate over females. When the dissection develops, haemorrhage occurs between the middle and outer thirds of the media. An intimal tear is considered if the tear is found in the ascending portion of the arch. This type of dissection extends proximally towards the heart, as well as distally, sometimes to the iliac and femoral arteries. A small portion of dissections do not have an obvious intimal tear. Extravasation may completely encircle the aorta or extend along one segment of its circumference, or it may rupture into any of the body cavities.

Types of Dissections

There are three classifications of aortic dissection. The first begins at the root of the aorta and may extend the entire length of the arch, descending to the aorta and

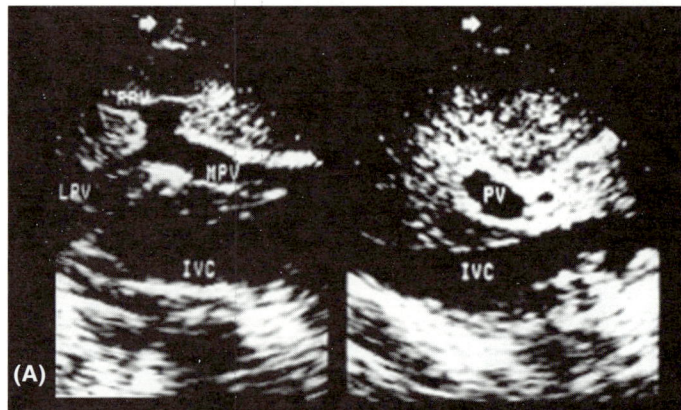

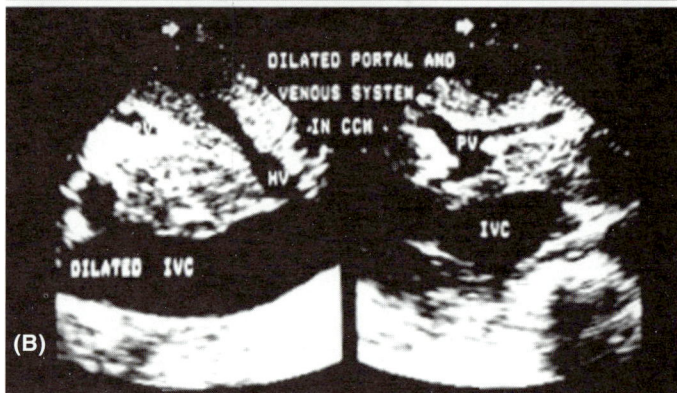

Fig. 22.24A and B: (A) Subcostal transverse dual scan showing anatomical localisation of portal venous system. **(B)** Dual scan showing extremely dilated inferior vena cava in patient with congestive cardiomyopathy

into the abdominal aorta. This is the most dangerous, especially if the dissection spirals around the aorta, cutting off the blood supply to the carotid, brachiocephalic, and subclavian vessels. The second type of dissection begins at or below the level of the left subclavian artery and extends down the descending aorta. It may or may not continue into the abdominal aorta. The third type of dissection begins at the lower end the descending aorta and extends into the abdominal aorta. This may be critical if the dissection spirals around to impede the flow of blood into the renal vessels (Figs 22.25 and 22.26).

Dissections of the aorta may be secondary to cystic medial necrosis (weakening of the arterial wall), to the inherited disease of Marfan's syndrome (individuals with this disorder are extremely tall, lanky, and double jointed; a progressive stretching disorder exists in all arterial vessels, especially in the aorta, causing abnormal dilation, weakened walls, and eventual dissection, rupture or both), or hypertension.

Ruptured Aortic Aneurysms

The classic symptoms of ruptured aortic aneurysm are excruciating abdominal pain, shock, and an expanding

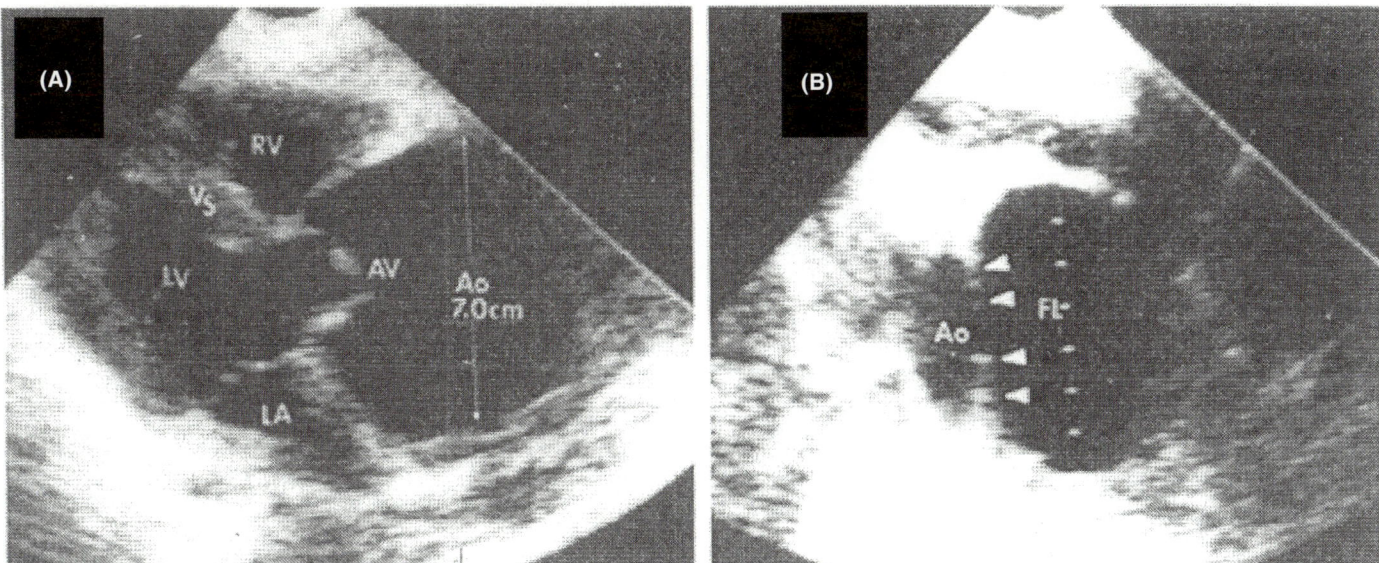

Fig. 22.25A and B: **(A)** Long axis **(B)** transthoracic echocardiogram of an elderly patient with type I aortic dissection. The long axis view shows only an abnormally dilated aortic root (7.0 cm). The short axis scan depicts an aortic dissection

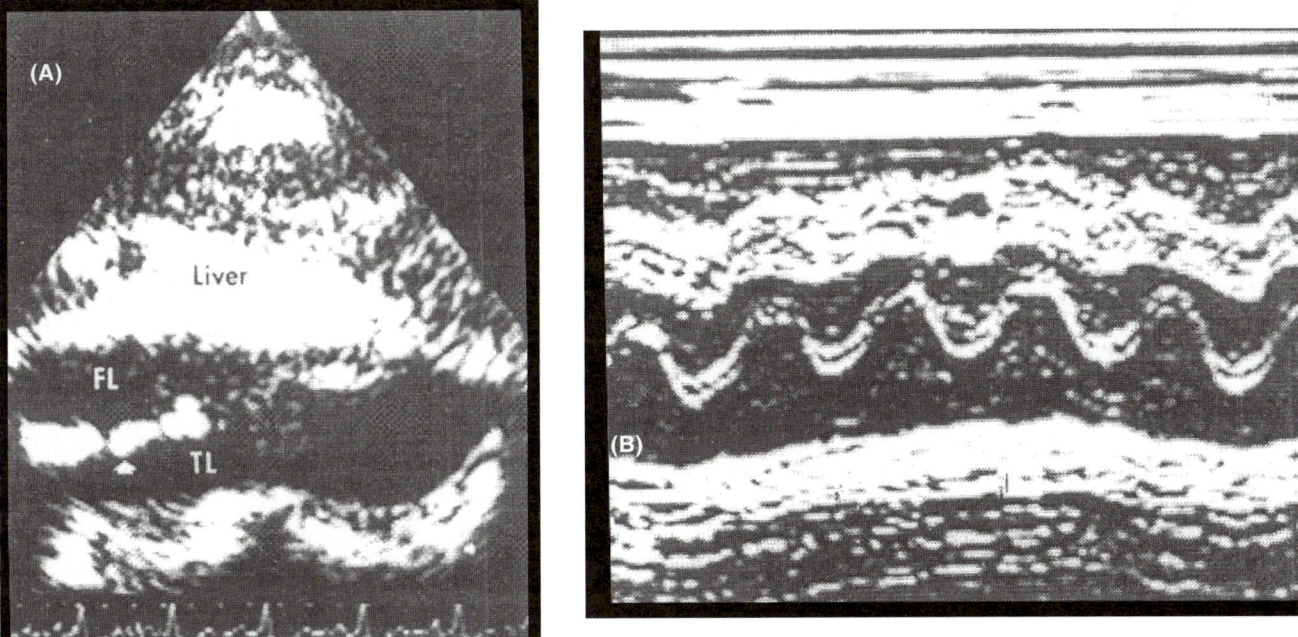

Fig. 22.26A and B: Subcostal two-dimensional and M-mode echoscans of abdominal aorta showing aortic dissection. The M-mode recording shows oscillations of intimal flap between the false lumen (FL) and the true lumen (TL)

abdominal mass. The operative mortality for such ruptures is 40% to 60%. The rupture may be into perirenal space with displacement of renal hilar vessels, and silhouetting of the lateral psoas border at the level of the kidney. The most common site is the lateral wall below the renal vessels. The haemorrhage into the posterior pararenal space accounts for a loss of lateral psoas muscle emerging inferior to the kidney and may also displace the kidney.

Other Complications of Aortic Aneurysms
A large aneurysm may compress the neighbouring structures (i.e. the common bile duct, causing obstruction, and the renal artery, causing hypertension and renal ischemia). Retroperitoneal fibrosis with aneurysm may involve the ureter.

Aortic Grafts
The abdominal aortic aneurysm may be surgically repaired with a flexible graft material.

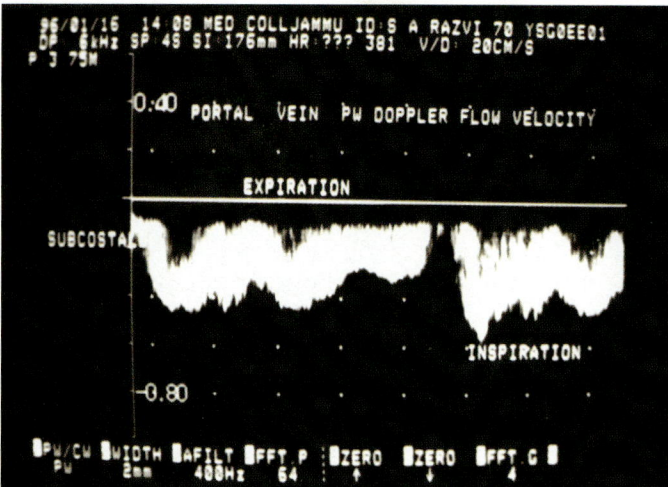

Fig. 22.27: Subcostal approach IVC showing normal inspiratory augmentation of pulsed Doppler velocity flow

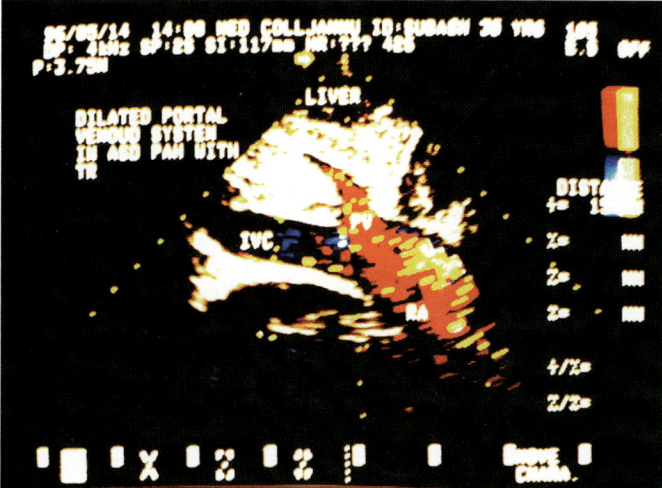

Fig. 22.28: Subcostal color transhepatic approach showing dilated IVC and portal venous system in patient with ASD secundum with PAH and tricuspid regurgitation

Pulsatile Abdominal Masses

Masses other than an aortic aneurysm that can simulate a pulsatile abdominal mass are retroperitoneal tumour, fibroid uterus, or paraortic nodes. After aneurysms, the most common etiology for a pulsatile abdominal mass is a node. This mass is usually the result of lymphoma in the middle aged patient. Symptoms include fever, weight loss, or malaise. On ultrasound, the nodes are homogeneous masses surrounding the aorta. The aortic wall may be poorly defined because of the close acoustic impedance of the nodes and the aorta. The sonographer should also look for splenomegaly.

Pancreatic carcinoma may appear as a hypoechoic mass and may displace the normal pancreas; biliary dilation with an enlarged gallbladder may be present.

A retroperitoneal sarcoma may present as a pulsatile mass; it may extend into the root of the mesentery and give rise to a large intraperitoneal component. The echodensity depends on the tissue type that predominates: Fatty lesions are more echo dense than fibrous or myomatous lesions.

Infrahepatic Interruption of the Inferior Vena Cava

This condition is the failure of union of the hepatic veins and the right subcardinal vein; with it there can be azygos or, less commonly hemiazygos continuation. It is associated with acyanotic and cyanotic congenital heart disease, abnormalities of cardiac position, and abdominal situs with asplenia and polysplenia.

Ultrasound Findings

In patients with an interruption of the inferior vena cava the azygos vein continuation is identical or larger than the inferior vena cava that passes along the aorta medial to the right crus of the diaphragm. The hepatic veins drain into an independent confluence that passes through the diaphragm to enter the right atrium. A membranous obstruction of the inferior vena cava may simulate infrahepatic interruption of the vena cava with azygos continuation. A web or membrane obstructs the inferior vena cava at the level of the diaphragm and leads to chronic congestion of the liver with centrilobular and periportal fibrosis.

There are three types of obstruction:

1. A thin membrane at the level of the entrance to the right atrium.
2. An absent segment of the inferior vena cava without characteristic conical narrowing.
3. Complete obstruction secondary to thrombosis. Clinically patients present in their third to fourth decade of life with portal hypertension.

Ultrasound shows obstruction at the diaphragm and dilation of the azygos system. On longitudinal scans it is very difficult to identify the presence of the inferior vena cava. The azygos system is dilated on the right side of the midline, acting as right inferior vena cava.

Inferior Vena Caval Tumour

It is important for the sonographer to identify the entire inferior vena cava; bowel gas can make the distal cava difficult to identify.

Hepatic Portion of Inferior Vena Cava

Masses posterior to the hepatic portion of the inferior vena cava are adrenal, neurogenic and hepatic. With enlargement of the liver, the cava is compressed rather than displaced. A localized liver mass would produce posterior, lateral, or medial displacement of the inferior

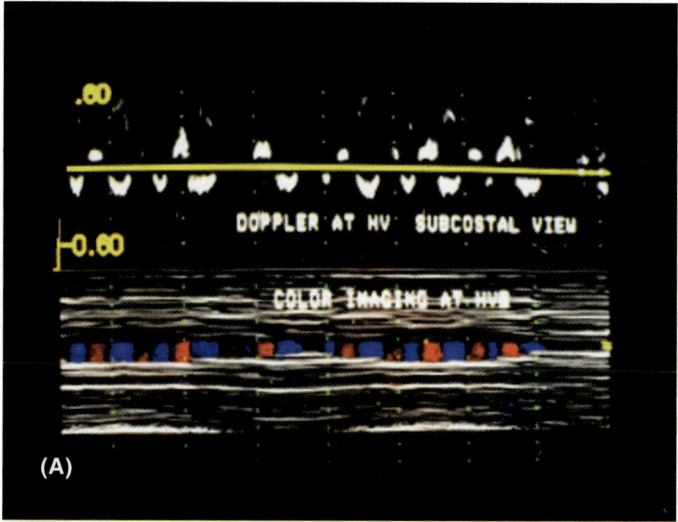

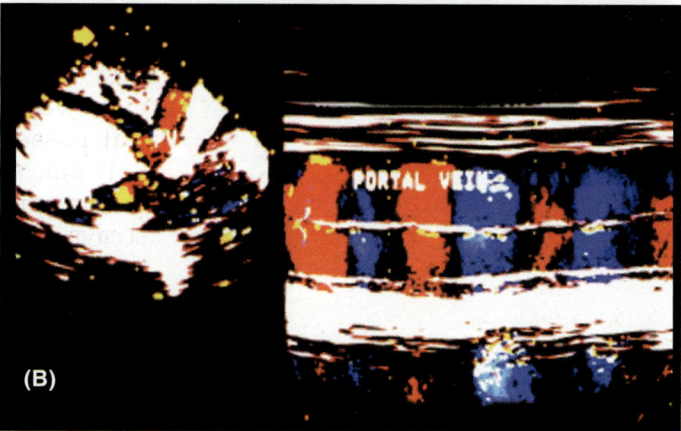

Fig. 22.29A and B: (A) Subcostal Doppler and color M-mode echoscan of normal main hepatic vein showing alternate blue and red color during inspiration and expiration. **(B)** Subcostal 2-D (left) and color M-mode scan (right) of portal vein showing exaggerated and admixture of colors in patient with ASD secundum with pulmonary arterial hypertension and TR

vena cava, whereas a mass in the posterior caudate lobe and right lobe may elevate the cava.

Middle or Pancreatic Portion of the Inferior Vena Cava

The middle or pancreatic portion of the inferior vena cava may elevate the cava from abnormalities of the right renal artery, right kidney, lumbar spine, or lymph node masses.

Inferior Vena Cava and Hepatic Veins (Fig. 22.27)

The inferior vena cava and hepatic veins present a complex waveform, which flows above and below the baseline, reflecting the reflux of blood from the right atrium during systole and variations with the respiratory cycle. Always look at the cava and renal veins for tumour invasion when you see a renal cell carcinoma.

Budd-Chiari Syndrome

Budd-Chiari syndrome is caused by thrombosis of hepatic veins. Duplex Doppler is an effective method for screening patients suspects of having Budd-Chiari syndrome. Sonographically, hepatic veins appear reduced in size and may contain echogenic thrombotic material. The presence of "typical" blood flow in the hepatic veins permits the exclusion of Budd-Chiari Syndrome. Budd-Chiari Syndrome is a rare disease; 30% of cases are idiopathic.

Portal Vein (Figs 22.28 and 22.29)

In the normal superior mesenteric vein and splenic vein, flow is hepatopetal (towards the liver). The portal vein shows a relatively continuous flow at low velocities, which may vary slightly with respirations. Portal vein thrombosis can be easily diagnosed with sonography. A direct sign is visualisation of thrombus. Indirect signs are the loss of normal portal venous landmarks, dilation of the superior mesenteric artery and splenic vein, and venous collaterals in the porta hepatic (cavernous transformation of the portal vein).

Pulsed Doppler adds to these findings; lack of Doppler signals from the lumen indicates absence of blood flow. In cirrhotic patients, thrombosis is often suspected when ascites suddenly worsens. Consequently, in these patients, special attention must be paid to the portal vein to identify thrombus. It is often difficult to visualise the portal vein in such patients.

Cavernous Transformation of the Portal Vein

Cavernous transformation of the portal vein demonstrates periportal collateral channels in patients with chronic portal vein obstruction. The Doppler analysis of the tubular structures is characteristic of portal venous flow-hepatopetal (towards the liver) with continuous low-velocity flow. Diagnosis can be made sonographically based on the following indications:

1. Extrahepatic portal vein is not visualised.

2. High level echoes produced by fibrosis are present in the porta hepatis.

3. Multiple tubular structures are present in the porta hepatis, representing periportal collaterals attached to the end of the remaining aorta. The synthetic material used for a graft produces bright echo reflections compared to those from the normal aortic walls. After surgery, the attached walls may swell at the site of the attachment and form another aneurysm or pseudoaneurysm. Other complications of prosthetic grafts include hematoma, infection, and degeneration of graft material.

Arteriovenous Fistulas

The development of an arteriovenous fistula is not a common finding with ultrasound. The majority of fistulas are acquired secondary to trauma. Some may develop as a complication of arteriosclerotic aortic aneurysms.

Clinical Signs

The patient may develop low back and abdominal pain, progressive cardiac decompensation, a pulsatile abdominal mass associated with a bruit, and massive swelling of the lower trunk and lower extremities. Clinical signs are explained on the basis of the altered hemodynamics produced by a high-velocity shunt leading to increased blood volume, increased venous pressure, and cardiac output with cardiac failure and cardiomegaly.

If there is lower trunk and leg edema and a dilated inferior vena cava, an arteriovenous fistula should be suspected. If the fistula is large, the vein becomes very distended. A normal inferior vena cava is less than 2.5 cm wide. Right sided heart disease or failure can also cause inferior vena cava distension.

Renal arteriovenous fistulas can be congenital or acquired. Congenital arteriovenous fistulas may be of the crisoid type or the aneurysmal type. Acquired fistulas are secondary to trauma, surgery, or inflammation or associated with a neoplasm such as renal cell carcinoma.

Ultrasound Findings

The sonographer finds multiple anechoic tubular structures feeding the malformation with an enlarged renal artery and vein, confirming increased blood flow to the kidney. It may look like hydronephrosis or a parapelvic cyst in association with a dilated inferior vena cava. The diagnosis is made by identifying one or more channels that enter the mass, suggesting that the lesion is related to the renal vasculature. The sonographer should look for pulsations. The crisoid type of fistula has a characteristic ultrasound appearance of a cluster of tubular anechoic structures within the kidney; it is supplied by an enlarged renal artery and drained by a dilated renal vein. In the aneurysmal type of fistula a vascular lesion should be suspected when the presence of thrombus is noted in the periphery of a mass with tubular anechoic lumen with pulsations. Occasionally renal cell carcinoma is associated with arteriovenous shunting resulting from invasion of larger arteries and venous structures.

Inferior Vena Cava Abnormalities
Congenital Abnormalities

The inferior vena cava is formed by three pairs of cardinal veins in the retroperitoneum; these veins

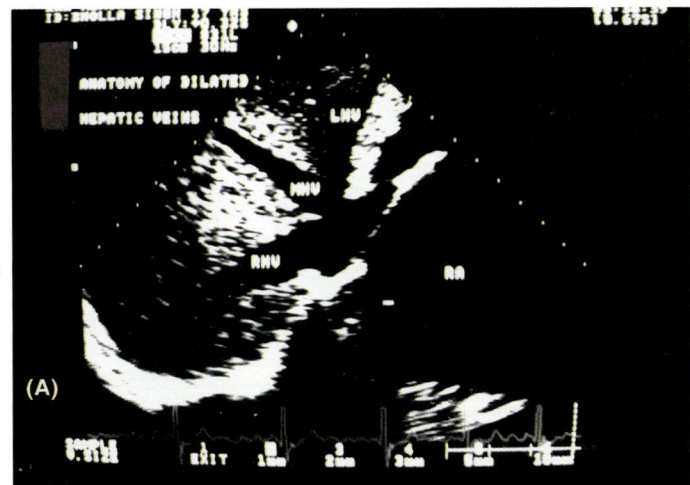

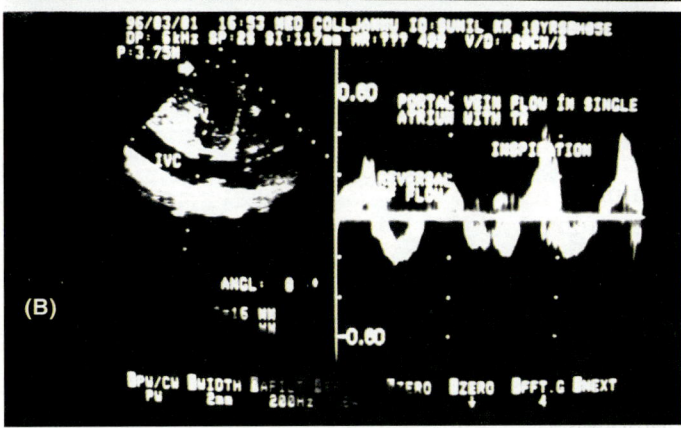

Fig. 22.30A and B: (A) Subcostal hepatic approach showing anatomical localisation of main hepatic vein and its left and right branches as it emerges out of portal venous system. **(B)** Subcostal hepatic approach showing reversal of Doppler flow velocity across portal vein in a patient with single atrium

undergo sequential development and regression. The posterior cardinal veins appear at 6 weeks and form no part of the cava but may be part of the anomalies. The subcardinal veins appear at 7 weeks to produce the prerenal segment of the inferior vena cava. The supracardinal system at 8 weeks produces the postrenal segment of the inferior vena cava. The subcardinal and supracardinal systems form the renal veins. The normal left cardinal system involutes and the right is composed of the posterior infrarenal vein, supracardinal vein, renal segment, anterior pararenal subcardinal vein, and the confluence of hepatic veins.

Double Inferior Vena Cava

This condition has an incidence of under 3%. The size of the two vessels can be the same or vary depending on the dominant side. The most common type is where the left inferior vena cava joins the left renal vein, which crosses the midline at its normal level to join the right inferior vena cava. There is no continuation of the left inferior vena cava above the left renal vein. Less commonly, the right inferior vena cava joins the left inferior vena cava to join the hemiazygos.

Lumbar spine abnormalities or lymph nodes would elevate the inferior vena cava.

Ultrasound Findings

The inferior vena cava may become obstructed by tumour formation. The ultrasound appearance of tumour is of a single or multiple echogenic nodules along the wall. The cava may be distended and filled with tumour. The most common tumour is renal cell carcinoma, usually from the right kidney. Wilms tumour is also seen to extend into the inferior vena cava and right atrium. Other less common tumours are retroperitoneal liposarcoma, leiomyosarcoma pheochromocytoma, osteosarcoma, and rhabdomyosarcoma. Benign tumours, such as angiomyolipoma, can have venous involvement.

Inferior Vena Caval Thrombosis

Complete thrombosis of the inferior vena cava is life threatening. Patients present with leg edema, low back pain, pelvic pain, gastrointestinal complaints, and renal and liver abnormalities.

Ultrasound Findings

Thrombosis within the inferior vena cava appears as homogeneous echo-mass. Colour Doppler is useful to determine if the vessel is occluded.

Inferior Vena Caval Filters

The most common origin of pulmonary emboli is venous thrombosis from the lower extremities. Surgical and angiographic placement of transvenous filters into the cava has been used to prevent recurrent embolisation in patients who cannot tolerate anticoagulants. The preferred location of the filter is in the iliac bifurcation below the renal veins.

Some filters can migrate cranially or caudally and perforate the cava, producing a retroperitoneal bleed. Filters can also perforate the duodenum, aorta, ureter and hepatic vein.

Renal Vein Obstruction

Renal vein obstruction is seen in the dehydrated or septic infant. It may also be seen in adults with multiple renal abnormalities (nephrotic syndrome, shock, renal tumour, kidney transplant, or trauma). Left renal vein obstruction may result from the spread of such non-renal malignancies as carcinoma of the pancreas or lung or lymphoma. A retroperitoneal tumour can occlude the left renal vein by direct extension to the vein lumen or compression of the lumen by a contiguous mass.

Ultrasound Findings

Ultrasound can be used to confirm that a palpable mass in kidney and to exclude hydronephrosis and multicystic kidney as causes of a nonfunctioning kidney. In infants with renal vein obstruction, enlarged kidneys without cysts are seen. Medium echoes or "clumps" of echoes may be randomly scattered within the kidney with surrounding echo-free spaces. The parenchymal anechoic areas are the result of hemorrhage and infarcts. The renal pattern progresses to atrophy over 2 months. Late findings are increased parenchymal echoes, loss of corticomedullary junction and decreased size.

Renal Vein Thrombosis

If the following are present on ultrasound, renal vein thrombosis can be diagnosed:

1. Direct visualisation of thrombi in the renal vein and inferior vena cava.
2. Demonstrated renal vein dilation proximal to the point of occlusion.
3. Loss of normal renal structure.
4. Increased renal size (acute phase).
5. Doppler shows decrease or no flow.

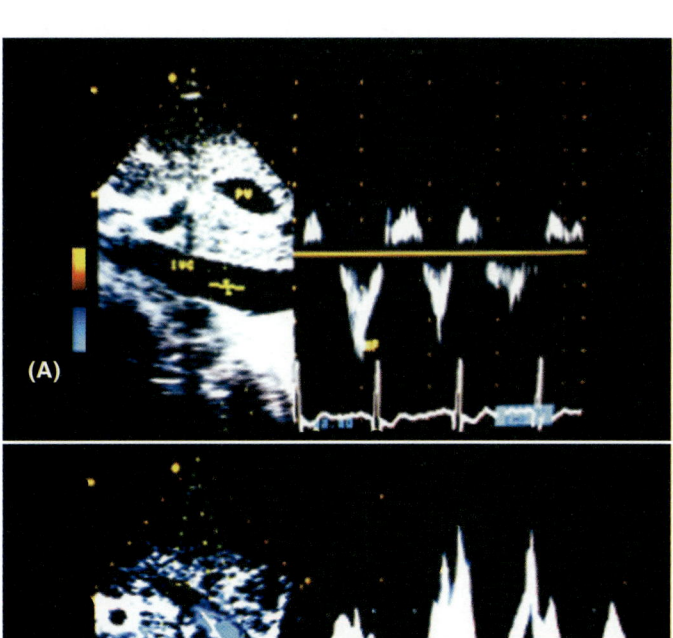

Fig. 22.31A and B: (A) Subcostal 2-D color Doppler scan showing reversal of Doppler flow in IVC in patient with pulmonary arterial hypertension. **(B)** There is also reversal of portal venous flow in patient with chronic obstructive lung disease with right heart failure

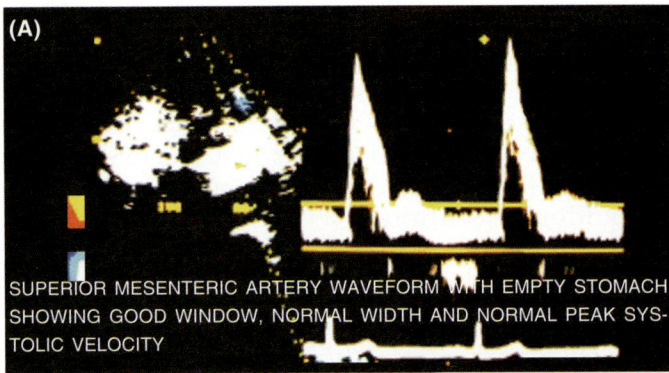

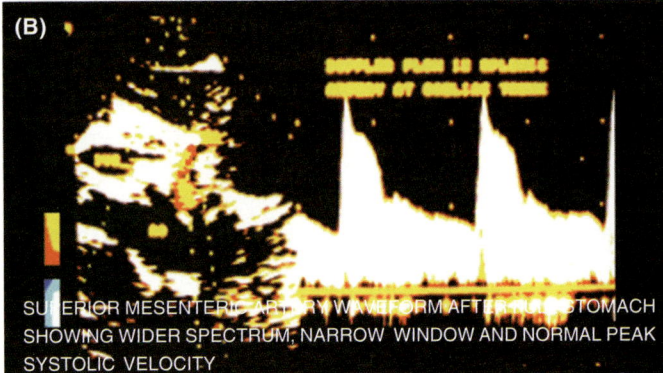

Fig. 22.32A and B: (A) Subcostal superior mesenteric artery waveform in person with empty stomach. **(B)** Subcostal color Doppler transhepatic scan showing arteries localisation of superior mesenteric and gastric arteries (left) and Doppler wider spectral waveforms of superior mesenteric artery after one hour taking his breakfast. It is to clarify that wider spectral waveform type of character can occur with full stomach in normal individual

Application of Abdominal Doppler
Techniques
Doppler ultrasound has been a clinically useful tool in diagnosing many disease processes. Doppler has helped detect the presence or absence of blood flow, the direction of blood flow, and flow disturbance patterns. It has also been used in tissue characterisation and waveform analysis.

Presence or Absence of Blood Flow
Doppler ultrasound frequently is used to differentiate vessels from nonvascular structures. For example, to distinguish the common bile duct from the hepatic artery, look for absence of flow in the common duct; to distinguish the hepatic artery from the splenic artery, look for direction of flow; to differentiate aneurysm from pancreatic pseudocyst, look for flow in the aneurysm; to differentiate dilated intrahepatic bile ducts and prominent hepatic artery, again look for absence of flow in the bile duct.

Direction of Blood Flow
In patients who develop portal venous hypertension, the portal blood flow becomes hepatofugal (away from the liver) instead of hepatopetal (towards the liver). This may be secondary to portal venous shunts of varices. The sonographer detects a high-velocity flow pattern at the site of the shunt with a turbulent flow pattern on colour Doppler.

Flow Disturbance
A flow disturbance (increased velocity or obstruction of flow) may result from the formation of an atheroma or aneurysmal dilation.

Tissue Characterisation
Research is currently underway in the area of tissue characterisation, Doppler is thought to be capable of characterizing tissue because of the specific perfusion patterns characteristic of some tissues or states or states of activity. Hepatocellular carcinomas of the liver appear to have a specific pattern. Pseudoaneurysms of peripancreatic arteries have turbulent flow patterns. Pancreatic tumours may have specific flow patterns.

Doppler Waveform Analysis
The shape of the waveform provides information on the vascular impedance of the organ the vessel supplies. Spectral analysis tells the velocity and turbulence of blood flow.

Nonresistive Versus Resistive: Nonresistive vessels have a high diastolic component and supply organs that need constant perfusion, such as the internal carotid artery, the hepatic artery, and the renal artery.

Resistive vessels have very little or even reversed flow in diastole and supply organs that do not need a constant blood supply, such as the external carotid and the iliac and brachial arteries.

Compare peak systole with minimum diastole to quantify a vessel's impedance. This ratio is the resistive index.

Plug flow is a pattern of blood flow, typically seen in large arteries, in which most cells are moving at the same velocity across the entire diameter of the vessel. In other vessels the different velocities are the result of friction between the cells and arterial walls. A "clear window" under systole is typical of plug flow. When plug flow is present, the volume of blood flow can be calculated.

Doppler Technique
Unlike visualisation of the heart, where high velocity flows are present, visualisation of abdominal vessels requires very sensitive Doppler instrumentation. Abdominal vessels generally have low velocity and flow.

Methods
Doppler is performed as part of the routine real-time examination. The patient should be fasting and suspend

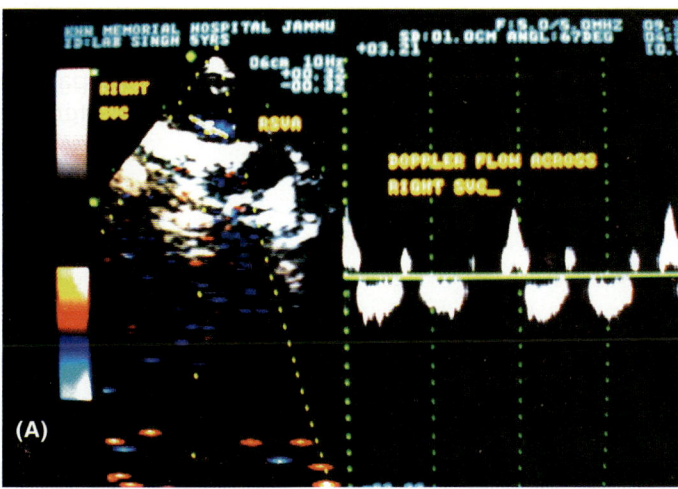
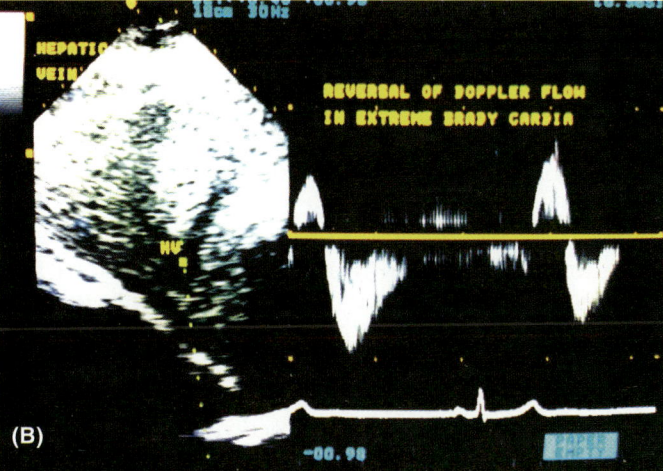

Fig. 22.33A and B: (A) Right supraclavicular approach showing normal blood flow velocity across right superior vena cava. **(B)** Subcostal transhepatic approach showing reversal of flow velocity across main hepatic vein in patient with extreme form of sinus bradycardia with heart rate less than 40 bpm

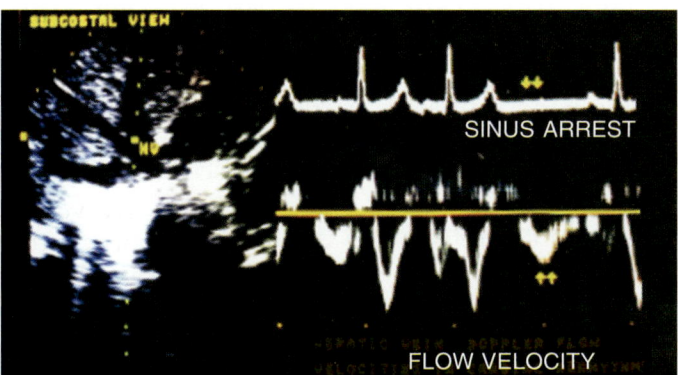
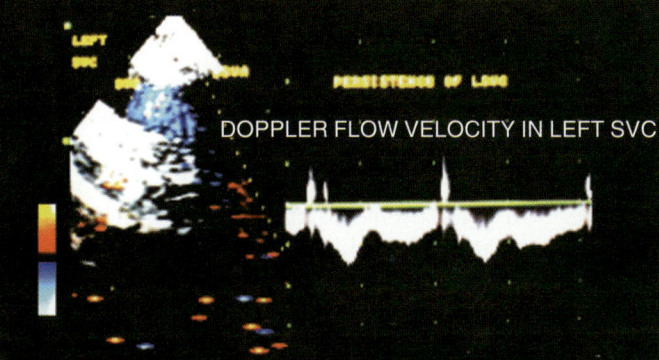

Fig. 22.34A and B: (A) Subcostal transhepatic approach showing normal blood flow in normal sinus rhythm and attenuated flow velocity during sinus arrest (arrow) in a patient with cardiac arrthythmia. **(B)** Left supraventricular approach showing Doppler blood flow in left superior vena cava

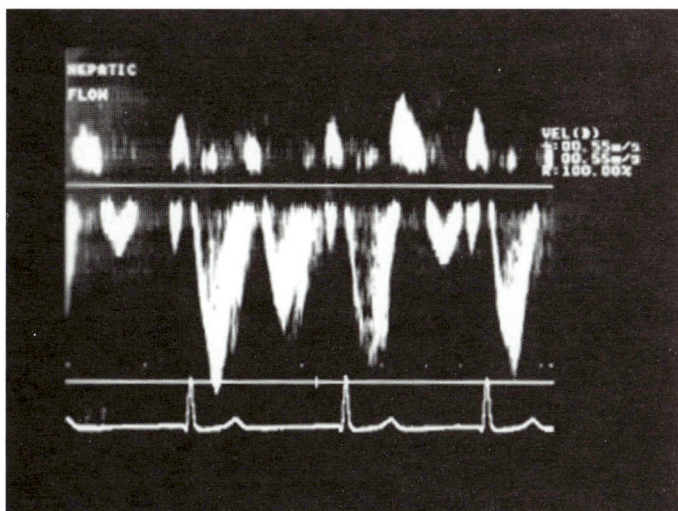
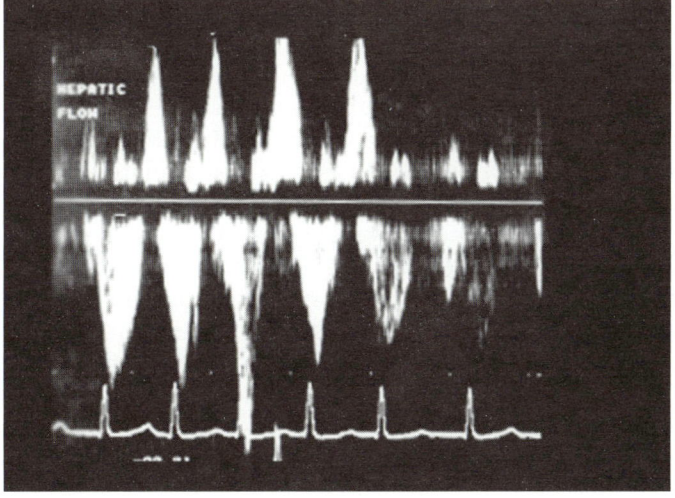

Fig. 22.35A and B: (A) Subcostal approach Doppler flow velocity across hepatic vein in bradycardia showing mild form of reversal of flow. **(B)** Hepatic blood flow showing typical reversal of flow in supraventricular tachyarrhythmia and reduced blood flow during sinus arrest in patient with brady-tachy syndrome

respirations for the best colour and pulsed Doppler sample volume to be obtained. The Doppler sample volume (sometimes referred to as the Doppler "gate") should be adjusted to encompass but not exceed the diameter, noise and ghost echoes may appear. This is because too wide a Doppler gate caused interference from the surrounding vessels and structures. The sonographer has the ability to control the velocity of the returning echoes to prevent the alias pattern. An other feature of Doppler is that the beam only records accurate velocity patterns when the beam is parallel to the flow (the angle of flow can be changed up to 60° and still be accurate). The more perpendicular the beam is to the flow, the less signal is recorded; it falls to zero velocity when the beam is directly perpendicular to flow. Thus Doppler caused the sonographer to be creative in attempting to record accurate velocity flow patterns. The patient must be rolled into various obliquities with different angulations of the transducer to be parallel to many vascular structures.

Colour Doppler is a relatively new and exciting modality that makes it easier to localize and identify smaller vessels from the biliary tree, lymphadenopathy, or other pathology. The colours are arbitrarily assigned on all equipment and refer to the direction of flow. If red is assigned as a positive flow signal, all the flow towards the transducer is coded in various shades of red, depending on their returning velocity. If blue is assigned a negative flow signal, the flow away from the transducer is coded in various shades of blue. The sonographer may select the particular colour scheme to be used; some labs choose to code all positive-flow patterns red and negative patterns blue. Other labs code all arterial flow red and venous flow blue.

Doppler Flow Patterns in the Abdominal Vessels
Aorta

The patient should be scanned in the longitudinal plane. The pattern of blood flow in the abdominal aorta differs with the level at which the vessel is scanned. The flow pattern of the proximal abdominal aorta above the renal arteries shows a high systole peak and a relatively low diastolic component. There is little spectral broadening. A clear window under systole means there is plug flow.

The distal abdominal aorta below the renal arteries shows flow with a small reversed component present during diastole. The closer one approaches the common iliac vessels, the greater the reverse component becomes. This is because of the high impedance of the peripheral circulation in the leg as it becomes triphasic, crossing the baseline three times (Fig. 22.19).

Celiac Axis

The sonographer should scan transversely to search for the segull sign, celiac trunk, hepatic artery, and splenic artery. If they can not be seen, scan longitudinally. Typically the spectral analysis of the celiac trunk shows some window under systole with spectral broadening (turbulence) in diastole. There is no chance in the flow pattern after meals.

Hepatic Artery

It has been reported that 1% of the population has replaced hepatic arteries arising from the superior mesenteric artery. Flow in diastole persists because of the low vascular impedance of the liver. Similar waveforms are seen in the main hepatic and intrahepatic arteries. Typically, there is more spectral broadening during both systole and diastole.

In a patient with a liver transplant, always document flow in the hepatic artery. Occlusion is one of the most dangerous complications, potentially resulting in death.

Splenic Artery

This vessel shows the most turbulence of all the celiac branches (probably because of its tortuosity). Aneurysms of the celiac branches have been described most commonly in the splenic branch. Patients with chronic pancreatitis are particularly prone to these. Always apply Doppler to pancreatic pseudocysts. Their appearance is very similar to that of vascular aneurysms.

Superior Mesenteric Artery (Fig. 22.32)

Typically the superior mesenteric artery is a highly resistive vessel (with decreased diastolic flow) in the fasting state with little or no flow in diastole. However, after a meal, the pattern of the superior mesenteric artery changes to a flow-resistive waveform demonstrating enhanced diastolic flow. Doppler analysis of the superior mesenteric artery has the potential to diagnose mesenteric arterial occlusion and abdominal angina.

Renal Artery (Fig. 22.16)

The main renal artery has a low impedance (non-resistive) pattern with significant diastole flow, usually 30% to 50% of peak systole. The continuous diastolic flow gives us continuous perfusion of the kidneys. There is spectral broadening in systole and diastole. The segmental interlobar, and arcuate arteries demonstrate a pattern similar to that of the main renal artery. However, the flow is progressively dampened in the periphery and shows reduced velocity patterns.

Renal Artery Stenosis

It is hard to demonstrate renal artery stenosis in a native kidney because of the difficulty in seeing the vessel at its origin and in its entirety. Renal artery occlusion can only be declared when the artery is unquestionably imaged. The sonographer should be careful because with complete obstruction of the native artery, collaterals may be mistaken for a patent renal artery. At least 30% of the population has multiple renal arteries, which makes it more difficult to rule out obstruction.

Renal Hydronephrosis

When there is even minimal separation of the renal pelvis, the sonographer should Doppler the area. Surprisingly, no hydronephrosis may be found, just prominent renal vessels in the renal pelvis.

Renal Transplants

In the main renal artery, there is turbulence near the anastomosis. Only 12% of patients develop renal artery stenosis after transplantation; it is characterized by a high-velocity jet with distal turbulence. Renal artery occlusion is easier to diagnose in transplants than in native kidneys, because there is no flow throughout the entire transplant.

Rejection

Normal transplants have a diastolic flow that is 30% to 50% of that of systole. During rejection, the vascular impedance increases, resulting in decrease or even reversal of the diastolic flow. There are a few methods to quantify the Doppler signals.

A resistive index (RI) is the most popular method in use. An RI of 0.7 or less indicates good perfusion, whereas an RI of 0.7 to 0.9 indicates possible rejection and over 0.9 indicates probable rejection.

Renal Vein

The renal vein shows variable flow like the inferior vena cava. The sonographer should closely evaluate the renal veins in any patient with a suspected tumour or renal obstructive lesion because they may be invaded by tumour or clot. In renal transplant patients, always look for a patent renal vein.

Bibliography

1. A comparison of six weeks with six months of oral anticoagulant therapy after a first episode of venous thromboembolism. Duration of Anticoagulation Trial Study Group: *N Engl J Med* 1995;332:1661.
2. Anand SS, Wells PS, Hunt D, *et al.* Does this patient have deep vein thrombosis? *JAMA* 1998;279:1094.
3. Anderson FA, Wheeler HB, Goldberg RJ, *et al.* The prevalence of risk factors for venous thromboembolism among hospital patients. *Arch Intern Med* 1992;152:1660.
4. Bernardi E, Prandoni P, Lensing AWA, *et al.* D-dimer testing as an adjunct to ultrasonography in patients with clinically suspected deep vein thrombosis: prospective cohort study. *BMJ* 1998; 317:1037.
5. Brandjes DPM, Buller HR, Heijboer H, *et al.* Randomised trial of effect of compression stockings in patients with symptomatic proximal-vein thrombosis. *Lancet* 1997; 349:759.
6. Brill-Edwards P, Ginsberg JS, Johnston M, *et al.* Establishing a therapeutic range for heparin therapy. *Ann Intern Med* 1993;119:104.
7. Cattaneo M: Hyperhomocysteinemia, atherosclerosis and thrombosis. *Thromb Haemost* 1999; 81:165.
8. Colwell CW, Collis DK, Paulson R, *et al.* Comparison of enoxaparin and warfarin for the prevention of venous thromboembolic disease after total hip arthroplasty. *J Bone Joint Surg Am* 1999; 81:932.
9. Decousus H, Leizorovicz A, Parent F, *et al.* A clinical trial of vena caval filters in the prevention of pulmonary embolism in patients with proximal deep-vein thrombosis. *N Engl J Med* 1998;338:409.
10. Dolovich LR, Ginsberg JS, Douketis JD, *et al.* A meta-analysis comparing low-molecular-weight heparins with unfractionated heparin in the treatment of venous thromboembolism. *Arch Intern Med* 2000; 160:181.
11. Eikelboom JW, Quinlan DJ, Douketis JD: Extended-duration prophylaxis against venous thromboembolism after total hip or knee replacement: a meta-analysis of the randomized trials. *Lancet* 2001;358:9.
12. Fedullo PF, Auger WR, Kerr KM, *et al.* Chronic thromboembolic pulmonary hypertension. *N Engl J Med* 2001; 345:1465.
13. Fraser DG, Moody AR, Morgan PS, *et al.* Diagnosis of lower-limb deep venous thrombosis: a prospective blinded study of magnetic resonance direct thrombus imaging. *Ann Intern Med* 2002; 136:89.
14. Geerts WH, Heit JA, Clagett P, *et al.* Prevention of venous thromboembolism. *Chest* 2001; 119 (suppl) : 1325.
15. Ginsberg JS, Kearon C, Douketis J, *et al.* The use of D-dimer testing and impedance plethysmographic examination in patients with clinical indications of deep vein thrombosis. *Arch Intern Med* 1997; 157:1077.
16. Ginsberg JS, Wells PS, Kearon C, *et al.* Sensitivity and specificity of a rapid whole-blood assay for D-dimer in the diagnosis of pulmonary embolism. *Ann Intern Med* 1998;129:1006.
17. Ginsberg JS: Management of venous thromboembolism. *N Engl J Med* 1996;335: 1816.
18. Grady D, Wenger NK, Herrington D, *et al.* Postmenopausal hormone therapy increases risk for venous thromboembolic disease. *Ann Intern Med* 2000; 132:689.
19. Harrison L, Johnston M, Massicotte MP, *et al.* Comparison of 5-mg and 10-mg loading doses in initiation of warfarin therapy. *Ann Intern* Med 1997;126:133.
20. Heijboer H, Brandjes DPM, Buller HR, *et al,* Deficiencies of coagulation-inhibiting and fibrinolytic proteins in outpatients with deep-vein thrombosis. *N Engl J Med* 1990;323:1512.
21. Heijboer H, Buller HR, Lensing AWA, *et al.* A comparison of real-time-compression ultrasonography with impedance plethysmography for the diagnosis of deep-vein thrombosis in symptomatic outpatients. *N Engl J Med* 1993;329:1365.
22. Heit JA, Silverstein MD, Mohr DN, *et al.* Risk factors for deep vein thrombosis and pulmonary embolism: a population-based case-control study. *Arch Intern Med* 2000;160:809.
23. Hirsh J, Dalen J, Anderson DR, *et al.* Oral anticoagulants: mechanism of action, clinical effectiveness, and optimal therapeutic range. *Chest* 2001;119:8S.

24. Hirsh J, Lensing A: Thrombolytic therapy for deep vein thrombosis. *Int J Angiol* 1996; 5:S22.

25. Hirsh J, Heparin. *N Engl J Med* 1991;324:1565.

26. Hoibraaten E, Qvigstad E, Arnesen H, *et al.* Increased risk of recurrent venous thromboembolism during hormone replacement therapy: results of the randomized, double-blind, placebo-controlled Estrogen in Venous Thromboembolism Trial (EVTET). Thromb Haemost 2000; 84:961.

27. Hull R, Delmore T, Genton E, *et al.* Warfarin sodium versus low-dose heparin in the long-term treatment of venous thrombosis. *N Engl J Med* 1979;301:855.

28. Hull RD, Raskob GE, Ginsberg JS, *et al.* A noninvasive strategy for the treatment of patients with suspected pulmonary embolism. *Arch Intern Med* 1994; 154:289.

29. Jerjes-Sanchez C, Ramírez-Rivera A, de Lourdes García M, *et al.* Streptokinase and heparin versus heparin alone in massive pulmonary embolism: a randomized controlled trial. *J Thromb Thrombolysis* 1995;2:227.

30. Kearon C, Crowther M, Hirsh J, *et al.* Management of patients with hereditary hypercoagulable disorders. *Annu Rev Med* 2000; 51:169.

31. Kearon C, Gent M, Hirsh J, *et al.* A comparison of three months of anticoagulation with extended anticoagulation for a first episode of idiopathic venous thromboembolism. *N Engl J Med* 1999; 340:901.

32. Kearon C, Ginsberg JS, Douketis J, *et al,* Management of suspected deep venous thrombosis in outpatients by using clinical assessment and D-dimer testing. *Ann Intern Med* 2001;135:108.

33. Kearon C, Ginsberg JS, Hirsh J: The role of venous ultrasonography in the diagnosis of suspected deep venous thrombosis and pulmonary embolism. *Ann Intern Med* 1998; 129:1044.

34. Kearon C, Julian JA, Newman TE, *et al,* Noninvasive diagnosis of deep venous thrombosis. *Ann Intern Med* 1998;128:663.

35. Kearon C, Salzman EW, Hirsh J: Epidemiology, pathogenesis, and natural history of venous thrombosis. *Hemostasis and Thrombosis: Basic Principles and Clinical Practice,* 4th ed. Colman RW, Hirsh J, Marder VJ, *et al.* Eds. JB Lippincott Co, Philadelphia, 2001.

36. Kearon C: Diagnosis of pulmonary embolism. *CMAJ* 2003;168:183.

37. Kearon C: Duration of therapy for acute venous thromboembolism. *Clin Chest Med* 2003 ;24:63.

38. Kearon C: Epidemiology of venous thromboembolism. *Semin Vascular Med* 2001;1:7.

39. Kearon C: Natural history of venous thromboembolism. *Semin Vascular Med* 2001;1:27.

40. Koopman MMW, Prandoni P, Piovella F, *et al.* Treatment of venous thrombosis with intravenous unfractionated heparin administered in the hospital as compared with subcutaneous low-molecular-weight heparin administered at home. *N Engl J Med* 1996; 334:682.

41. Kyrle P, Minar E, Hirschl M, *et al.* High plasma levels of factor VIII and the risk of recurrent venous thromboembolism. *N Engl J Med* 2000;343:62.

42. Lagerstedt CI, Olsson CG, Fagher BO, *et al.* Need for long-term anticoagulant treatment in symptomatic calf-vein thrombosis. *Lancet* 1985;2:515.

43. Lane DA, Mannucci PM, Bauer KA, *et al.* Inherited thrombophilia (Pt 1). *Thromb Haemost* 1996;76:651.

44. Lane DA, Mannucci PM, Bauer KA, *et al.* Inherited thrombophilia (pt 2). *Thromb Haemost* 1996;76:824.

45. Lee AY, Ginsberg JS: Laboratory diagnosis of venous thromboembolism. *Baillieres Clin Haematol* 1998; 11:2461.

46. Levine M, Gent M, Hirsh J, *et al.* A comparison of low-molecular-weight heparin administered primarily at homewith unfractionated heparin administered in the hospital for proximal deep-vein thrombosis. *N Engl J Med* 1996; 334:677.

47. Levine M, Raskob G, Landerfeld S, *et al.* Hemorrhagic complications of antithrombotic therapy. *Chest* 2001; 119 (suppl):108S.

48. Levine MN, Hirsh J, Gent M, *et al,* Optimal duration of oral anticoagulant therapy: a randomized trial comparing four weeks with three months of wafarin in patients with proximal deep vein thrombosis. *Thromb Haemost* 1995;74:606.

49. Low-molecular-weight heparin in the treatment of patients with venous thromboembolism. The Columbus Investigators: *N Engl J Med* 1997;337:657.

50. Meijers JCM, Tekelenburg WLH, Bouma BN, *et al.* High levels of coagulation factor XI as a risk factor for venous thrombosis. *N Engl J Med* 2000;342:696.

51. Miniati M, Prediletto R, Formichi B, *et al.* Accuracy of clinical assessment in the diagnosis of pulmonary embolism. *Am J Respir Crit Care Med* 1999;159:864.

52. Mullins MD, Becker DM, Hagspiel KD, *et al.* The role of the spiral volumetric computed tomography in the diagnosis of pulmonary embolism. *Arch Intern Med* 2000;160:293.

53. Musset D, Parent F, Meyer G, *et al.* Diagnostic strategy for patients with suspected pulmonary embolism: a prospective multi-centre outcome study. *Lancet* 2002;360:1914.

54. Optimum duration of anticoagulation for deep-vein thrombosis and pulmonary embolism. Research Committee of the British Thoracic Society: *Lancet* 1992;340:873.

55. Perrier A, Desmarais S, Miron MJ, *et al.* Non-invasive diagnosis of venous thromboembolism in outpatients. *Lancet* 1999;353:190.

56. Perrier A, Howarth N, Didier D, *et al.* Performance of helical computed tomography in unselected outpatient with suspected pulmonary embolism. *Ann Intern Med* 2001; 135:88.

57. Pinede L, Ninet J, Duhaut P, *et al.* Comparison of 3 and 6 months of oral anticoagulant therapy after a first episode of proximal deep vein thrombosis or pulmonary embolism and comparison of 6 and 12 weeks of therapy after isolated calf deep vein thrombosis. *Circulation* 2001;103:2453.

58. Poort SR, Rosendaal FR, Reitsma PH, *et al.* A common genetic variation in the 3Á untranslated region of the prothrombin gene is associated with elevated plasma prothrombin levels and an increase in venous thrombosis. *Blood* 1996;88:3698.

59. Prandoni P, Lensing AW, Piccioli A, *et al.* Recurrent venous thromboembolism and bleeding complications during anticoagulant treatment in patients with cancer and venous thrombosis. *Blood* 100:3484, 2002

60. Prandoni P, Lensing AWA, Cogo A, *et al.* The long-term clinical course of acute deep venous thrombosis. *Ann Intern Med* 1996; 125:1.

61. Prevention of pulmonary embolism and deep vein thrombosis with low dose aspirin. Pulmonary Embolism Prevention (PEP) Trial Collaborative Group: *Lancet* 2000; 355:1295.

62. Prins MH, Hirsh J: A critical review of the evidence supporting a relationship between impaired fibrinolytic activity and venous thromboembolism. *Arch Intern Med* 1991; 151:1721.

63. Rathbun SW, Raskob GE, Whitsett TL: Sensitivity and specificity of helical computed tomography in the diagnosis of pulmonary embolism: a systematic review. *Ann Intern Med* 2000;132:227.

64. Rosendaal FR: High levels of factor VIII and venous thrombosis. *Thromb Haemost* 2000;83:1.

65. Rossouw JE, Anderson GL, Prentice RL, *et al,* Risks and benefits of estrogen plus progestin in healthy postmenopausal women: principal results from the Women's Health Initiative randomized controlled trial. *JAMA* 2002;288:321.

66. Simonneau G, Sors H, Charbonnier B, *et al,* A comparison of low-molecular-weight heparin with unfractionated heparin for acute pulmonary embolism. *N Engl J Med* 1997;337:663.

67. Turpie AG, Bauer KA, Eriksson BI, *et al.* Fondaparinux vs enoxaparin for the prevention of venous thromboembolism in major orthopedic surgery: a meta-analysis of 4 randomized double-blind studies. *Arch Intern Med* 162:1833, 2002.

68. van den Belt AGM, Prins MH, Huisman MV, *et al.* Familial thrombophilia: a review analysis. *Clin Appl Thromb Hemost* 1996;2:227.

69. Vandenbrouke JP, Koster E, Briet E, *et al.* Increased risk of venous thrombosis in oral contraceptive users who are carriers of factor V Leiden mutation. *Lancet* 1994; 344:1453.

70. Weitz JI, Crowther M: Direct thrombin inhibitors. *Thromb Res* 2002;106:V275.

71. Weitz JI, Stewart RJ, Fredenburgh JC: Mechanism of action of plasminogen activators. *Thromb Haemost* 1999;82:974.

72. Weitz JI: Low-molecular-weight heparins. *N Engl J Med* 1997;337:688.

73. Wells PS, Anderson DR, Rodger M, *et al.* Derivation of a simple clinical model to categorize patients' probability of pulmonary embolism: increasing the model's utility with the Simplified D-dimer. *Thromb Haemost* 2000;83:416.

74. Wells PS, Anderson DR, Rodger M, *et al.* Excluding pulmonary embolism at the bedside without diagnostic imaging: management of patients with suspected pulmonary embolism presenting to the emergency department by using a simple clinical model and D-dimer. *Ann Intern Med* 2001;135:98,

75. Wells PS, Ginsberg JS, Anderson DR, *et al,* Use of a clinical model for safe management of patients with suspected pulmonary embolism. *Ann Intern Med* 1998;129:997.

76. Wells PS, Hirsh J, Anderson DR, *et al.* A simple clinical model for the diagnosis of deep vein thrombosis combined with impedance plethysmography: potential for an improvement in the diagnostic process. *J Intern Med* 1998;243:15.

77. Wells PS, Hirsh J, Anderson DR, *et al.* Accuracy of clinical assessment of deep vei n thrombosis. *Lancet* 1995; 345:1326.

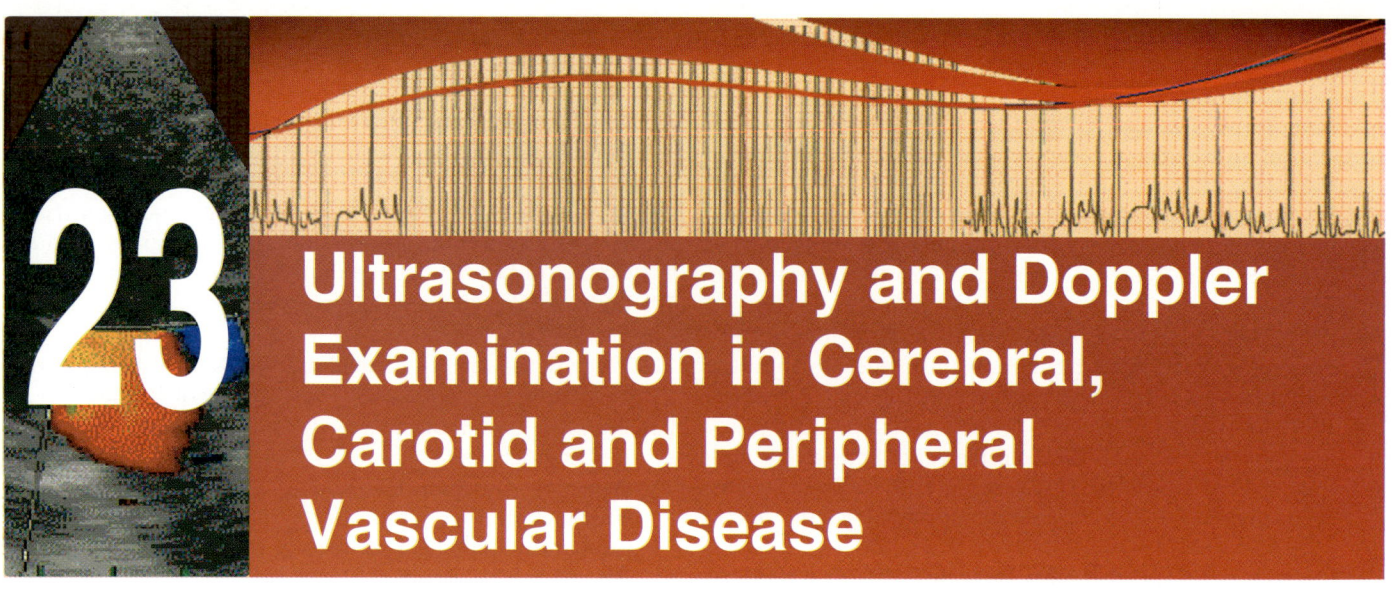

23

Ultrasonography and Doppler Examination in Cerebral, Carotid and Peripheral Vascular Disease

Transcranial Doppler and Transcranial Duplex Imaging

Newer developments in Doppler and sonographic technology have enabled examiners to assess the flow and circulatory anatomy of the intracranial vault directly, using thinner areas of the skull as acoustic windows to the circle of Willis, basilar artery, terminal internal carotid, anterior cerebral, and middle cerebral and posterior cerebral arteries. The methods used to evaluate these intracranial vessels are transcranial Doppler (TCD) and transcranial Duplex imaging (often abbreviated TCI). Although the Doppler method (a nonimaging approach) may ultimately give way to the duplex imaging method, more experience and data are currently available from transcranial Doppler than from the more recent and evolving transcranial imaging modality. Knowledge and familiarity with both techniques are important, since they are complementary (Figs 23.1, 23.2, 23.10 and 23.11).

Transcranial Doppler

Transcranial Doppler was introduced by Rune Aaslid in 1982 and had developed and advanced, remarkably since that time. The technique is related to blind Doppler assessment (such as with direct continuous wave Doppler), and many of the examination techniques are similar to those used in the periorbital Doppler examination, although somewhat more challenging. Even though the user has no 2-dimensional image to guide sample placement, transcranial Doppler's ability to diagnose and define the intracerebral hemodynamic state has made it a very well accepted technique.

Equipment: The device used is a bi-directional pulsed Doppler with a 2-MHz transducer, which

has sufficient ability to penetrate bony structures. The original maximum allowable power levels of 100 MW/cm^2 (SPTA) and small sample volume have recently been expanded by the FDA to allow these instruments a much greater sensitivity and diagnostic capability than was previously available. The sample volume size can be adjusted as necessary and the sample focal depth is variable on these devices, since they by necessity must be range-gated. Depth increments range from 2 to 5 mm per step to a maximum depth of about 150 mm. The pulse-repetition rates are also adjustable, since cerebrovascular velocities are usually quite high (especially in cases of abnormality). The Doppler velocities assume an angle of 0 to 30°, since the beam intercepts arterial flow at nearly that angle because of the anatomic vascular pathways. A spectrum analysis display is incorporated into these units, and external displays and computer interfaces are supported as well. The focal depth, peak and mean velocity, flow direction, pulse repetition frequency (PRF), and sample volume size are all displayed on the analysis screen, as is the spectral waveform. Some computer-based packages also allow for individual display and wave length profile analysis of the peak and mean velocities, as well as calculating a form of relative volume flow and cross-sectional vessel area (the usefulness and accuracy of volume flow in all vascular applications is still under investigation by numerous companies and institutions). Transcranial Doppler devices are easily portable and can be used for bedside evaluations or can be transported to surgery for intraoperative monitoring. Many duplex scanner manufacturers are currently supplementing their transcranial duplex imaging packages with the capability to perform additional blind transcranial Doppler evaluations.

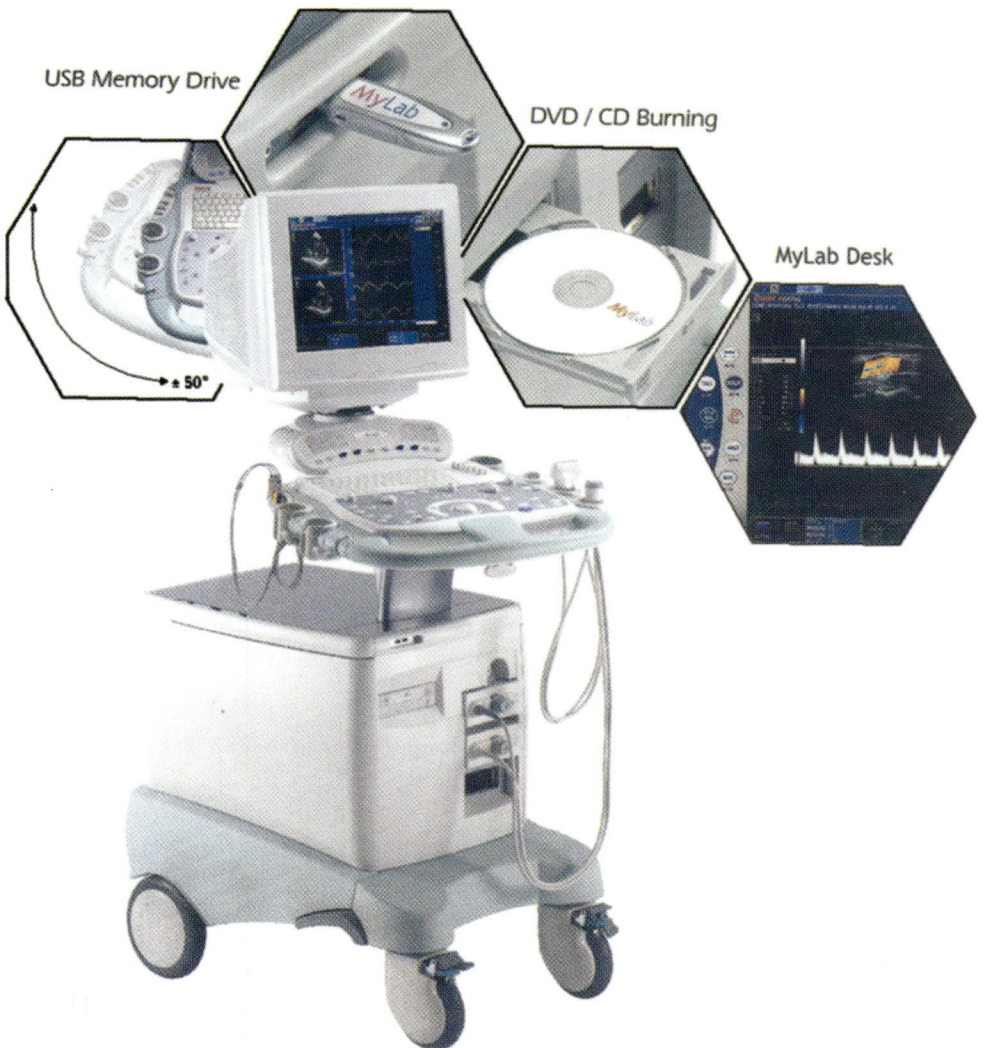

Fig. 23.1: Latest version of ultrasound machine used for study of both intracranial and extracranial vessels including Duplex imaging

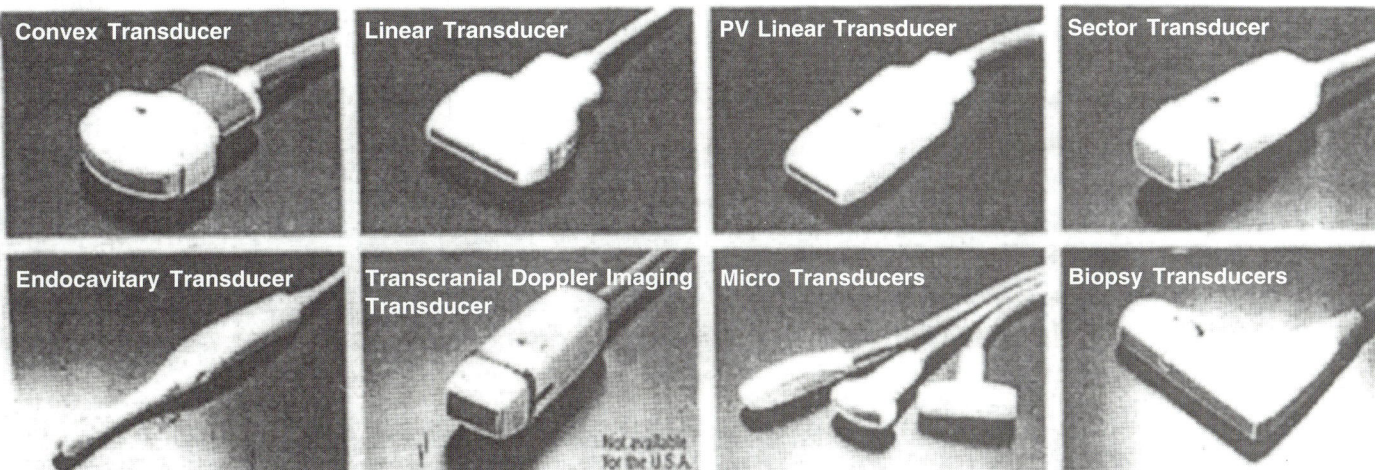

Fig. 23.2: Different types of transducers being employed in the assessment of cerebral, carotid and peripheral vasculature including transacranial Doppler imaging transducer

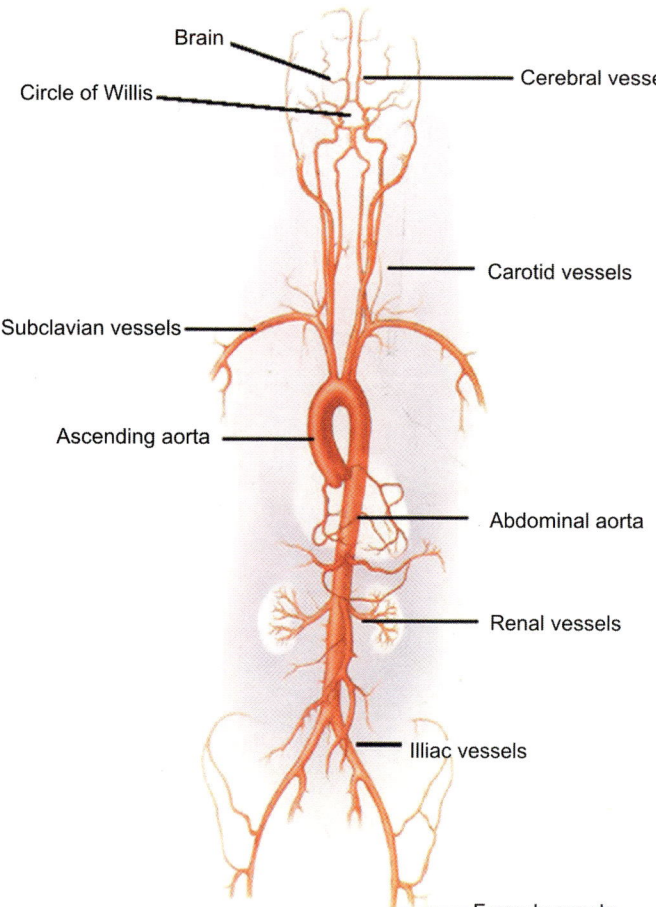

Fig. 23.3: Anatomical localization of cerebral, carotid and peripheral vascular system in human body

Anatomy of the Intracranial Cerebrovascular Circulation (Figs 23.3 and 23.4)

The arteries of the circle of Wills and posterior circulation that are accessible to transcranial Doppler include the following:

1. Middle cerebral artery (MCA)
2. Anterior cerebral artery (ACA)
3. Posterior cerebral artery (PCA)
4. Terminal internal carotid artery (TICA)
5. Internal carotid artery (Carotid siphon)
6. Ophthalmic artery (OA)
7. Basilar artery (BA)
8. Vertebral arteries (VA)
9. Anterior communicating artery (AcoA)
10. Posterior communicating artery (PcoA)

To gain access to these arteries, the ultrasound beam must penetrate the skull in some fashion. This is best accessed in each approach as identified by the following:

1. The sample volume depth;

2. The direction of blood flow in relation to the transducer beginning at the middle and anterior cerebral bifurcation, increasing the sample depth by about 5 mm, then angling posteriorly and inferiorly. Flow is towards the transducer and may occasionally be confused with the (towards or away from);
3. Spatial relationships to other Doppler spectra;
4. Response to common carotid artery compressions and vertebral artery compression. Common carotid compression is routinely used to isolate and define collateral flow (much in the Doppler periorbital study); its use is considered an important part of the examination despite controversies in the past.

As stated previously, the examiner should still use caution; the CCA should be straddled between two closely placed fingertips low in the neck and still should be compressed for only about beats (which should be sufficient time to determine the effect on the monitored Doppler signal). The vertebral artery is compressed to determine collateral effect or flow direction in the basilar artery or posterior circulation; this is accomplished along the atlantal portion by palpating the mastoid process behind the ear and compressing in the mastoid notch.

The transorbital approach is used to evaluate the ophthalmic artery and the intercranial carotid siphon segments of the internal carotid artery. Power levels should be set very low (about 10 MW/cm^2) to avoid overexposure of the lens and eye tissues to excessive acoustic power levels. The eye is closed, and the transducer is gently placed over the eyelid and coupled with gel. The beam is oriented anteroposteriorly with a slight tilt to the midline.

The QA is evaluated at a sample depth of 40 to 50 mm. The sample depth is increased slowly as adjustments are made to keep to opthalmic artery in the Doppler beam. At 55 to 70 mm the carotid siphon area is located and is easily discerned by the higher diastolic velocity compared with the ophthalmic signal. The different curved segments of the intracranial internal carotid artery where it exits the carotid canal and before it joins the circle of Willis (proximal, parasellar, curve, genu, distal and posterior, supraclinoid) are detected by flow direction. The parasellar (near the sella turcica) portion is found by angling inferiorly, and flow is towards the transducer. The flow in the anterior curve (genu section) is bi-directional (since the beam is entering perpendicular to the flow). Locating the genu section first, can help locate the other two segments. The supraclinoid segment is found by angling superiorly and flow is away from the transducer.

The transtemporal approach is used to evaluate the middle cerebral artery, anterior cerebral artery, terminal portion of the internal carotid, posterior cerebral artery,

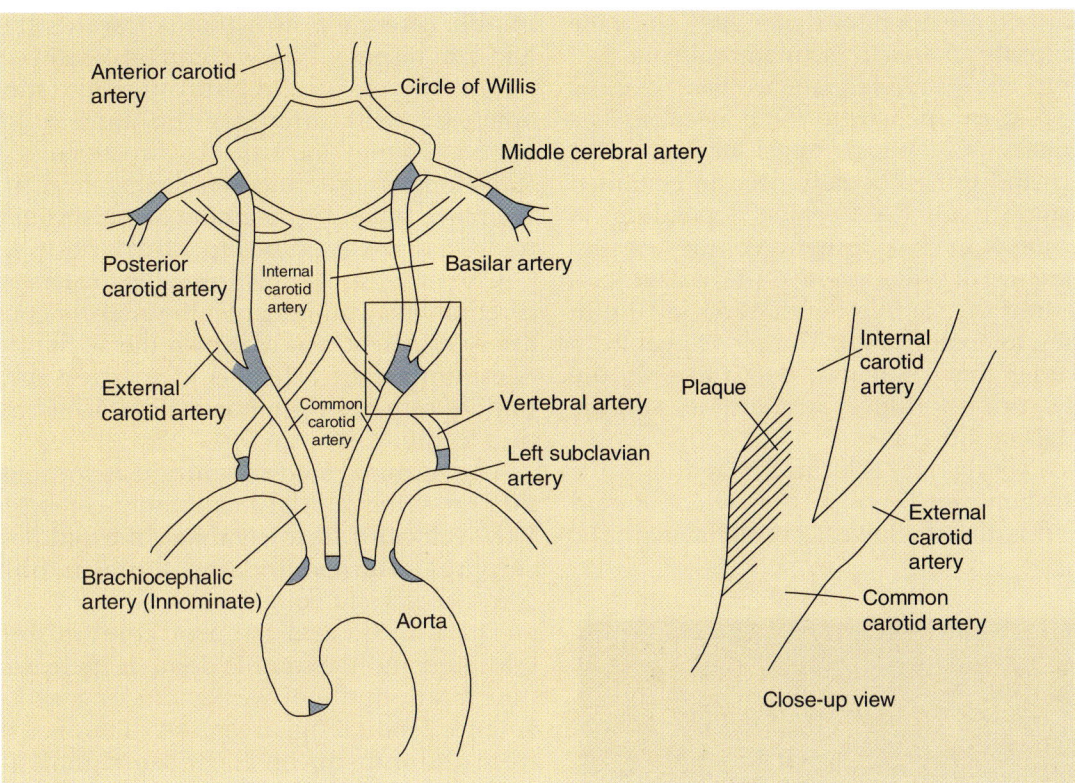

Fig. 23.4: Normal anatomy of aortic arch, great vessels, and circle of wills. The shaded area predicts the areas most prone for the development of atherosclerosis

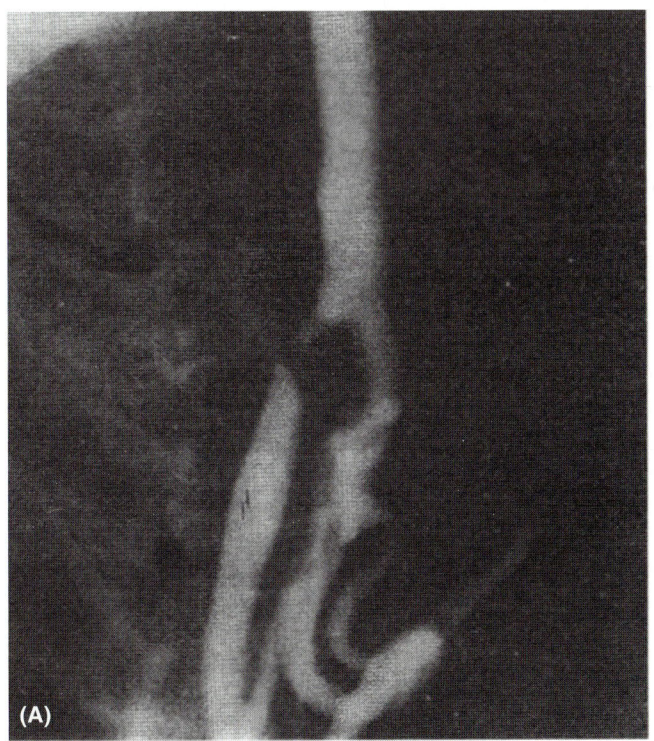

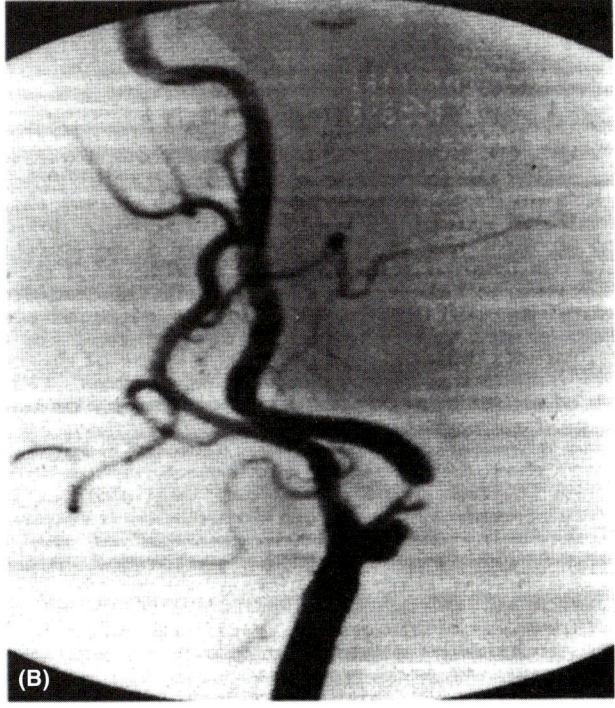

Fig. 23.5 A and B: (A) Severe stenosis at the origin of the interval carotid artery on carotid angiogram. **(B)** Arterial DSA in unilateral carotid artery stenosis

and the anterior and are operator dependent, since the examiner must locate an area in the temporal bone that is thin enough to allow an adequate acoustic window where the Doppler can penetrate the bone well. The location for transtemporal insonation is superior to the zygomatic arch, and the probe may need to be aimed anteriorly, posteriorly, or dead center, depending on which window allow the best reception of the Doppler signals from the circle of Willis arteries. The best location is found by setting the sample depth at 55 to 60 mm and then moving to obtain a clear Doppler signal from any of the arteries that lie at that depth usually the anterior, middle, or posterior cerebral arteries and the terminal internal carotid artery.

The middle cerebral artery is located by reducing the sample depth by between 25 and 50 mm, which should detect it, since it is the shallowest arterial signal. The

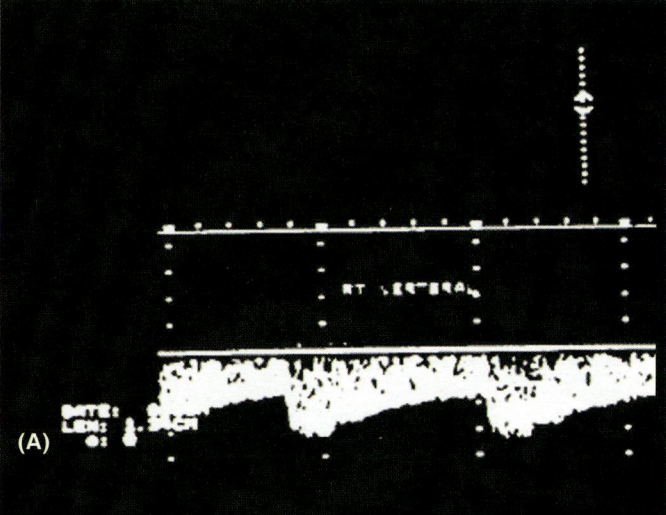

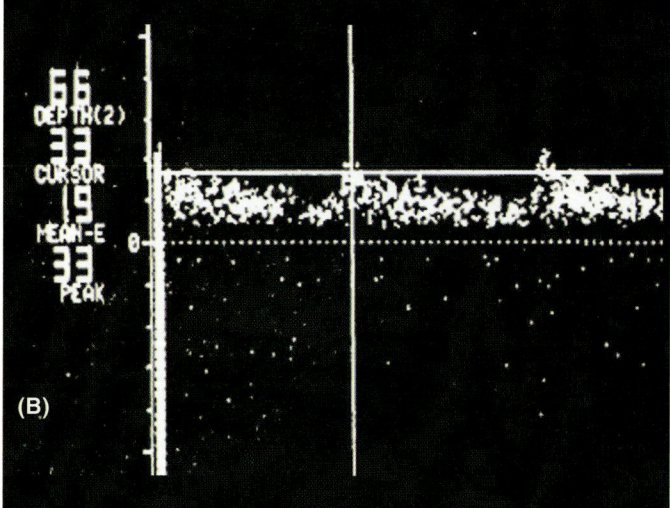

Fig. 23.6: (A) Normal vertebral artery signal from the transoccipital approach with flow traveling away from the transducer. (B) Normal posterior cerebral artery spectrum

middle cerebral flow signal is towards the transducer and diminishes with low common carotid compressions.

The internal carotid bifurcation into the middle and anterior cerebral arteries can be found at a sample depth of 55 to 65 mm and has a bi-directional signal. The bi-directional middle and anterior cerebral bifurcation is a reference point for obtaining signals from the anterior, middle, and posterior cerebral arteries.

Common carotid compressions reserve the anterior cerebral flow component if the anterior communicating artery is patent and diminish the signal if the anterior communicating artery is obstructed or absent. The middle cerebral component diminished as mentioned previously.

The terminal internal carotid is located by angling inferior to the middle and anterior cerebral bifurcation. Flow velocities are lower than if the middle and anterior cerebral arteries, and the signal is obliterated by common carotid compression.

The middle and anterior cerebral bifurcation is relocated and the sample depth is increased to 70 to 80 mm (brain midline) while adjusting and keeping the anterior cerebral signal centered. Flow is normally away from the transducer. Reversed signals imply cross-channel collateral flow from the opposite side, and this may occur when the ipsilateral internal carotid is severely stenosed, and the contralateral anterior cerebral exhibits increased flow velocities. Common carotid compression normally reverses the anterior cerebral signal or diminished flow in absence of a patent anterior communicating artery. The anterior communicating artery is not normally detected unless it is acting as a collateral, when high velocities and turbulence will be noted at the 70 to 80 mm level.

The posterior cerebral artery signal is located by beginning at the middle and anterior cerebral bifurcation, increasing the sample depth by about 5 mm, then angling posteriorly and inferiorly. Flow is towards the transducer and may occasionally be confused with the middle cerebral, but the posterior cerebral artery cannot be tracked at any depth shallower than 55 mm, whereas the middle cerebral artery can be visualised distal to posterior cerebral artery flow signal, since the anatomic course of the posterior cerebral changes in relation to the transducer window and the beam sweeps across the curve.

The posterior communicating artery is seldom located but appears as turbulent, high-velocity signal when acting as a collateral and is found in a manner similar to that used for the posterior cerebral artery.

The trans occipital approach is used for the evaluation of the intracranial vertebral arteries and basilar artery. The head is slightly flexed forward and the probe is placed in the center of the suboccipital area with a simple depth of 60 to 70 mm. The probe is angled laterally right

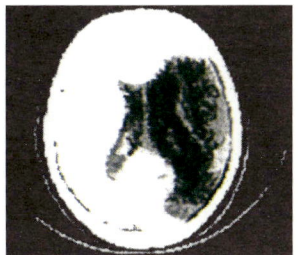

Fig. 23.7: Cerebral CT scan showing extensive area of ischaemic infarction in the territory of the left middle cerebral artery (dark black area)

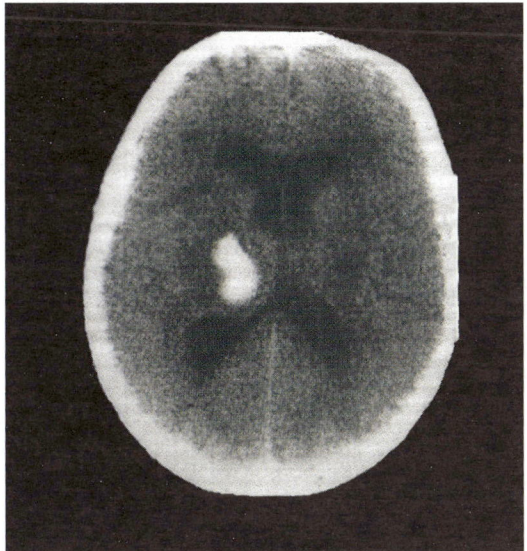

Fig. 23.8: Cerebral CT scan showing intracranial hemorrhage in the right hemisphere (white area)

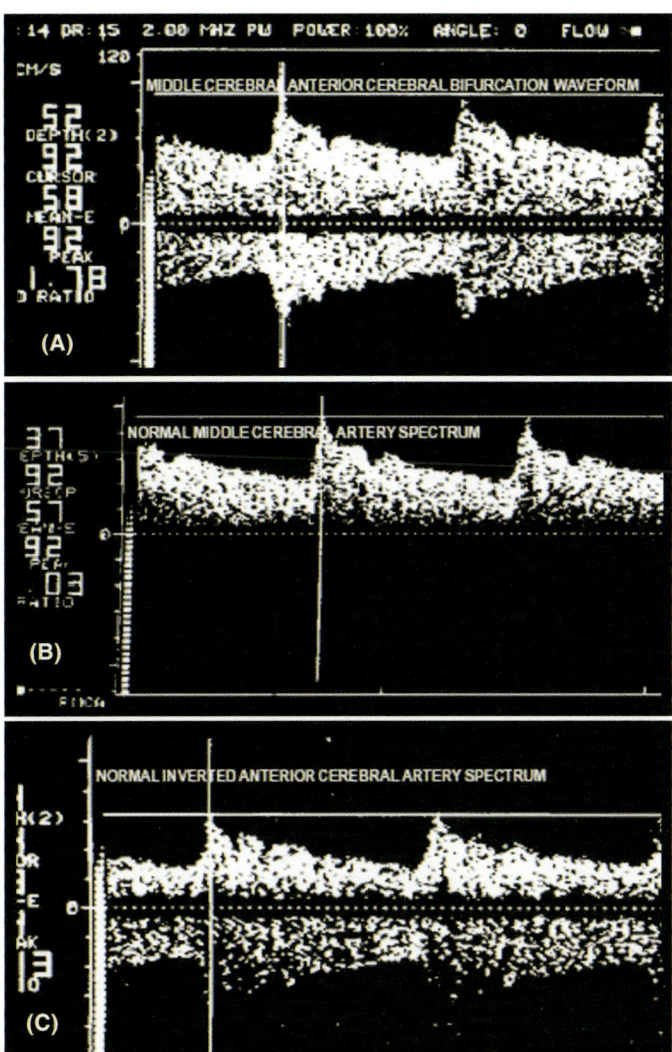

Fig. 23.9: (A) Normal middle cerebral anterior cerebral bifurcation spectrum. **(B)** Normal middle cerebral artery spectrum. **(C)** Normal inverted anterior cerebral artery spectrum

and left of midline across the individual vertebra. The sample depth is then increased until the vertebrobasilar junction is located (85 to 100 mm) and the single basilar artery signal is accessed. The probe may need to be elevated superiorly when following the arteries. The flow in the vertebral and basilar will be away from transducer normally. A reversed signal in one vertebral or other with turbulence at the basilar junction is indicative of a subclavian steal, and evidence to this effect should already have been gained from earlier extracranial duplex carotid assessments.

Characteristics of Doppler Intracranial Arterial Waveforms (Figs 23.2 and 23.3)

The normal appearance of the intracranial waveform is similar to that of the extracranial internal carotid artery, since the intracranial arterial system is also a low-resistance system. The diastolic component of the spectral waveform does not normally go below the baseline and the concentration of frequencies follows the envelope contour, as in the normal internal carotid signal.

Transcranial Doppler Diagnostic Interpretation Criteria

The primary measurement factor used in quantifying the intracranial Doppler spectral signal is the peak systolic velocity, which is measured in the same location as on waveforms from the extracranial Doppler examination, or the mean velocity, which is time averaged over several waveforms. Most transcranial Doppler devices automatically calculate and display the mean velocity in real time based on the placement of the cursor along the peak (on some displays, cursor indicates the peak systolic frequency at placement). Most investigators, as well the ICA VL Essentials and Standards, recommend the use of mean velocities rather than peak velocities. The reason for using mean velocities is that the precise Doppler angle of insonation is not known but is assumed to be $0°$ and no more than $30°$.

Abnormal Flow Criteria

As in the extracranial carotid duplex examination, increased flow velocities occur across a significant stenosis, in the presence of arterial spasm, or in collateral arteries. As stated previously, the increase in velocity is usually proportional to the degree of luminal reduction. Diminished waveforms and dampened pulsatility also occur distal to a severe stenosis, just as in the extracranial system or the peripheral arteries. The direction of flow within the artery being examined is also a diagnostic factor, as are the presence and degree of flow disturbance and turbulence. Since the intracranial arteries are of small caliber, turbulent signals manifest as squeaking or whining bruit sounds with prominent harmonics; these bruits often are almost musical in nature. Some spectral broadening occurs naturally in intracranial arteries because of the many branches bifurcation's, and small overall calibers, spectral broadening criteria therefore do not apply, with the exception of baseline turbulence and envelope disturbance. Certain velocity and directional findings are often consistent with specific types of intracerebral pathology; these abnormal value and findings are discussed in their appropriate subtopics.

Application of Transcranial Doppler and Respective Abnormal Diagnostic Criteria

Transcranial Doppler has been found to be useful in numerous applications:

1. Detecting the presence of severe, greater than 65% stenosis in the major basal intracranial arteries;
2. Assessing the patterns and extent of collateral circulation in patients with known severe stenosis or occlusion;
3. Evaluating and following patients with vasospasm or vasoconstriction, especially after a subarachnoid haemorrhage;
4. Determining arteriovenous malformation (A–VMs) and documenting their supply vessels and flow patterns; and
5. Assessing patients with suspected brain death.

The following section addresses the utility of TCD in some of the areas and discusses diagnostic criteria used in evaluating these conditions.

Intracranial Artery Stenosis Detection

Transcranial Doppler can be used effectively to evaluate stroke patients for high grade stenosis or occlusion in the cerebral vasculature, and to assess the success or failure of thrombolysis or cerebral percutaneous transluminal angioplasty (using protocols defined in the NACPT AR trials). The Doppler criteria for severe stenosis in the cerebral arteries are very similar to those used for internal carotid stenosis, but no accepted universal value for categorizing degree of abnormality for grading percentage have been published. Detection of stenosis should therefore be subjectively based on documented velocity increases, turbulence, waveform diminution distal to the stenosis, and comparisons to the normal velocity values.

Indirect Evaluation of Extracranial Disease and Collateralization

When used as an adjunct to carotid duplex sonography, transcranial Doppler can also function as an indirect study for carotid disease detection in the manner of the periorbital examination but with much more detail regarding the intracranial collateral pathways and distal

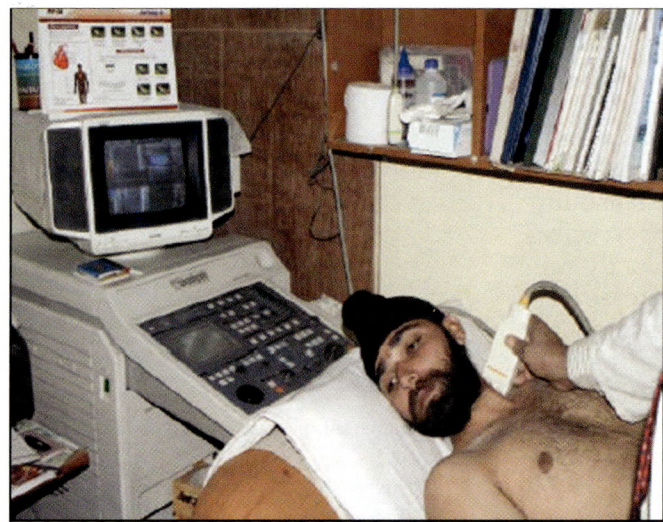

Fig. 23.10: Duplex color Doppler probe in left lateral position in the region of neck for obtaining signatures of left vertebral artery

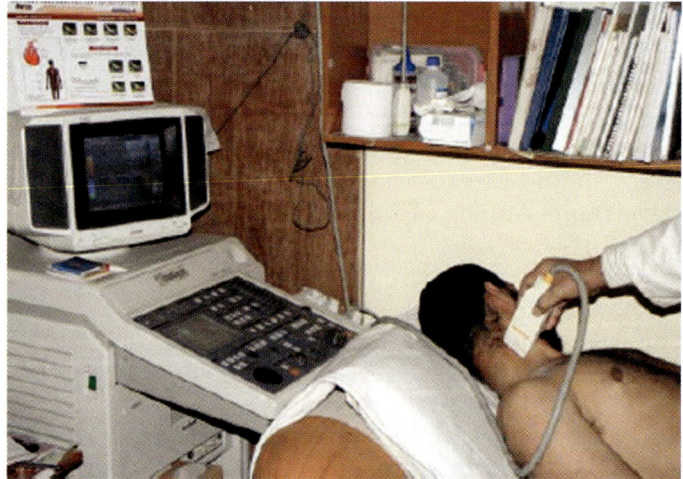

Fig. 23.11: Duplex color Doppler probe in left lateral position in the region of neck for obtaining signatures of right vertebral artery

effects of proximal ICA stenosis or occlusion. Flow changes, in the terminal ICA may indicate the severity of the stenosis, as does reversed flow in the ophthalmic artery (the basis for the periorbital Doppler examination). Decreased velocities, diminished flow patterns, and distal branches in the middle cerebral artery often can occur as an indirect result of severe ICA stenosis, but these characteristics are not generally quantifiable. Collateral patterns through the anterior and posterior communicating arteries, however, are detectable and can be characterized by direct assessment of the anterior and posterior communicating arteries as described previously (when possible) or by using the following supporting criteria: Collateral flow through the anterior communicating artery is confirmed by reversed flow in the ipsilateral anterior cerebral artery on the side with the ICA obstruction and an increase in the contralateral anterior cerebral artery velocity on the same side by 150%. The ipsilateral MCA also has reversed flow during ipsilateral CCA compression or decreased flow velocities during contralateral CCA compression if the anterior communicating artery is patent. Collateral flow through the posterior communicating artery is confirmed by an increase in the ipsilateral proximal posterior cerebral artery velocity that exceeds the middle cerebral artery velocity on the same side by 125%. There is also an increase in the ipsilateral posterior cerebral artery during compression of the ipsilateral common carotid artery if the posterior communicating artery is patent. Transcranial Doppler also has applications in evaluating patients with subclavian steal; flow around the vertebrobasilar junction, can be evaluated and directional effect established from the transoccipital window. Any cross-collateralization (including reversed flow in the basilar artery or retrograde filling of the internal carotid artery across collaterals in innominate occlusion and/or carotid steal can also be traced and documented. Individual vertebral artery compression (accomplished by applying digital pressure at the posterior slope of the mastoid) is sometimes used to determine the flow direction in the basilar artery and enhance the degree of collateral or contributing flow from the circle of Willis to the posterior circulation.

Intracranial Vasospastic Disorders

Cerebral artery spasm often follows subarachnoid hemorrhage and is a major contributing factor to stroke deaths. Angiography is the most accurate means of assessing vasospasm but is impractical for the follow-up period required to determine a spasm's onset and resolution. Mean velocity interpretation criteria published by Seiler and Aaslid were developed by correlated TCD results with angiographic comparisons of the MCA diameter velocities correspondingly increase as the vessel diameter reduces.

Normal	30 to 80 cm/sec
Mild spasm	120 to 140 cm/sec
Moderate spasm	140 to 200 cm/sec
Severe spasm	$\geq$ 200 cm/sec

Progression of spasm also has been followed by noting day-to-day changes in velocities; they have been observed to increase by more than 2 cm/sec per day patients who later progress to severe vasospasm. Transcranial Doppler's clinical value in evaluating vasospasm is in its ability to detect the flow velocity changes in evolving vasospasm before the onset of ischemic neurologic defects; this forewarning enables clinical mangement and prophylactic treatment to be given before severe problems occur.

Evaluation of Arteriovenous Malformations (AVM)

Like techniques used to evaluate arteriovenous fistulas in extremity arteries and grafts, transcranial Doppler can help locate feeding branch vessels and occasionally the AVM itself. The flow pattern in feeding arteries are similar to those seen in arteriovenous fistulas in the extremities; there is high-velocity, turbulent flow, sometimes with decreased pulsatility. In the AVM itself the flow may be bi-directional in nature and more prominently disturbed.

In a series published by Lindegaard *et al.* the average remote MCA mean velocity was between 44 to 94 cm/sec, tapering AVM feeder vessels had mean velocities of 75 to 124 cm/sec, and nontapering AVM feeder vessels had mean velocities of 90 to 237 cm/sec among 22 patients with cerebral AVMs.

Three-Dimensional Transcranial Doppler Scanning

In addition to the standard conventional transcranial Doppler method, another supplemental technique has been developed that combined standard transcranial Doppler with a mapping method similar to that used in the older ultrasonic arteriograph. The older technique was used to map flow presence and obtain samples in carotid bifurcation by cathode ray tube (CRT) recodings of audible traces during back-and-forth sweeps of Doppler probe over the cervical carotid arteries.

Three-Dimensional Colour Transcranial Doppler

It uses the same insonation techniques and protocols as conventional transcranial Doppler. Instead of a hand-held probe, however, this device uses a unique headpiece with integral 2-MHz transducers, fixed to a series of position registering X-Y-Z potentiometers (similar to B-scan arms) located on both sides of the headpiece. The patient is examined supine and the patient's head is carefully and correctly positioned so that it is straight within the headpiece. Insonation is performed via the windows described above. The sample volume's distance from the glabella and bregma and its location relative to the transducer are tracked in space by the computer software, allowing its location to be shown in a three-dimensional representation. As the sample is advanced or relocated and waveforms and samples are stored, colour-coded velocity indicators representing the flow direction and velocity at the evaluation point are manually plotted on the screen.

The colour map assigns specific shades to the sample point in 15 cm/sec steps based on the flow patterns at the sample site. Zero flow is grey. Flow towards the probe is shown (in ascending velocity order) as brown ($\geq$15 cm/sec), orange ($\geq$30 cm/sec), yellow ($\geq$45 cm/sec), and red ($\geq$60 cm/sec). Flow away from the probe is shown (in ascending velocity order) as dark blue ($\geq$15 cm/sec). Medium blue ($\geq$30 cm/sec), light blue ($\geq$45 cm/sec), and white (60 cm/sec). The Doppler waveforms and velocities at the sample site are stored at the plotted point for later recall. As the vessels are examined and the insonation sample points are plotted, an image is built up on the computer display that ultimately forms a colour-coded image map of the cerebral arteries and the hemodynamic characteristics alongwith their courses. Coronal, sagittal, and horizontal views of the resulting map can be displayed.

Colour-coded waveform spectra can be recalled from any point along the map and can also be displayed for hard-copy purposes.

This three-dimensional device is still widely used and has been beneficial in localizing and evaluating intracerebral artery stenosis, AVMs aneurysms, and potential occlusions. The mapping technique enables the abnormalities and their relations to significant portions of the circle of Willis to be compared and isolated, and the point-by-point Doppler waveform storage ability allows recall of flow dynamics and other calculations to be performed in a concise manner. This device also makes learning and performing TCD easier because of the simultaneous feedback provided by the combination of the visual spatial orientation map and the audio spectra. Despite its utility, this device will probably ultimately be supplemented by transcranial duplex imaging as that technology improves much as ultrasonic arteriography was made obsolete by the duplex scanner.

Transcranial Duplex Imaging

Although blind transcranial Doppler can show the intracranial hemodynamics, it does not provide a two-dimensional image of the cerebral relationships and vasculature. Transcranial duplex imaging is the next logical step and has recently become practical through technological advances and improvements in transducer technology.

The internal landmarks of the brain and intracranial vault can enable the examiner to obtain excellent images of the circle of Willis and can guide placement of the Doppler sample volume for precise measurement of the flow velocities in the arteries. An additional benefit is that angle correction can be used for (theoretically) more accurate velocity calculations.

In many ways, transcranial imaging is an evolution of real time neonatal echoencephalographic techniques applied as in adults.

Equipment: Transcranial imaging is performed with colour-flow duplex instrumentation equipped with transcranial-specific annotation and waveform analysis software. Imaging is accomplished through a phased array multielement sector transducer, usually at a 2 to 2.5 MHz image and 1.9 to 2.25 MHz Doppler transmit frequency. Most equipment displays the output power as a cranial thermal index per American Institute of Ultrasound in Medicine (AIUM) output display standards, especially given the recent approval of higher transmission power levels. The device is nonimaging 2-MHz pulsed Doppler transducer for additional blind TCD evaluations; the sample volume depth is graphically and numerically represented on the image in some systems for ease in tracking. Most of the spectral display features associated with transcranial Doppler devices are duplicated on transcranial imaging system.

Transcranial Imaging Techniques

Transcranial imaging requires a thorough knowledge of the appearance of intracranial vessels and the hemodynamics. Before attempting imaging, the reader should become completely familiar with the intracerebral anatomy and the transcranial Doppler examination principles described previously; transcranial imaging is an extension of almost the principles and technique covered. Unlike in TCD, once the arteries have been visualised, the examiner can move the sample directly to the identified artery of interest and sample at any point along the visualised artery or circle of Willis branch. An additional advantage of transcranial imaging is that the contralateral vascular anatomy is also seen deep in the same view, so that flow reversals in cross collateralization or areas of stenosis can be instantly identified with colour-flow imaging.

Transcranial imaging is accomplished through the same access windows into the cranium as in transcranial Doppler; the transtemporal, transoccipital (transforamenal or transunchal) and transorbital windows. The vessels that can be seen and monitored in each of the planes were described previously.

Transtemporal: ACA, MCA, PCA, and AcoA and PcoA.

Transoccipital: VA and BA and PCAs (Fig. 23.6).

Transorbital: OA and TICA (Figs 23.2 and 23.3).

When beginning the examination, the e-aminer should initially maximize the acoustic power (to the upper limit of 397 MW/cm^2 SPTA) until penetration is achieved and the arteries are seen, then should lower the power to the minimum levels needed to maintain good visualisation and colour filling. The PFR should be adjusted as low as possible to maintain sensitivity but avoiding aliasing of frequencies. Colour-flow and Doppler directional assignments should be set so that flow towards the transducer is coded as red and flow away from the transducer is coded as blue. This reflects the normal cerebral arterial flow characteristics and flow travels from the inner circle vessels outward. Vessels that are seen deep have opposite colour direction shades compared with arteries in the superficial area of the image. In the transtemporal approach (over the temporal bone above the zygomatic arch and anterior to the ear) the examiner should orient the transducer so that the scanning plane is in an axial orientation, with the transducer rotated so that the trailing edge to see the posterior circulation. Landmarks used to identify the proper insonation level and scan plane rotation included the mesencephalon, the lesser wing of the sphenoid, and the petrous pyramid of the temporal bone. Once the proper orientation is achieved, slight angulation and rotation may be needed to visualise the arteries; the MCA usually is seen paralleling to lesser wing of the sphenoid, and the PCA is seen near the mesencephalon. The P1 segment of the PCA (the segment proximal to the PcoA insertion) usually appears red, and the P2 segment (distal to the PcoA) appears blue. Although this plane shows the circle of Willis in its entirety in certain patients, this result is not to be expected. Even though the contralateral vascular anatomy may periodically be seen deep in the image, the examiner should scan both sides in each temporal windows to clearly and fully evaluate the vessels in an optimal fashion. In the transoccipital approach (with the transducer in the posterior neck aiming superiorly through the foramen magnum) an angled oblique coronal orientation should be obtained by having the patient pull the chin in, placing the transducer in the nuchal area at the junction of the skull and neck, and aiming the transducer towards the nasion (the dent above the bridge of the nose). The brain stem and spinal cord are the primary soft-tissue landmarks and the vertebral arteries are seen on either side wrapping anteriorly around them. The vertebro-basilar confluence and basilar artery are seen by angling upward, aiming more anteriorly, and using the posterior border of the foramen magnum (the base of occipital bone) as a bony landmark. Normally, image orientation shows the vertebral arteries as superficial on the image and the basilar artery as deep, with flow travelling away from the transducer. If the duplex scanner enables horizontal flipping of the image so that the transducer main bang can be shown at the bottom of the display, this may help the examiner orient the vertebrobasilar junction so that the vertebrals are on the bottom and the basilar on the top, as in life. The colour-flow in this plane may be inverted if the flipped display mode is adopted. Because the vertebrals and basilar are seldom symmetric, some angulation or rotation may be required to image and evaluate them; both vertebrals and the basilar junction are not always seen in the same plane. A perfect Y vertebrobasilar image is not to be expected, just as the Y of the carotid bifurcation is seldom obtained in carotid duplex examination. In the transorbital approach the examiner has the patient close the eye, then places the transducer over the eyelid and adjusts the output power to as low level as possible, again to avoid overexposing the lens of the eye. By angling posteriorly and tilting and rotating the transducer, the ophthalmic artery can be seen; the carotid canal portion of the ICA, the genu, and the TICA all can be seen from this approach by angling the transducer more towards the back of the head, then pivoting inferiorly and superiorly. The proximal ICA as red-coded flow is detected travelling anteriorly. Blue-coded flow is detected travelling away from the transducer in the TICA segment.

This examination should be repeated over each eye to ensure that both distal ICAs and ICAs are fully evaluated.

Table 23.1: *Ranges in transcranial Doppler diagnostic velocity criteria*

Cerebral vessel	Sample depth	PSV (cm/sec)	MV (cm/sec)	MF (KHz)
Middle cerebral artery	50–55 mm	95 ± 23	62 ± 12	1.4 ± 0.45
Anterior cerebral artery	65 mm	71 ± 18	51 ± 12	1.85 ± 0.35
Posterior cerebral artery	70 mm	56 ± 12	44 ± 11	1.53 ± 0.34
Terminal internal Carotid artery	55–70 mm	89 ± 23	37 ± 6.5	
Ophthalmic artery	40–55 mm	—	24 ± 8	
Basilar artery	85–100 mm	56 ± 13	41 ± 10	1.63 ± 0.33
Vertebral artery	60–80 mm	45 ± 18	36 ± 9	

PSV, peak systolic velocity; MV, mean velocity; MF, mean frequency.

Interpretation of Transcranial Image Data and Doppler Findings

The hemodynamics of the intracranial arteries have been throughly described. In keeping with this, anticipated normal colour-flow imaging patterns are described. Areas of stenosis or spasm should be seen as higher velocity streamline concentrations, with possible bruits in severely stenotic regions centering at the stenosis (just as in the carotid duplex examination).

The appearances of normal and abnormal Doppler directional waveforms obtained with transcranial imaging are identical to those obtained with blind transcranial Doppler. Although common carotid compressions are freely used to enhance or isolate collateral pathways in transcranial duplex should alert the examiner to the presence of occlusions and the existence of retrograde flow patterns. Compressions, however may augment these pathways for onscreen confirmation and VCR recordings. Transcranial imaging gives instant feedback on the presence and hemodynamic effect of subclavian and vertebrobasilar steal, since colour-flow directional changes are dramatically seen around the vertebrobasilar junction.

Velocity Criteria and Angle Correction

It would be expected that angle-corrected velocities would be more accurate than those specified for an assumed 0 to 30° angle of insonation and that new criteria would have to be developed.

Interestingly enough, a study by Fujioka, *et al.* found that angle corrected velocities were comparable with velocities established in previously existing TCD criteria tables with little if any clinical variation angles of insonation of less than 30° in all visualised vessels. Fujioka, *et al.* reached the conclusion that an examiner can confidently use established TCD criteria when the corrected angle is less than 30° in the cerebral arteries but cautions against using corrected velocities in cases where corrected angles are greater than 30°.

Carotid Duplex Sonography

Carotid duplex sonography should be the primary method used to evaluate the cerebrovascular system, with other methods used adjunctively. Although arteriography is still considered the gold standard by many, duplex correlation with surgical findings has proved quite accurate in many institutions and many surgeons perform endarterectomies based solely on the results of the carotid duplex examination. Carotid duplex sonography does not eliminate arteriography, however, for evaluating structures above the mandible or intracranially, especially regarding the many small cerebral vessels inaccessible to conventional Doppler imaging. Arteriograpy is also too risky and invasive for routine screening of patients with suspected carotid

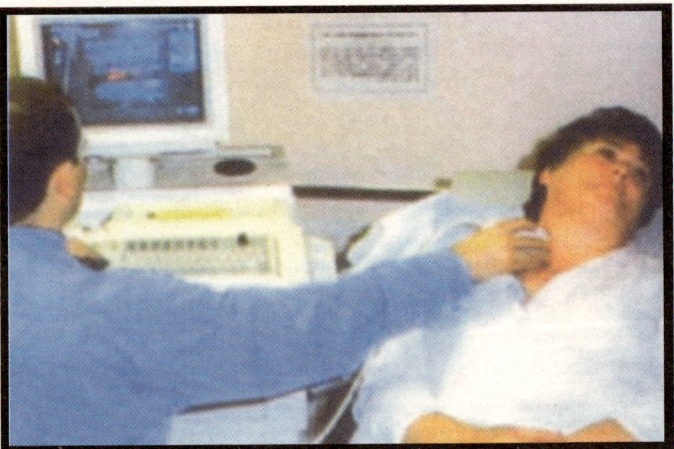

Fig. 23.12: Sonographer is performing Duplex carotid scan in patient with transient ischaemic attacks (recurrent)

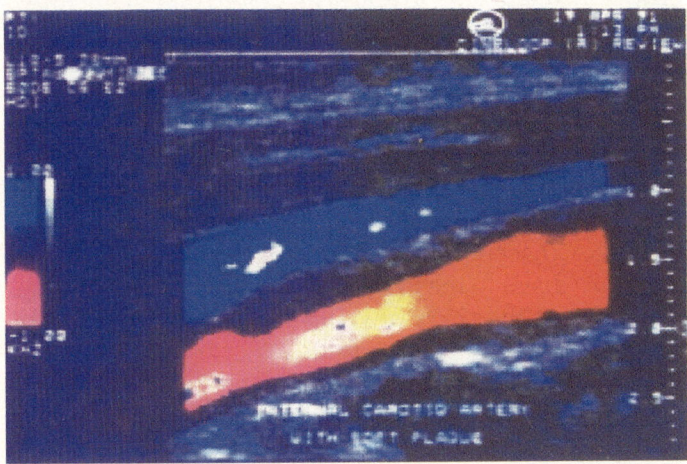

Fig. 23.13: Colour Duplex image showing internal carotid artery in red with a moderate stenosis characterised as soft plaque which carries a prognostic chemical value

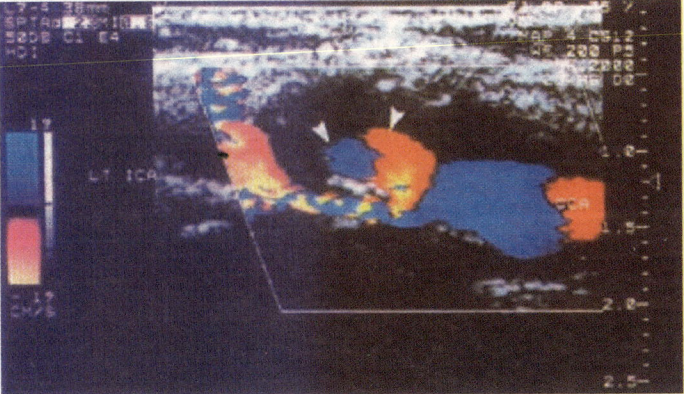

Fig. 23.14: Colour duplex scan of the carotid artery. The common carotid artery (CCA) is normal but there is severe stenosis of the internal carotid artery (ICA). It also shows increase in velocities across the stenosis and flow pattern is turbulent. There is also deep ulcer with in the plaque (arrow) just proximal to the stenosis

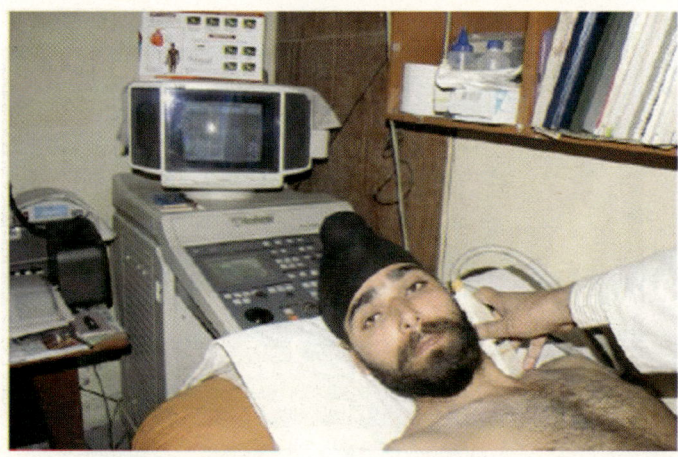

Fig. 23.15: Duplex color Doppler probe in the supraclavicular region for obtaining signatures of left subclavian artery

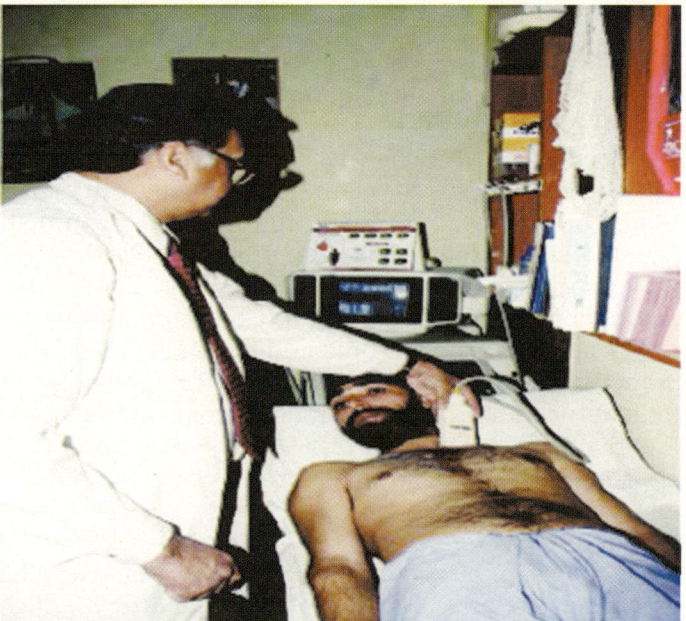

Fig. 23.16: Duplex color Doppler probe in the supraclavicular region for obtaining signatures of common cartoid artery

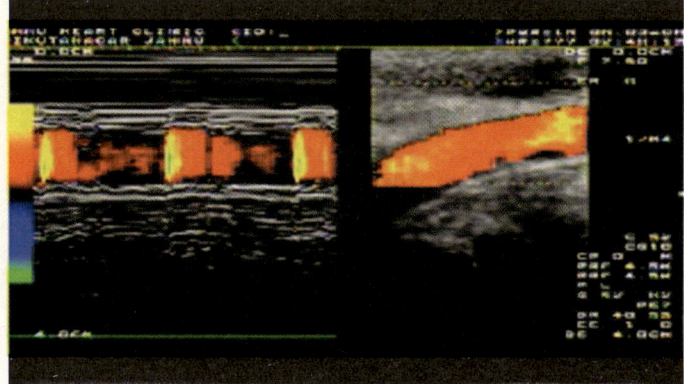

Fig. 23.17: M-Mode and color flow across normal common carotid artery and color flow across normal common carotid artery

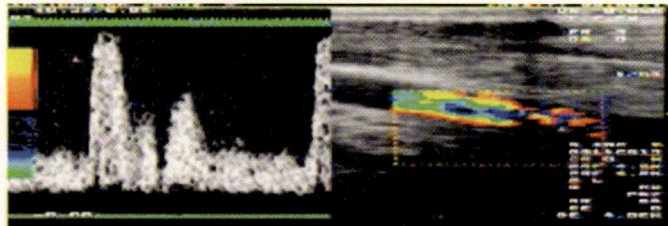

Fig. 23.18: Color flow and Doppler velocity across common carotid artery showing normal color flow and normal spectral waveforms

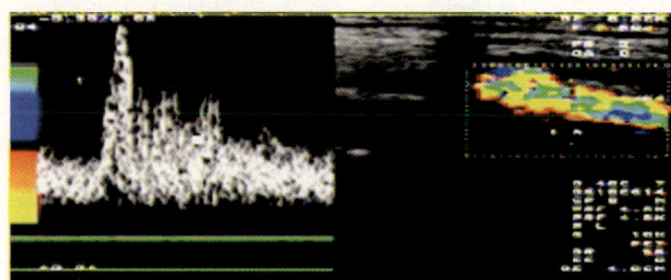

Fig. 23.19: Color flow and Doppler velocity across internal carotid artery showing normal color flow and normal spectral waveforms

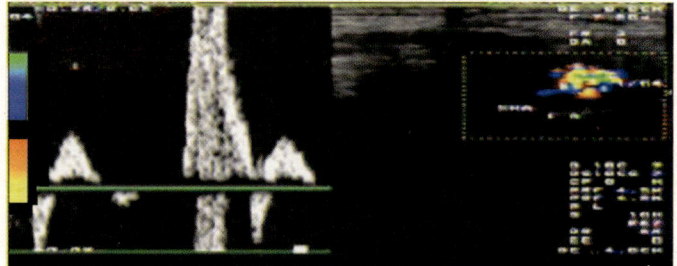

Fig. 23.20: Color flow and Doppler velocity across subclavian artery showing normal color flow and normal spectral waveforms

stenosis. In general, carotid imaging should never be performed without either duplex or direct carotid Doppler assessment, since imaging alone can miss a surprising number of carotid stenosis (Fig. 23.5A and B).

Description of the Carotid Duplex Real-Time Gray-Scale Image (Figs 23.10–23.14 and 23.17)

Before performing or interpreting an examination, the technologists or sonographer must have a thorough knowledge of the appearance and anatomy of the carotid system.

The common, internal, and external carotids appear to have sonolucent fluid-filled lumina bordered by two bright reflections on the arterial walls. The walls are lined with a low-level grey layer bordered by a fine, slightly brighter echo, thought to represent the intima of the arteries.

Orientation of the image can vary, depending on the make of duplex scanner, but commonly cephalad is to

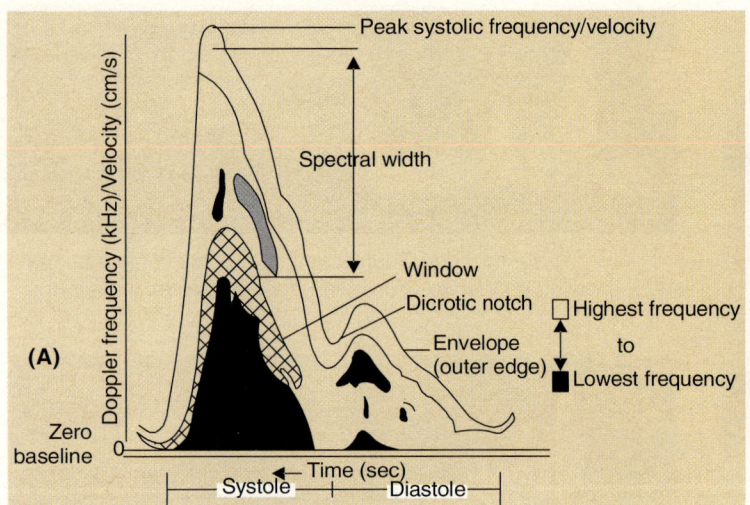

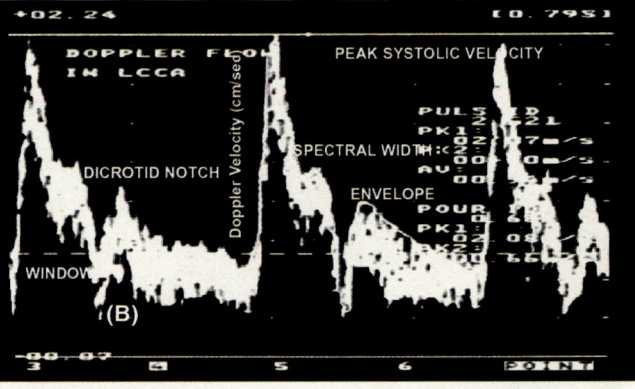

Prototype Configuration of Different Hemodynamic Points

Systole — Diastole — Systole — Diastole

Fig. 23.21A and B: (A) Graphic representation of various prototype hemodynamic points on carotid system. **(B)** Clinical application of these different points for derivation of hemodynamic data of left common carotid artery of normal approach

the left and cauded to right of the image in the longitudinal axis, with medial side of the body to the left of the image in transverse.

The common carotid artery can be followed superiorly from the supraclavicular area and lies medial to the trachea. The even parallel echoes of the common carotid wall can be traced distally.

Usually an irregular vessel without the thicker-walled characteristics of an artery is seen either anterior to or on one side of the common carotid. The internal jugular vein can be distinguished by its lack of pulsatility, its phasic dilation and collapse with respiration, its tendency to be irregularly shaped and to widen out at the base, and the ease with which it is collapsed by light pressure from the transducer. This is much more apparent when compared with the even diameter, thicker walls, regular pulsatility, and much more stable appearance of the common carotid.

As the transducer moves up the neck, the carotid is seen to widen out into the area of the carotid bulb. The bulb is the most common site of plaque and intimal thickening, which is usually seen to extend into the internal and/or external carotids directly above the bulb.

Contrary to what some believe, a perfect Y appearance of the carotid bifurcation is infrequently seen. The bifurcation tends to be rotated differently in certain individuals, and the appearance depends on the ability to obtain both vessels in the same view. For evaluation the internal and external carotids are best examined individually.

Longitudinally the internal carotid can be seen by moving the transducer in a posterior direction from the area of the bulb. It is a vessel generally of slightly larger diameter than the external carotid, tapering into regularly spaced walls that come off the bulb, a slight counterclockwise rotation of the probe (on the right side

of the neck) or clockwise rotation (on the left side of the neck) using the fingers should bring in the internal carotid origin.

The external carotid is seen by moving anteriorly and rotating the transducer central (Z) axis in a direction opposite that used to locate the internal carotid. It usually has a smaller diameter without the prominent widening frequently seen at the takeoff of the internal carotid. Branches (most commonly the superior thyroid artery near the origin or bulb and the lingual and facial branches above that) can usually be seen arising from the external carotid; finding branches confirms the visual identity of the external carotid since there are normally no branches off the internal carotid artery within the neck.

As stated several rare internal carotid branches of persistent fetal circulatory origin can occasionally be present. These are ascending pharyngeal artery (which comes off distal to the bifurcation), the proatlantal artery, the hypoglossal artery, and the trigeminal artery (the latter three of which come off high in the neck between the C-1 and C-3 vertebrae). The ascending pharyngeal may be seen by duplex scanning in those rare cases where it occurs at the bifurcation, since it may be mistaken for the superior thyroid artery. The internal and external are often transposed, the internal carotid lies medially and the external carotid laterally. The internal and external carotids also may be anterior and posterior, respectively, in one patient and inverted in another.

If there is doubt as to which artery is the internal and which is the external, several techniques can be used to assist in identification:

1. Look at the colour-flow imaging pattern. The internal carotid normally has a lower intensity of colour present throughout diastole, the external

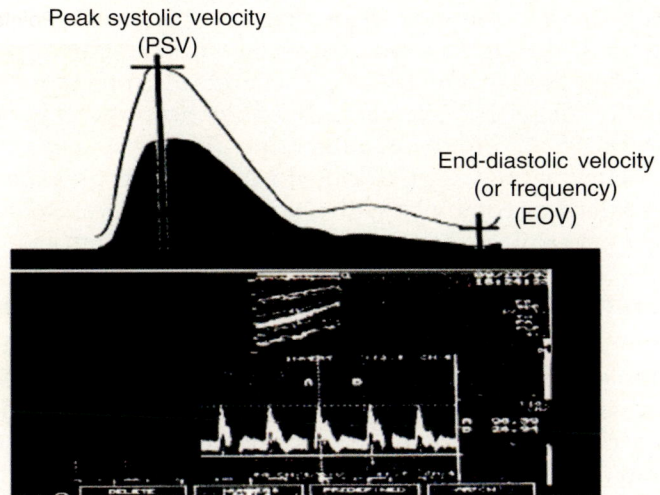

Peak systolic velocity
(PSV)

End-diastolic velocity
(or frequency)
(EOV)

Fig. 23.22: Normal Doppler spectral waveform from the common carotid artery

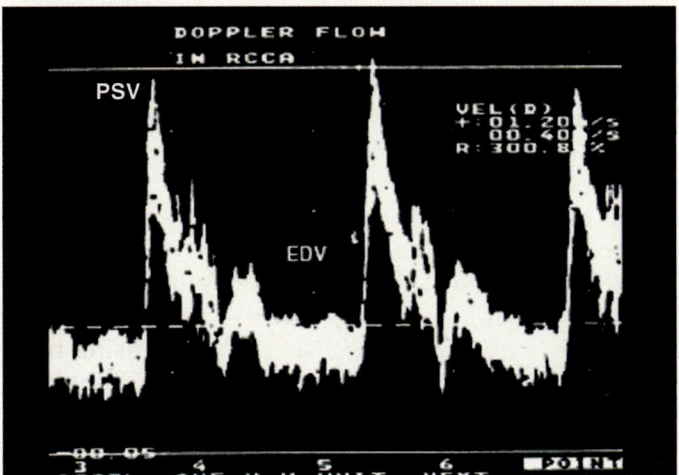

Fig. 23.23: Normal flow velocities as peak systolic and end-diastolic velocities in right common carotid artery in normal person

carotid often has more of an 'on-off' appearance as flow drops to near zero in diastole because of the higher resistance in the external carotid from the branches (Figs 23.15–23.17 and 23.20).

2. Obtain Doppler spectra from each vessel; again, a lower-resistance pattern with flow above the baseline in diastole normally characterizes the internal carotid artery (ICA) and a higher-resistance waveform similar to that of an extremity artery waveform normally characterizes the external carotid artery (ECA) (Figs 23.18–23.20).

3. In cases of distal disease or vertebral insufficiency, it is possible for the external carotid to become "internalized." Flow patterns adopt a lower resistance pattern as cerebral collateral demands increase.

Occlusion of either the internal or external carotid in these cases can make absolute visual identification nearly impossible by gray-scale, colour-flow imaging, or Doppler. The examiner can perform temporal artery percussion to identify the external carotid. This technique is performed by first monitoring the arterial signal in the questioned bifurcation vessel using duplex and Doppler spectral waveforms; the examiner next should palpate the ipsilateral superficial temporal artery on the temple in front of the ear lobe and feel for the pulse. Once located, the examiner should rhythmically and rapidly compress and release (vibrate) the temporal artery and determine if there is any audible and visible effect on the signal in the artery being examined. If the artery being examined is the internal carotid, no effect on the signal occurs. If the artery is the external carotid, the rhythmic compressions cause short peaks in the signal (most visible in distole) from brief flow reversal through the branch. The technique cannot be used reliably, if the external carotid is occluded or the temporal artery pulse cannot be palpated.

When evaluating transversely, the common carotid appears as a rounded lumen posterior or lateral to the irregularly shaped jugular vein. The normal carotid retains its round appearance to the level of the bulb, where the diameter of the vessel becomes larger and begins to elongate as the bifurcation approaches.

The internal and the external carotids are seen as two separate round lumina emerging from the bulb as the transducer moves superiorly. The internal is larger than the external and positioned slightly posterior to the smaller round lumen of the external.

Disease in the carotid appears as low to moderate gray, soft and smooth to irregularly edged deformations of the intima extending into the lumen. Calcific plaque is a bright echo with sonic dropout extending past the lesion. Calcific plaque can be incorporated into a "soft" (medium-to-low echogenic) plaque and is troublesome when the area of dropout obscures the deep wall and a superficial wall plaque is present. Ulcerated plaque can be seen as indentations or erosions in either soft-tissue plaque or the intima.

Description of Carotid Duplex
Colour-Flow Characteristics (Figs 23.15–23.25)

The normal colour-flow pattern in the carotid artery system appears as uniform shades of red with a concentrated flow streamline. An area of blue flow reversal or flow separation normally occurs at the carotid bulb, but the appearance of shades of blue within the normal red colour pattern indicative of turbulence or flow disturbance, with the exception of some artifacts. Sometimes this disturbance is an expected normal variation, such as in the post-endarterectomy vessel. In

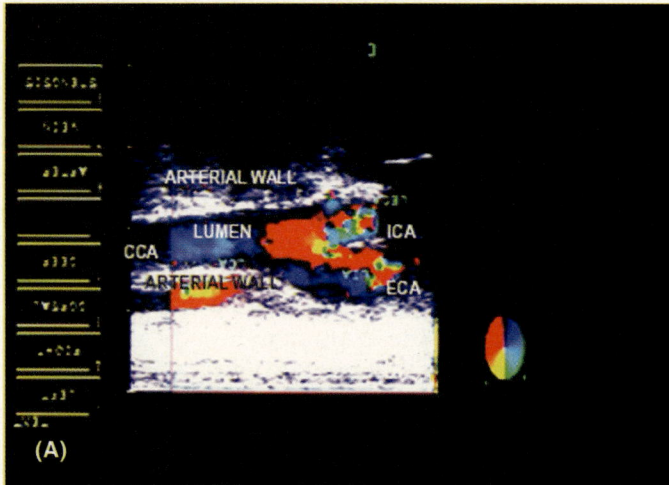

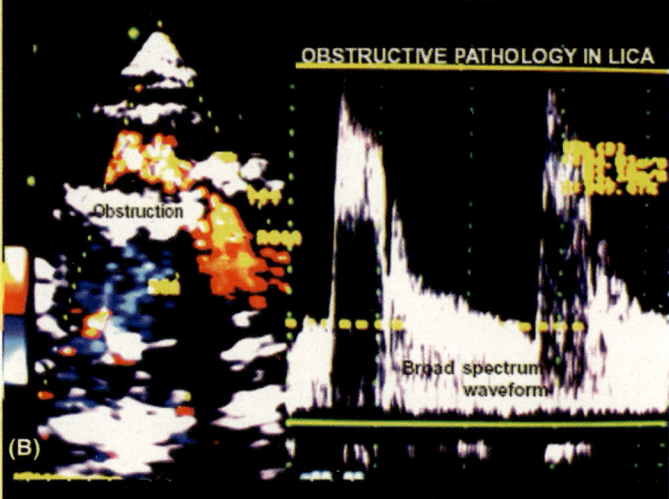

Fig. 23.24A and B: (A) Color flow supraclavicular approach with hyperextended neck in lateral position showing normal anatomical localisation of carotid arterial system, i.e. CCA = Common carotid artery, ECA = External carotid artery, ICA = Internal carotid artery. (B) Color Doppler flow velocity across left internal carotid artery showing marked obstructive pathology with irregular lumen (left scan) with increased in flow velocity >4.0 m/sec and broadened spectral waveforms (right)

factors in angle correction, because flow is seldom laminar through a stensosis. Axial and tangential flow jets can exist that might affect accurate alignment of the vector alone. The examiner must not, however, rely on colour-flow alone to determine flow velocities or patency of the vessel; colour-flow is most accurate and useful when combined with Doppler spectral waveforms and gray-scale evaluation with the colour turned off.

Examination Technique in Carotid Duplex Sonography

There are as many ways of holding and guiding the duplex transducer as there are types of transducers the vascular technologist may encounter. In spite of this the approach to imaging the carotids and vertebrals and obtaining duplex Doppler information from them is basically the same for all machines.

The patient should lie supine with the head and shoulders lying on a pillow and the neck extended back to allow the examiner full access to the neck and supraclavicular area. The examiner requires the duplex scanner, a video-type recorder, a hardcopy printer or camera, and, optionally, a continuous-wave Doppler for blood-pressure measurement and periorbital examination (Figs 23.12–23.14).

In the majority of duplex scanners, the image display should be oriented so that when imaging longitudinally, the head of the patient is to the left of the screen. Following standard ultrasound imaging protocol on duplex scanner, however, orients the image sideways so that the patient's head may be at the top of the screen when the right side is being examined, and inverts the image when the left side is being examined. Some of the images accompanying the text are in this format and are so noted. When imaging transversely, the medial side of the patient should be towards the left as well. Older biosound units place the medial side at the top of the image when examining the right side and at the bottom when examining the left side.

Initially, the carotids should be examined in the longitudinal plane. Three longitudinal approaches, or positions, afford optimal visualisation of the neck vessels and allow almost the entire visible circumference of the carotids to be evaluated. Although the technologist should eventually synthesize all these positions into one smooth longitudinal examination, each of the approaches is discussed individually.

The first position used is the anterior position. The patient should turn his or her head to the left side to expose the right side of the neck, and the vice versa when examining the left carotid. The sagittal plane of the head should be at about a 45° angle to the surface of the bed. The neck is oriented for long-axis imaging. To obtain as true anterior view as possible, the examiner should come in directly parallel with the sagittal plane of the neck.

most cases, however, it implies the presence of stenosis and can occur on the downstream side of an obstruction within ulcerated areas, or along irregular plaque surfaces.

If colour becomes regularly absent in the common or internal carotid artery at some point in the cardiac cycle as is seen in diastole—an "on-off" pattern, a distal occlusion may be implied. Absence of colour in diastole may, however, normally occur in the external carotid artery, since this finding characterizes a high-resistance vascular structure.

The streamline can be useful guide to the examiner, not only in determining the presence, location, and degree of stenosis, but also in size adjustment and placement of the simple volume for Doppler spectral waveform acquisition. Streamlines are also important

The examiner then examines the common carotid from the base to the bifurcation in long axis, being careful to show the artery continuously. Slight side-to-side motion of the transducer is used to pick up plaque, which may project from a lateral wall parallel the plane of the examination. It is noted, recorded on the videotape, or photographed for later reference.

On reaching the bifurcation, the examiner moves the transducer anteriorly and posteriorly to determine the takeoffs of the external and internal carotids at the bifurcation.

When the position and identification of each artery are determined, the examiner checks to see if any disease is present in the common carotid, bulb, and bifurcation areas. The transducer is moved accordingly to show the extent and degree of occlusion of the disease. Areas of disease are documented and the positioning described.

The examiner then determines the position of the internal carotid and moves the transducer posteriorly toward the ear, while rotating it slightly along the plane of the long axis of the artery. The ICA is followed up as high as practicable.

The transducer next is moved anteriorly and rotated or angled to demonstrate the external carotid. As much of the artery as possible should be demonstrated. The anterior view is not the best, since the probe comes against the mandible within the area of the bifurcation. It can, however, show disease that is not well seen in the other long-axis views.

The patent should turn his or her head a little more to facilitate the lateral position. The transducer is

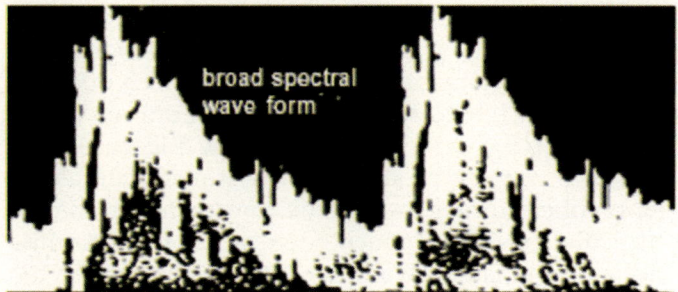

Fig. 23.27: Moderate (50–75% luminal reduction) there is broader spectral and diastolic velocity is less than width, more filling of window, turbulence systolic velocity is more than 120 cm/sec and diastolic velocity is less than 100 cm/sec

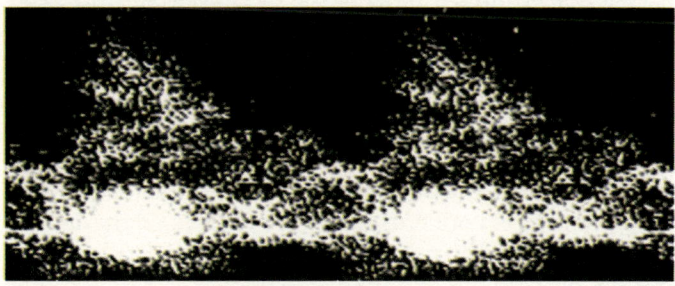

Fig. 23.28: Severe (75–99% luminal reduction) there is severe turbulence, concentration is towards baseline window is absent, peak systolic velocities exceed 150 cm/sec and end-diastolic velocity more than 100 cm/sec

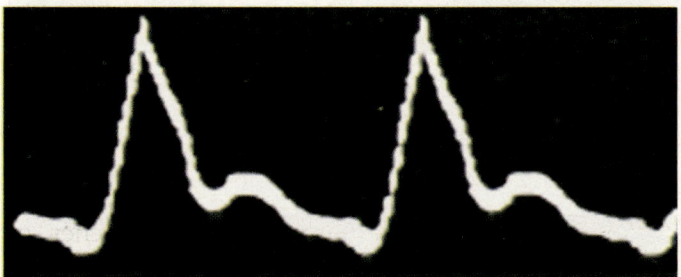

Fig. 23.25: Narrow spectral width, window clear using pulsed Doppler velocity peak does not exceed 100 cm/sec

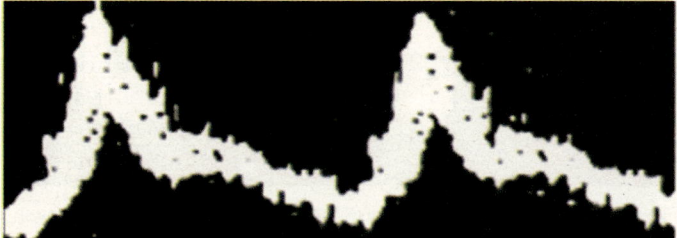

Fig. 23.26: Mild (15–50% luminal reduction) there is increased in spectral width. Window is less clear. The peak velocity still remains within normal limits

brought around so that the beam intersects the artery perpendicular to sagittal plane of the head.

The patient should then turn his or her head as far as possible. In the posterior position the transducer is brought in from behind the sternocleidomastoid muscle and angled towards the anterior side of the patient. The arteries are located and examined as above. The common and bifurcation vessels may be deep in this view and not readily visualised. The Y appearance of the bifurcation tends to be seen in this position more often than in any other (Fig. 23.24A and B).

As stated previously, these three positions can be combined into one smooth scan with the examiner compensating and instinctively turning the transducer, rocking the transducer, and shifting planes. When videotaping, the examiner should be certain to note position, where the transducer is being moved, what vessels are being imaged, the nature of the plaque and vessel walls, and the orientation of the vessel (e.g. cephalad is to the left of the image).

The carotid should appear as one continuous parallel structure and it is important to show continuity (i.e. common carotid artery (CCA) to bulb, ECA connections to bulb, ICA origin, and bulb) even in case of tortuosity, since the jugular vein is located close to the carotid; maladjusted technical factors or slip of the probe by an inattentive sonographer can often make the jugular seem to be part of the carotid (or even to be mistaken for it).

Some tips may help when imaging the carotids in the longitudinal plane. A common mistake of sonographers is to hold the wrist rigid when scanning, which does not allow him or her to follow the natural curves of the carotid. Keep the wrist loose, and use the fingers as pivot joints. Do not try to strangle the transducer. Also, sonographers forget to rock the transducer or change planes and positions, which often causes them to miss plaque on the lateral wall. In contrast, some move too much, sweeping past the very structures in the carotids are very small and that you are imaging a vessel that is less than a centimeter in diameter to adjustments involve minimal motions of the transducer.

When scanning the neck, the examiner should hold the transducer around the body of the housing so that the little finger is actually in contact with the neck, this allows greater control and eliminates some of the hand and wrist fatigue that can result from holding it at the base end. This position also stabilises the transducer better, and thus the probe is less likely to wander when the examiner is concentrating on controls or the image display. At the bifurcation, this position also helps in that the examiner can anchor the heel of the transducer where the little finger is at the bifurcation point and rotate the transducer along the Y-axis, using the thumb and fingers for more precise definition of the internal and external carotids. Remember that the common carotid is major landmark; if you get lost while searching for the internal or external, reorient the transducer to the common carotid and begin moving cephalad again.

When using colour-flow imaging, optimal colour filling and saturation are obtained by setting the thresholds so that colour ends at the vessel walls and does not "bleed" over into the intima or neck tissues. In longitudinal imaging the examiner may have to use a heal-toe technique along the longitudinal axis of the transducer to increase or decrease the Doppler angle and improve colour-flow resolution. In transverse imaging the transducer should be angled slightly cephalad along the transverse axis to evoke a Doppler shift and ensure that flow away from the transducer appears in the proper colour. In tortuous vessels the examiner may have to periodically invert the colour assignments in the artery.

The arteries should be completely evaluated with grey scale only and colour-flow off, if any areas of increased colour-flow intensity are seen that cannot be accounted for by the joint colour-flow grey scale image; colour-flow can obscure important grey-scale pathology if the flow patterns cross lateral wall lesions. Turning colour-flow imaging off also increases the grey-scale sensitivity of the system. It is a good idea to perform one scanning pass with the colour-flow off and another with colour flow to ensure that significant pathology has not been obscured.

Once the longitudinal images are obtained, the examiner should turn the probe 90° to image the carotid arteries in the transverse plane. Although there is only one position here, the transducer can be directed at angles around the circumference of the neck.

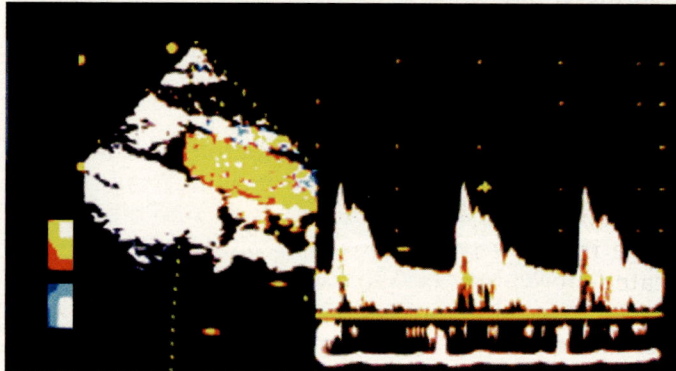

Fig. 23.29: Color Doppler scan of left internal carotid artery showing increased peak velocity, wider spectral width, very narrow window in 50–75% intraluminal obstruction

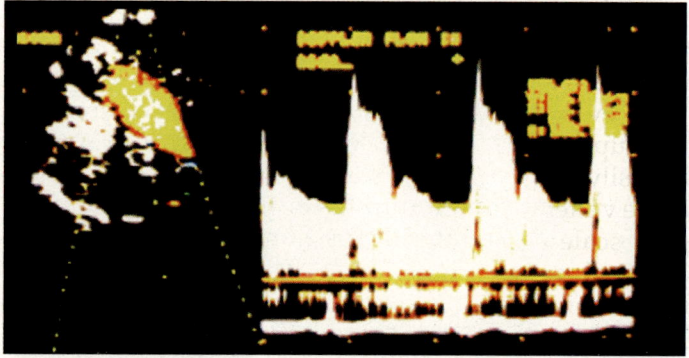

Fig. 23.30: Color Doppler scan of right internal carotid artery showing increased peak velocity, almost negligible window, wider spectral width in 75% intraluminal stenosis

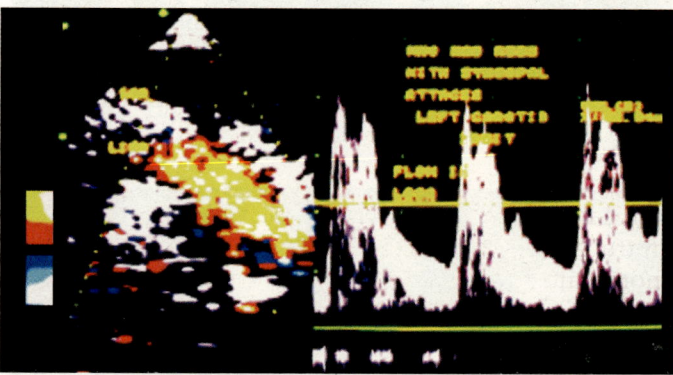

Fig. 23.31: Color Doppler scan of left internal carotid artery showing roughed and irregular luminal morphology, enhanced peak velocity, visible spectral width, mosaic color in nearly 50% intraluminal stenosis in a patient who had left carotid bruit associated with recurrent syncopal attacks

The transducer should be placed at the clavicle level and slowly moved cephalad, following the common carotid to the bulb and bifurcation. Special attention should be given to documenting any plaque formations in the longitudinal views.

The area of the bifurcation should be evaluated for circumferential or partly obstructive plaques that may be at the origins, but not extending into the internal or external carotids. The transducer can then be moved cephalad further to image the internal and external carotids. They should be followed cephalad as far as practicable. In cases where the internal and external carotids bifurcate at odd angles or run deep to the transducer, accurate evaluation may not be possible.

The internal carotid is generally but not always located posterior to the external carotid, with the external carotid positioned superficially to the deeper internal carotid on the duplex image. The examiner should bear in mind that anatomic variations frequently occur where the external carotid appears as the deeper vessel and may actually be posterior on the neck to the internal carotid. Again, the best ways to isolate and identify the bifurcation vessels are by using Doppler waveforms, colour-flow pattern recognition, and temporal artery percussion in conjunction with the image appearance.

The vertebral arteries should always be included in the duplex evaluation of the carotids because they can be easily evaluated in the longitudinal plane. The origins of the vertebral arteries are often easier to evaluate using grey scale duplex to rule out disease of the origins although some individuals do not have satisfactory body habitus to enable easy visualisation of the origins. The main trunks of the verterbral arteries can be imaged between the transverse processes of the cervical vertebrae; they are especially easy to see using colour-flow imaging.

The transducer is placed in long axis lateral to the common carotid and above the clavicle, then moved laterally and slightly cephalad. Look for regularly spaced areas of shadowing with what appear to be vessel walls between them, then attempt to follow the vessel to its origin at the subclavian. Following the subclavian artery laterally starting at the carotid area and looking for the vertebral origin. The vertebral is often easier to find on the right side, since the examiner can trace the origin of the right common carotid to the innominate artery and then follow the subclavian artery laterally from the innominate-carotid bifurcation to the vertebral origin.

Duplex Doppler Spectral Waveform Acquisition

Greyscale and colour-flow imaging evaluation of the carotid system can demonstrate the presence of disease and allow approximate degree of stenosis to be ascertained, but these modalities alone are insufficient to accurately grade the percentage and hemodynamic significance of the stenosis. Examiner must acquire duplex Doppler spectral waveforms from appropriate sites to document the flow states at each level of the carotid system (Figs 23.25–23.31).

During the imaging portion of the examination, the duplex Doppler should be used primarily for vessel identification and initial estimates of flow so that the examiner can concentrate on identifying the presence, location, and extent of any disease present. Once the examiner has become familiar with the location of visible plaque or stenosis, a systematic evaluation of the Doppler hemodynamics should be performed.

Duplex Doppler Spectral Waveforms should be Routinely Taken and Recorded from the Following

1. The proximal common carotid artery.
2. The distal common carotid artery, just below the bulb (Figs 23.21–23.23).
3. The internal carotid artery about 1 cm distal to its origin, away from the flared takeoff.
4. The external carotid artery about 1 cm distal to its origin.
5. The vertebral artery, either in the proximal pre-cervical segment or between two vertebral interspaces.

The above waveforms are sufficient in a normal carotid system. If prominent plaque is present and appears to comprise a significant stenosis either by visual estimation or with colour-flow imaging, then additional waveforms should be obtained:

1. At the point of maximum stenosis, where velocities appear to be the highest.
2. Downstream to the stenosis, to document the hemodynamic effect distally.

These additional waveforms should be obtained at all stenotic sites within the common, internal, and external carotids, preferably in the longitudinal scan plane.

As each spectral waveform is obtained, the examiner should angle correct the flow vector, using colour-flow imaging to align the vector along the streamline. Electronic calipers should then be used on the spectral waveforms to measure two specific velocity factors for documentation and later interpretation. These factors are the peak systolic velocity (or frequency) and the end-diastolic velocity (or frequency). Bear in mind that Doppler velocities obtained in a transverse position cannot be angle corrected because the precise angle of flow insonation is unknown. If some estimation of flow is required in these cases, frequency criteria should be used rather than velocity criteria.

The peak systolic velocity (PSV) or frequency is measured at the peak of the systolic component of the

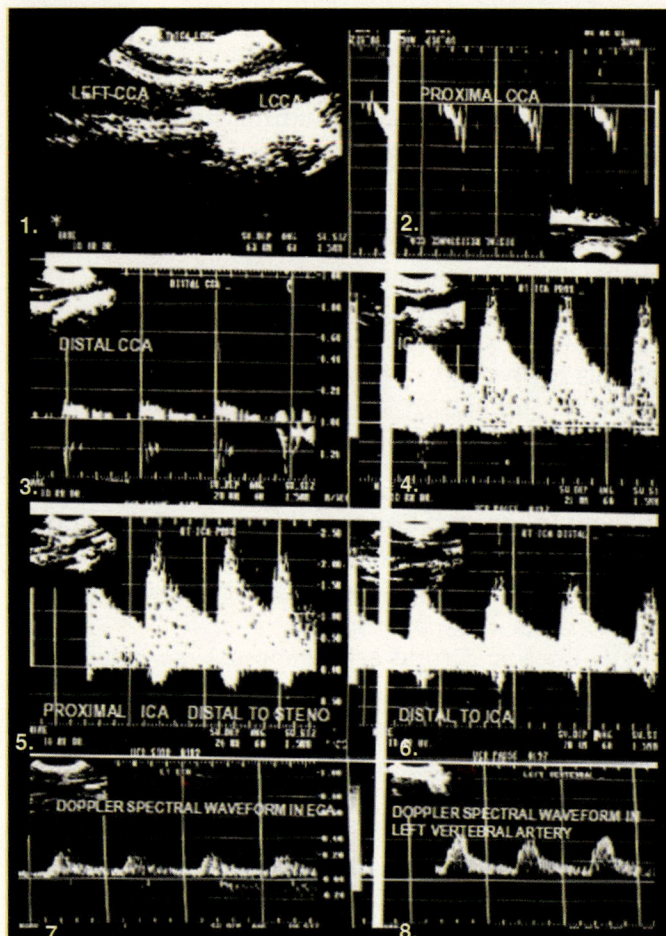

Fig. 23.32: 1. Ultrasonic scan of distal left CCA and proximal ICA, 2. High resistance Doppler spectral waveform in proximal CCA, 3. Preocclusive disturbed Doppler spectral waveform in distal CCA, 4. High velocity Doppler spectral waveform across ICA stenosis, 5. High velocity Doppler spectral waveform in proximal ICA just distal to stenosis with severe baseline turbulence, 6. Disturbed stenotic Doppler spectral waveform in distal ICA, 7. Doppler spectral waveform in the ECA, 8. Antergrade Doppler spectral waveform in vertebral artery

waveform. The end-diastolic velocity (EDV) or frequency is measured at the lowest point to diastole, usually at the end of the cardiac cycle just before the initial upslope of another systolic peak.

Carotid Duplex Examination Protocol

The following is a sample examination protocol that summarizes the technique used to evaluate the carotid system:

1. Begin in a longitudinal position and evaluate the common, internal, and external carotid arteries with grey scale and colour-flow imaging, evaluating the vessels for plaque and the presence of stenosis. Use the anterior, lateral and posterior imaging planes as needed to optimally visualise the vessels. If the common carotid origin and subclavian area can be seen, include these in the examination.
2. Obtain routine Doppler spectral waveforms from sample sites. In the proximal and distal CCA, the proximal and distal ICA, and the ECA. Additional waveforms should be obtained distal to areas of stenosis.
3. Rotate the transducer to a transverse position and evaluate the common carotid from the base of the neck, scanning cephalad to evaluate the entire cervical carotid system to above the mandible level, if possible. Be certain that image orientation is consistent and demonstrate the bulb, ICA, and ECA as completely as possible.
4. Evaluate the vertebral artery from the origin and within the cervical segment, and document flow direction and appearance.
5. Repeat steps 1 to 4 for the contralateral side. (Some institutions, incidentally, prefer to switch steps 1 and 3, starting in transverse.)

Interpretation of the Carotid Duplex Image

Interpretation of the image result, must take into account the Doppler spectral findings and those of colour-flow imaging. Making a diagnosis based on the image alone can result in a partial and often inaccurate diagnosis, especially if colour-flow imaging is not available.

By the same token, direct carotid Doppler studies or periorbital examination performed with continuous-wave probes and are only diagnostic when a stenosis is severe enough to cause significant hemodynamic alteration or turbulence.They also do not permit exact identification of the location of the stenosis and cannot generally isolate multiple stenosed segments.

Criteria for Defining and Localizing Carotid Disease

Characterizing and categorizing the visual data obtained in the cerebrovascular system can vary highly subjective and often open to variation in individual interpretation.

Although many investigators have attempted to determine what morphologic processes are taking place in a plaque (e.g., hemorrhage calcification), atherosclerotic plaque that is visualised is generally characterized as homogeneous in appearance. The presence of distinct ulceration should not be diagnosed unless the ulcer is deep and can be documented in both longitudinal and transverse images. Plaque surfaces are best classified as either smooth or irregular.

Plaque Morphology and Sonographic Characteristics
(Figs 23.13 and 23.14)

The progressive changes in morphology and categories of plaque can be distinguished by certain patterns of appearance. The fatty streak plaque as a low-to moderate-level grey homogeneous thickening or elevations of the intima, extending into the lumen from one or both walls. The intima normally follows the vessel walls closely, making intimal thickening or plaque dramatically obvious when well visualised. This appearance is also typical of so-called soft plaque and thrombus.

The fibrous plaque appear as a moderate to highly echogenic luminal irregularity or focal plaque, "mixed plaque". Low-level grey areas often are found alongside areas of higher echogenicity. These appear as elevations and focal enlargements into the lumen.

The calcified plaque is bright with high echogenicity and sonic dropout extending deep and parallel with the beam path. The inability of the ultrasound beam to penetrate calcific plaque often obscures areas deep to the plaque and can obliterate the lumen, making stenosis calculation almost impossible across the plaque area. Relocation of the transducer may be necessary to look around the area of calcification. If colour-flow imaging is used, flow windows can be detected more easily between shadows for Doppler sample volume placement. The colour-flow streamline and presence or absence of turbulence on the distal side of a plaque shadow can also help the examiner determine whether the calcific shadow obscures a hemodynamically significant lesion.

The complex plaque may have a speckled appearance, with areas of calcification. The calcium and denser-appearing areas are often the result of necrosis or intraplaque hemorrhage. The lesion also may have an extremely irregular and pock-marked appearance on the intimal side; in some cases the fine line of the intimal lining can appear disrupted in places. Although a cratered appearance may be noted and even the occasional ulceration, ulcers should not be identified as such unless they are deep enough to be shown clearly in longitudinal and transverse planes; colour-flow imaging also may confirm the presence of a flow pocket within the plaque.

Complete arterial occlusion usually is identified by one of the following distinctive image appearances:

1. A lumen completely filled with soft specular echoes distal to a patent vessel.
2. A lumen completely filled with bright, hetero-geneous echoes distal to a patent vessel.
3. A chronically atrophied vessel distal to a dense echogenic plaque at the origin. The artery often tapers abruptly and may appear smaller than an accompanying vessel, especially in the transverse plane.

In some cases the artery segment distal to a complete occlusion reconstitutes from collaterals or from retrograde flow through the external carotid system. There is usually a distinct border between the occluded and patent segments of the vessel, often at the origin of the occluded artery. Colour-flow imaging demonstrates this well.

Flow is not detectable within the occluded artery using Doppler spectral waveforms proximal to an occlusion become characteristic of high resistance and colour-flow imaging changes and can also alert the examiner to the presence of a distal occlusion.

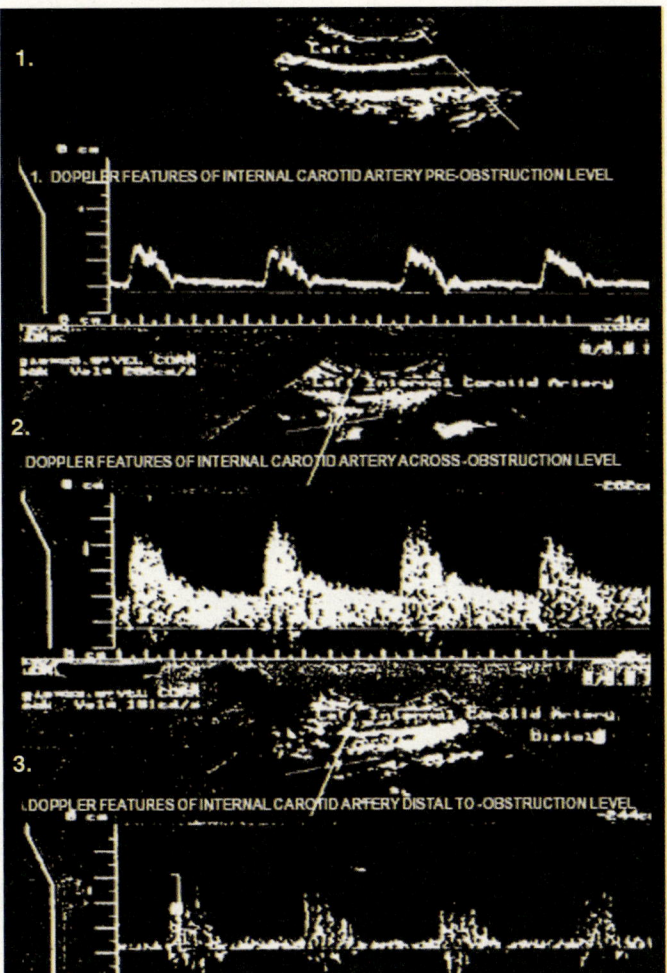

Fig. 23.33: 1. Doppler characteristics pre-stenosis are normal peak velocity, good window and no wider spectral width in the internal carotid artery, 2. Alternations across to the obstruction are higher peak velocity, wider spectral waveform width and least window 3. Distal to the obstruction are, least peak velocity, tubulance, least spectral width, no window and even retrograde flow can be seen

Atypical Sonographic Abnormalities of the Carotid Artery

Carotid Aneurysms

Aneurysms appear as widely dilated or ectatic areas of the common carotid, bulb, internal carotid, or external carotid but occur more frequently in the bulb or area of the internal carotid. Plaque formation, mural thrombus, calcification, and occasionally dissection of the artery may occur in combination with an aneurysm. Aneurysmal dilation usually is quite distinct compared with the normal widening of the carotid bulb area or origin of the internal carotid. It is important to note that patients are referred for suspected aneurysm in the low neck or supraclavicular region, with a prominent pulsatile mass noted. These pulsatile masses very often turn out to be prominent normal, subclavian arteries or common carotid origins, which are usually superficial and project into the supraclavicular fossa, thus the examiner should evaluate any suspected aneurysm carefully.

Carotid Dissection

Carotid dissection is not common but may manifest sonographically as a characteristic "extra lumen" within the confines of a relatively uniform-appearing carotid artery. Colour-flow patterns usually make this diagnosis easier because retrograde flow may be seen in the false channel and regular antegrade flow in the true channel. Grey scale imaging at an angle perpendicular to the dissection may help visualise the septumlike dissected inner wall. Careful evaluation with grey-scale, colour-flow imaging, and Doppler spectral sampling may help reveal the inflow point. In some cases a flow entrance and a flow exit may also be detected.

Unstable Lesions

The examiner should be alert to the existence of any number of unstable lesions that may occasionally be detected during the course of the carotid duplex examination. These are distinct dynamic intravascular phenomena that move or have motion within, as opposed to the typical stationary plaque. These lesions can, among other forms, manifest as loose intimal flaps; free-floating moving thrombus, pseudovalves, or partially organized liquefied thrombus within an ulcerated plaque. The main concern, is that of a potential embolic event occuring, should part or all of the visualised material break free and travel cephalad. The examiner may initially see something unusual moving within the lumen or some unaccounted for colour-flow pattern, if this occurs, turn the colour off and optimize the grey scale image and focal transmit zones to allow the clearest image possible. The examiner may need to change imaging planes to catch the phenomenon at the best angle of incidence.

Extracarotid Lesions

Extracarotid lesions, such as carotid body tumors may be detected on a carotid duplex examination; these appear as soft-tissue homogeneous masses resembling the sonographic texture of the thyroid gland but with tumor neovasculature often defined within the parenchyma of the mass. These benign or malignant masses may appear in between the internal and external carotid as outgrowths of the carotid body chemoreceptor and may expand to encompass both vessels at the bifurcation. Although the artery walls may appear to be incorporated into the mass, the lumens usually remain patent. Colour-flow imaging can greatly assist the branching colour-flow patterns of the tumor, since the branching colour-flow patterns of the tumor neovasculature are easily recognizable.

Method of Calculating Luminal Reduction

Stenoses that are visualised can be measured using the scanners integrated calipers. Two types of measurements are generally obtained on carotid artery images. Diameter calculations are performed on longitudinal images; the examiner first measures the diameter of the artery from superficial wall to deep wall with one set of calipers, and then measures the diameter of the residual lumen at the point of maximal stenosis. The residual luminal diameter is divided by the vessel diameter to give an estimated percentage of diameter stenosis.

Residual Lumen Diameter/Vessel Diameter = Percentage of Diameter Stenosis.

This calculation is not always accurate because it depends on assuming that the plaque is symmetric in the sagittal plane being evaluated; eccentric stenoses thus cannot always be accurately measured. Direct diameter measurements compare well with area of stenosis measurements but, because of the technique, seldom agree with arteriographic diameter measurements. Arteriographic diameter stenosis measurements assume that the true lumen diameter is in the straight portion distal to the dilated origin of the internal carotid; the point of maximal narrowing is then measured and again calculated (Figs 23.22 and 23.23).

The potential discrepancy is that angiograms only provide a physiologic image of a filled vessel lumen and do not show soft tissue architecture, so what may appear as a 50% or more sonographic stenosis may not calculate as a significant stenosis by arteriogram. If, ultimately, measurement correlations with arteriograms are desired, the examiner should perform diameter calculations on the ultrasound image at the same estimated locations that an arteriographer uses on an arteriographic image. The examiner should be aware, however, that interobserver and intraobserver interpretations of angiographic results vary widely and correlation may not be consistent. Area stenosis measurements are made using electronic calipers on transverse images; the examiner first traces the inner circumference of the residual lumen. The resulting area measurements are usually provided in square millimeters. The residual lumen area is divided by the vessel area, then that result is subtracted from 1; the result, multiplied by 100, equals the estimated percentage of area stenosis.

Area stenosis calculations can reliably assess asymmetric stenoses and often correlate very accurately with corresponding Doppler velocity criteria. One problem with area stenosis calculations, however, is that there is no similar cross-sectional arteriographic measurement; the closest arteriographic equivalent requires biplaner arteriography and summary estimation of the cross-sectional diameter.

Diameter and area stenosis measurement of the plaque and the vessel can often give a better luminal reduction estimate than by visual estimations but if they are obtained, these physical measurements should be correlated and combined with the hemodynamic criteria for estimated stenosis.

Identification and Interpretation of Abnormal Carotid Colour-Flow Imaging Patterns (Figs 23.32 and 23.33)

As mentioned, colour-flow imaging patterns in the carotid system correspond well to the flow patterns shown by Doppler. The normal colour-flow pattern in the carotid artery system appears as uniform shades of red with a concentrated flow streamline throughout systole and diastole; no colour-flow reversal is normally seen in the carotid system in diastole.

The normal common carotid has colour patterns that appear as described. The internal carotid normally has higher velocities and colour intensities during systole. Some normal elevation of the diastolic intensities may occur with more intense white or yellow shades than in the common carotid because of the low-resistance hemodynamics. Note that an area of blue flow reversal or flow separation may normally occur at the carotid bulb, but may be considered normal only if no significant plaque development is present.

The external carotid artery normally has a higher-resistance flow pattern, with a characteristic on-off pattern isolated to that vessel; absence of colour in diastole normally occurs in the external carotid artery, since this finding characterizes a high-resistance hemodynamic state.

There are no criteria applicable at the time of writing to categorize the degree of stenosis by the hemodynamic changes seen in colour-flow imaging. Such classification is best done using Doppler spectral waveform acquisition, since velocity changes in colour Doppler imaging and duplex Doppler are often related. Certain easily detectable changes in the saturation, flow-streamlines, and velocity levels, however, occur at certain degrees of luminal reduction:

1. The normal streamline usually concentrate towards the center or slightly to the side distal to flow divider. Broadening of the streamline where instead of a bright gradient in the center, the intensities are diffusely spread within the vessel may suggest a proximal turbulent phenomenon, such as a proximal CCA stenosis. This is analogous to a disturbance of the envelope deformation in a Doppler spectral waveform.
2. Highly concentrated narrow streamlines indicate a flow jet, usually appearing distal to a stenosis; there usually is a clearly defined area of blue flow separation beneath the jet directly distal to the stenotic plaque.
3. Diastole-persistent streamlines are indicative of a severe stenosis; they are analogous to the elevated and high velocity diastolic flow seen within Doppler waveforms across high-grade stenoses.
4. If colour becomes regularly absent in diastole in the common or internal carotid artery, the existence of a distal occlusion may be implied.
5. Mixed colour-flow patterns indicate turbulence within the arterial segment, often distal to a stenosis; this finding is very useful in cases where an extensively calcified plaque prevents determination of the underlying degree of stenosis. By evaluating the colour-flow patterns distal to the calcified plaque, an examiner can find out whether the "hidden" stenosis is hemodynamically significant.
6. A visible bruit is an indicator of stenosis causing a luminal reduction of greater than 60%; note that the bruit may disappear if the luminal reduction approaches the high ninetieth percentile.
7. Completely retrograde (blue) flow in the right carotid or either vertebral artery, flickering patterns (for example, the colour pattern in the right internal carotid goes blank or absent during systole rather than in diastole as in number 4), or alternating blue-red patterns (with blue occurring during systole and red during diastole) are signs of pending or active subclavian steal; if seen in the vertebral arteries and carotid steal in innominate stenosis or occlusion if seen in the right carotid artery.

The hemodynamics of subclavian steal, colour-flow, and Doppler waveform appearances in the vertebral artery and the examination technique; the hemodynamics of carotid steal are closely related brief description of carotid steal phenomenon is as follows:

If the innominate artery is severely stenosed or occluded proximal to the origin of the right common carotid artery which arises from the innominate rather than the aortic arch, it is possible for flow to shunt around the circle of Willis and travel in a retrograde fashion through both the vertebral and the internal carotid—common carotid to compensate the right arm. This phenomenon is very dramatic (especially with colour-flow) and may manifest with flow pattern in an

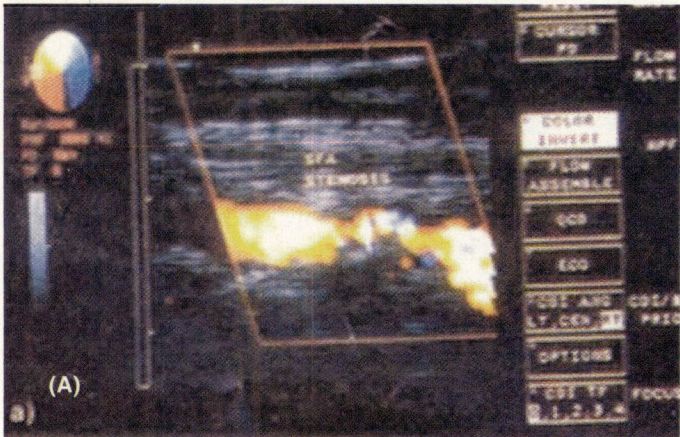

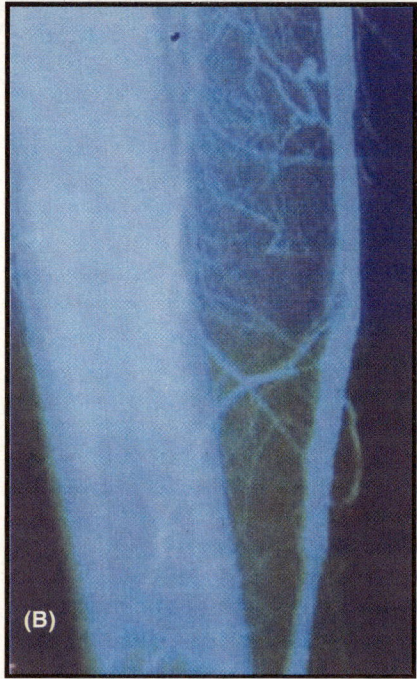

Fig. 23.34A and B: (A) Colour Duplex scan of superficial femoral showing stenosis which was confirmed by angiography **(B)**

identical pattern to those seen in subclavian steal in the vertebral artery. Retrograde flow of this type should not ever occur in the left carotid system.

The degree of steal, as in the vertebral, can be determined by the following particular patterns of systolic reversal in the carotid:

1. If systolic flow goes to baseline but does not fully reverse, a flickering internal carotid colour pattern may occur which may not reflect into the common carotid if innominate pressure is still substantial. Usually a normal common carotid antegrade colour pattern persists.
2. If flow reverses in systole but becomes antegrade in diastole, an alternating blue-red pattern occurs. This parallels the latent or transitional steal pattern.
3. Finally, if flow is completely retrograde throughout

all of the cardiac cycle which is rare in carotid steal, a fully blue pattern is seen.

Some investigators have attempted to use velocity tagging not only to localize the point of maximum frequency and velocity shift but attempt to quantify the velocities; the examiner must remember that most colour Doppler systems display mean velocities in colour, not peak velocities (system with time colour-flow processing are an exception). The examiner should not, therefore, expect the trigged velocity to correlate exactly with peak velocities obtained from the Doppler spectral waveform. Tagged velocities can, however, serve as a guide to where the sample volume should optimally be placed for accurate Doppler spectral sampling.

Interpretation of Carotid Duplex Doppler Spectral Waveforms
Normal Carotid Waveform Patterns

Many of the criteria about interpreting the spectral display previously discussed apply to diagnosis of carotid hemodynamics and interpreting the duplex Doppler spectral waveform.

The normal common carotid waveform has a clearly defined envelope and an uncluttered spectral window with a narrow spectral width, i.e. little if any spectral broadening. Peak systolic internal carotid frequencies generally are under 4 kHz, and velocities are under 125 cm/sec. Some mild turbulence or flow disturbance may occur within the bulb area around the bifurcation, which is normal. Diastolic flow is clearly defined above the baseline, and there is normally no retrograde flow.

The normal internal carotid waveform is of a low-resistance quality, with most of the same characteristics as in the common carotid—a uniform envelope, little or no spectral broadening, but slightly more elevated systolic and diastolic flow. Peak systolic common carotid frequencies also are under 4 kHz with peak velocities under 125 cm/sec.

The normal external carotid waveforms, however, is of a higher resistance quality because of the numerous branches. Again there is a uniform envelope and little or no spectral broadening. Flow generally still remains above the baseline, but systolic flow has a more rapid and sharp upstroke and flow in end-diastole generally goes close to the baseline. A mildly prominent third diastolic component is sometimes seen. Peak frequencies and velocities vary; in general, they still are less than or equal to 4 KHz or 130 cm/sec.

Abnormal Waveform Patterns
(Figs 23.27, 23.28, 23.35 and 23.36)

In the presence of hemodynamically significant disease the Doppler spectral waveforms in the carotid arteries develop many qualitative changes.

These waveform characteristics are directly proportional to the severity of the stenosis (or stenoses) and not only alert the examiner to the presence of an abnormality but also aid in classifying the disease into one or more categories of severity. These characteristic flow-pattern changes have been correlated accurately with arteriographically documented luminal reduction measurements and have become reliable indicators of the approximate degree of stenosis.

In general, few hemodynamic changes (except some increase in spectral broadening) are seen in the carotid waveform until a stenosis produces a luminal reduction of about 60%. At this point, several quantifiable things happen to the blood-flow waveform:

1. The spectral broadening increases proportionally with the degree of luminal reduction, approaching a spread of greater than 40 cm/sec, and the window may fill in or become absent as a stenosis increase;

2. The waveform of outer envelope begins to lose its definition, with significant disruption proportional to the degree of flow turbulence;

3. The peak systolic velocity (frequency) elevates above 120 to 130 cm/sec or 4 kHz; the end-diastolic velocity begins to elevate above 40 cm/sec. The more severe the stenosis and flow disruption, the higher both of these values will be.

Partial or complete retrograde flow in one vertebral artery suggests the presence of subclavian steal which can be confirmed with brachial systolic pressure comparisons.

If proximal innominate artery stenosis or occlusion is present, the carotid waveform on the right may become transitionally or completely retrograde as carotid steal occurs.

Doppler spectral waveforms obtained proximal to an occlusion or stenoses approaching the high ninetieth percentile become characteristic of high resistance, appearing similar to an extremity artery with a loss of diastolic flow which may drop to a velocity of zero at end-diastole.

Doppler Spectral Velocity Criteria for Classifying Carotid Artery Disease (Figs 23.22 and 23.23)

As mentioned, the Doppler velocity and spectral broadening criteria measured during the examination are used by the interpreter to classify the degree of stenosis based on where the velocity and waveform criteria from the internal carotid artery fit into a specific diagnostic category. One or more of the following parameters are used in published classification tables to determine the category:

1. Peak-systolic velocity (PSV) (frequency);
2. End-diastolic velocity (EDV) (frequency);
3. Internal carotid—common carotid peak systolic velocity ratio;
4. Internal carotid—common carotid peak systolic velocity ratio;
5. Spectral broadening in cm/sec.

The PSV or peak systolic frequency is measured at the peak of the systolic component of the waveform. This is considered by some investigators to be one of the most sensitive parameters for identifying a critical stenosis (70% to 80% luminal reduction or higher), although alone it may not accurately distinguish between 60% to 80% and 80% to 99% stenosis grades.

The EDV or end-diastolic frequency is measured at the lowest point of diastole, usually at the end of the cardiac cycle just before the initial upslope of another systolic peak. Evaluation of EDV is a very sensitive indicator for stenosis, especially when it is over 80%.

The internal carotid/common carotid (IC/CC) peak systolic velocity ratio (PSVR) is calculated by dividing the peak systolic velocity number of the internal carotid by the peak systolic velocity number of the ipsilateral common carotid.

Internal PSV/Common PSV = IC/CC Ratio

This value normally is less than 1.8; low values generally are not considered significant. This is because the internal carotid systolic velocity may occasionally be lower than average, such as in a dilated, patched vessel after end arterectomy. Evaluated ratio occur at greater than 60% stenosis, and higher values are usually diagnostic for severe stenosis in combination with the other factors.

The IC/CC end-diastolic velocity ratio (EDVR) is calculated by dividing the peak end-diastolic velocity number of the internal carotid by the peak end-diastolic velocity number of the ipsilateral common carotid.

Internal carotid EDV/Common carotid EDV=lC/CC Ratio.

This value normally is less than 2.5. The end-diastolic velocity ratio begins to elevate at a 60% stenosis; as with the PSVR, it caliber a specific indicator of higher-grade stenoses (generally those over 70%) and may help confirm the severity of the stenosis in combination with the other factors. Study by Moneta, *et al.* indicated that an end-diastolic velocity ratio of greater than 4.0 is significant for the presence of a 70% or greater stenosis. Quantificaton of spectral broadening is more often done visually than by acutal caliper measurement, but the spectral bandwidth can be measured at peak systole distal to a severe stenosis using electronic calipers. One marker should be placed at the peak of the waveform and a second at the top edge of any visible window (at the baseline if a window is not present). Most velocity calipers measure from the baseline to the marker location, so the examiner should subtract the second

Table 23.2: *Diameter reduction in terms of peak systolic frequency ranges*

Diameter reduction (normal)	Peak-systolic frequency (4.5 kHz between 30 and 60 decibels)
1% to 50%	<4 KHz
50% to 60%	4 to 5 KHz
60% to 80%	5 to 6 KHz
80% to > 95%	>6
100%	(occluded)

Table 23.3: *Percentage reduction in diameter according to PSV and EDV*

Diameter reduction	PSV	EDV
0% to 29%	<110 cm/sec	<100 cm/sec
30% to 49%	≥110 cm/sec	<100 cm/sec
50% to 79%	≥130 cm/sec	<100 cm/sec
80% to 99%	≥130 cm/sec	<100 cm/sec
100%		occluded

PSV, peak systolic volume; EDV, end-diastolic volume

Table 23.4: *Diameter stenosis according to PSV, EDV and spectral broading bandwidth*

Diameter stenosis	PSV	EDV	IC/CC PSVR	IC/CC EDVR	SB
0% (normal)	<110 cm/sec	<40 cm/sec	<1.8	<2.4	<30cm/sec
01% to 39% (mild)	<110 cm/sec	<40 cm/sec	<1.8	<2.4	<40cm/sec
40% to 59% (moderate)	<130 cm/sec	40 cm/sec	<1.8	<2.4	<40cm/sec
60% to 79% (severe)	>130 cm/sec	40 cm/sec	>1.8	>2.4	>40cm/sec
80% to 99% (critical)	>I30 cm/sec	>100 cm/sec	>3.7	>5.5	>80cm/sec
100% (occlusion)	N/A	N/A	N/A	N/A	N/A

PSV, peak-systolic velocity; EDV, end-diastolic velocity ratio; SB, spectral broadening bandwidth measurement

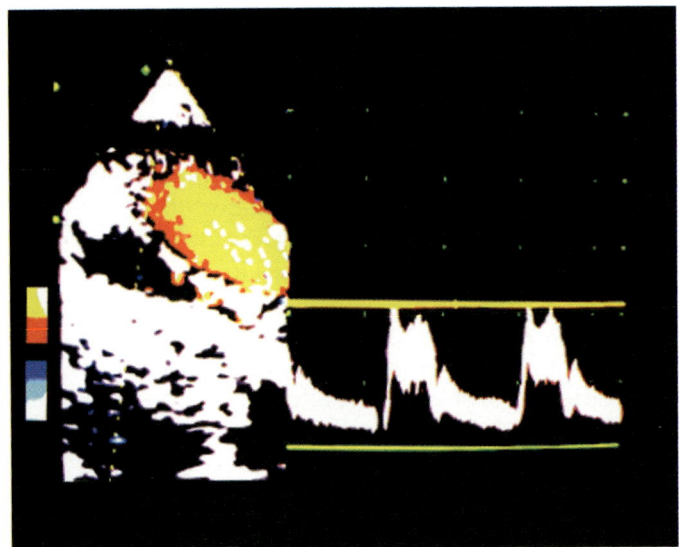

Fig. 23.35: Color Doppler scan of left internal carotid artery showing post-stenotic dilatation wider spectral width, visible widow normal peak systolic and end-diastolic velocities in mild-luminal obstruction in a patient with left carotid bruit and recurrent syncopal attacks

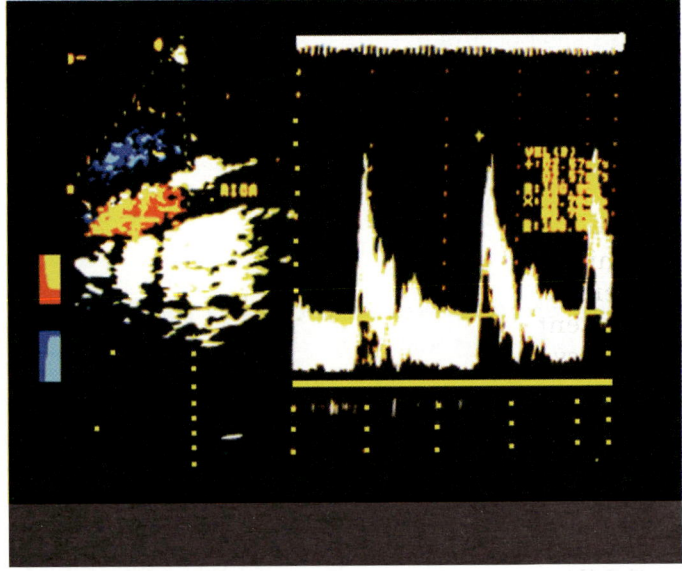

Fig. 23.36: Color Doppler scan of right internal carotid artery showing normal peak systolic and diastolic velocities, narrow spectral width and good window in normal person

measurement from the peak measurement ; the result will be in centimeters per second and should represent the spectral bandwidth (SW), PSV – PWV = SW.

Peak systolic velocity (PSV) – Velocity at top of window (PWV) = spectral width (SW) in cm/sec.

A spectral width of 40 cm/sec or less is considered normal by some criteria. This parameter is less sensitive than the others mentioned but may be useful in supporting findings from one or more of the other four calculations (Tables 23.1–23.4).

Some specific makes of ultrasound equipment include a capability to automatically calculate a range of spectral broadening based on the range of velocities at the 50% amplitude of a spectral power histogram or to determine a percentage of window from a comparison of maximum and minimum frequency values. In theory the lower the percentage window number, the more spectral broadening is present; this factor, however, can sometimes be affected by improperly set Doppler gain and threshold settings. These capabilities are not present on the majority of currently manufactured systems and therefore have no universal application.

Measurement aside, the best assessment of spectral broadening is probably qualitative rather than quantitative; if the window appears to be filled in, there is probably a significant stenosis over 60%. If not, the stenosis is probably less than 60%.

Velocity versus Frequency

Throughout this chapter reference to both velocity and frequency are made; frequency values can be converted to velocity values provided the transducer frequency and angle of insonation are known. Although most ultrasound duplex scanners perform this calculation automatically, it may help the reader to know how to convert kHz to cm/sec: the frequency in kHz is multiplied by 78, then this product is divided by the cosine of the angle (cos θ- you may need to use a scientific calculator to get this figure) time the transducer frequency in MHz, resulting in the velocity in cm/sec.

Velocity in cm/sec = 78 (frequency in kHz)/ (transducer frequency 111 MHz) (cos θ)

While reporting results as velocity is currently preferred, since velocity values are universally consistent regardless of the transducer transmit frequency; frequency measurements (e.g., on follow-up studies) unless Doppler transducer frequency and insonation angle are identical to those used in the original study. It is important to make the distinction that this refers to Doppler transmit frequency; for example, a transducer that images at 7.5 MHz may perform pulsed Doppler at a lower frequency (such as at 5 MHz). The peak-frequency criteria limitations described here refer to the Doppler transmit frequency and not the imaging frequency.

Over the years many investigators have developed duplex velocity/frequency criteria for quantifying and categorizing internal carotid artery stenosis. All of the criteria use peak systolic and end-diastolic velocities or frequencies, some use the IC/CC PSV ratios and EDV ratios study.

The sonographic image of the carotids after endarterectomy can vary; if a straightforward endarterectomy was done, the artery generally appears very similar to a normal carotid bifurcation with perhaps a thinner wall, no defined intimal echoes in the operated area, and a step-off where the normal artery ends and the endarterectomy begins. If a patch angioplasty was performed, the repaired area will additionally appear enlarged and dilated; sometimes the suture line or patch borders can be imaged along the walls. If the artery was patched to enlarge the vessel around a recurrent stenosis, residual stenotic material may be seen and should be monitored on subsequent follow-up examinations.

Fibrotic or hyperplastic stenosis often appear as narrow vessels without evidence of intraluminal stenosis, as if the vessel itself has shrunk in diameter. Neointimal stenoses adopt typical appearance of stenosis plaque within the endarterectomy site. Thrombus can also occasionally form a reaction to wall trauma.

Colour-flow and Doppler patterns can vary in endarterectomized vessels. In nonpatched arteries the flow hemodynamics generally do not differ from those seen in normal arteries. In patched vessels a significant amount of flow disturbance and multicolour swirling or kaleidoscopic flow is seen within the endarterectomy area. Doppler spectral flow patterns should not be obtained in these areas because of the turbulent, nondiagnostic waveform patterns. At the distal margin of the endarterectomy where the artery tapers and resumes a normal, unoperated caliber, some colour-flow acceleration may be seen, especially if a large, dilated endarterectomy terminates into a small native artery.

Doppler patterns are often best obtained either within straight, non disturbed segments distal to the bifurcation or in the native artery distal to the margins of the endarterectomy. Low velocities may be seen in the vessel if it is enlarged after surgery; such velocities are often normal. Elevated velocities that occur within an otherwise normal artery distal to the endarterectomy may result from the acceleration caused by diameter change (provided no distinct focal stenosis is identified). Since the margins of the endarterectomy often can be sites of recurrent stenosis, careful longitudinal and transverse evaluation of these area should be performed to determine the significance of any flow acceleration.

If metal clips are used during an endarterectomy, these may occasionally show up as bright echoes with acoustic dropout below them, similar to calcified plaque shadows. Repositioning the transducer may help the examiner obtain an image around them.

Percutaneous Transluminal Angioplasty

Percutaneous transluminal angioplasty is periodically being used for dilation of extracranial and intracranial lesions. Angioplasty is performed frequently on subclavian and vertebral arteries, and at the common carotid origin but varying success has occurred with focal, short lesions that are not heavily calcified or rigid.

The sonographic appearance and Doppler/colour-flow patterns of an internal carotid artery after angioplasty are not very different from routine imaging and flow findings; the vessel may have an apparent stretched or dilated shape and plaque may still be present, depending on the severity of the lesion. The objective of duplex in these cases is to determine whether a hemodynamic improvement or increase in the residual luminal diameter has occurred compared with the pre-angioplasty state.

Carotid Bypass Grafts

Bypass grafts or reconstructive procedures are used in cases where endarterectomy will not suffice or may be inappropriate (e.g. severely stenoses with multiple repairs). Grafts can be either of synthetic material (e.g. GoreTex, Decron) or of autogenous venous origin. Bypasses used to connect two separate arteries are usually synthetic, whereas saphenous vein is preferred for interposition grafts.

Some examples of bypass grafts that may be encountered by the examiner include the following:

1. **Caroto-subclavian:** The carotosubclavian graft connects the subclavian artery to the ipsilateral proximal common carotid artery and is used to either restore flow to the subclavian and vertebral artery in cases of proximal subclavian stenosis, occlusion and/or subclavian steal or to restore flow to the common carotid artery in cases of severe origin stenosis. The subclavian anastomosis may be difficult to see, but the carotid anastomosis is usually easily visualised. Colour-flow and Doppler assessment can help the examiner determine the correct flow direction in the graft, evaluated the hemodynamics and patency of the graft.

2. **Carotocarotid:** The carotocarotid graft connects the common carotid to the contralateral common carotid across the low neck, usually inferior to the thyroid cartilage. It shares flow from one carotid with the other. It is easily palpated and followed with duplex and colour-flow, and waveforms can be taken within. The anastomoses should be easily visualised.

This type of bypass is infrequently performed and is seldom seen.

3. **Interposition Graft:** An interposition graft is usually performed when a carotid aneurysm is present or when common carotid disease is so extensive that replacement, excision, or exclusion, rather than endarterectomy, is indicated. Usually an end-to end anastomosis of a vein is performed between the native common carotid and the distal native internal carotid artery. The external carotid may be reimplanted into the graft but sometimes is excluded. The sonographic appearance is usually that of a normal carotid bifurcation or of one continuous vessel from base to mandible. The graft may be large or small, depending on the vein segment used; a shadow or diameter irregularity may mark the anastomosis points of the graft and native arteries. Colour-flow and Doppler patterns are consistent as with normal vessels and generally have no distinct characteristics that the examiner need to be aware of image.

Reimplantation

Reimplantation or transposition procedures may occasionally be performed to restore normal flow through the vertebral, common carotid, or subclavian arteries; some examples include the following:

1. Reimplantation of a vertebral artery into an ipsilateral proximal common carotid artery.
2. Implantation of a subclavian artery into an ipsilateral proximal common carotid artery.
3. Transposition of a proximal common carotid artery to the ipsilateral subclavian artery.

Many of these reconstructions lie infraclavicularly and may require a sector transducer to visualise them, although vertebrocarotid and carotosubclavian reimplantations can usually be easily seen and evaluated.

General Comments on Evaluating Patients after Surgery

The examiner needs to thoroughly evaluate any operative notes that may be available before performing a duplex examination; these notes not only describe the type of surgery performed and the date of the operation but also provide exact descriptions of the extent of the endarterectomy or type of repair procedure that was done. Patients who are referred as outpatients may not have operative notes available and do not always volunteer that they have had surgery; the examiner should look for scars on the neck and ask the patient what procedure was done. Endarterectomy scars typically appear as either fairly long scars on one side of the neck along the border of the sternocleidomastoid muscle (often in a neck fold), or sometimes as transverse scars midway up the neck. Physical signs of other procedures may appear as scars in the supraclavicular or infraclavicular areas.

There are generally no contraindications to evaluating patients after surgery with duplex either within the immediate postoperative period or a long-term followup. The examiner should note, however, that duplex studies may have poor visualisation of the carotid anatomy if they are routinely performed within the first 4 weeks, because of local edema and hematoma formation. Increased penetration with lower-frequency transducers may be required, if emergent evaluation is necessary to rule out a postoperative restenosis or thrombosis. If an acute postoperative occlusion is suspected, as supplemental periorbital Doppler examination may help determine whether hemodynamically significant changes with frontal artery flow reversal have occurred.

Upper-Extremity Arterial Examination Techniques

Evaluation of the upper-extremity arteries differs little from the examination in the lower extremities; the same Doppler, segmental pressure, plethysmographic, and duplex sonography techniques can be used with similar diagnostic criteria. The specifics of upper-extremity evaluation are covered in some detail here. Upper-extremity examinations are performed less often in general vascular laboratories than are lower-extremity studies, but there are subtleties in technique and diagnoses of conditions unique to the arms and hands that all vascular technologists and sonographers should know. Some of the techniques and conditions described here also have a bearing on the cerebrovascular evaluation, and the examiner should be aware of those appropriate relationships.

Arterial Anatomy of the Upper-Extremities

This section covers Doppler-related anatomy in the upper extremity and upper thorax (Fig. 23.37).

The subclavian artery is the last major artery to arise from the aortic arch. It has different origin on each side. On the right it arises from the brachiocephalic (innominate) artery, and on the left directly from the aortic arch. The last branch of the subclavian artery is the vertebral artery.

Many other arteries are given off between the arch and the shoulder. At the level of the last rib, the subclavian becomes the axillary artery. The axillary artery tends to run superficially through the axilla and then slightly more deeply at the tendon of the teres major. Here it becomes the brachial artery.

The brachial artery runs medially along the arm to the elbow. Approximately 1 cm distal to the elbow, it bifurcates into the radial and ulnar arteries.

These continue on to the wrist on the anterior surface of the arm, the radial on the radial side and the ulnar on the ulnar side. The ulnar artery gives off a medial interosseus branch, which may occasionally be seen between the radial and ulnar. Each artery passes into the hand and terminates at respective radial and ulnar palmar arches, which are connected by collaterals.

Basic Upper-Extremity Examination Techniques

The same basic primary techniques and instrumentation used for lower-extremity evaluation are applied to the upper-extremities (Figs 23.38 and 23.39).

The last step is again to take a detailed history from the patient with emphasis on upper-extremity occlusive disease. The classic symptoms consist of claudication of the arm that occurs with lifting objects or holding the arms raised over the head for short periods. The afflicted arm also feels colder to the touch than the unobstructed arm, and occasionally numbness and discolouration of the fingers occur. Systolic blood pressures usually show a discrepancy between the two sides. Microembolic activity, digital artery or palmar arch stenosis, or vasospastic. phenomena can be suspected in cases of digital discolouration when the rest of the arm is normal. Note should be made also of whether the patient notices discolouration with exposure to cold or temparature changes.

A patient with dizziness accompanying the extremity problems can be suspected of having subclavian steal syndrome. This is always a possibility when there is a pressure difference of greater than 20 to 40 mm Hg between the two arms.

After the history is taken, the patient should lie supine on the examination table prior to the examination.

Doppler Velocity Waveform Analysis (Fig. 23.40A–E)

Doppler waveform characteristics in the arms are no different than those in the legs. A triphasic waveform is obtained in a normal individual, and the waveform loses amplitude of the second and third components and deteriorates progressively distal to a stenosis.

As in the lower-extremities, the waveforms can be obtained and recorded in any order. An examiner should listen to any record signals from the following vessels..

Both Subclavian Arteries

The subclavian artery can be heard by one of two methods. The probe can be placed in the supraclavicular fossa angling medially, slightly anteriorly, and downward. The probe can also be placed just beneath the clavicle but medial to the shoulder and angled deep, medially, and slightly superiorly towards the clavicle. A strong triphasic signal should be heard, but slight angle adjustments may have to be made to eliminate venous interference (Figs 23.42, 23.43 and 23.44).

Both Axillary Arteries

The axillary artery can be best heard by having the patient raise the upper arm and then placing the probe into the axilla, angling medially and cephalad with the probe against the axillary surface of the upper arm. The axillary artery can also be accessed by listening at the fleshy part of the shoulder below the clavicle and shoulder joint, angling the probe medially.

Both Brachial Arteries

The brachial artery is heard best in the antecubital fossa, usually on the medial side of the fossa, angling the probe cephalad. Some side-to-side searching may have to be done since the artery location can vary slightly in some individuals.

Both Radial Arteries

The radial artery is found on the lateral, or radial side of the wrist (with the palm turned out in the anatomic position).

Both Ulnar Arteries

The ulnar artery is accessed on the medial, or ulnar side of the wrist.

The Vertebral Arteries

The vertebral arteries should be included in the evaluation when there is an ipsilateral significant blood pressure difference between the two arms (of more than 20 mm Hg), an abnormal (monophasic or biphasic) signal in the subclavian artery on one side, or both. This is important to role out subclavian steal syndrome and also to determine whether the stenosis is proximal or distal to the vertebral origin. The vertebral arteries can be evaluated with a continuous-wave probe but are most easily examined with a duplex scanner and spectral Doppler. Colour-flow imaging is very beneficial because direction of flow in the vertebral artery and its degree of patency are immediately apparent.

If using a continuous-wave Doppler, place the probe on the proximal neck just above the supraclavicular fossa but just posterior to the sternocleidomastoid muscle. Angling medially and caudally, listen for a distinct low-resistance waveform that is similar to a carotid waveform but is not in the same area as the common carotid. It is possible to be insonating on top of a vertebra, so it is important to move up and down to try to get a signal proximal to C-6 or between the vertebral interspaces. A triphasic signal more than likely represents subclavian artery and not the vertebral. Biphasic signals or high-resistance signals may indicate distal vertebral stenosis or occlusion.

The best way to obtain the vertebral signals is by using a duplex scanner. The examiner should seat himself or herself at the patient's head, and turn the head slightly away from the side being examined. Imaging should be done with the head of the patient oriented towards the left side of the image per general ultrasound convention. The examiner needs to locate the common carotid artery lost by scanning in a longitudinal and anterior plane, then the examiner should slowly angle laterally until the bright echoes from the cervical vertebral bodies give way to a series of interrupted bony echoes with vessels identified between them (the transverse processes). Colour-flow imaging normally shows pulsatile red flow from the vertebral artery and phasic blue flow from the vertebral vein. Spectral pulsed Doppler waveforms should be obtained from the vertebral artery to indicate the direction and velocity of flow. Retrograde or reversed flow in one vertebral artery is suggestive of subclavian steal.

Interpretation of Upper-Extremity Doppler Velocity Waveforms

Waveform interpretation in stenosis follows the same guidelines in the lower-extremities Doppler waveform criteria.

1. Normal flow at all sites will be triphasic; if spectral pulsed Doppler is used, there will be little or no spectral broadening.
2. Triphasic patterns in the subclavian, axillary, and brachial arteries with abnormal waveforms in the

Sites for placement of Doppler probe for obtaining flow velocities in neck and upper limb vessels

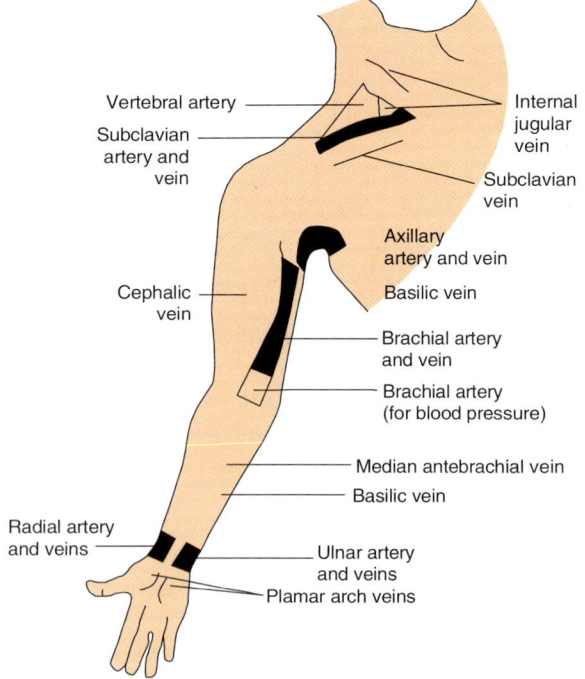

Vertebral artery
Subclavian artery and vein
Cephalic vein
Radial artery and veins

Internal jugular vein
Subclavian vein
Axillary artery and vein
Basilic vein
Brachial artery and vein
Brachial artery (for blood pressure)
Median antebrachial vein
Basilic vein
Ulnar artery and veins
Plamar arch veins

Fig. 23.37: Diagrammatic representation of various sites shown in shaded areas for obtaining color flow and Doppler flow velocity across neck and upper limb vessels

radial and/or ulnar arteries indicate focal stenosis or occlusion of the respective radial or ulnar vessels.

3. Normal waveforms in the subclavian and axillary arteries with abnormal brachial, radial, and ulnar artery waveforms suggest a brachial artery stenosis or occlusion.

4. A normal subclavian waveform with abnormal waveforms at the axillary artery and distal to it implies a stenosis or occlusion of the distal subclavian and/or axillary artery.

5. Abnormal waveforms from the subclavian distally indicate a probable subclavian artery stenosis or occlusion; if the vertebral artery is antegrade with normal flow, the obstruction is probably distal to the vertebral origin.

Segmental Pressures

The same techniques for cuff placement and obtaining pressures in the lower extremities are applicable in the arms.

1. Pressure cuffs are applied to the upper arm and fore-arm.

2. Doppler signals are monitored in the brachial artery and a systolic pressure is obtained and recorded bilaterally.

3. Signals are located in the radial artery at the wrist, and a systolic pressure is obtained and recorded using the forearm cuff then a systolic pressure is obtained and recorded from the brachial cuff bilat-erally.

4. Signals are located in the ulnar artery, and a systolic pressue is obtained and recorded again using the forearm cuff then a systolic pressure is obtained and recorded from the brachial cuff bilaterally.

5. The highest of the two brachial artery systolic pressures is divided into the systolic pressures at each wrist artery to obtain-forearm brachial indices for each forearm artery.

   Forearm brachial index = radial pressure/highest brachial pressure or ulnar pressure/highest brachial pressure

   Do not use the brachial cuff segmental pressure that were taken using the radial or ulnar artery; use the ones obtained from the brachial cuff with the probe at the brachial artery in the antecubital fossa.

Interpretation of Upper-Extremity Segmental Pressures

The same criteria for comparing pressure differences in the legs applies to the study in the arms. A pressure drop of more than 30 mmHg implies the presence of a significant focal stenosis in the arteries between the two cuffs; a difference between sides implies a stenosis or occlusion on the side with the lower brachial pressure.

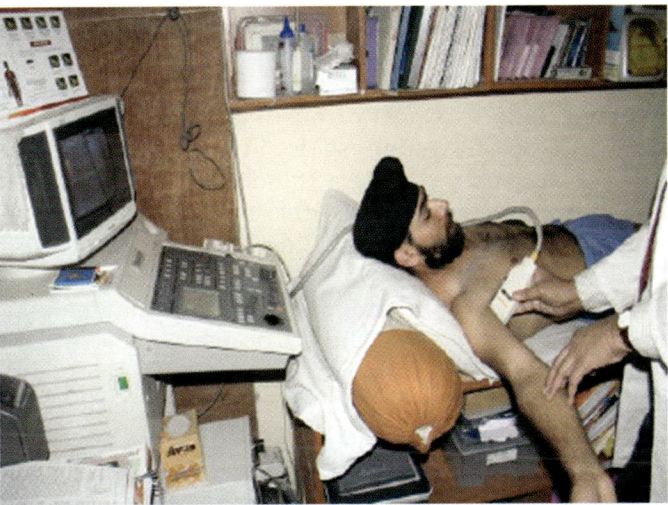

Fig. 23.38: Duplex color Doppler probe in the right axillary region for obtaining color flow and Doppler flow velocity across right axiliary vessels

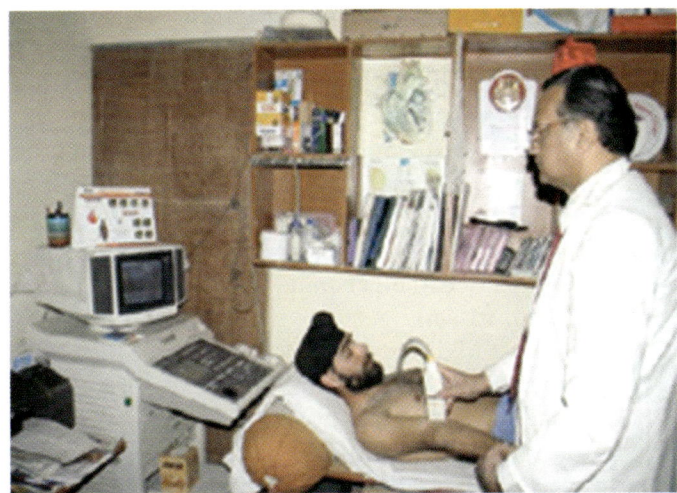

Fig. 23.39: Duplex color Doppler probe over the right brachial region for obtaining color flow and Doppler flow velocity across right brachial vessels

It is possibe for both arms to have equal or comparable pressures with normal forearm-brachial indices. But abnormal can occur when there is an aortic arch problem or bilateral subclavian or axillary stenosis or occlusions. The waveforms must be relied on in this case, so segmental pressures should not be performed without using some method of obtaining waveform patterns for segment comparison.

Arterial Duplex Sonography

Duplex sonography and colour-flow imaging are less frequently used in the upper-extremity arteries than in the cerebrovascular system or lower-extremity arteries, except to evaluate renal dialysis access fistulas, pseudoaneurysm, or aneurysm.

All arteries in the upper-extremity can be evaluated with colour-flow imaging and grey-scale duplex sonography, but the main requirement in the arm is that the transducer's near-field focal zone be able to show structures within the top centimeter of the visual display. Higher-frequency transducers should be used. Transducers with wedges seldom have a problem, but other devices may require a standoff or gel pad to see such superficial structures. Arteries in the shoulder and infraclavicular areas may be best imaged with lower-frequency transducers.

The best use of duplex and colour-flow imaging may be as an adjunctive study to a Doppler waveform and segmental pressure evaluation. It is important, however, to know the sonographic appearance and patterns in normal arteries in the arm. If an examiner is uncertain as to the identity of a vessel, colour-flow imaging can easily enable identification by colour and flow pattern, as can be the use of spectral pulsed Doppler.

1. The subclavian artery is accessed in the longitudinal plane by scanning beneath the clavicle and rotating and angling the transducer until the artery and vein are visualised. The artery can be more readily identified and distinguished from the vein using colour-flow imaging.

2. Following the subclavian artery laterally across the anterior shoulder into the arm brings the axillary artery into view. This can be traced into the upper arm distally into the biceps groove, where the brachial artery can be visualised, and tracked to the antecubital fossa.

3. Just below the inner bend of the elbow, the radial and ulner bifurcation of the brachial artery can be identified and examined.

4. The radial artery is found laterally in the forearm and can be followed to the wrist.

5. The ulnar artery can be traced medially and usually dives deep before moving superficially to the wrist. At about the upper third of the forearm, the bifurcation of the median volar interosseous branch off the ulnar is visualised and, if desired, the artery can be followed distally in the center of the forearm.

Images of each artery should be obtained in both longitudinal and transverse planes.

Spectral pulsed Doppler waveforms will be triphasic and should be obtained from each artery as necessary.

Any given segment can be measured using electronic calipers in longitudinal and transverse planes if attempting to rule out ectasia or aneursym.

Hemodialysis grafts are generally loop like graft easily visible under the skin of the forearm (a common placement site), connecting a superficial vein or the brachial vein with the brachial artery. The basic techniques for evaluating them are the same as for evaluating any other artery, but there is a focus on identifying any stenoses or kinks by grey-scale imaging,

colour-flow imaging, and Doppler spectral analysis. The normal colour-flow and Doppler patterns are pulsatile but have a characteristic high-velocity turbulent and disturbed quality similar to those found in other non-surgically created arteriovenous fistulas.

The graft should be followed in longitudinal and transverse planes from one anastomosis to the other, and areas of stenosis, occlusion, kinking, or flow decrease should be identified and documented.

Upper-Extremity Arterial Duplex Interpretation Criteria (Figs 23.42–23.44)

The same interpretation criteria concerning plaque identification, stenosis determination, waveform appearances and flow velocities in the lower-extremities can be applied to the upper-extremities.

No velocity criteria can be applied to dialysis graft because of the extreme turbulence and high velocities normally seen. Efforts to quantity and grade flow volume in milliliters per minute by calculations of velocity compared with cyclic wall diameter are, however, being done for future potential applications.

Aneurysmal dilation is diagnosed by comparing segment size, often with accepted norms. In general, if maximal arterial diameter is 1.5 times that of a straight, uniform normal segment, it may be classed as ectatic or mildly aneurysmal; if greater than one, it may be aneurysmal.

Thoracic Outlet Syndrome Examination

Patients often show completely normal resting upper-extremity pressures even though they have difficulty only when their arms are raised or placed at an unusual angle. These patients usually complain of numbness, tingling, and discolouration if the arm is abducted, or held over the head. Changing the position of the arm to a more forward or neutral position resolves the symptoms completely. In these patients a routine upper-extremity examination should be performed and then a more specialized examination of the thoracic outlet (Fig. 23.41).

Photoplethysmography can be used as a waveform monitoring device in the thoracic outlet examination, as well as a Doppler probe; the photocell can be taped with double-sided cellophane tape to a digit or strapped on using a Velcro strip. The tracing should be calibrated before the testing maneuver are performed. A benefit of using a photocell is that both of the examiner's hands are free to support the patient's arm during the examination. If a Doppler probe is used, it must be held against the brachial artery with one hand while the arm is supported with the other.

Thoracic outlet syndrome occurs when the arteries, veins, and/or nerves supplying the arm are obstructed by compression between the clavicle and last rib, a cervical rib and the scalene muscles, or the pectoralis minor with hyperabduction of the arm. The vessels usually involved are the subclavian artery and vein and the brachial nerve plexus where it leaves the chest and goes to the arm.

In the thoracic outlet examination the patient should sit either in a chair or on the edge of the examination table with the arms completely relaxed. The examiner takes a tracing from the brachial artery with a Doppler probe (or from the digit if a PPG is used) with the arm in a neutral position. Then the patient's arm is raised to a 45° angle. A tracing is taken from the arm in this position and is marked accordingly. With the arm in this position the patient then is instructed to pull the shoulders back into a military posture and perform a Valsalva maneuver. The examiner keeps the probe in place during the Valsalva and records any changes that occur.

The arm is raised to 90° angle, and the procedure is repeated. A tracing is made both neutrally and with the patient in military posture performing a position and the same steps are repeated. The arm can also be raised to a 180° angle if symptoms warrant.

Additional maneuvers can include hyperabduction, hyperadduction, and Adson's test. In Adson's test, the patient hyperabducts the arm over the head and turns the head towards the side being examined. This position can help reveal the presence of a cervical rib.

Positive findings in thoracic outlet syndrome will be a reduction or cessation of flow at or above a specific degree of elevation or abduction, diminution or cessation with military posturing, and with the application of Adson's test. Any comments the patient makes concerning the onset of symptoms with the assumption of a particular position should be noted on the report form.

Subclavian Steal Syndrome (Fig. 23.30)

Subclavian steal syndrome occurs when there is an obstruction in the subclavian or innominate artery, which is proximal to the vertebral origins. If flow to the arm is compromised significantly enough, flow from the contralateral patent vertebal is "stolen" around the vertebrobasilar junction reversing down the ipsilateral vertebral artery into the subclavian artery to help supply the arm. In complete steal a fully retrograde flow pattern is seen in the vertebral artery a pulsatile blue pattern is seen in the vertebral artery with an antegrade pattern in the opposing vertebral in this condition. In latent steal (where the subclavian stenosis may be moderate) flow reverses in systole but recovers antegrade in diastole (an alternating blue-red-blue-red pattern in colour-flow).

If the proximal innominate artery becomes severely stenosed or occluded, it is possible for carotid steal to occur, where flow from the left vertebral is shunted via the circle of Wills to the right side of the body and travels retrograde in both the vertebral and carotid systems; this occurs rarely but knowledge of its characteristics helps the examiner if it is encountered. In a patient with vertebral steal, a well-defined reversed vertebral signal on the side with a subclavian stenosis is often more than sufficient to imply a probable steal. In patient presenting with questionably reversed or weak but antegrade vertebral flow, steal presence should be verified. To check for steal syndrome, the examiner asks the patient to lie supine and place a pressure cuff on the arm with the occlusion. The vertebral artery is monitored with either Doppler or colour-flow duplex scanner with the cuff inflated to at least 10 mm Hg above the systolic pressure to occlude flow to the arm and induce hyperemia. The monitoring continues with the cuff inflated for 3 minutes. At the end of the time, the cuff pressure is released. The chart recorder or spectrum analyzer display should be running before release of the cuff to show any changes that occur.

In a patient with vertebral steal a reversed signal augment for the short period. An antegrade monitoring reverses below the zero line for several beats within the last 5–15 seconds; if monitored longer, the examiner sees the waveform return to its preocclusive state.

Doppler Lower-extremity Arterial Examination (Figs 23.45, 23.55 and 23.56)
Arterial Anatomy of the Lower-Extremities

To understand the Doppler lower-extremity examination, thorough knowledge of the vascular anatomy as it pertains to the Doppler examination is necessary.

Flow to the extremities comes from the abdominal aorta. The aorta bifurcates above the level of the umbilicus to form the common iliac arteries. The common iliac vessels then bifurcate into the internal and external iliac arteries. The internal iliac (hypogastric) supplies the buttock and genital area. The external iliac supplies the leg and becomes the common femoral artery at approximately the level of the inguinal ligament. Several branches are given off, of which the profunda femoris is the most important. It comes of about 2 to 3 cm below the inguinal ligament and supplies the bone and muscles of the thigh (Figs 23.47, 23.48 and 23.51).

At this point the common femoral becomes the superficial femoral artery. It runs along the medial surface of the thigh and curves posteriorly behind the knee to become the popliteal artery (Figs 23.57 and 23.58)

The popliteal artery continues behind the knee joint and gives off the anterior tibial artery 3 to 6 cm below

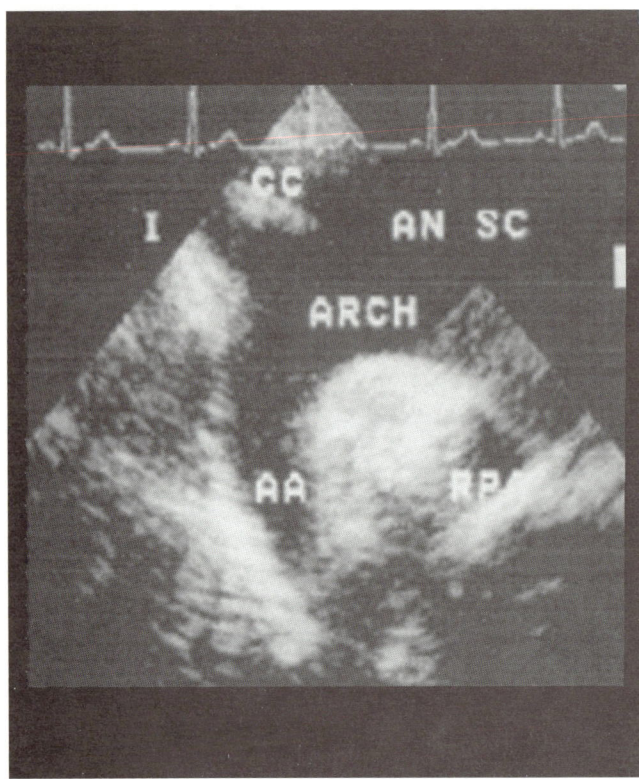

Fig. 23.40A: Suprasternal approach showing dilated left subclavian artery

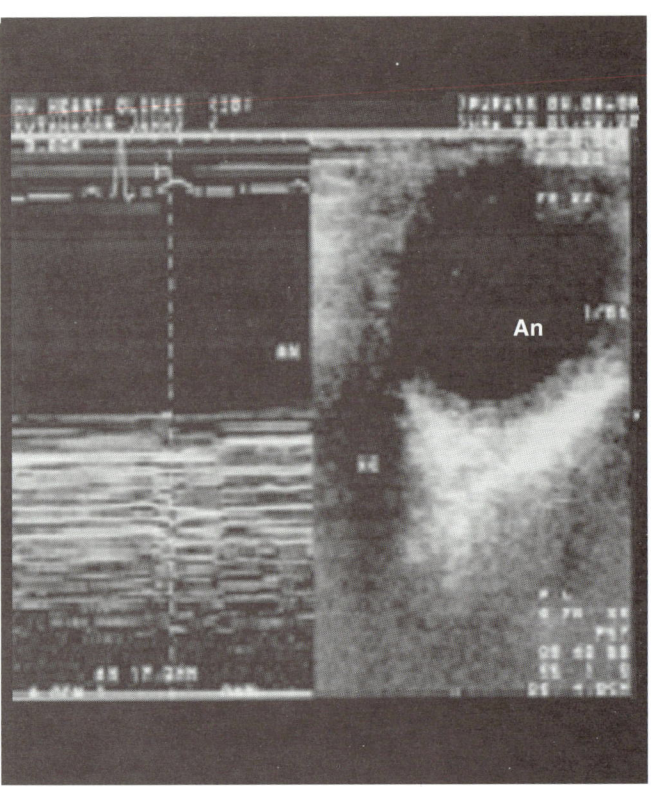

Fig. 23.40B: Short axis Duplex scan at left subclavian artery showing aneurysm (An) of the vessel

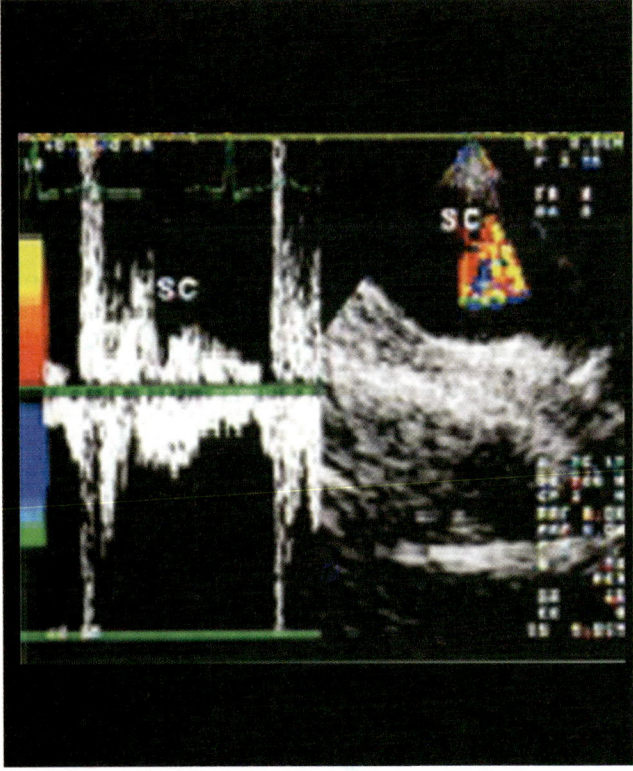

Fig. 23.40C: 2-D and Color Doppler scan showing signatures of aneurysmally dilated left subclavian artery

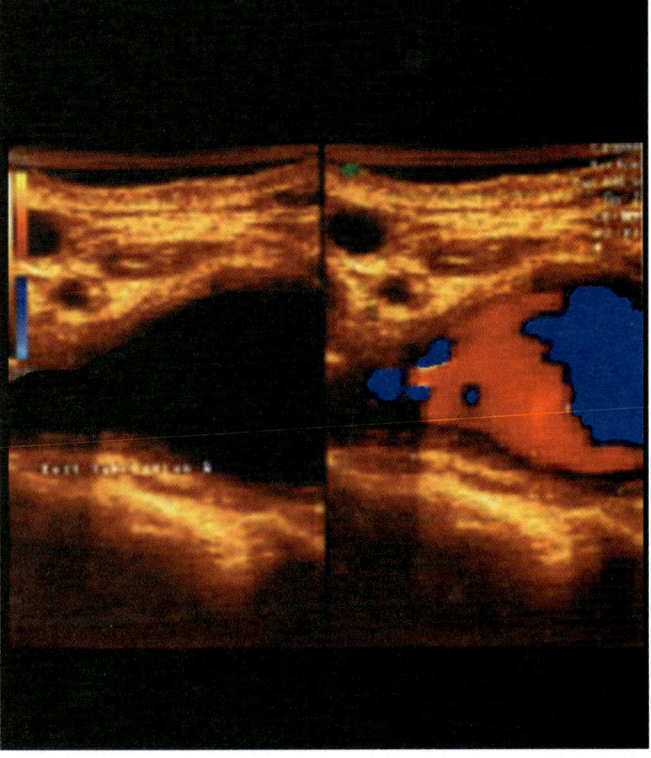

Fig. 23.40D: Color Duplex scan of left subclavian artery showing hugely dilated vessel with disturbed intraluminal blood flow

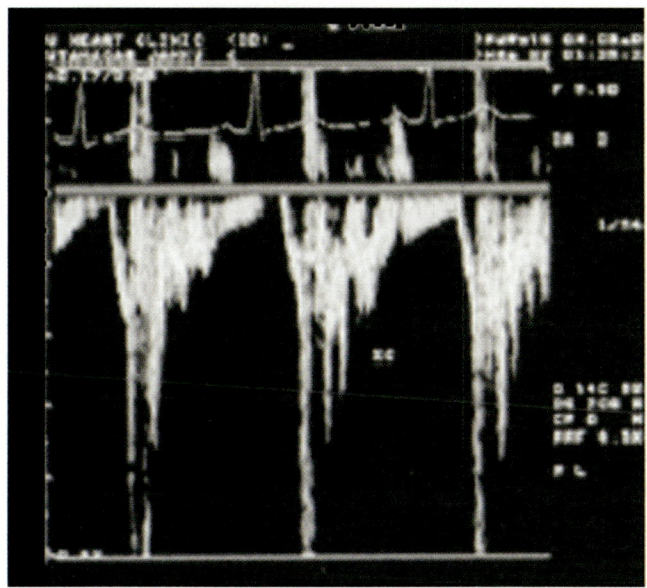

Fig. 23.40E: Doppler flow velocity across aneurysm of left subclavian artery

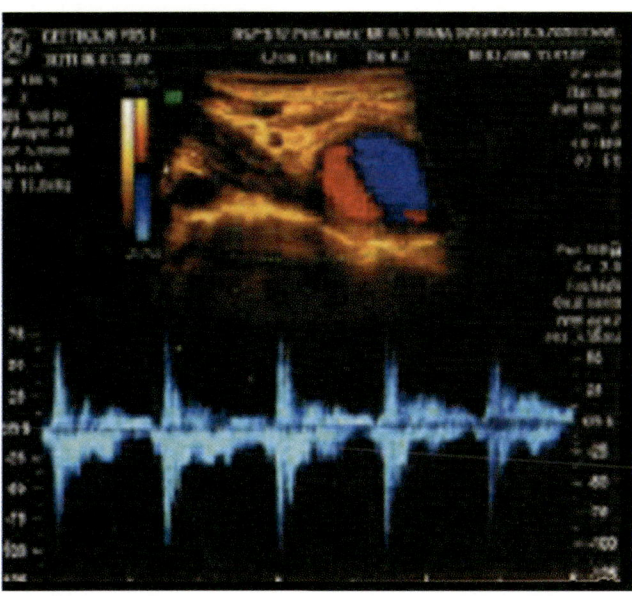

Fig. 23.40F: Color Doppler study of an aneurysmally dilated left subclavian artery

120°

90°

Military posture

Relaxed

Front

Neutral

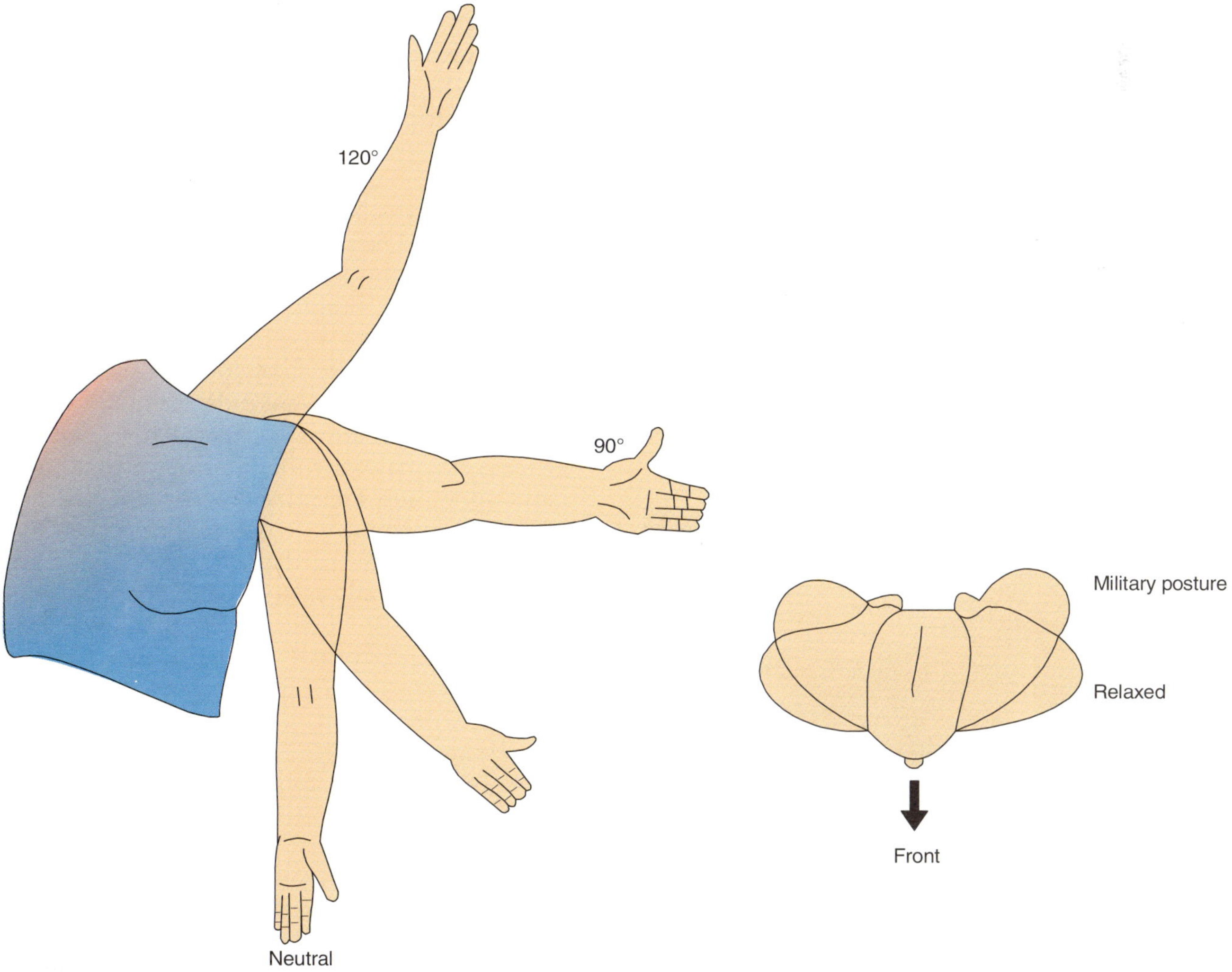

Fig. 23.41: Different positions employed for demonstration of thoracic outlet syndrome

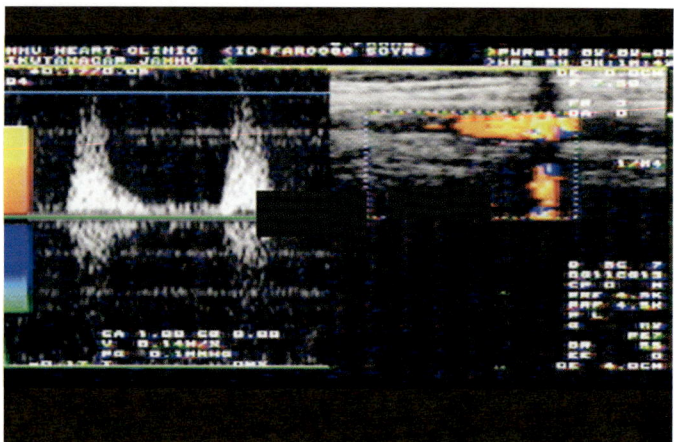

Fig. 23.42: Color flow in left subclavian artery (right) and Doppler flow velocity (left) showing diminished flow and reduced velocity in patient with angiographically diagnosed left subclavian artery obstruction

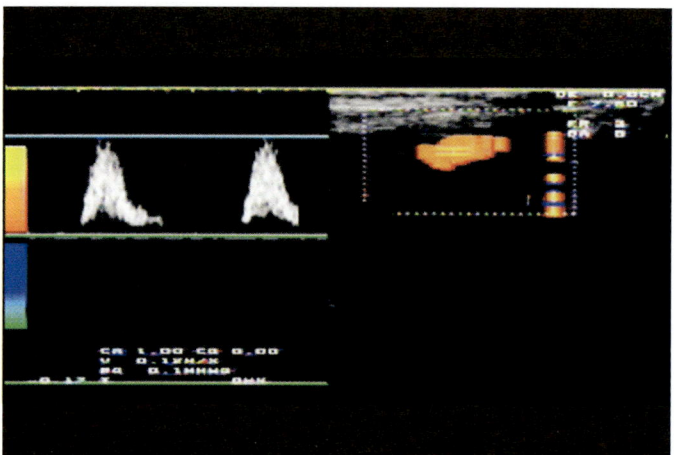

Fig. 23.43: Color flow in left axillary artery (right) and Doppler flow velocity (left) showing diminished flow and reduced velocity in patient with angiographically diagnosed left subclavian artery obstruction

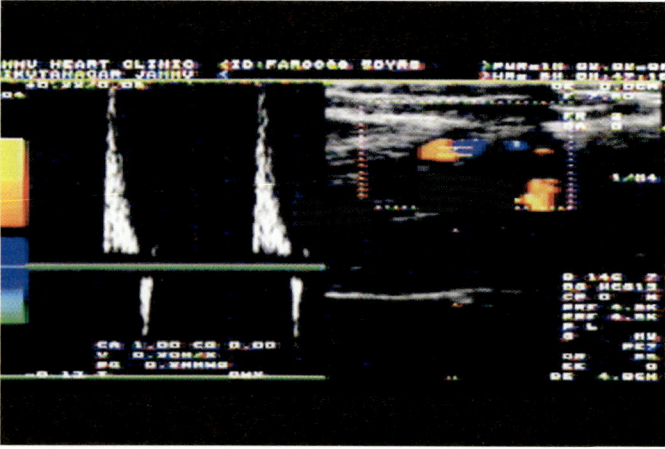

Fig. 23.44: Color flow in left brachial artery (right) and Doppler flow velocity (left) showing truncated flow and reduced velocity in patient with angiographically diagnosed left subclavian artery obstruction

the popliteal fossa. The popliteal then terminates as the posterior tibial and peroneal arteries.

The anterior tibial descends through muscles along the tibia and becomes the dorsalis pedis at the level of the ankle. The dorsalis pedis then runs superficially and dorsally on the medial side of the foot to terminate in the deep planter arch between the first and second metatarsals.

The peroneal tibial artery descends along the posterior surface of the tibia to run posterior to the medial malleolus.

The peroneal artery descends deeply on the fibular side of the leg and becomes accessible anterior to the lateral malleolus.

Lower-Extremity Arterial Examination Techniques

Before beginning any examination of the lower-extremities, the first step is to obtain as complete a history as possibly from the patient, the patient's chart, or both. The emphasis should be placed on the following information (Figs 23.49, 23.50 and 23.54):

1. If the patient is claudicating, note whether one or both legs are affected, where the pain is felt (e.g., calf, thigh, hip), and if it is a tiring or a cramp in the muscle. The distance due to the patient can ambulate before stopping, the pain should be noted and whether the symptoms are relieved by rest.
2. Palpate the pulses at the femoral, popliteal, posterior tibial, and dorsalis pedis arteries. Weak or absent pulses should be noted.
3. Check for night cramping or ischemic rest pain. Remember that simple aching or pain at rest may not constitute the specific diagonsis of rest pain unless the other criteria of critical ischemia are met (e.g. skin changes, absent pulses, limited mobility).
4. Note the skin colour and condition. Check for dry skin, erythema of the toes, thickened nails, gangrenous spots, and unhealed ulcers.
5. Check for known vascular diseases, past bypass surgeries, diabetes, cardiac disease, smoking, hypertension, and family history of these atherosclerotic risk factors. Also, when a patient states that he or she has had a "bypass," enquire further as to whether this means a peripheral arterial bypass in the extremity or a coronary bypass. This is important, since scars from the harvesting of saphenous veins for coronary artery bypass grafting often appear identical to those encountered in peripheral arterial bypassing.

Several different component methods can make up an evaluation of the lower-extremity arterial system. Usually one or more of these is used in combination with segmental pressure measurement. The four techniques described here are considered.

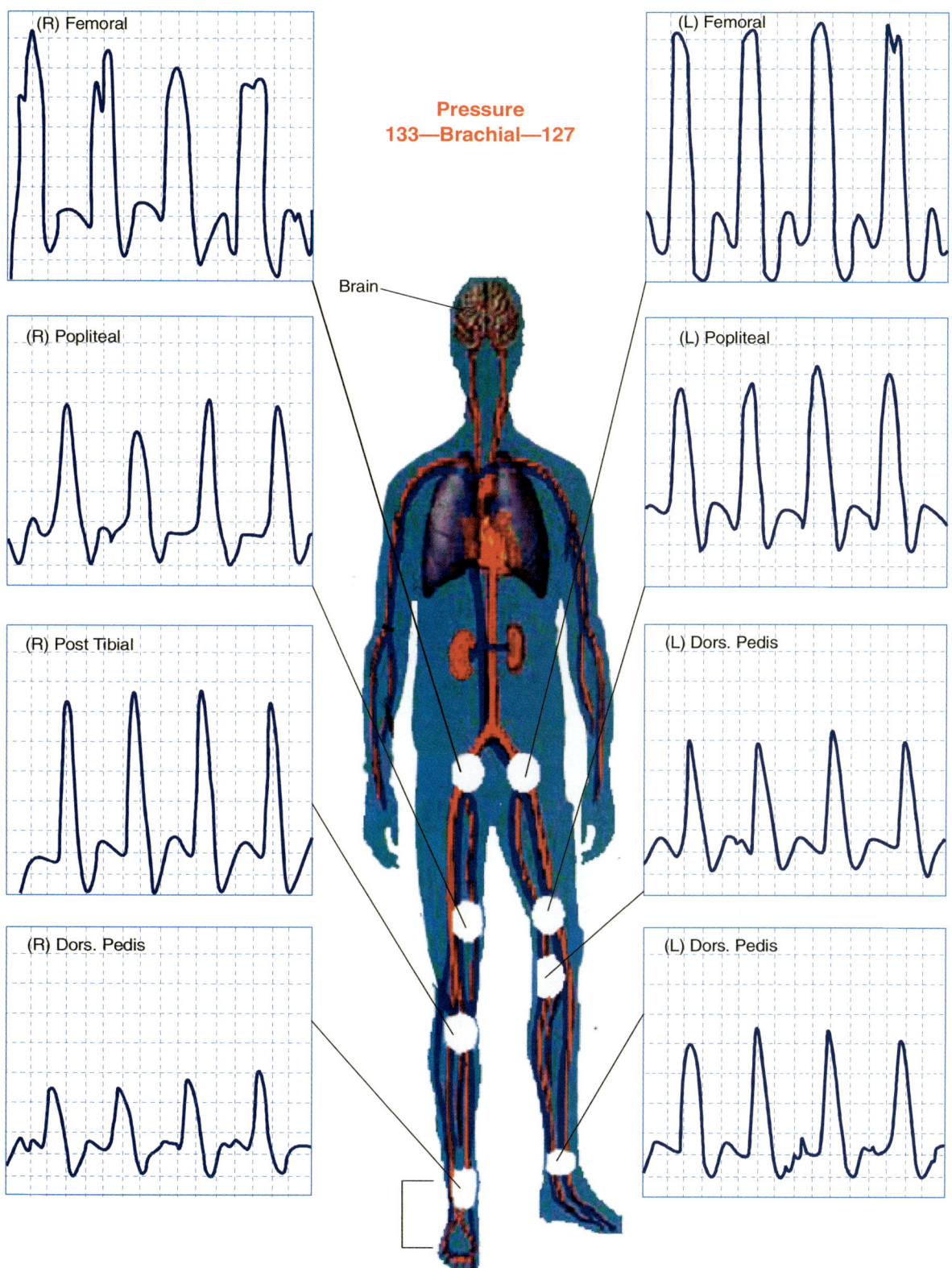

Fig. 23.45: Representation of various sites for probe placement for obtaining normal Doppler waveforms in lower extremity

Doppler Velocity Wave Analysis

Continuous-wave Doppler waveforms can be taken in any order and at any time or can be integrated with the segmental pressure technique. The procedure below follows one logical progression (Figs 23.52 and 23.53).

The patient should lie supine and be made comfortable. The femoral arteries are first accessed by palpating the superior border of the inguinal ligament and placing the probe in position just above the ligament to determine the proper site for monitoring of the femoral artery. The external iliac is actually being monitored at this level rather than the common femoral, but it is better to obtain the signal here than to listen below the ligament, where the bifurcation of the profunda femoris can cause confusion. The common femoral arteries are then monitored and recorded bilaterally. Some pressure on the probe may be needed to obtain a clear signal. The signals are found lateral to

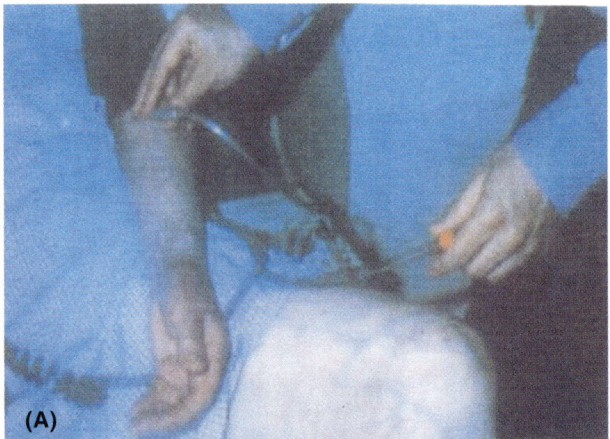

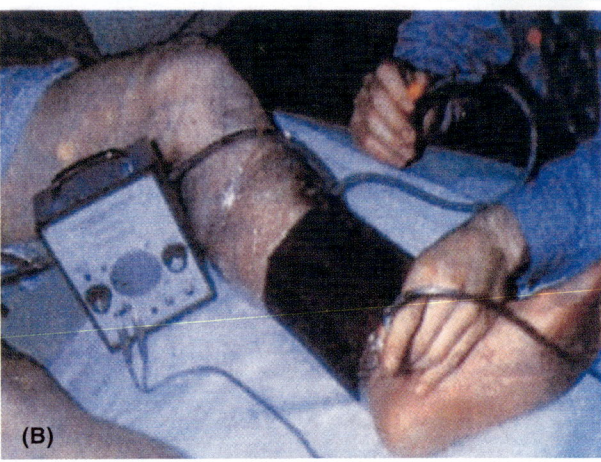

Fig. 23.46: **(A)** Hand-held Doppler and pneumatic cuff for determining the ankle-branchial index (ABPI). The cuff is first placed around the upper arm and the branchial artery signal identified with the Doppler. The cuff is then inflated until the branchial artery signal disappears. **(B)** The procedure is repeated for the posterior tibial or dorsalis pedis signals with the cuff. The ABPI is then calculated as the highest ankle to branchial pressure

the common femoral venous signals (heard as a "windstorm" sound). An arterial signal found medial to the vein is probably the hypogastric artery and must not be mistaken for the femoral. If, in doubt, move the probe laterally and medially to locate the vein and determine the vessel's relationship. The hypogastric artery also may appear as retrograde signal when the probe is angled cephalad.

The popliteal arteries are next to be examined and are found at their sites behind the knees. There are two methods of examining the popliteal arteries: supine and prone.

In the supine position the knees are bent to about a 75° angle and are relaxed laterally ('frog-leg" position) and the probe is placed in the popliteal fossa and angled cephalad. An ample quantity of gel is required to ensure good probe-skin contact. Firm pressure may be needed to displace fat and tissue. Be careful not to occlude the artery. The probe should be angled to obtain the clearest signal with distinct waveform pattern. This segment of the study requires an accurate tracing, since the popliteal signal may be the determining factor in deciding whether an occlusion exists above the knee or in the trifurcation vessels below the knee. The best signal is obtained with the probe more toward the calf than toward the knee.

In the prone position the patient's legs are elevated 30 to 45° and are supported with a bolster or pillow. The same basic examination technique is used as in the supine position, and the probe is angled cephalad. The advantage of this position is the ability actually to see the relationship of the popliteal fossa and the probe. It is a good position to use for the examiner-in-training.

Both positions give excellent results. A major advantage of the supine position is that the patient does not need to move after the initial portion of the examination has been completed. This is especially beneficial to the postoperative or invalid patient who cannot turn over. The choice of examination positions is best left to the examiner's preference.

If there is a discrepancy in the signal quality between the femoral and popliteal sites, the superficial femoral artery can be examined by palpating the femur on the anterior aspect of the leg and placing the probe medial to it in the muscle groove, angling cephalad. This can help localize the level of stenosis more accurately.

To Summarize the Technique

1. Obtain Doppler waveforms from the femoral artery above the inguinal ligament.
2. Obtain waveforms from the popliteal artery behind the knee, either with the patient in a supine position with knee, bent (preferred) or with the patient prone, knee flexed, and with the lower leg supported by a bolster or pillow.

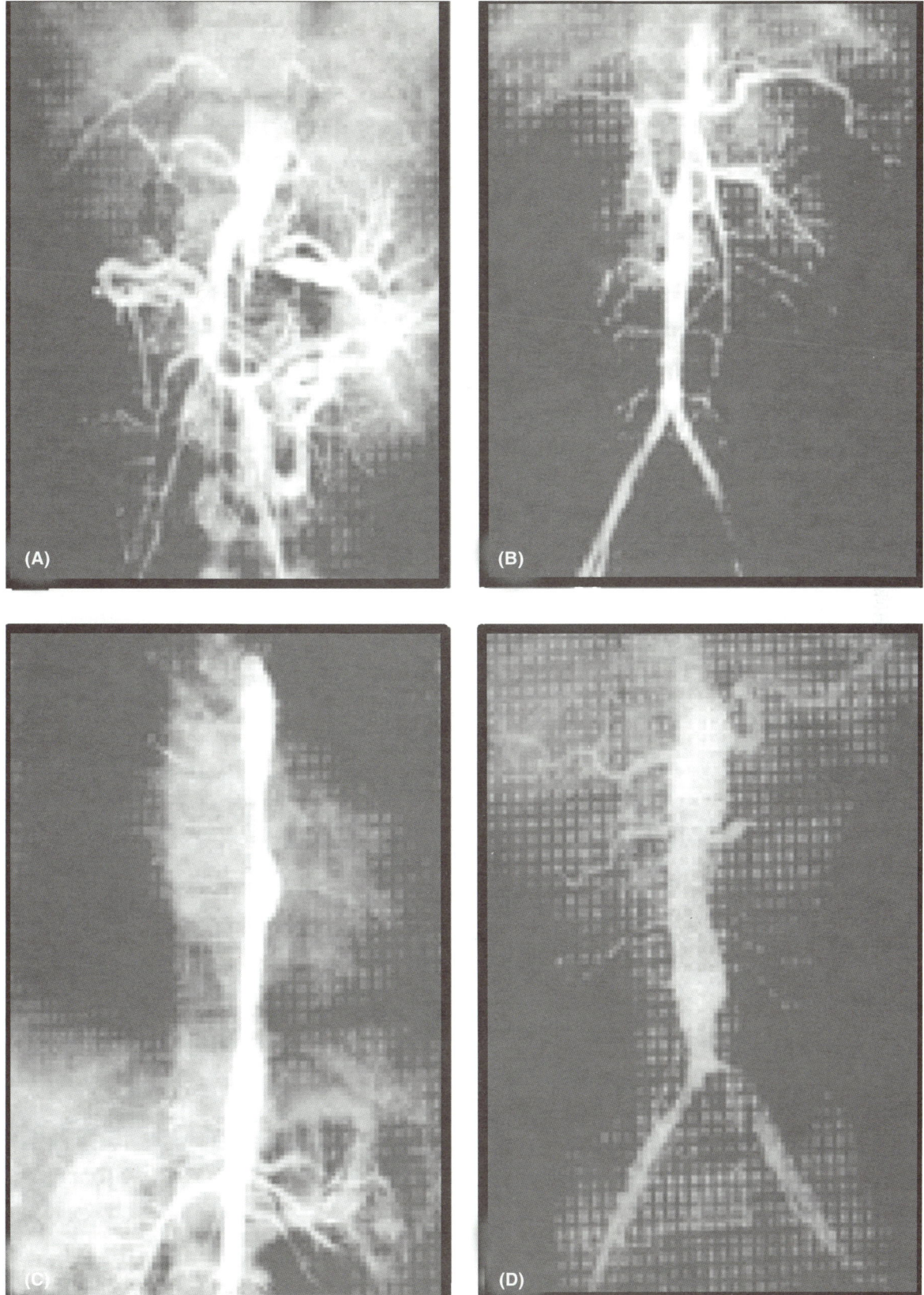

Fig. 23.47A to D: **(A)** Aortogram showing reduced blood flow in celiac vessels of abdominal aorta. **(B)** reduced blood flow in right illiac artery. **(C)** Beaded appearance of abdominal aorta. **(D)** Reduced blood flow in renal and illiac vessels in patient with non-specific aorta-arteries syndrome

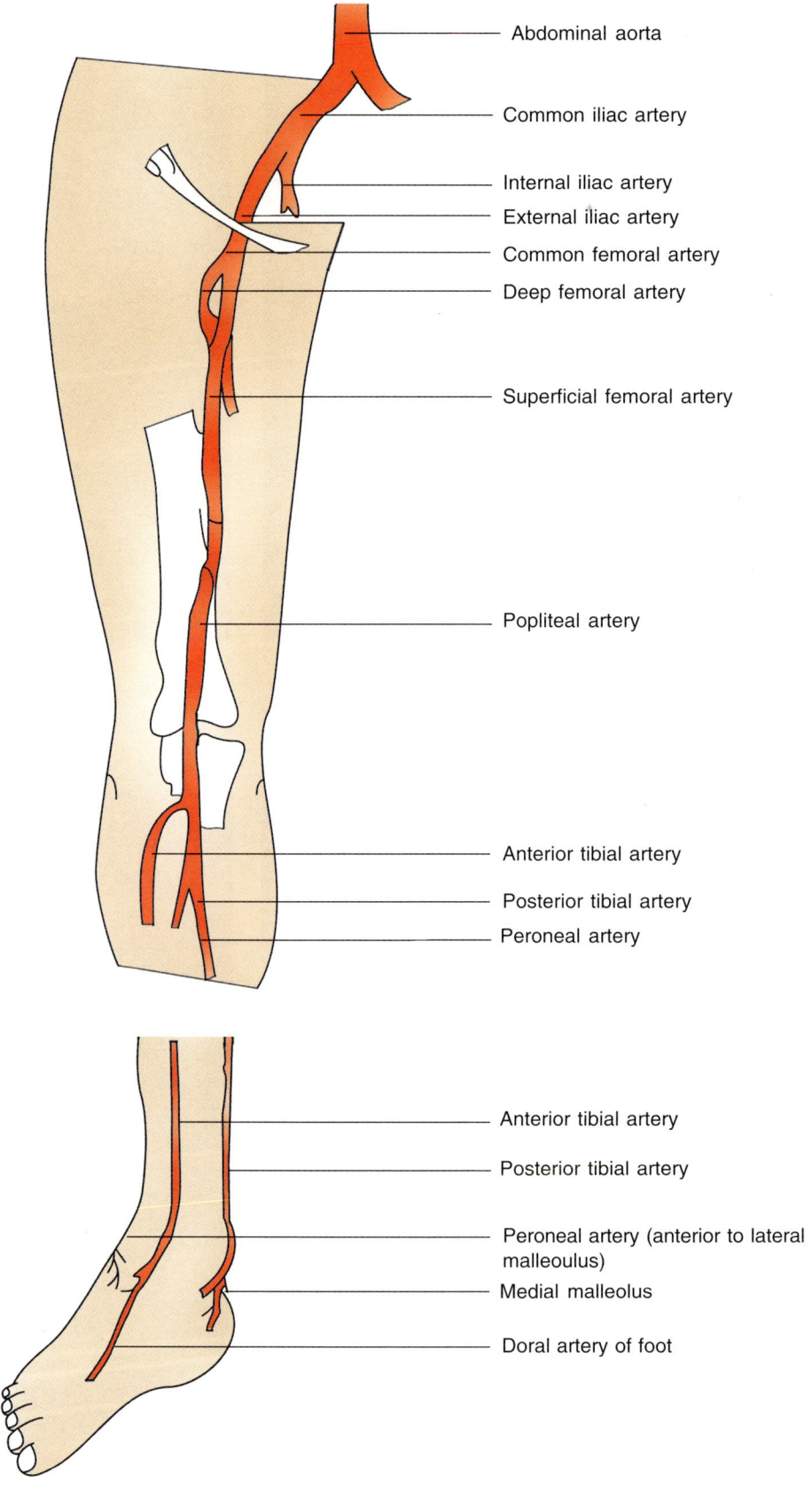

Abdominal aorta

Common iliac artery

Internal iliac artery
External iliac artery
Common femoral artery
Deep femoral artery

Superficial femoral artery

Popliteal artery

Anterior tibial artery

Posterior tibial artery

Peroneal artery

Anterior tibial artery

Posterior tibial artery

Peroneal artery (anterior to lateral malleoulus)

Medial malleolus

Doral artery of foot

Fig. 23.48: (A) Diagrammatic representation of arterial blood supply to the lower limb. **(B)** Blood flow through the ankle arteries which are easily accessible to the Doppler probe

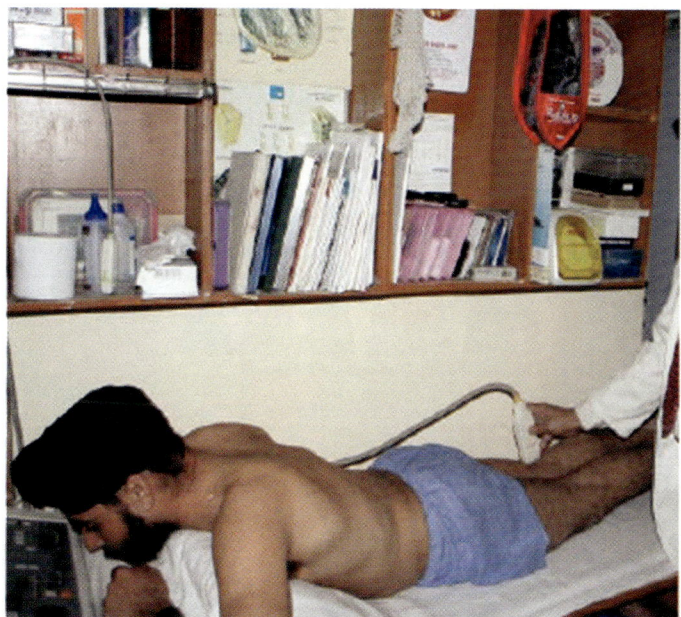

Fig. 23.49: Color Doppler duplex probe over the poplitial vessel for assessment of vascular diseases

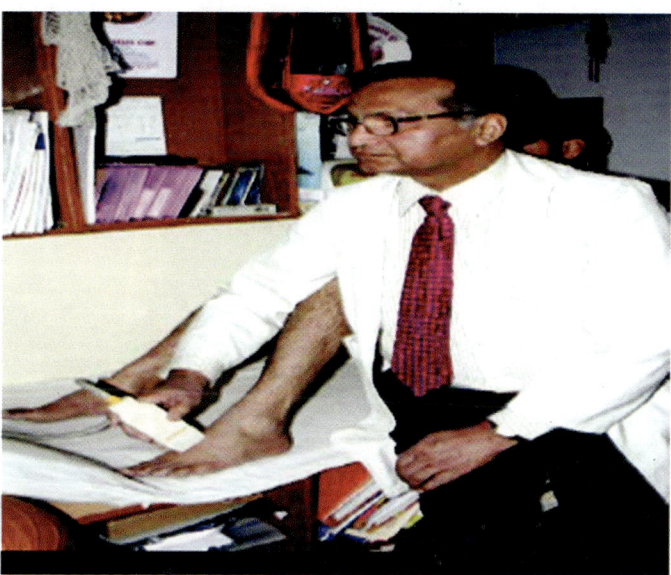

Fig. 23.50: Color Doppler duplex probe over the Dorsails pedis vessel for assessment of vascular diseases

Accessible sites for probe placement for obtaining blood flow velocities in lower limbs

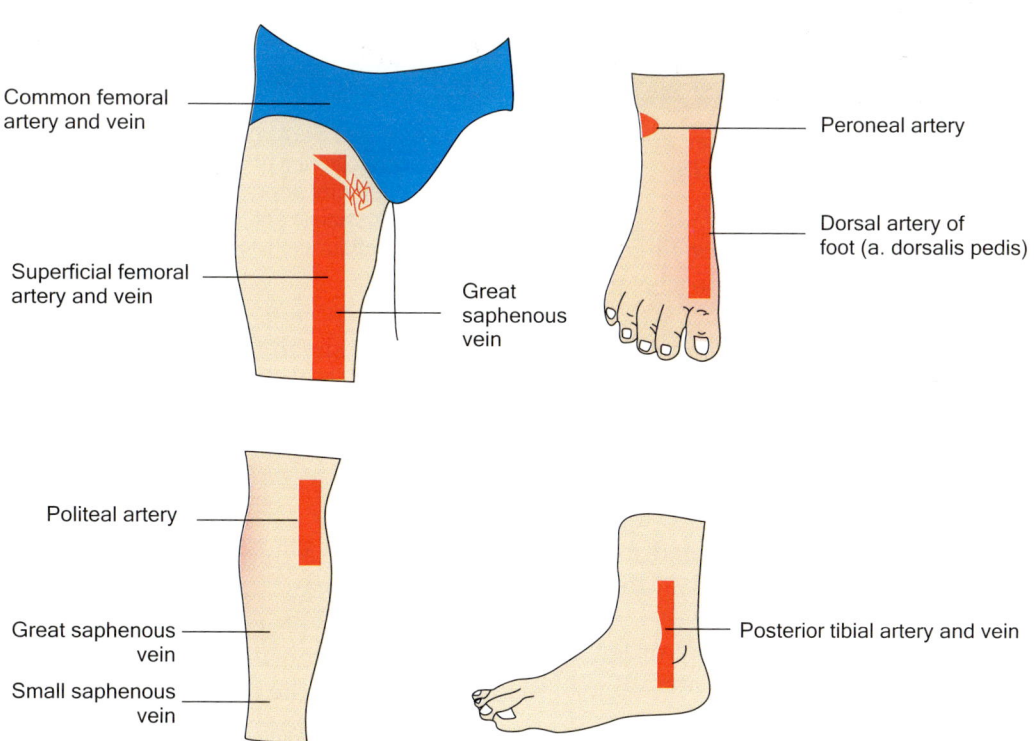

Fig. 23.51: Diagrammatic representation of various sites for probe placement for obtaining color flows and Doppler velocities of vascular system in the lower limb

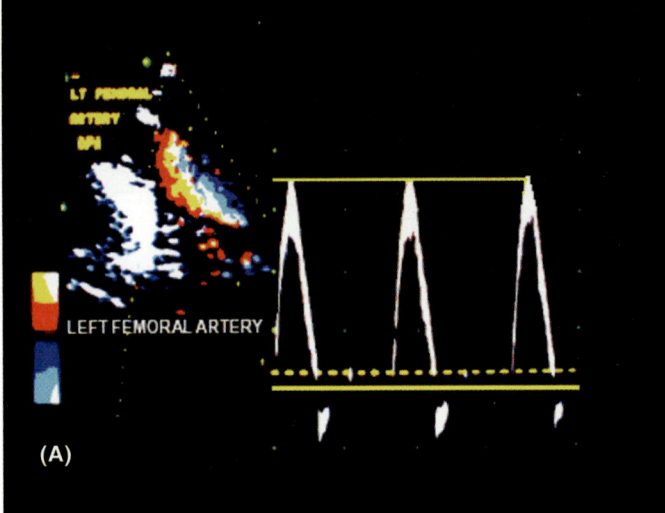

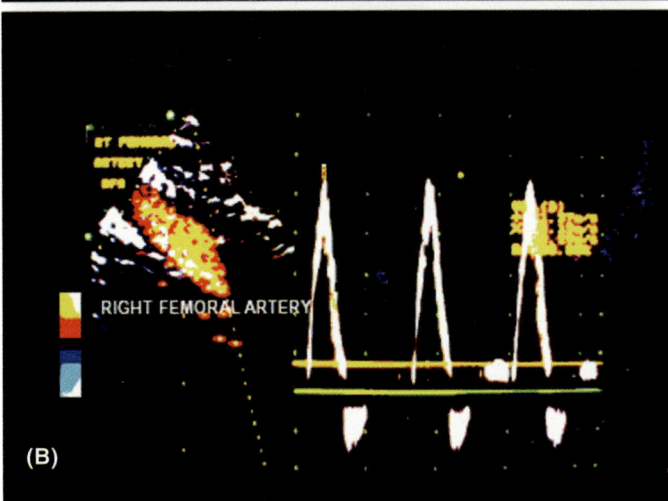

Fig. 23.52A and B: Color Doppler flow velocities in normal left femoral artery **(A)** and normal right femoral artery **(B)**

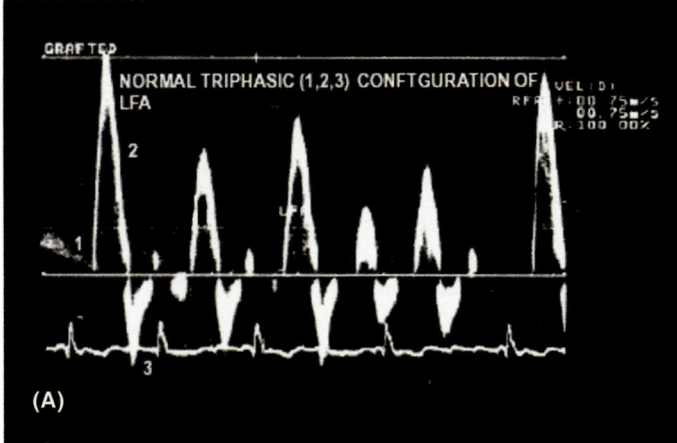

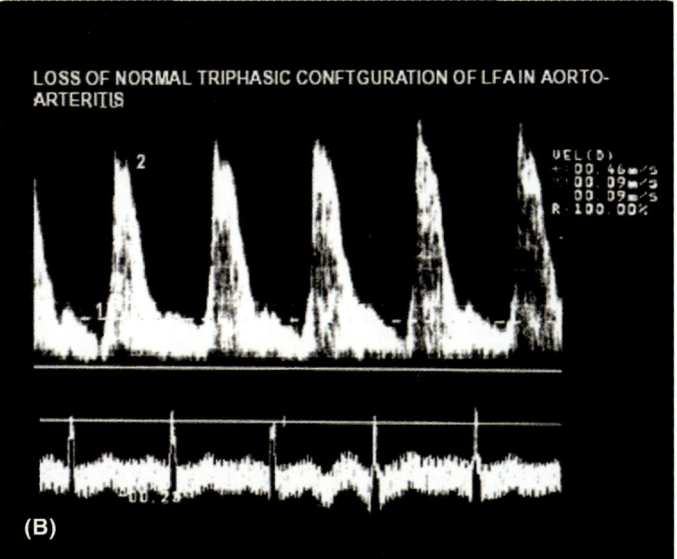

Fig. 23.53A and B: (A) Doppler flow velocity in a person with normal triphasic configuration of left femoral artery. **(B)** Doppler flow velocity across left femoral artery showing wide spectrum, less window and normal peak systolic and diastolic flow velocities and loss of normal triphasic configuration in patient with wide spread aorto-arteritis syndrome

3. Obtain waveforms from the posterior tibial artery at its site medial and posterior to the medial malleolus.
4. Obtain waveforms from the dorsalis pedis artery along the midpoint of the volar surface of the foot, in line with the space between the first two toes and the ankle.
5. If necessary, obtain a waveform from the peroneal artery anterior to the lateral malleolus at the ankle.
6. Optionally, a waveform can be obtained from the superficial femoral artery medially along the sartorius groove.

The waveforms can be obtained in any order, and each of the steps should be performed bilaterally when possible.

Interpretation of Doppler Waveforms

A normal arterial signal is triphasic. Diminution or loss of any of the components implies obstruction proximal to the probe site. If flow is triphasic at the ankle, it must be triphasic at all sites above the ankle. The absence of a triphasic pattern in the popliteal artery in the presence of a normal triphasic pattern in the femoral and ankle areas implies technical error, and the artery should be rechecked.

Following is a guide to interpretation of the waveforms in cases of disease:

1. If the waveforms are triphasic in the femoral, popliteal, dorsalis pedis, and posterior tibial arteries, the flow in the leg is within normal limits.
2. If the waveforms are triphasic in the femoral and popliteal but biphasic or monophasic in either of the ankle vessels where the other is triphasic, the abnormal artery is probably the only one diseased.

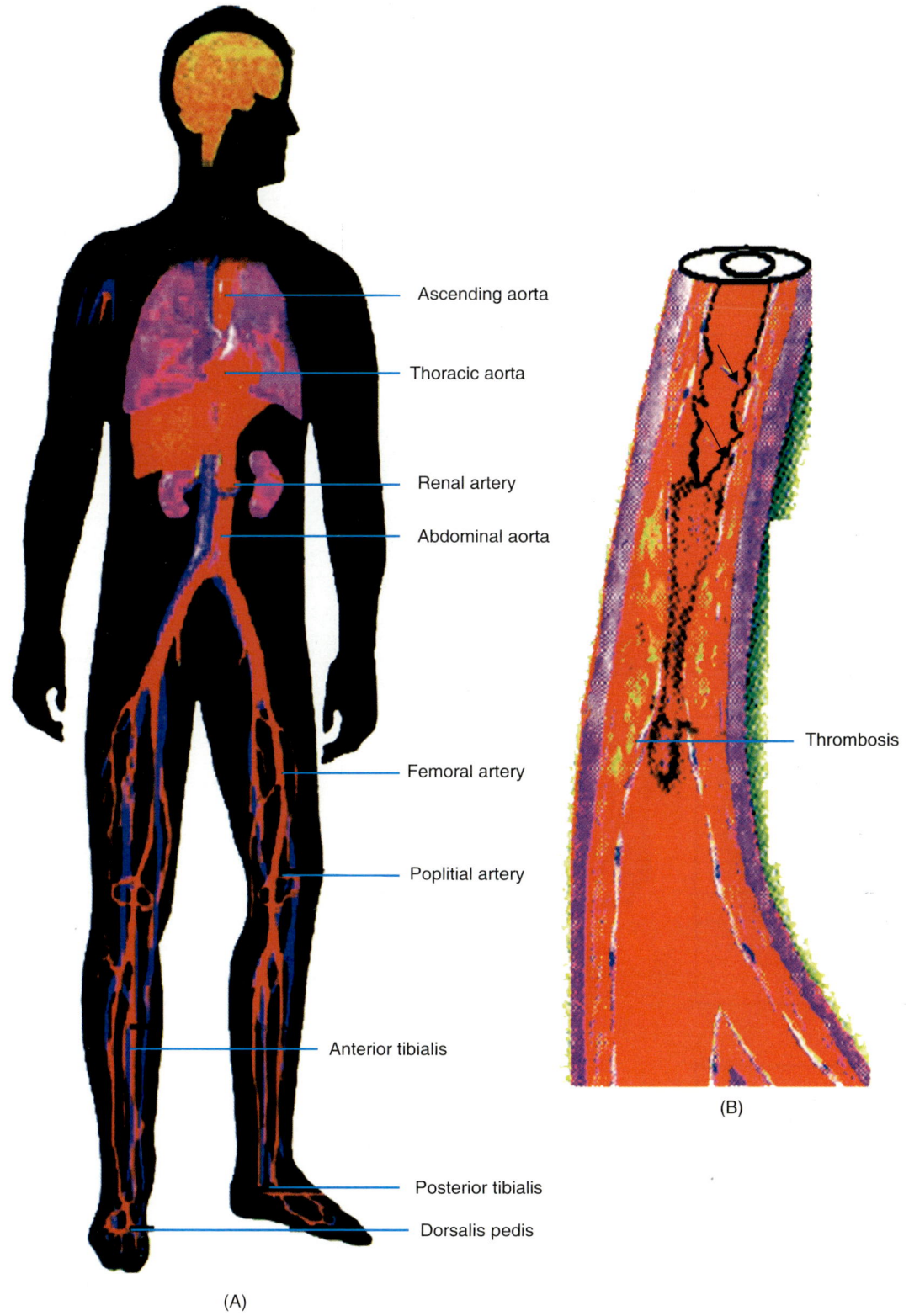

Fig. 23.54: **(A)** Peripheral vascular system in human. **(B)** Thrombotic obstruction in femoral artery (arrow) along with atherosclerotic lesion (arrow)

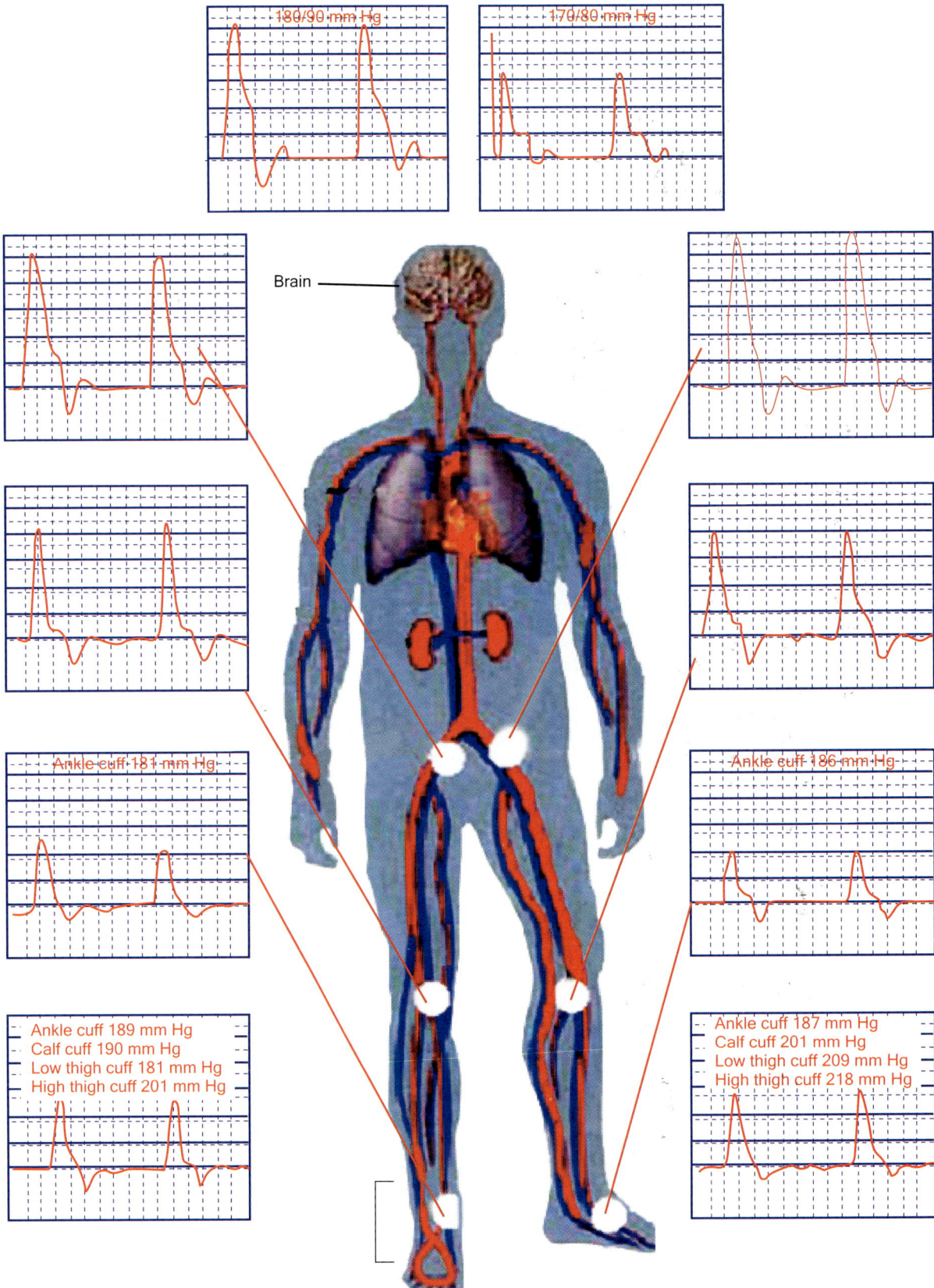

Fig. 23.55: Normal Doppler examination of lower extremities

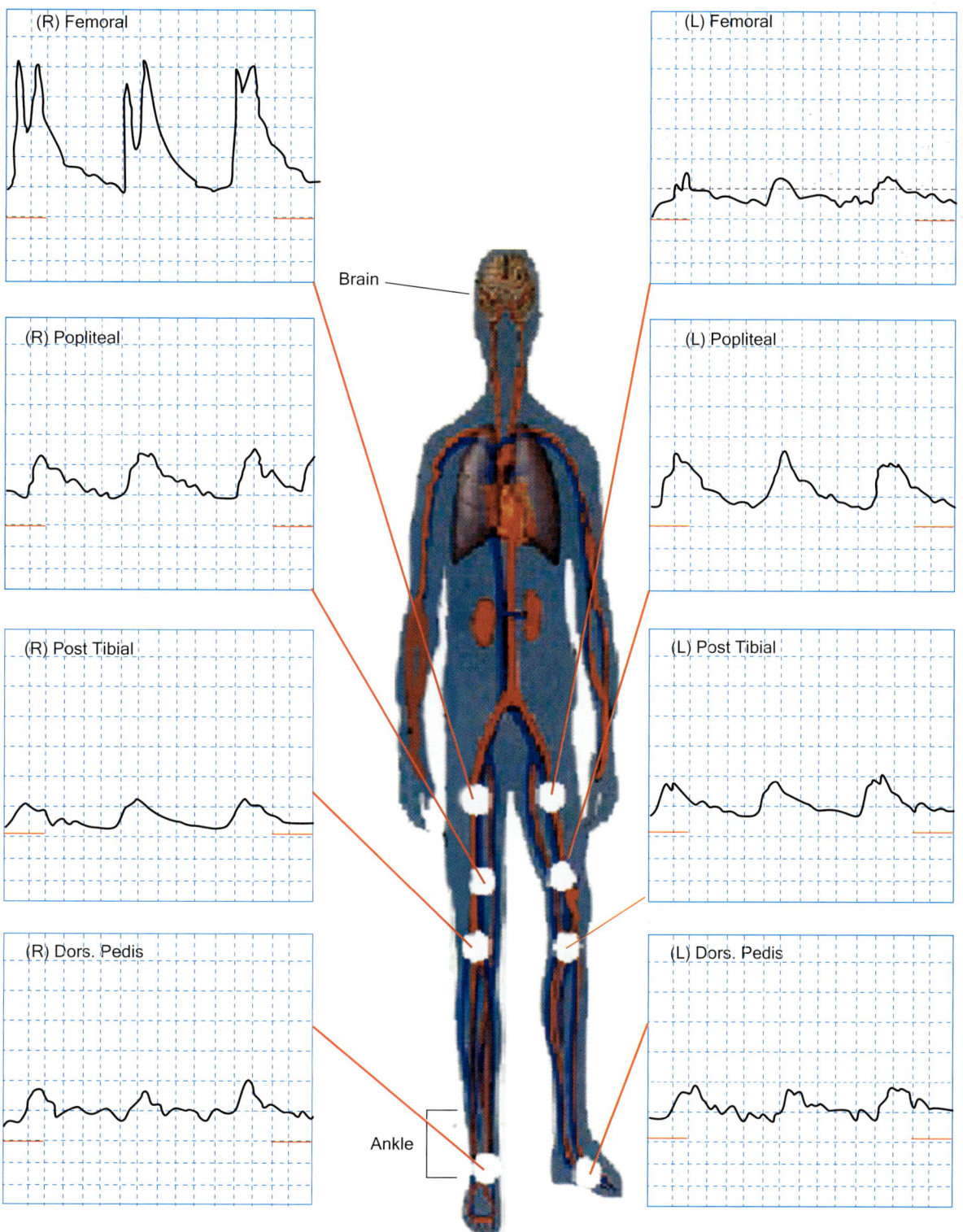

Fig. 23.56: Doppler waveforms in bilateral illiac occlusion showing turbulence in right femoral signal and diminished left femoral signal

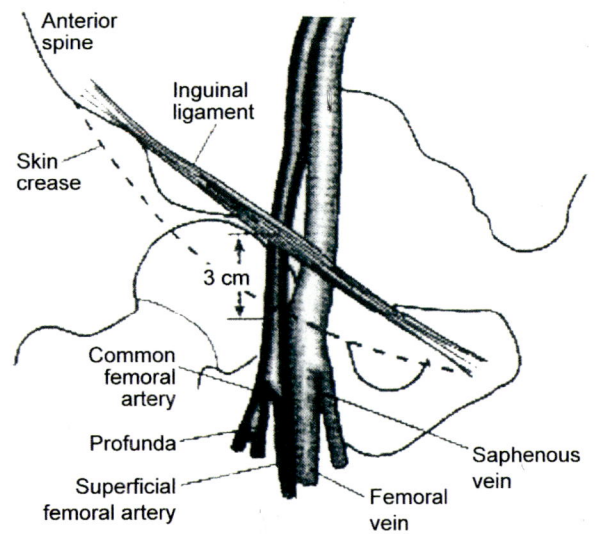

Fig. 23.57: Anatomy of the inguinal canal, the femoral vein lies medial to the femoral artery. It also shows the placement of common femoral artery, profunda and superficial femoral artery

3. If flow is triphasic in the femoral and popliteal but biphasic or monophasic in both ankle arteries, there is probably disease within the distal popliteal or below the popliteal involving the trifurcation vessels.

4. If flow is triphasic in the femoral but biphasic or monophasic at the popliteal and ankle vessels, this implies superficial femoral artery or popliteal artery stenoses or occlusions. Examination of the proximal and distal superficial femoral artery can help locate the level of obstruction.

5. Biphasic or monophasic flow at the femoral and all sites below implies an iliac artery or distal aortic stenosis or occlusion.

6. Finally, absence of a signal in any artery with no detectable distal flow implies a complete occlusion or thrombosis of the artery. This diagnosis can be made most reliably in trifurcation vessels.

The additional use of segmental pressures compared with the waveform read out and audible information is quite accurate in helping to determine the relative flow status of the extremity. However, error in interpretation can occur and are often the result of poor examination technique.

Interpretation of Segmental Pressure Measurements

To determine the flow status of the extremities, one must calculate ratios of the ankle systolic pressures divided by the brachial systolic pressures. The ankle-brachial index is thus obtained. The higher systolic pressure of the two arteries examined at the ankle is divided by the higher systolic pressure of the two arms. This is done for each leg. The higher brachial pressure should be used for both legs to ensure uniformity.

In normal individuals the ankle-brachial index should be greater than 1, patients who are asymptomatic or with slight symptoms have indices from 0.90 to 1 patients with claudication showing indices of 0.4 to 0.85. Anything less than 0.4 implies rest pain or severe ischemia.

Using this criteria, the ankle-brachial ratio also can be used in categorizing the severity of flow impairment to the distal extremity.

- Indices running between 0.85 and 1 imply mild to moderate impairment.
- Indices running between 0.4 and 0.85 imply moderate impairment.
- Indices running between 0.1 and 0.4 imply severe impairment.

Reading falling on the borderline between categories are often interpreted as "mild to moderate," "moderate to severe," and so on.

Experience with follow-up studies has shown that in normal individuals the ankle-brachial index can vary from 0.85 to as much as 1.1. This factor seems to depend on the relative blood pressure that a patient may have on the day of examination and whether it may change between the time, the arm is checked and when the ankle pressures are taken. Therefore the examiner and interpreting physician should not expect the same index in a normal patient to be completely reproducible from examination to examination and should be aware that a lower index may not imply disease if a strong triphasic signal is found (Fig. 23.46A and B).

It should also be noted that patients with calcific arteries often have abnormally or unusually high ankle-brachial indices, such as 1.2 to 3. In these individuals the quality of the waveform is the best indicator of occlusion, since the vessels are incompressible. Patients with extremely obese legs or diabetes also may have abnormally high indices.

Further information about the circulation may be obtained by comparison of the segmental pressures. In a normal patient, there is usually no greater than 40 mm Hg of difference between any two cuffs. The pressure reading increases as the circumference of the extremity increases.

An accurate pressure at the thigh could be obtained only with an extremely wide cuff, but it is unnecessary for Doppler readings because the difference between cuffs is used as an indicator of a pressure drop. The upper thigh pressure should not exceed 50 mm Hg above the brachial pressure.

As mentioned, extremely high pressures (as in noncompressible arteries or other situations with

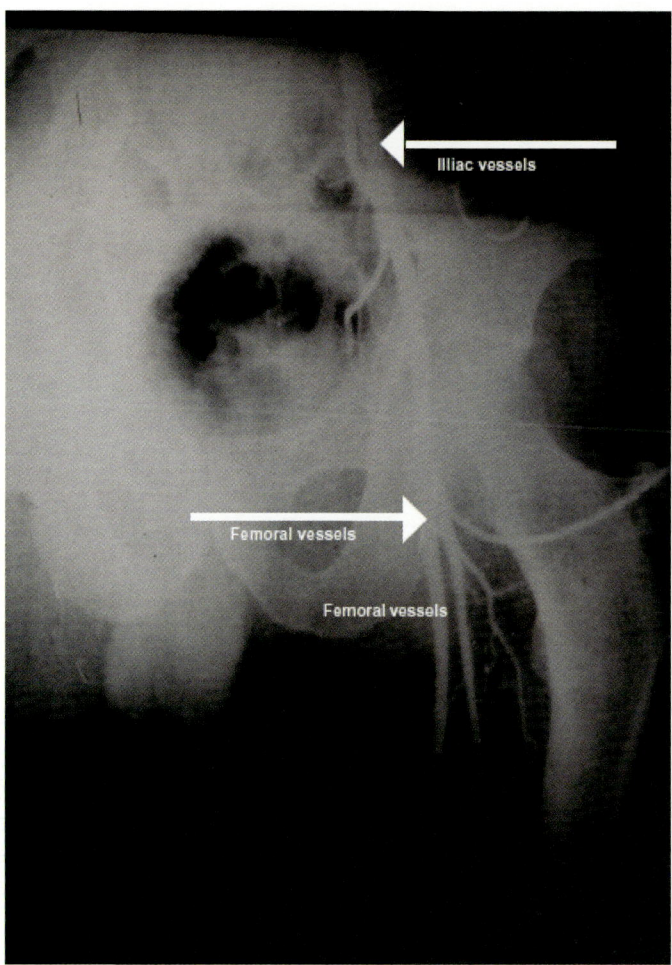

Fig. 23.58: Aortogram depicting reduced luminal size and truncated blood flow in both illiac and femoral vessels in patient with non-specific type of aorta-arteritis syndrome

pressures greater than 300 mm Hg) in the ankle or calf imply a calcified segment. This should be noted on the report form so there will be no confusion during interpretation.

If an upper thigh pressure is significantly less than the brachial pressure, this implies iliac artery stenosis.

If there is a significant pressure drop between the lower and upper thigh cuffs, this implies a superficial femoral artery obstruction.

If there is a significant pressure drop between the lower thigh and calf cuffs, a popliteal artery stenosis is implied.

If there is a significant pressure drop between the ankle and calf cuffs, this implies stenosis of the anterior tibial, posterior tibial, or peroneal arteries. Marked pressure drops between metatarsal-toe pressure and ankle pressure may indicate small-vessel disease in the forefoot or digits. This finding is not uncommon in cases of diabetes or Buerger's disease.

It is important to correlate segmental pressure findings with the results of duplex, Doppler velocity waveform analysis, or volume pulse recording, if available, to obtain a more complete picture of hemodynamic and perfusion conditions in the leg.

Arterial Duplex Sonography

Arterial duplex sonography involves direct imaging of the arterial structures in the leg, with an emphasis on visualising or occlusions and detecting their location. The hemodynamic effect of any stenoses can additionally be measured by colour-flow imaging, spectral Doppler, of both aneurysmal vessels, arteriovenous fistulas, and iatrogenic arterial injuries (e.g., pseudoaneurysms) can be evaluated. Assessing patency and flow in arterial reconstructions and bypass grafts is also an important application of duplex.

The duplex examination of the lower extremities, whether of arteries or veins, demands a great deal from the examiner. He or she must have a very thorough knowledge of the normal arterial anatomy and hemodynamics and be familiar with what would constitute an abnormal finding. It is also important to know how the vessels are oriented in the calf to avoid misinterpreting the image (Fig. 23.57).

Interpretation of the Lower Extremity Arterial Duplex Sonography Examination

The arterial images should be evaluated for the presence of plaque formations and the degree of luminal reduction. Stenoses can occur at almost any location and it is possible that several stenoses can cause a severe reduction of flow to the lower leg. The best way to determine the significance of a stenosis is to look for filling defects in the colour-flow pattern and evaluate the colour-flow streamlines to see if areas of increased turbulence and velocity increase are occurring. Once an area of increased velocity is isolated, a Doppler spectrum should be obtained at that site. The sample volume should be sized accordingly and then placed within the streamline slightly distal to the most reduced portion of the lumen. Please note that greyscale or colour-flow imaging alone is insufficient to diagnose hemodynamically significant stenoses and pulsed Doppler spectrum analysis must be used in conjunction. Area of suspected stenosis must be evaluated in transverse as well as longitudinal planes to check for asymmetry and irregularities that may not be seen directly in the longitudinal plane (Fig. 23.34A and B).

Luminal-reduction caliper measurements can be obtained but are generally not pertinent because of difficulty correlating these measurements with angiography.

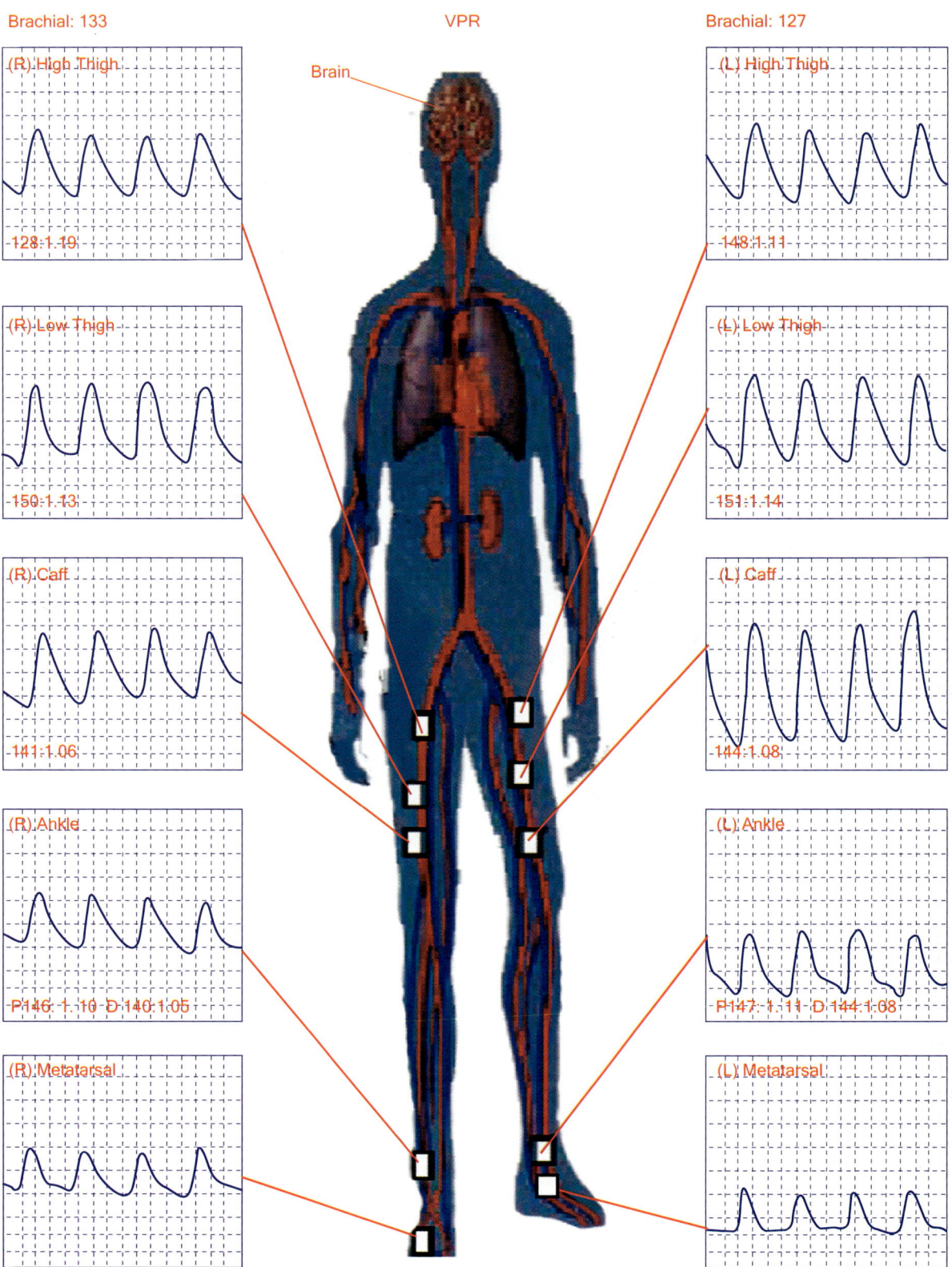

Brachial: 133

VPR

Brachial: 127

(R) High Thigh

128:1.19

(L) High Thigh

148:1.11

(R) Low Thigh

150:1.13

(L) Low Thigh

151:1.14

(R) Calf

141:1.06

(L) Calf

144:1.08

(R) Ankle

P146:1.10 D 140:1.05

(L) Ankle

P147:1.11 D 144:1.08

(R) Metatarsal

(L) Metatarsal

Brain

Fig. 23.59: Abnormal volume pulse waveforms showing roughly equal perfusion levels and loss of dicrotic notch in brachial arteries

Diagnostic Velocity Criteria

Diagnosis of the degree of stenosis is based on velocity increases at the stenotic site with turbulence and disturbed flow downstream. Many published diagnostic criteria base estimates of stenotic significance on spectrally demonstrated hemodynamic changes, with a luminal reduction of greater than 50% corresponding to an increase in the peak systolic velocity is double that of the segment proximal to the stenosis. Increased spectral broadening, disruption of the envelope, and progressive loss of waveform components can occur distal to the stenosis as severity increases (Fig. 23.54).

Total occlusion of a segment manifests as homogeneous or heterogeneous echogenic material filling the entire lumen; colour-flow imaging shows flows abruptly stopping with some retrograde flow turbulence at the point where the flow stream hits "a dead end". An occluded segment may not cause proximal loss of diastolic flow if collateralization has occurred. Colour-flow imaging often enables the actual collateral branches and pathways to be traced around the blockage and then followed distally to a patent, reconstituted segment.

Occluded segments with no collaterals show an abrupt flash of systolic colour on colour-flow imaging with no colour in diastole; this is seen mostly in tibial vessels or in bypass grafts. Spectral Doppler waveforms show a high-resistance "whipcrack" waveforms in patent segments proximal to the occlusion in these cases.

Summary of Diagnostic Criteria

1. Stenoses appear as homogeneous or heterogeneous echogenic areas projecting into the lumen; a stenosis may not have a significant effect on the hemodynamics of the artery, until a 50% to 60% luminal reduction occurs. The presence of a stenosis can be identified more easily at times with colour-flow imaging, as can be the presence of hemodynamic streamline effects and turbulence caused by the stenosis. Colour-flow imaging and grey-scale imaging alone are not sufficient to grade the significance of a stenosis.
2. Hemodynamic changes can be determined by pulsed Doppler and spectral analysis. Stenosis of greater than 50% have a doubling of the peak segment proximal to the stenosis. Flow distal to the stenosis shows a decrease in peak velocity with rounding and blunting of the peak and progressive loss of the second and third components as the severity increases.

Arterial Aneurysm Evaluation

Aneurysms and ectasia of arterial segments can occur without significant stenosis. Although the basic techniques of imaging, colour-flow, and Doppler acquisition apply, it is important to evaluate the arterial segment in longitudinal and transverse planes and take respective images of segments at the proximal, central, and distal portions of the area in question. Electronic calipers should be used to record the anteroposterior and lateral diameters for comparison.

In general, peripheral arteries are normally smaller than 1 cm in diameter, although this varies; a segment with a slight measurable dilation compared with a proximal or distal segment may be classed as ectatic; and a focal enlargement approximately double the size of a normal proximal or distal segment may be considered true aneurysm. Aneurysms can be additionally classed as saccular (where they appear as a focal bulging central to the proximal and distal segments of normal caliber) or fusiform (where the aneurysm appears to be a gradual tapered expansion of the vessel over several centimeters). Examiners should be aware that arterial segments that have had balloon angioplasty have focally dilated segments because of the expansion of the balloon and compression of the plaque. These do not represent aneurysms.

Evaluation of the Postoperative Patient

This section deals with the variations in the examination needed to provide adequate results in the patients who has recently undergone vascular surgery. The basic format's of the routine Doppler waveform and segmental pressure examinations are adhered to by the sonographer. The brachial arteries are examined as in the routine examination, unless an arterial monitor line or IV prevents it. One of the two arms is required for the ankle-brachial index determination, especially since the success or failure of the surgery often depends on the results obtained by the examiner. Again, either the higher of the two arm pressures or the single arm pressure is used. Note, however, that if the only available brachial artery signal appear stenosed or occluded, the index will be inaccurate.

The history is taken, and the type of surgery and graft material (either the patient's own vein or a synthetic) is noted. If possible, a drawing of the surgical connections should be made for future reference if included in the patient's chart, showing the vessels that were resected or ligated, the levels where the graft is attached to the artery, and the course of the graft in the extremity. It is often beneficial to review the surgeon's operative notes. When the procedure was performed and exactly what was done. These also can help the examiner determine where the proximal and distal anastomoses actually are located and what type of graft materials were used.

There are many different methods of bypass grafting and types of graft materials, materials used for grafts are either of organic or synthetic origin. Organic graft include human allografts, human prepared umbilical vein, and a patient's own autogenous superficial veins.

The purpose of the graft is to shunt the main bloodflow around the obstructed area to the patent sections of the artery at a lower level.

Types of graft and the surgical conditions for which they are used include the following:

1. **Aortoiliac:** Commonly a synthetic bifurcated graft, employed in cases of abdominal aortic aneurysm at the bifurcation of the common iliac arteries.

2. **Aortofemoral:** Also synthetic, either unilateral or bilateral, used to bypass iliac obstructions or aneurysms expanding, past the common iliac regions.

3. **Femorofemoral:** Synthetic, placed subcutaneously across the lower abdomen to shunt flow from a patent femoral to point distal to the obstruction in the opposite femoral artery.

4. **Femoropopliteal:** Synthetic graft, or preferred autogenous saphenous vein. In the latter case the patient's own greater or lesser saphenous veins are used in the following ways:

   (a) The great saphenous is physically removed, the small branches are ligated, and the vein is turned backward and then anastomosed to the native artery above and below the obstruction. It is often placed deep in an anatomic tunnel or routed through the tissues to protect it (reversed saphenous vein).

   (b) The great saphenous is physically removed and has the small branches ligated, a valvulotome (valve cutter) is passed through, then the vein is anastomosed to the native artery above and below the obstruction without being reversed. It is sometimes relocated deep in the leg (non-reversed translocated saphenous vein).

   (c) Sections of greater or lesser saphenous vein from either leg, or basilic or cephalic vein from the arm, may be attached to each other end to end to form a longer bypass (composite vein).

   (d) The great saphenous vein is left *in situ*; in this method the vein is not removed from the thigh, but the proximal and distal ends needed for anastomosis are exposed, a valvulotome is passed through and feeding branched are ligated. The proximal and distal ends are then reanastomosed to the native artery above and below the obstruction (*in situ* vein).

5. **Femorotibial:** The same materials are used as in the femoropopliteal graft, but insertion is in either the anterior or the posterior tibial arteries; it is often passed subcutaneously on the medial (in frequently the lateral) surface of the leg and may be palpated easily at the knee area; used to bypass obstructions extending through the popliteal artery or involving the trifurcation vessels.

6. **Femoroperoneal:** Used in the same circumstances as the femorotibial graft but may be passed through the popliteal fossa rather than the medial side of the knee.

7. **Axillofemoral:** Usually synthetic, passed from the axillary artery subcutaneously across the chest and lower abdomen to the ipsilateral femoral artery can also be palpated along its length.

There are many variation on these methods. To avoid confusion, the examiner should be aware of the extent and exact type of surgery performed.

There is a definite rule to follow in postoperative examination, and although this suggestion is not often followed in many institutions, it is sound nevertheless. Never put a pressure cuff over a graft whether new or old, because you might occlude the graft. It is far safer to use just the ankle and calf cuffs or just the ankle cuff if the graft extends that far down (as in femorotibial bypass). If ankle cuffs has not been used (as in cases of femorotibial bypasses that anastomose in the foot area or to the dorsalis pedis), then velocity waveforms should be obtained. One factor that is not often considered is the patient's potential reaction to postoperative pressure cuffs. A patient tends to be somewhat protective of the graft, especially considering that he or she has already undergone a traumatic procedure and may have noted a marked improvement. If the graft fails or complications with it develop, it is not uncommon for the patient to believe (albeit probably incorrectly) that the use of a pressure cuff occluded the graft; this can lead to a number of uncomfortable situations for the examiner and laboratory alike. Using velocity measurements and duplex sonography can obviate this reaction and still obtain more diagnostic information about the graft.

In addition, many synthetic graft materials, such as PTFE or Goretex, can be obtained with rigid rings spaced evenly along the length of the graft to prevent inadvertent compression or kinking of the graft and to preserve the lumen shape. These grafts are usually used in stress or flexible points, such as at knee joints, or when added protection is required (such as an axillofemoral segments along the superficial abdominal wall). These grafts often resist compression and do not yield accurate results in any case.

Only the ankle pressure is required for the ankle-brachial index. The use of segmental cuffs is not actually necessary in the immediate postoperative period since in most patients a prior examination or arteriogram has confirmed the occlusion preoperatively. If the patient has undergone an endarterectomy or embolectomy rather than a bypass, the same guidelines should be observed.

Duplex Evaluation of Vein Bypass Grafts

Graft surveillance is a common application of duplex sonography, and one that has been very successful. Vein graft have their own set of idiosyncrasies, any of which can cause failure or perfusion problems.

1. Arteriovenous fistulas can occur *in situ* grafts when one or more feeder branches of the saphenous vein have not been ligated. These fistulas can cause local varicosities and discomfort and sometimes "steal" flow from the graft causing a decrease in distal perfusion and runoff.
2. Valve cups that have been insufficiently cut can act as sites for thrombus formation and can cause focal stenotic changes.

To evaluate the graft, the examiner should adjust the technical factors as described earlier. The examiner then locates the native artery proximal to the graft (above the incision) longitudinally and progresses distally until the proximal anastomosis is visualised. The anastomosis should be evaluated for the presence of stenosis, then the graft itself should be steadily followed, moving distally until the distal anastomosis is reached. When examining the graft, the transducer should be moved from side to side to look for tell tale signs of arteriovenous fistulas or intact valve cusps; colour-flow imaging is extremely beneficial in these cases. Once the distal anastomosis has been evaluated, the distal native vessel should also be briefly examined to check for extension of plaque. Spectral Doppler velocity measurements should be taken in the native vessels above and below the graft anastomoses, and (at minimum) proximally and distally within the graft. If areas of suspected stenosis or cusps are detected, velocity measurements must be recorded at the stenotic area and downstream from it. Transverse images should also be obtained if necessary.

If an arteriovenous fistula in the graft is detected, the patent branch should be followed in both longitudinal and transverse planes into the leg, and spectral Doppler velocities should be obtained in the graft above the fistula, below the fistula, and within the fistula branch itself. Sometimes it is even possible to track a branch to its insertion in major vein. Fistulas planned for focal surgical ligation can be marked by this using a waterproof surgical dye once the origin has been identified.

Since graft imaging is usually performed along with Doppler waveforms and an ankle-brachial ratio, the examination can sometimes be abbreviated to just a proximal and distal graft waveform coupled with an ankle-brachial ratio if ankle flow appears to be within normal limits.

Graft Stenosis and Velocity Criteria

The duplex criteria for evaluating *in situ* grafts is the some as that for the rest of the arterial system. One difference, however, is that a graft velocity of less than 45 cm/sec in the smallest-diameter graft segment has been suggested to predict potential graft failure if it is obtained after a 2-month postoperative period. (Normal graft velocities of less than 45 cm/sec can occur, however, if grafts are large in diameter). Occluded grafts with a graft lumen filled with echogenic thrombotic material, and a high-resistance waveform with a complete absence of diastolic flow may be present in a segment either proximal to an occlusion or in cases of outflow obstruction distal to a graft.

Procedure Summary

The following procedure for the postsurgical patient can be used:

1. Obtain the patient's history, concentrating on the operative notes (if available) and incisional locations to determine the levels and extents of any bypass grafts.
2. Obtain Doppler velocity waveforms from all sites as in a routine study. Take waveforms from specific axillofemoral segments, femorofemoral segments, and peripheral grafts.
   Note: If evaluating a below-knee femoropopliteal or femorotibial graft, do not try to obtain a popliteal waveform at the conventional site behind the knee unless the graft has been routed through the popliteal fossa. Waveforms obtained otherwise do not reflect the true hemodynamic state of the lower leg, since it is possible for a patent native popliteal artery to be monophasic from collaterals although triphasic flow reaches the rest of the leg through the graft.
3. Apply pressure cuffs to the arms and the ankle (when possible). Obtain ankle pressure and brachial pressures and calculate the ankle brachial indices.
4. If a vein graft is in place, perform Duplex and/or colour-flow imaging of the graft and obtain spectral Doppler waveforms and velocities from the proximal and distal sections, anastomoses, stenotic areas, and native vessels.

If dressing, skin closures, surgical clips, or other interfering items are present, the examination may have to be abbreviated. Some waveforms or images may not be taken in these cases, and the presence of these limiting factors should be noted on the report forms.

Examination of the Patient after percutaneous balloon angioplasty, balloon thrombectomy, atherectomy, or endarterectomy.

The Doppler examination after endarterectomy angioplasty, thrombectomy, or atherectomy does not differ from the normal examination, except that thigh cuffs and tracings in the region of the catherization site may be omitted if the patient is feeling tenderness in that area or if a cutdown wound interfere with cuff or transducer placement.

Bibliography

1. A randomised, blinded, trial of clopidogrel versus aspirin in patients at risk of ischemic events (CAPRIE). CAPRIE Steering Committee: *Lancet* 1996; 348:1329.
2. Abbott WM, Green RM, Matsumoto T, *et al.* Prosthetic above-knee femoropopliteal bypass grafting: results of a multicenter randomized prospective trial. Above-Knee Femoropopliteal Study Group. *J Vasc Surg* 1997;25:19.
3. Algra A, van Gijn J. Aspirin at any dose above 30 mg offers only modest protection after cerebral ischaemia. *J Neurol Neurosurg Psychiatry.* 1996; 60:197–199.
4. Anderson DE, McLane MP, Reichman OH, Origitano TC. Improved cerebral blood flow and CO_2 reactivity after microvascular anastomosis in patients at high risk for recurrent stroke. *Neurosurgery.* 1992;31:26–34.
5. Armstrong WF, Bach DS, Carey L, *et al.* Spectrum of acute dissection of the ascending aorta: a transesophageal echocardiographic study. *J Am Soc Echocardiogr* 1996;9:646.
6. Armstrong WF, Bach DS, Carey LM, *et al.* Clinical and echocardiographic findings in patients with suspected acute aortic dissection. *Am Heart J* 1998;136:1051.
7. Ashton HA, Buxton MJ, Day NE, *et al.* The Multicentre Aneurysm Screening Study (MASS) into the effect of abdominal aortic aneurysm screening on mortality in men: a randomised controlled trial. *Lancet* 2002;360:1531.
8. Atherosclerotic disease of the aortic arch as a risk factor for recurrent ischemic stroke. The French Study of Aortic Plaques in Stroke Group: *N Engl J Med* 1996;334:1216.
9. Ausman JI, Diaz FG. Critique of the Extracranial-Intracranial Bypass Study. *Surg Neurol* 1986;26:218–221.
10. Ballard DJ, Fowkes FG, Powell JT: Surgery for small asymptomatic abdominal aortic aneurysms. *Cochrane Database Syst Rev* (2):CD001835, 2000.
11. Banning AP, Ruttley MST, Musumeci F, *et al.* Acute dissection of the thoracic aorta: transesophageal echocardiography is the investigation of choice. *BMJ* 1995; 310:72.
12. Bansal RC, Chandrasekaran K, Ayala J, *et al.* Frequency and explanation of false negative diagnosis of aortic dissection by aortography and transesophageal echocardiography. *J Am Coll Cardiol* 1995; 25:1393.
13. Baquis GD, Pessin MS, Scott RM. Limb shaking: a carotid TIA. *Stroke.* 1985;16:444–448.
14. Barnett HJM, Fox A, Hachinski V, Haynes B, Peerless SJ, Sackett D, Taylor DW. Further conclusions from the Extracranial-Intracranial Bypass Trial. *Surg Neurol* 1986; 26:227–235.
15. Barnett HJM, Peerless SJ, Kaufmann JCE. 'Stump' of internal carotid artery: a source for further cerebral embolic ischemia. *Stroke* 1978;9:448–456.
16. Barnett HJM. Delayed cerebral ischemic episodes distal to occlusion of major cerebral arteries. *Neurology* 1978;28:769–774.
17. Baron JC, Bousser MG, Rey A, Guillard A, Comar D, Castaigne P. Reversal of focal misery-perfusion *Surg* 1987; 74:802–804.
18. Bladin CF, Chambers BR. Clinical features, pathogenesis, and computed tomographic characteristics of intervere stenosis of the internal carotid artery. *Stroke* 1996;27:2026–2032.
19. Boger RH, Bode-Boger SM, Thiele W, *et al.* Restoring vascular nitric oxide formation by L-arginine improves the symptoms of intermittent claudication in patients with peripheral arterial occlusive disease. *J Am Coll Cardiol* 1998;32:1336.
20. Bogousslavsky J, Regli F, Hungerbuhler J, Chrzanowski R. Transient ischemic attacks and external carotid artery: a retrospective study of 23 patients with an occlusion of the internal carotid artery. *Stroke* 1981;12:627–630.
21. Bogousslavsky J, Regli F. Borderzone infarctions distal to internal carotid artery occlusion: prognostic implications. *Ann Neurol.* 1986;20:346–350.
22. Bogousslavsky J, Regli F. Unilateral watershed cerebral infarcts. *Neurology* 1986;36:373–377.
23. Bojar RM, Payne DD, Murphy RE, *et al.* Surgical treatment of systemic atheroembolism from the thoracic aorta. *Ann Thorac Surg* 1996;61:1389.
24. Bosch JL, Hunink MG: Meta-analysis of the results of percutaneous transluminal angioplasty and stent placement for aortoiliac occlusive disease. *Radiology* 1997; 204:87.
25. Bradac GB, Kaden B, Oppel F, Hirner A. Occlusion of internal carotid artery: further clinical, angiographic, and therapeutic considerations. *Neuroradiology* 1984;26:445–450.
26. Brevetti G, Diehm C, Lambert D: European multicenter study on propionyl-L-carnitine in intermittent claudication. *J Am Coll Cardiol* 1999;34:1618.
27. Brown MM, Wade JPH, Bishop CCR, Ross Russell RW. Reactivity of the cerebral circulation in patients with carotid occlusion. *J Neurol Neurosurg Psychiatry* 1986;49:899–904.
28. Bullock R, Mendelow AD, Bone I, Patterson J, Macleod WN, Allardice G. Cerebral blood flow and CO_2 responsiveness as an indicator of collateral reserve capacity in patients with carotid arterial disease. *Br J Surg* 1985;72:348–351.
29. Burns J, Satiani B, Vasko JS. Long-term survival following total carotid artery occlusion. *Cardiovasc Rev Rep* 1984;5:903–911.
30. Cambria RP, Davison JK, Zannetti S, *et al.* Clinical experience with epidural cooling for spinal cord protection during thoracic and thoracoabdominal aneurysm repair. *J Vasc Surg* 1997;25:234.
31. Cantore GP, Santoro A, Delfini R, Mariottini A, Palma L. Stenosis of one carotid artery with occlusion of the contralateral carotid. *Acta Neurochir (Wien)* 1989;101:42–45.
32. Cao P, Giordano G, De Rango P, Ricci S, Zanetti S, Moggi L. Carotid endarterectomy contralateral to an occluded carotid artery: a retrospective case-control study. *Eur J Vasc Endovasc Surg.* 1995;10:16–22.
33. Caplan LR, Sergay S. Positional cerebral ischemia. *J Neurol Neurosurg Psychiatry* 1976;39:385–391.
34. Capon A, de Rood M, Verbist A, Fruhling J. Action of vasodilators on regional cerebral blood flow in subacute or chronic cerebral ischemia. *Stroke* 1977;8:25–29.
35. Carter JE. Chronic ocular ischemia and carotid vascular disease. *Stroke* 1985;16:721–728.
36. Carter JE. Panretinal photocoagulation for progressive ocular neovascularization secondary to occlusion of the common carotid artery. *Ann Ophthalmol* 1984;16:572–576.

37. Coady MA, Rizzo JA, Hammond GL, *et al.* What is the appropriate size criterion for resection of thoracic aortic aneurysm? *J Thorac Cardiovasc Surg* 1997;113:476.

38. Collaborative overview of randomised trials of antiplatelet therapy. II: Maintenance of vascular graft or arterial patency by antiplatelet therapy. Antiplatelet Trialists' Collaboration. *BMJ* 1994;308:159.

39. Collaborative overview of randomised trials of antiplatelet therapy. I: Prevention of death, myocardial infarction, and stroke by prolonged antiplatelet therapy in various categories of patients. Antiplatelet Trialists' Collaboration. *BMJ* 1994;308:81.

40. Coselli JA, LeMaire SA, deFigueiredo LP, *et al.* Paraplegia after thoracoabdominal aortic aneurysm repair: is dissection a risk factor? *Ann Thorac Surg* 1997 ;63:28.

41. Coselli JS, Buket S, Djukanovic B: Aortic arch operation: current treatment and results. *Ann Thorac Surg* 1995;59:19.

42. Cote R, Barnett HJM, Taylor DW. Internal carotid occlusion: a prospective study. *Stroke.* 1983;14:898–902.

43. Crawford ES, Cohen ES: Aortic aneurysm: a multifocal disease. *Arch Surg* 1982;117:1393.

44. Criqui M, Langer RD, Fronek A, *et al.* Mortality over a period of 10 years in patients with peripheral arterial disease. *N Engl J Med* 326:381, 1992

45. Dake MD, Kato N, Mitchell RS, *et al.* Endovascular stent-graft placement for the treatment of acute aortic dissection. *N Engl J Med* 1999;340:1546.

46. Dapunt OE, Galla JD, Sadeghi AM, *et al.* The natural history of thoracic aortic aneurysms. *J Thorac Cardiovasc Surg* 1994;107:1323.

47. Dawson DL, Cutler BS, Hiatt WR, *et al.* A comparison of cilostazol and pentoxifylline for treating intermittent claudication. *Am J Med* 2000;109:523.

48. Day AL, Rhoton AL, Little JR. The Extracranial-Intracranial Bypass Study. *Surg Neurol* 1986;26:222–226.

49. De Vries SO, Hunink MG: Results of aortic bifurcation grafts for aortoiliac occlusive disease: A meta-analysis. *J Vasc Surg* 1997;26:558.

50. Deeb GM, William DM, Bolling SF, *et al.* Surgical delay for acute type A dissection with malperfusion. *Ann Thorac Surg* 1997;64:1669.

51. Demetriades D, Gomez H, Velmahos CG, *et al.* Routine helical computed tomographic evaluation of the mediastinum in high-risk blunt trauma patients. *Arch Surg* 1998; 133:1084.

52. Deriu GP, Franceschi L, Milite D, Calabro A, Saia A, Grego F, Cognolato D, Frigatti P, Diana M. Carotid artery endarterectomy in patients with contralateral carotid artery occlusion: perioperative hazards and late results. *Ann Vasc Surg.* 1994;8:337–342.

53. Dobkin BR. Orthostatic hypotension as a risk factor for symptomatic occlusive disease. *Neurology.* 1989;39:30–34.

54. Dormandy JA, Rutherford RB: Management of peripheral arterial disease (PAD). TASC Working Group. *J Vasc Surg* 31:S1, 2000.

55. Drinkwater JE, Thompson SK, Lumley JSP. Cerebral function before and after extra-intracranial carotid bypass. *J Neurol Neurosurg Psychiatry.* 1984;47:1041–1043.

56. Dyken M, Klatte E, Kolar OJ, Spurgeon C. Complete occlusion of common or internal carotid arteries: clinical significance. *Arch Neurol.* 1974;30:343–346.

57. Eagle KA, Brundage BH, Chaitman BR, *et al.* Guidelines for perioperative cardiovascular evaluation for noncardiac surgery. Report of the American College of Cardiology/ American Heart Association Task Force on Practice Guidelines. Committee on Perioperative Cardiovascular Evaluation for Noncardiac Surgery. *Circulation* 1996;93: 1278.

58. Edwards MS, Chater NL, Stanley JA. Reversal of chronic ocular ischemia by extracranial-intracranial arterial bypass: case report. *Neurosurgery.* 1980; 7:480–483.

59. Eggleston TF, Bohling CA, Eggleston HC, Hershey FB. Photocoagulation for ocular ischemia associated with carotid artery occlusion. *Ann Ophthalmol.* 1980; 12:84–87.

60. Elefteriades JA: Natural history of thoracic aortic aneurysms: indications for surgery, and surgical versus nonsurgical risks. *Ann Thorac Surg* 2002; 74:S1877.

61. Elkayam U, Ostzega E, Shotan A, *et al.* Cardiovascular problems in pregnant women with the Marfan syndrome. *Ann Intern Med* 1995;123:177.

62. Endo M, Tomizawa Y, Nishida H, *et al.* Angiographic findings and surgical treatments of coronary artery involvement in Takayasu arteritis. *J Thorac Cardiovasc Surg* 2003;125:570.

63. Ernst CB: Abdominal aortic aneurysm. *N Engl J Med* 1993; 328:1167.

64. Evangelista A, Garcia-del-Castillo H, Gonzales-Alujas T, *et al.* Diagnosis of ascending aortic dissection by transesophageal echocardiography: utility of M-mode in recognizing artifacts. *J Am Coll Cardiol* 1996;27:102.

65. Evans JM, O'Fallon WM, Hunder GG: Increased incidence of aortic aneurysm and dissection in giant cell (temporal) arteritis: a population-based study. *Ann Intern Med* 1995;122:502.

66. Evine RL, Lagreze HL, Dobkin JA, Hanson JM, Satter MR, Rowe BR, Nickles RJ. Cerebral vasocapacitance and TIA's *Neurology.* 1989;39:25–29.

67. Fann JI, Smith JA, Miller C, *et al.* Surgical management of aortic dissection during a 30-year period. *Circulation* 1995;92:II113.

68. Faries PL, Brener BJ, Connelly TL, *et al.* A multicenter experience with the Talent endovascular graft for the treatment of abdominal aortic aneurysms. *J Vasc Surg* 2002;35:1123.

69. Fein JM. Prognosis of internal carotid occlusion. In: Fein JM, Spetzler RF, Carter LP, Selman WR, Martin NA, eds. *Cerebral Revascularization for Stroke.* New York, Thieme-Stratton; 1985:45–47.

70. Ferguson CG, Peerless SJ. Extracranial-intracranial bypass in the treatment of dementia and multiple extracranial arterial occlusion. *Stroke.* 1976; 7:13.

71. Ferrari E, Vidal R, Chevallier T, *et al.* Atherosclerosis of the thoracic aorta and aortic debris as a marker of poor prognosis: benefit of oral anticoagulants. *J Am Coll Cardiol* 1999;33:1317.

72. Fields WS, Lemak NA. Joint study of extracranial arterial occlusion, X: internal carotid artery occlusion. *JAMA.* 1976;235:2734–2738.

73. Finklestein S, Kleinman GM, Cuneo R, Baringer JR. Delayed stroke following carotid occlusion. *Neurology* 1980; 30:84–88.

74. Fisher CM. Concerning recurrent transient cerebral ischemic attacks. *Can Med J.* 1962;86:1091–1099.

75. Fisher CM. Senile dementia: a new explanation for its causation. *Can Med Assoc J* 1951;65:1–7.

76. Fisher M, Sotak CH, Minematsu K, Li L. New magnetic resonance techniques for evaluating cerebrovascular disease. *Ann Neurol* 1992; 32:115–122.

77. Fowkes FG, Housley E, Riemersma RA, *et al.* Smoking, lipids, glucose intolerance, and blood pressure as risk factors for peripheral atherosclerosis compared with ischemic heart disease in the Edinburgh Artery Study. *Am J Epidemiol* 135:331, 1992.

78. Frame PS, Fryback DG, Patterson C: Screening for abdominal aortic aneurysm in men ages 60 to 80 years: a cost-effectiveness analysis. *Ann Intern Med* 1993;119:411.

79. Freedman RR, Baer RP, Mayes MD: Blockade of vasospastic attacks by alpha 2-adrenergic but not alpha 1-adrenergic antagonists in idiopathic Raynaud's disease. *Circulation* 1995;92:1448.

80. Friedman SG, Lamparello PJ, Riles TS, Imperato AM, Sakwa MP. Surgical management of the patient with bilateral internal carotid artery occlusion. *J Vasc Surg* 1987;5:715–718.

81. Fritz VU, Voll CL, Levien LJ. Internal carotid artery occlusion: clinical and therapeutic implications. *Stroke* 1985;16:940–944.

82. Persson AV, Griffey EE. The natural history of total occlusion of the internal carotid artery. *Surg Clin North Am* 1985;65:411–416.

83. Furlan AJ, Whisnant JP, Baker HLJ. Long-term prognosis after carotid occlusion. *Neurology* 1980;30:986–988.

84. Furlan AJ, Whisnant JP, Kearns TP. Unilateral visual loss in bright light: an unusual symptom of carotid artery occlusive disease. *Arch Neurol* 1979;36:675–676.

85. Gadowski GR, Pilcher DB, Ricci MA: Abdominal aortic aneurysm expansion rate: effect of size and beta-adrenergic blockade. *J Vasc Surg* 1994;19:727.

86. Gardner AW, Poehlman ET: Exercise rehabilitation programs for the treatment of claudication pain: A meta-analysis. *JAMA* 1995;274:975.

87. Gasecki AP, Eliasziw M, Ferguson GG, Hachinski V, Barnett HJM, for the North American Symptomatic Carotid Endarterectomy Trial Collaborators. Long-term prognosis and effect of endarterectomy in patients with symptomatic severe carotid stenosis and contralateral carotid stenosis or occlusion: results from NASCET. *J Neurosurg* 1995;83:778–782.

88. Georgiadis D, Grosset DG, Lees KR. Transhemispheric passage of microemboli in patients with unilateral internal carotid artery occlusion. *Stroke.* 1993;24:1664–1666.

89. Gertler JP, Cambria RP. The role of external carotid endarterectomy in the treatment of ipsilateral internal carotid occlusion: collective review. *J Vasc Surg* 1987; 6:158–167.

90. Gibbs JM, Frackowiak RSJ, Legg NJ. Regional cerebral blood flow and oxygen metabolism in dementia due to vascular disease. *Gerontology* 1986;32(suppl 1):84–88.

91. Gibbs JM, Wise RJ, Leenders KL, Herold S, Frackowiak RSJ, Jones T. Cerebral haemodynamics in occlusive carotid-artery disease. *Lancet* 1985; 1:933–934.

92. Gibbs JM, Wise RJS, Leenders KL, Jones T. Evaluation of cerebral perfusion reserve in patients with carotid occlusion. *Lancet* 1984;1:310–314.

93. Gibbs JM, Wise RJS, Thomas DJ, Mansfield AO, Ross Russell RW. Cerebral haemodynamic changes after extracranial-intracranial bypass surgery. *J Neurol Neurosurg Psychiatry* 1987;50:140–150.

94. Goldhaber SZ, Manson JE, Stampfer MJ, *et al.* Low-dose aspirin and subsequent peripheral arterial surgery in the Physicians' Health Study. *Lancet* 1992;340:143.

96. Graham IM, Daly LE, Refsum HM, *et al.* Plasma homocysteine as a risk factor for vascular disease. The European Concerted Action Project. *JAMA* 1997;277:1775.

97. Gravanis MB: Giant cell arteritis and Takayasu aortitis: morphologic, pathogenetic and etiologic factors. *Int J Cardiol* 2000;75:S21.

98. Grillo P, Patterson RHJ. Occlusion of the carotid artery: prognosis (natural history) and the possibilities of surgical revascularization. *Stroke* 1975;6:17–20.

99. Hachinski VC. Vascular dementia: a radical redefinition. *Dementia* 1994;5:130–132.

100. Hagan PG, Nienaber CA, Isselbacher EM, *et al.* The international registry of aortic dissection (IRAD): new insights into an old disease. *JAMA* 2000; 283:897.

101. Hardy WG, Lindner DW, Thomas LN, Gurdjian ES. Anticipated clinical course in carotid occlusion. *Arch Neurol* 1962;6:64–76.

102. Harrison MJG, Marshall J. Prognostic significance of severity of carotid atheroma in early manifestations of cerebrovascular disease. *Stroke* 1982;13:567–569.

103. Hayreh SS, Zimmerman B: Management of giant cell arteritis: our 27-year clinical study: new light on old controversies. *Ophthalmologica* 2003;217:239.

104. Herold S, Brown MM, Frackowiak RSJ, Mansfield AO, Thomas DJ, Marshall J. Assessment of cerebral haemodynamic reserve: correlation between PET parameters and CO_2 reactivity measured by the intravenous 133 xenon injection technique. *J Neurol Neurosurg Psychiatry* 1988;51:1045–1050.

105. Hiatt WR, Hoag S, Hamman RF: Effect of diagnostic criteria on the prevalence of peripheral arterial disease. The San Luis Valley Diabetes Study. *Circulation* 91:1472, 1995.

106. Hollier LD, Taylor LM, Ochsner J: Recommended indications for operative treatment of abdominal aortic aneurysms: report of a subcommittee of the Joint Council of the Society for Vascular Surgery and of the North American Chapter of the International Society for Cardiovascular Surgery. *J Vasc Surg* 1992;15:1046.

107. Hunink MG, Wong JB, Donaldson MC, *et al.* Revascularization for femoropopliteal disease: A decision and cost-effectiveness analysis. *JAMA* 1995;274:165.

108. Hupperts RMM, Lodder J, Heuts-van Raak EPM, Kessels AGH, Wilmink JT. Borderzone brain infarcts on CT taking into account the variability in vascular supply areas. *Cerebrovasc Dis* 1996; 6:294–300.

109. Hurwitz BJ, Heyman A, Wilkinson WE, Haynes CS, Utley CM. Comparison of amaurosis fugax and transient cerebral

ischemia: a prospective clinical and arteriographic study. *Ann Neurol* 1985;18:698–704.

110. Intensive blood-glucose control with sulphonyl ureas or insulin compared with conventional treatment and risk of complications in patients with type 2 diabetes (UKPDS 33). UK Prospective Diabetes Study (UKPDS) Group: *Lancet* 1998; 352:837.

111. Ishikawa K: Diagnostic approach and proposed criteria for the clinical diagnosis of Takayasu's arteriopathy. *J Am Coll Cardiol* 1988;12:964.

112. Isner JM, Baumgartner I, Rauh G, *et al.* Treatment of thromboangiitis obliterans (Buerger's disease) by intramuscular gene transfer of vascular endothelial growth factor: preliminary clinical results. *J Vasc Surg* 1998;28:964.

113. Jacobs NA, Ridgway AEA. Syndrome of ischaemic ocular inflammation: six cases and a review. *Br J Ophthalmol.* 1985;69:681–687.

114. Juvonen T, Ergin MA, Galla JD, *et al.* Risk factors for rupture of chronic type B dissections. *J Thorac Cardiovasc Surg* 1999;117:776.

115. Kaji S, Nishigama K, Akasada T, *et al.* Prediction of progression or regression of type A aortic intramural hematoma by computed tomography. *Circulation* 1999;100:II281,

116. Kamata T, Yokota T, Furukawa T, Tsukagoshi H. Cerebral ischemic attack caused by postprandial hypotension. *Stroke* 1994;25:511–513.

117. Kato M, Matsuda T, Kaneko M, *et al.* Outcomes of stent-graft treatment of false lumen in aortic dissection. *Circulation* 1998 1998;98:II305.

118. Kawaguchi S, Sakaki T, Kamada K, Iwanaga H, Nishikawa N. Effects of superficial temporal to middle cerebral artery bypass for ischaemic retinopathy due to internal carotid artery occlusion/ stenosis. *Acta Neurochir (Wien).* 1994; 129:166–170.

119. Keane MG, Wiegers SE, Yang E, *et al.* Structural determinants of aortic regurgitation in type A dissection and the role of ventricular resuspension as determined by intraoperative transesophageal echocardiography. *Am J Cardiol* 2000;85:604.

120. Kearns TP, Hollenhorst RW. Venous stasis retinopathy of occlusive disease of the carotid artery. *Proc Staff Meeting Mayo Clinic.* 1963;38:304–312.

121. Kearns TP. Differential diagnosis of central retinal vein obstruction. *Ophthalmology.* 1983;90:475–480.

122. Kiser WD, Gonder J, Magargal LE, Sanborn GE, Simeone F. Recovery of vision following treatment of the ocular ischemic syndrome. *Ann Ophthalmol* 1983;15:305–310.

123. Kleiser B, Krapf H, Widder B. Carbon dioxide reactivity and patterns of cerebral infarction in patients with carotid artery occlusion. *J Neurol.* 1991;238:392–394.

124. Koelemay MJ, Lijmer JG, Stoker J, *et al.* Magnetic resonance angiography for the evaluation of lower extremity arterial disease: a meta-analysis. *JAMA* 285:1338, 2001.

125. Kuroda S, Kamiyama H, Abe H, Houkin K, Isobe M, Mitsumori K. Acetazolamide test in detecting reduced cerebral perfusion reserve and predicting long-term prognosis in patients with internal carotid artery occlusion. *Neurosurgery* 1993;32:912–919.

126. Lang EW, Daffertshofer M, Daffertshofer A, Wirth SB, Chesnut RM, Hennerici M. Variability of vascular territory in stroke: pitfalls and failure of stroke pattern interpretation. *Stroke* 1995;26:942–945.

127. Lazarous DF, Unger EF, Epstein SE, *et al.* Basic fibroblast growth factor in patients with intermittent claudication: results of a phase I trial. *J Am Coll Cardiol* 2000;36:1239.

128. Lederle FA, Johnson GR, Wilson SE, *et al.* Rupture rate of large abdominal aortic aneurysms in patients refusing or unfit for elective repair. *JAMA* 2002;287:2968.

129. Lederle FA, Wilson SE, Johnson GR, *et al.* Immediate repair compared with surveillance of small abdominal aortic aneurysms. *N Engl J Med* 2002;346:1437.

130. Lederle FA, Wilson SE, Johnson GR, *et al.* Variability in measurements of abdominal aortic aneurysms. *J Vasc Surg* 1995;21:945.

131. Leng GC, Lee AJ, Fowkes FG, *et al.* Incidence, natural history and cardiovascular events in symptomatic and asymptomatic peripheral arterial disease in the general population. *Int J Epidemiol* 25:1172, 1996.

132. Lievre M, Morand S, Besse B, *et al.* Oral beraprost sodium, a prostaglandin I(2) analogue, for intermittent claudication: a double-blind, randomized, multicenter controlled trial. Beraprost et Claudication Intermittente (BERCI) Research Group. *Circulation* 2000;102:426.

133. Lindgarde F, Labs KH, Rossner M: The pentoxifylline experience: exercise testing reconsidered. *Vasc Med* 1996;1:145.

134. Maraj R, Rerkpattanapipat P, Jacobs LE, *et al.* Meta-analysis of 143 reported cases of aortic intramural hematoma. *Am J Cardiol* 2000;86:664.

135. Markus HS, Harrison MJH, Adiseshiah M. Carotid endarterectomy improves haemodynamics on the contralateral side: implications for operating contralateral to an occluded artery. *Br J Surg* 1993;80:170–172.

136. Matsunaga N, Hayaski K, Sakamoto I, *et al.* Takayasu arteritis: MR manifestations and diagnosis of acute and chronic phase. *J Magn Reson Imaging* 1998;8:406.

137. Mattos MA, Barkmeier LD, Hodgson KJ, Ramsey DE, Sumner DS. Internal carotid artery occlusion: operative risks and long-term stroke rates after contralateral carotid endarterectomy. *Surgery* 1992;112:670–680.

138. McDowell FH, Potes J, Groch S. The natural history of internal carotid and vertebral-basilar artery occlusion. *Neurology* 1961;11:153–157.

139. Mehdorn HM, Nau HE, Forster M. Carotid occlusion and ocular ischemia: therapy control using evoked potentials. *Neurosurgery* 1986; 19:1031–1034.

140. Mehta RH, O'Gara PT, Bossone E, *et al.* Acute type A aortic dissection in the elderly: Clinical characteristics, management, and outcomes in the current era. *J Am Coll Cardiol* 2002;40:685.

141. Mehta RH, Suzuki T, Hagan PG, *et al.* Predicting death in patients with acute type A aortic dissection. *Circulation* 2002;105:200.

142. Mitchell RS, Miller DC, Dake MD, *et al.* Thoracic aortic aneurysm repair with an endovascular stent graft: the "first generation." *Ann Thorac Surg* 1999;67:1971.

143. Mortality results for randomised controlled trial of early elective surgery or ultrasonographic surveillance for small abdominal aortic aneurysms. The UK Small Aneurysm Trial Participants: *Lancet* 1998;352:1649.

144. Movsowitz H, Levine RA, Hilgenberg AD, *et al.* Transesophageal echocardiographic description of the mechanisms of aortic regurgitation in acute type A aortic dissection: implications for aortic valve repair. *J Am Coll Cardiol* 2000;36:884.

145. Muller M, Schimrigk K. Vasomotor reactivity and pattern of collateral blood flow in severe occlusive carotid artery disease. *Stroke* 1996;27:296–299.

146. Murabito JM, D'Agostino RB, Silbershatz H, *et al.* Intermittent claudication: a risk profile from The Framingham Heart Study. *Circulation* 96:44, 1997.

147. Nicholls SC, Kohler TR, Bergelin RO, Primozich JF, Lawrence RL, Strandness DE. Carotid artery occlusion: natural history. *J Vasc Surg* 1986;4:479–485.

148. Nienaber CA, Fattori R, Lund G, *et al.* Nonsurgical reconstruction of thoracic aortic dissection by stent-graft placement. *N Engl J Med* 1999;340:1539.

149. Nienaber CA, von Kodolitsch Y, Petersen B, *et al.* Intramural hemorrhage of the thoracic aorta: diagnostic and therapeutic implications. *Circulation* 1995;92:1465.

150. Nienaber CA, vonKodolitsch Y, Nicolas V, *et al.* The diagnosis of thoracic aortic dissection by noninvasive imaging procedures. *N Engl J Med* 1993;328:1.

151. Norrving B, Nilsson B, Risberg J. rCBF in patients with carotid occlusion: resting and hypercapnic flow related to collateral pattern. *Stroke* 1982; 13:155–162.

152. Norrving B, Nilsson B. Carotid artery occlusion: acute symptoms and long term prognosis. *Neurol Res* 1981;3:229–236.

153. Numano F, Kobayashi Y: Takayasu arteritis—beyond pulselessness. *Intern Med* 1999;38:226.

154. Okita Y, Takamoto S, Ando M, *et al.* Mortality and cerebral outcome in patients who underwent aortic arch operations using deep hypothermic circulatory arrest with retrograde cerebral perfusion: no relation of early death, stroke, and delirium to the duration of circulatory arrest. *J Thorac Cardiovasc Surg* 1998;115:129.

155. Olin JW: Thromboangiitis obliterans (Buerger's disease). *N Engl J Med* 2000;343:864.

156. Ouriel K, Veith FJ, Sasahara AA: A comparison of recombinant urokinase with vascular surgery as initial treatment for acute arterial occlusion of the legs. Thrombolysis or Peripheral Arterial Surgery (TOPAS) Investigators. *N Engl J Med* 1998;338:1105.

157. Palma JH, Almeida DR, Carvalho AC, *et al.* Surgical treatment of acute type B aortic dissection using an endoprosthesis (elephant trunk). *Ann Thorac Surg* 1997;63:1081.

158. Patel NH, Stephens KE, Mirvis SE, *et al.* Imaging of acute thoracic aortic injury due to blunt trauma: a review. *Radiology* 1998;209;335.

159. Paulson GW, Kapp J, Cook W. Dementia associated with bilateral carotid artery disease. *Geriatrics* 1966;11:159–166.

160. Persky JM, Kempczinski RF, Fowl RJ: Entrapment of the popliteal artery. *Surg Gynecol Obstet* 1991;173:84.

161. Petersen MJ, Cambria RP, Kaufman JA, *et al.* Magnetic resonance angiography in the preoperative evaluation of abdominal aortic aneurysms. *J Vasc Surg* 1995;21:891.

162. Poldermans D, Boersma E, Bax JJ, *et al.* The effect of bisoprolol on perioperative mortality and myocardial infarction in high-risk patients undergoing vascular surgery. Dutch Echocardiographic Cardiac Risk Evaluation Applying Stress Echocardiography Study Group. *N Engl J Med* 1999;341:1789.

163. Powers WJ, Tempel LW, Grubb RL. Influence of cerebral hemodynamics on stroke risk: one-year follow-up of 30 medically treated patients. *Ann Neurol* 1989;25:325–330.

164. Powers WJ. Cerebral hemodynamics in ischemic cerebrovascular disease. *Ann Neurol* 1991;29:231–240.

165. Prostanoids for chronic critical leg ischemia: a randomized, controlled, open-label trial with prostaglandin E1. The ICAI Study Group. Ischemia Cronica degli Arti Inferiori: *Ann Intern Med* 1999;130:412.

166. Provinciali L, Ceravolo MG, Minciotti P. A transcranial Doppler study of vasomotor reactivity in symptomatic occlusion. *Cerebrovasc Dis* 1993;3:27–32.

167. Radack K, Deck C: Beta-adrenergic blocker therapy does not worsen intermittent claudication in subjects with peripheral arterial disease: A meta-analysis of randomized controlled trials. *Arch Intern Med* 1991;151:1769.

168. Results of a prospective randomized trial evaluating surgery versus thrombolysis for ischemia of the lower extremity. The STILE trial. *Ann Surg* 1994;220:251.

169. Riles TS, Imparato AM, Kopelman I. Carotid artery stenosis with contralateral internal carotid occlusion: long-term results in fifty-four patients. *Surgery* 1980;87:363–368.

170. Rodin MB, Daviglus ML, Wong GC, *et al.* Middle age cardiovascular risk factors and abdominal aortic aneurysm in older age. *Hypertension* 2003;42:61.

171. Rojo-Leyva F, Ratliff NB, Cosgrove DM, *et al.* Study of 52 patients with idiopathic aortitis from a cohort of 1,204 surgical cases. *Arthritis Rheum* 2000;43:901.

172. Ross Russell RW, Page GR. Critical perfusion of brain and retina. *Brain* 1983;106:419–434.

173. Ruff RL, Talman WT, Petito F. Transient ischemic attacks associated with hypotension in hypertensive patients with carotid artery stenosis. *Stroke* 1981;12:353–355.

174. Rutherford RB, Baker JD, Ernst C, *et al.* Recommended standards for reports dealing with lower extremity ischemia: revised version. *J Vasc Surg* 1997;26:517.

175. Rutherford RR: Standards for evaluating results of interventional therapy for peripheral vascular disease. *Circulation* 1991;83(suppl I):1.

176. Sacquegna T, De Carolis P, Pazzaglia P, Andreoli A, Limoni P, Testa C, Lugaresi E. The clinical course and prognosis of carotid artery occlusion. *J Neurol Neurosurg Psychiatr* 1982;45:1037–1039.

177. Samson D, Watts C, Clark K. Cerebral revascularization for transient ischemic attacks. *Neurology* 1977;27:767–771.

178. Satiani B, Das BM, Vasko JS. Reconstruction of the external carotid artery. *Surg Gynecol Obstet* 1987;164:105–110.

179. Schmiedek P, Piepgras A, Leinsinger G, Kirsch C, Einhaupl K. Improvement of cerebrovascular reserve capacity by EC-IC arterial bypass surgery in patients with ICA occlusion

and hemodynamic cerebral ischemia. *J Neurosurg* 1994; 81:236–244.

180. Schmiedek P. Zerebrale ischamie: Neuansatz fur die mikrochirurgische Behandlung. *Dtsch Artzebl.* 1990;87:1518–1523.

181. Shores J, Berger KR, Murphy EA, *et al.* Progression of aortic dilatation and the benefit of long-term beta-adrenergic blockade in Marfan's syndrome. *N Engl J Med* 1994; 330:1335.

182. Smith MD, Cassidy JM, Souther S, *et al.* Transesophageal echocardiography in the diagnosis of traumatic rupture of the aorta. *N Engl J Med* 1995;332:356.

183. Sommerville ER. Orthostatic transient ischemic attacks. *Stroke* 1984;15:1066–1067.

184. Song JK, Kim HS, Song JM, *et al.* Outcomes of medically treated patients with aortic intramural hematoma. *Am J Med* 2002;113:181.

185. Standefer M, Little JR, Tomsak R, Furlan AJ, Zegarra H, Williams G. Improvement in the retinal circulation after superficial temporal to middle cerebral artery bypass. *Neurosurgery* 1985;16:525–529.

186. Sterpetti AV, Feldhaus RJ, Schultz RD, Farina C. Operative strategies in patients with symptomatic internal carotid artery occlusion. *Surgery* 1989;105:632–637.

187. Sundt TM. Was the international randomized trial of extracranial-intracranial arterial bypass representative of the population at risk? *N Engl J Med* 1987;316:814–816.

188. Suzuki T, Katoh H, Kurabayashi M, *et al.* Biochemical diagnosis of aortic dissection by raised concentrations of creatine kinase BB-isozyme. *Lancet* 1997;350:784.

189. Suzuki T, Katoh H, Tsuchio Y, *et al.* Diagnostic implications of elevated levels of smooth-muscle myosin heavy-chain protein in acute aortic dissection. The smooth muscle myosin heavy chain study. *Ann Intern Med* 2000; 133:537.

190. Tatemichi TK, Desmond DW, Mayeux R, Paik M, Stern Y, Sano M, Remien RH, Williams JB, Mohr JP, Hauser WA, Figueroa M. Dementia after stroke: baseline frequency, risks, and clinical features in a hospitalized cohort. *Neurology* 1992;42:1185–1193.

191. Tatemichi TK, Desmond DW, Paik M, Figueroa M, Gropen TI, Stern Y, Sano M, Remien R, Williams JB, Mohr JP, Mayeaux R. Clinical determinants of dementia related to stroke. *Ann Neurol* 1993; 33:568–575.

192. Tatemichi TK, Desmond DW, Prohovnik I, Eidelberg D. Dementia associated with bilateral carotid occlusions: neuro-psychological and haemodynamic course after extracranial to intracranial bypass surgery. *J Neurol Neurosurg Psychiatry* 1995;58:633–636.

193. Tatemichi TK, Young WL, Prohovnik I, Gitelman DR, Correll JW, Mohr JP. Perfusion insufficiency in limb-shaking transient ischemic attacks. *Stroke* 1990;21:341–347.

194. Tetteroo E, van der Graaf Y, Bosch JL, *et al.* Randomised comparison of primary stent placement versus primary angioplasty followed by selective stent placement in patients with iliac-artery occlusive disease. DutcIliac Stent Trial Study Group. *Lancet* 1998;351:1153.

195. The EC/IC Bypass Study Group. Failure of extracranial-intracranial arterial bypass to reduce the risk of ischemic stroke: results of an international randomized trial. *N Engl J Med* 1985;313:1191–1200.

196. Torvik A. The pathogenesis of watershed infarcts in the brain. *Stroke* 1984;15:221–223.

197. Transesophageal echocardiographic correlates of thromboembolism in high-risk patients with nonvalvular atrial fibrillation. The Stroke Prevention in Atrial Fibrillation Investigators Committee on Echocardiography: *Ann Intern Med* 1998;128:639.

198. Tsuda Y, Yamada K, Hayakawa T, Ayada Y, Kawasaki S, Matsuo H. Cortical blood flow and cognition after extracranial-intracranial bypass in a patient with severe carotid occlusive lesions: a three year follow-up study.nal watershed infarction. *Stroke* 1993;24:1925-1932.

199. Tulleken CAF, Verdaasdonk RM, Berendsen W, Mali WPTM. Use of the Excimer laser in high-flow bypass surgery of the brain. *J Neurosurg.* 1993;78:477–480.

200. Tulleken CAF, Verdaasdonk RM, Mansvelt Beck RJ, Mali WPTM. The modified Excimer laser assisted high flow bypass operation. *Surg Neurol.* 1996;46:424–429.

201. Umana JP, Miller DC, Mitchell RS: What is the best treatment for patients with acute type B aortic dissections—medical, surgical, or endovascular stent-grafting? *Ann Thorac Surg* 2002;74:S1840.

202. Van der Zwan A, Hillen B, Tulleken CAF, Dujovny M, Dragovic L. Variability of the territories of the major cerebral arteries. *J Neurosurg* 1992;77:927–940.

203. Van Rij AM, Solomon C, Packer SG, *et al.* Chelation therapy for intermittent claudication: a double-blind, randomized, controlled trial. *Circulation* 1994;90:1194.

204. Vilacosta I, San Román JA, Aragoncillo P, *et al.* Penetrating atherosclerotic aortic ulcer: documentation by transesophageal echocardiography. *J Am Coll Cardiol* 1998;32:83.

205. Vilacosta I, San Roman JA, Ferreiros J, *et al.* Natural history and serial morphology of aortic intramural hematoma: a novel variant of aortic dissection. *Am Heart J* 1997; 134:495.

206. Von Kodolitsch Y, Csosz SK, Koschyk DH, *et al.* Intramural hematoma of the aorta: predictors of progression to dissection and rupture. *Circulation* 2003;107:1158.

207. Vorstrup S, Brun B, Lassen NA. Evaluation of the cerebral vasodilatory capacity by the acetazolamide test before EC-IC bypass surgery in patients with occlusion of the internal carotid artery. *Stroke* 1986;17:1291–1298.

208. Vorstrup S, Lassen NA, Henriksen L, Haase J, Lindewald H, Boysen G, Paulson OB. CBF before and after extra-intracranial bypass surgery in patients with ischemic cerebrovascular disease studied with 133 Xe inhalation tomography. *Stroke* 1985;16:616–626.

208. Vorstrup S, Paulson OB. Extracranial-intracranial bypass revisited. *Cerebrovasc Dis* 1992;2:61–262.

210. Vorstrup S. Tomographic cerebral blood flow measurements in patients with ischemic cerebrovascular disease and evaluation of the vasodilatory capacity by the acetazolamide test. *Acta Neurol Scand* 1988;77(suppl 114):1–48.

211. Wade JPH, Wong W, Barnett HJM, Vandervoort P. Bilateral occlusion of the internal carotid arteries. *Brain* 1987; 110:667–682.

212. Webster MW, Makaroun MS, Steed DL, Smith HA, Johnson DW, Yonas H. Compromised cerebral blood flow reactivity *Echocardiogr* 1996;9:646.

213. Webster MW, Makaroun MS, Steed DL, Smith HA, Johnson DW, Yonas H. Compromised cerebral blood flow reactivity is a predictor of stroke in patients with symptomatic carotid artery occlusive disease. *J Vasc Surg* 1995;21:338–345.

214. Weiller C, Ringelstein EB, Reiche W, Buell U. Clinical and hemodynamic aspects of low flow infarcts. *Stroke* 1991; 22:1117–1123.

215. Widder B, Paulat K, Hackspacher J, Mayr E. Transcranial Doppler CO_2 test for the detection of hemodynamically critical carotid artery stenoses and occlusions. *Eur Arch Psychiatry Neurol Sci* 1986;236:162–168.

216. Wigley FM, Wise RA, Seibold JR, *et al.* Intravenous iloprost infusion in patients with Raynaud phenomenon secondary to systemic sclerosis: a multicenter, placebo-controlled, double-blind study. *Ann Intern Med* 1994;120:199.

217. Willens HJ, Kessler KM: Transesophageal echocardiography in the diagnosis of diseases of the thoracic aorta: part II—atherosclerotic and traumatic diseases of the aorta. *Chest* 2000;117:233.

218. Wolf YG, Fogarty TJ, Olcott C, *et al.* Endovascular repair of abdominal aortic aneurysms: eligibility rate and impact on the rate of open repair. *J Vasc Surg* 2000 ;32:519.

219. Yamashita C, Okada M, Ataka K, *et al.* Cerebral complications and distal false lumen in the repair of aortic dissection with retrograde cerebral perfusion. *J Cardiovasc Surg* 1997;38:581.

220. Yamauchi H, Fukuyama H, Nagahama Y, Nabatame H, Nakamura K, Yamamoto Y, Yonekura Y, Konishi J, Kimura J. Evidence for misery perfusion and risk for recurrent stroke in major cerebral arterial occlusive diseases from PET. *J Neurol Neurosurg Psychiatry* 1996;61:18–25.

221. Yanagihara T, Klass DW. Rhythmic involuntary movement as a manifestation of transient ischemic attacks. *Trans Am Neurol Assoc* 1981;106:46–48.

222. Yanagihara T, Marsh WR, Piepgras DG, Ivnik RJ. Dementia in bilateral carotid occlusive disease. *Stroke* 1990;21(suppl I): I–99.

223. Yanagihara T, Piepgras DG, Klass DW. Repetitive involuntary movement associated with episodic. *Ann Neurol* 1985; 18:244.

224. Yonas H, Smith HA, Durham SR, Pentheny SL, Johnson DW. Increased stroke risk predicted by compromised cerebral blood flow reactivity. *J Neurosurg* 1993;79:483.

225. Younkin D, Hungerbuhler JP, O'Connor M, Goldberg H, Burke A, Kushner M, Hurtig H, Obrist W, Gordon J, Gur R, Reivich M. Superficial temporal-middle cerebral artery anastomosis: effects on vascular, neurologic, and neuropsychological functions. *Neurology.* 1985; 35: 462–469.

226. Yusuf S, Sleight P, Pogue J, *et al.* Effects of an angiotensin-converting-enzyme inhibitor, ramipril, on cardiovascular events in high-risk patients. The Heart Outcomes Prevention Evaluation Study Investigators. *N Engl J Med* 2000;342:145.

227. Zeman RK, Berman PM, Silverman PM, *et al.* Diagnosis of aortic dissection: value of helical CT with multiplanar reformation and three-dimensional rendering. *AJR Am J Roentgenol* 1995;164:1375.

228. Smith MD, Cassidy JM, Souther S, *et al.* Transesophageal echocardiography in the diagnosis of traumatic rupture of the aorta. *N Engl J Med* 1995;332:356.

229. Demetriades D, Gomez H, Velmahos CG, *et al.* Routine helical computed tomographic evaluation of the mediastinum in high-risk blunt trauma patients. *Arch Surg* 1998 ;133:1084.

230. Patel NH, Stephens KE, Mirvis SE, *et al.* Imaging of acute thoracic aortic injury due to blunt trauma: a review. *Radiology* 1998; 209:335.

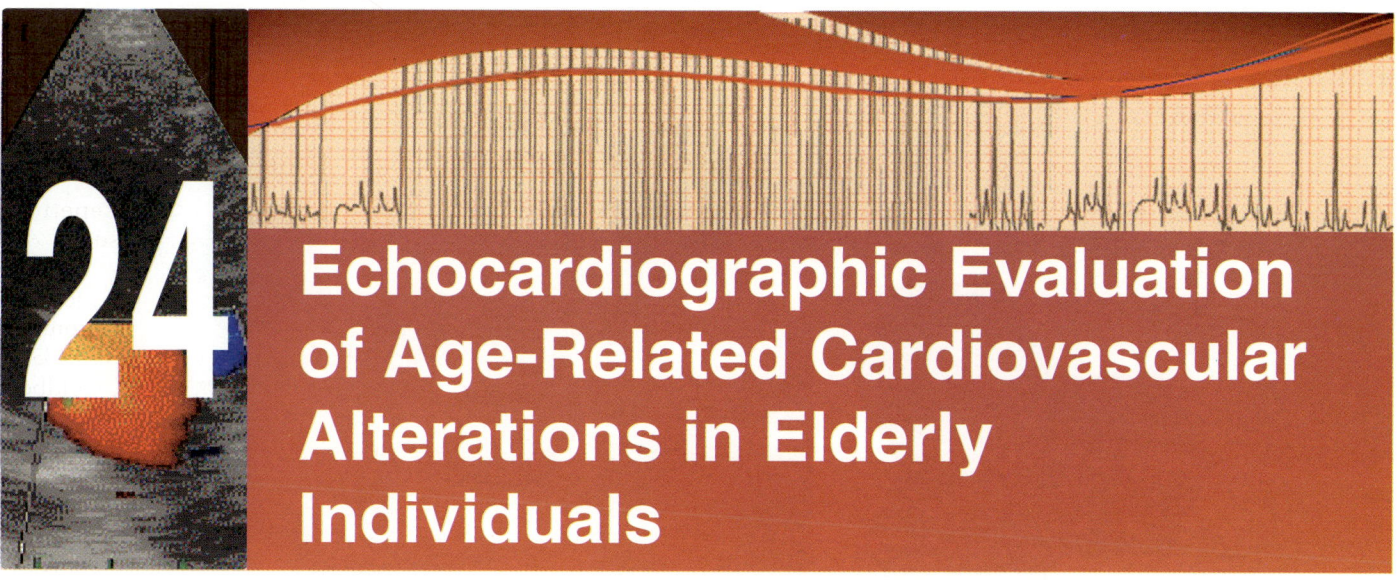

24 Echocardiographic Evaluation of Age-Related Cardiovascular Alterations in Elderly Individuals

There is no precise definition of **'the aged'**, 'the elderly' or **'advanced age'**. This is hardly surprising, because there is no specific clinical marker of the 'geriatric' patient, and ageing does not occur abruptly but represents a continuum. In fact, the 'geriatric population' is unique for its nonhomogeneity: physical and medical heterogeneity increase with advancing age. Nevertheless, data analysis by age quintiles supports the clinical relevance of usually defining patients aged > 64 year as the elderly. Approximately 15% of the Western population, and about 25% of surgical patients are aged 65 yr. Half of these will undergo surgery in the remainder of their lifetime.

Age itself is an independent morbidity and mortality risk factor for a long list of diseases and injuries, hospitalization, length of hospitalization, and adverse drug reactions. With very few exceptions, age has been shown to be an independent predictor of perioperative outcome. If we are to successfully reduce age-related perioperative cardiovascular morbidity and mortality (the main contributor to overall adverse perioperative outcome we need to define the factors that increase perioperative cardiovascular risk age-dependently. Although we might not always be able to improve underlying conditions, awareness of such additional risk factors may modify our perioperative anaesthetic management in a way that will ultimately improve outcome.

Accordingly, this review will first address the question of what constitutes perioperative cardio-vascular risk, independent of age. It will then focus on factors that might affect perioperative cardiovascular outcome age-dependently. Such factors include age-related changes in cardiovascular structure and function,

altered cardiovascular response to increased flow demands in the elderly, coexisting cardiovascular and other disease with advancing age, and drug therapy in older people. Finally, anaesthetic implications will be discussed.

Age-Related Cardiovascular Changes in Heart

Ageing is associated with numerous molecular, ionic, biophysical and biochemical changes in the heart. These changes affect protein function, mitochondrial oxidative phosphorylation, Ca^{2+} kinetics, excitation-contraction coupling, myofilament activation, contractile response, matrix composition and regeneration, cell growth and size, and apoptosis.

Age-related changes in cardiac morphology are mostly the result of alterations of intracellular molecular and biochemical pathways. In turn, many of the changes in cardiac function with advancing age develop in response to underlying alterations in morphology. Ultimately, cardiac ageing results in decreased mechanical and contractile efficiency, prolongation of the relaxation phase, stiffening of myocardial cells, mural connective tissue and valves, decreased number of myocytes, increased myocyte size, increased rate of myocyte apoptosis and blunted β-adrenoceptor-mediated contractile and inotropic response (Fig. 24.7).

Vasculature

Ageing affects various aspects of vascular morphology and function. The large arteries dilate, their walls thicken, the wall matrix changes, elastolytic and collagenolytic activity increases and smooth muscle tone increases. As a result, vascular stiffness increases with advancing age.

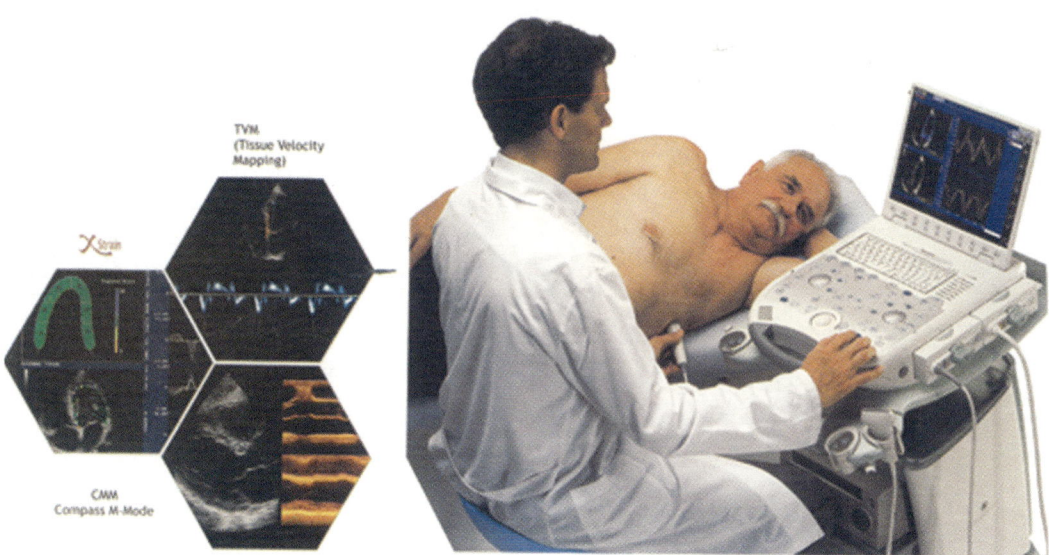

Fig. 24.1: Photograph of both operator and ultrasound machine employed for obtaining CMM, 2D-Doppler, tissue mapping, colour Doppler and Duplex colour imaging in the assessment cardiac and peripheral vascular disease in elderly patient

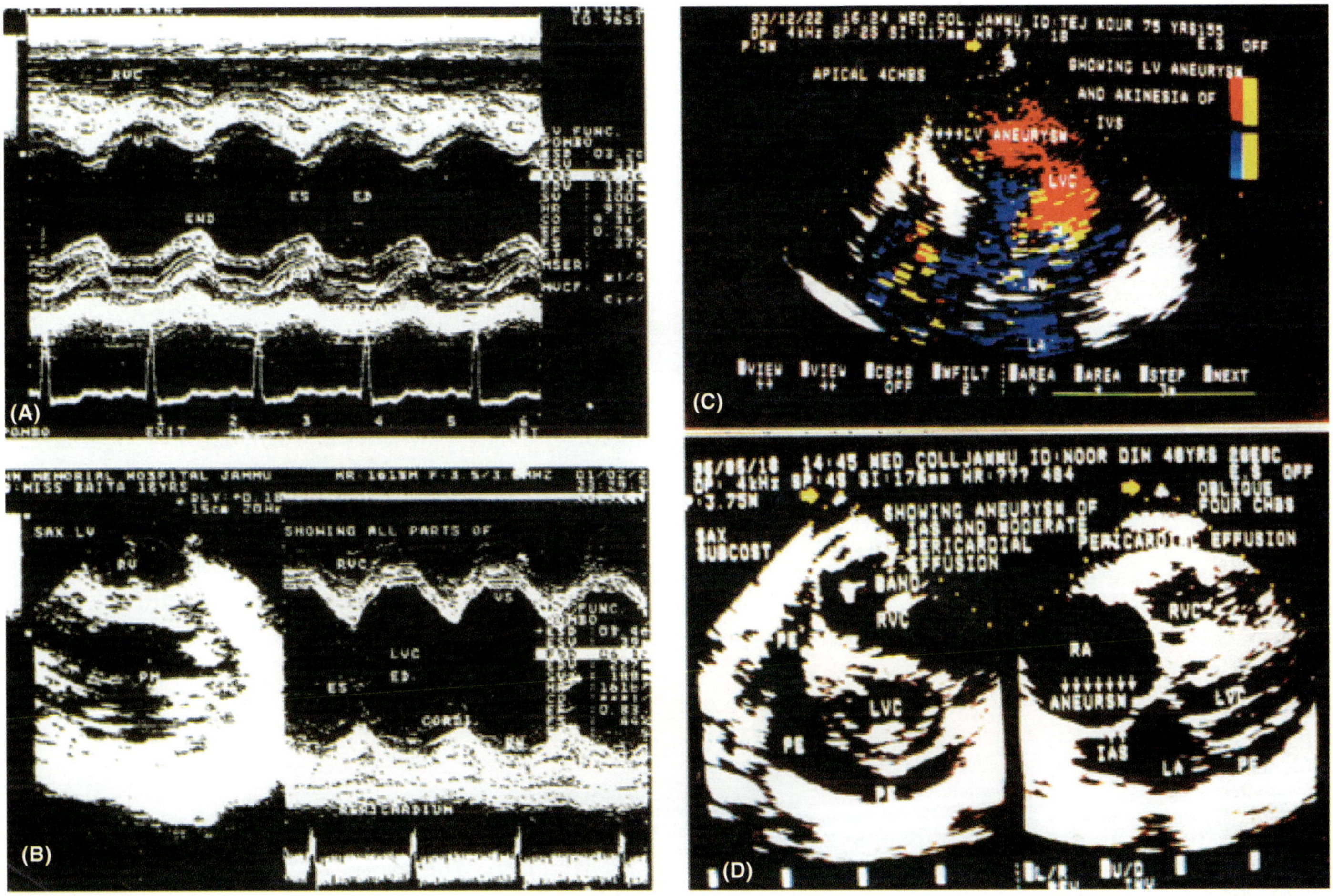

Fig. 24.2A to D: (A) M-Mode echocardiogram showing systolic and diastolic cycles and pomb method of automatic calculating endsystolic (ES), enddiastolic (ED) volumes and left ventricular ejection fraction (LVEF%). This scan also showing various parts of heart, i.e. anterior wall RV, IVS, endocardium and posterior left ventricular wall. **(B)** M-Mode echo showing dilated LV with raised cardiac volumes and low LVEF in patient with chronic ischemic cardiomyopathy. **(C)** Apical 4C view color flow showing LV aneurysm in patient with three vessels CAD. **(D)** Subcostal approach showing aneurysm of IAS in patient with chronic rheumatic heart disease

Tissue Doppler Imaging in CAD

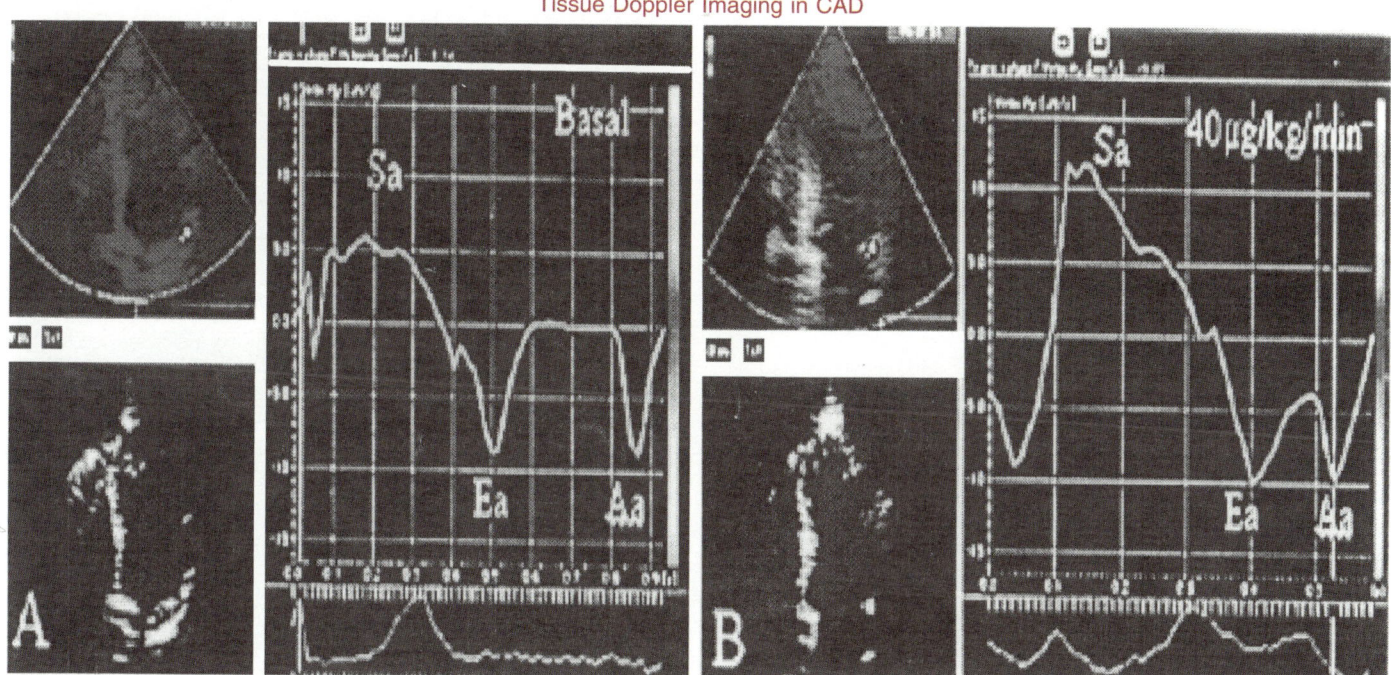

Fig. 24.3A: Myocardial velocities in normal person during dobutamine stress echocardiography taken from the lateral corner of the mitral annulus

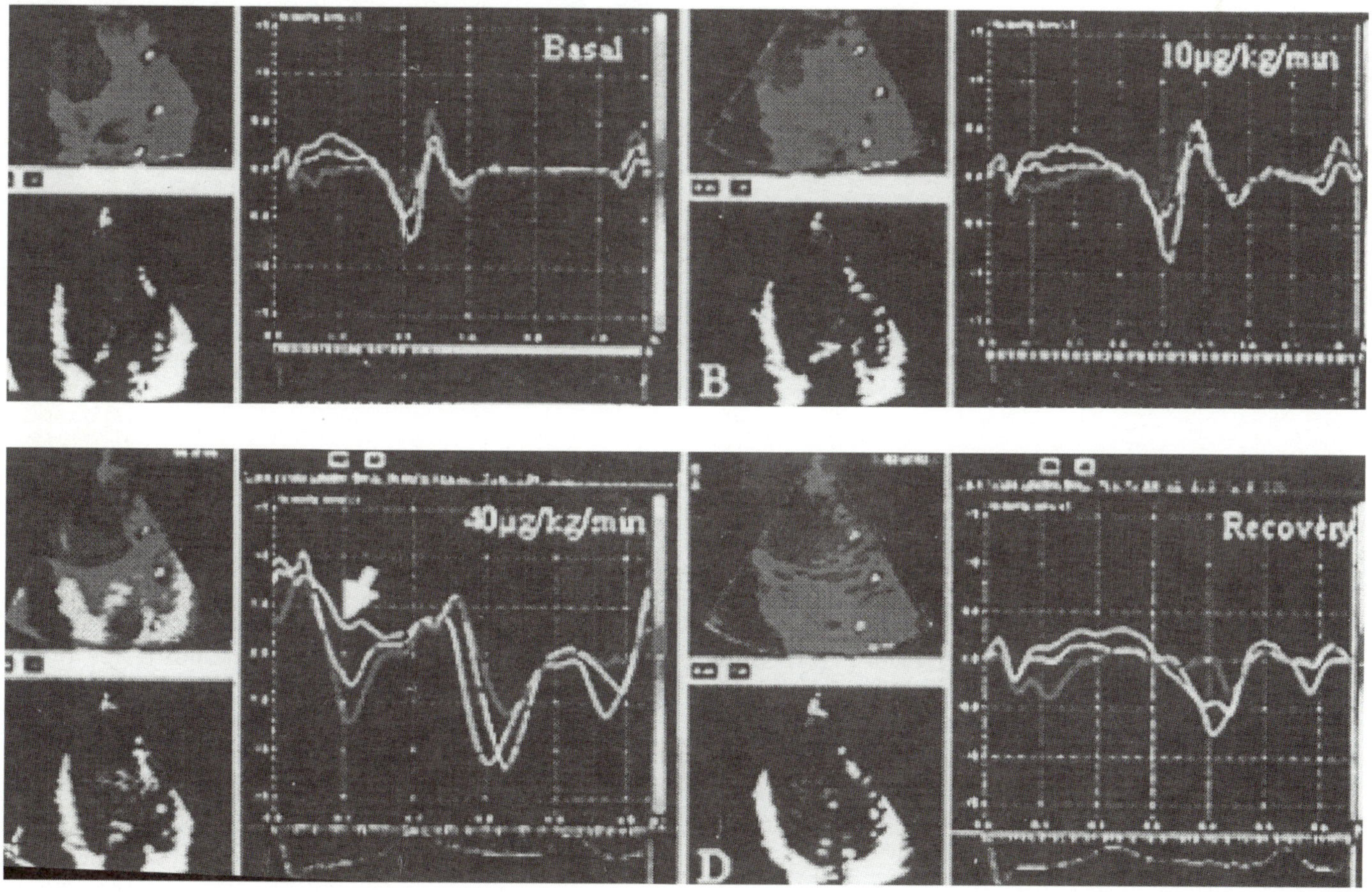

Fig. 24.3B: TDI during stress echocardiography in a patient with coronary artery disease showing systolic myocardial velocities in the ejection period (S$_2$) are recorded normal during resting period. (A) but attenuated response observed during peak stress (C) and normalised during recovery period (D). He showed 90% ostial lesion of left circumflex artery and 95% proximal lesion in the first obtuse marginal artery

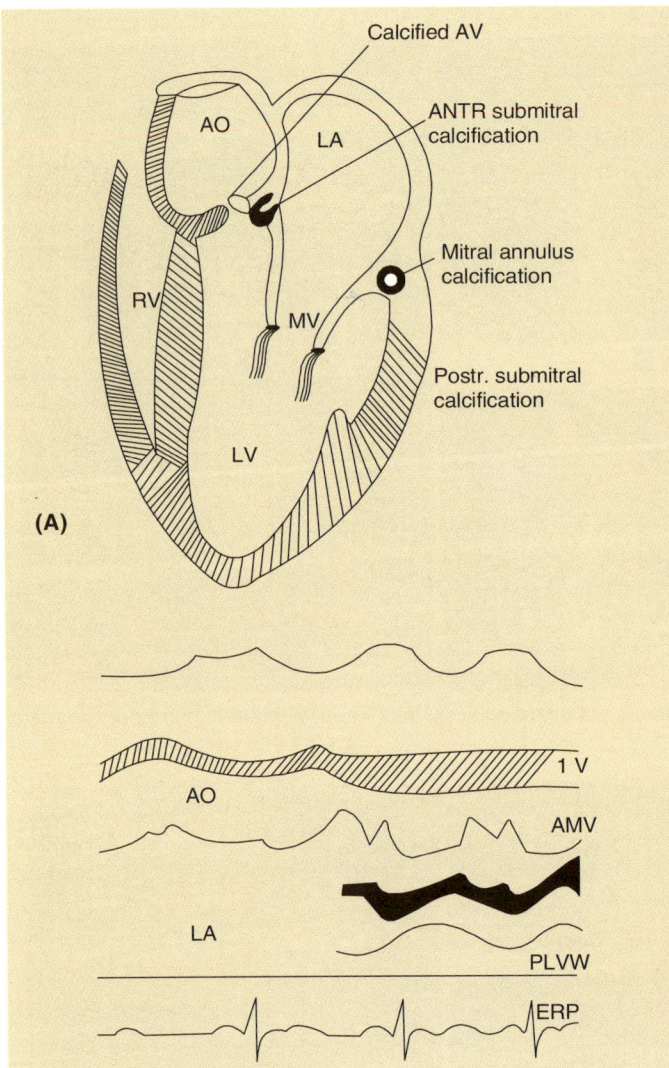

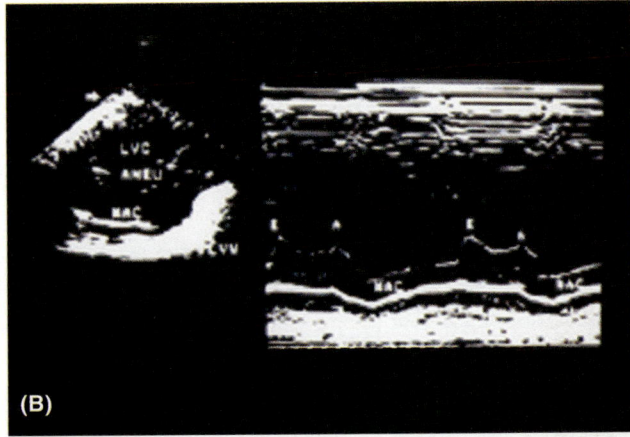

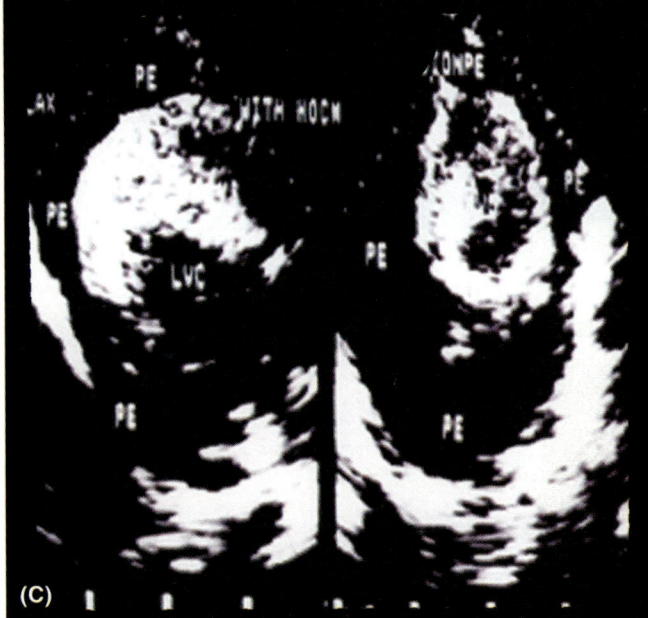

Fig. 24.4A to C: **(A)** Diagrammatic depiction of sites of localization of calcification including mitral annular calcification. **(B)** M-Mode echocardiogram showing mitral annular calcification in elderly individual with normal anterior and posterior mitral leaflets. **(C)** Short axis view showing both anterior and posterior moderate pericardial effusion in patient with tubercular pericarditis

Cardiac Adaptations (Fig. 24.2)

Increased vascular stiffness leads to elevated systolic arterial pressure and pulse-wave velocity, and to early reflected pulse pressure waves and late peak systolic pressure, thereby augmenting aortic impedance and cardiac mechanical load. In this way, arterial stiffening triggers a variety of cardiac adjustments. Some of these adjustments are additional and are similar to the age-related intrinsic changes in cardiac morphology and may, therefore, be expected to worsen cardiac performance.

The chronically elevated left ventricular afterload ultimately causes left ventricular wall thickening, which is largely a result of an increase in the size of cardiac myocytes. The combination of late augmentation of aortic impedance (through early reflected pulse

waves) and left ventricular hypertrophy (partly adaptive) prolongs myocardial contraction. The prolonged myocardial contraction time could contribute to preserve left ventricular pump function, as it prolongs the time available to eject blood from the heart into the stiffened vasculature. On the other hand, prolonged myocardial contraction delays ventricular relaxation at the time of mitral valve opening, as reflected by reduced early left ventricular filling rate in older individuals. In addition to the purely mechanical reason (i.e. prolonged contraction time), the decrease in early diastolic filling rate may, in part, be caused by a prolonged isovolumetric relaxation time between aortic valve closure and mitral valve opening, possibly because of a reduced rate of Ca^{2+} sequestration from the myoplasm to the sarcoplasmic reticulum. An in-

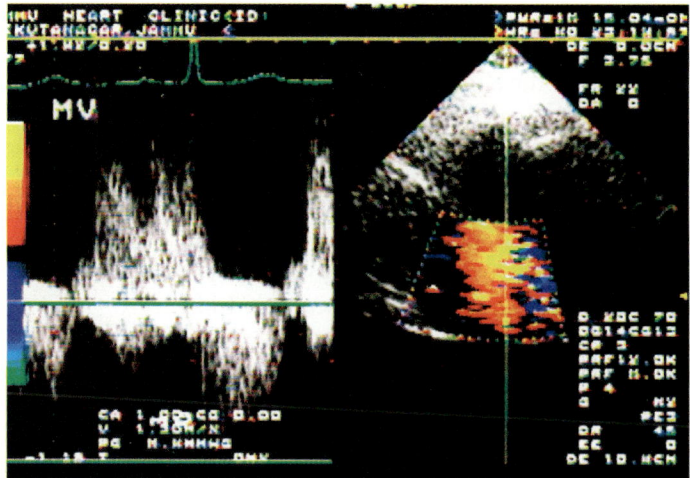

Fig. 24.5: Color Doppler dual echoscan showing Doppler velocity across normal mitral valve with mild type of mitral regurgitation (MR)

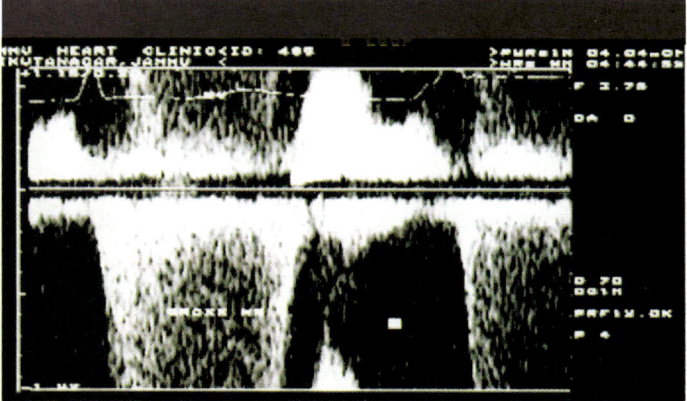

Fig. 24.6: Doppler flow velocity across mitral valve showing gross mitral regurgitation in an elderly patient with chronic rheumatic mitral valvular dysfunction

crease in late diastolic filling partly compensates for the decrease in early diastolic filling rate and helps to maintain end-diastolic volume and stroke volume in the elderly. However, this compensatory mechanism is dependent on the effective atrial contribution to late diastolic filling. The importance of atrial activity is reflected by an age-related increase in left atrial size and enhanced atrial contribution to late ventricular filling. The latter explains the greater dependency of stable haemodynamics on sinus rhythm with advancing age. Left atrial enlargement may contribute to the greater likelihood of lone atrial fibrillation in the elderly.

In ageing men, an elevated end-diastolic volume maintains cardiac output by increasing stroke volume in the presence of an age-related decline in heart rate. As there is no comparable increase in end-diastolic volume in women, cardiac output decreases modestly in ageing females.

The heterogeneity in filling among left ventricular segments increases with age. The normal ageing process seems to have similar effects on right and left ventricular diastolic performance. At rest, mild diastolic dysfunction has little adverse effect on systolic myocardial performance in healthy elderly people, as reflected by maintained ejection fraction, stroke volume and stroke work, and only marginally elevated end-systolic volume in men. At times of cardiovascular stress, however, the limited cardiac reserve capacity of the elderly becomes apparent.

An age-related increase in left ventricular systolic stiffness (as determined by the end-systolic elastance, Ea_{es} seems to accompany the age-related increase in vascular stiffness (as determined by the effective arterial elastance, E_a), even in the absence of cardiac hypertrophy. Comparable increases in E_a and Ea_{es} with age maintain the Ea/Ea_{es} ratio, an index of ventricular-arterial coupling. Ageing increases E_a principally by its effects on pulsatile loading, with an additional but smaller age-dependent effect from mean resistance.

Although the increase in E_{es} maintains the E_a/E_{es} ratio with age, the increase in both parameters imposes a limitation on net ventricular-arterial interaction, in as much as systolic arterial pressure becomes more sensitive to changes in ventricular filling. Even small blood volume shifts from heart to peripheral vessels can result in considerable changes in arterial pressure (Fig. 24.3).

Since contractile reserve is also linked to increase in E_{es}, age-related elevation of baseline E_{es} might limit some of this contractile reserve and may contribute to the blunting of end-systolic volume decline during exercise. Furthermore, the age-related increase in ventricular stiffness may contribute to the increased prevalence of hypotension with normal physiological stresses like postural shift, and enhanced pressure changes with excess sodium intake or restriction and diuretics. Thus, ventricular and arterial stiffening may well amplify the adverse effects of diastolic, autonomic and baroreflex dysfunction on cardiovascular compensatory mechanisms.

Coronary Circulation

Ageing is associated with structural and functional changes in the coronary vasculature, which could affect myocardial perfusion with advancing age. The gradual age-related decline in coronary flow reserve may be a result of elevated baseline cardiac work and myocardial blood flow or abnormal vasodilator capacity. Such a reduced dilator reserve may be the result of impaired endothelium-dependent dilation of large epicardial and resistance coronary vessels, decreased basal and stimulated release of nitric oxide by the coronary endothelium, or increased coronary vasoconstrictor effect of endothelin-1 (ET-1). Endothelin plasma concentrations increase with increasing age.

Autonomic Nervous System

Ageing is accompanied by a variety of neurohumoral changes. Increased basal sympathetic outflow and norepinephrine plasma concentrations suggest an up-regulation of sympathetic outflow. Such sympathetic overactivity leads to desensitization of β-adrenoceptors, which may account for the blunted postsynaptic responsiveness to β-adrenergic stimuli with ageing.

Whereas the vasodilatory response to β-adrenoceptor stimulation decreases with age, the contractile response to adrenoceptor stimulation appears to be unaltered, or may even increase with age. The precise mechanism for this observation remains uncertain. It may be related to an age-related increase in arterial (but not venous) 1-adrenoceptor density.

Ageing affects autonomic cardiovascular control mechanisms in different ways. Attenuated respiratory sinus arrhythmia with advancing age suggests a decrease in parasympathetic influence on sinus node function. Age-related increases in catecholamine plasma concentrations and in the basal rate of sympathetic neural firing reflect increased sympathetic nerve activity and suggest blunted sinoaortic baroreflex sensitivity that reduces the restraint on sympathetic outflow. Preservation of the sympathetic limb of the baroreflex (i.e. sympathetic reflex response to changes in the peripheral circulation) with advancing age would suggest reduced tonic baroreceptor function (i.e. less inhibitory afferent signals at a given arterial pressure) but maintained gain during arterial pressure pertubations. In contrast, the heart rate reflex response to alterations in arterial pressure is clearly impaired with advancing age.

Age-related autonomic and baroreflex dysfunction may compromise arterial pressure homeostasis in response to diuretic therapy, altered fluid intake and postural stress. Age-related changes in heart rate response to posture, hypotension and various other physiological stimuli have also been reported. Blunted baroreceptor reflex response may contribute to sinus node depression, carotid sinus syndrome and syncope in the elderly.

Response to Increased Oxygen Demand

The haemodynamic response to cardiovascular stress is influenced by various factors, including the nature of the cardiovascular stimulus, the posture in which the cardiovascular system is challenged, gender, fitness and cardiovascular health. Besides these factors, age plays a significant role.

In healthy, sedentary individuals, maximum work capacity and oxygen consumption (VO_2 max) decrease by approximately 10% per decade after the age of 20 yr. At a given VO_2 max, increases in heart rate and ejection fraction, and peripheral vasodilation are blunted in the elderly. The decrease in maximum physical capacity may not result solely from limitations in the central circulation (i.e. cardiac reserve capacity), but may also be related to peripheral factors (i.e. redistribution of blood to working muscles, impaired ability of muscle to extract and use oxygen). The cardiac element of the diminished VO_2 max in healthy individuals is caused primarily by an age-related decline in the maximum heart rate.

One of the major age-associated alterations in the cardiovascular response to exercise is a striking decrease in heart rate and contractile response, as reflected by decreases in peak heart rate and peak ejection fraction, and by a progressively blunted exercise-induced decrease in end-systolic volume with advancing age. The Frank–Starling mechanism is the major mechanism that maintains stroke volume in the elderly: peak end-diastolic volume during exercise increases progressively with advancing age and is considerably (.30%) larger in old than in young individuals. The augmentation of end-diastolic volume preserves stroke volume but attenuates the increase in ejection fraction.

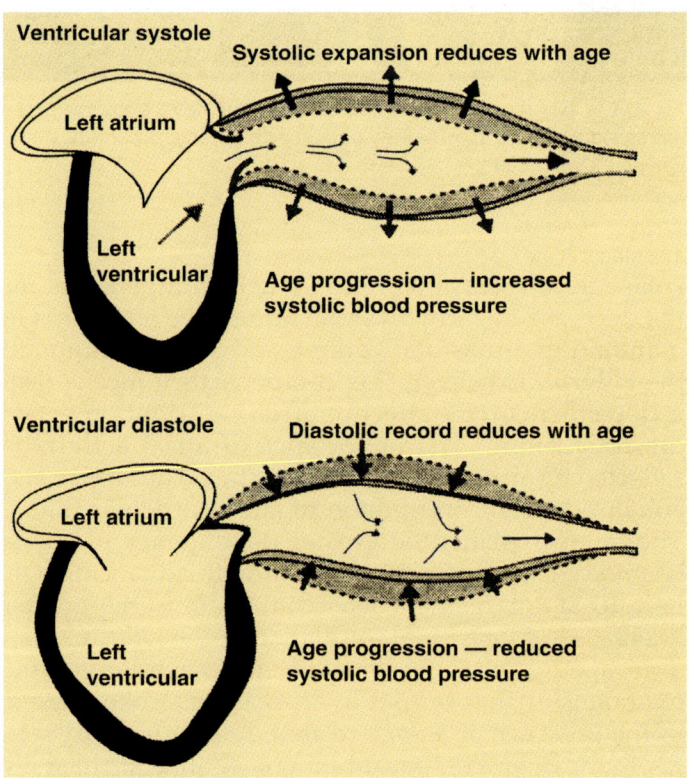

Fig. 24.7: Mechanism as to how age progression leads to increase in systolic blood pressure and decrease in diastolic blood pressure

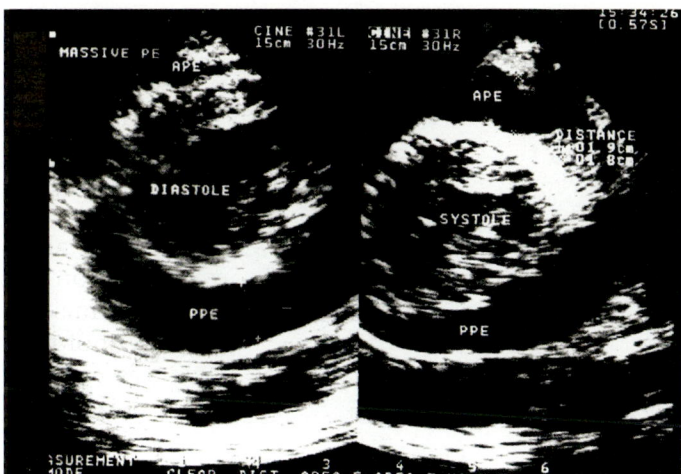

Fig. 24.8: Short axis view LV showing both pleural and pericardial effusion in an elderly patient with pulmonary tuberculosis and pericarditis

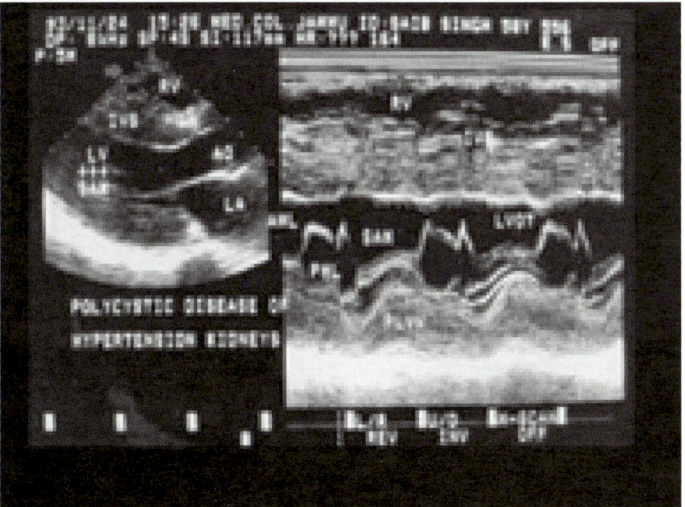

Fig. 24.9: M-Mode and 2D echocardiogram showing non-obstructive concentric LVH in an elderly individual with systemic hypertension

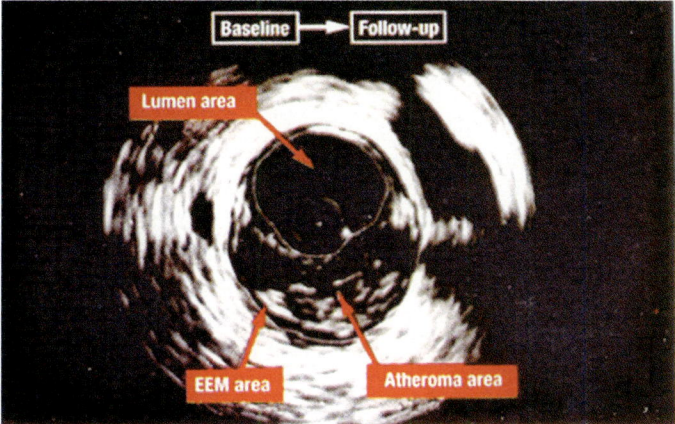

Fig. 24.10: Intravascular ultrasonography (IVUS) showing characterization of atheroma (5° clock) along with identification of external elastic membrane (EEM) and lumen area in an elderly individual

The age-associated decline in maximal heart rate and left ventricular contractility during vigorous exercise probably reflects diminished β-adrenergic modulation of contractility, chronotropy and vasomotor tone with advancing age. β-Adrenoceptor blockade effectively converts the haemodynamic profile of young men to that more typical of older men across submaximal work rates. This finding supports the hypothesis that blunted β-adrenoceptor responsiveness underlies the attenuated increases in heart rate and myocardial contractility, and the cardiac dilation that occur during exhaustive exercise in older individuals.

The clinical implications of blunted β-adrenoceptor responsiveness with advancing age are considerable. The young respond to increased flow demands primarily with sympathoadrenergic activation, followed by β-adrenoceptor-mediated modulation of cardio-vascular performance. Such a mechanism maintains heart size despite increases in heart rate, venous return and systolic arterial pressure. As preload reserve is preserved, additional flow demands can be met by activation of the Frank-Starling mechanism, i.e. by increasing end-diastolic volume.

In contrast, in the elderly, the increased peripheral flow demand is met primarily by activation of the pre-load reserve. As no further compensatory mechanism exists, additional flow demands may result in cardiovascular insufficiency. Such reduced cardiovascular reserve capacity explains the higher incidence of acute and chronic heart failure in the elderly. The cardiovascular response to exercise in the elderly is comparable to disease states such as congestive heart failure. It emphasizes the importance of peripheral vasodilation.

The clinically most relevant alterations in cardiovascular physiology with ageing are increased myocardial and vascular stiffness, blunted β-adrenoceptor-mediated modulation of inotropy, chronotropy and vasomotor tone, and autonomic reflex dysfunction. The increase in myocardial stiffness decreases left ventricular compliance which, in turn, impairs diastolic function. These changes are reflected by reduced early diastolic filling rate, elevated end-diastolic volume in elderly men and a tendency for higher cardiac filling pressures. Despite maintained stroke volume and ejection fraction, the increase in end-systolic volume in elderly men reflects an age-dependent decline in intrinsic myocardial contractility.

Although the cardiac adaptation to arterial stiffening will help to maintain systolic function and myocardial oxygen supply/demand balance, diastolic function will be impaired even further. In general, however, despite evidence of impaired diastolic and systolic function in elderly males, overall cardiac performance is adequately maintained at rest during advancing age. Despite arterial stiffening, pump function is maintained via

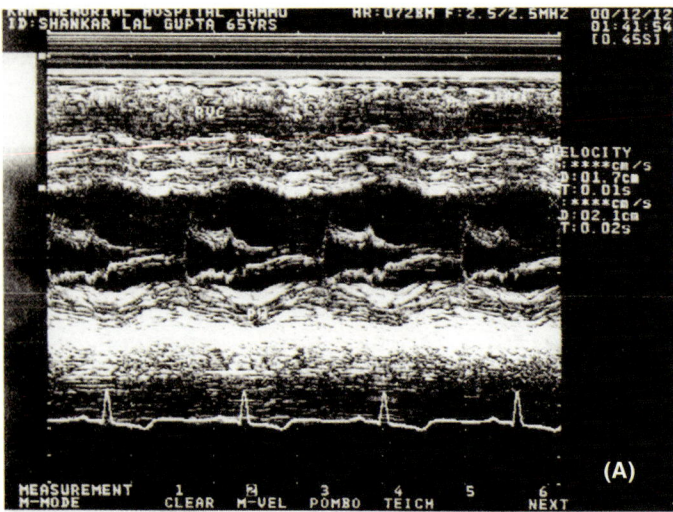

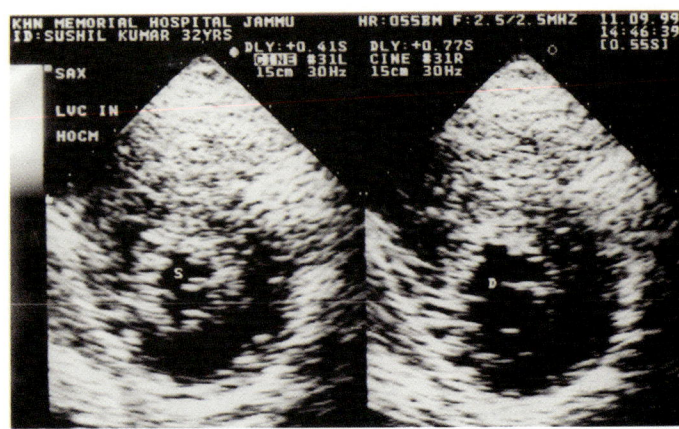

Fig. 24.12: 2D Short axis view in a dual scan showing marked concenteric LV hypertrophy including IVS in both systole and diastole

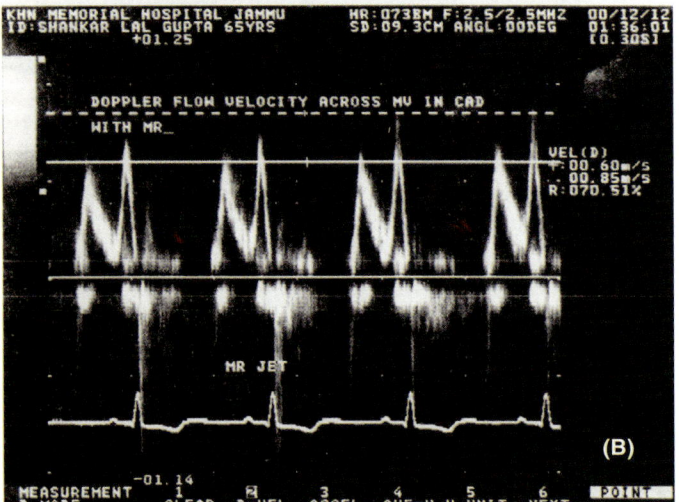

Fig. 24.11: (A) Panel showing marked hypokinesia of both IVS and posterior LV wall. **(B)** Increased A velocity with E/A ratio of less than 1.0 (defect in LV relaxation) in an elderly patient with CAD, HT and NIDDM

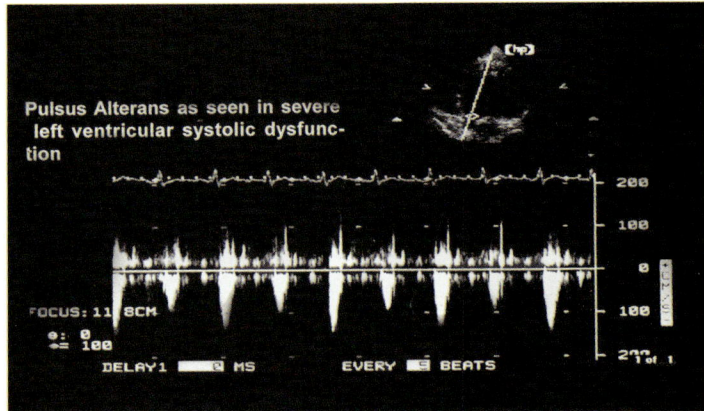

Fig. 24.13: Doppler flow study across valve in 5C view showing alternate weak and strong systolic contraction in patient with severe LV systolic dysfunction. Note: Pulsus alterans is a physical finding characterized by a regular alteration of the force of the arterial pulse (pulse pressure). It is due to alternating strong and weak contractions of the LV and it almost invariably indicates the presence of severe LV systolic dysfunction

various adaptations which include a moderate increase in left ventricular wall thickness, prolonged contraction, atrial enlargement, enhanced atrial contribution to left ventricular filling and elevated end-diastolic volume in males. The age-related alteration in cardiovascular response to a change in posture or exercise is probably caused more by autonomic reflex dysfunction and blunted β-adrenoceptor responsiveness with advancing age than by impaired myocardial function.

Aging of Heart Function in Man

In normal subjects at rest neither heart rate nor ejection volume are influenced by age. The loss of elasticity of the great arteries, and in particular the aorta which becomes tortuous and wider, results in an increase of impedance at ejection. As systole time pressure rises in the whole cardiovascular system, the left ventricle is subjected to an increase of parietal tension to which it adapts itself by hypertrophy which normalizes this tension. Ejection fraction and end-systolic volume are thus preserved, and the systolic function at rest globally remains unmodified by age. The delay and slowing down of relaxation due to hypertrophy of the left ventricle, to the reflection waves and to other changes in cardiac muscle physical properties during senescence reduce the importance of the initial phase of left ventricular filling. This major modification of diastolic dynamics at rest is compensated, at the end of diastole, by a more vigorous contraction of the left atrium, which increases its contribution to left ventricular filling. The global filling volume is thus preserved and the end-diastolic volume remains appropriate, these two conditions being necessary to start off a normal ejection. In normal subjects at exercise the cardiac function is also modified by age. Maximum heart rate is reduced in the elderly, whereas the ejection volume increases more than in younger subjects, which maintains the appropriate cardiac output. This adaptation takes place owing to an increase of cardiac volume and through Starling's mechanism which ensures a greater ejection volume. Only the maximum exercise level (VO_2 max) decreases with age, mainly because of the decrease of skeletal muscle mass. Filling of the left ventricle seems to continue to rely, at rest as at exercise, on atrial compensation. Cardiac output therefore is globally maintained with age during a dynamic effort. During isometric exercise, which in the elderly results in a

higher rise in blood pressure, the ejection fraction decreases, the end-systolic volume increases and the initial filling decreases but is compensated by a greater contribution of the atrium. Thus, cardiac work at rest and during exercise is well preserved in the ageing man, due to secondary homeostatic adaptations which counterbalance the primary age-related changes. The principal primary changes are loss of elasticity of the great vessels and reduction of efficacy in response to adrenergic stimulation. The principal secondary adaptations are left ventricular hypertrophy, increased atrial contribution and, during exercise, intervention of Starling's mechanism.

In the elderly, **echocardiography** (Fig. 24.1) is useful for assessing left ventricular chamber size and function after diagnosis of heart failure or after acute MI; for assisting in the differential diagnosis of systolic murmurs, especially those grade 3/6 or higher in loudness; for measuring left atrial size and assessing left ventricular function in patients with new atrial fibrillation; for determining pulmonary artery pressures in patients with heart failure; for confirming the presence of pericardial effusion or tamponade; and for detecting a left ventricular aneurysm (Figs 24.8,24..9, 24.20, 24.21, 24.32–24.34)

Echocardiography can detect thickened aortic or mitral valve leaflets or a calcified mitral annulus, which are the most common sources of systolic murmurs in the elderly. Atrial myxomas, left ventricular thrombi, and valvular vegetations are best detected by echo-cardiography (Figs 24.30 and 24.31).

Echocardiography performed immediately after treadmill or pharmacologic stress testing may be used instead of radionuclide perfusion imaging to detect

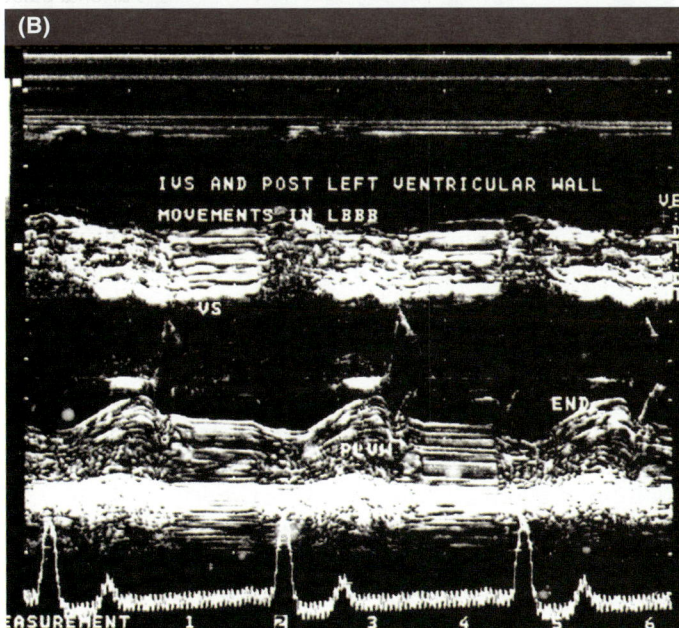

Fig. 24.14A and B: M-Mode echocardiograms showing systolic notch along IVS an elderly individual with LBBB and systemic hypertension

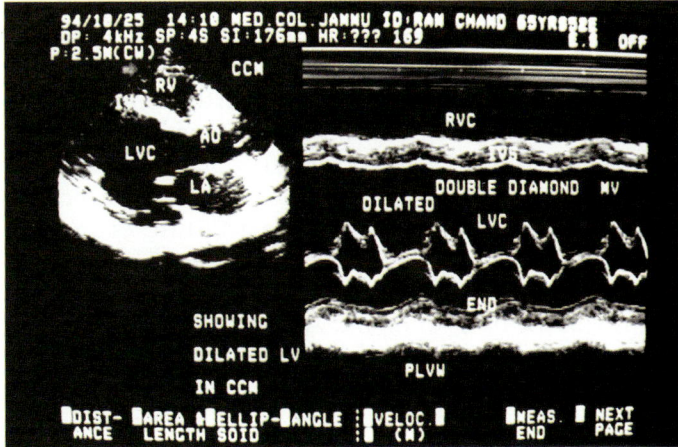

Fig. 24.15: 2D and M-mode echocardiogram showing marked hypokinesia of both IVS and posterior left ventricular wall,diamond shaped deformity of MV along with increased dimension between E point of mitral valve and septum (EPSS) in an elderly patient with 3-vessels disease of coronary artery presenting as ischemic cardiomyopathy

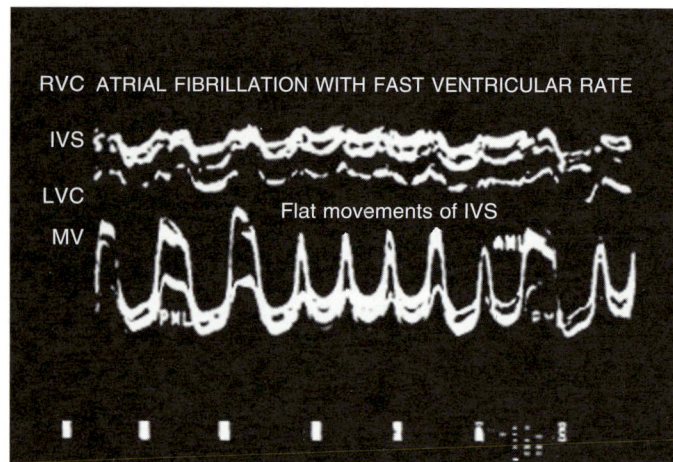

Fig. 24.16: M-Mode echocardiogram showing incomplete opening of mitral valve (almost atrial A waves only) with fast ventricular response (beats 3–7) in patient with rheumatic mitral valvular stenosis with atrial fibrillation. Note also the minimal to flat movements of interventricular septum (IVS) from beats 3–7 followed by normal thickening of IVS in cycle 1 and 8 which showed restricted opening of valve due to mitral stenosis

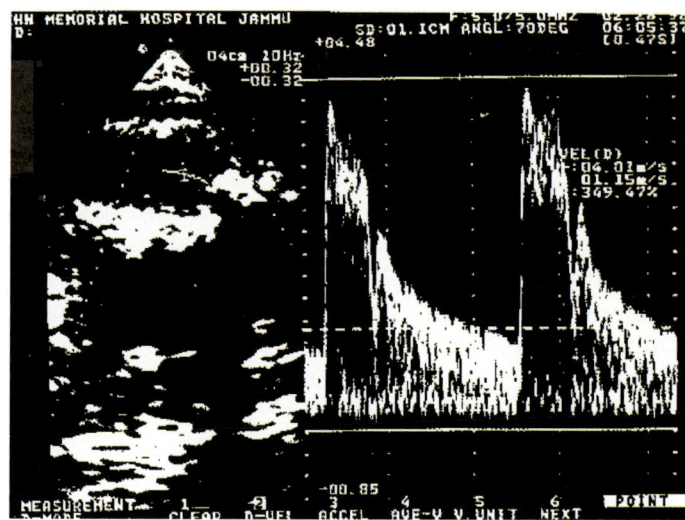

Fig. 24.17: Ultrasonography of internal carotid artery showing obstruction of the vessel with peak systolic velociy of more than 4.0 m/s and wide spectral waveforms in 80yrs. old patient with recurrent syncopal attacks, with ischemic cerebral infarct

myocardial ischemia (which is indicated by wall motion abnormalities) and to determine prognosis. For patients ≥ 70 years, dobutamine stress echocardiography, which is the preferred noninvasive test for the elderly by many clinicians, has a sensitivity of 87%, a specificity of 84%, and an accuracy of 86% for the diagnosis of CAD. Adenosine stress echocardiography has a sensitivity of 66%, a specificity of 90%, and an accuracy of 73%. Exercise echocardiography has a sensitivity of 85% and a specificity of 77%.

M-mode echocardiography can detect age-related changes such as small increases in aortic root and left atrial dimensions, an increase in left ventricular wall thickness with no change in cavity size, and a decrease in mitral valve E-F closure slope (the rate of mitral valve closure in early diastole). Despite these changes, values for elderly persons usually remain within the limits of what is considered normal for younger persons.

Doppler echocardiography is used to quantify aortic valve stenosis. It is also used to assess diastolic dysfunction, particularly in patients with heart failure of unclear etiology. Doppler echocardiography can be used to predict length of survival for elderly patients with heart failure on the basis of E- and A-wave velocity measurements. Colour Doppler echocardiography, with flow mapping, is useful for detecting and estimating the severity of valvular regurgitation. Mild multivalvular regurgitation is common among otherwise healthy elderly persons, so regurgitation is significant only if it is moderate or severe (Fig. 24.17).

Transesophageal echocardiography is safe for elderly patients and should be considered for those with suspected heart disease if transthoracic echocardio-

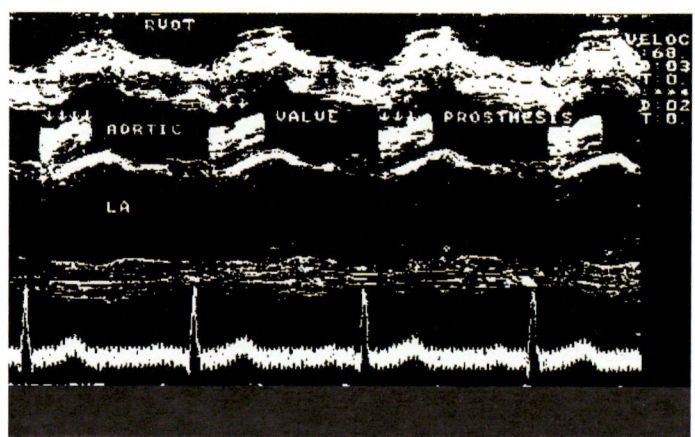

Fig. 24.18: M-Mode echocardiogram showing prosthetic aortic valve fitted in an elderly patient with chronic rheumatic severe type of native aortic valvular stenosis

graphy is not diagnostic. Transesophageal echocardiography is particularly useful for detecting aortic dissection, valvular vegetations, thrombi in the left atrium or left atrial appendage, and prosthetic valve dysfunction in patients who have the appropriate clinical presentation. Elderly patients with intraaortic atherosclerotic debris detected by transesophageal echocardiography are at increased risk of thromboembolic events during cardiac surgery.

Intravascular ultrasonography allows detailed morphologic assessment of CAD but is expensive and invasive. This procedure may be useful for determining the suitability of a specific intervention (e.g., balloon angioplasty, laser therapy, stent placement) for patients with CAD (Fig. 24.10).

Cardiovascular Changes in Physiologic Aging

It is important to differentiate the cardiac manifestations of normal aging which do not require medical management from cardiac disease in the older patient. A rationale for greater utilization of diagnostic techniques can be made in the older patient who may present with atypical symptoms, multiple confounding medical problems, and age-related alterations in physical findings of some cardiac diseases. The management of most cardiac diseases in the older patient is similar to that of the younger patient, with the important recognition of the need to reduce medication dosages and be aware of the increased risk of adverse effects or drug interactions. Age should not be a contraindication to invasive procedures or surgical procedures or thrombolytic therapy, since when properly selected, they benefit older patients to the same or greater degree as younger patients. For several diseases unique to aging (i.e. diastolic heart failure or atrial fibrillation), optimal therapeutic strategies are still evolving.

Rhythm

Heart Rate

Resting heart rate is not generally affected by ageing; however, decreased heart rate in response to exercise and stress (especially beta-adrenergically mediated) is characteristic of healthy aging. The clinical consequence of this is that maximal heart rate on treadmill is decreased (220-age) and the heart rate response to fever, hypovolemia, and postural stress is also decreased with healthy aging. The response to beta-adrenergic blockade (as well as stimulation) is also reduced with healthy aging. Daytime bradycardia with heart rates < 40 bpm and sinus pauses of over 3 seconds are not seen with healthy aging.

Atrioventricular Conduction (Fig. 24.41A and B)

The time for conduction through the atrioventricular (AV) node is increased with healthy aging. Therefore, the P-R interval on the ECG increases with age and the upper limit of normal for people>65 is 210–220 milliseconds (not 200 ms). Second and third degree AV block are not normal consequences of aging. Right bundle branch block is seen more frequently in older compared to younger populations but has not been shown to identify increased risk for further conduction abnormalities. A gradual leftward shift of the QRS axis is observed with aging and left anterior hemiblock is seen with increasing frequency in older populations. Isolated left anterior hemiblock is not an independent predictor of cardiovascular morbidity or mortality in otherwise healthy elderly. Combined right bundle branch block and left anterior fascicular block is

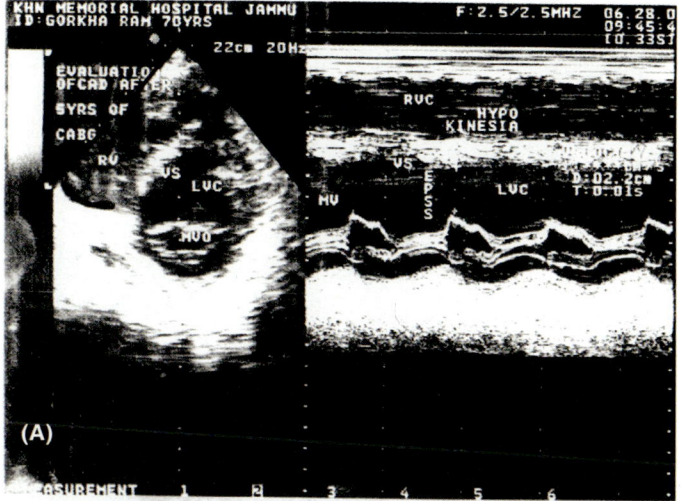

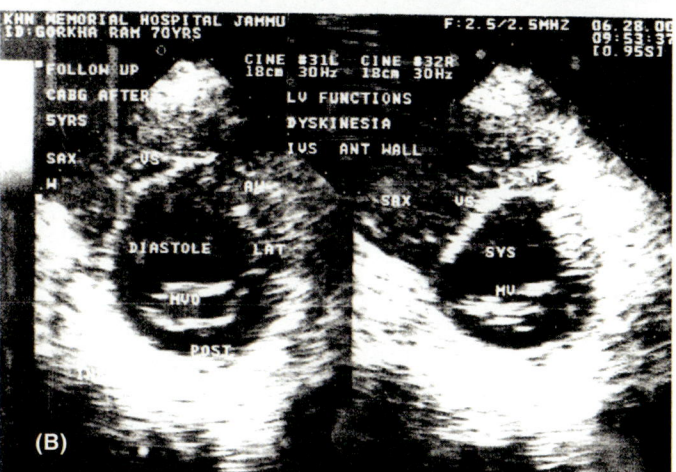

Fig. 24.19A and B: **(A)** 2D and M-mode echocardiogram, showing dilated LV,sclerosed MV and hypokinesia of both IVS and posterior left ventricular wall. **(B)** 2D LV view showing dyssynergy at IVS in patient with wide spread atherosclerosis including coronary arteries

associated with cardiovascular disease in 75% of older patients and only 25% with this finding have otherwise normal hearts. Left bundle branch block is not associated with normal aging and is associated with cardiovascular disease and risks for cardiac events.

Arrhythmias (Fig. 24.16)

Atrial premature contractions increase with age and are frequent in up to 95% of older healthy volunteers at rest and during exercise in the absence of detectable cardiac disease. Atrial fibrillation is usually associated with coronary, hypertensive, valvular, sinus node disease or thyrotoxicosis but may occur in older patients with no other detectable diseases (1/5 of older men and 1/20 of older women with atrial fibrillation). Similarly, isolated and even multiform ventricular ectopy has been reported in up to 80% of older men and women without detectable cardiac disease.

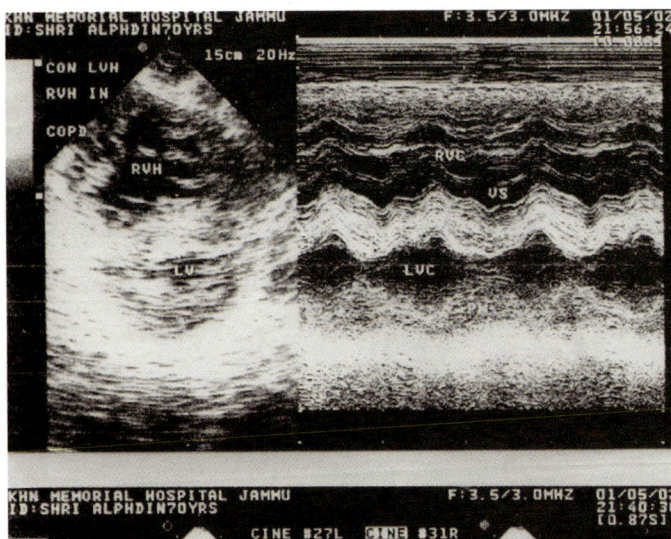

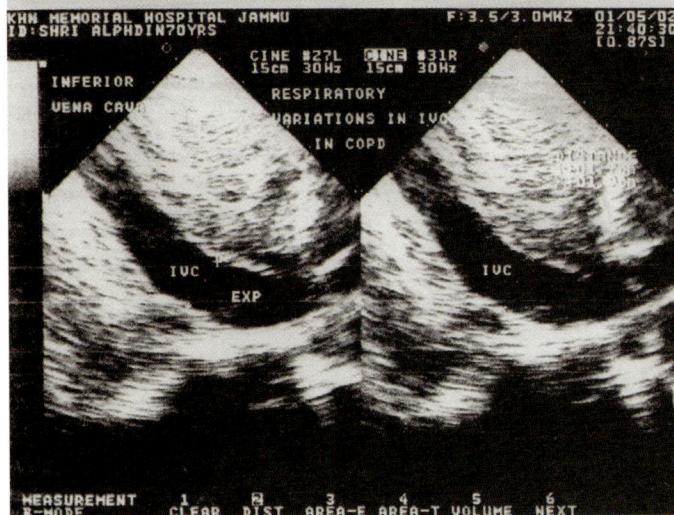

Fig. 24.20: Upper panel 2D and M-mode echo showing hypertrophic RV, compressed small LV. Lower panel subcostal approach showing dilated inferior vena cava with no inspiratory collapse in patient with chronic obstructive lung disease with right heart failure

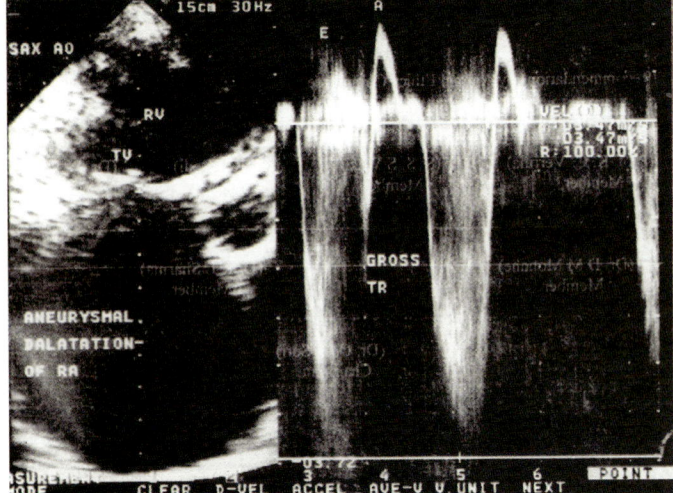

Fig. 24.21: Doppler flow at TV showing hugely dilated RA with moderately severe tricuspid regurgitation in patient with COPD and severe pulmonary hypertension

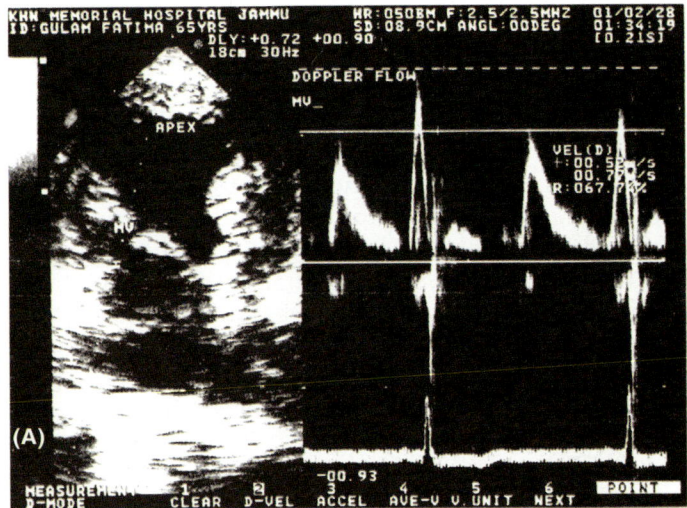

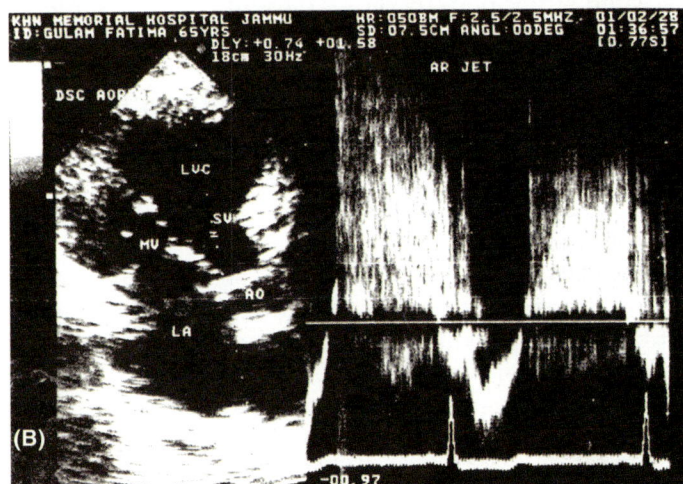

Fig. 24.22A and B: (A) 2-D and Doppler flow velocity across MV showing A velocity > E a defect in relaxation of LV. **(B)** 2-D Doppler flow across aortic valve showing moderate regurgitation without significant stenosis in patient with atherosclerotic heart disease.

Cardiac Contractility/Left Ventricular Function at Rest and during Exercise

In contrast to the decline in skeletal muscle mass seen with aging in healthy populations, left ventricular mass is preserved or increased with age.

Systolic Function (Fig. 24.13)

Resting left ventricular systolic function (ejection fraction and/or stroke volume) is not altered by aging in most studies of subjects rigorously screened to exclude coronary artery disease; however, a few studies report declines of stroke volume with sedentary older populations. Cardiac output is equal to stroke volume × heart rate. So, resting cardiac output and left ventricular ejection fraction do not usually decrease with normal

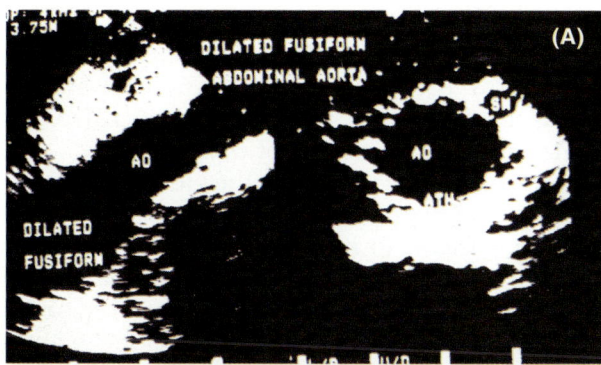

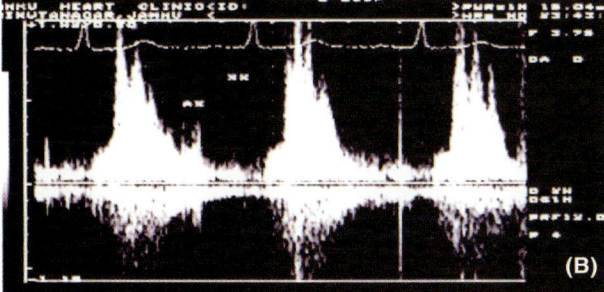

Fig. 24.23A and B: (A) Subcostal transverse and short axis views of abdominal aorta showing dilated, thickened and irrregular wall of aorta. **(B)** Suprasternal approach shows increased velocity of aortic flow with mild to moderate aortic stenosis in patient with atherosclerotic heart disease

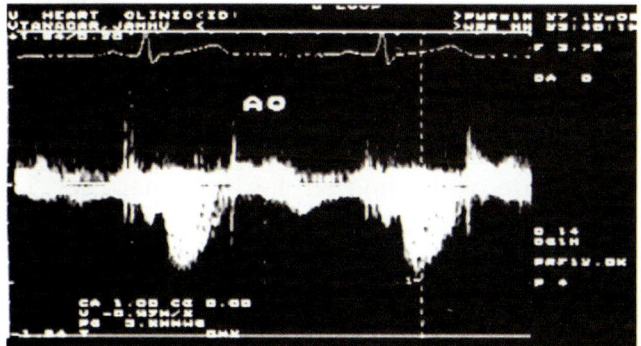

Fig. 24.24: Doppler flow velocity across aortic valve showing mild enhancement of aortic velocity in patient with aortic valvulitis

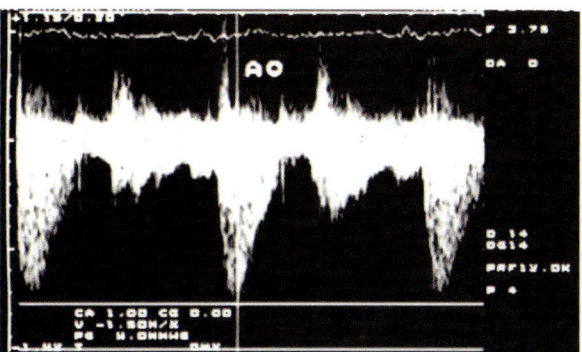

Fig. 24.25: Doppler flow velocity across aortic valve showing mild to moderate enhancement of aortic flow veloctiy in patient with rheumatic mild aortic valvular stenosis

aging. Contractile responses to beta-adrenergic responses are decreased with aging. Therefore, exercise cardiac output may be reduced due to both the decrease in maximal heart rate and a limit to the ability to increase contractility (stroke volume) in response to beta-adrenergic blockade in the elderly. The age-associated decline in maximal cardiac output and cardiovascular reserve capacity may not limit usual ability in otherwise healthy elderly because the vast majority of daily activities are performed at low and submaximal workloads. In addition, the age-related decline in exercise capacity can be attenuated by physical conditioning.

Diastolic Function (Fig. 24.11)

The time for cardiac relaxation and for ventricular filling are prolonged with aging leading to altered early diastolic filling times on echocardiography and nuclear studies. The etiology of the prolonged time for relaxation may be multifactorial—increased ventricular mass, collagen infiltration, or altered myocardial calcium handling. Prolonged filling times may limit cardiac output with increased heart rates. While altered diastolic function accompanies aging, congestive heart failure is not a normal consequence of the prolonged times required for cardiac relaxation or diastolic filling.

Common Cardiovascular Diseases Prevalent in Older Patients

Atrial Fibrillation (Fig. 24.16)

The prevalence of chronic atrial fibrillation rises from <1 per 1000 people at 25–35 years of age to about 40 per 100 at ages 80–90 years (Framingham data, Baltimore Longitudinal Study, Cardiovascular Health Study). Chronic atrial fibrillation has been shown to be an important risk factor for cerebrovascular accidents (strokes) and control of rate is associated with better exercise tolerance. The goals of therapy in an individual patient may vary and include rate control, prevention of stroke or restoration of sinus rhythm.

Hypertension (Fig. 24.9)
Systolic

The prevalence of hypertension increases with aging in North American men and women. This increase in systolic pressure is thought to be due to thickening of the arterial wall which makes it less distensible and less able to buffer the rise in pressure that occurs with cardiac ejection. These changes result in an elevated systolic blood pressure with a relatively unchanged diastolic blood pressure. A large body of data have now demonstrated that cardiovascular morbidity and mortality increase with increasing systolic as well as **diastolic blood pressure** in the elderly. Furthermore, treatment of both diastolic and isolated systolic hypertension has been shown to decrease mortality and morbidity in both older men and women—there is a decrease in adverse events for every degree of blood pressure reduction towards the normal range. Treatment goals are now the same for older patients as they are for younger patients (Fig. 24.12).

Systolic blood pressure <140 mm Hg **Diastolic** pressure < 90 mm Hg.

Coronary Artery Disease (Fig. 24.14)

It has long been recognized that the prevalence of coronary artery disease rises with increasing age and that multivessel disease in older patients with coronary artery disease is more common. The age-related increase in coronary artery disease occurs in women as well as men but begins at a later age in women. The same risk factors that predict atherosclerosis in younger adults (lipid abnormalities, smoking, hypertension, diabetes) are predictive in older individuals as well. Modification

of these risk factors is effective in reducing the risk of atherosclerosis in older patients. Therefore, preventive strategies for the older patient include stopping smoking, blood pressure control, control of lipid abnormalities, and treatment of diabetes.

The approach to diagnosis in the elderly is similar to that in the younger patient. The history may be somewhat more difficult to interpret because exercise may be limited by other factors (arthritis, pulmonary disease, etc.) and chest discomfort may be atypical because of the prevalence of diabetes (10% of the elderly) and the greater preponderance of women in the older populations. ECG criteria for the diagnosis of coronary artery disease are also not as reliable in women of any age as in men. Nuclear imaging (usually thallium) with or without pharmacologic stress is often used to overcome the limits of ECG interpretation, but again is not as good in women as men (estimated 20% false positives). Because the prevalence of coronary artery disease is high in the elderly, the goal of diagnostic testing may be to quantify the amount of ischemia rather than to diagnose its presence and perfusion imaging allows localization, quantification, and differentiation between infarcted and ischemic myocardium. Pharmacologic stress testing combined with echocardiography may also have some advantages in the older patient since it can provide assessment of valvular function, left ventricular function, and the presence and extent of wall motion abnormalities indicative of ischemia or infarction. Angiography is of value for both assessment and as a preclude to interventions. Slightly greater complications are seen in older patients than in younger patients (local bleeding, stroke) but remain low. This should be recognized but should not preclude procedures.

Myocardial Infarction

The older patient with myocardial infarction also benefits from the same therapies as the younger patient and age >75 years alone should not be a contraindication to thrombolytic therapy. Beta blockers and aspirin should be administered post infarction. ACE inhibitors are also of probable benefit if given in lower doses and not during the immediate acute MI period. However, goals of the post-MI period may differ for the older patient versus the younger patient. All physiologic processes related to healing and stress appear to be attenuated with aging, so timing for diagnostic testing after the acute event may need to be slightly later in older patients. In addition, the probability of post-MI ischemia is greater in the older patient because of the higher incidence of multivessel disease. No studies of predominantly older patients have been performed to identify the best post-MI strategy for further risk stratification and to guide in clinical decision making

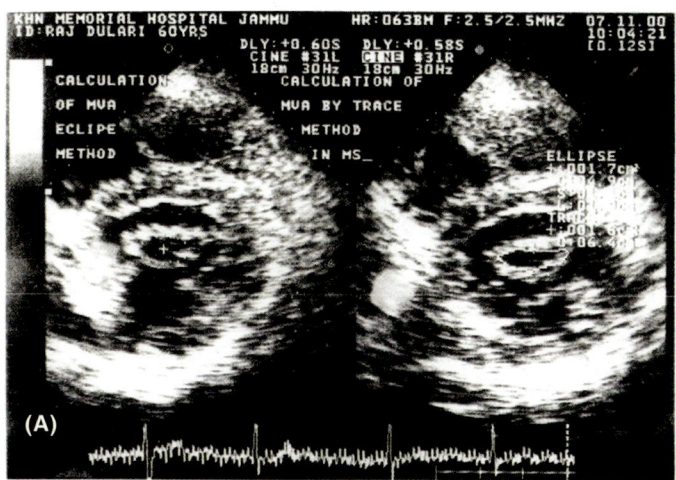

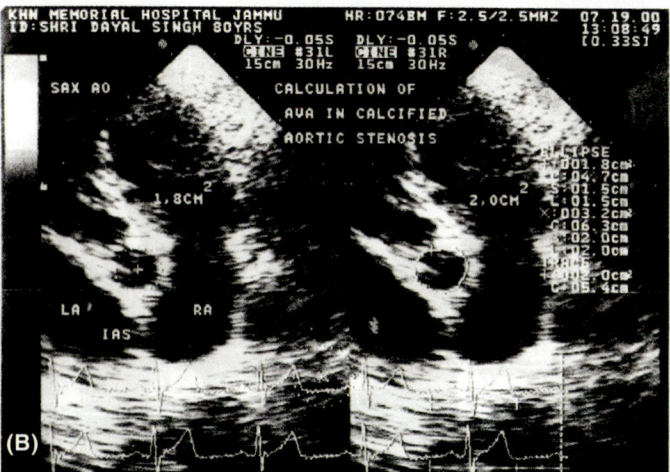

Fig. 24.26A and B: (A) Short axis dual scan view of LV showing thickened mitral valve without significant mitral valve stenosis. **(B)** Short axis view aorta showing dilated main pulmonary artery in patient with atherosclerotic heart disease

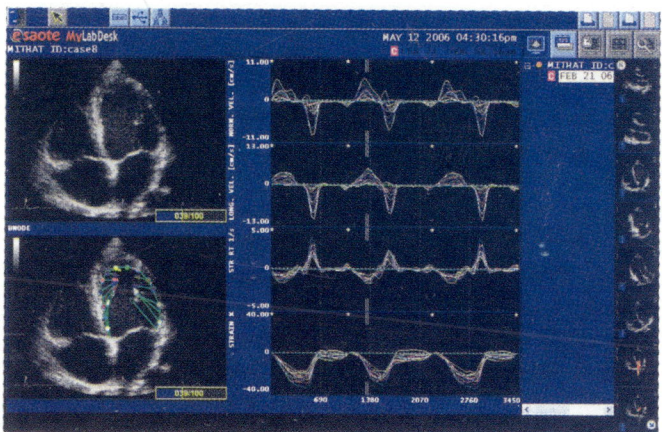

Fig. 24.27: New imaging method to estimate and quantify endocardial velocities of contractions and relaxation and estimate and quantity deformation of the heart (strain and strain rate)

regarding medical versus revascularization strategies. Therapy should therefore be individualized and it is not appropriate to consider the older patient, especially in the presence of multiple diseases, as a "routine" post-MI pathway patient (Fig. 24.15).

Ageing affects cardiovascular risk factors, incidence and clinical manifestation of cardiac disease, treatment strategies and prognosis. Cardiovascular disease is superimposed on age-associated changes in cardiac and vascular characteristics. The final pathophysiological mechanism and clinical presentation result from an interaction between age-related changes in cardiovascular physiology and cardiovascular disease.

Chronic Ischemic Heart Disease

The diagnosis of ischaemic heart disease may be more difficult in the elderly. Reduced physical activity with age limits the occurrence of demand angina. Possibly related to the age-related changes in myocardial compliance and diastolic relaxation, dyspnea, rather than pain, may dominate the clinical picture of myocardial ischemia and infarction. The predictive value of a negative exercise stress test is low in a population with a high prevalence of ischemic heart disease. As many elderly people are unable to exercise to 85–90% of their predicted maximum heart rate, a pharmacological stress test with thallium scan or echocardiogram is often of greater diagnostic accuracy.

Although the goal and choice of anti-ischemic treatment are generally similar in young and old patients, the elderly must be expected to be more sensitive to the hypotensive effects of certain anti-ischaemic drugs because of blunted baroreceptor reflex activity and sympathetic responsiveness, and increased myocardial and vascular stiffness. As a result of the same age-related decrease in sympathetic responsiveness, myocardial

ischemia is less likely to be provoked by adrenergic-mediated increases in myocardial oxygen demand and the benefit derived from treatment with β-adrenoceptor blockers may be reduced (Fig. 24.14).

Congestive Heart Failure (Fig. 24.27)

Systolic

The therapy of congestive heart failure due to systolic dysfunction does not differ in the older patient. The mainstay of therapy are digoxin, diuretics, and especially angiotensin converting enzyme inhibitor drugs. Renal function and potassium may need to be monitored more closely in the older patient because of the likely concomitant administration or ingestion of nonsteroidal anti-inflammatory drugs (high incidence of arthritis in the older population) and the additive effects of NSAID's to lower renal perfusion and potassium excretion. The role of beta blockers in the management of patients with congestive heart failure is just emerging and there are no data regarding the older patient.

Diastolic

Congestive heart failure with preserved left ventricular systolic function is termed "diastolic heart failure" and is more prevalent in the older population, may account for one half of the older population with congestive heart failure, and may be more common in women than men. The prognosis of patients with CHF due to diastolic dysfunction is less ominous than in patients with systolic dysfunction, yet the morbidity can be high with frequent treatment failures and hospital readmissions. No long-term studies of drug therapies for diastolic congestive heart failure have been performed. Drugs which selectively affect diastolic filling and relaxation (calcium channel antagonists or beta-adrenergic blockers) can alter these parameters after short-term administration and might provide a specific therapy. However, one of the more surprising findings from a recent trial was the lower incidence of recurrent hospitalizations and death in patients with congestive heart failure who received digoxin (vs. placebo) in combination with diuretics and ACE inhibitors. This was true for CHF patients with both decreased and preserved systolic function. Thus, optimal management of the older patient with diastolic congestive heart failure is evolving. Control of hypertension, prevention of myocardial ischemia, treatment of congestive heart failure symptoms, and maintenance of normal sinus rhythm have received emphasis. It appears that digoxin and diuretics do play a role and that beta blockers and/or calcium blockers may also play a role. Treatment of acute exacerbation of congestive heart failure or pulmonary edema in the setting of diastolic heart failure focuses on diuretics and, if needed, positive inotropes on a short-term basis. The

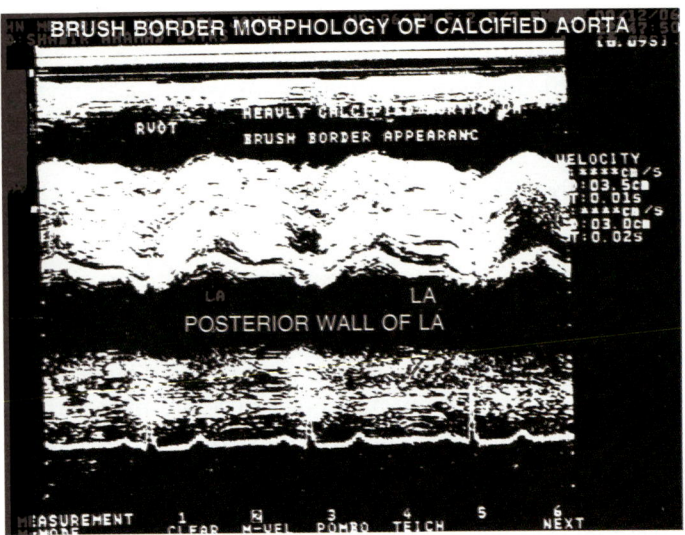

Fig. 24.28: M-Mode echocardiogram of aorta showing heavily calicified aorta resembling imprints of borders of paint brush, also called *brush border appearance* of aorta

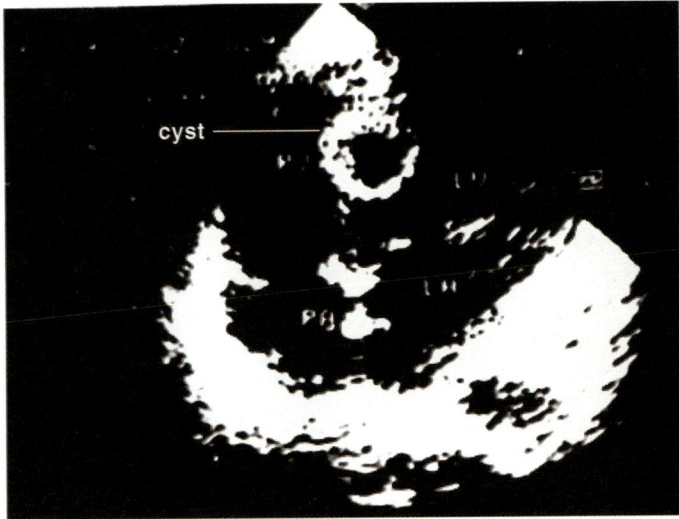

Fig. 24.30: Apical 4C view showing a big hydatid cyst in the region of apical septum in patient with complete heart block

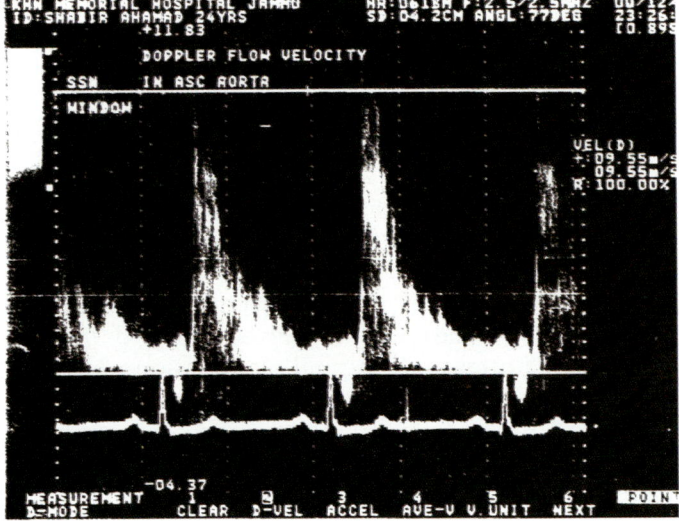

Fig. 24.29: Suprasternal notch window at ascending aorta showing Doppler signatures of aortic valvular stenosis in the same patient as Fig. 24.23. Note high velocity jet exceeding 9.0 m/s

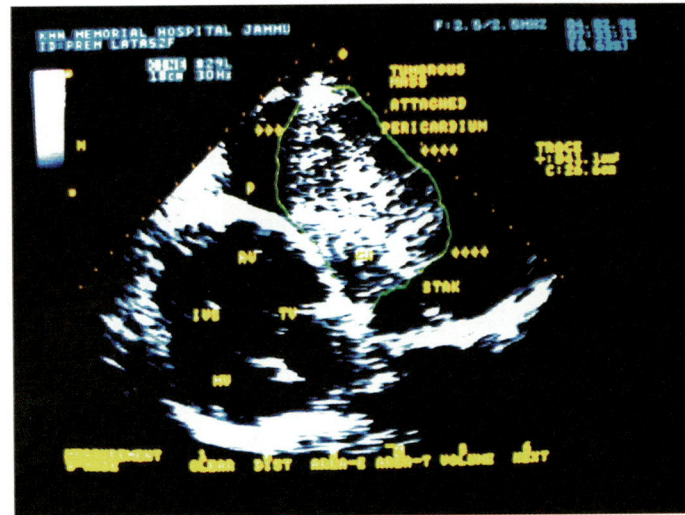

Fig. 24.31: Apical 4C view showing a big mass (encircled) attached to pericardium with compression on the anterior wall of the left ventricle

role of ACE inhibitors is unclear unless used for the treatment of hypertension or to attempt regression of hypertrophy.

Valvular Diseases

Degenerative calcification (leading to sclerosis) and myxomatous degeneration (which can lead to regurgitation) affect the aortic and mitral valves with aging. These changes are considered secondary to aging and differ from the primary changes due to rheumatic heart disease or congenital valve abnormalities. These changes can progress to impair the function of the valve; then the changes are considered pathologic and no longer "normal aging".

Aortic Stenosis (Figs 24.18, 24.23–24.25, 24.28 and 24.29)

The frequency of aortic stenosis increases with age and it is the most clinically significant valvular lesion in the elderly. Progressive degenerative calcification is now the most common cause, as opposed to rheumatic disease. The calcification occurs along the margins of the valve leaflet (vs. commisural fusion in rheumatic fever) and thus does not affect valve opening or closing during the early stages but will produce a murmur. Because of the stiffened peripheral arteries in the older patient, the carotid pulse may feel normal to palpation even in the presence of significant aortic stenosis. Other physical findings associated with critical aortic stenosis due to rheumatic heart disease are often absent with

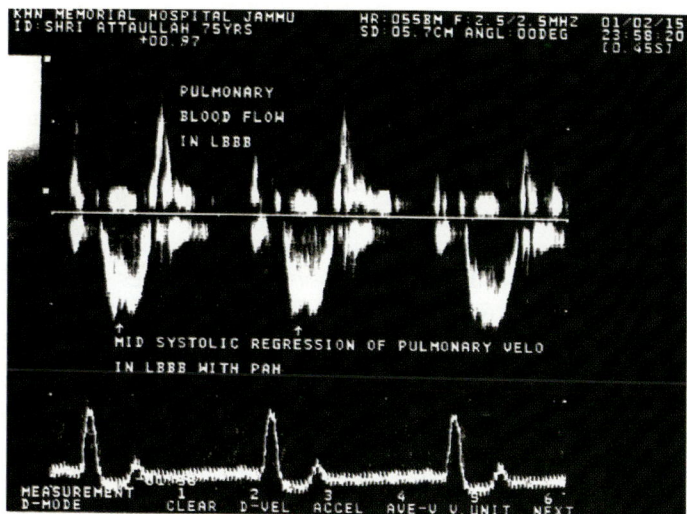

Fig. 24.32: Doppler flow velocity across pulmonary valve showing systolic regression of peak flow velocity in elderly patient with COPD and severe pulmonary arterial hypertension

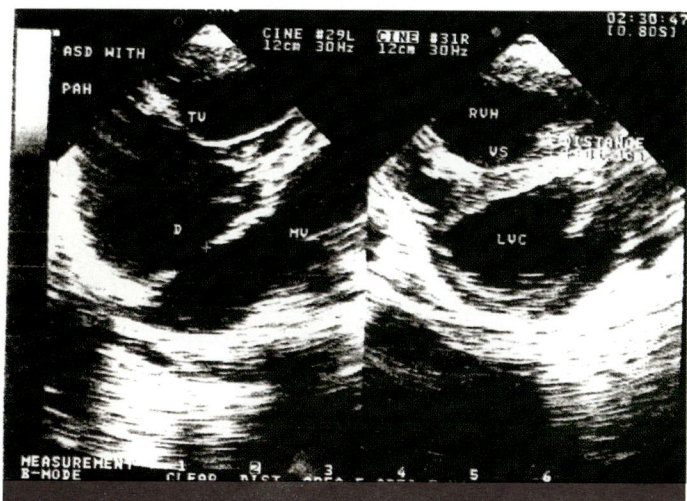

Fig. 24.33: Subcostal approach with biatrial and ventricular views respectively shows ASD secundum (D) hypertrophy and dilatation along with crescent shaped LV configuration in patient with ASD with severe pulmonary arterial hypertension

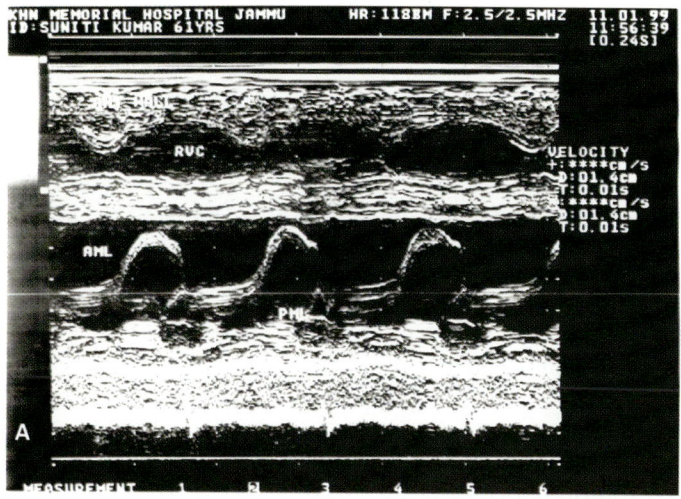

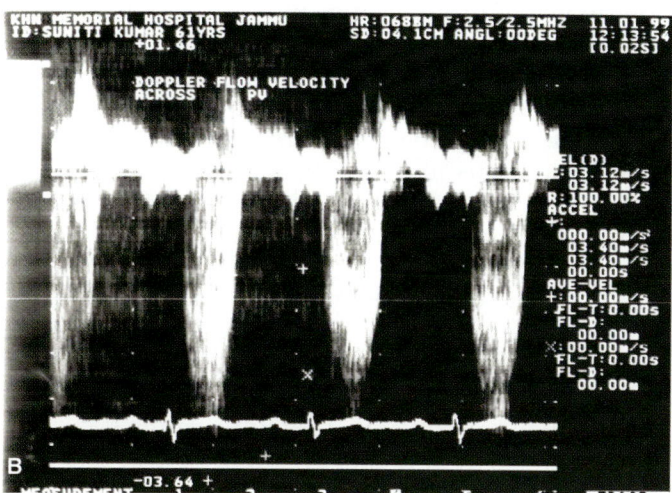

Fig. 24.34: (A) M-Mode echocardiogram showing reduction in EF slope and thikened tricuspid valve. **(B)** Increased peak systolic Doppler flow velocity (>3.12 m/s) in a 61 yrs old patient with congenital infundibular pulmonary stenosis

calcific aortic stenosis (decreased S_1 and S_2). The intensity of the murmur does not correlate with the severity of stenosis. Progression to critical aortic stenosis is often gradual but is unpredictable. Therefore, diagnostic testing is essential for the diagnosis or evaluation of a symptomatic elderly patient with an aortic systolic murmur. Fortunately, noninvasive echocardiographic and Doppler testing can now accurately assess the severity of obstruction as well as define the aortic valve. About 20% of elderly patients with aortic disease have a rheumatic etiology—these patients usually have associated mitral valve disease and should receive antibiotic prophylaxis before all invasive procedures including dental procedures. The only effective treatment for critical aortic stenosis is surgical. Aortic valve replacement, even in older patients, improves survival and quality of life. Experience with aortic balloon valvuloplasty shows that re-stenosis occurs frequently within months and it has thus been largely abandoned.

Aortic Regurgitation (Fig. 24.22B)

The most common cause of aortic regurgitation in the elderly is aortic root dilation secondary to the age-related rise in blood pressure and increased peripheral resistance. With the advent of widespread echocardiography, mild degrees of aortic regurgitation are diagnosed frequently and are usually not of clinical significance. Aortic regurgitation due to rheumatic valvular disease or associated with disease of a bicuspid valve is more likely to progress to clinically significant disease. When significant aortic regurgitation is present, therapy is aimed at afterload reduction and clinical symptom relief with monitoring for definitive surgical intervention prior to left ventricular failure.

Mitral Valve Disease (Figs 24.4A and B and 24.26A)

Mitral regurgitation accounts for 2/3 of mitral valve disease in the elderly. The etiologies include rheumatic disease (usually with concomitant aortic disease), papillary muscle dysfunction due to ischemia or infarction, calcification of the mitral annulus (more common in women than men), and myxomatous degeneration causing mitral valve prolapse. Medical management centers on maintenance of sinus rhythm or control of atrial fibrillation, afterload reduction and prevention of infection by use of prophylactic antibiotic regimens before all invasive procedures (including dental). The subset of patients with significant mitral regurgitation and mitral valve prolapse may have an increased risk for stroke and should be considered for anticoagulation. Acute symptoms may also benefit from diuretics. As disease progresses, the ventricle dilates and pulmonary hypertension develops and medical treatment is no longer effective. Surgical interventions have the best results prior to the development of ventricular dysfunction or marked dilation. Operative results to date show return towards normal pressures and ventricular size, but improvement is not as marked as that seen after aortic valve replacement. Therefore, optimal surgical timing has not been identified but morbidity and mortality are high, when once left ventricular failure occurs. Surgical repair as opposed to replacement is currently being used and evaluated for patients with regurgitation and noncalcified, nonstenotic valves. This may preclude the need for anticoagulation with mechanical valves, which could potentially be of clinical advantage in the older patient since surgical mitral valve replacement (whether it is a tissue or mechanical valve) requires lifelong high intensity anticoagulation. The management of the less common mitral stenosis in the elderly also targets control of heart rate and symptoms (digiorin and diuretics), anticoagulation to prevent emboli, and antibiotic prophylaxis to prevent infections. Surgical therapy is the only definitive therapy. Valvuloplasty is seldom of long-term benefit (Figs 24.5 and 24.6).

Summary

It is mostly acknowledged that 'normal' or 'healthy' aging of the cardiovascular system is distinct from the increasing incidence and severity of cardiovascular disease with advancing age (e.g. hypertension, ischemic heart disease and congestive heart failure). It is also recognized that chronological and biological age may differ considerably. Nevertheless, even in the absence of overt coexisting disease, advanced age is always accompanied by a general decline in organ function, and specifically by alterations in structure and function of the heart and vasculature that will ultimately affect cardiovascular performance. Actual biological age is thus the net result of the interaction between age-related and concomitant disease-associated changes in organ function. As cardiovascular performance at a given moment is the net result of interactions between heart rate, intrinsic contractility, diastolic and systolic function, ventricular afterload and coronary perfusion, it is important to be aware of the age-related changes in each of these variables, independent of disease, as they determine cardiac performance at rest and its response to stress in the elderly.

The most relevant age-related changes in cardiovascular performance for perioperative management are the stiffened myocardium and vasculature, blunted β-adrenoceptor responsiveness and impaired autonomic reflex control of heart rate. These changes are of little clinical relevance at rest, but may have considerable consequences during superimposed cardiovascular stress. Such stress can take the form of increased flow demand (as in exercise or postoperatively), demand for acute autonomic reflex control (as in change of posture) or severe disease (as during myocardial ischemia, tachyarrhythmias or uncontrolled hypertension). It may interfere with diastolic relaxation (i.e. ventricular filling), systolic contraction (i.e. ventricular emptying) and vasomotor control (i.e. arterial pressure homeostasis).

Three factors contribute most to the increased perioperative risk related to advanced age. First, physiological ageing is accompanied by a progressive decline in resting organ function. Consequently, the reserve capacity to compensate for impaired organ function, drug metabolism and added physiological demands is increasingly impaired. Functional disability will occur more quickly and take longer to be cured.

Second, aging is associated with progressive manifestation of chronic disease which further limits baseline function and accelerates loss of functional reserve in the affected organ. Some of the age-related decline in organ function (e.g. impaired pulmonary gas exchange, diminished renal capacity to conserve and eliminate water and salt, or disturbed thermoregulation) will increase cardiovascular risk. The unpredictable interaction between age-related and disease-associated changes in organ functions, and the altered neurohumoral response to various forms of stress in the elderly may result in a rather atypical clinical presentation of a disease. This may, in turn, delay the correct diagnosis and appropriate treatment and, ultimately, worsen outcome.

Third, related to the increased intake of medications and altered pharmacokinetics and pharmacodynamics, the incidence of untoward reactions to medications, anaesthetic agents, and medical and surgical interventions increases with advancing age.

On the basis of various clinical studies and observations, it must be concluded that advanced age is an independent predictor of adverse perioperative cardiac outcome. It is to be expected that the aged cardiovascular risk patient carries an even higher perioperative cardiac risk than the younger cardiovascular risk patient. Although knowledge of the physiology of aging should help reduce age-related complications, successful prophylaxis is hindered by the heterogeneity of age-related changes, unpredictable physiological and pharmacological interactions and diagnostic difficulties.

Bibliography

1. Alfonso F, Azcona L, Perez-Vizcayno MJ, *et al.* Initial results and long-term clinical and angiographic implications of coronary stinting in elderly patients. *Am J Cardiol* 1999; 83: 1483–7.

2. Amrani M, Goodwin AT, Gray CC, Yacoub MH. Ageing is associated with reduced basal and stimulated release of nitric oxide by the coronary endothelium. *Acta Physiol Scand* 1996; 157: 79–84.

3. Ashton CM, Petersen NJ, Wray NP *et al.* The incidence of perioperative myocardial infarction in men undergoing noncardiac surgery. *Ann Intern Med* 1993; 118: 504–10.

4. Barakat K, Wilkinson P, Deaner A, Fluck D, Ranjadayalan K, Timmis A. How should age affect management of acute myocardial infarction? A prospective cohort study. *Lancet* 1999; 353: 955–9.

5. Baron JF, Mundler O, Bertrand M *et al.* Dipyridamole-thallium scintigraphy and gated radionuclide angiography to assess cardiac risk before abdominal aortic surgery. *New Engl J Med* 1994; 330: 663–9.

6. Batchelor WB, Jollis JG, Friesinger GC. The challenge of health care delivery to the elderly patient with cardiovascular disease. Demographic, epidemiologic, fiscal, and health policy implications. *Cardiol Clin* 1999; 17: 1–15.

7. Berthoud MC, McLaughlan GA, Broome IJ, Henderson PD, Peacock JE, Reilly CS. Comparison of infusion rates of three i.v. anaesthetic agents for induction in elderly patients. *Br J Anaesth* 1993; 70: 423–7.

8. Bonow RO, Vitale DF, Bacharach SL, Maron BJ, Green MV. Effect of aging on asynchronous left ventricular regional function and global ventricular filling in normal human subjects. *J Am Coll Cardiol* 1988; 11: 50–58.

9. Bovill JG, Boer F. Opioids in cardiac anesthesia. In: Kaplan JA, Reich DL, Konstadt SN, eds. *Cardiac Anesthesia,* 4th Edn. Philadelphia, PA: W.B. Saunders, 1999; 573–609.

10. Browner WS, Li J, Mangano DT, for the Study of Perioperative Ischemia Research Group. In-hospital and long-term mortality in male veterans following non-cardiac surgery. *J Am Med Assoc* 1992; 268: 228–32.

11. Buhre W, Hoeft A. Anaesthesia and the cardiovascular system. In: Priebe H-J, Skarvan K, eds. *Cardiovascular Physiology,* 2nd Edn. London: BMJ Publishing Group, 2000; 331–73.

12. Carli R, Emery PW, Freemantle CAJ. Effect of preoperative normothermia on postoperative protein metabolism in elderly patients undergoing hip arthroplasty. *Br J Anaesth* 1989; 63: 276–82.

13. Carpo RO, Campbell EJ. Aging of the respiratory system. In: Fishman AP, ed. *Pulmonary Diseases and Disorders.* New York, NY: McGraw-Hill, 1998: 251–64.

14. Chen C-H, Nakayama M, Nevo E, Fetics BJ, Maughan WL, Kass DA. Coupled systolic-ventricular and vascular stiffening with age. Implications for pressure regulation and cardiac reserve in the elderly. *J Am Coll Cardiol* 1998; 32: 1221–7.

15. Chobanian A. Pathophysiologic considerations in the treatment of the elderly hypertensive patient. *Am J Cardiol* 1983; 52: 490–539.

16. Classen DC, Pestotnik SL, Evans RS, Lloyd JF, Burke JP. Adverse drug events in hospitalized patients: excess length of stay, extra costs, and attributable mortality. *J Am Med Assoc* 1997; 277: 301–6.

17. Cohen G, David TE, Ivanov J, Armstrong S, Feindel CM. The impact of age, coronary artery disease, and cardiac comorbidity on late survival after bioprosthetic aortic valve replacement. *J Thorac Cardiovasc Surg* 1999; 117: 273–84.

18. Czernin J, Müller P, Chan S *et al.* Influence of age and hemodynamics on myocardial blood flow and flow reserve. *Circulation* 1993; 88: 62–9 .

19. Detsky AS, Abrams, HB, McLaughlin JR *et al.* Predicting cardiac complications in patients undergoing non-cardiac surgery. *J Gen Intern Med* 1986; 1: 211–19.

20. Eagle KA, Coley CM, Newell JB *et al.* Combining clinical and thallium data optimizes preoperative assessment of cardiac risk before major vascular surgery. *Ann Intern Med* 1989; 110: 859–66.

21. Ebert TJ, Harkin CP, Muzi M. Cardiovascular responses to sevoflurane: a review. *Anesth Analg* 1995; 81: S11–22.

22. Ebert TJ, Kanitz DD, Kampine JP. Inhibition of sympathetic neural outflow during thiopental anesthesia in humans. *Anesth Analg* 1990; 71: 319–26.

23. Ebert TJ, Morgan BJ, Barney JA, Denahan T, Smith JJ. Effects of aging on baroreflex regulation of sympathetic activity in humans. *Am J Physiol* 1992; 263: H798–803.

24. Ebert TJ, Muzi M, Berens R, Goff D, Kampine JP. Sympathetic responses to induction of anesthesia in humans with propofol or etomidate. *Anesthesiology* 1992; 76: 725–33.

25. Egashira K, Inou T, Hirooka Y *et al.* Effects of age on endothelium-dependent vasodilation of resistance coronary artery by acetylcholine in humans. *Circulation* 1993; 88: 77–81.

26. Esler MD, Turner AG, Kaye DM *et al.* Aging effects on human sympathetic neuronal function. *Am J Physiol* 1995; 268: R278–85.

27. Fishman RF, Kuntz RE, Carrozza JP Jr. Friedrich. Acute and long-term results of coronary stents and atherectomy in women and the elderly. *Coronary Artery Disease* 1995; 6(2):159–68.

28. Fleg J, Lakatta EG. Role of muscle loss in the age-associated reduction in VO2 max. *J Appl Physiol* 1988; 65: 1147–51.

29. Fleg JL, O'Connor F, Gerstenblith G, *et al.* Impact of age on the cardiovascular response to dynamic upright exercise in healthy men and women *J Appl Physiol* 1995; 78: 890–900

30. Fleg JL, O'Connor FC, Gerstenblith G, *et al.* Impact of age on the cardiovascular response to dynamic upright exercise in healthy men and women. *J Appl Physiol* 1995;78: 890–900.

31. Fleg JL, Schulman S, O'Connor F, *et al.* Effects of acute β-adrenergic receptor blockade on age-associated changes in cardiovascular performance during dynamic exercise. *Circulation* 1994; 90: 2333–41.

32. Fletcher GF, Balady G. Froelicher VF, Hartley LH, Haskell WL, Pollock ML. Exercise standards: A statement for healthcare professionals from the American Heart Association: writing Group. *Circulation* 1995; 91: 580–615

33. Folkow B, Svanborg A. Physiology of cardiovascular aging. *Physiol Rev* 1993; 73: 725–64.

34. Frank SM, Beattie C, Christopherson R, *et al.* The Perioperative Ischemia Randomized Anesthesia Trial Study Group. Unintentional hypothermia is associated with postoperative myocardial ischemia. *Anesthesiology* 1993; 78: 468–76.

35. Frank SM, Shir Y, Raja SN, Fleisher L, Beattie C. Core hypothermia and skin-surface temperature gradients. Epidural versus general anesthesia and the effects of age. *Anesthesiology* 1994; 80: 502–8[ISI][Medline]

36. Franklin SS, Gustin W IV, Wong ND, *et al.* Hemodynamic patterns of age-related changes in blood pressure. The Framingham Heart Study. *Circulation* 1997; 96: 308–15[Abstract/Free Full Text].

37. Friedl LP, Kronmal RA, Newman AB, *et al.* Risk factors for 5-year mortality in older adults: the cardiovascular health study. *J Am Med Assoc* 1998; 279: 585–92[Abstract/Free Full Text].

38. Gajraj RJ, Doi M, Mantzaridis H, Kenny GNC. Comparison of bispectral EEG analysis and auditory evoked potentials for monitoring depth of anaesthesia during propofol anaesthesia. *Br J Anaesth* 1999; 82: 672–8.

39. Gardin JM, Arnold AM, Bild ED, *et al.* Left ventricular diastolic filling in the elderly: the cardiovascular health study. *Am J Cardiol* 1998; 82: 345–51.

40. Gold MI, Abello D, Herrington C. Minimum alveolar concentration of desflurane in patients older than 65 yr. *Anesthesiology* 1993;79: 710–14.

41. Goldman L, Caldera DL, Nussbaum SR, *et al.* Multifactorial index of cardiac risk in noncardiac surgical procedures. *New Engl J Med* 1977; 297: 845–50.

42. Gooding JM, Weng JT, Smith RA, Berninger GT, Kirby RR. Cardiovascular and pulmonary responses following etomidate induction of anesthesia in patients with demonstrated cardiac disease. *Anesth Analg* 1979; 58: 40–41.

43. Goodwin AT, Amrani M, Marchbank AJ, Gray CC, Jayakumar J, Yacoub MH. Coronary vasoconstriction to endothelin-1 increases with age before and after ischaemia and reperfusion. *Cardiovasc Res* 1999; 41: 554–62.

44. Groenink M, Langerak SE, Vanbavel E, *et al.* The influence of aging and aortic stiffness on permanent dilation and breaking stress of the thoracic descending aorta. *Cardiovasc Res* 1999; 43: 471–80.

45. Guidelines for Perioperative Cardiovascular Evaluation for Noncardiac Surgery. Report of the American College of Cardiology/American Heart Association Task Force on Practice Guidelines (Committee on Perioperative Cardiovascular Evaluation for Noncardiac Surgery). *Circulation* 1996; 93: 1278–317.

46. Hall WJ. Update in geriatrics. *Ann Intern Med* 1997; 127: 557–64.

47. Heier T, Caldwell JE, Sessler DI, Miller RD. Mild intraoperative hypothermia increases duration of action and spontaneous recovery of vecuronium blockade during nitrous oxide-isoflurane anesthesia in humans. *Anesthesiology* 1991; 74: 815–19.

48. Hlatky MA, Boineau RE, Higginbotham MB, *et al.* A brief self-administered questionnaire to determine functional capacity (the Duke activity status index). *Am J Cardiol* 1989; 64: 651–4.

49. Holmes DR Jr, White HD, Pieper KS, Ellis SG, Califf RM, Topol EJ. Effect of age on outcome with primary angioplasty versus thrombolysis. *J Am Coll Cardiol* 1999; 33: 412–19.

50. Ikeda T, Doi M, Morita K, Ikeda K. Effects of midazolam and diazepam as premedication on heart rate variability in surgical patients. *Br J Anaesth* 1995; 73: 479–83.

51. Jacobs JR, Reves JG, Marty J, White WD, Bai SA, Smith LR. Aging increases pharmacodynamic sensitivity to the hypnotic effects of midazolam. *Anesth Analg* 1995; 80: 143–8.

52. Kampmann JP, Sinding J, Moller-Jorgensen I. Effect of age on liver function. *Geriatrics* 1975; 30: 91–5.

53. Kannel WB. Framingham study insights into hypertensive risk of cardiovascular disease. *Hypertension Research* 1995; 18(3):181–96. *Cardiol* 1995; 423A–4A.

54. Katoh T, Bito H, Sato S. Influence of age on hypnotic requirement, bispectral index, and 95% spectral edge frequency associated with sedation induced by sevoflurane. *Anesthesiology* 2000; 92: 55–61.

55. Kazama T, Ikeda K, Morita K, *et al.* Comparison of the effect-site KeOs of propofol for blood pressure and EEG bispectral index in elderly and younger patients. *Anesthesiology* 1999; 90: 1517–27.

56. Kazmers A, Perkins AJ, Jacobs LA. Outcomes after abdominal aortic aneurysm repair in those 80 years of age: Recent Veterans Affairs experience. *Ann Vasc Surg* 1998; 12: 106–12.

57. Kennedy HL. Long-term prognostic significance of ambulatory electrocardiographic findings in apparently healthy subjects > 60 years of age. *Am J Cardiol* 1992;70: 748–51.

58. Kirkpatrick T, Cockshott D, Douglas EJ, Nimmo WS. Pharmacokinetics of propofol (Diprivan) in elderly patients. *Br J Anaesth* 1988; 60: 146–50.

59. Kitzman DW, Sheikh KH, Beere PA, *et al.* Age-related alterations of Doppler left ventricular filling indices in normal subjects are independent of left ventricular mass, heart rate, contractility and loading conditions. *JACC* 1991; 18:1243–50.

60. Klein AL, Leung DY, Murray RD, Urban LH, Bailey KR, Tajik AJ. Effects of age and physiologic variables on right ventricular filling dynamics in normal subjects. *Am J Cardiol* 1999; 84: 440–48.

61. Kuo TBJ, Lin T, Yang CH, Li C-L, Chen C-F, Chou P. Effect of aging on gender differences in neural control of heart rate. *Am J Physiol* 1999; 277: H2233–9.

62. Kurz A, Plattner O, Sessler DI, Huemer G, Redl G, Lackner F. The threshold for thermoregulatory vasoconstriction during nitrous oxide/isoflurane anesthesia is lower in elderly than in young patients. *Anesthesiology* 1993; 79: 465–9.

63. Kurz A, Sessler DI, Lenhardt R, for the Study of Wound Infection and Temperature Group. Perioperative normothermia to reduce the incidence of surgical wound infection and shorten hospitalization. *New Eng J Med* 1996; 334: 1209–15.

64. Lakatta E. Aging effects on the vasculature in health: risk factors for cardiovascular disease. *Am J Geriatr Cardiol* 1994; 3: 11–17.

65. Lakatta EG, Gerstenblith G, Weisfeldt ML. The aging heart: structure, function, and disease. In: Braunwald E, ed. *Heart Disease: A Textbook of Cardiovascular Medicine*, 5th Edn. Philadelphia, PA: W. B. Saunders, 1997; 1687–703.

66. Lakatta EG. Cardiovascular aging research: the next horizons. *J Am Geriatr Soc* 1999; 47: 613–25.

67. Lakatta EG. Cardiovascular regulatory mechanisms in advanced age. *Physiol Rev* 1993; 73: 413–67.

68. Lakatta EG. Changes in cardiovascular function with aging. *Eur Heart J* 1990;11 (Suppl C): 22–9

69. Lakatta EG. Deficient neuroendocrine regulation of the cardiovascular system with advancing age in healthy humans. *Circulation* 1993; 87: 631–6.

70. Lee TH. Reducing cardiac risk in noncardiac surgery. New Engl J Med 1999; 341: 1838–40.

71. Lindeman RD. Renal physiology and pathophysiology of aging. *Contrib Nephrol* 1993; 105: 1–12.

72. Mangano DT, Layug EL, Wallace A, Tateo I. Effect of atenolol on mortality and cardiovascular morbidity after noncardiac surgery. *New Engl J Med* 1996; 335: 1713–20. (Erratum: *New Engl J Med* 1997; 336: 1039.

73. Mangano DT. Perioperative cardiac morbidity. *Anesthesiology* 1990;72: 153–84.

74. Manolio, TA, Furberg CD, Rautaharju, PM. Cardiac arrhythmias on 24-hr ambulatory electrocardiography in older women and men: The Cardiovascular Healthy Study. *JACC* 1994; 23:916–25.

75. McKinney MS, Fee JPH, Clarke RSJ. Cardiovascular effects of isoflurane and halothane in young and elderly adult patients. *Br J Anaesth* 1993; 71: 696–701.

76. Minto CF, Schnider TW, Egan TD, *et al.* Influence of age and gender on the pharmacokinetics and pharmacodynamics of remifentanil. I. Model development. *Anesthesiology* 1997; 86: 10–23.

77. Miyauchi T, Yanagisawa M, Iida K, *et al.* Age- and sex-related variation of plasma endothelin-1 concentration in normal and hypertensive subjects. *Am Heart J* 1992;123: 1092–3.

78. Montamat SC, Cusack BJ, Vestal RE. Management of drug therapy in the elderly. *New Engl J Med* 1989; 321: 303–9[ISI][Medline]

79. MRC Working Party. Medical Research Council trial of treatment of hypertension in older adults: principal results. *Br Med J* 1992; 304: 405–12 [ISI] [Medline]

80. Murabito JM. Women and cardiovascular disease: contributions from the Framingham Heart Study. *Journal of the American Medical Women's Association.* 50(2):35–9, 55.

81. Nakajima R, Nakajima Y, Ikeda K. Minimum alveolar concentration of sevoflurane in elderly patients. *Br J Anaesth* 1993; 70: 273–5.

82. O'Keefe JH Jr., Sutton MB, McCallister BD, Vacek JL, Piehler JM, Ligon RW, Hartzler GO. Coronary angioplasty versus bypass surgery in patients > 70 years old matched for ventricular function. *Journal of the American College of Cardiology.* 24(2):425–30.

83. Ogawa T, Spina RJ, Mahia WH III, *et al.* Effects of aging, sex and physical training on cardiovascular responses to exercise. *Circulation* 1992; 86: 494–503.

84. Olivetti G, Melissari M, Capasso JM, Anversa P. Cardiomyopathy of the aging human heart. Myocyte loss and reactive cellular hypertrophy. *Circ Res* 1991;68:1560–68.

85. Ooi WL, Barrett S, Hossain M, Kelley-Gagnon MM, Lipsitz LA. Patterns of orthostatic blood pressure change and their clinical correlates in a frail, elderly population. *J Am Med Assoc* 1997; 277: 1299–1304.

86. Oskvig RM. Special problems in the elderly. *Chest* 1999; 115: 158S–164.

87. Palka P, Lange A, Nihoyannopoulos P. The effect of long-term training on age-related left ventricular changes by Doppler myocardial velocity gradient. *Am J Cardiol* 1999; 84: 1061–71.

88. Park KW, Haering JM, Reiz S, Lowenstein E. Effects of inhalation anesthetics on systemic hemodynamics and the coronary circulation. In: Kaplan JA, Reich DL, Konstadt SN, eds. *Cardiac Anesthesia*, 4th Edn. Philadelphia, PA: W.B. Saunders 1999; 537–72.

89. Pashos CL, Newhouse JP, McNeil BJ. Temporal changes in the care and outcomes of elderly patients with acute myocardial infarction, 1987 through 1990. *JAMA.* 270(15):1832–6.

90. Paul SD, O'Gara PT, Mahjoub ZA. Geriatric patients with acute myocardial infarction: cardiac risk factor profiles, presentations, thrombolysis, coronary interventions and prognosis. *Am Heart J* 1996; 131:710–15.

91. Peterson ED, Batchelor WB. Percutaneous intervention in the very elderly: weighing the risks and benefits. *Am Heart J* 1999; 137:585–7.

92. Pocock SJ, Henderson RA, Seed P, Treasure T, Hampton JR. Quality of life, employment status, and anginal symptoms after coronary angioplasty or bypass surgery. 3-year follow-up in the Randomized Intervention Treatment of Angina (RITA) Trial. *Circulation.* 94(2):135–42.

93. Poldermans D, Boersma E, Bax JJ, *et al.* for the Dutch Echocardiographic Cardiac Risk Evaluation Applying Stress Echocardiography Study Group. The effect of bisoprolol on perioperative mortality and myocardial infarction in high-risk patients undergoing vascular surgery. *New Engl J Med* 1999; 341: 1789–94.

94. Practice Guidelines for Perioperative Transesophageal Echocardiography. A Report by the American Society of Anesthesiologists and the Society of Cardiovascular Anesthe-siologists Task Force on Transesophageal Echocardiography. *Anesthesiology* 1996;84: 986–1006.

95. Practice Guidelines for Pulmonary Artery Catheterization. A Report by the American Society of Anesthesiologists Task Force on Pulmonary Artery Catheterization. *Anesthesiology* 1993; 78: 380–94.

96. Priebe HJ. Anesthesia and the heart. In: Dalla Volta S, de Luna AB, Brochier M, *et al.*, eds. *Cardiology.* London: McGraw-Hill, 1999; 815–23.

97. Priebe HJ. Effects of anesthetic agents on the heart and circulation. In: Foex P, Harrison GG, Opie LH, eds. *Cardiovascular Drugs in the Perioperative Period.* New York, NY: Authors' Publishing House, 1999; 33–57.

98. Reilly DF, McNeely MJ, Doerner D, *et al.* Self-reported exercise tolerance and the risk of serious perioperative complications. *Arch Intern Med* 1999; 159: 2185–92.

99. Reves JG, Hill S, Berkowitz D. Pharmacology of intravenous anesthetic induction drugs. In: Kaplan JA, Reich DL, Konstadt SN, eds. *Cardiac Anesthesia,* 4th edn. Philadelphia, PA: W.B. Saunders, 1999; 611–34 .

100. Rich MW, Beckham V, Wittenberg C, Leven CL, Freedland KE, Carney RM. A multidisciplinary intervention to prevent the readmission of elderly patients with congestive heart failure. *N Engl J Med* 1995;333:1190–95.

101. Rudner XL, Berkowitz DE, Booth JV, *et al.* Subtype specific regulation of human vascular 1-adrenergic receptors by vessel bed and age. *Circulation* 1999; 100: 2336–43.

102. Schnider TW, Minto CF, Shafer SL, *et al.* The influence of age on propofol pharmacodynamics. *Anesthesiology* 1999;90:1502–16.

103. Schulman SP, Fleg JL, Goldberg AP, *et al.* Continuum of cardiovascular performance across a broad range of fitness levels in healthy older men. *Circulation* 1996; 94: 359–67.

104. Schulman SP, Lakatta EG, Fleg IL, *et al.* Age-related decline in left ventricular filling at rest and exercise. *Am J Physiol* 1992; 263: H1932–8.

105. Seals DR, Taylor JA, Ng AV, Esler MD. Exercise and aging: autonomic control of the circulation. *Med Sci Sports Exerc* 1994; 26: 568–76.

106. Sellgren J, Ponten J, Wallin BG. Characteristics of muscle sympathetic nerve activity during general anaesthesia in humans. *Acta Anaesthesiol Scand* 1992; 36: 336–45.

107. Selzer A. Changing aspects of the natural history of valvular aortic stenosis. *N Engl J of Med* 1987; 317(2):91–8.

108. Shannon RP, Minaker KL, Rowe JW. The influence of age on water balance in man. *Semin Nephrol* 1984; 4: 346–52.

109. Shannon RP, Wei JY, Rosa RM, Epstein FH, Rowe JW. The effect of age and sodium depletion on cardiovascular response to orthostasis. *Hypertension* 1986;8:438–43.

110. Shipton EA. The perioperative care of the geriatric patient. *S Afr Med J* 1983; 63: 855–60.

111. Sleigh JW, Donovan J. Comparison of bispectral index, 95% spectral edge frequency and approximate entropy of the EEG, with changes in heart rate variability during induction of general anaesthesia. *Br J Anaesth* 1999; 82: 666–67.

112. Stanski DR, Maitre PO. Population pharmacokinetics and pharmacodynamics of thiopental: The effect of age revisited. *Anesthesiology* 1990; 72: 412–22.

113. Taddai CFG, Weintraub WS, Douglas JS Jr, *et al.* Influence of age on outcome after percutaneous transluminal coronary angioplasty. *Am J Cardiol* 1999; 84: 245–51.

114. Tresch DD, McGough MF. Heart failure with normal systolic function: A common disorder in older people. *J Am Geriatr Soc* 1995; 43: 1035–42.

115. Valeri RC, Cassidy G, Khuri S, Feingold H, Ragno G, Altschule MD. Hypothermia-induced reversible platelet dysfunction. *Ann Surg* 1987; 205: 175–81.

116. Vaughan MS, Vaughan RW, Cork RC. Postoperative hypothermia in adults: relationship of age, anesthesia, and shivering to rewarming. *Anesth Analg* 1981; 60:746–51 .

117. Wagner JA, Robinson S, Marino RP. Age and temperature regulation of humans in neutral and cold environments. *J Appl Physiol* 1974; 37: 562–5.

118. Wallace A, Layug B, Tateo I, *et al.* Prophylactic atenolol reduces postoperative myocardial ischemia. *Anesthesiology* 1998; 88: 7–17.

119. Wei JY. Age and the cardiovascular system (review article). *New Engl J Med* 1992;327: 1735–9.

120. Weinberger MH, Fineberg NS. Sodium and volume sensitivity of blood pressure. Age and pressure change over time. *Hypertension* 1991;18: 67–71.

121. Wennberg DE, Makenka DJ, Sengupta A, *et al.* Percutaneous transluminal coronary angioplasty in the elderly: epidemiology, clinical risk factors and in-hospital outcomes. *Am Heart J* 1999; 137: 639–45.

122. White M, Roden R, Minobe W, *et al.* Age-related changes in beta-adrenergic neuroeffector systems in the human heart. *Circulation* 1994; 90: 1225–38.

123. Wilson PW. Established risk factors and coronary artery disease: The Framingham Study. *American Journal of Hypertension* 1994; 7(Pt 2):7S–12S.

124. Woodhouse KW, Mutch E, Williams FM, Rawlins MD, James OF. The effect of age on pathways of drug metabolism in human liver. *Ageing* 1984;13: 328–34.

125. Yang B, Larson DF, Watson R. Age-related left ventricular function in the mouse: analysis based on in vivo pressure-volume relationships. *Am J Physiol* 1999;46: H1906–13.

126. Younis LT, Melin JA, Robert AR, Detry JMR. Influence of age and sex on left ventricular volumes and ejection fraction during upright exercise in normal subjects. *Eur Heart J* 1990; 11: 916–24.

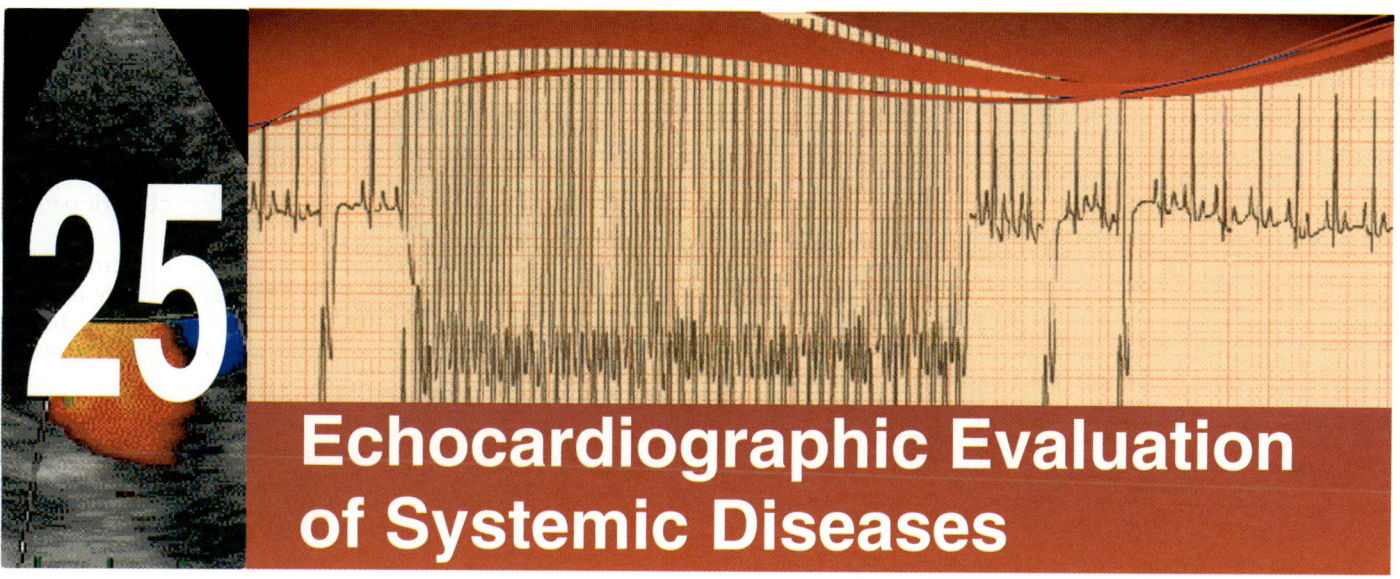

25

Echocardiographic Evaluation of Systemic Diseases

Mitral Valve Prolapse (MVP)

Prolapse of the mitral valve is usually caused by the myxomatus degeneration of the tissue including mitral apparatus leading to sagging of anterior mitral leaflet beyond the mitral annulus into the left atrial cavity. Barlow, *et al.* had given an excellent account of MVP and had demonstrated mid systolic click and late systolic murmur, commonly described as click murmur syndrome in such cases. Click systolic murmur due to MVP is usually caused by billowing or prolapse of the mitral leaflet into the left atrial cavity during systole. It is also called as Barlow's syndrome. The patients usually have mitral regurgitation in the later part of the systole due to mitral valve prolapse and anatomical changes of MV apparatus (Table 25.1).

The prolapsed leaflet generally becomes elongated, redundant, and thickened by the myxomatous degeneration. The chordae become elongated and thus allow the mitral apparatus to buckle into the left atrium (producing the click on auscultation). The timing and intensity of the click and murmur (of mitral regurgitation) vary with volume changes of the left ventricle induced by posture changes, with the Valsalva maneuver, or with amyl nitrite.

The major complications of prolapse include mitral regurgitation, spontaneous chordal rupture, increased tendency to develop infective endocarditis, or infrequently, sudden death. Echocardiography perhaps is the only sensitive method of diagnosis of mitral valve prolapse, provided certain parameters are met. The systolic posterior displacement of the anterior or posterior leaflet is one of the primary findings in prolapse. Prolapse can occur throughout systole (holosystolic or pansystolic), in midsystole, or in late systole. Normally the C-D segment of the mitral apparatus moves slightly anterior

in systole. However, in prolapse the D point stays 2 to 3 mm behind the C point into the left atrial cavity. The midsystolic click coincides with this posterior movement.

Table 25.1: *Systemic diseases with cardiovascular manifestations*

Hypertension
Diabetes mellitus
Pregnancy
Chronic renal insufficiency
Connective tissue disease
Systemic lupus erythematosus
Scleroderma
Marfan syndrome
Chronic hepatic disease
Pulmonary arterial hypertension

Miscellaneous diseases

Thyroid disease
Sarcoidosis
Hemochromatosis
Muscular dystrophies
Friedreich ataxia
Carcinoid syndrome
Ergotamine toxicity

Clinical presentations

Congestive heart failure
Dyspnea
Pulmonary embolus
Atrial fibrillation
Cardioembolic disease
Radiation therapy
Syncope
Athletic screening

The mitral valve may reveal several echoes throughout systole and diastole that may represent thickening, degeneration, or redundancy of the leaflet. The holosystolic bowing of the mitral apparatus has been demonstrated by De Maria, *et al.* (1980) as a collapse of the mitral leaflet to the back wall of the left atrium. In the diagnosis of MVP, the entire mitral apparatus should be scanned by an experienced echographer. If recordings are made at the tip of the leaflet with the beam exiting through the left atrial wall, the abnormal valve movement will more likely be recorded. The transducer must be perpendicular to the mitral apparatus. If it is too high on the chest and angled down towards the feet, a "pseudo" prolapse can be constructed.

Clinical symptoms can be augmented in MVP and patients should be examined in different postures such as supine, semidecubitus, upright, standing or squatting but some patients who present with MVP in the upright and squatting positions appear completely normal at rest. Two dimensional imaging allows a more precise evaluation of mitral prolapse. The parasternal long axis, short axis, and apical four-chamber views of the heart provide an opportunity to visualize the mitral apparatus as it prolapses into the left atrial cavity. The posterior leaflet can also be seen more clearly with two-dimensional imaging, as can be chordal structures and papillary muscles. Prolapse of both AV valves (mitral and tricuspid) lead to varying grades of mitral and tricuspid regurgitations, which can accurately be assessed by Doppler and colour Doppler echocardiography by placing the transducer in the apical four chamber view at the level of annulus of the valve. The jet is visualised as a posterior displacement during systole on the spectral tracing. The probe is then moved towards the left atrial cavity and carefully "swept" from a lateral to medial direction to record the presence of regurgitation (Figs 25.1–25.3).

If jet is seen, the flow is "mapped" or followed by the range-gated probe to see its extent into atrial cavity. Colour-flow Doppler guides to find out the exact direction of the regurgitant flow.

Marfans' Syndrome

Marfan's syndrome is an autosomal-dominant metabolic condition that involves the skeletal system including joints and abnormalities of the connective tissues. Clinical manifestations of the patients with which this syndrome presents are tall stature along with long and slender fingers with abnormal metacarpal index. They may reveal various cardiovascular abnormalities. The vision may be affected with dislocation of lens due to abnormalities in supporting ligaments of the eyes (Fig. 25.4A and B).

The cardiac changes noted on the echocardiogram may include a dilated aortic root (with extension into

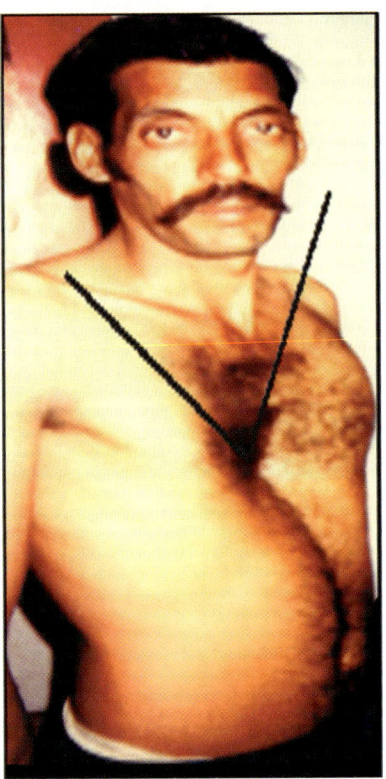

Fig. 25.1: Xiphisternal regression as a somatic anomaly in a patient with mitral valve prolapse (MVP)

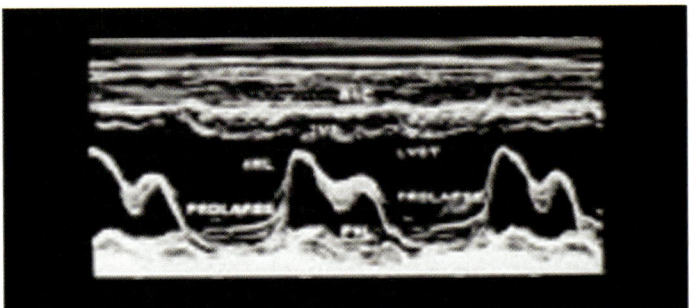

Fig. 25.2: M-Mode echocardiogram showing systolic sagging of both anterior and posterior mitral leaflets in the above-said patient with MVP

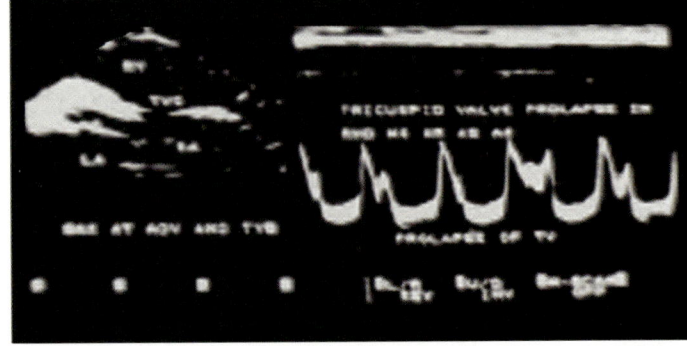

Fig. 25.3: M-Mode echocardiogram showing systolic sagging of anterior tricuspid leaflet in patient with tricuspid valvular prolapse

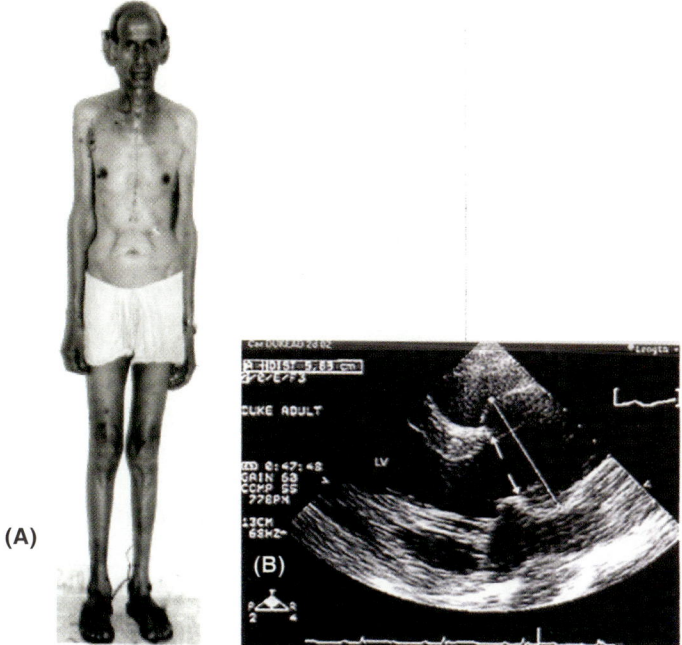

(A)

(B)

Fig. 25.4A and B: (A) 69 years old male was suffering from chronic aortic regurgitation with dilated ascending aorta and marfanoid habitus, aortography revealed annuloaortic ectasia with gross aortic regurgitation. He was managed with patch annuloplasty and his subseqent follow up showed neglegible/trace aortic regurgitation. **(B)** Echoscan, long axis view of LV showing dilated ascending aorta in patient with chronic aortic regurgitation and Marfan's syndrome

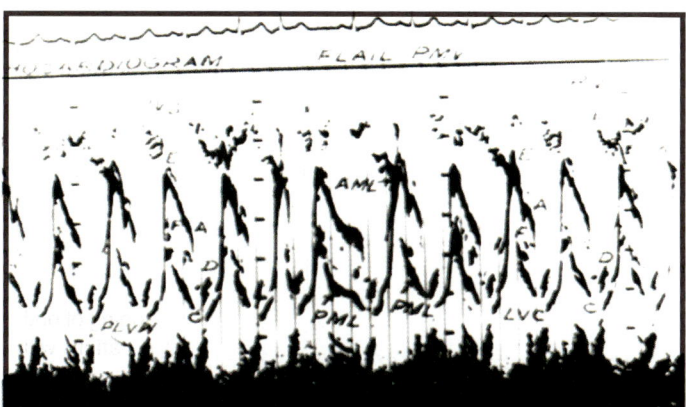

Fig. 25.5: M-Mode echocardiogram showing free floating/fluttering movements of ruptured posterior papillary muscle in patient with rheumatic carditis

the ascending aorta in more severe cases) and myxomatous degeneration of the aortic and mitral valves with resulting into redundancy, prolapse, and insufficiency. As the insufficient valve becomes more severe, the left ventricle dilates to accommodate the hemodynamic overload, and subsequently give rise to left ventricular dysfunction. The dilated aortic root may become very thin with increased dimensions and may lead to a dissection of the aorta.

Flail Mitral Apparatus or Ruptured Papillary Muscle

Myocardial infarction may lead to rupture to the papillary muscle or it may occur due to chest trauma. The rupture of papillary muscle will lead to gross acute mitral regurgitation and if not managed surgically, the patient may die due to acute left ventricular failure. It may also be the part of infective endocarditis of mitral valve. With auscultation, a gross mitral regurgitation murmur is heard at the apex of the heart. The left atrial size will be normal because the regurgitation is in an acute stage.

Echocardiographic Features

Rupture may be visualised echocardiographically in with a coarse, erratic and irregular flutter throughout the diastole. There may be a systolic dropout with the flail leaflet dipping far posteriorly into the left atrial cavity and then moving anteriorly in diastole. A ruptured chordae may be seen to "fly" throughout the mitral valve apparatus and may appear as a pseudo-SAM (systolic anterior motion) in systole.

Cardiac involvement occurs in upto 50% of patients with primary amyloidosis. Diffuse amyloid deposits lead to impairment of papillary muscle dysfunction.

This type of abnormality usually occurs in patients suffering from either dilated cardiomyopathy or ischemic heart disease affecting the mitral apparatus. In papillary muscle dysfunction the papillary or adjacent ventricular muscle may be scarred, dyskinetic, or merely dilated; thus the leaflet to which the muscle is attached, may not be able to close fully with resultant incomplete closure of the valve. The papillary muscle dysfunction clinically present with varying grades of mitral regurgitation which can be accurately diagnosed by M-mode and 2-dimensional echocardiography by placing the sample volume in apical view where mitral leaflets line up in a plane approximately parallel to the mitral annulus (Fig. 25.5).

Calcified Mitral Annulus

Echocardiographically MAC is recognised as a band of very dense, coarse, and highly reflective echoes posterior to the mitral valve apparatus. Often the calcification of the annulus obscures visualization of the posterior mitral leaflet or the endocardial surface of the posterior heart wall. Moreover, the bright echo of the MAC should be differentiated critically from that of the posterior heart wall or the echo of the heart wall with that of the pericardium (Fig. 25.6).

A false diagnosis of pericardial effusion will probably not be made if careful sweeps from the left atrium to the apex of the heart are performed. Besides the involvement of mitral annulus, the calcification may extend into other areas of the heart, especially

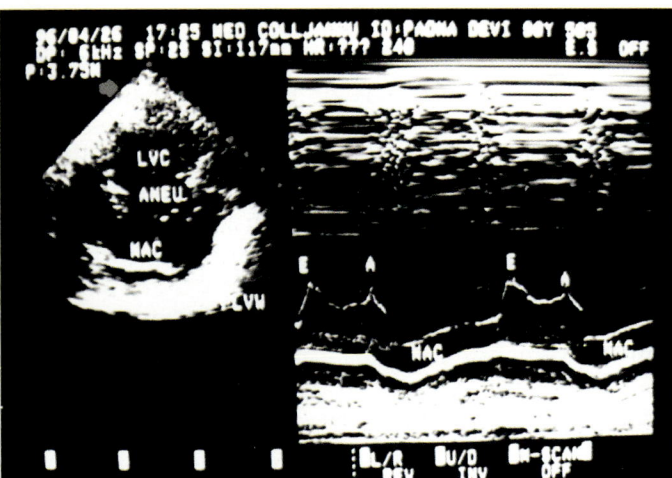

Fig. 25.6: M-Mode echocardiogram and 2-D scans showing normal anterior mitral leaflet and calcified mitral annulus in patient with CAD IDDM and HT

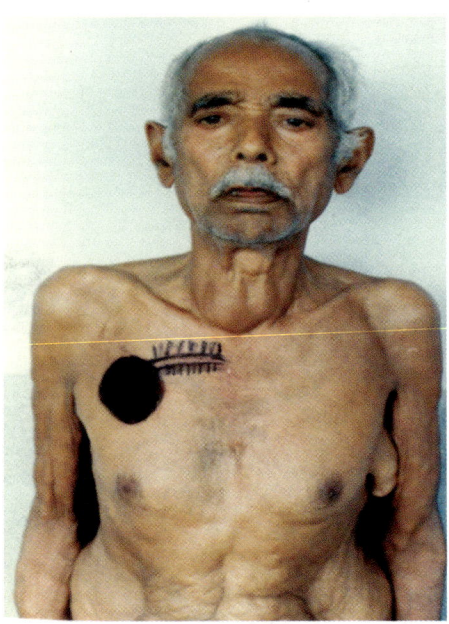

Fig. 25.8: 75 years old male was suffering from complete heart block for which PPI done by the author for the management of block (shown battery in right infraclavicular region) with non-compation type of cardiomyopathy

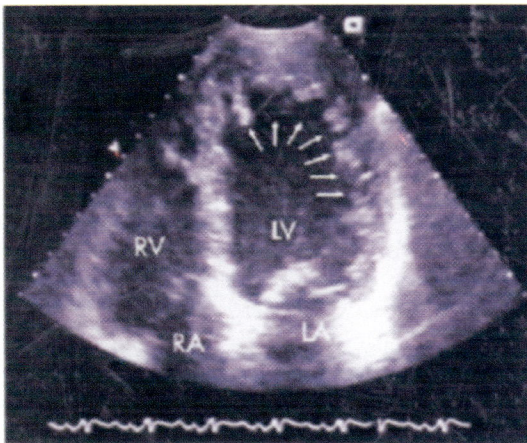

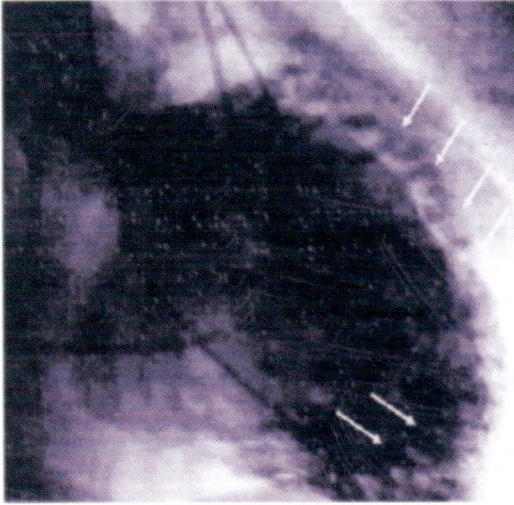

Fig. 25.7A and B: (A) Echoscan 4C view of LV and **(B)** LV angiography reveal a dilated hypocontractile left ventricle with a two tailored wall; the inner zones of heavily spongious, trabecularised endocardial layers with deep intertrabecular recesses (arrows) can be distinguished from thin outer zones of compacted myocardium in patient with non-compaction of LV

throughout the base of the left atrium. It may also extend into both the mitral and the aortic valves, into the root of the aorta, and into the left ventricle (along the chordae and papillary muscles).

MAC is associated with number of other diseases like calcific aortic stenosis, mitral valve prolapse, and hypertrophic subaortic stenosis. The calcified mitral annulus may impair the normal function of the mitral valve apparatus and frequently produces mitral regurgitation. It is frequently mixed with calcification of posterior mitral leaflet, but 2-dimensional or transesophageal or 3-dimensional echocardiography usually separates the two conditions with greater confidence of the echocardiographer.

Isolated Noncompaction of the Ventricular Myocardium (INVC) (Fig. 25.7)

Noncompaction of the ventricular myocardium is a rare congenital disorder characterised by the presence of numerous prominent trabeculation and deep intertrabecular recesses which communicate with the left ventricular cavity. The disease uniformly affects the left ventricle, and sometimes also affects the right ventricle.

Echocardiographic findings are important clues for the diagnosis. Clinical symptoms include signs of left ventricular systolic dysfunction even to the point of heart failure, ventricular arrhythmias, and embolic events remains critical.

Diagnosis of INVC by echocardiography using strict criteria is feasible. Its mortality and morbidity are high, including heart failure, thromboembolic events and ventricular arrhythmias.

Risk stratification includes heart failure therapy, oral anticoagulation, heart transplantation and implantation of an automated defibrillator/cardioverter. As IVNC is a distinct entity, its classification as a specific cardiomyopathy seems to be more appropriate.

Progressive Systemic Sclerosis (Scleroderma)

Systemic sclerosis is a multi system disorder characterised by fibrosis of skin and internal organs. Cardiac involvement in the form of myocardial fibrosis and pericarditis occurs frequently in systemic sclerosis,

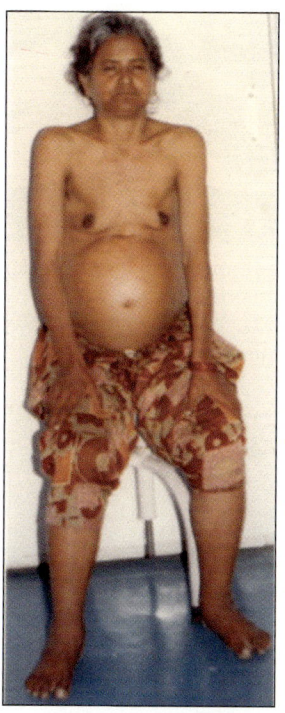

Fig. 25.10: 55 years old female was suffering from chronic renal failure and who had in addition severe HT, anasarca and echocardiographically revealed moderate pericardial effusion and diastolic LV dysfunctions

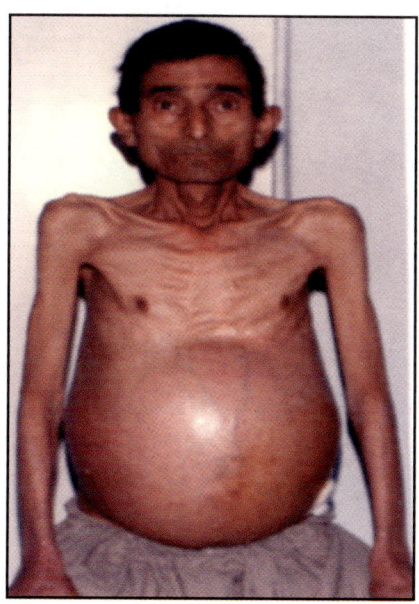

Fig. 25.9: 50 years old man with h/o chronic alcohalism with cirrhosis of liver and who in addition had echocardiographic proved dilated cardiomyopathy

while valvular involvement has been reported only sporadically. Adenocarcinoma of left breast pulmonary hypertension, gangrene of toes, and stenotic mitral valve disease have been reported rarely.

Echocardiography is the most important diagnostic tool in patients with suspected pulmonary hypertension. Other noninvasive tools such as electrocardiograms or radiographs are less sensitive and accurate. Echocardiography should be used as a screening tool in patients at high risk for the development of pulmonary hypertension; in systemic sclerosis, CREST syndrome.

Usefulness of Dobutamine Stress Echocardiography in Detecting Coronary Artery Disease in End-stage Renal Disease (Fig. 25.10)

The cardiovascular evaluation of patients with end-stage renal disease (ESRD) has been hampered by the suboptimal sensitivity and specificity of currently employed diagnostic tests. Dobutamine stress echocardiography (DSE) is a technique which is accurate for the diagnosis of coronary artery disease (CAD) in general populations.

Echocardiography in Chronic Liver Disorder

Prevalence of hepatopulmonary syndrome in cirrhosis and extrahepatic portal venous obstruction has been reported by various workers. Hepatopulmonary syndrome (HPS) is characterised by arterial hypoxemia in patients with chronic liver disease caused by abnormal intrapulmonary vasodilations (Fig. 25.9).

Intrapulmonary vascular dilatations (IPVD) are extrahepatic complications of acute and chronic liver disorders that can result in severe hypoxemia. Contrast-enhanced (CE) echocardiography provides a noninvasive method to detect right-to-left shunting associated with IPVD.

Left Ventricular Morphology in Chronic Renal Failure by Echocardiography (Fig. 25.10)

M-mode, two-dimensional, and Doppler echocardiography in chronic renal failure (CRD) has showed that the incidence of hypertension, left ventricular (LV) end diastolic volume, LV end systolic volume, and LV mass

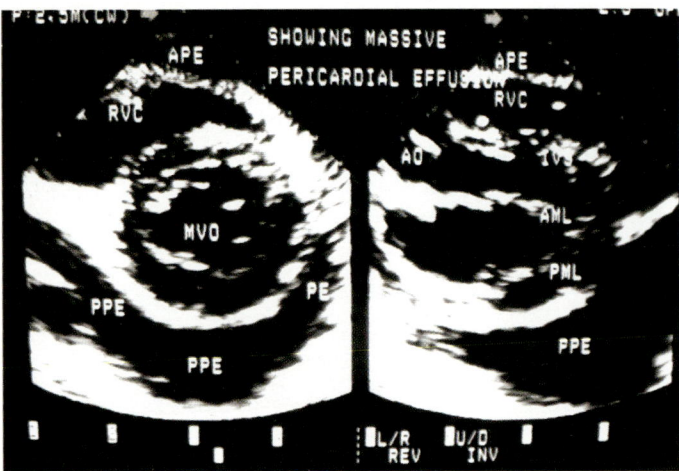

Fig. 25.11: 32 years young driver by profession, was suffering from progressive deterioration of general health investigations revealed that he had AIDS and echocardiography showed moderate pericardial effusion with dilated LV cavity

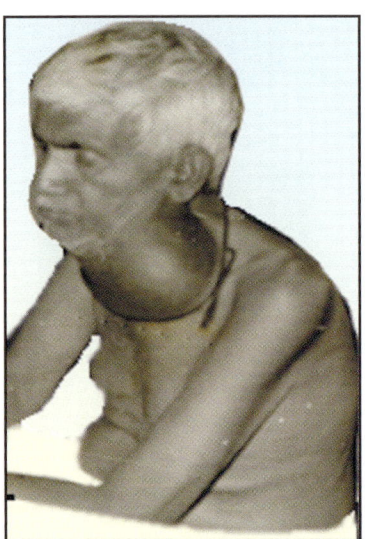

Fig. 25.12: 60 years old male had goitrous hypothyroidism and echocardiography revealed LV hypertrophy with diastolic LV dysfunctions

index are significantly higher in patients on hemodialysis compared to the controls. The LV parameters in the predialysis patients are not significantly different from the controls, except the LV end systolic internal dimensions are significantly higher in the CRF patients. Multiple regression analysis underscores the strong association between increase in LV mass index (LVMI) and hypertension. The diabetic patients with renal failure have large LV internal diameter and end diastolic volume compared to non-diabetics. Systolic function are well preserved even in hypertensive and diabetic patients with uremia. The incidence of diastolic dysfunction and asymmetrical septal hypertrophy are not significantly different in the patients.

Echocardiography Detects Myocardial Damage in AIDS

Few data are available about cardiac involvement in AIDS. Cardiac abnormalities are common in AIDS. Impairment in LV contractility as assessed from fractional shortening appears to be the most common echocardiographic finding, followed by LV wall thinning, pericardial effusion and eventually by LV cavity dilation. This evolution is suggestive of myocardial damage and supports the hypothesis that dilated cardiomyopathy may be a cardiac complication of AIDS.

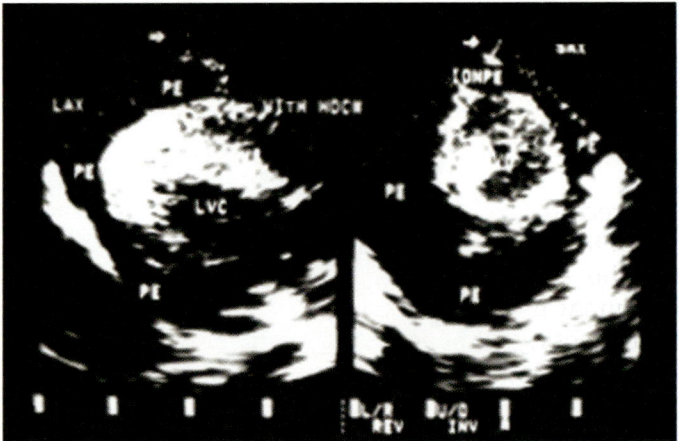

Fig. 25.13: Long and short axis views of LV showing LV hypertrophy and moderate pericardial effusion in patient with longstanding hypothyroidism

Cardiovascular Complications in Thyroid Disease

Hypothyroidism and hyperthyroidism are both associated with clinically significant cardiovascular derangements. In hypothyroidism, these include pericardial effusion, heart failure, and the complex interrelationship between hypothyroidism and ischemic heart disease. Cardiovascular disorders associated with hyperthyroidism include atrial tachyarrhythmias, mitral valve dysfunction, and heart failure. Although these usually occur in individuals with intrinsic heart disease, thyroid dysfunction alone rarely causes serious but reversible cardiovascular dysfunction.

In hypothyroidism a measurable abnormality of the left ventricle is the lengthened duration of contraction and relaxation, normalizing after restoration of euthyroidism. The ejection fraction and cardiac reserve are only slightly diminished. There is reversible diastolic dysfunction. Diastolic hypertension due to hypothyroidism is the most frequent cause of endocrine hypertension, more often in an asymptomatic stage because of more frequent or routine determinations of thyroid function tests, especially in the elderly. The incidence of pericardial effusion is only 3% to 6%.

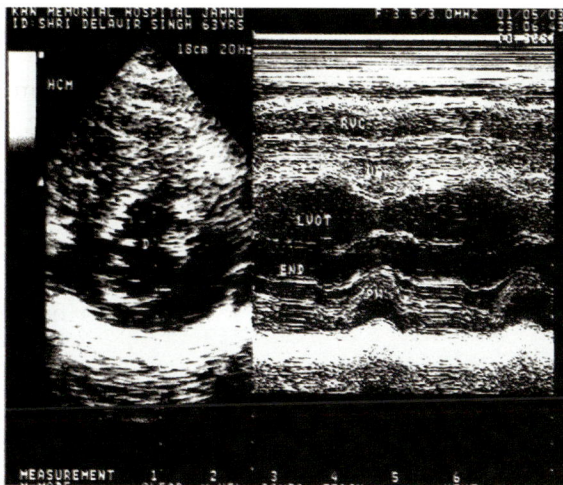

Fig. 25.14: Young man of 25 years old with atheletic built regular exercise performer, had HO atypical chest pain of recent onset, M-mode echocardiography revealed concenteric LV hypertrophy

Moreover, the occurrence of pericardial effusion in hypothyroidism appears to be dependent on the severity of the disease. Thus pericardial effusion may be a frequent manifestation in myxedema, because of the timeliness with which the latter condition is nowadays detected. Hypothyroidism produces a decrease in myocardial contractility and an increase in left ventricular mass, both related to the severity of hormone deficiency. Pericardial effusion is mainly related to thyrotrophin plasma levels. Most of cardiac manifestations of hypothyroidism reverse with thyroid replacement (Figs 25.12 and 25.13).

Cardiovascular Studies in the Mucopolysaccharidoses

The main echocardiographical findings are thickening of the interventricular septum and left ventricular posterior wall in the absence of ECG evidence of ventricular hypertrophy. Moreover, reduced QRS voltages are present in the majority of the patients (77%) and some have reduced shortening fraction (33%). These findings are suggestive of infiltrative cardiomyopathy owing to mucopolysaccharide deposition as a cause of the cardiac thickening rather than true ventricular hypertrophy. Thickening of the mitral valve and the aortic valve is a common finding, however, other heart valves are affected very rarely. Echocardiography is the best means of detecting valvular involvement in patients with mucopolysaccharidosis.

Echocardiography in Athletes Heart (Fig. 25.14)

Cardiac ultrasound will frequently reveal a modest uniform increase in wall thickness seldom to more than 1.6 cm and usually less than 1.3 cm. Mild left ventricular cavity dilatation is also observed. Trivial regurgitation of mitral and tricuspid valves is reported more

frequently. Indices of systolic and diastolic function are normal. In some extreme cases, however, a pattern indistinguishable from hypertrophic cardiomyopathy is observed, even though exhaustive further investigations of the subject and immediate family yield no confirmatory evidence. Echocardiographic features of other confounding conditions may be present. Transoesophageal echocardiography has a role in excluding a patent foramen ovale in scuba divers.

The Evaluation of Left Ventricular Systolic and Diastolic Functions in Patients with Friedreich Ataxia

Friedreich's ataxia (FRDA), the most common subtype of early onset hereditary ataxia, is an autosomal recessive neurodegenerative disorder caused by

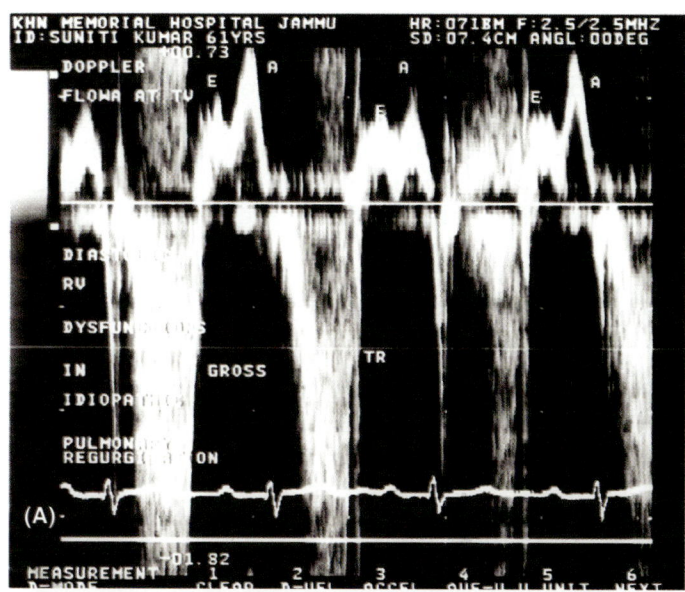

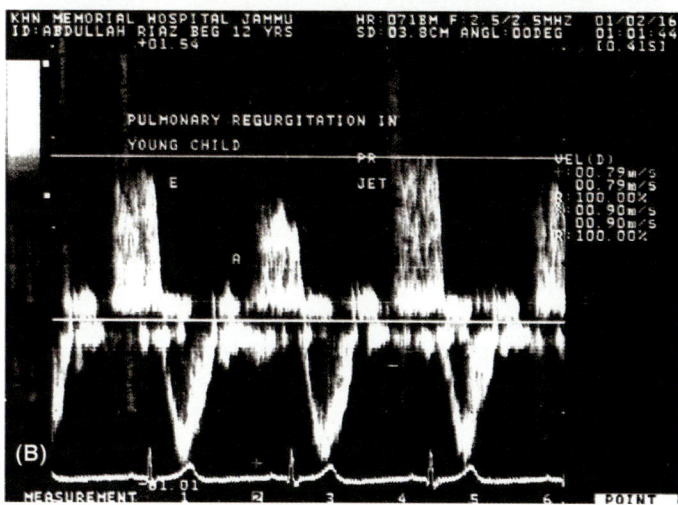

Fig. 25.15A and B: (A) Doppler flow velocity across PV showing enhanced pulmonary velocity with significant pulmonary regurgitation. **(B)** Doppler flow velocity across TV showing gross tricuspid valvular regurgitation due to raised RV pressure in primary pulmonary arterial hypertension

unstable GAA expansions. Two-dimensional, pulse, and pulse tissue Doppler echocardiographic examinations were performed on 21 patients with GAA expansion. There was no association between left ventricle ejection fraction, tissue Doppler systolic wave, and left ventricle diastolic functions examined by pulse and tissue Doppler. The septum thickness of patients with Friedreich's ataxia was significantly increased when compared with that of the control group and wall thickness was found to be associated with GAA repeats. In patients with FRDA, despite a correlation between genetic abnormality with left ventricular early and late diastolic parameters, global diastolic functions were preserved when examined by tissue Doppler. The cardiomyopathy of FRDA is associated with asymmetrical LV hypertrophy, a decrease in LV cavity size, and a reduction in both systolic and early diastolic MVGs. The strongest relationship was found between the size of the smaller GAA triplet repeat expansion and early diastolic MVG and interventricular septal thickness. Tissue Doppler echocardiographically derived MVG technique offers an additional means of assessing structural and functional changes in inherited myocardial disease.

Primary Pulmonary Hypertension

Primary pulmonary hypertension (PPH) is a rare disorder characterised by raised pulmonary-artery pressure in the absence of secondary causes. Precapillary pulmonary arteries are affected by medial hypertrophy, intimal fibrosis, microthrombosis, and plexiform lesions. Most individuals present with dyspnea or evidence of right heart failure.

The pathogenesis is not completely understood, but recent investigations have revealed many possible candidate modifier genes. Without treatment, the disorder progresses in most cases to right heart failure and death. With current therapies such as epoprostenol, progression of disease is slowed, but not halted. Many promising new therapeutic options, including prostacyclin analogues, endothelin-1-receptor antagonists, and phosphodiesterase inhibitors, improve clinical function and haemodynamic measures and may prolong survival.

Echocardiography is the best noninvasive test to screen for suspected pulmonary hypertension. The discovery of mutations in the coding region of the gene for bone morphogenetic protein receptor 2 in patients with familial and sporadic PPH may help not only to elucidate pathogenesis but also to direct future treatment options (Fig. 25.15 A and B).

Heart Failure in Beta-Thalassemia Syndromes

The thalassemia are common monogenic disorders of hemoglobin synthesis. Beta-thalassemias are the most

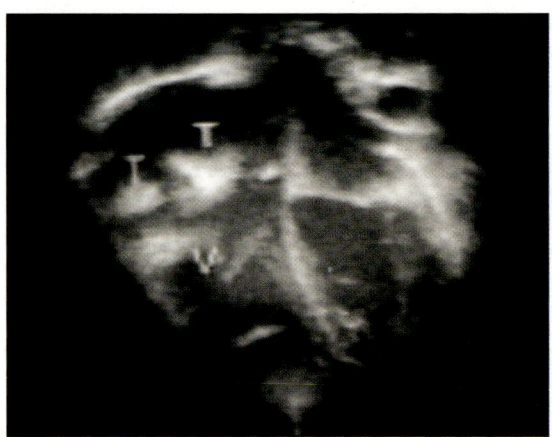

Fig. 25.16: Inverted scan in apical 4C view showing multiple tumor masses (T) over TV and right ventricular cavity in patient with beta-thalassemia syndrome

important among the thalassemia syndromes and have become a worldwide clinical problem due to an increasing immigrant population. In beta-thalassemia major, regular blood transfusions are necessary early in life. Beta-thalassemia intermedia refers to a less severe phenotype, whereas beta-thalassemia/hemoglobin E disease encompasses a broad phenotypic spectrum. Blood transfusions and increased gastrointestinal iron absorption result in iron overload and tissue damage. Among patients with beta-thalassemia major, biventricular, dilated cardiomyopathy remains the leading cause of mortality. In some patients, a restrictive type of left ventricular cardiomyopathy or pulmonary hypertension is noted. The clinical course, although variable and occasionally fulminant, is more benign in recent than in older series. Myocarditis has been described as a cause of left-sided heart failure in younger patients. Pulmonary arterial hypertension is the principal cause of heart failure in beta-thalassemia intermedia. Chelation therapy has improved prognosis in beta-thalassemia major, both by reducing the incidence of heart failure and by reversing cardiomyopathy. Estimation of the patient's cardiac risk is mainly based on clinical criteria and serial echocardiography. A new cardiovascular magnetic resonance technique will probably fulfil the need for more precise risk stratification in beta-thalassemia syndromes. By increasing the proportion of patients on optimal chelation, survival in beta-thalassemia major may further improve. Recent advances in gene therapy are expected to result in the long-awaited cure of this disease (Fig. 25.16).

Obstructive Sleep Apnea Coexisting with Treated Systemic Hypertension and Subendocardial Ischemia

Left ventricular (LV) hypertrophy is a common consequence of systemic hypertension (SH) and

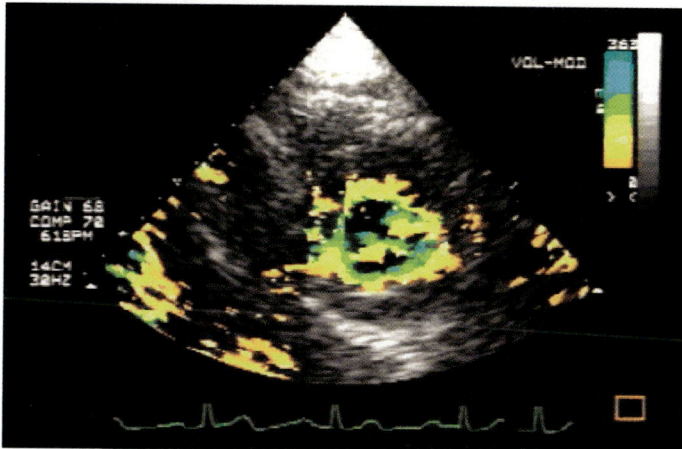

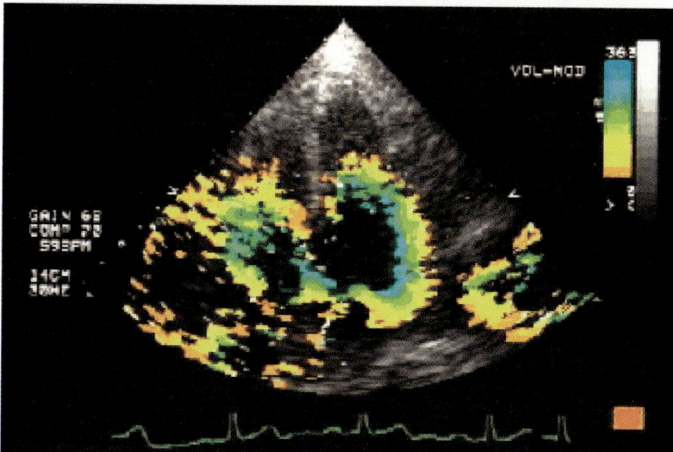

Fig. 25.17: Upper and lower panels showing apical hypokinesia and aneurysm folowing anterior myocardial infarction in long and short axis views of LV

obstructive sleep apnea (OSA). However, little is known about the degree of LV involvement in patients with OSA coexisting with treated SH.

LVED correlated positively with the apnea-hypopnea index and desaturation index. LV eccentric hypertrophy was the commonest type of LV geometry in newly-diagnosed OSA patients. Relatively moderate degree of LV involvement in hypertensive OSA patients may depend on the cardioprotective effect of concomitant antihypertensive therapy, ameliorating OSA-dependent neurohumoral abnormalities.

Noticeable asynergy in the apex view despite the absence of asynergy in the short axis at the same segment is **a sign of subendocardial ischemia** that has not been reported previously. The subendocardium is the area of the myocardium initially most vulnerable to ischemic damage. Because subendocardial ischemia is a forerunner of more serious complications, early detection of a subendocardial ischemic sign is important to improve the prognosis of patients with this disease.

Cardiac Involvement in Systemic Lupus Erythematosus

Pericarditis is the most common cardiac abnormality in systemic lupus erythematosus (SLE) patients, but lesions of the valves, myocardium and coronary vessels may all occur.Echocardiography is a sensitive and specific technique in detecting cardiac abnormalities, particularly mild pericarditis, valvular lesions and myocardial dysfunction. Therefore, echocardiography should be performed periodically in SLE patients. Vascular occlusion, including coronary arteries, may develop due to vasculitis, premature atherosclerosis or antiphospholipid antibodies associated with SLE. Premature atherosclerosis is the most frequent cause of coronary artery disease (CAD) in SLE patients. Efforts should be made to control traditional risk factors as well as all other factors which could contribute to atherosclerotic plaque development.

Cardiac Toxicity in Cancer Therapy

Cardiac toxicity associated with chemotherapy and radiotherapy may be life threatening, can limit the dose and duration of the treatment and certainly adversely affect short-term and long-term quality of life. A development of new strategies for reduction and prophylaxis of cardiac toxicity has great clinical impact. Chemotherapeutic agents may cause acute myocardial injury or chronic complications (e.g. congestive heart failure). Among cardiotoxic agents anthracyclines cause most serious cumulative, dose-limiting and dose-related cardiomyopathy. Most of them are subclinical changes. The frequency of cardiomyopathy may be reduced by modifying the schedule of administration, patients selection considering risk factors, careful cardiac monitoring during chemotherapy, using less toxic doxorubicin analogues and liposomal formulation. The use of pharmacological protection with dexrazoxane remains controversial. A substantial risk of cardiotoxicity may be associated with radiotherapy of the chest and mediastinum. Moreover, radiotherapy may have an additive affect to chemotherapy-induced toxicity. However, with the use of modern treatment techniques radiation cardiomyopathy is uncommon. A group of patients at risk of cardiac complication are patients with breast cancer, Hodgkin's and non-Hodgkin's lymphomas and soft tissue sarcomas.

Echocardiographic Abnormalities in Sickle Cell Disease

Echocardiographic abnormalities in patients with sickle cell disease (SCD) are found to be dilated atrium, dilated ventricle, and ventricle dysfunction. There is an increased incidence of abnormal flow across the valves on Doppler analysis. A majority of patients with SCD have evidence of pulmonary hypertension, which correlated with older age and history of acute chest syndrome common.

Late Cardiac Toxicity in Hodgkin's Disease

Maximal and integrated early (E, E_i) and late (A, A_i) diastolic flow velocities and their ratio (E/A, E_i/A_i) are measured by pulsed Doppler over the mitral and tricuspid valves. Although on two-dimensional echo are found to have valvar thickening, pericardial thickening

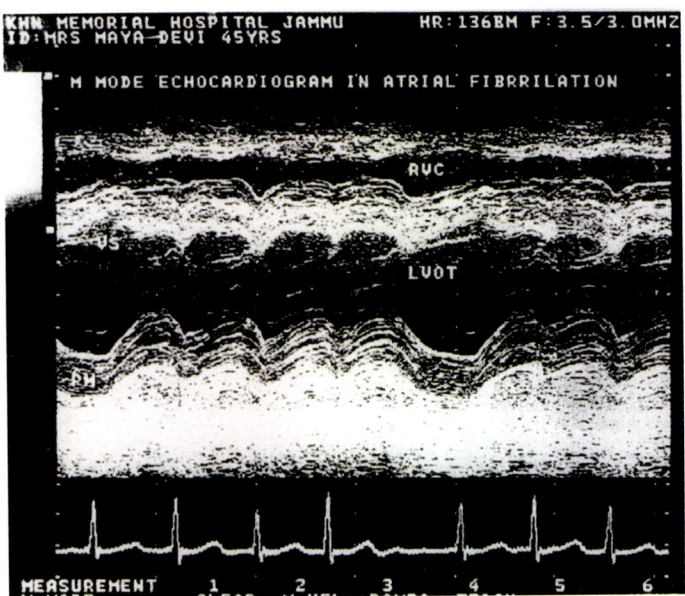

Fig. 25.18: M-Mode echocardiogram showing concenteric LVH and atrial fibrillation in patient with hypertension and obstructive sleep apnea

and a reduced fibre shortening fraction, the Doppler indices are statistically not significantly different from those with normal hearts. These echocardiographic data of functional and morphological parameters indicate that there is no effect on various measurements of diastolic function after chemotherapy with or without mediastinal radiation. In successfully treated patients with Hodgkin's disease, the described changes are of minor significance.

Echocardiographic Abnormalities Following Cardiac Radiation

The abnormalities detected included pericardial thickening in 70%, thickening of the aortic and/or mitral valves in 28%, right ventricular dilatation or hypokinesis in 39%, and left ventricular dysfunction. The incidence of right ventricular abnormalities and valvular thickening is significantly lower than in patients treated with modified techniques.

Usefulness of Transoesophageal Echocardiography Prior to Cardioversion in Patients with Atrial Fibrillation

To evaluate the prevalence of atrial thrombi in patients with atrial fibrillation and different anticoagulation regimens prior to cardioversion (CV) transoesophageal (TOE) guided cardioversion to prevent thromboembolic complications was employed to correlate the presence of atrial thrombi to clinical and echocardiographic data.

The prevalence of atrial thrombosis before CV despite different anticoagulant therapies is approximately 7% and a TOE-guided approach may prevent the risk of embolic events.

Left Ventricular Diastolic Function in Pregnancy in Patients with Arterial Hypertension: A Prospective Study with M-mode Echocardiography and Doppler echocardiography

Hypertensive pregnant women may show a delayed relaxation at the beginning of pregnancy and 50% developed early signs of restrictive cardiomyopathy. These changes may predispose to critical complications during pregnancy.

Assessment of Left Ventricular Systolic and Diastolic Function in Juvenile Rheumatoid Arthritis

Juvenile rheumatoid arthritis (JRA) is the commonest cause of chronic inflammatory arthritis in childhood. Cardiac (pericardial, myocardial or endocardial) involvement is known to occur in patients with JRA, as it does in adults with rheumatoid arthritis (RA). Though pericarditis is identifiable in nearly 45% cases at autopsy, clinical manifestations of pericardial involvement are much less commonly observed. Endocardial involvement leads to aortic and mitral

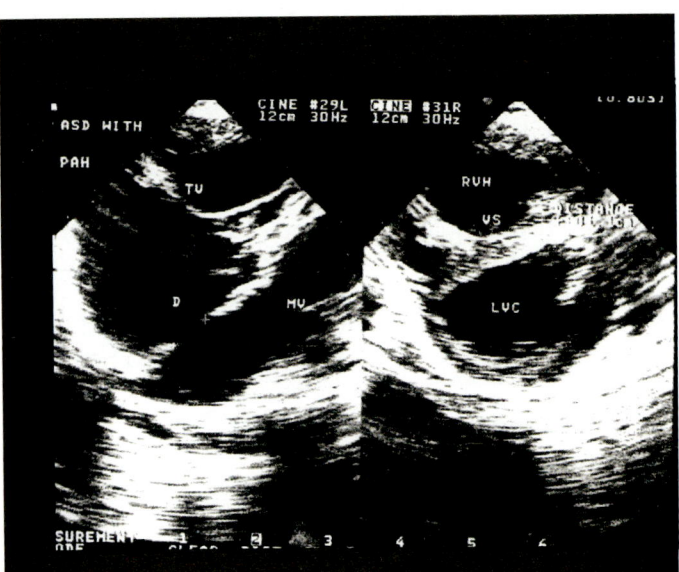

Fig. 25.19: Subcostal approach showing foramen ovale, compressed LV cavity and hypertrophic and dilated right ventricle in patient with chronic obstructive lung disease

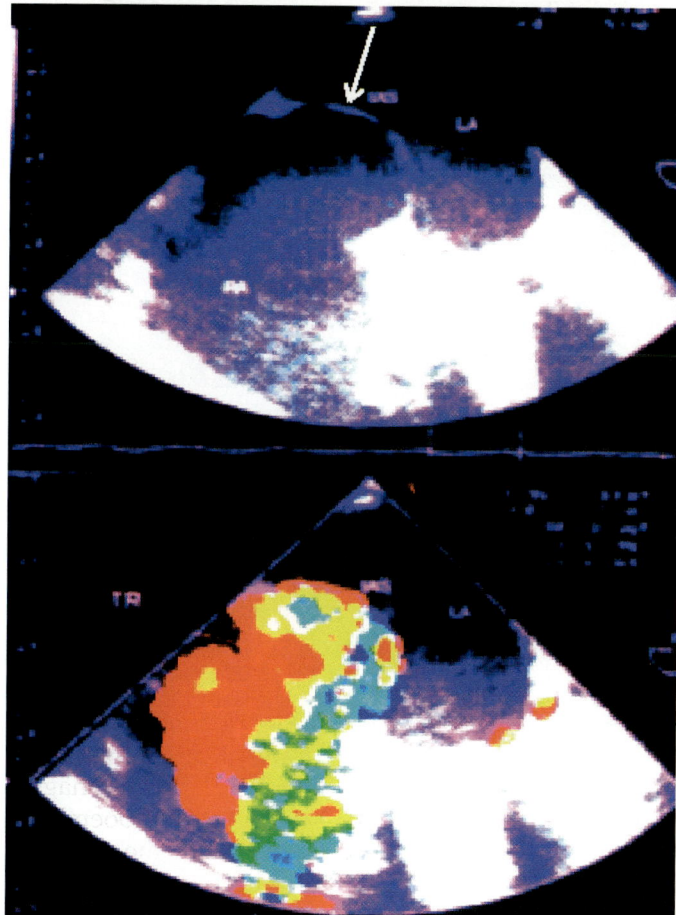

Fig. 25.20: Upper panel TEE biatrial scan showing aneurysm of interatrial septum (arrow). Lower panel color Doppler flow depicting tricuspid regurgitation (arrow) in interatrial septum aneurysm

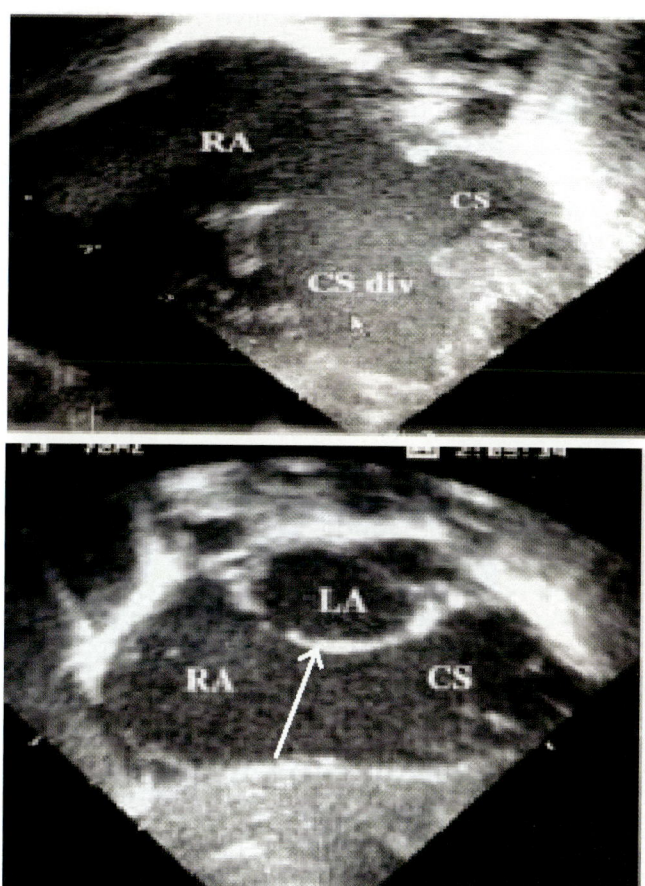

Fig. 25.21: Upper panel inverted 2D scan showing hugely dilated right atrium (RA) and coronary sinus (CS). Lower panel shows aneurysm of interatrial septum, hugely dilated RA and CS

valve incompetence, and usually occurs in late onset oligoarthritis type of JRA. Clinical manifestations are usually mild and surgery is rarely required. Myocardial involvement may present as congestive heart failure or arrhythmias.

Patients with JRA have significantly higher LV systolic and diastolic dimensions and volumes as compared to controls. Diastolic dysfunction is also common in the form of lower transmitral E velocity, higher A velocity and prolonged IVRT. The presence of these despite an asymptomatic cardiac status highlights the importance of early diagnosis and detection of these abnormalities.

Congenital Absence of the Pericardium: Echocardiography as a Diagnostic Tool

The echocardiographic features in order of frequency (a) unusual echocardiographic windows, (b) cardiac hypermobility in patients, (c) abnormal ventricular septal motion and (d) abnormal swinging motion of the heart.

Valve Morphology in Antiphospholipid Antibody Syndrome: Echocardiographic Features

This entity presents with a variety of clinical manifestations including cardiac valvular lesions. Transesophageal echocardiographic features are focal, symmetrical, nodular thickening at the leaflet's coaptation point.

Subepicardial Aneurysm of the Left Ventricle

The patients are presented with subepicardial aneurysm as a complication of a myocardial infarction. The aneurysm of the left ventricle is unusual and has 3 distinctive traits: an abrupt interruption of the myocardium that comprises the mouth and typically a narrow neck of the aneurysm; aneurysmal wall comprised of epicardium with or without a thin myocardial layer; and a propensity to rupture spontaneously regardless of the wall components or stage of development. Echocardiography is the best means of diagnosis of this condition and most helpful for undergoing surgical aneurysmectomy (Fig. 25.17).

Role of Emergency Intraoperative Transesophageal Echocardiography

Transesophageal echocardiography (TEE) has a definitive role in the diagnosis and management of critically ill patients with cardiovascular disease and patients undergoing cardiac operations. It is therefore, recommended that TEE be considered as the diagnostic tool of choice when surgical patients have unexplained hemodynamic instability, when time does not permit complete preoperative evaluation, when cardiovascular injury is suspected in a trauma patient, and to evaluate unexplained hypoxemia.

Pericardial Thickness Measured with Transesophageal Echocardiography: Feasibility and Potential Clinical Usefulness

Transthoracic echocardiography cannot reliably detect thickened pericardium. The superior resolution achieved with transesophageal echocardiography should allow better pericardial definition. Measurement of pericardial thickness with transesophageal echocardiography is reproducible and should be a valuable adjunct in assessing constrictive pericarditis.

An aneurysm of the interatrial septum and cerebral embolic events

Previous reports have described an association between atrial septal aneurysm and cerebral embolic events. We report the case of 68-year old woman who was referred for evaluation of two syncopal episodes that had occurred within the previous three months. Physical examination, 12-Lead ECG and exercise stress test were unremarkable; a 24-hour Holter monitoring did not show cardiac arrhythmias, and carotid ultrasonography excluded atherosclerotic lesions. Magnetic resonance imaging of the brain revealed multiple areas of decreased tissue density. Two-dimensional transthoracic echocardiography showed an atrial septal aneurysm that was confirmed by transesophageal imaging, which improved its morphologic characterisation and ruled out the possibility of other atrial abnormalities with embolic potential. In conclusion, the syncopal episodes observed in our patient were likely due to cerebral embolism. This observation confirms the relation between atrial septal aneurysm and cerebrovascular ischemic events. As previously indicated, the presence of this abnormality dictates the need for anticoagulant therapy.

Early Detection of Left Ventricular Diastolic Dysfunction in Hypertensive Heart Disease by Colour Doppler Myocardial Imaging (Fig. 25.22A and B)

To determine if colour Doppler myocardial imaging could provide evidence of diastolic dysfunction in patients with hypertension whose pulse-wave Doppler parameters are normal. Conventional Doppler parameters indicated relaxation disturbances in patients

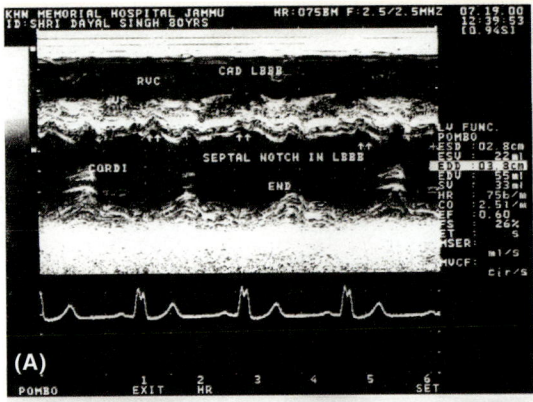
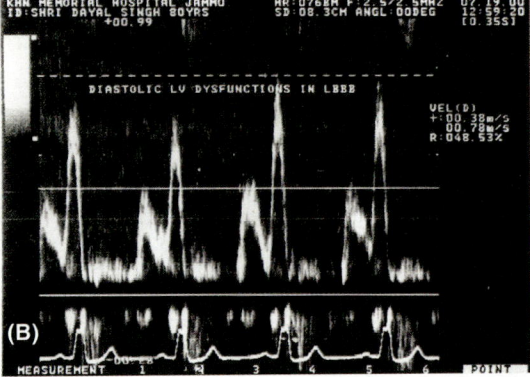

Fig. 25.22A and B: (A) Hypokinesia of IVS and posterior; left ventricular wall. **(B)** Defect in diastolic relaxation of LV

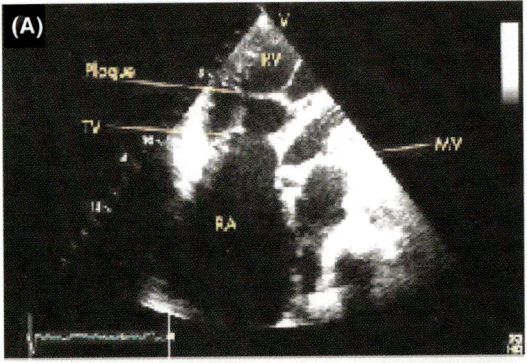
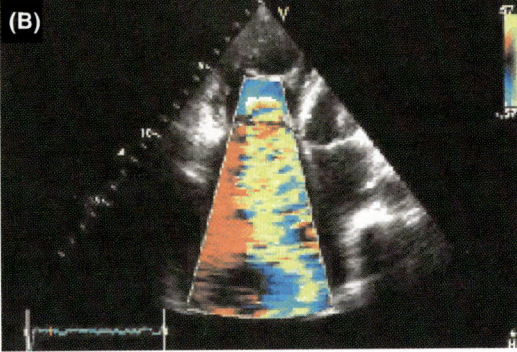

Fig. 25.23: (A) Apical 2 chambers view showing thickened tricuspid valve and dilated right atrium in idiopathic dilatation of right atrium. **(B)** Color flow showing gross tricuspid regurgitation in patient with idiopathic enlargement of right atrium

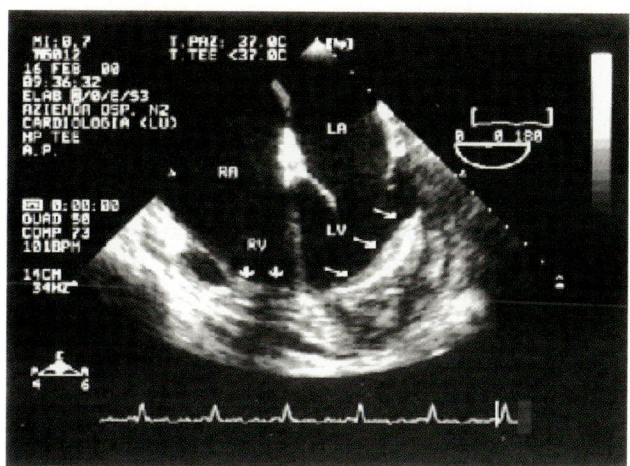

Fig. 25.24: Apical 4C view showing mural thrombus in LV, thickening of MV and roughening of endocardial surface in patient with idiopathic hypereosinophilic syndrome

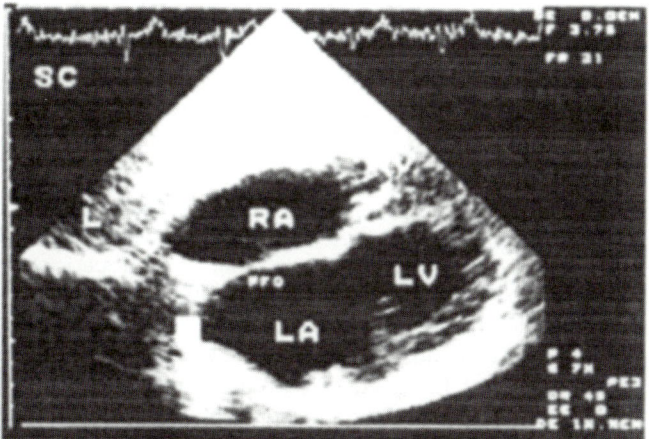

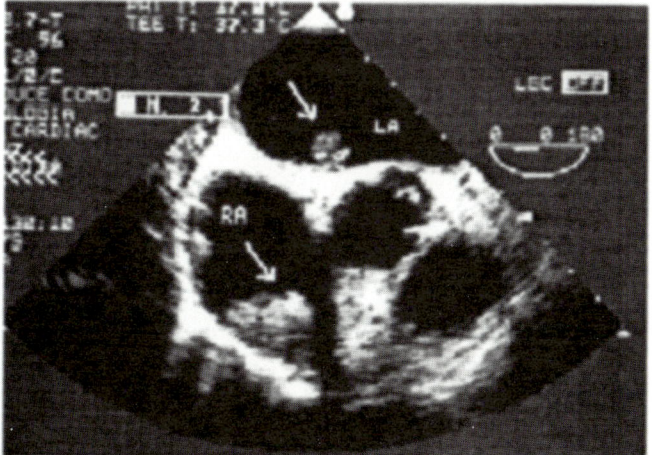

Fig. 25.25: M-Mode echocardiogram and 2D scans showing normal anterior mitral leaflet and calcified mitral annulus in patient with CAD IDDM and HT

with uncontrolled hypertension, but were within a normal range in patients with controlled hypertension at baseline and follow-up. Parameters of global diastolic function measured by colour Doppler myocardial

imaging revealed that E/A, the ratio between E'-wave (early filling phase) and A'-wave plays a central role in the diagnostic and prognostic evaluation of this condition.

Congenital Malformations of the Right Atrium and the Coronary Sinus (Figs 25.20 and 25.21)

Congenital malformations of the RA and the CS frequently are associated with arrhythmias. SVT and sudden cardiac death have been reported in a significant percentage of patients with diverticula of the CS.

Idiopathic Enlargement of the Right Atrium (IERA)

Severe IERA induced atrial fibrillation, systemic embolism, and symptoms of heart failure without systolic dysfunction. Mild IERA seems to become manifest during middle age and may be followed by gradual progression to clinically relevant disease (Fig. 25.23A and B).

Cardiac Amyloidosis (Fig. 25.25A and B)

Infiltrative cardiomyopathy is a term used for a group of diseases, many of which are metabolic in nature, whereby the cardiac muscle is infiltrated by abnormal substances. These abnormalities reported to produce myocardial changes that can be detected with echocardiography include amyloidosis, iron over load from multiple transfusions, hemochromatosis, thalassemia, sarcoidosis, glycogen storage disease or Pompeis, disease and mucolipidosis. The amyloid apparently infiltrates all parts of heart; therefore, thickening of all myocardial walls and valves noted.

It also lead to hypertrophy of interventricular septum and posterior left ventricular walls and can also present with thickening of interatrial septum, though rarely. One may find small pericardial effusion. One may also encounter multiple infracavitory masses in rare instances.

Bibliography

1. Agmon Y, Khandheria BK, Meissner I, *et al.* Frequency of atrial septal aneurysms in patients with cerebral ischemic events. *Circulation* 1999;99: 1942–1944.
2. Alizad A, Seward JB. Echocardiographic features of genetic diseases: Part 4. Connective tissue, *J Am Soc Echocardiogr* 2000;13:325–330.
3. Alizad A, Seward JB. Echocardiographic features of genetic diseases: part 2. Storage disease. *J Am Soc Echocardiogr* 2000;13:164–170.
4. Applefeld MM, Wiernik PH. Cardiac disease after radiation therapy for Hodgkin's disease: analysis of 48 patients. *Am J Cardiol* 1983;51:1679–1681.
5. Appleton CP, Hatle LK, Popp RL. Relation of transmitral flow velocity patterns to left ventricular diastolic function; new insights from a combined haemodynamic and

Doppler echocardiographic study. *J Am Coll Cardiol* 1988;12:426–40.

6. Asinger RW, Koehler J, Pearce LA, *et al.* Pathophysiologic correlates of thromboembolism in nonvalvular atrial fibrillation: II. Dense spontaneous echocardiographic contrast (The Stroke Prevention in Atrial Fibrillation [SPAF-III] study). *J Am Soc Echocardiogr* 1999;12; 1088–1096.

7. Aurigemma GP, Gottdiener JS, Shemanski L, *et al.* Predictive value of systolic and diastolic function for incident congestive heart failure in the elderly: the cardiovascular health study. *J Am Coll Cardiol* 2001;37:1042–1048.

8. Baigent C, Burbury K, Wheeler D. Premature cardiovascular disease in chronic renal failure. *Lancet* 2000;356:147–152.

9. Barbaro G, Di Lorenzo G, Grisorio B, *et al.* Cardiac involvement in the acquired immunodeficiency syndrome. A multicenter clinical-pathological study. *AIDS Res Hum Retroviruses* 1998;14:1071–107.

10. Barbaro G, Di Lorenzo G, Grisorio B, *et al.* Incidence of dilated cardiomyopathy and detection of HIV in myocardial cells of HIV positive patients. *N Engl J Med* 1998;339:1093–109.

11. Barbaro G, Di Lorenzo G, Soldini M, *et al.* Clinical course of cardiomyopathy in HIV-infected patients with or without encephalopathy related to the myocardial expression of TNF- and iNOS. *AIDS* 2000;14:827–838.

12. Barbaro G, Di Lorenzo G, Soldini M, *et al.* The intensity of myocardial expression of inducible nitric oxide synthase influences the clinical course of human immunodeficiency virus-associated cardiomyopathy. *Circulation* 1999;100:633–639.

13. Barbaro G. Cardiovascular manifestations of HIV infection. *Circulation* 2002;106:1420–1425.

14. Berk JL, Falk RH, *et al.* Tolerability and efficacy of thalidomide for the treatment of patients with light chain-associated (AL) amyloidosis. *Clin Lymphoma* 2003; 3: 241–246.

15. Bernstein B, Takahashi M, Hanson V. Cardiac involvement in juvenile rheumatoid arthritis. *J Pediatr* 1974;85:313–7.

16. Brewer EJ Jr, Bass J, Baum J, Cassidy IT, Fink C, Jacobs J, *et al.* Current Proposed Revisions of JRA Criteria. *Arthritis Rheum* 1977;20:195–9.

17. Cabell CH, Tiichon BH, Velazquez EJ, *et al.* Importance of echocardiography in patients with severe nonischemic heart failure: the second Prospective Randomised Amlodipine Survival Evaluation (PRAISE-2) echocardiographic study. *Am Heart J* 2004;147:151–157.

18. Charra B, Calemard M, Laurent G. Importance of treatment time and blood pressure control in achieving long-term survival on dialysis. *Am J Nephrol* 1996;16:35–44.

19. Collis T, Devereux RB, Roman, *et al.* Relations of stroke volume and cardiac output to body composition: the Strong Heart study. *Circulation* 2001; 103:820–825.

20. Corrao S, Salli L, Arnone S, Scaglione R, Pinto A, Licata G. Echo Doppler left ventricular filling abnormalities in patients with rheumatoid arthritis without clinically evident cardiovascular disease. *Eur J Clin Invest* 1996;26:293–7.

21. Currier JS. How to manage metabolic complications of HIV therapy: what to do while we wait for answers. *AIDS Read* 2000;10:162–169.

22. Curtis JP, Sokol SI, Wang Y, *et al.* The association of left ventricular ejection fraction, mortality, and cause of death in stable outpatients with heart failure. *J Am Coll Cardiol* 2003;42:736–742.

23. Dhodapkar MV, Hussein MA, Rasmussen E, .Solomon A, Larson RA, Crowley JJ, *et al.* Clinical efficacy of high-dose dexamethasone with maintenance dexamethasone/alpha interferon in patients with primary systemic amyloidosis: Results of United States intergroup trial southwest oncology group (SWOG) S9628. *Blood;* 2004.

24. Di Salvo TG, Mathiel' M, Semigran MJ, *et al.* prestenosed right ventricular ejection fraction predicts exercise capacity and survival in advanced heart failure. *J Am Coll Cardiol* 1995;25:tl43–1153.

25. Dube MP, Sprecher D, Henry WK, *et al.* Preliminary guidelines for the evaluation and management of dyslipidemia in adults infected with human immunodeficiency virus and receiving antiretroviral therapy: Recommendations of the adult AIDS clinical trial group cardiovascular disease focus group. *Clin Infect Di* 2000;31:1216–1224

26. Dubrey S, Simms RW, Skinner M, Falk RH. Recurrence of primary (AL) amyloidosis in a transplanted heart with four-year survival. *Am J Cardiol* 1995; 76: 739–741.

27. Dubrey SW, Burke MM, Khaghani A, Hawkins PN, Yacoub MH, Banner NR. Long term results of heart transplantation in patients with amyloid heart disease. *Heart* 2001; 85: 202–207.

28. Dujardin KS, Tei C, Yeo TC, *et al.* Prognostic value of a Doppler index combining systolic and diastolic performance in idiopathic-dilated cardiomyopathy. *Am J Cardiol* 1998; 82:1071–1076.

29. Eckel RH, Barouch WW, Ershow AG. Report of the National Heart, Lung, and Blood institute-National Institute of Diabetes and Digestive and Kidney Diseases Working Group on the pathophysiology of obesity-associated cardiovascular disease. *Circulation* 2002; 105:2923–2928.

30. Fang ZY, Yuda S, Anderson V, *et al.* Echocardiographic detection of early diabetic myocardial disease. *J Am Coll Cardiol* 2003; 41:611–617.

31. Faris R, Coats AJ, Henein MY. Echocardiography-derived-miable-predict outcome in patients with nonischemic dilated cardiomyopathy with or without a restrictses filling pattern. *Am Heart J* 2002; 144:343–350.

32. Florea VG, Henein MY, Cicoira M, *et al.* Echocardiographic determinants of mortality in patients >67 years of age with chronic heart failure. *Am J Cardiol* 2000;86:158–160.

33. Foley RN, Parfrey PS, Sarnak MJ. Clinical epidemiology of cardiovascular disease in chronic renal disease. *Am J Kidney Dis* 1998; S112–S119.

34. Gardin JM, Schumacher O, Constantine G, *et al.* Valvular abnormalities and cardiovascular status following exposure to dexfenfluramine orphenterminelfenfluramine. *JAMA* 2000; 283:1703–1709.

35. Gardin JM, Weissman NJ, Leung C, *et al.* Clinical and echocardiographic follow-up of patients previously treated with dexfenfluramine or phenterminelfenfluramine. *JAMA* 2001;286:2011–2014.

36. Ghio S. Gavazzi A, Campana C, *et al.* Independent and additihoe prognostic value of right ventricular systolic

function and pulmonary artery pressure in patients with chronic heart failure. *J Am Coli Cardiol* 2001;37:183–188.

37. Goldman ME, Pearce LA, Hart RG, *et al.* Pathophysiologic correlates of thromboembolism in nonvalvular atrial fibrillation: I. Reduced flow velocity in the left atrial appendage (The Stroke Prevention in Atrial Fibrillation Study). *J Am Soc Echocardiogr* 1999;12: 1080–1087.

38. Grimm RA, Stewart WJ. Arheart K, *et al.* Left atrial appendage stunning after electrical cardioversion of atrial flutter: an attenuated response compared with atrial fibrillation as the mechanism for lower susceptibility to thromboembolic events. *J Am Coll Cardiol* 1997;29: 582–589.

39. Gullestad L, Aass H, Fjeld J G, *et al.* Immunomodulating therapy with intravenous immunoglobulin in patients with chronic heart failure. *Circulation* 2001; 103:220–225.

40. Heidenreich PA, Hancock SL, Lee BK, *et al.* Asymptomatic cardiac disease following mediastinal irradiation. *J Am Coll Cardiol* 2003;42: 743–749.

41. Hogg K, Swedberg K, McMurray J. Heart failure with preserved left ventricular systolic function: epidemiology, clinical characteristics, and prognosis. *J Am Coli Cardiol* 2004:43:317–327.

42. Hrncic R, Wall J, Wolfenbarger DA, Murphy CL, Schell M, Weiss DT, *et al.* Antibody-mediated resolution of light chain-associated amyloid deposits. *Am J Pathol* 2000; 157: 1239–1246.

43. Huppertz H, Voigt I, Müller-Scholden J, Sandhage K. Cardiac manifestation in patients with HLA B27-associated juvenile arthritis. *Pediatr Cardiol* 2000; 21:1417.8.

44. Hussein MA, Juturi JV, Rybicki L, Lutton S, Murphy BR, Karam MA. Etanercept therapy in patients with advanced primary amyloidosis. *Med Oncol* 2003; 20: 283–290.

45 Jollis JG, Landolfo CK, Kisslo J, *et al.* Fenfluramine and phentermine and cardiovascular findings: effect of treatment duration on prevalence of valve abnormalities. *Circulation* 2000; 101 :2071–2077.

46. Kasiske BL, Chakkera HA, Roel J. Explained and unexplained ischaemic heart disease after renal transplantation. *J Am Soc Nephrol* 2000;11:1735–174.

47. Kasiske BL, Chakkera HA, Roel J. Explained and unexplained ischaemic heart disease after renal transplantation. *J Am Soc Nephrol* 2000;11:1735–174.

48. Kasiske BL, Chakkera HA, Roel J. Explained and unexplained ischaemic heart disease after renal transplantation. *J Am Soc Nephrol* 2000;11:1735–174.

49. Katz R. KarlineI' JS, Resnik R. Effects of a natural volume overload state (pregnancy) on left ventricular performance in normal human subjects. *Circulation* 1978;58:434–441.

50. Kimura BJ, Bocchicchio, Willis CL, *et al.* Screening cardiac ultrasonographic examination in patients with suspected cardiac disease in the emergency department. *Am Heart J* 2001;142:324–330.

51. Klein AL, Grimm RA, Murray RD, *et al.* Use of transesophageal echocardiography to guide cardioversion in patients with atrial fibrillation. *N Engl J Med* 2001; 344:1411–1420.

52. Klein AL, Munay RD, Grimm RA. Role of transesophageal echocardiography-guided cardioversion of patients with atrial fibrillation. *J Am Coll Cardiol* 2001;37:691–704.

53. Koelling TM, Aaronson KD, Cody RJ, *et al.* Prognostic significance of mitral regurgitation and tricuspid regurgitation in patients with left ventricular systolic dysfunction. *Am Heart J* 2002;144:524–529.

54. Kumar N, Rasheed K, Gallo R, Al Halees Z, Duran CM. Rhematic involvement in all four heart valves-preoperative echocardiographic diagnosis and successful surgical management. *Eur J Cardiothorac Surg* 1995;9:713–4.

55. Kuperstein R, Hanly P. Niroumand M, *et al.* The importance of age and obesity on the relation between diabetes and left ventricular mass. *J Am Coll Cardiol* 2001;37:1957–1962.

56. Leibowitz D. Role of echocardiography in the diagnosis and treatment of acute pulmonary thromboembolism. *J Am Soc Echocardiogr* 2001; 14:921–926.

57 Meacham RR 3rd, Headley AS, Bronze MS, *et al.* Impending paradoxical embolism. *Arch Intern Med* 1998;158:438–448.

58. Lewis EJ, Hunsicker LG, Bain RP, *et al.* The effect of angiotensin converting enzyme inhibition on diabetic nephropathy. *N Engl J Med* 1993;329:1456–1462

59. Lewis EJ, Hunsicker LG, Bain RP, *et al.* The effect of angiotensin converting enzyme inhibition on diabetic nephropathy. *N Engl J Med* 1993;329:1456–1462.

60. Lietman PS, Bywaters EG. Pericarditis in juvenile rheumatoid arthritis. *Pediatrics* 1963;32:855–60.

61. Lipshultz SE, Easley KA, Orav EJ, *et al.* Cardiac dysfunction and mortality in HIV-infected children. The prospective P2C2 HIV multicenter study. *Circulation* 2000;102:1542–1548.

62. Lipshultz SE, Orav EJ, Sanders SP, *et al.* Immunoglobulins and left ventricular structure and function in pediatrics HIV infection. *Circulation* 1995;92:2220–2225.

63. Lipshultz SE. Dilated cardiomyopathy in HIV-infected patients [editorial]. *N Engl J Med* 1998; 339:1153–1155.

64. Lust JA, Lacy MQ, *et al.* Long-term survival (10 years or more) in 30 patients with primary amyloidosis. *Blood* 1999; 93: 1062–1066.

65. McLaughlin K, Jardine AG. Clinical management of diabetic nephropathy. *Diabetes, Obesity & Metabolism* 1999; 1:307–315.

66. Miniati M, Monti S, Pratali L, *et al.* Value of transthoracic echocardiography in the diagnosis of pulmonary embolism: results of a prospective-study in unselected patient. *Am J Med* 2001;110:528-535.

67. Mody GM, Stevens JE, Meyers OL. The heart in rheumatoid arthritis-a clinical and echocardiographic study. *Q J med* 1987;65:921–8.

68. Naschitz JE, Slobodin G, Lewis RJ, *et al.* Heart diseases affecting the liver and liver diseases affecting the heart. *Am Heart J* 2000;140:111–120.

69. Oguz D, Ocal B, Ertan U, Narin H. Kardemir S, Senocak F. Left ventricular diastolic function in juvenile rheumatoid arthritis. *Paediatr Cardiology* 2000;21:374.

70. Olofsson BO, Backman C, Karp K, Suhr OB. Progression of cardiomyopathy after liver transplantation in patients with familial amyloidotic polyneuropathy, Portuguese type. *Transplantation* 2002; 73: 745–751.

71. Opelz G, Wujciak T, Ritz E. Association of chronic kidney graft failure with recipient blood pressure. *Kidney Int* 1998;53:217–222 Coronary artery calcification in young adults with 1978; 58:1072–83.

72. Opelz G, Wujciak T, Ritz E. Association of chronic kidney graft failure with recipient blood pressure. *Kidney Int* 1998;53:217–222.

73. Paton P, Tabib A, Loire R, *et al.* Coronary artery lesions and human immunodeficiency virus infection. *Res Virol* 1993;144:225–231.

74. Pelliccia A, Maron BJ, Spataro A, *et al.* The upper limit of physiologic cardiac hypertrophy in highly trained elite athletes. *N Engl J Med* 1991 ;324:295–301.

75. Penzak SR, Chuck SK, Stajich GV. Safety and efficacy of HMG-CoA reductase inhibitors for treatment of hyperlipidemia in patients with HIV infection. *Pharmacotherapy* 2000;20:1066–20.

76. Peterson LR, Waggoner AD, Schechtman KB, *et al.* Alterations in left ventricular structure and function in young healthy obese women: assessment by echocardiography and tissue Doppler imaging. *J Am Coll Cardiol* 2004; 43: 1399-1404.

77. Pinamonti B, Di Lenarda A, Sinagra G, *et al.* Restrictive left ventricular filling pattern in dilated cardiomyopathy assessed by Doppler echocardiography: clinical, echocardiographic and hemodynamic correlations and prognostic implications. Heart Muscle Disease Study Group. *J Am Coll Cardiol* 1993; 22:808-815.

78. Pinamonti B, Zecchin M, Di Lenarda A, *et al.* Persistence of restrictive left ventricular filling pattern in dilated cardiomyopathy: an ominous prognostic sign. *J Am Coll Cardiol* 1997;29:604–612.

79. Pluim BM. Zwinderman AH, van del' Laarse A, *et al.* Correlation of heart rate variability with cardiac functional and metabolic variables in cyclists with training induced left ventricular hypertrophy. *Heart* 1999;81:612–617.

80. Rahman JE. Helyou EF. Gelzer-Bell R, *et al.* Noninvasive diagnosis of biopsy-proven cardiac amyloidosis. *J Am Coll Cardiol* 2004;43:410–415.

81. Raymond RJ, Hinderliter AL, Willis PW, *et al.* Echocardiographic predictors of adverse outcomes in primary pulmonary hypertension. *J Am Coll Cardiol* 2002;39:1214–1219.

82. Rerkpattanapipat P, Wongpraparut N, Jacobs LE, *et al.* Cardiac manifestations of acquired immunodeficiency syndrome. *Arch Intern Med* 2000;160:602–608.

83. Ribeiro A, Lindmarker P, Johnsson H, *et al.* Pulmonary embolism: one-year follow-up with echocardiography Doppler and five-year survival analysis. *Circulation* 1999; 99:1325–1330.

84. Ribeiro A, Lindmarker P, Juhlin-Dannfelt A, *et al.* Echocardiography. Doppler in pulmonary embolism: Right ventricular dysfunction as apredictor of mortality rate. *Am Heart J* 1997; 134:479–487.

85. Rihal CS, Nishimura RA, Hade LK, *et al.* Systolic and diastolic dysfunction in patients with clinical diagnosis of dilated cardiomyopathy. Relation to symptoms and prognosis. *Circulation* 1994;90:2772–2779.

86. Rubler S, Damani PM, Pinto ER. Cardiac size and performance during pregnancy estimated with echocardiography. *Am J Cardiol* 1977;40: 534–540.

87. Sahn DJ, Maciel BCM: Physiological valvular regurgitation: Doppler echocardiography and the potential for iatrogenic heart disease, *Circulation* 1988; 78:1075.

88. San Roman JA, Vilacosta I, Zamorano JL, *et al.* Transesophageal echocardiography in right-sided endocarditis, *J Am Coll Cardiol* 1993; 21:1226.

89. Sanfilippo AJ, Harrigan P, Popovic AD, *et al.* Papillary muscle traction in mitral valve prolapse: quantitation by two-dimensional echocardiography, *J Am Coll Cardiol* 1992;19:564.

90. Sanfilippo AJ, Picard MH, Newell JB, *et al.* Echocardiographic assessment of patients with infectious endocarditis: prediction of risk for complications. *J Am Coll Cardiol* 1991;18:1191.

91. Savage DD, Levy D, Dannenberg AL, *et al.* Association of echocardiographic left ventricular mass with body size, blood pressure and physical activity (the Framingham Study). *Am J Cardiol* 1990;65: 371–376.

92. Schillaci G, Reboldi G, Verdecchia P. High normal serum creatinine concentration is a predictor of cardiovascular risk in essential hypertension. *Arch Intern Med* 2001;161:886–89.

93. Schillaci G, Reboldi G, Verdecchia P. High normal serum creatinine concentration is predictor of cardiovascular risk in essential hypertension. *Arch Intern Med* 2001;161:886–89.

94. Schwinger ME, Tunick PA, Freedberg RS, and Kronzon I: Vegetations on endocardial surfaces stuckregurgitant jets: *Am Heart J* 1990; 119:1212.

95. Silverman DI, Manning WJ. Role of echocardiography in patients undergoing elective cardioversion of atrial fibrillation. *Circulation* 1998; 98:479–486.

96. Svenungsson E, Jensen-Urstad K, Heimburger M, *et al.* Risk factors for cardiovascular disease in systemic lupus erythematosus. *Circulation* 2001; 104:1887–1893.

97. Temporelli PL, Corra U, Imparato A, *et al.* Reversible restrictive left ventricular diastolic filling with optimised oral therapy predicts a more favorable prognosis in patients with chronic heart failure. *J Am Coll Cardiol* 1998;31:1591–1597.

98. Tsang TS, Barnes ME, Gersh BJ, *et al.* Prediction of risk for first age-related cardiovascular events in an elderly population: the incremental value of echocardiography. *J Am Coli Cardiol* 2003;42: 1199–1205.

99. Weihs W, Homer S, *et al.* The association between the diameter of a patent foramen ovale and the risk of embolic cerebrovascular events. *Am J Med* 2000; 109:456–462.

100. Whalley GA, Doughty RN, Gamble GD, *et al.* Pseudonormal mitral filling pattern predicts hospital re-admission in patients with congestive heart failure. *J Am Coil Cardiol* 2002;39:1787–1795.

101. Woo YM, Jardine AG, Clark AF, *et al.* The influence of early graft function on patient survival following renal transplantation. *Kidney Int* 1999; 55:692–699.

102. Zabalgoitia M. Halperin JL, Pearce LA, *et al.* Transesophageal echocardiographic correlates of clinical risk of thromboembolism in nonvalvular atrial fibrillation. Stroke Prevention in Atrial Fibrillation III Investigators. *Am Coll Cardiol* 1998;31:1622–1626.

103. Zaroff JG, Rordorf GA, Ogilvy CS, *et al.* Regional patterns of left ventricular systolic dysfunction after subarachnoid hemorrhage: evidence for neurally mediated cardiac injury. *J Am Soc Echocardiogr* 2000;13:774–779.

Appendix

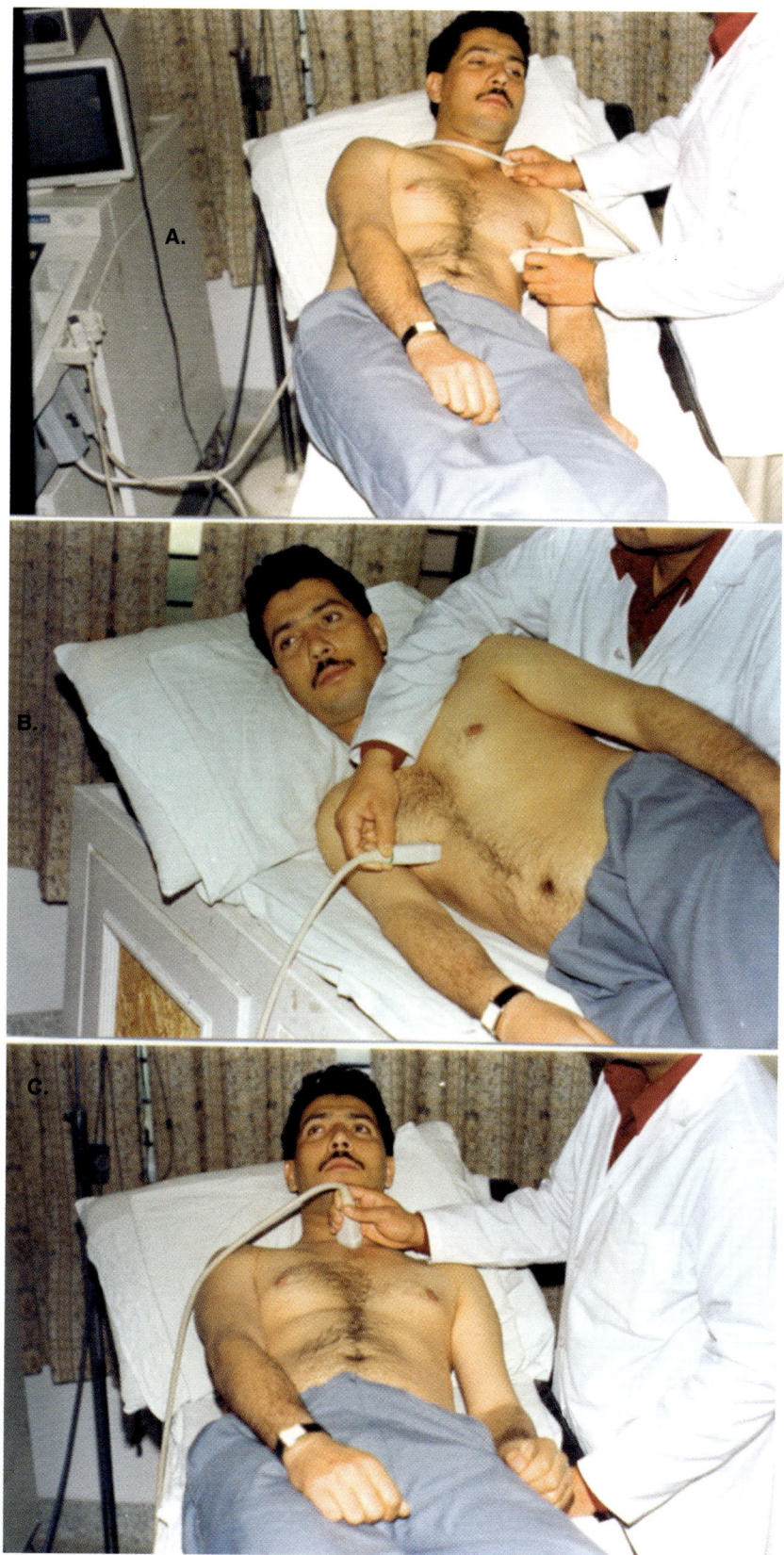

Fig. A1 (A to C): (A) Bedside left lateral position of the model and hand-held transducer. This is an ideal posture for obtaining apical 4.5 and 2 chambers view in M-mode, 2-D B/W and color Doppler scans. **(B)** Right lateral posture for aortic valve and ascending aorta. **(C)** Supine position with head and neck tilted backward in suprasternal notch for obtaining scans of ascending aorta and its valve, arch of aorta, descending aorta, right pulmonary artery, LA and carotid vessels including superior vena cava

Table A-1: *Normal measurements in adults**

RV dimension, supine (R)	0.7–2.3 cm
RV dimension, left lateral (R)	0.9–2.6 cm
LV dimension, supine (R)	3.7–5.6 cm
LV dimension, left lateral (R)	3.5–5.7 cm
LV posterior wall thickness (R)	0.6–1.1 cm
LV posterior wall excursion	0.7–1.7 cm
Ventricular septal thickness (R)	0.6–1.1 cm
Ventricular septal excursion	0.3–0.8 cm
LV outflow tract dimension (beginning S)	2.0–3.5 cm
Left atrial dimension (end-s)	1.9–4.0 cm
Aortic root diameter (R)	2.0–3.7 cm
Aortic cusp separation (early S)	1.5–2.6 cm
LV fractional shortening or % ΔMD	0.25–0.42
LV ejection fraction	45%–84%
Mean V_{cf} (LV)	1.02–1.94 circ/sec
Ventricular septal thickening	0.30–0.65
Ventricular septal velocity (S)	3.3–7.0 cm/sec
LV posterior wall thickening	0.36–0.95
Mean LV posterior wall velocity (S)	3.0–7.1 cm/sec
Max. LV posterior wall velocity (S)	3.0–8.3 cm/sec
Max. LV posterior wall velocity (D)	9.1–28 cm/sec

* Data from Feigenbaum, H.: Echocardiography, ed. 2, Philadelphia, 1976, Lea and Febiger and Felner, J.M. and Schlant, R.C.: Echocardiography, a teaching atlas, New York 1976, Grune and Stratton, Inc.

R, measurement taken at the R wave of ECG; RV, right ventricle; LV, left ventricles; S, ventricular systole; D, ventricular diastole; V_{ef}, velocity of circumferential fiber shortening, circ. circumferences.

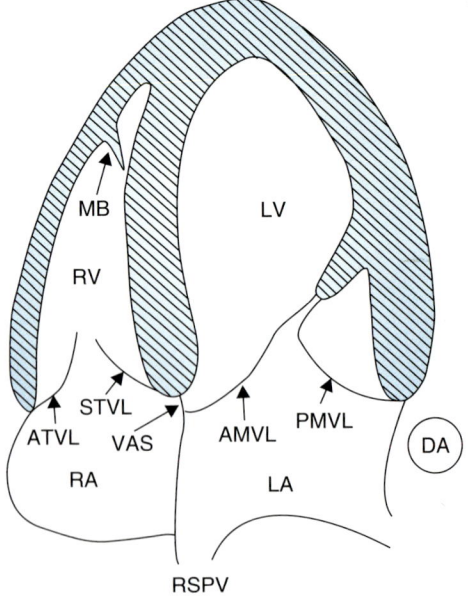

Fig. A2: Schematic diagram of the apical four-chamber view. AMVL, anterior mitral leaflet; ATL, anterior tricuspid leaflet; DA, descending aorta; PMVL, posterior mitral leaflet; LA, left atrium; LV, left ventricle; ME, moderate band; RA, right atrium; RUPV, right upper pulmonary vein; RV, right ventricle; STL, septal tricuspid leaflet

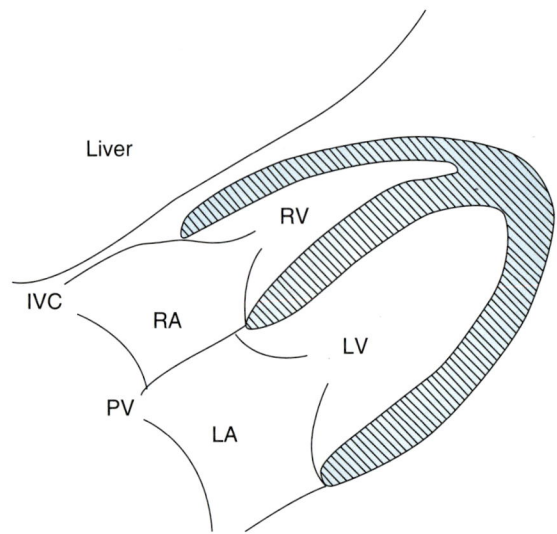

Fig. A3: Schematic diagram of the four-chamber view from the subcoastal approach. IYC, inferior vena cava; LA, left atrium; LV, left ventricular; RA, right atrium; RV, right ventricle

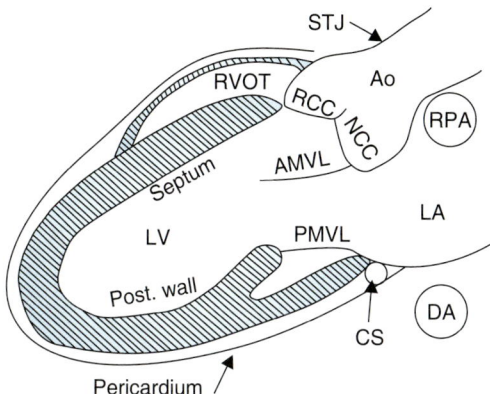

Fig. A4: Schematic diagram of the parasternal long-axis view in diastole. AML, anterior mitral leaflet; AO, aorta; CS, coronary sinus; DA, descending aorta; LA, left atrium; LV, left ventricle; NCC, noncoronary cusp; PMVL, posterior mitral leaflet; PW, posterior wall; RCC, right coronary cusp; RPA, right pulmonary artery; RVOT, right ventricular outflow tract; STJ, sinotubular junction

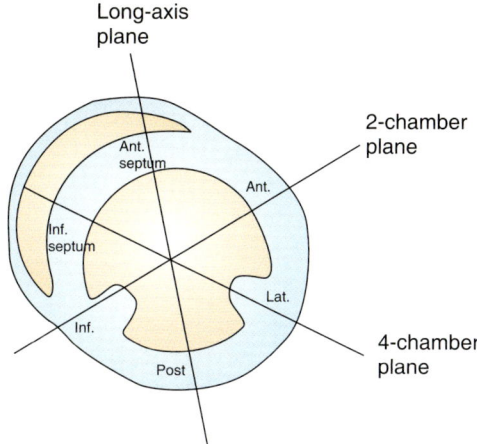

Fig. A5: Schematic diagram of the parasternal short-axis view at the level of papillary muscles. Ant. Septum, anterior septum; Ant., anterior wall; Inf. Septum, inferior septum; Inf., inferior wall; Lat., lateral wall; Post., posterior wall

Table A-2: *Normal measurements: left ventricular outflow tract**

Weight (lbs.)	Left ventricular outflow tract dimension (cms) (beginning systole)
In normal newborns	0.9–1.5
0–25	0.9–1.7
26–50	1.8–2.3
51–75	2.0–2.8
76–100	2.4–3.4
101–125	2.5–3.5
126–200	2.0–3.3

* Data from Nanda, N.C. and Gramiak, R.: Clinical Echocardiography. The C.V. Mosby Company, Saint Louis, p. 432, 433, 1978 (James Powers).

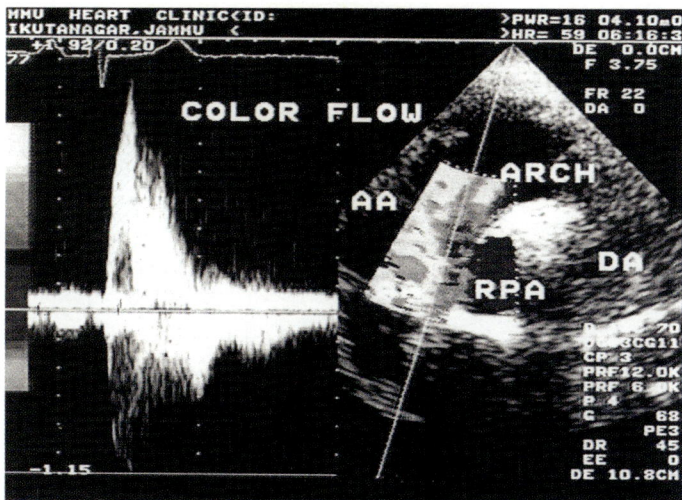

Fig. A6: Color Doppler flow velocity across ascending aorta (left) visualising ascending aorta (RA) in mosaic color and right pulmonary artery (RPA) in blue color (centre)

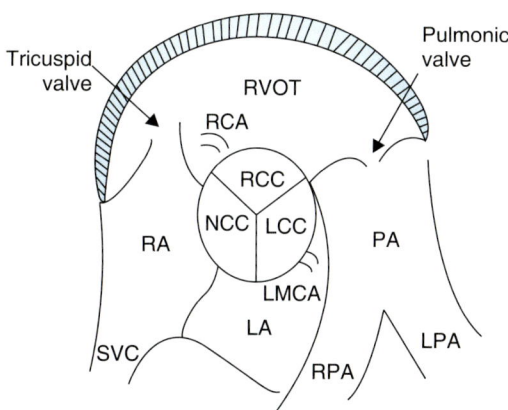

Fig. A7: Schematic diagram of the parasternal short-axis view at the aortic valve level. LA, left atrium; LCC, left coronary cusp; LMT, left main trunk; LPA, left pulmonary artery; NCC, non-coronary cusp; PA, pulmonary artery; PV, pulmonary valve; RA, right atrium; RCA, right coronary artery; RCC, right coronary cusp; RPA, right pulmonary artery; RVOT, right ventricular outflow tract; SVC, superior vena cava, TV, tricuspid valve

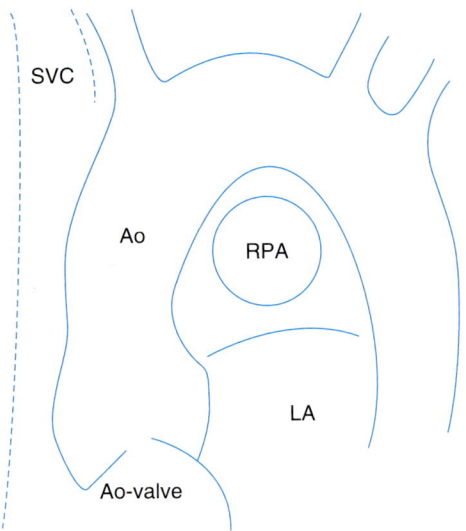

Fig. A8: Schematic diagram of the arota and right pulmonary artery from the suprasternal notch window. AO,aorta; AV, aortic valve; LA, left atrium; RPA, right pulmonary artery; SVC, superior vena cava

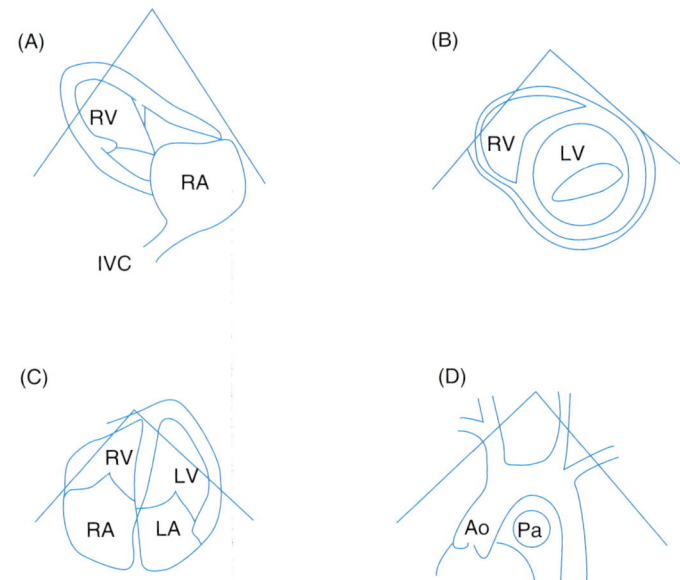

Fig. A9 (A to D): (A) Parasternal long axis view (RV inflow). **(B)** Parasternal short axis (mitral valve level). **(C)** Apical 4 chamber view. **(D)** Superasternal long axis

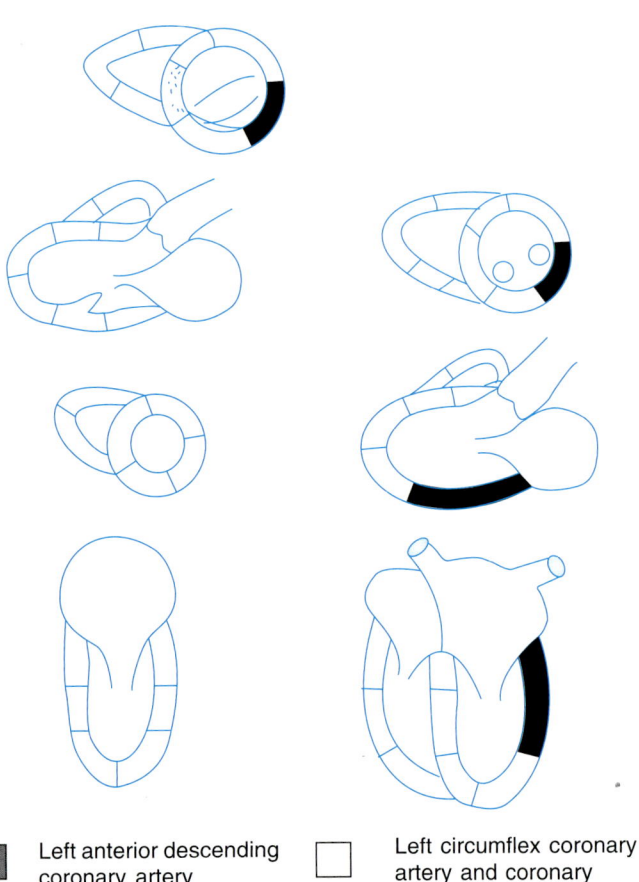

Left anterior descending coronary artery

Right coronary arterty

Left circumflex coronary artery and coronary artery

Left circumflex coronary artery

Fig. A10

Fig. A11 (A and B): (A) Parasternal long axis view. **(B)** Parasternal short axis view (aortic level)

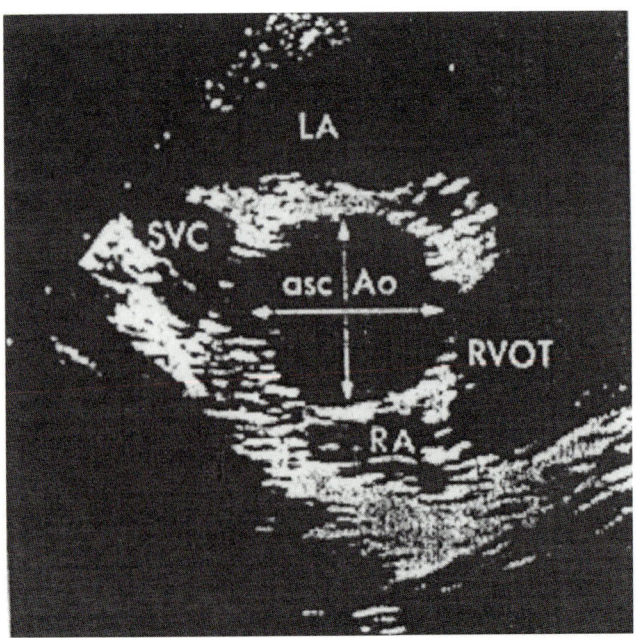

Fig. A12: TEE examination of the base of the heart showing measurements of ascending aorta (Asc AO)

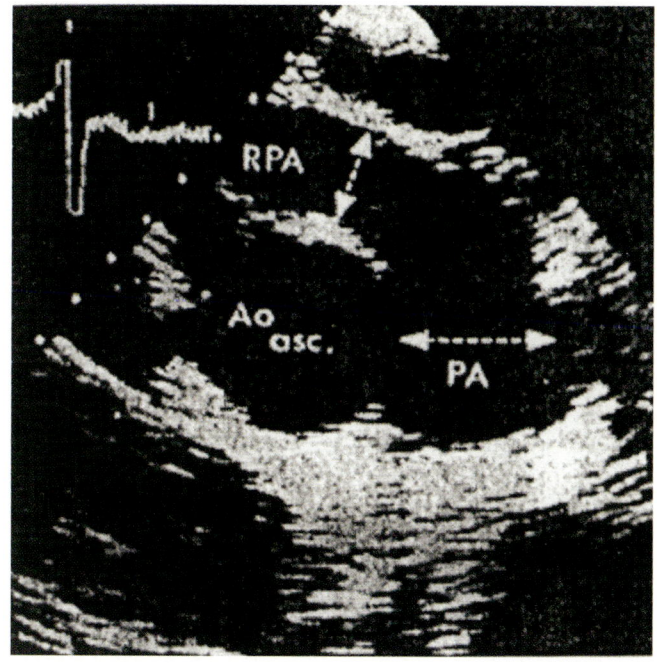

Fig. A13: TEE examination of right pulmonary artery

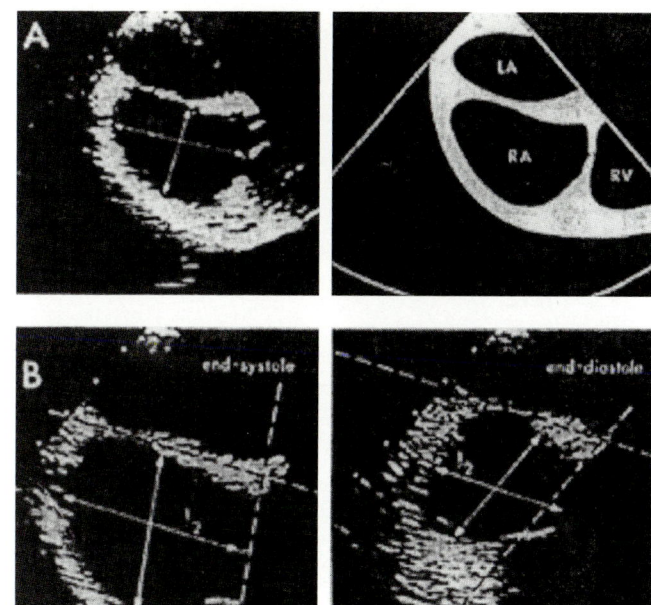

Fig. A14 (A and B): End-systolic and end-diastolic measurement of right atrium (RA)

Table A-3: *Adult normal values, corrected for body surface area**

	Range (cm)	Mean (cm)	Number
RVD/M²–flat	0.4–1.4	0.9	76
RVD/M²–left lateral	0.4–1.4	0.9	79
LVID.M²–flat	2.1–3.2	2.6	77
LVID/M²–left lateral	1.9–3.2	2.6	81
LAD/M²	1.2–2.2	1.6	127
Aortic root/M²	1.2–2.2	1.5	115

* Data from Feigenbaum, H.: Echocardiography, ed. 2, Philadelphia, 1976, Lea and Febiger.

Table A-4: *Normal measurements from the suprasternal transducer position**

Aortic arch lumen diameter	24 ± 1.1 mm
Right pulmonary artery lumen diameter	20 ± 1.2 mm
Left atrial cephalocaudal diameter	52 ± 12.7 mm
Left atrial anteroposterior diameter	42 ± 7.3 mm

* From Golberg, B.B.: Ultrasonic measurement of the aortic arch, right pulmonary artery and left atrium, Radiology 101:383–390, 1971.

Table A-5: *Left ventricular filling dynamics in normal subjects*

	<50 years (n = 61)	≥50 (n = 56)	P value
Left ventricular inflow			
Peak E (cm/sec)	72 ± 14	62 ± 14	<0.01
Peak A (cm/sec)	40 ± 10	59 ± 14	<0.01
E/A	1.9 ± 0.6	1.1 ± 0.3	<0.01
DT (msec)	179 ± 20	210 ± 36	<0.01
IVRT (msec)	76 ± 11	90 ± 17	<0.01
Pulmonary	(n = 44)	(n = 41)	
Peak S (cm/sec)	48 ± 9	71 ± 9	<0.01
Peak D (cm/sec)	50 ± 10	38 ± 9	<0.01
Peak AR (cm/sec)	19 ± 4	23 ± 14	<0.01

Table A-6: *Right ventricular filling dynamics in normal subjects*

	<50 years (n = 61)	≥50 (n = 56)	P value
Right ventricular			
Peak E (cm/sec)	51 ± 7	41 ± 8	<0.01
Peak A (cm/sec)	27 ± 8	33 ± 8	<0.01
E/A	2.0 ± 0.5	1.34 ± 0.4	<0.01
DT (msec)	188 ± 22	198 ± 23	<0.01
IVRT (msec)	76 ± 11	90 ± 17	<0.01
Superior vena cava	(n = 59)	(n = 53)	
Peak S (cm/sec)	41 ± 9	42 ± 12	Non significant
Peak D (cm/sec)	22 ± 5	22 ± 5	Non significant
Peak AR (cm/sec)	13 ± 3	16 ± 3	<0.01

Table A-7: *Normal maximal velocities, Doppler measurements*

	Mean	Range	Mean	Range
Mitral flow	1.00 m/sec	0.8–1.3 m/sec	0.90 m/sec	0.6–1.3 m/sec
Tricuspid flow	0.60 m/sec	0.5–0.8 m/sec	0.50 m/sec	0.3–0.7 m/sec
Pulmonary artery	0.90 m/sec	0.7–1.1 m/sec	0.75 m/sec	0.6–0.9 m/sec
Left ventricle	1.00 m/sec	0.7–1.2 m/sec	0.90 m/sec	0.7–1.1 m/sec
Aorta	1.50 m/sec	1.2–1.8 m/sec	1.35 m/sec	1.0–1.7 m/sec

(From Hatle, L; and Angelsen, B.: Doppler Ultrasound in Cardiology, Second Edition. Philadelphia, Lea and Febiger, 1985.)

Table A-8: *Normal Doppler velocities in children*

Site	Mean	Range
SVC	51 cm/sec	28–80 cm/sec
RA (peak)	47	38–74
RV inflow	62	41–84
MPA	76	50–105
LA (peak)	58	45–80
LV inflow	78	44–128
AA	97	60–154

SVC, superior vena cava; RA, right atrium; RV, Right ventricle; MPA, main pulmonary artery; LA, left atrium; LV, left ventricle; AA, ascending aorta. (From: Goldberg, S.J., Allen, H.D., Marx, G.R. and Flinn, C.J.: Doppler Echocardiography. Philadelphia, Lea and Febiger, 1985)

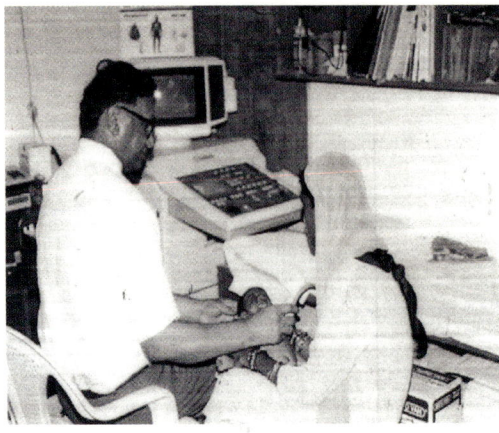

Fig. A15: Operator performing echocardiography in a young child for mesurement of various Doppler velocities of native values and other hemodynamic values

Table A-9: *Normal values for children arranged by weight**

	Weight (lbs.)	Mean (cm.)	Range (cm.)	Number of subjects
RVD	0–25	0.9	0.3–1.5	26
	26–50	1.0	0.4–1.5	26
	51–75	1.1	0.7–1.8	20
	76–100	1.2	0.7–1.6	15
	101–125	1.3	0.8–1.7	11
	126–200	1.3	1.2–1.7	5
LVID	0–25	2.4	1.3–3.2	26
	26–50	3.4	2.4–3.8	26
	51–75	3.8	3.3–4.5	20
	76–100	4.1	3.5–4.7	15
	101–125	4.3	3.7–4.9	11
	126–200	4.9	4.4–5.2	5
LV and IV septal wall thickness	0–25	0.5	0.4–0.6	26
	26–50	0.6	0.5–0.7	26
	51–75	0.7	0.6–0.7	20
	76–100	0.7	0.7–0.8	15
	101–125	0.7	0.7–0.8	11
	126–200	0.8	0.7–0.8	5
LA dimension	0–25	1.7	0.7–2.3	26
	26–50	2.2	1.7–2.7	26
	51–75	2.3	1.9–2.8	20
	76–100	2.4	2.0–3.0	15
	101–125	2.7	2.1–3.0	11
	126–00	2.8	2.1–3.7	5
Aortic root	0–25	1.3	0.7–1.7	26
	26–50	1.7	1.3–2.2	26
	51–75	2.0	1.7–2.3	20
	76–100	2.2	1.9–2.7	15
	101–125	2.3	1.7–2.7	11
	126–200	2.4	2.2–2.8	5
Aortic valve opening	0–25	0.9	0.5–1.2	26
	26–50	1.2	0.9–1.6	26
	51–75	1.4	1.2–1.7	20
	76–100	1.6	1.3–1.9	15
	101–125	1.7	1.4–2.0	11
	126–200	1.8	1.6–2.0	5

* Data from Feigenbaum, H.: Echocardiography, ed. 2, Philadelphia, 1976, Lea and Febiger.
RVD, right ventricular dimension, LVID, left ventricular internal dimension.

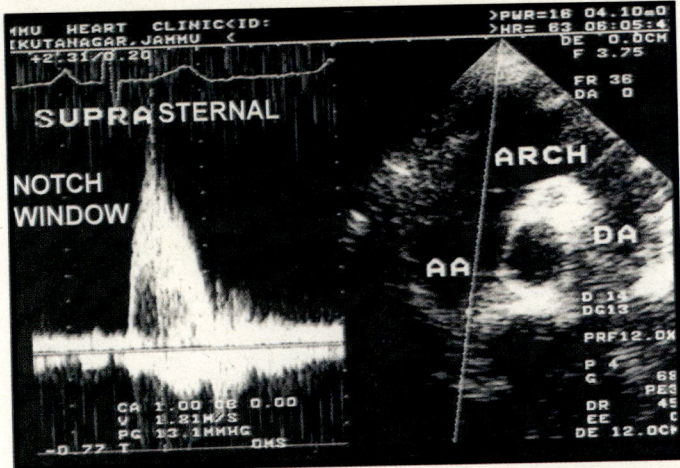

Fig. A16: Doppler flow velocity across ascending aorta showing blood flow in normal individual (left) and visualising anatomic placement of ascending arch and descending aorta (right)

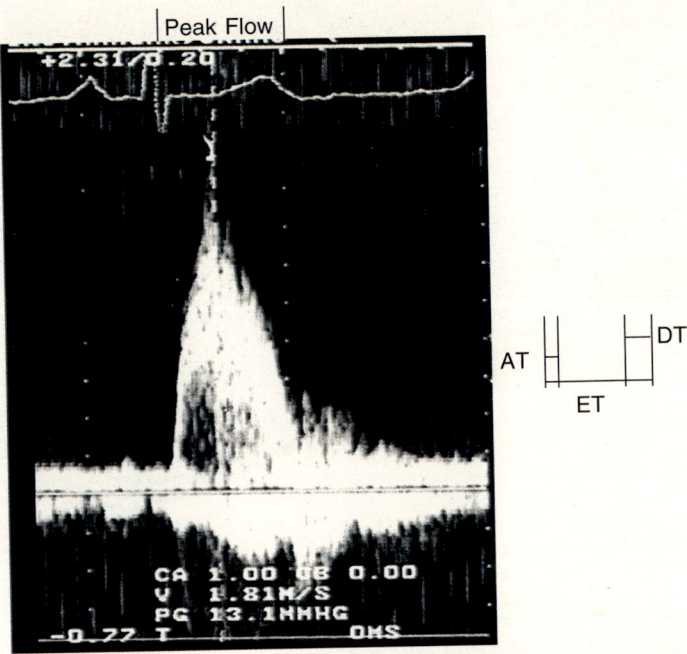

Fig. A17: Pulsed Doppler recording of aortic blood flow velocity showing how ejection time, peak flow velocity, acceleration time (AT) and deceleration time (DT) are measured

Table A-10: *Normal values for children arranged by body surface area**

	BSA (m²)	Mean (cm.)	Range (cm.)	Number of subjects
RVD	0.5 or less	0.8	0.3–1.3	24
	0.6 to 1.0	1.0	0.4–1.8	39
	1.0 to 1.5	1.2	0.7–1.7	29
	Over 1.5	1.3	0.8–1.7	11
LVID	0.5 or less	2.4	1.3–3.2	24
	0.6 to 1.0	3.4	2.4–4.2	39
	1.0 to 1.5	4.0	3.3–4.7	29
	Over 1.5	4.7	4.2–5.2	11
LV and IV Septal wall thickness	0.5 or less	0.5	0.4–0.6	24
	0.6 to 1.0	0.6	0.5–0.7	39
	1.0 to 1.5	0.7	0.6–0.8	29
	Over 1.5	0.8	0.7–0.8	11
LA dimension	0.5 or less	1.7	0.7–2.4	24
	0.6 to 1.0	2.1	1.8–2.8	39
	1.0 to 1.5	2.4	2.0–3.0	29
	Over 1.5	2.8	2.1–3.7	11
Aortic root	0.5 or less	1.2	0.7–1.5	24
	0.6 to 1.0	1.8	1.4–2.2	39
	1.0 to 1.5	2.2	1.7–2.7	29
	Over 1.5	2.4	2.0–2.8	11
Aortic valve opening	0.5 or less	0.8	0.5–1.0	24
	0.6 to 1.0	1.3	0.9–1.6	39
	1.0 to 1.5	1.6	1.3–1.9	29
	Over 1.5	1.8	1.5–2.0	11

* Data from Feigenbaum, H.: Echocardiography, ed. 2, Philadelphia, 1976, Lea and Febiger.

RVD - right ventricular dimension.
LVID - left ventricular internal dimension.

Table A-11: *Echocardiographic values in normal newborns (from Moss et al)**

Age of patient weight	1½ hr. – 1 mo. 1.9 – 4.9 kg.	Age of patient weight	1½ hr. – 1 mo. 1.9 – 4.9 kg.
No. of cases	(633)	No. of cases	(633)
MVD	22 – 47 mm	LAD	4 – 13.5 mm
MVTE	6.5 – 1.4 mm	IST	1.8 – 4.5 mm
MVDE	6 – 12 mm	LVPW (S)	2.5 – 6 mm
MVVS	36 – 130 mm	LVPW (D)	1.6 – 4.6 mm
TVD	13 – 32 mm	LVD (S)	8 – 18.6 mm
TVTE	8 – 14.2 mm	LVD (D)	12 – 24.1 mm
TVDE	7 – 14 mm	RVAW (S)	3.3 – 7.3 mm
TVVS	34 – 11 mm/sec	RVAW (D)	1.1 – 4.7 mm
ARD	7 – 13.6 mm	RVD (S)	5.5 – 11.4 mm
AVO	4 – 6.8 mm	RVD (D)	6.1 – 17.7 mm
PRD	9.2 – 15.8 mm	MVCF	0.92 – 2.2 circ/sec
PVO	5.8 – 9.9 mm		

MVD, mitral valve depth;

MVTE, mitral valve total excursion;

MVDE, mitral valve diastolic excursion;

MVVS, mitral valve velocity slope;

TVD, tricuspid valve depth,

TVTE, tricuspid valve total excursion,

TVDE, tricuspid valve diastolic excursion;

TVVS, tricuspid valve velocity slope;

ARD, aortic root diameter;

AVO, aortic valve opening;

PRD, pulmonary root diameter;

(S), systole;

(D), diastole;

PVO, pulmonary valve opening;

LAD, left atrial dimension;

IST, interventricular septal thickness;

LVPW, left ventricular septal thickness;

LVD, left ventricular posterior wall;

RVAW, right ventricular anterior wall;

RVD, right ventricular dimension;

MVCF, mean velocity circumferential fiber shortening

* Moss, A. J., Gussoni, C.C., Isabel-Jones, J.: Echocardiography in congenital heart disease. Western Journal of Medicine, 124, 102–121, 1976. Quoted by Feigebaum, H.: Echocardiography, second edition, Lea and Febiger, Philadelphia, 1976.

Bernoulli equation

$$\Delta p = 1/2\, p(v_2^2 - v_1^2) + p\,\{(dv/dt)\,{}^*ds + R(\mu)$$
$$\Delta p = 4(v_2^2 - v_1^2)$$
$$\Delta p = 4(v_2^2 - v_1^2)$$
$$\Delta p = 4v^2$$

Doppler echocardiography pressure drop or gradient measurement

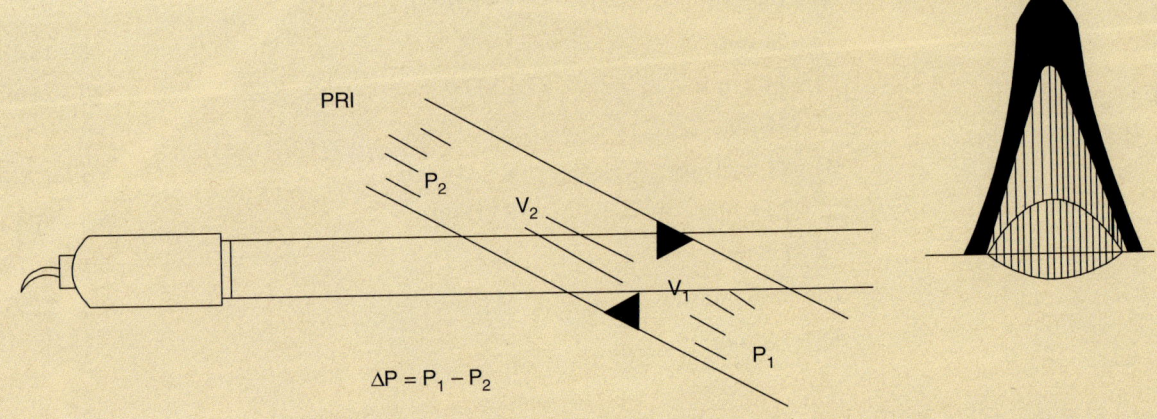

PRI

P_2 V_2 V_1 P_1

$$\Delta P = P_1 - P_2$$

Bernoulli equation

$$P_1 - P_2 = \underbrace{\tfrac{1}{2}\rho\,(V_2^2 + V_1^2)}_{\substack{\text{Convective}\\\text{Acceleration}}} + \rho \underbrace{\int_1^2 \frac{\overrightarrow{DV}}{DT}\,DS}_{\substack{\text{Flow}\\\text{Acceleration}}} + \underbrace{R(\overrightarrow{V})}_{\substack{\text{Viscous}\\\text{Friction}}}$$

$$P_1 - P_2 = \tfrac{1}{2}\rho\,(V_2^2 - V_1^2)$$

V_1 Much $< V_2 \therefore$ Ignore V_1

$$\rho = \text{Mass density of blood} = 106.10^3\ \text{kg/m}^3$$

$$\therefore \quad \Delta P = 4V_2^2$$

Clinical application of the Bernoulli equation

Application	*Clinical utility*
Peak velocity through a stenotic valve	Aortic stenosis maximal gradient
TRjet velocity	RV systolic pressure
LV outflow tract contour and velocity	HOCM gradient
Peak velocity across VSD	RV systolic pressure
End-diastolic velocity of PR jet	Pulmonary artery diastolic pressure
Velocity through a PDA	Pulmonary artery systolic pressure
MR contour and velocity	Left ventricular dp/dt

HOCM, hypertrophic obstructive cardiomyopathy; LV, left ventricle; MR, mitral regurgitation;

PDA, patent ductus arteriosus; PR, pulmonic regurgitation; RV, right ventricular;

VSD, ventricular septal defect; TR, tricuspid regurgitation.

Fig. A18

Table A-12: Normal values of mechanical prostheses in mitral position

Prosthesis	References	No. of patients	Peak velocity	Peak gradient	Mean velocity	Mean gradient	Half-time	MVA	Regurgitant valves	
									No.	%
Starr-Edwards	32	3	1.80 ± 0.20	13.00 ± 5.00	1.12 ± 0.22	5.00 ± 2.00	105 ± 32.5	2.10 ± 0.50	1	33
	33	12	2.00	17.00	NI	NI	105	2.10	5	42
	34	10	1.58	10.00	NI	NI	110 ± 19.4	2.00 ± 0.30	3	30
	35	18	1.97 ± 0.42	15.50 ± 5.80	1.06 ± 0.29	4.47 ± 2.42	113 ± 29	1.95 ± 0.50	NI	NI
Total		43	1.88 ± 0.40	14.56 ± 5.50	1.07 ± 0.28	4.55 ± 2.40	109.5 ± 26.6	2.01 ± 0.49	9	36
St. Jude	36	13	1.38 ± 0.33	7.62 ± 0.64	0.73 ± 0.16	2.30 ± 290	61.2 ± 16.9	3.60 ± 0.99	NI	NI
	32	44	1.60 ± 0.30	11.00 ± 4.00	1.12 ± 0.22	5.00 ± 2.00	73.3 ± 14.7	3.00 ± 0.60	14	32
	35	56	1.63 ± 0.27	10.63 ± 3.52	0.76 ± 0.18	2.32 ± 1.10	78.0 ± 16.0	2.93 ± 0.60	NI	NI
	37	10	1.73 ± 0.32	12.00 ± 4.40	1.8 ± 0.22	5.60 ± 2.10	71.0 ± 18.3	3.10 ± 0.80	2	20
	38	33	1.40 ± 0.30	7.84 ± 3.36	0.80 ± 0.10	3.30 ± 1.10	86.0 ± 21.0	2.56 ± 0.62	NI	NI
Total		156	1.56 ± 0.29	9.98 ± 3.62	0.88 ± 0.19	3.49 ± 1.34	76.5 ± 17.1	2.88 ± 0.64	16	30
Bjork-Shiley	39	9	NI	NI	NI	NI	13.3 ± 32.7	2.13 ± 0.72	NI	NI
	32	8	1.60 ± 0.30	10.00 ± 3.00	1.12 ± 0.22	5.00 ± 2.00	100.0 ± 18.8	2.20 ± 0.40	NI	NI
	34	36	1.58	10.00	NI	NI	88.0 ± 28.2	2.50 ± 0.80	3	38
	40	17	1.27 ± 0.39	6.41 ± 3.30	0.71 ± 0.28	2.00 ± 1.56	102.8 ± 12.5	2.14 ± 0.26	4	11
	35	40	1.57 ± 0.24	9.86 ± 2.78	0.79 ± 0.22	2.47 ± 1.36	82.0 ± 17.0	2.68 ± 0.26	3	19
	41	6	NI	NI	1.17 ± 0.28	5.50 ± 2.65	NI	NI	NI	NI
	42	12	2.36 ± 0.33	22.30 ± 5.82	NI	NI	NI	NI	NI	NI
Total		128	1.61 ± 0.30	10.72 ± 2.74	0.84 ± 0.24	2.90 ± 1.61	90.2 ± 22.4	2.44 ± 0.62	10	16
Lillehei-Kaster	35	10	1.84	13.54	0.92	3.35	125.0 ± 29.0	1.88 ± 0.56	NI	NI
Beall	32	13	1.80 ± 0.2	13.40 ± 4.0	1.22 ± 0.20	6.00 ± 2.00	129.4 ± 15.2	1.70 ± 0.20	NI	NI

MVA = mittal valve area; NI = no information. (From Reisner, S.A. and Meltzer, R.S.: Normal values of prosthetic valve Doppler echocardiographic parameters: A review. J. Am. Soc. Echocardiogr., 1:201, 1988.)

Table A-13: Normal values of tissue prostheses in mitral position

Prosthesis	References	No. of patients	Peak velocity	Peak gradient	Mean velocity	Mean gradient	Half-time	MVA	Regurgitant valves No.	%
Ionescu-Shiley	43	17	1.39 ± 0.20	7.73 ± 2.00	0.94 ± 0.11	3.54 ± 0.80	93.5 ± 23.0	2.35 ± 0.77	NI	NI
	35	12	1.56 ± 0.35	9.73 ± 3.87	0.84 ± 0.27	2.90 ± 1.60	93.0 ± 28.0	2.37 ± 0.71	NI	NI
Total		29	1.46 ± 0.24	8.53 ± 2.91	0.90 ± 0.19	3.28 ± 1.19	93.5 ± 25.0	2.36 ± 0.75	NI	NI
Carpentier-Edwards	44	38	1.60 ± 0.20	10.24 ± 2.40	NI	NI	90.0 ± 23.0	2.44 ± 0.84	NI	NI
	37	25	2.10 ± 0.37	17.30 ± 5.30	1.37 ± 0.22	7.50 ± 0.20	84.6 ± 31.2	2.60 ± 0.70	NI	NI
	43	12	1.55 ± 0.24	9.63 ± 2.74	1.04 ± 0.26	4.36 ± 1.93	100.0 ± 16.7	2.20 ± 0.44	NI	NI
Total		75	1.76 ± 0.24	12.49 ± 3.64	1.26 ± 3.64	6.48 ± 2.12	89.8 ± 25.4	2.45 ± 0.74	NI	NI
Hancock	39	8	NI	NI	NI	NI	157.0 ± 76.3	1.40 ± 0.68	NI	NI
	45	14	NI	NI	1.54 ± 0.3	6.50 ± 1.4	142.9 ± 27.9	1.54 ± 0.30	NI	NI
	33	29	1.90	14.00	NI	NI	91.7	2.40 ± 0.80	12	42
	40	23	1.21 ± 0.27	5.83 ± 2.48	0.77 ± 0.19	2.39 ± 1.16	141.0 ± 30.8	1.56 ± 0.34	3	14
	46	28	1.38 ± 0.24	7.62 ± 2.65	NI	4.60	136.0 ± 18.0	1.62 ± 0.27	1	4
	47	5	NI	NI	10.70		NI	NI	NI	NI
	7	7	1.80 ± 0.30	12.96 ± 4.32	1.10 ± 0.30	5.90 ± 3.00	150.0 ± 80.0	1.47 ± 0.78	NI	NI
Total		114	1.54 ± 0.26	9.70 ± 3.20	1.07 ± 0.25	4.29 ± 2.14	128.6 ± 30.9	1.71 ± 0.41	16	20

MVA, mitral valve area; NI, no information. (From Reisner, S.A. and Meltzer, R.S.: Normal values of prosthetic valve Doppler echocardiographic parameters: A review. J. AM. Soc. Echocardiogr., 1:201, 1988.)

Table A-14: *Normal values for mechanical prostheses in aortic position*

Prosthesis	References	No. of patients	Peak velocity	Peak gradient	Mean velocity	Mean gradient	Regurgitant valves No.	%
St. Jude	32	38	2.30 ± 0.60	22.0 ± 12.0	1.73 ± 0.57	12.0 ± 7.00	22	58
	36	7	1.97 ± 0.52	15.5 ± 8.2	1.23 ± 0.25	6.0 ± 2.50	NI	NI
	48	12	2.70 ± 0.40	30.0 ± 9.0	1.80 ± 0.30	16.0 ± 5.60	NI	NI
	37	13	2.50 ± 0.50	26.5 ± 9.1	2.00 ± 0.35	16.0 ± 5.60	4	30
Total		70	2.37 ± 0.27	25.5 ± 5.12	1.69 ± 0.47	12.5 ± 6.35	26	51
Bjork-Shiley	32	8	2.60 ± 0.50	17.0 ± 9.00	1.87 ± 0.40	1.48 ± 6.00	5	62
	40	20	2.35 ± 0.28	22.0 ± 5.31	1.80 ± 0.36	13.0 ± 5.20	3	17
	49	20	2.17 ± 0.40	18.8 ± 6.94	NI	NI	2	10
	34	33	3.29 ± 0.50	21.5 ± 10.0	NI	NI	8	26
	48	21	2.70 ± 0.40	30.0 ± 9.00	1.80 ± 0.30	16.0 ± 5.00	NI	NI
Total		102	2.62 ± 0.42	23.8 ± 8.80	1.82 ± 0.34	14.3 ± 5.25	18	22
Starr-Edwards	32	4	3.20 ± 0.20	40.0 ± 3.0	2.45 ± 0.20	24.0 ± 4.0	3	75
	49	12	3.35 ± 0.45	45.0 ± 12.0	NI	NI	6	50
	33	34	3.10	40.0	NI	NI	18	53
	34	6	2.71 ± 0.61	29.3 ± 13.3	NI	NI	2	33
Total		56	3.10 ± 0.47	38.6 ± 11.7	2.45 ± 0.20	24.0 ± 4.0	29	52

NI, no information. (From Reisner, S.A. and Meltzer, R.S.: Normal values of prosthetic valve Doppler echocardiographic parameters: A review. J. Am. Soc. Echocardiogr., 1:201, 1988.)

Table A-15: *Normal values for tissue protheses in aortic position*

Prosthesis	References	No. of patients	Peak velocity	Peak gradient	Mean velocity	Mean gradient	Regurgitant valves No.	%
Carpentier-Edwards	44	24	2.44 ± 0.48	23.81 ± 9.37	NI	NI	2	8
	49	43	2.17 ± 0.49	18.84 ± 8.51	NI	NI	9	22
	48	7	2.70 ± 0.70	31.00 ± 15.0	1.90 ± 0.5	18.0 ± 9.0	NI	NI
	37	41	2.50 ± 0.40	26.10 ± 7.70	1.95 ± 0.31	15.2 ± 4.8	11	26
	43	28	2.34 ± 0.40	23.10 ± 8.20	1.75 ± 0.42	12.3 ± 5.9	NI	NI
Total Hancock		143	2.37 ± 0.46	23.18 ± 8.72	1.87 ± 0.37	14.4 ± 5.7	22	20
	40	22	2.00 ± 0.19	16.0 ± 2.97	1.66 ± 0.17	11.40 ± 2.29	5	22
	49	32	2.56 ± 02.3	26.2 ± 4.71	NI		7	22
	33	10	2.70	30.0	NI	NI	5	50
	34	27	2.37 ± 0.53	22.4 ± 10.1	NI	NI	8	26
Total Ionescu-Shiley		91	2.38 ± 0.35	23.0 ± 6.71	1.66 ± 0.17	11.0 ± 2.29	25	27
	37	16	2.60 ± 0.50	27.0 ± 9.10	2.00 ± 0.33	16.40 ± 5.3	NI	NI
	43	16	3.37 ± 0.31	21.96 ± 5.86	1.70 ± 0.21	11.57 ± 2.9	NI	NI
Total		32	2.49 ± 1.71	24.68 ± 7.65	1.85 ± 0.29	13.99 ± 4.3	NI	NI

NI, no information. (From Reisner, S.A. and Meltzer, R.S.: Normal values of prosthetic valve Doppler echocardiographic parameters: A review. J. Am. Soc. Echocardiogr., 1:201, 1988.)

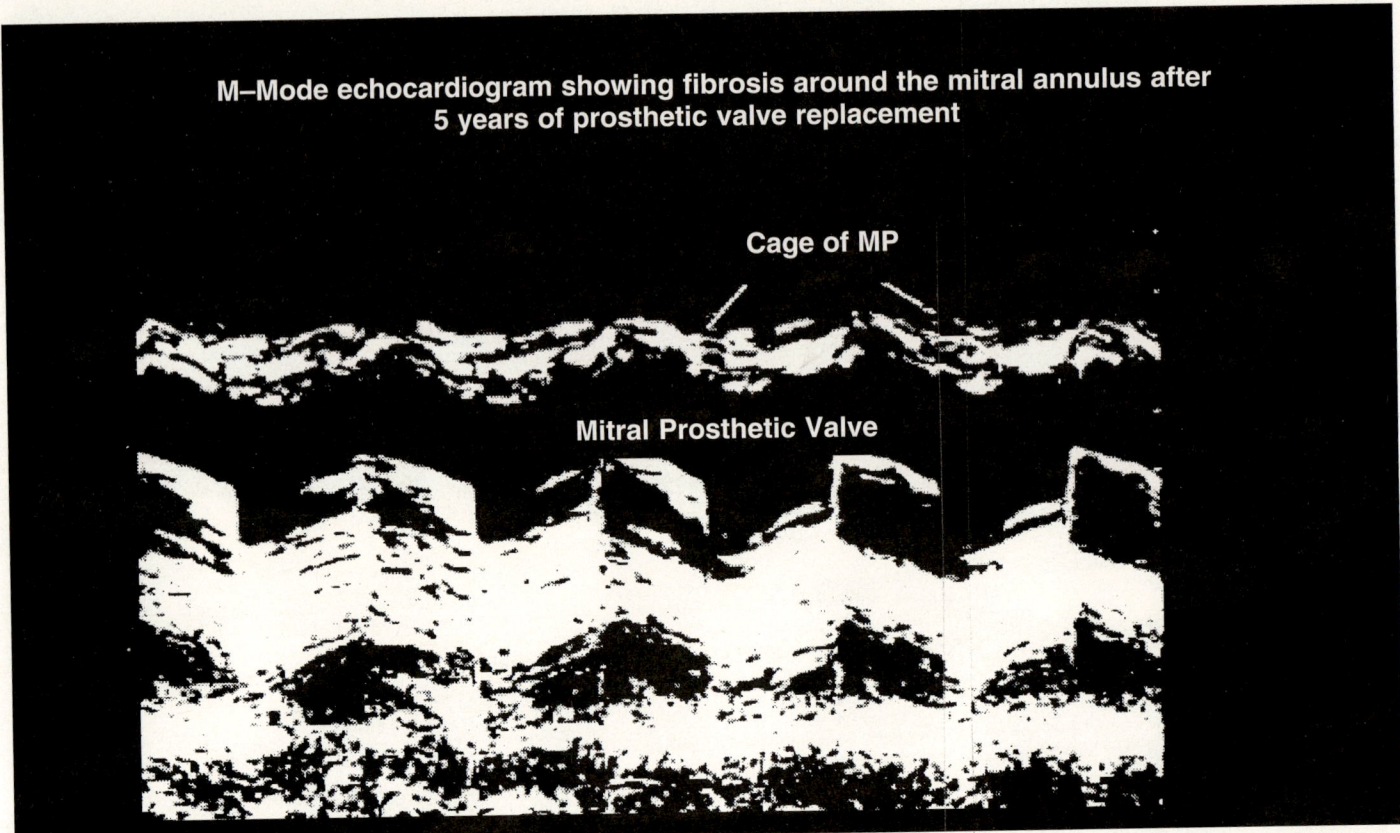

Fig. A19 (A): A–M-Mode echoscan of prosthetic mitral valve (Bjork-Shiley) showing fibrosis around the place of sutures and mitral annulus

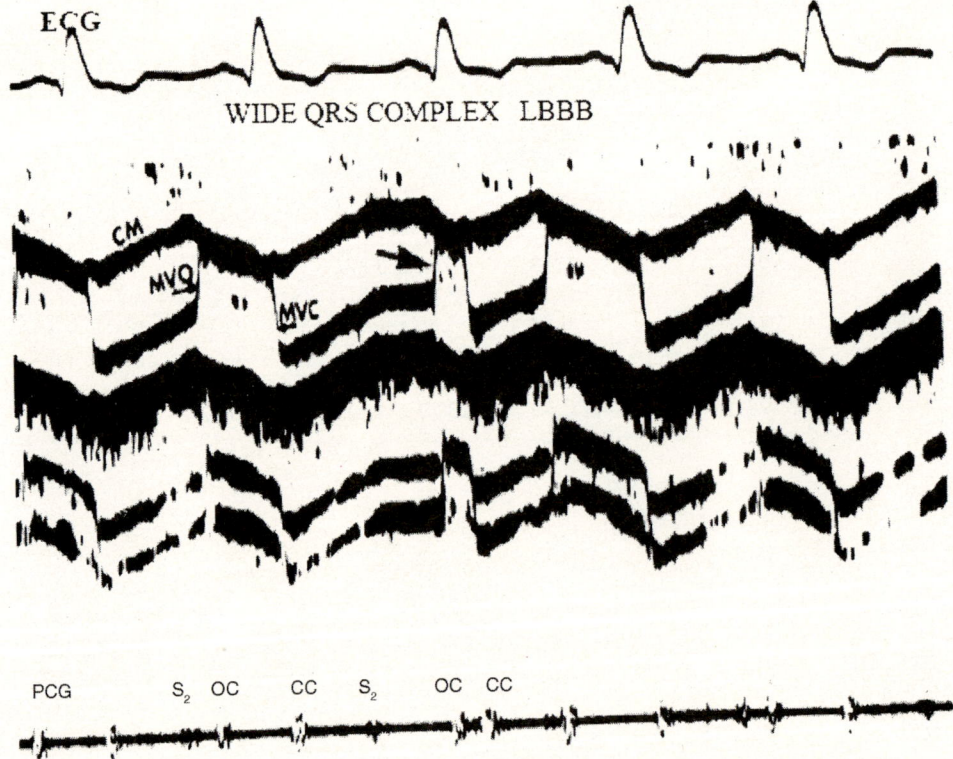

Fig. A19 (B): M-Mode echocardiogram showing a delayed mitral valve opening (MVO) in the third cardiac complex (arrow) in patient with malfunctioning mitral prosthetic valve, CM = cage of mitral valve, MVC = mitral valve closing, S_2 = second heart sound, OC = opening click, CC = closing click

Table A-16: *Measurements in normal young adult subjects by transesophageal echocardiography*

Patient	Age (yrs)	Body Surface (m²)	Left Ventricular Short axis (cm/m²) D↔	D↕	S↔	S↕	Fractional shortening D(%)↔	D(%)↕	Right ventricular Right axis (cm/m²) D↔	D↕	S↔	S↕	Left atrium (cm/m²) D↕	D↔	S↕	S↔	Right ventricular Long axis (cm/m²) D↔	D↕	S↔	S↔	Right atrium (cm/m²) D↗	D↖	S↗	S↕
1	24	2.09	2.5	2.6	1.5	1.7	40	34	—	—	—	—	1.0	2.0	1.7	2.5	—	—	—	—	—	—	—	—
2	29	2.12	—	—	—	—	—	—	2.6	3.6	1.8	2.7	0.8	1.7	1.1	2.4	—	—	—	—	—	—	—	—
3	24	1.65	2.5	2.6	1.6	1.6	37	37	—	—	—	—	0.8	1.7	1.4	2.5	—	—	—	—	—	—	—	—
4	23	1.91	—	—	—	—	—	—	2.8	3.9	2.0	.3	1.4	1.4	1.9	2.1	2.5	1.5	2.0	1.0	1.8	2.4	2.4	2.6
5	26	2.22	—	—	—	—	—	—	2.4	3.1	1.6	2.4	—	—	—	—	2.7	1.7	2.3	1.2	—	—	—	—
6	22	1.79	2.4	2.4	1.6	1.6	35	34	2.5	3.1	1.6	2.4	0.7	1.7	1.4	2.3	2.6	1.3	2.2	1.0	1.9	1.8	2.5	1.9
7	30	2.08	3.0	2.7	1.8	1.7	42	36	2.4	3.4	1.6	2.7	1.3	1.8	1.9	2.6	2.7	1.6	2.2	1.2	2.2	2.2	2.4	2.4
8	22	2.05	—	—	—	—	—	—	—	—	—	—	—	—	—	—	—	—	—	—	—	—	—	—
9	22	1.67	—	—	—	—	—	—	2.8	3.5	2.2	3.0	0.4	1.1	1.1	2.2	2.8	1.8	2.5	1.2	1.8	1.9	2.5	1.8
10	22	1.89	—	—	—	—	—	—	2.7	3.1	1.8	2.7	—	—	—	—	2.5	1.3	2.0	1.0	1.8	1.8	2.0	2.0
11	19	1.67	2.5	2.5	1.5	1.5	41	38	2.3	3.0	1.7	2.4	0.8	1.7	1.4	2.3	2.7	1.2	2.4	0.8	1.9	1.7	2.4	1.8
12	27	1.55	2.9	2.9	1.8	1.9	38	34	2.9	3.4	2.0	2.5	0.4	1.5	1.4	2.8	—	—	—	—	—	—	—	—
13	24	1.87	2.5	2.6	1.7	1.9	31	27	—	—	—	—	—	—	—	—	2.8	1.6	2.3	0.9	—	—	—	—
14	23	2.00	—	—	—	—	—	—	—	—	—	—	—	—	—	—	3.1	1.6	2.6	1.1	1.9	2.4	2.8	2.3
15	26	2.06	2.8	2.6	1.8	1.9	35	27	—	—	—	—	0.6	1.3	1.2	2.1	2.8	1.5	2.2	0.9	—	—	—	—
16	22	1.84	2.7	2.6	1.7	1.7	35	36	—	—	—	—	—	—	—	—	—	—	—	—	1.7	2.2	2.3	2.1
17	22	1.83	2.4	2.4	1.6	1.6	34	31	—	—	—	—	—	—	—	—	2.7	1.3	2.3	1.1	1.7	2.0	2.3	2.2
18	22	1.73	2.6	2.6	1.9	1.8	28	30	—	—	—	—	—	—	—	—	2.4	1.3	2.1	0.9	1.7	1.9	2.3	2.0
19	23	1.82	2.5	2.5	1.6	1.7	35	33	2.6	2.9	1.9	2.5	0.5	1.7	1.2	2.3	2.9	1.6	2.2	1.0	1.9	2.4	2.7	2.7
20	25	1.61	—	—	—	—	—	—	2.4	3.7	1.7	2.8	0.9	1.4	1.8	2.5	2.9	1.6	2.3	1.0	1.8	2.1	2.7	1.9
21	23	1.86	—	—	—	—	—	—	2.5	3.1	1.7	2.6	0.8	1.5	1.4	2.1	3.0	1.4	2.6	1.1	1.4	1.7	2.2	1.9
22	22	1.53	2.5	2.3	1.7	1.6	29	42	2.6	3.7	1.9	2.8	1.2	1.8	2.0	2.7	3.0	1.3	2.4	1.0	2.2	1.9	3.0	2.0
23	20	1.55	2.6	2.5	1.5	1.7	38	37	—	—	—	—	—	—	—	—	—	—	—	—	—	—	—	—
24	23	2.07	2.6	2.4	1.8	1.6	30	31	2.5	3.0	2.0	2.3	—	—	—	—	2.6	1.3	1.9	0.8	1.9	2.4	2.2	2.4
25	22	1.83	2.3	2.2	1.5	1.5	39	31	2.5	3.7	1.9	2.9	1.4	1.5	2.1	2.8	2.9	2.0	2.4	1.0	1.7	2.1	2.3	2.0
Mean			2.6	2.5	1.7	1.7	35	34	2.6	3.4	1.8	2.7	0.9	1.6	1.5	2.4	2.8	1.6	2.3	1.0	1.8	2.1	2.4	2.1
±2 SD			0.4	0.3	0.3	0.3	8	8	0.4	0.6	0.4	0.5	0.7	0.4	0.6	0.5	0.4	0.3	0.4	0.2	0.4	0.5	0.4	0.6
Tolerance			2.1– 3.1	2.1– 2.9	1.3– 2.1	1.3– 2.1	25– 31	23– 43	2.1– 3.1	2.7– 4.1	1.3– 2.3	2.1– 3.3	0.1– 1.8	1.1– 2.1	0.9– 2.1	1.8– 3.0	2.3– 3.3	1.2 2.0	1.8 2.8	0.8– 1.2	1.3 2.3	1.6 2.6	1.9 2.9	1.5 2.7

Mean values and double standard deviation (x ± 2SD) and tolerance limits for all cardiac and extracardiac structures and dimensions measured by transesophageal echocardiography. D = end-systole; ↔, ↗ = lateral axes; ↕, ↖ = sagittal axes; ↔ = lateral axes; = cross-sectional area. (From Drexler M., Erbel, R., Muller, U., Wittlich, N., Mohr-Kahyl, S., and Meyer, J.: Measurement of intracardiac dimensions and structures in normal young adult subjects by transesophageal echocardiography, Am. J. Cardiol., 65:1491, 1990).

Aortic valve cm/M² D↕	D↔	cm/m² •	Asc aorta cm²/m² D↕	D↔	cm/m² •	Desc aorta cm²/m² D↕	D↔	cm/m² •	Tricuspid ring (cm²/m²) D	S	Mitral ring cm/m² ○	Atrial septum (cm) D	S	Right main Pulmonary Artery (cm) ○	○
1.6	1.8	4.5	1.3	1.8	3.7	0.8	1.3	1.8	—	—	1.8	—	—	—	—
1.3	1.7	3.3	1.3	1.7	3.7	0.8	1.1	1.6	—	—	1.8	—	—	—	—
1.7	2.0	4.8	1.6	1.9	4.1	—	—	—	—	—	2.2	—	—	—	—
1.3	1.7	3.4	—	—	—	1.0	1.3	2.1	1.8	1.4	1.9	1.6	2.1	1.2	1.8
1.4	1.7	4.1	1.5	1.9	5.1	1.0	1.2	2.3	1.7	1.4	1.5	—	—	—	—
1.3	1.7	2.8	1.5	1.7	3.5	0.9	1.4	1.8	1.6	1.0	1.5	1.6	2.1	1.2	2.1
1.5	1.9	4.5	—	—	—	0.9	1.4	2.1	1.8	1.3	1.8	1.6	2.1	1.4	2.1
1.4	1.8	4.0	1.3	1.7	3.6	0.9	1.2	1.7	—	—	1.8	—	—	—	—
1.5	1.7	3.4	—	—	—	—	—	—	1.7	1.2	1.7	1.4	1.8	1.2	1.8
—	—	—	1.3	1.8	3.8	—	—	—	1.5	1.5	1.5	1.6	2.2	1.1	1.6
1.5	2.0	3.9	1.6	1.8	4.0	0.8	1.3	1.5	1.3	1.2	1.5	1.7	2.2	1.4	—
1.3	1.9	3.3	1.3	1.8	3.1	1.0	1.3	1.6	—	—	1.9	—	—	—	—
1.5	1.7	4.6	—	—	—	1.0	1.4	2.2	—	—	—	—	—	—	—
1.3	1.8	3.5	1.3	1.6	3.3	0.9	1.5	2.2	1.7	1.5	1.9	1.6	2.1	1.0	2.0
1.5	1.8	4.4	1.2	1.5	3.1	0.9	1.3	1.9	2.0	1.5	1.9	—	—	—	—
1.4	2.0	4.1	—	—	—	1.0	1.5	2.6	—	—	—	1.6	1.7	1.1	2.1
1.6	2.1	4.8	—	—	—	0.9	1.4	1.4	1.7	1.4	—	1.4	1.7	1.2	2.2
1.4	1.9	3.7	1.4	1.7	3.7	0.8	1.4	1.7	1.5	1.3	—	1.6	2.0	1.1	2.3
1.5	2.1	4.7	1.3	1.6	3.1	0.9	1.2	1.6	1.8	1.4	1.7	1.2	1.8	1.2	2.0
1.5	2.2	5.1	1.5	1.9	3.7	0.9	1.4	2.3	1.7	1.5	2.0	1.9	2.6	1.0	2.0
—	—	—	1.3	1.6	3.3	0.8	1.2	1.3	1.6	1.2	1.7	1.5	2.0	1.3	—
1.6	2.1	4.8	1.7	1.9	4.2	0.8	1.3	1.8	1.5	1.4	2.1	1.9	2.7	1.0	—
1.4	1.9	3.4	1.5	1.7	3.3	0.9	1.6	1.9	—	—	—	1.4	1.7	—	—
—	—	—	—	—	—	1.1	1.5	2.7	1.8	1.4	—	1.4	1.7	—	—
1.7	1.9	3.6	1.4	1.6	3.4	0.9	1.5	2.0	1.8	1.3	2.0	1.6	1.5	1.3	—
1.5	1.9	4.0	1.4	1.7	3.6	0.9	1.3	1.9	1.7	1.4	1.8	1.6	2.1	1.2	2.0
0.3	0.3	1.2	0.3	0.3	1.0	0.2	0.3	0.8	0.3	0.3	0.4	0.4	0.7	0.2	0.4
1.2– 1.8	1.6– 2.2	2.8– 5.2	1.0– 1.8	1.4– 2.1	2.4– 4.8	0.7– 1.1	1.0– 1.6	1.1– 2.7	1.3– 2.1	1.0– 1.8	1.3– 2.3	1.1– 2.1	1.2– 3.0	0.9– 1.3	1.5– 2.5

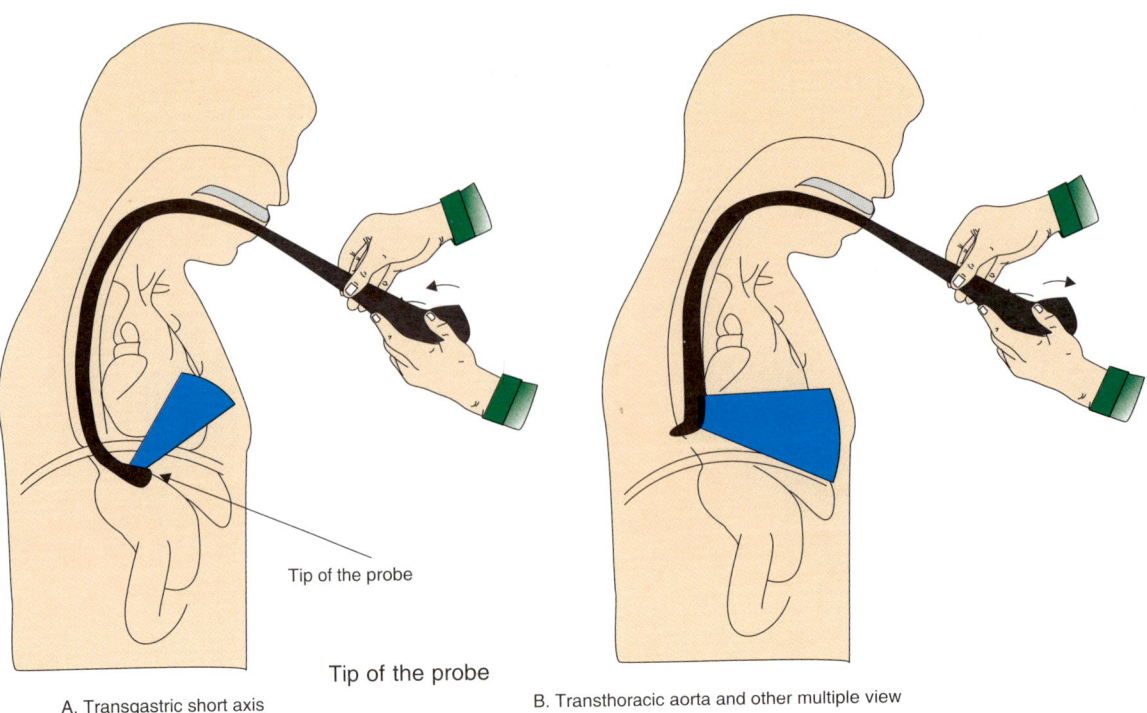

Tip of the probe

Tip of the probe

A. Transgastric short axis

B. Transthoracic aorta and other multiple view

Fig. A20

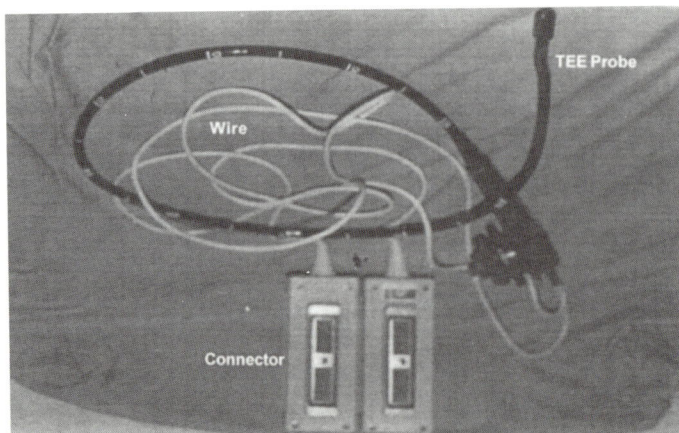

Fig. A21: Two connectors at the bottom of TEE probe which are to be fitted with the basic color Doppler echocardiographic machine to make it fully functional for obtaining TEE graphs

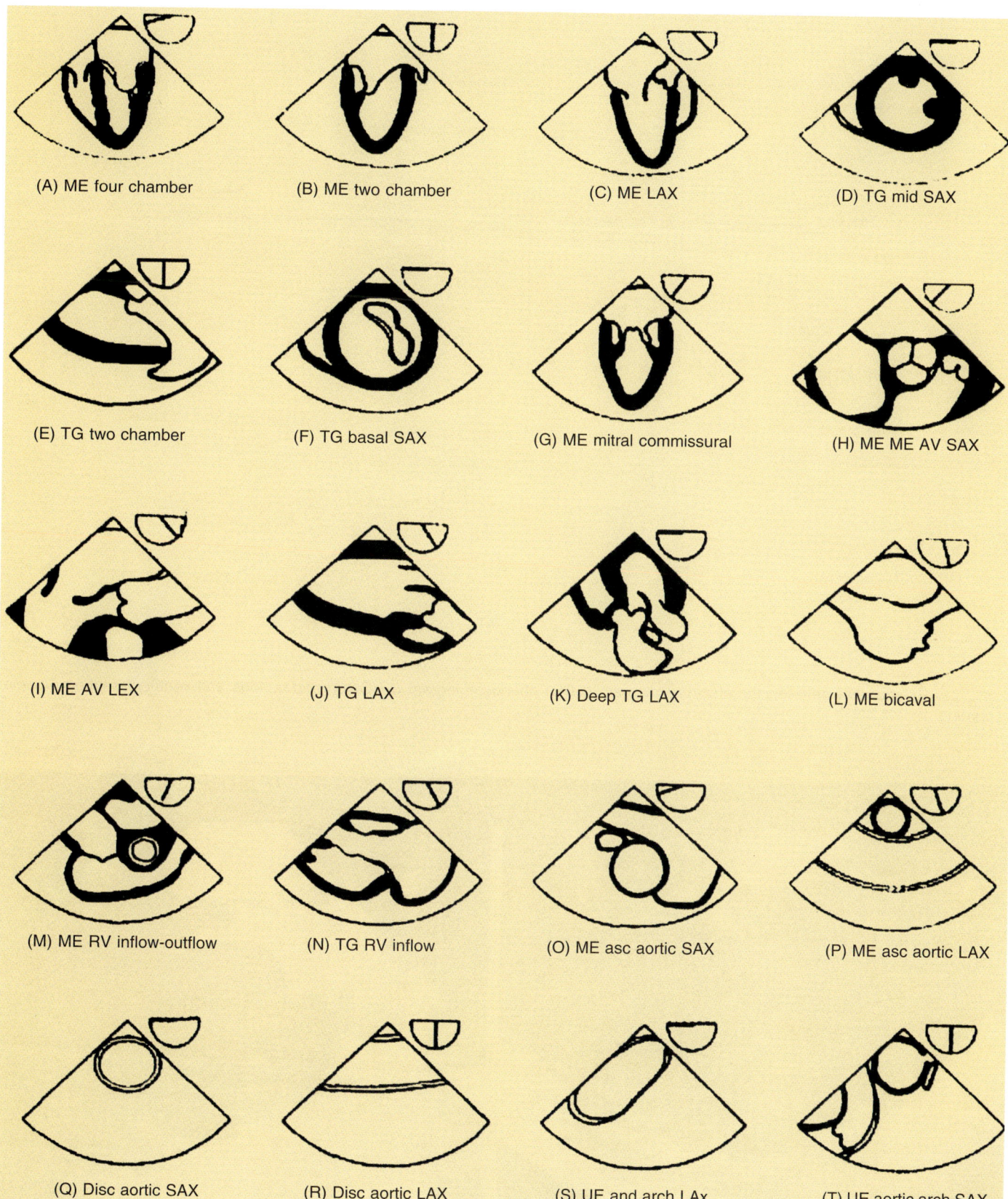

Fig. A22: Standard TOE views, ME, mid oesophageal; CAX, long axis; TLs, transgastric, SAX, short-axis; AV, aortic valve; RV, right ventricular

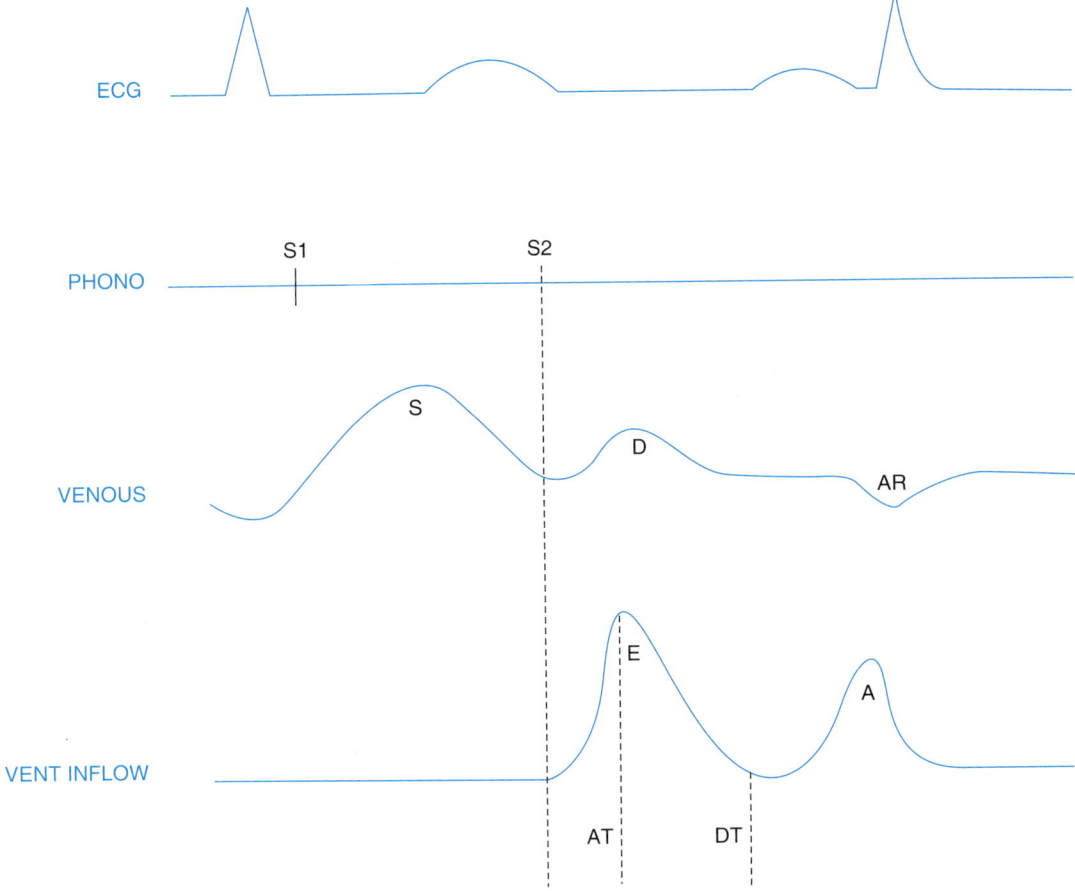

Fig. A23: Relationship between the electrocardiogram (ECG) phonocardiogram (PHONO) and venous and ventricular inflow Doppler recording

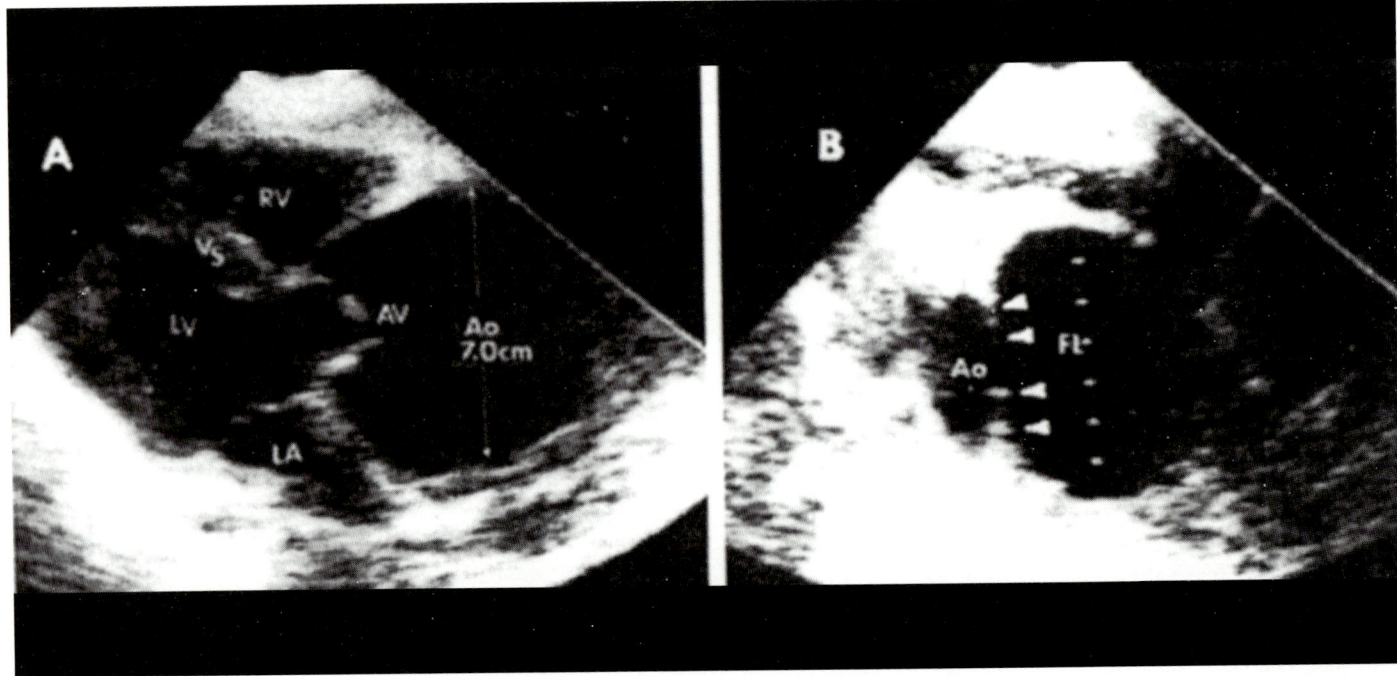

Fig. A24: Long axis (A) and short axis (B) transthoracic echocardiogram showing type I aortic dissection in patient with acute chest pain

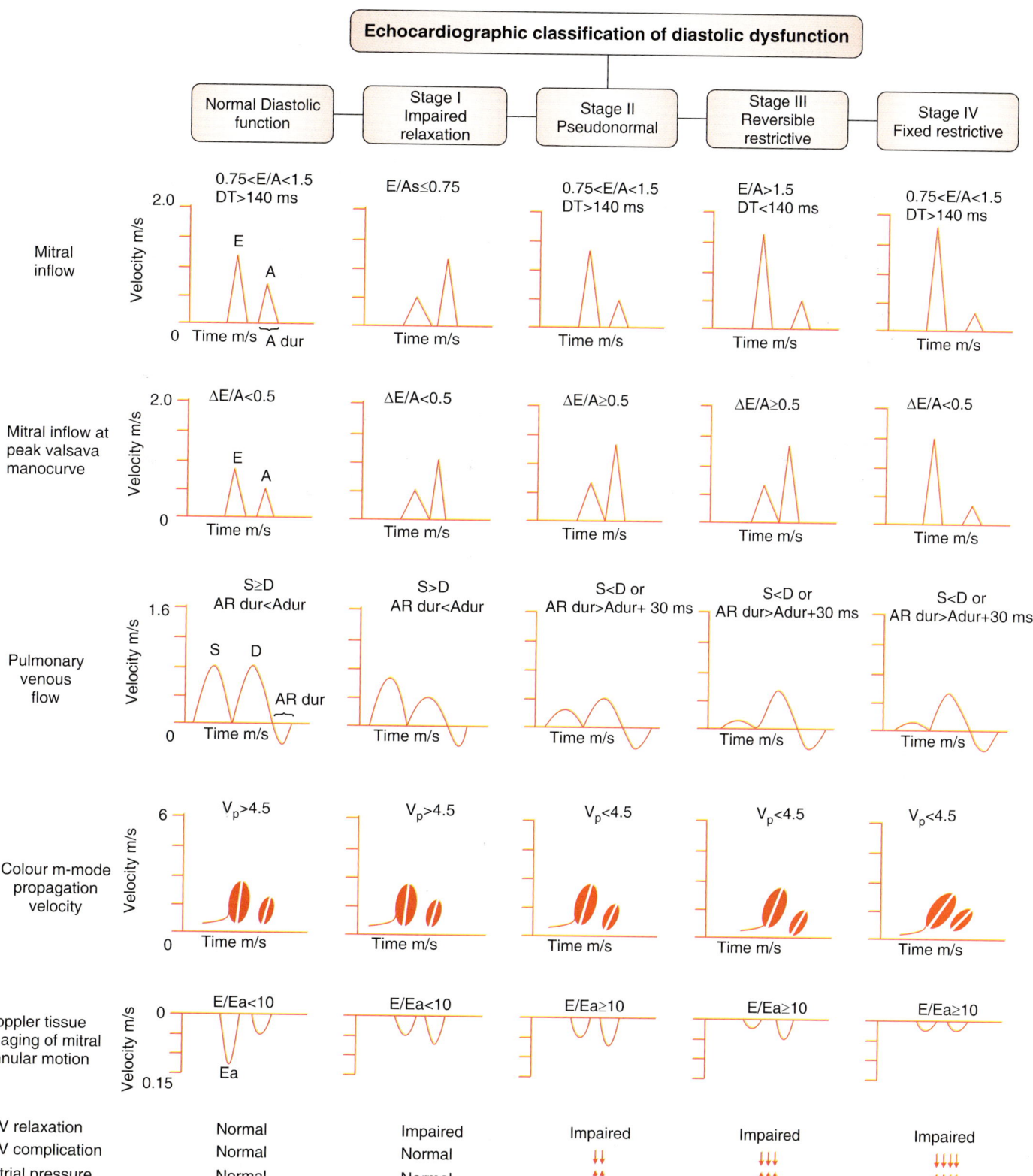

Fig. A25: Echocardiographic features of mitral inflow velocities, at peak valsalva, pulmonary venous flow, colour. M-mode propagation velocity, Doppler tissue imaging of mitral annular motion, LV relaxation, LV compliance and atrial pressures

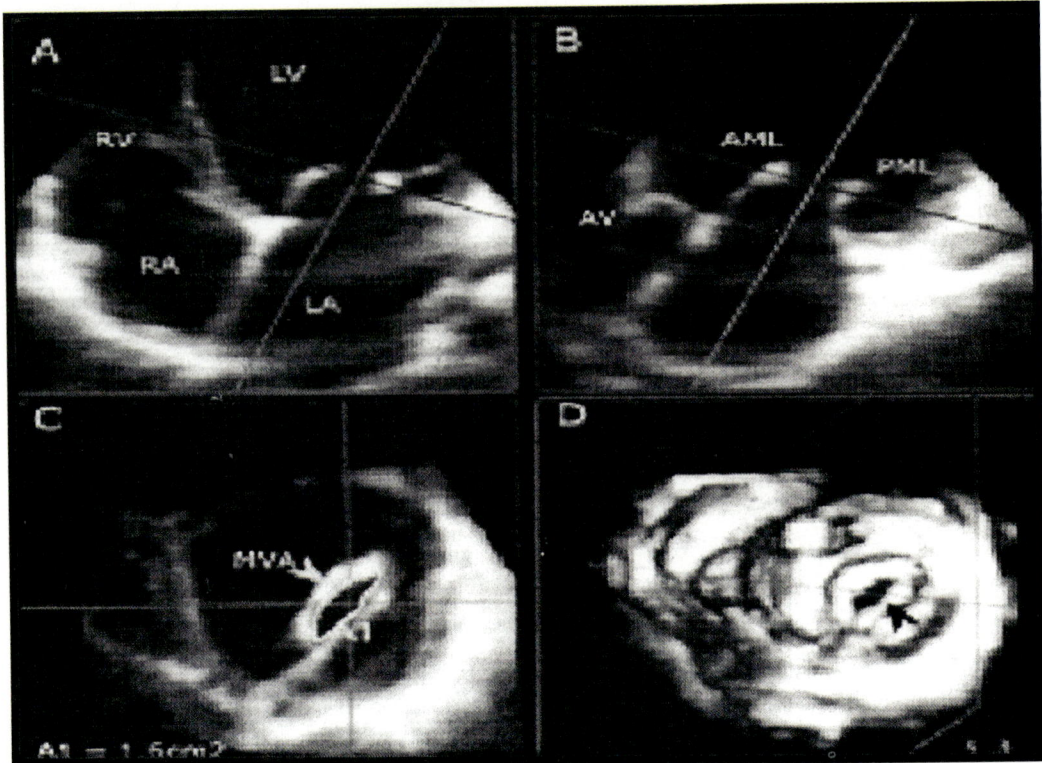

Fig. A26 (A to D): Full volume 3DTT data set has been obtained from apical window shown with three orthogonal cutting planes (D) along with contemporary two dimensional images in the respective planes A, B, C. The C cutting plane is aligned to the opening plane of mitral valve in A and B images to visualize the shortest mitral valve opening area in image C for measurement

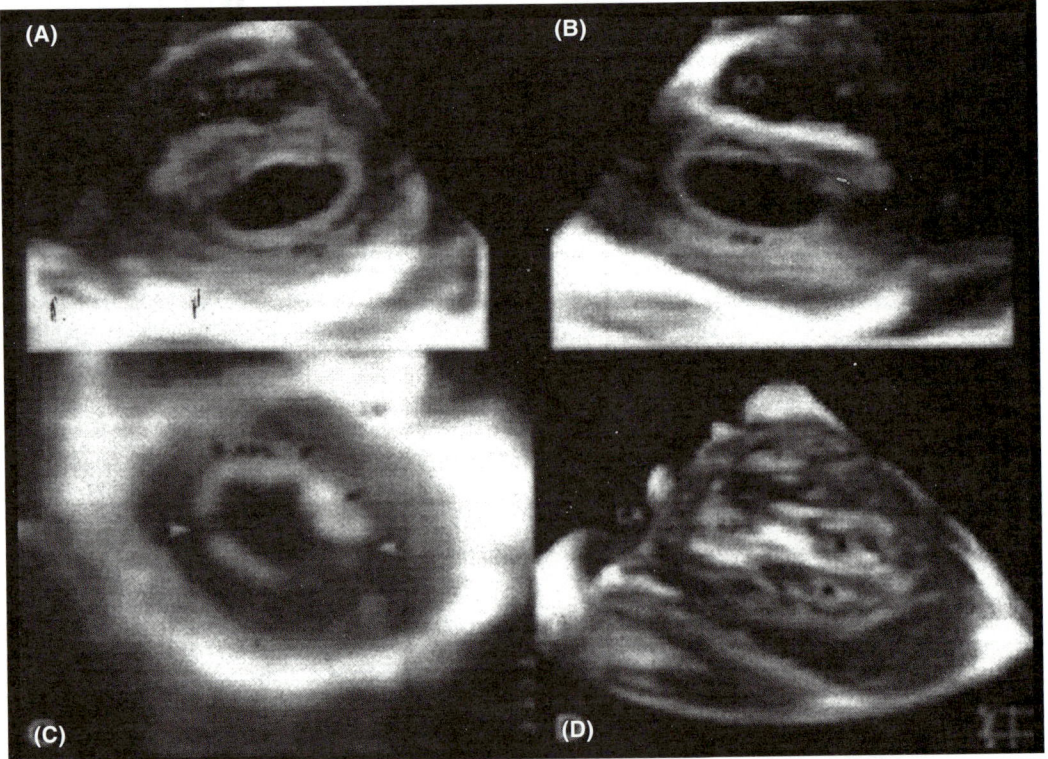

Fig. A27 (A to D): Real time 3DTTE data set taken from parasternal window showing mitral valve viewed from LV side (A) and LA side (B) showing the surface of the thickened anterior and posterior mitral leaflet. (C) Full volume 3D data set acquired from parasternal window. Anterolateral left ventricular wall has been cropped to visualize mitral apparatus with subvalvular structures

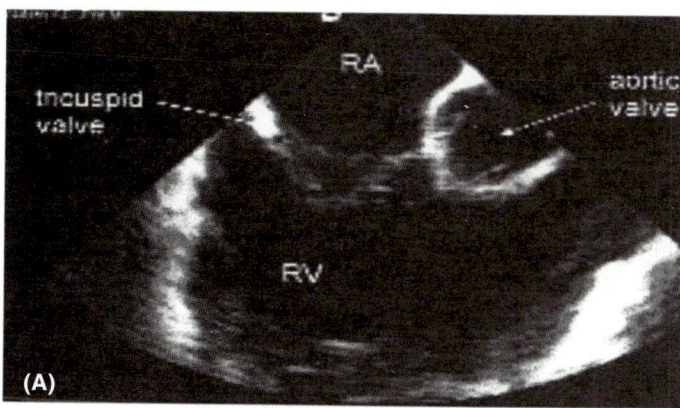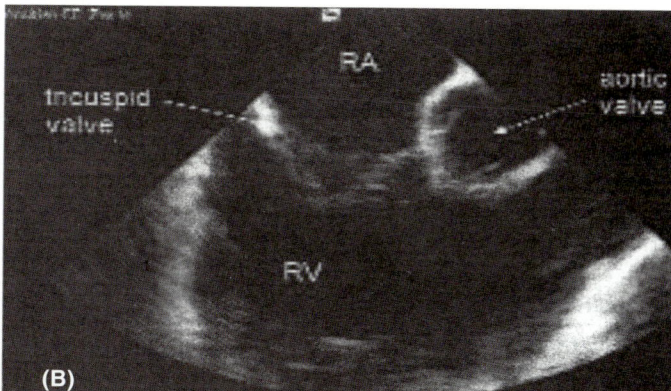

Fig. A28 (A and B): The intracardiac echocardiography (ICE) catheter advanced to the mid right atrium (RA). This provides views of the tricuspid and aortic valves

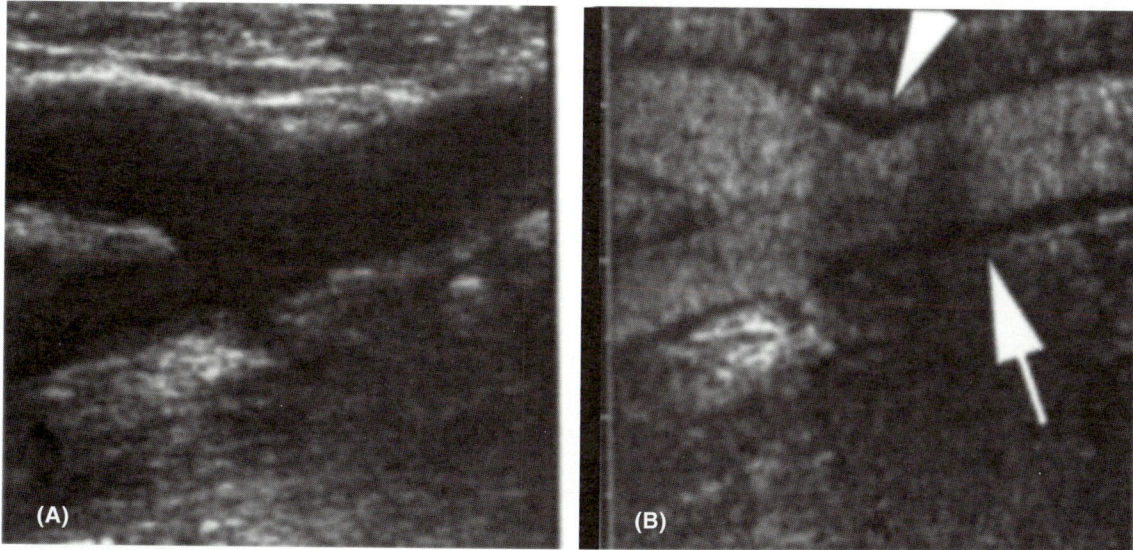

Fig. A29 (A and B): Carotid Duplex imaging of a common carotid artery, bulb and bifurcation panel A, shows images without contrast, panel B. shows images with contrast agent. Note the dramatic ability to detect intimal and medial thickness arrows accurately which has been underestimated by non-contrast imaging (Y-configuration of carotid arteries)

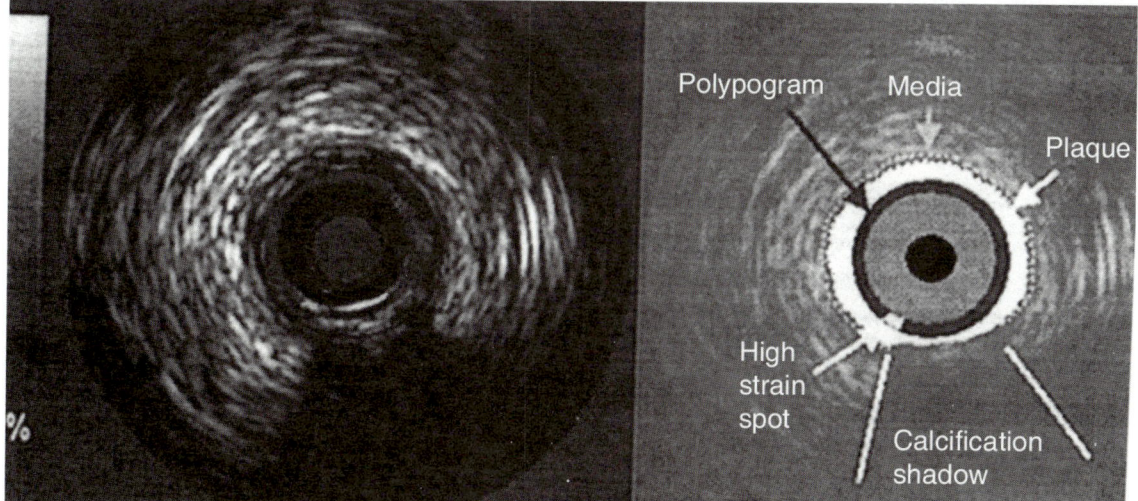

Fig. A30: The polypogram shows an eccenteric plaque with a big calcification. On the left shoulder there is a high strain spot of an otherwise less deformable plaque; probably representing a vulnerable plaque

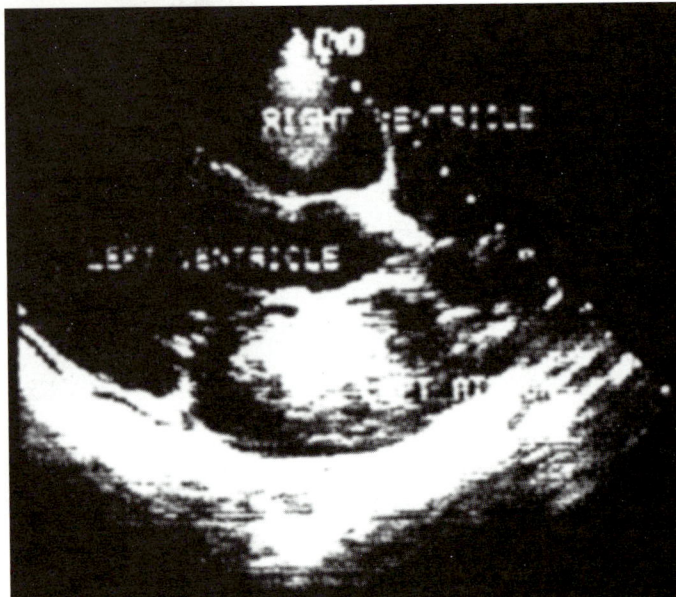

Fig. A31: Long axis view of LV showing tumor mass in both the right and left ventricles in patient with cardiac amyloidosis

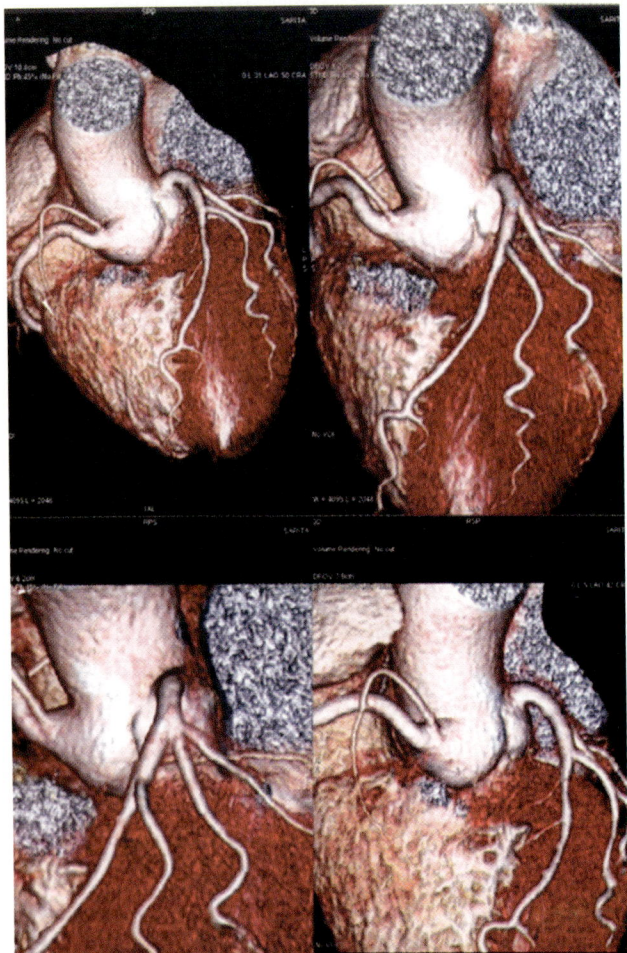

Fig. A32: Two and three-dimensional views of the anatomical location of right and left coronary arteries as imaged by 65 slices/ sec multidetector computerised cardiac scan

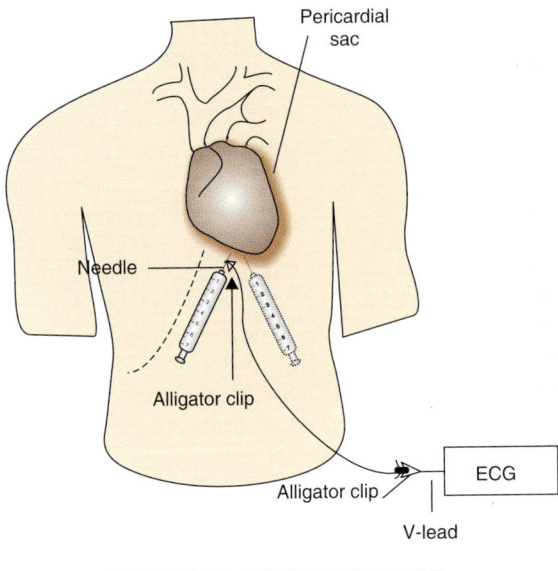

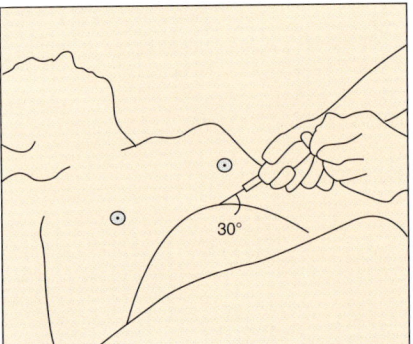

Fig. A33: Proper positioning of pericardiocentesis needle

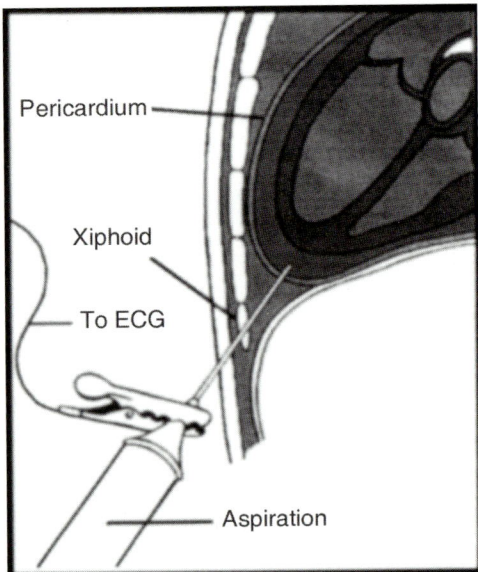

Fig. A34: Technique of pericardiocentesis. Needle is inseted 2–4 cm below the junction of subxiphoid process and the left costal margin at an angle of 15–30 so that it passes along the posterior aspect of the sternum until it enters the pericardial sac. The chest lead of the ECG is connected in the hub of the needle and monitored during insertion to determine if the needle touches the myocardium

Bibliography

1. Henry WL, Ware J, Gardin JM, Hepner SI, McKay J, Weiner M: Echocardiographic measurements in normal subjects: Growth-related changes that occur between infancy and early adulthood. *Circulation,* 1978, 52:278.

2. Gardin JM, Henry WL, Savage DD, Ware JH, Burn C, Borer JS: Echocardiographic measurements in normal subjects: Evaluation of an adult population without clinically apparent heart diseases. *JCU,* 1979,7:439.

3. Goldberg SJ, Allen HD, Sahn DJ: *Pediatric and Adolescent Echocardiography,* Chicago, Yearbook Medical Publishers, 1975.

4. Moss AJ, Gussoni CC, Isabel-Jones J: Echocardiography in congenital heart disease. *West J Med,* 1976, 124:102.

5. Hagan AD, Deely WJ, Sahn DJ, Karliner J, Friedman WF, O'Rourke R: Ultrasound evaluation of systolic anterior septal motion in patients with and without right ventricular volume overload. *Circulation,* 1973, 50:1221.

6. Meyer RA, Kaplan S: Echocardiography in the diagnosis of hypoplasia of the left or right ventricle in the neonate. *Circulation,* 1972, 46:55.

7. Solinger R, Elbl F, Minhas K: Echocardiography in the normal neonate, *Circulation* 1973, 47:108.

8. Godman MJ, Tham P, Kidd BSL: Echocardiography in the evaluation of the cyanotic newborn infant. *Br Heart J* 1974, 36:154.

9. Lunjdstrom NR, Elder I: Ultrasound cardiography in infants and children. *Acta Paediatr Scand,* 1971, 60:117.

10. Winsberg F: Echocardiography of the fetal and newborn heart. *Invest Radiol,* 1972, 7:152.

11. Sahn DJ, Deely WJ, Hagan AD, Friedman WF: Echocardiographic assessment of left ventricular performance in normal newborns. *Circulation,* 1974, 49:232.

12. Gordon EP, Schnittger I, Fitzgerald PJ, Williams P, Popp RL: Reproducibility of left ventricular volumes by two-dimensional echocardiography. *J Am Coll Cardiol* 1983, 2:506.

13. Erbel R, Schweizer P, Herrn G, Mayer J, Effert S: Apical two-dimensional echocardiography: Normal values for single and bi-plane determination of left ventricular volume and ejection fraction. *Dtsch Med Wochenschr,* 1982, 107:1872.

14. Nidorf SJ, Picard MH, Triulizi MO, Thomas JD, Newell J, King ME, Weyman AE: New perspectives in the assessment of cardiac chamber dimensions during development and adulthood. *J Amk Coll Cardiol,* 1992, 19:983.

15. Drexler M, Erbel R, Muller U, Wittlich N, Mohr-Kehaly S, Meyer J: Measurement of intracardiac dimensions and structures in normal young subjects by transesophageal echocardiography. *Am J Cardiol,* 1990, 65:1491.

16. Rijsterborgh H, Romdoni R, Vletter W, Bom N, Roelandt J: Reference ranges of left ventricular cross-sectional echocardiographic measurements in adult men. *J Am Soc Echocardiogr,* 1989, 2:415.

17. Pearlman JD, Triulzi MO, King ME, Abascal VM, Newell J, Weyman AE: Left atrial dimensions in growth and development: Normal limits for two-dimensional echocardiography. *J Am Coll Cardiol,* 1990, 16:1168.

18. Foale R, Nihoyannopoulos P, McKenna W, Kliene-benne A, Nadazdin A, Rowland E, Smith G: Echocardiographic measurement of the normal adult right ventricle. *Br Heart J,* 1986, 56:33.

19. Ichida F, Aubert A, Denef B, Dumoulin M, vanDer Hauwaert LG: Cross sectional echocardiographic assessment of great artery diameters in infants and children. *Br Heart J* 1987, 58:627.

20. Daniels SR, Meyer RA, Liang Y, Bove KE, Echocardiographically determined left ventricular mass index in normal children, adolescen and young adults, *J Am Coll Cardiol,* 1988 12:703.

21. Hatle L, Angelsen B: *Doppler Ultrasound in Cardiology,* Second edition. Philadelphia, Lea and Febiger, 1985.

22. Gardin JM, Burn CS, Childs WJ, Henry WL: Evaluation of blood flow velocity in the ascending aorta and main pulmonary artery of normal subjects by Doppler echocardiography, *Am Heart J* 1984, 107:310.

23. Goldberg SJ, Allen HD, Marx GR, Flinn CJ: *Doppler Echocardiograhy.* Philadelphia, Lea and Febiger, 1985.

24. Davidson WR, Pasquale MJ, Fanelli C: A Doppler echocardiographic examination of the normal aortic valve and left ventricular outflow tract. *Am J Cardiol,* 1991, 67:547.

25. Klein AC, Cohen GI: Doppler echocardiographic assessment of constrictive pericarditis, cardiac amyloidosis, and cardiac tamponade. *Cleve Clin J Med* 1992, 59:281.

26. Benjamin EJ, Levy D, Anderson KM, Wolf PA, Plehn JF, Evans JC, Comai K, Fuller DL, St. John Sutton M: Determinants of Doppler indexes of left ventricular diastolic function in normal subjects (the Framingham Heart Study). *Am J Cardiol,* 1992, 70:508.

27. Meijburg JWJ, Visser CA, Westerhof PW, Kasteleyn I, van der Twell I, deMedina EOR: Normal pulmonary venous flow characteristic as assessed by transesophageal pulsed Doppler echocardiography. *J Am Soc Echocardiogr,* 1992, 5:588.

28. Kitzman DW, Sheikh KW, Beere PA, Philips JL, Higginbotham MB: Age-related alterations of Doppler left ventricular filling indexes in normal subjects are independent of left ventricular mass, heart rate, contractility and loading conditions. *J Am Coll Cardiol,* 1991, 18: 1243.

29. Lernfelt B, Wiksterand J, Svanborg A, Landahl S: Aging and left ventricular function in elderly healthy people. *Am J Cardiol,* 1991, 68:547.

30. Pye MP, Pringle SD, Cobbe SJ: Reference values and reproducibility of Doppler echocardiography in the assessment of the tricuspid valve and right ventricular diastolic function in normal subjects *Am J Cardiol,* 1991, 67: 269.

31. Reisner SA, Meltzer RS: Normal values of prosthetic valve Doppler echocardiographic parameters: A review. *J Am Soc Echocardiogr,* 1988, I:201.

32. Panidis IP, Ross J, Mintz GS: Normal and abnormal prosthetic valve function as assessed by Doppler echocardiography. *J Am Coll Cardiol,* 12986, 8:317.

33. Rothbart RM, Smucker MK, Gibson RS: Overestimation by Doppler echocardiography of pressure gradients across Starr-Edwards prosthetic valves in the aortic position. *Am J Cardiol,* 1988, 61:465.

34. Williams GA, Labovitz AJ: Doppler hemodynamic evaluation of prosthetic (Starr-Edwards and bjork-Shiley) and bioprosthetic (Hancock and Carpentier-Edwards) cardiac valves. *Am J Cardiol*, 1985, 56:325.

35. Cruitus JM, Pawelzik H, Mittmann B, Breuer HW, Loogen F: Doppler echocardiography normal values in various types of mitral valve prostheses, *Z Kardiol*, 1987, 76:25.

36. Weinstein IR, Marbarger JP, Perez JE: Ultrasonic assessment of the St. Jude prosthetic valve: M-mode two-dimensional and Doppler echocardiography. *Circulation*, 1983, 68:897.

37. Cooper DM, Stewart WJ, Schiavone WA, Lombardo HP, Lytle BW, Loop FO, Salcedo EE: Evaluation of normal prosthetic valve function by Doppler echocardiography. *Am Heart J*, 1987, 114:576.

38. Kisanuki A, Tei C, Arikawa K, Natsugoe K, Otsuji Y, Kawazoe Y, Tanaka H, Morishita Y, Maruko M, Taira A: Continuous wave Doppler assessment of prosthetic valves in the mitral position: Comparison of the St. Jude medical mechanical valve and the porcine xenograft valve. *J Cardiogr*, 1985, 15:1119.

39. Holen J, Joie J, Semb B: Obstructive characteristics of Bjork-Shiley, Hancock, Lillehei-Kaster prosthetic mitral valves in the immediate postoperative period. *Acta Med. Scand*, 1978, 204:5.

40. Sagar KB, Wann S, Paulsen WHJ, Rombhilt DW: Doppler echocardiographic evaluation of Hancock and Bjork-Shiley prosthetic valves. *J Am Coll Cardiol*, 1986, 7:681.

41. Holen J, Simonsen S, Froysaker T: An ultrasound Dopler technique for the noninvasive determination of the pressure gradient in the Bjork-Shiley mitral valve. *Circulation*, 1979, 59:436.

42. Dubach-Reber PA, Vargus-Barron J: Velocidad maxima del flujo en la prostesis mitrale de Bjork-Shiley normo-function-ante. *Arch Inst Cardiol Mex* 1986, 56:57.

43. Lesbre JP, Chassat C, Lesperance J, Petitelerc R, Bonan R, Dyrda I, Pasternac A, Bourassa M: Evalution of new pericardial bioprostheses by pulsed and continuous Doppler ultrasound. *Arch Mal Coeur*1986, 79:1439.

44. Gibbs JC, Wharton GA, Williams GJ: Doppler echocardiographic characteristics of the Carpentier Edwards xenograft. *Eur Heart J*, 1986, 7:353.

45. Fawzy ME, Halim M, Ziady G, Mercer E, Phillips R, Andaya W: Hemodynamic evaluation of porcine bioprostheses in the mitral position by Doppler echocardiography, *Am J Cardiol*, 1987, 59:643.

46. Ryan T, Armstrong WF, Dillon JC, Feigenbaum H: Doppler echocardiographic evaluation of patients with porcine mitral valves. *Am Heart J* 1986, 111:237.

47. Holen J, Simonsen S, Froysaker T: Determination of pressure gradient in the Hancock mitral valve from noninvasive ultrasound Doppler data. *Scand J Clin Lab Invest*, 1981, 41:177.

48. Kisanuki A, Tei C, Arikawa K, Otsuji Y, Kawazoe Y, Natsugoe K, Tanaka H, Morishita Y, Taira A: Continuous wave Doppler echocardiographic assessment of prosthetic aortic valves. *J Cardiogr*, 1986, 16:121.

49. Ramirez ML, Wong M, Sadler N, Shah PM: Doppler evaluation of bioprosthetic and mechanical aortic valves: Data from four models in 107 stable, ambulatory patients. *Am Heart J*, 1988, 115:418.

50. Nihoyannopoulos P, Kambouroglou D, Athanassopoulos G, Nadazdin A, Smith P, Oakley CM: Doppler hemodynamic profiles of clinically and echocardiographically normal mitral and aortic valve prostheses. *Eur Heart J*, 1992, 13:348.

51. Heldman D, Gardin JM: Evaluation of prosthetic valves by Doppler echocardiography, *Echcardiography*, 1989, 6:63.

52. Goldrath N, Zimes R, Vered Z: Analysis of Doppler-obtained velocity curves in functional evaluation of mechanical prosthetic valves in the mitral and aortic positions. *J Am Soc Ecocardiogr*, 1988, l:211.

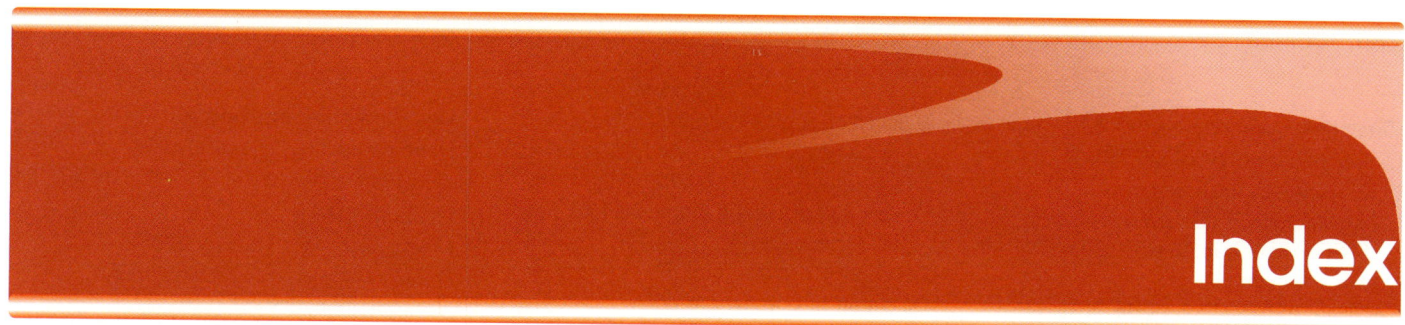

Index